Anticancer Agents

Anticancer Agents: Design, Synthesis and Evaluation

Editor

Qiao-Hong Chen

MDPI • Basel • Beijing • Wuhan • Barcelona • Belgrade • Manchester • Tokyo • Cluj • Tianjin

Editor
Qiao-Hong Chen
California State University
USA

Editorial Office
MDPI
St. Alban-Anlage 66
4052 Basel, Switzerland

This is a reprint of articles from the Special Issue published online in the open access journal *Molecules* (ISSN 1420-3049) (available at: https://www.mdpi.com/journal/molecules/special_issues/anticancer_agents_design_synthesis_evaluation).

For citation purposes, cite each article independently as indicated on the article page online and as indicated below:

LastName, A.A.; LastName, B.B.; LastName, C.C. Article Title. *Journal Name* **Year**, *Volume Number*, Page Range.

ISBN 978-3-0365-0140-6 (Hbk)
ISBN 978-3-0365-0141-3 (PDF)

Contents

About the Editor

Qiao-Hong Chen (Associate Professor) Dr. Qiao-Hong Chen received her PhD degree in Medicinal Chemistry from Sichuan University, China. Appointed as a Lecturer in 2001, she was promoted to the position of Full Professor in 2003 at Sichuan University. She was a Postdoctoral Fellow for three years at the University of Alberta in Canada and a Senior Research Fellow for six years at Virginia Tech. She joined Fresno State in 2012 and is currently an Associate Professor in the Chemistry Department. Her research interests focus on natural product-based anticancer agents. She has published 151 peer-reviewed scientific publications, as well as 5 book chapters.

Preface to "Anticancer Agents: Design, Synthesis and Evaluation"

Current cancer therapies still have various limitations, such as multi-drug resistance, undesired off-target effects, and unpredictable efficacies. The cancer-related mortality rate remains high. The development of novel anticancer agents thus continues to be imperative to combat various deadly cancers. The emerging molecular targets and signal pathways enable the development of novel strategies for the rational design of new anticancer agents. Numerous well-established synthetic methods and biological screening assays have paved the way for the discovery and development of new anticancer agents. This Special Issue of Molecules is devoted to all aspects of recent studies searching for new anticancer agents. Both original research and review articles focusing on the rational design, synthesis, and/or biological evaluation of various agents (including small molecules, natural products, intrinsic molecules, antibodies, and vaccines) as potential cancer therapeutics are welcome to be submitted for publication in this Special Issue.

Qiao-Hong Chen
Editor

molecules

MDPI

Review

Mimicking Strategy for Protein–Protein Interaction Inhibitor Discovery by Virtual Screening

Ke-Jia Wu [1,†], Pui-Man Lei [1,†], Hao Liu [2], Chun Wu [2], Chung-Hang Leung [1,*] and Dik-Lung Ma [2,*]

1 State Key Laboratory of Quality Research in Chinese Medicine, Institute of Chinese Medical Sciences, University of Macau, Macao 999078, China; Yb67513@um.edu.mo (K.-J.W.); Mb85817@um.edu.mo (P.-M.L.)
2 Department of Chemistry, Hong Kong Baptist University, Kowloon Tong, Hong Kong 999077, China; yjhxliuhao@163.com (H.L.); ccwuchem@gmail.com (C.W.)
* Correspondence: duncanleung@um.edu.mo (C.-H.L.); edmondma@hkbu.edu.hk (D.-L.M.); Tel.: +(853)-8822-4688 (C.-H.L.); +(852)-3411-7075 (D.-L.M.)
† These authors contributed equally to this work.

Academic Editor: Qiao-Hong Chen
Received: 29 October 2019; Accepted: 28 November 2019; Published: 4 December 2019

Abstract: As protein–protein interactions (PPIs) are highly involved in most cellular processes, the discovery of PPI inhibitors that mimic the structure of the natural protein partners is a promising strategy toward the discovery of PPI inhibitors. In this review, we discuss recent advances in the application of virtual screening for identifying mimics of protein partners. The classification and function of the mimicking protein partner inhibitor discovery by virtual screening are described. We anticipate that this review would be of interest to medicinal chemists and chemical biologists working in the field of protein–protein interaction inhibitors or probes.

Keywords: protein–protein interactions; virtual screening; mimetics; drug discovery

1. Introduction

Protein–protein interactions (PPIs) are involved in the regulation of biological processes, including cell proliferation, signal transduction, transcription, and apoptosis [1]. Since numerous ailments are associated with abnormal PPIs, the inhibition of PPIs is an attractive approach for the generation of new therapeutics. However, because of their large and amorphous interfaces, targeting PPIs is a great challenge in pharmaceutical and academic research.

In recent years, computer-aided approaches became useful tools to assist scientists in drug discovery. In particular, virtual screening emerged as a complementary technique to aid high-throughput screening (HTS) in pharmaceutical development. Virtual screening can reduce the number of compounds to be screened in bioassays, leading to a large reduction of time and cost [2,3]. Virtual screening strategies can be traditionally classified into two broad types: ligand-based virtual screening (LBVS) and structure-based virtual screening (SBVS). LBVS strategies include approaches such as pharmacophore-based methods, quantitative structure–activity relationships (QSAR), and three-dimensional shape matching [4]. On the other hand, SBVS techniques mainly revolve around the docking of molecules to three-dimensional (3D) structures of the biological target as determined by X-ray crystallography, nuclear magnetic resonance (NMR), or homology modeling.

Recently, virtual screening found increasing use for identifying inhibitors against various targets. Sun et al. constructed QSAR models of Sirtuin 1 (SIRT1) ligands and discovered 12 compounds as inhibitors of SIRT1 through ligand-based virtual screening [5]. Yang et al. identified a potent and selective KDM5A inhibitor using structure-based virtual screening [6]. Wu et al. reported mitoxantrone as an inhibitor of NAE using virtual screening of an approved drug database [7]. Virtual screening was also used to develop inhibitors of PPIs. Yang et al. described a compound as an inhibitor of the VHL–HIF1α interaction using structure-based virtual screening [8]. Zhong et al. utilized structure-based virtual screening and identified a cytosine alkaloid compound as an inhibitor that inhibited the menin–MLL interaction and another compound as a potential inhibitor of TLR1–TLR2 heterodimerization [9,10]. However, virtual screening still has many challenges and limitations that need to be overcome, especially its high false positive rate, which limits virtual screening to initial screening only [11].

The rational design of compounds that mimic key interactions at the protein–protein interface is another successful strategy for PPI inhibitor discovery [12]. Compared with low-molecular-weight compounds, mimetics can be more selective and show lower toxicity. Modification and optimization of peptide mimetics can also improve structural stability, resulting in increased oral availability [13]. For example, Groß et al. designed and synthesized a soluble peptide mimicking CXCR4 to interrupt the gp-120 and CXCR4 interaction [14]. In this context, the combined utilization of mimicking strategies and virtual screening has broad application prospects for drug discovery (Figure 1). Based on this strategy, many mimetics targeting cancer-related PPIs were discovered using virtual screening, such as p53 mimetics for the MDM2–p53 interaction [15–20], BH3 mimetics for the Bcl-2–BH3 interaction [21–26], and SMAC mimetics for the IAP–SMAC interaction [1,27–29]. Knowledge of the 3D structures of proteins allows the use of different approaches for mimetics design. For the interruption of PPIs, inhibitors may be larger in size than traditional drug compounds. Peptides and proteins mimetics are increasingly considered to be viable therapeutics for PPI inhibitor discovery [30]. However, there are still some challenges in protein or peptide mimetics design. For example, we still do not fully understand folding and the physical forces that stabilize protein structures. Moreover, sequences with many degrees of freedom can complicate the sequence search, which leads to a requirement for effective methods to find sequences related to a particular structure and measure essential protein folding criteria.

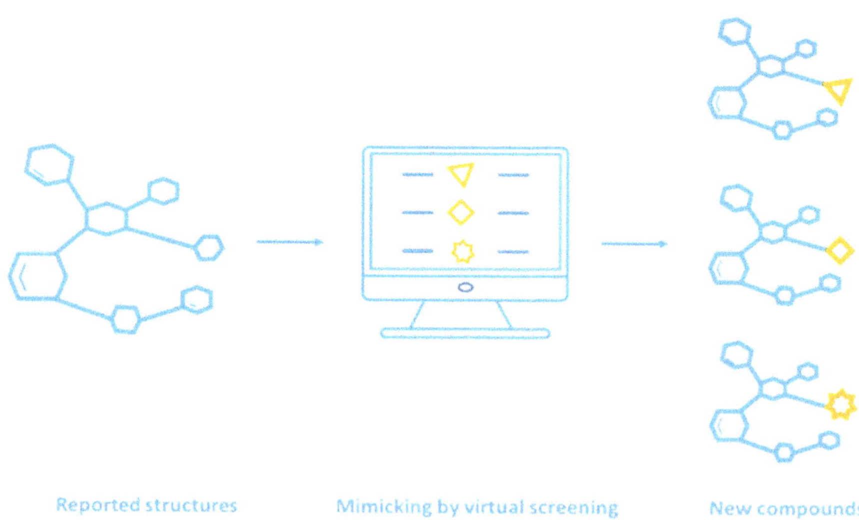

Figure 1. Mimicking strategy for inhibitor discovery by virtual screening [31]. (Reprinted with permission from Copyright (2015) Wiley—VCH Verlag GmbH & Co. KGaA.).

In this review, we discuss the recent advances in the application of virtual screening to design protein or peptide mimetics for PPI inhibitor discovery, and we summarize different methods for virtual screening. The classification of mimicking strategies and the function of the mimicking protein partner inhibitors discovered using virtual screening techniques are also described.

2. Integrating Mimicking and Virtual Screening Strategy for Protein–Protein Interaction Inhibitor Discovery

Recent studies indicated that certain types of PPIs are amenable for targeting by small molecules, which can block the interaction between a protein and its peptide or protein partner via binding at the proteinous interface [7,32–38]. As key residues of the protein or peptide may serve as a beginning point for PPI inhibitor design, the effective mimicking of peptides in their biologically active conformation and the development of mimicking ligands are important goals in science beyond the development of PPI modulators. Meanwhile, virtual screening emerged as a complementary technique to aid mimicking strategy in pharmaceutical development, complementing high-throughput screening (HTS) techniques. Integrating mimicking and virtual screening is a potentially viable strategy for protein–protein interaction inhibitor discovery. In this section, we describe the application of virtual screening and a mimetic strategy for PPI inhibitor discovery and discuss their merits and drawbacks.

2.1. *Virtual Screening for PPI Inhibitor Discovery*

Virtual screening is a kind of computer-aided technique that is usually considered as an initial step in the lead discovery process in order to enrich the library with active compounds and predict experimental activity [11]. Usually, based on the information about the target or the ligands of reported compounds, virtual screening is usually classified into two types: ligand-based virtual screening (LBVS) and structure-based virtual screening (SBVS). LBVS strategies depend on the similarity or dissimilarity of the compounds of interest, and they require a large amount of structure–activity data from a large chemical compound library. One of the ligand-based approaches is QSAR modeling, which focuses on achieving a correlation between the physicochemical and structural properties of the ligands and their biological function and potency. QSAR modeling includes two-dimensional (2D-QSAR) and three-dimensional QSAR (3D-QSAR). Scientists use 2D-QSAR and 3D-QSAR properties of ligands to build up a model of biological activity, which can be applied to predict the activity of some new compounds [39]. Compared with 3D-based algorithms, 2D-based algorithms are usually faster but may be less accurate; moreover, 2D-based algorithms cannot find new active compounds with dissimilar chemical structures [40]. Moreover, 2D- and 3D-QSAR do not consider ligand conformations, protein structure and flexibility, or solvation effects. Another LBVS approach is based on the similarity of compounds, which is a simple computational method with low cost, focusing on obtaining compounds that are similar to known ligands. However, this method is easily influenced by human users because it is difficult to objectively select the input molecules [41]. It is usually carried out by using common chemical features from the 3D structures of some known ligands that represent interactions between the ligands and the target. Pharmacophore modeling is another approach for LBVS. Based on analyzing the structures of known inhibitors against a target, a ligand-based pharmacophore can be generated that describes the spatial arrangement of chemical features of active compounds. However, under many circumstances, it is hard to find a library with functionally and structurally diverse molecules with quantitative activity data for a given protein. More importantly, the lack of publications with negative results hinders the identification of inactive molecules, resulting often in the development of qualitative common feature pharmacophores only from active compounds [41,42]. Finally, as LBVS applications are generally based on the properties of the known ligands, the diversity of the hits discovered are generally limited.

In contrast, SBVS techniques do not require knowledge of the biological activity of known compounds. Instead, 3D structures of the protein must be known or inferred. Protein-ligand docking is widely applied to identify compounds that are predicted to bind tightly to the active sites of the target. During the SBVS process, the 3D structure of a target protein and a set of ligands are considered as starting points and screened by virtual filtering, followed by docking and scoring to identify potential lead candidates. Many algorithms were developed to perform SBVS, such as DOCK, GOLD, And AUTODOCK, which can be used for identifying the binding mode and binding affinity between protein and ligand [43]. After docking and scoring, a set of compounds with the highest predicted binding affinity against the target can be obtained [44]. One relatively new strategy that falls within the purview of SBVS is the binding site comparison approach. This strategy, which can be utilized for drug repurposing and polypharmacology, relies on the recognized fact that many different proteins have similar binding sites [45]. Thus, binding sites in any given protein can be searched and matched with specific chemical structures. Finally, the pharmacophoric approach can also be employed within SBVS. If a high-resolution 3D structure of the target is available, a structure-based pharmacophore of the binding site can be generated based on the structural features of the binding site. In this case, a library of known inhibitors against the target is not needed. Compared to LBVS (Table 1), SBVS is more likely to identify new scaffolds because it is based on physical interactions calculated in silico, rather than relying on the similarity/dissimilarity of known ligand compounds. Thus, SBVS may be able to identify inhibitors with unique mechanisms of action [11,46]. Another difference is that, unlike LBVS, the docking model obtained by SBVS can be used for interaction analysis, in order to further enhance the affinity or selectivity of the compounds.

Table 1. The advantages and limitations of structure-based virtual screening (SBVS) and ligand-based virtual screening (LBVS). QSAR—quantitative structure–activity relationships.

Types		Pros	Cons
SBVS	1) Pharmacophore-based models	Uses protein structure	Increased screening time
	2) Molecular docking	Not biased toward existing ligand structures	Higher false positives
	3) Binding site comparisons	Takes protein flexibility into consideration	Oversimplification of scoring functions
LBVS	1) Similarity methods	Simple and fast	Requires existing ligands
	2) QSAR modeling	Less computationally intensive	Poor accuracy
	3) Pharmacophore-based models	Protein structure information may remain unknown	Lack of consideration of protein structural framework

Receptor and ligand flexibility is crucial for predicting drug binding and evaluating thermodynamic and kinetic properties. Molecular dynamics (MD) simulation is a technique for investigating atomic and molecular motion, and it is widely and effectively used for analyzing the relationship between the structure and function of molecules [47,48]. The main advantage of MD simulations is that they can thoroughly sample the conformational space around both the protein and the ligand under realistic conditions, accommodating both structural flexibility and entropic effects, thus allowing the thermodynamics and kinetics of the drug–target interaction to be more accurately calculated [47]. Therefore, MD simulation can be combined with SBVS or LBVS to further understand the binding mode of candidate molecules, thus accelerating the process of drug development [49]. Additionally, MD simulations can be used to identify potential pockets and binding hotspots of PPIs [50]. Saez et al. used MD simulations to predict the atomic interactions of the PcTx1–cASIC1 interaction and the hotspot residues of their interface, which could be beneficial for designing therapeutically useful PcTx1 mimetics [51]. By combining structural information, MD, and functional experiments, they obtained detailed insight into the molecular basis of this PPI. The TRAF6–Basigin interaction is implicated in melanoma metastasis. Biswas et al. used MD simulations to study the interactions between individual proteins and TRAF6–Basigin complexes, revealing conformation changes in the PPI and the adoption of a helical conformation [52].

In terms of the chemical library used for SBVS or LBVS, different filters can be used. For fragment-sized compounds, Congreve et al. described a "rule of three" with molecular weight < 300, $\log P < 3$, number of hydrogen bond donors and acceptors < 3, and number of rotatable bonds < 3 [53]. Alternatively, based on physicochemical properties, the "Pfizer's Rule of 3/75" can be applied to predict the toxicology of compounds. Compounds with calculated partition coefficient (ClogP) < 3 and topological polar surface area (TPSA) > 75 are approximately 2.5 times more likely to be safe in in vivo assays [54]. However, overly strict application of filters may introduce bias, leading to the exclusion of potentially active compounds. To assess the potency of the hits derived from virtual screening, IC_{50}, EC_{50}, K_i, or K_d values can be calculated. Ripphausen considered four subdivisions of potency (<1, >1–10, >10–100, and >100 μM), and suggested that docking hits are generally weakly potent, falling into the 1–100 μM range [55].

As virtual screening is often used as first stage of the primary screening process, false positives are a common problem. Based on six cases, Schierz et al. reported that the average percentage of false positives from the high-throughput primary screen is quite high at 64% [56]. To eliminate false positives, cross-referencing between primary and confirmatory screening assays is required. On the other hand, selectivity is a crucial aspect for developing potent PPI inhibitors. Off-target effects can arise when the compounds bind to other protein targets rather than their intended target, leading to side effects [57]. Virtual screening can be used for resigning, repositioning, and predicting side effects or toxicity of drugs, which can significantly decrease the time and cost of development compared to the traditional drug discovery process [58,59]. In one example, Spahn et al. used a computational simulation to create chemical modifications of fentanyl, an opioid pain killer with severe adverse effects due to off-target effects throughout the body. The newly discovered compound, named NFEPP, possesses a lower pKa and eliminates pain by selectively activating the MOR pathway in the inflamed acidic area without causing side effects [60].

Taken together, virtual screening greatly decreases the time and money costs by processing thousands of compounds in a short time in silico, thereby reducing the number of compounds to be synthesized or purchased [61]. However, because virtual screening relies on analyzing the physicochemical properties of compounds rather than biological activity directly, it has a high rate of false positives or false negatives compared to cellular or phenotypic screens [62].

In order to improve the efficiency of screening for more bioactive PPI lead inhibitors, the mimicking peptide strategy can be used. Virtual screening can be employed to target PPI surfaces or to mimic "hotspot" residues. Peptide mimetics that mimic the bioactivity of the parent peptides can also show improved pharmacokinetic and pharmacodynamic properties, such as bioavailability and stability [63]. It should be noted that the mimicking protein domain can be achieved with protein backbone scaffolds or small molecules [30,31].

2.2. *Structure-Based Mimicking Peptide Strategy for PPI Inhibitor Discovery*

Peptides are utilized as feasible molecules to mimic protein binding sites [64]. Peptidomimetics are non-peptide compounds that mimic the conformation and characteristics of peptide molecules to interrupt PPIs [63]. In general, chemical synthetic, screening, and structure design approaches are usually used for designing and extending the diversity of peptide-derived chemical structures, as well as enhancing their metabolic stability [64]. Synthetic strategies can explore and expand the chemical space for peptidomimetics. Screening strategies, including high-throughput screening and fragment screening, are often used to identify hot hits and discover peptidomimetics based on reported compounds [65]. Meanwhile, design strategies can use hotspot residues as starting points to design analogues by mimicking key secondary-structure motifs involved in the PPI interface. Design strategies can be subdivided into sub-structure search, *de novo* design, and bioisostere design [65]. As peptides usually contain secondary structures such as α-helices and β-sheets, peptidomimetics for inhibiting PPIs should be able to mimic these structures in order to be able to displace the natural peptides [66]. Therefore, peptides that mimic α-helices or β-sheets of proteins are attractive targets for drug discovery. α-helix structures are indispensable secondary structural elements which constitute most structured protein domains and contribute greatly to the protein–protein interface. Main strategies for synthesizing α-helix mimetics include (i) cross-linking of peptide side chains and the incorporation of stabilizing caps at the N-terminus, (ii) use of foldamers to modulate backbone variations, and (iii) introduction of projecting rod-like elements that mimic the side chains of an α-helix [31,67]. For example, Ernst et al. designed a polyamide foldamer as an α-helix mimetic, leading to the synthesis of inhibitors of the Bak BH3/Bcl-xL complex [68]. Meanwhile, a β-strand is an extended structural element between three and 10 amino acids long, and adjacent β-strand structures can be connected laterally backbone hydrogen bonds, forming a twisted or pleated sheet. β-sheets play key roles in maintaining the tertiary and quaternary structures of proteins, as well as PPIs. A number of strategies were utilized to design β-strand and β-sheet mimetics: (i) incorporation of turn mimetics to nucleate β-sheet generation, (ii) macrocyclization via covalent or noncovalent linkages, and (iii) introduction of β-strand-enforcing residues [31]. In addition to α-helix structures and β-strand structure mimetics, mimicking the turn structure of peptides is another potential approach for PPI inhibitor discovery. Turn structures are anomalous secondary structures that differ from α-helix and β-sheet structures due to the non-repetitive dihedral angles of the main chains. Turn motifs allow a peptide chain to fold back, and are important for forming globular proteins [31,69,70]. For instance, Bartfai et al. designed a β-turn mimetic that interrupted the interaction between IL-1RI and MyD88 in the TIR domains [71].

Gimeno and co-workers developed a classification of peptide mimetics depending on the extent of similarity to the native peptide. Class A mimetics contain the parent peptide amino-acid sequence, with the side chains being arranged to closely mimic the active conformation of the native peptide. Class B mimetics possess further modification of the native sequence, including the introduction of non-natural amino-acid residues, other small molecular motifs, or changes of the backbone sequence. Class B mimetics include foldamers, β- and α/β-peptides, and peptoids. Class C mimetics are highly modified structures with small molecular motifs and changes in the main chains of the peptide. Class D mimetics mimic the method of action of the native peptide rather than through structural mimicry of the side chains, and they can be developed via affinity optimization of class C mimetics or, alternatively, they can be identified by virtual screening [31]. An alternative classification of peptide mimetics was also described in the past two decades. Type I mimetics are short peptide sequences that mimic the α-helical motif of a PPI interface. Type II mimetics are functional mimetics that are based on a small molecular scaffold rather than a peptide scaffold. Type III mimetics include non-peptide templates that mimic the topography of the original helix by retaining the spatial arrangement of key binding residues [31,72,73]. In peptide mimetics design, one of the main challenges is that the topological shapes of proteins are complex, leading to variations in the types of interactions, binding pockets, and recognition sites formed [74]. This variability of PPIs is a crucial aspect that has to be mastered for the design of peptide mimetics targeting PPIs.

2.3. Integration of Mimicking Strategies with VS for PPI Inhibitor Discovery

Effectively mimicking the bioactive conformation of a peptide is a critical part of developing mimics as PPI inhibitors. However, developing mimetics with appropriate pharmacokinetic properties is a key challenge to overcome [31]. To strike a balance for these two properties, applying virtual screening can allow for simultaneous optimization of affinity and pharmacokinetic properties [75–77]. Thus, the integration of mimicking strategies and virtual screening is a complementary strategy for efficiently developing PPI inhibitors. In this section, we introduce and classify mimicking strategies using different virtual screening approaches (Figure 2).

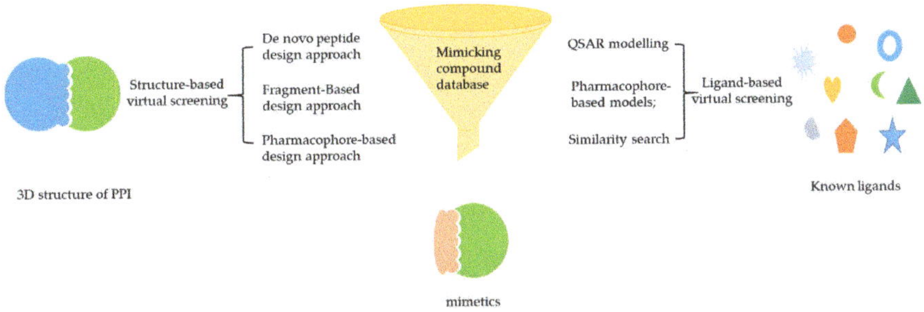

Figure 2. Different approaches for mimetics discovery based on structure-based virtual screening (SBVS) and ligand-based virtual screening (LBVS) [78]. (Reprinted with permission from Copyright (2002) Elsevier Science B.V.).

2.3.1. *De Novo* Peptide Design Approach

De novo peptide design is an attractive approach for constructing designed peptides with desired structures and functions, including peptide mimetics targeting PPIs. *De novo* design can create novel molecules that do not exist in known compound databases. This method only requires a scaffold library and a few key anchor residues as a starting point. By knowledge of the structural features of the native peptide, new inhibitors with the desired secondary structural characteristics can be built up *de novo* according to the targeted binding site. The virtual *de novo* peptide design method can be considered to comprise the following stages: (i) documentation of key anchor residues and the preparation of the scaffold library, (ii) virtual screening to find scaffold fragments that the anchor residues can be attached to, (iii) sequence design and structure refinement, and (iv) experimental validation [79]. There are several advantages of *de novo* peptide design to developing protein mimics. The first one is that the backbone of the natural protein sequence can be utilized as a template to initiate the design. Another advantage is that knowledge of sequence/structure relationships and/or statistical forcefields from native proteins can be used to guide the sequences of the designed peptides [80]. Therefore, *de novo* peptide design approach is a complementary strategy for peptide mimetics discovery.

Using the joint application of the *de novo* peptide design approach and peptide mimetics design, Li et al. designed PD-1-binding peptides by mimicking five residues (Y56, R113, A121, D122, and Y123) of the ligand PD-L. The most potent peptide Ar5Y_4 had a K_D value of 1.38 ± 0.39 μM, which was comparable to the binding affinity of the PD-L1. Ar5Y_4 showed the ability to interrupt the binding of PD-L1 to PD-1, providing a potential strategy for further optimization of PD-L1 peptide mimetics [74,81]. Smadbeck et al. used a three-stage *de novo* peptide design approach to design EZH2 inhibitory peptides. The approach comprises a sequence selection stage, a fold specificity calculation stage, and an approximate binding affinity calculation stage. The novel peptide SQ037 showed the highest in vitro response, with an IC_{50} of 13.5 μM. Compared to the native and K27A mutant control peptides, SQ037 had greater potency as an inhibitor and showed higher specificity to EZH2 [79]. Ruiz-Gómez et al. optimized the *de novo* design approach for small scaffolds mimicking protein recognition epitopes of large, non-structured, and discontinuous PPIs. They applied this novel re-scaffolding approach to the *de novo* design of potent interleukin 10 (IL-10) ligands that mimic the high-affinity receptor IL-10R1 [82]. Overall, these studies demonstrate that computer-aided *de novo* design is an effective strategy for peptide mimetics discovery.

2.3.2. Fragment-Based Design Approach

The fragment-based design approach uses fragments with low molecular weight and small size as starting points for modifying into high-affinity compounds. Compared with HTS, the fragment-based design approach can result in higher hit rates and a higher probability of synthesizing an efficient binding compound [83]. Hence, fragment-based approaches are particularly effective for generating small molecules or peptides targeting PPIs. The most common biophysical screening techniques for the fragment-based design method include differential scanning calorimetry (DSF), ligand- or protein-based nuclear magnetic resonance (NMR), surface plasmon resonance (SPR), isothermal titration calorimetry (ITC), or X-ray crystallography [1,74]. The fragment-based design approach is widely applied to mimetics design. For example, Petros et al. discovered a high-affinity ligand for the anti-apoptotic protein Bcl-X_L using fragment-based screening. From NMR-based structural studies and parallel synthesis, a potent BH3 mimetic ligand was obtained, which bound to Bcl-xL with an inhibition constant (K_i) of 36 ± 2 nM [22,23]. Using NMR-based screening, parallel synthesis, and structure-based design, further modification of this ligand was achieved by Oltersdorf and co-workers. They discovered ABT-737, a small-molecule inhibitor of the anti-apoptotic proteins Bcl-2, Bcl-X_L, and Bcl-w, which showed two to three orders of magnitude more potent affinity than previously reported compounds [24]. Although ABT-737 showed great antitumor activity in murine tumor xenograft models, it lacked oral bioavailability. Park et al. reported that targeted modifications at three positions of ABT-737 led to a 20-fold improvement in the pharmacokinetic/pharmacodynamic relationship (PK/PD). The resulting compound ABT-263 was orally available in a xenograft model of human small-cell lung cancer, and induced complete tumor regressions in all animals [25]. Based on ABT-263, Souers et al. redesigned and reported the first-in-class orally bioavailable Bcl-2-selective inhibitor with potent anticancer activity in vitro and in vivo [26]. Fragment-based design, in concert with computational approaches, show high promise for peptide mimetic design and discovery.

2.3.3. Pharmacophore-Based Design Approach

Pharmacophore-based approaches enables the virtual screening of large numbers of peptide mimetics using a conventional pharmacophore broadly derived either using structure-based or ligand-based methods, depending on whether a 3D structure of the target is available or not [74,84]. The pharmacophore-based approach can be divided into four steps: (i) atom typing, (ii) conformational sampling, (iii) hypothetical pharmacophore construction, and (iv) virtual screening of candidate ligands against the hypothetical pharmacophore [85]. Using the pharmacophore approach, Hansen et al. synthesized small beta-peptidomimetics with anti-staphylococcal activity. Their research showed that small β-peptidomimetics can mimic the antimicrobial activity of much larger antimicrobial peptides (AMPs), making them promising candidates for treating bacterial infections [74,86]. Caporuscio et al. developed compounds that showed micromolar potency against replication of HIV-1 in cells via a target-based pharmacophore model mapping the CD4-binding site on HIV-1 gp-120 [87]. Hall et al. conducted a two-round computational screening of potential peptide mimetic compounds in order to develop inhibitors of the αvβ3 integrin receptor. Biological testing revealed that the peptide mimetic molecules potently inhibited hantavirus with two thousand times more potency than the natural cyclic peptide (cyclo-[CPFVKTQLC]). The second round of screening furnished molecules with improved chemical diversity by building up the pharmacophore models [74,88]. Atatreh et al. started with a 3D pharmacophore and performed virtual screening to discover a series of MDM2–p53 interaction inhibitors with inhibition activity at the submicromolar level, which showed anticancer activities against different breast cancer cell lines [89]. Overall, the pharmacophore-based design approach is a suitable method for peptide mimetics discovery when the target protein structure is unavailable.

2.3.4. Integration of Mimicking Strategies with LBVS for PPI Inhibitor Discovery

In contrast to structure-based approaches, LBVS uses the structures of known binders as templates to discover and identify diverse bioactive compounds with high affinity. In general, LBVS methods depend on the application of computational descriptors of molecular structure, properties, or pharmacophore features, and they analyze relationships between active and database or test compounds in various defined chemical descriptor spaces [90,91]. Three major methods are usually utilized for LBVS: QSAR modeling, pharmacophore modeling, and the efficient similarity method. QSAR modeling can be broadly divided into three steps: (i) collect compound data, (ii) develop and validate QSAR models, and (iii) use the models to identify compounds from a chemical library. QSAR approaches are not computationally intensive, so they can be performed relatively quickly [92]. However, ligand-based 2D- and 3D-QSAR models do not consider ligand conformations, protein structure and flexibility, or solvation effects, which may lead to poor accuracy. When the three-dimensional (3D) structure of a target is unknown, pharmacophore modeling can be utilized to identify biologically active compounds via chemical features such as hydrogen bonding and lipophilicity as the input data for flexible alignment. Ligand-based virtual screening involves two different methods: (i) flexible alignment of molecules by considering only the atomic contributions, and (ii) use of other chemical features that are unrelated to 3D pharmacophore representations, such as hydrogen bonding and lipophilicity [84,93]. In the similarity method, compounds with similar structures are assumed to have similar activities, allowing the topological, steric, electronic, and/or physical properties of compounds to be predicted by comparison with known molecules [94]. Six types of similarity are exploited: chemical similarity, molecular/2D similarity, 3D similarity, biological similarity, global similarity, and local similarity [95]. In recent years, LBVS was increasingly applied to identify active compounds as PPI inhibitors [96]. Švajger et al. used two parallel virtual screening methods targeting the TLR4–MD-2 interface by mimicking interactions with MD-2 to discover novel TLR4 antagonists. They identified a potent hit compound with an IC_{50} value of 16.6 μM and no cytotoxic properties, which may be a potential agent to treat sepsis and neuropathic pain [97]. Varney et al. previously reported the interaction of Lipid II with defensins, based on the 3D structure of the human defensin peptide HNP1–Lipid II complex. They designed a pharmacophore model and used it for screening for defensin mimetics, leading to the first Lipid II-targeted low-molecular-weight compound, BAS00127538 [98]. Ambaye et al. used the co-crystal structure of a lead peptide antagonist and combined a shape-based similarity search, molecular docking, and 2D-similarity searches to identify nine novel phenylbenzamide-based antagonists of the Grb7 SH2 domain as potential Grb7 anticancer therapeutics [99].

3. Conclusions

Due to the critical roles of PPIs in disease, targeting PPIs is a potential therapeutic strategy. High-throughput screening is a widely used technique in drug discovery; however, a large investment into compounds and screening assays is required. Virtual screening is an emerging technology for drug discovery because there is no need for physical compounds and bioassays for screening. As we highlighted in this review, virtual screening is used for discovering mimetics of PPIs based on different approaches, such as *de novo* peptide design approach, fragment-based design approach, pharmacophore-based design approach, and ligand-based design approach. We anticipate that the integration of virtual screening with mimicking strategies will become a powerful tool in cancer research and that that this review could arouse the interest of chemical and biological scientists working in the field of PPI inhibitors.

Author Contributions: Writing—original draft preparation, K.-J.W. and P.-M.L.; writing—review and editing, C.W. and H.L., writing—review and editing, project administration, D.-L.M. and C.-H.L.

Funding: This research was funded by the Hong Kong Baptist University (FRG2/17-18/003), the Health and Medical Research Fund (HMRF/14150561), the National Natural Science Foundation of China (201575121and 21775131, China), the Hong Kong Baptist University Century Club Sponsorship Scheme 2018 (China), the Interdisciplinary Research Matching Scheme (RC-IRMS/16-17/03, China), the Interdisciplinary Research Clusters Matching Scheme (RC-IRCs/17-18/03, China), the Collaborative Research Fund (C5026-16G, China), the SKLEBA and HKBU Strategic Development Fund (SKLP_1718_P04, China), the Science and Technology Development Fund, the Macau SAR (File no. 0072/2018/A2 and SKL-QRCM-2017-2019), and the University of Macau (MYRG2018-00187-ICMS, China).

Conflicts of Interest: The authors declare no conflicts of interest.

References

1. Scott, D.E.; Bayly, A.R.; Abell, C.; Skidmore, J. Small molecules, big targets: Drug discovery faces the protein–protein interaction challenge. *Nat. Rev. Drug Discov.* **2016**, *15*, 533. [CrossRef] [PubMed]
2. Basile, L. Virtual screening in the search of new and potent anti-alzheimer agents. In *Computational Modeling of Drugs against Alzheimer's Disease*; Springer: Totowa, NJ, USA, 2018; pp. 107–137.
3. Lionta, E.; Spyrou, G.; Vassilatis, D.K.; Cournia, Z. Structure-based virtual screening for drug discovery: Principles, applications and recent advances. *Curr. Top. Med. Chem.* **2014**, *14*, 1923–1938. [CrossRef] [PubMed]
4. Villoutreix, B.O.; Renault, N.; Lagorce, D.; Sperandio, O.; Montes, M.; Miteva, M.A. Free resources to assist structure-based virtual ligand screening experiments. *Curr. Protein Pept. Sci.* **2007**, *8*, 381–411. [CrossRef] [PubMed]
5. Sun, Y.; Zhou, H.; Zhu, H.; Leung, S.-W. Ligand-based virtual screening and inductive learning for identification of SIRT1 inhibitors in natural products. *Sci. Rep.* **2016**, *6*, 19312. [CrossRef]
6. Yang, G.-J.; Ko, C.-N.; Zhong, H.-J.; Leung, C.-H.; Ma, D.-L. Structure-Based Discovery of a Selective KDM5A Inhibitor that Exhibits Anti-Cancer Activity via Inducing Cell Cycle Arrest and Senescence in Breast Cancer Cell Lines. *Cancers* **2019**, *11*, 92. [CrossRef]
7. Wu, K.-J.; Zhong, H.-J.; Li, G.; Liu, C.; Wang, H.-M.D.; Ma, D.-L.; Leung, C.-H. Structure-based identification of a NEDD8-activating enzyme inhibitor via drug repurposing. *Eur. J. Med. Chem.* **2018**, *143*, 1021–1027. [CrossRef]
8. Yang, C.; Wang, W.; Chen, L.; Liang, J.; Lin, S.; Lee, M.-Y.; Ma, D.-L.; Leung, C.-H. Discovery of a VHL and HIF1α interaction inhibitor with in vivo angiogenic activity via structure-based virtual screening. *Chem. Commum.* **2016**, *52*, 12837–12840. [CrossRef]
9. Zhong, H.-J.; Lee, B.R.; Boyle, J.W.; Wang, W.; Ma, D.-L.; Chan, P.W.H.; Leung, C.-H. Structure-based screening and optimization of cytisine derivatives as inhibitors of the menin–MLL interaction. *Chem. Commum.* **2016**, *52*, 5788–5791. [CrossRef]
10. Zhong, Z.; Liu, L.-J.; Dong, Z.-Q.; Lu, L.; Wang, M.; Leung, C.-H.; Ma, D.-L.; Wang, Y. Structure-based discovery of an immunomodulatory inhibitor of TLR1–TLR2 heterodimerization from a natural product-like database. *Chem. Commum.* **2015**, *51*, 11178–11181. [CrossRef]
11. Leung, C.-H.; Zhang, J.-T.; Yang, G.-J.; Liu, H.; Han, Q.-B.; Ma, D.-L. Emerging Screening Approaches in the Development of Nrf2–Keap1 Protein–Protein Interaction Inhibitors. *Int. J. Mol. Sci.* **2019**, *20*, 4445. [CrossRef]
12. Mullard, A. Protein–protein interaction inhibitors get into the groove. *Nat. Rev. Drug Discov.* **2012**, *11*, 173–175. [CrossRef] [PubMed]
13. Mason, J.M. Design and development of peptides and peptide mimetics as antagonists for therapeutic intervention. *Future Med. Chem.* **2010**, *2*, 1813–1822. [CrossRef] [PubMed]
14. Groß, A.; Möbius, K.; Haußner, C.; Donhauser, N.; Schmidt, B.; Eichler, J. Mimicking protein–protein interactions through peptide–peptide interactions: HIV-1 gp120 and CXCR4. *Front Immunol.* **2013**, *4*, 257. [CrossRef] [PubMed]
15. Carry, J.-C.; Garcia-Echeverria, C. Inhibitors of the p53/hdm2 protein–protein interaction—path to the clinic. *Bioorg. Med. Chem. Lett.* **2013**, *23*, 2480–2485. [CrossRef] [PubMed]
16. Ding, K.; Lu, Y.; Nikolovska-Coleska, Z.; Qiu, S.; Ding, Y.; Gao, W.; Stuckey, J.; Krajewski, K.; Roller, P.P.; Tomita, Y. Structure-based design of potent non-peptide MDM2 inhibitors. *J. Am. Chem. Soc.* **2005**, *127*, 10130–10131. [CrossRef] [PubMed]
17. Lin, J.; Chen, J.; Elenbaas, B.; Levine, A.J. Several hydrophobic amino acids in the p53 amino-terminal domain are required for transcriptional activation, binding to mdm-2 and the adenovirus 5 E1B 55-kD protein. *Genes Dev.* **1994**, *8*, 1235–1246. [CrossRef] [PubMed]
18. Ray-Coquard, I.; Blay, J.-Y.; Italiano, A.; Le Cesne, A.; Penel, N.; Zhi, J.; Heil, F.; Rueger, R.; Graves, B.; Ding, M. Effect of the MDM2 antagonist RG7112 on the P53 pathway in patients with MDM2-amplified, well-differentiated or dedifferentiated liposarcoma: An exploratory proof-of-mechanism study. *Lancet Oncol.* **2012**, *13*, 1133–1140. [CrossRef]
19. Rew, Y.; Sun, D.; Gonzalez-Lopez De Turiso, F.; Bartberger, M.D.; Beck, H.P.; Canon, J.; Chen, A.; Chow, D.; Deignan, J.; Fox, B.M. Structure-based design of novel inhibitors of the MDM2–p53 interaction. *J. Med. Chem.* **2012**, *55*, 4936–4954. [CrossRef]

20. Vassilev, L.T.; Vu, B.T.; Graves, B.; Carvajal, D.; Podlaski, F.; Filipovic, Z.; Kong, N.; Kammlott, U.; Lukacs, C.; Klein, C. In vivo activation of the p53 pathway by small-molecule antagonists of MDM2. *Science* **2004**, *303*, 844–848. [CrossRef]
21. Opydo-Chanek, M.; Gonzalo, O.; Marzo, I. Multifaceted anticancer activity of BH3 mimetics: Current evidence and future prospects. *Biochem. Pharm.* **2017**, *136*, 12–23. [CrossRef]
22. Petros, A.M.; Dinges, J.; Augeri, D.J.; Baumeister, S.A.; Betebenner, D.A.; Bures, M.G.; Elmore, S.W.; Hajduk, P.J.; Joseph, M.K.; Landis, S.K. Discovery of a potent inhibitor of the antiapoptotic protein Bcl-xL from NMR and parallel synthesis. *J. Med. Chem.* **2006**, *49*, 656–663. [CrossRef] [PubMed]
23. Park, C.-M.; Oie, T.; Petros, A.M.; Zhang, H.; Nimmer, P.M.; Henry, R.F.; Elmore, S.W. Design, synthesis, and computational studies of inhibitors of Bcl-XL. *J. Am. Chem. Soc.* **2006**, *128*, 16206–16212. [CrossRef] [PubMed]
24. Oltersdorf, T.; Elmore, S.W.; Shoemaker, A.R.; Armstrong, R.C.; Augeri, D.J.; Belli, B.A.; Bruncko, M.; Deckwerth, T.L.; Dinges, J.; Hajduk, P.J. An inhibitor of Bcl-2 family proteins induces regression of solid tumours. *Nature* **2005**, *435*, 677. [CrossRef] [PubMed]
25. Park, C.-M.; Bruncko, M.; Adickes, J.; Bauch, J.; Ding, H.; Kunzer, A.; Marsh, K.C.; Nimmer, P.; Shoemaker, A.R.; Song, X. Discovery of an orally bioavailable small molecule inhibitor of prosurvival B-cell lymphoma 2 proteins. *J. Med. Chem.* **2008**, *51*, 6902–6915. [CrossRef] [PubMed]
26. Souers, A.J.; Leverson, J.D.; Boghaert, E.R.; Ackler, S.L.; Catron, N.D.; Chen, J.; Dayton, B.D.; Ding, H.; Enschede, S.H.; Fairbrother, W.J. ABT-199, a potent and selective BCL-2 inhibitor, achieves antitumor activity while sparing platelets. *Nat. Med.* **2013**, *19*, 202. [CrossRef] [PubMed]
27. Cekay, M.J.; Roesler, S.; Frank, T.; Knuth, A.-K.; Eckhardt, I.; Fulda, S. Smac mimetics and type II interferon synergistically induce necroptosis in various cancer cell lines. *Cancer Lett.* **2017**, *410*, 228–237. [CrossRef]
28. Bai, L.; Smith, D.C.; Wang, S. Small-molecule SMAC mimetics as new cancer therapeutics. *Pharmacol. Ther.* **2014**, *144*, 82–95. [CrossRef]
29. Derakhshan, A.; Chen, Z.; Van Waes, C. Therapeutic small molecules target inhibitor of apoptosis proteins in cancers with deregulation of extrinsic and intrinsic cell death pathways. *Clin. Cancer Res.* **2017**, *23*, 1379–1387. [CrossRef]
30. Modell, A.E.; Blosser, S.L.; Arora, P.S. Systematic targeting of protein–protein interactions. *Trends Pharm. Sci.* **2016**, *37*, 702–713. [CrossRef]
31. Pelay-Gimeno, M.; Glas, A.; Koch, O.; Grossmann, T.N. Structure-based design of inhibitors of protein–protein interactions: Mimicking peptide binding epitopes. *Angew Chem. Int.* **2015**, *54*, 8896–8927. [CrossRef]
32. Wu, K.-J.; Liu, X.; Wong, S.-Y.; Zhou, Y.; Ma, D.-L.; Leung, C.-H. Synthesis and Evaluation of Dibenzothiophene Analogues as Pin1 Inhibitors for Cervical Cancer Therapy. *ACS Omega* **2019**, *4*, 9228–9234. [CrossRef] [PubMed]
33. Yang, Y.; Tse, A.K.; Li, P.; Ma, Q.; Xiang, S.; Nicosia, S.V.; Seto, E.; Zhang, X.; Bai, W. Inhibition of androgen receptor activity by histone deacetylase 4 through receptor SUMOylation. *Oncogene* **2011**, *30*, 2207. [CrossRef] [PubMed]
34. Sang, W.; Zhong, Z.; Linghu, K.; Xiong, W.; Tse, A.K.W.; San Cheang, W.; Yu, H.; Wang, Y. Siegesbeckia pubescens Makino inhibits Pam 3 CSK 4-induced inflammation in RAW 264.7 macrophages through suppressing TLR1/TLR2-mediated NF-κB activation. *Chin. Med.* **2018**, *13*, 37. [CrossRef] [PubMed]
35. Cheng, B.C.Y.; Yu, H.; Su, T.; Fu, X.Q.; Guo, H.; Li, T.; Cao, H.-H.; Tse, A.K.-W.; Kwan, H.-Y.; Yu, Z.-L. A herbal formula comprising Rosae Multiflorae Fructus and Lonicerae Japonicae Flos inhibits the production of inflammatory mediators and the IRAK-1/TAK1 and TBK1/IRF3 pathways in RAW 264.7 and THP-1 cells. *J. Ethnopharmacol.* **2015**, *174*, 195–199. [CrossRef] [PubMed]
36. Zhang, E.; Song, X.; Yin, S.; Fan, L.; Ye, M.; Hu, H. Glycycoumarin prevents hepatic steatosis through activation of adenosine 5,-monophosphate (AMP)-activated protein kinase signaling pathway and up-regulation of BTG1/Tob-1. *J. Funct. Foods* **2017**, *34*, 277–286. [CrossRef]
37. Liu, L.-J.; Wang, W.; Huang, S.-Y.; Hong, Y.; Li, G.; Lin, S.; Tian, J.; Cai, Z.; Wang, H.-M.D.; Ma, D.-L. Inhibition of the Ras/Raf interaction and repression of renal cancer xenografts in vivo by an enantiomeric iridium (III) metal-based compound. *Chem. Sci.* **2017**, *8*, 4756–4763. [CrossRef]
38. Zhong, H.-J.; Lu, L.; Leung, K.-H.; Wong, C.C.; Peng, C.; Yan, S.-C.; Ma, D.-L.; Cai, Z.; Wang, H.-M.D.; Leung, C.-H. An iridium (III)-based irreversible protein–protein interaction inhibitor of BRD4 as a potent anticancer agent. *Chem. Sci.* **2015**, *6*, 5400–5408. [CrossRef]

39. Verma, J.; Khedkar, V.M.; Coutinho, E.C. 3D-QSAR in drug design-a review. *Curr. Top. Med. Chem.* **2010**, *10*, 95–115. [CrossRef]
40. Stumpfe, D.; Ripphausen, P.; Bajorath, J. Virtual compound screening in drug discovery. *Future Med. Chem.* **2012**, *4*, 593–602. [CrossRef]
41. Drwal, M.N.; Griffith, R. Combination of ligand-and structure-based methods in virtual screening. *Drug Discov. Today Technol.* **2013**, *10*, e395–e401. [CrossRef]
42. Leach, A.R.; Gillet, V.J.; Lewis, R.A.; Taylor, R. Three-dimensional pharmacophore methods in drug discovery. *J. Med. Chem.* **2009**, *53*, 539–558. [CrossRef] [PubMed]
43. Andricopulo, A.D.; Guido, R.V.; Oliva, G. Virtual screening and its integration with modern drug design technologies. *Curr. Med. Chem.* **2008**, *15*, 37–46. [CrossRef] [PubMed]
44. Ghosh, S.; Nie, A.; An, J.; Huang, Z. Structure-based virtual screening of chemical libraries for drug discovery. *Curr. Opin. Chem. Biol.* **2006**, *10*, 194–202. [CrossRef] [PubMed]
45. Konc, J. Binding site comparisons for target-centered drug discovery. *Expert Opin. Drug Discov.* **2019**, *14*, 445–454. [CrossRef]
46. Yasuo, N.; Sekijima, M. Improved Method of Structure-Based Virtual Screening via Interaction-Energy-Based Learning. *J. Chem. Inf. Model.* **2019**, *59*, 1050–1061. [CrossRef]
47. Fischer, M.; Coleman, R.G.; Fraser, J.S.; Shoichet, B.K. Incorporation of protein flexibility and conformational energy penalties in docking screens to improve ligand discovery. *Nat. Chem.* **2014**, *6*, 575. [CrossRef]
48. Hospital, A.; Goñi, J.R.; Orozco, M.; Gelpí, J.L. Molecular dynamics simulations: Advances and applications. *Adv. Appl. Bioinform. Chem AABC* **2015**, *8*, 37.
49. De Vivo, M.; Masetti, M.; Bottegoni, G.; Cavalli, A. Role of molecular dynamics and related methods in drug discovery. *J. Med. Chem.* **2016**, *59*, 4035–4061. [CrossRef]
50. Perricone, U.; Gulotta, M.R.; Lombino, J.; Parrino, B.; Cascioferro, S.; Diana, P.; Cirrincione, G.; Padova, A. An overview of recent molecular dynamics applications as medicinal chemistry tools for the undruggable site challenge. *MedChemComm* **2018**, *9*, 920–936. [CrossRef]
51. Saez, N.J.; Deplazes, E.; Cristofori-Armstrong, B.; Chassagnon, I.R.; Lin, X.; Mobli, M.; Mark, A.E.; Rash, L.D.; King, G.F. Molecular dynamics and functional studies define a hot spot of crystal contacts essential for PcTx1 inhibition of acid-sensing ion channel 1a. *Br. J. Pharm.* **2015**, *172*, 4985–4995. [CrossRef]
52. Biswas, R.; Ghosh, S.; Bagchi, A. A structural perspective on the interactions of TRAF6 and B asigin during the onset of melanoma: A molecular dynamics simulation study. *J. Mol. Recognit* **2017**, *30*, e2643. [CrossRef]
53. Rees, D.C.; Congreve, M.; Murray, C.W.; Carr, R. Fragment-based lead discovery. *Nat. Rev. Drug Discov.* **2004**, *3*, 660. [CrossRef] [PubMed]
54. Hughes, J.D.; Blagg, J.; Price, D.A.; Bailey, S.; DeCrescenzo, G.A.; Devraj, R.V.; Ellsworth, E.; Fobian, Y.M.; Gibbs, M.E.; Gilles, R.W. Physiochemical drug properties associated with in vivo toxicological outcomes. *Bioorg. Med. Chem. Lett.* **2008**, *18*, 4872–4875. [CrossRef] [PubMed]
55. Ripphausen, P.; Stumpfe, D.; Bajorath, J. Analysis of structure-based virtual screening studies and characterization of identified active compounds. *Future Med. Chem.* **2012**, *4*, 603–613. [CrossRef] [PubMed]
56. Schierz, A.C. Virtual screening of bioassay data. *J. Cheminf.* **2009**, *1*, 21. [CrossRef] [PubMed]
57. Thorne, N.; Auld, D.S.; Inglese, J. Apparent activity in high-throughput screening: Origins of compound-dependent assay interference. *Curr. Opin.Chem. Biol.* **2010**, *14*, 315–324. [CrossRef] [PubMed]
58. Xu, X.; Huang, M.; Zou, X. Docking-based inverse virtual screening: Methods, applications, and challenges. *Biophys. Rep.* **2018**, *4*, 1–16. [CrossRef] [PubMed]
59. Ma, D.-L.; Chan, D.S.-H.; Leung, C.-H. Drug repositioning by structure-based virtual screening. *Chem. Soc. Rev.* **2013**, *42*, 2130–2141. [CrossRef]
60. Spahn, V.; Del Vecchio, G.; Rodriguez-Gaztelumendi, A.; Temp, J.; Labuz, D.; Kloner, M.; Reidelbach, M.; Machelska, H.; Weber, M.; Stein, C. Opioid receptor signaling, analgesic and side effects induced by a computationally designed pH-dependent agonist. *Sci. Rep.* **2018**, *8*, 8965. [CrossRef]
61. Gimeno, A.; Ojeda-Montes, M.J.; Tomás-Hernández, S.; Cereto-Massagué, A.; Beltrán-Debón, R.; Mulero, M.; Pujadas, G.; Garcia-Vallvé, S. The light and dark sides of virtual screening: What is there to know? *Int. J. Mol. Sci.* **2019**, *20*, 1375. [CrossRef]
62. Malo, N.; Hanley, J.A.; Cerquozzi, S.; Pelletier, J.; Nadon, R. Statistical practice in high-throughput screening data analysis. *Nat. Biotechnol.* **2006**, *24*, 167. [CrossRef] [PubMed]

63. Farhadi, T.; Hashemian, S.M. Computer-aided design of amino acid-based therapeutics: A review. *Dru Des. Devel. Ther.* **2018**, *12*, 1239. [CrossRef] [PubMed]
64. Eichler, J. Peptides as protein binding site mimetics. *Curr. Opin. Chem. Biol.* **2008**, *12*, 707–713. [CrossRef] [PubMed]
65. Sheng, C.; Dong, G.; Miao, Z.; Zhang, W.; Wang, W. State-of-the-art strategies for targeting protein–protein interactions by small-molecule inhibitors. *Chem. Soc. Rev.* **2015**, *44*, 8238–8259. [CrossRef]
66. Fletcher, S.; Hamilton, A.D. Targeting protein–protein interactions by rational design: Mimicry of protein surfaces. *J. R. Soc. Interface* **2006**, *3*, 215–233. [CrossRef]
67. Toniolo, C.; Bonora, G.M.; Bavoso, A.; Benedetti, E.; di Blasio, B.; Pavone, V.; Pedone, C. Preferred conformations of peptides containing α, α-disubstituted α-amino acids. *Biopolym. Orig. Res. Biomol.* **1983**, *22*, 205–215.
68. Ernst, J.T.; Becerril, J.; Park, H.S.; Yin, H.; Hamilton, A.D. Design and application of an α-helix-mimetic scaffold based on an oligoamide-foldamer strategy: Antagonism of the bak BH3/Bcl-xL complex. *Angew Chem. Int.* **2003**, *42*, 535–539. [CrossRef]
69. Venkatachalam, C. Stereochemical criteria for polypeptides and proteins. V. Conformation of a system of three linked peptide units. *Biopolym. Orig. Res. Biomol.* **1968**, *6*, 1425–1436. [CrossRef]
70. Chou, K.-C. Prediction of tight turns and their types in proteins. *Anal. Biochem.* **2000**, *286*, 1–16. [CrossRef]
71. Bartfai, T.; Behrens, M.M.; Gaidarova, S.; Pemberton, J.; Shivanyuk, A.; Rebek, J. A low molecular weight mimic of the Toll/IL-1 receptor/resistance domain inhibits IL-1 receptor-mediated responses. *Proc. Natl. Acad. Sci.* **2003**, *100*, 7971–7976. [CrossRef]
72. Azzarito, V.; Long, K.; Murphy, N.S.; Wilson, A.J. Inhibition of α-helix-mediated protein–protein interactions using designed molecules. *Nat. Chem.* **2013**, *5*, 161. [CrossRef] [PubMed]
73. Ripka, A.S.; Rich, D.H. Peptidomimetic design. *Curr. Opin. Chem. Biol.* **1998**, *2*, 441–452. [CrossRef]
74. Floris, M.; Moro, S. Mimicking peptides ... in silico. *Mol. Inf.* **2012**, *31*, 12–20. [CrossRef] [PubMed]
75. Jansen, J.M.; Martin, E.J. Target-biased scoring approaches and expert systems in structure-based virtual screening. *Curr. Opin. Chem. Biol.* **2004**, *8*, 359–364. [CrossRef]
76. Leung, K.-H.; Liu, L.-J.; Lin, S.; Lu, L.; Zhong, H.-J.; Susanti, D.; Rao, W.; Wang, M.; Che, W.I.; Chan, D.S.-H. Discovery of a small-molecule inhibitor of STAT3 by ligand-based pharmacophore screening. *Methods* **2015**, *71*, 38–43. [CrossRef]
77. Zhong, H.-J.; Liu, L.-J.; Chan, D.S.-H.; Wang, H.-M.; Chan, P.W.H.; Ma, D.-L.; Leung, C.-H. Structure-based repurposing of FDA-approved drugs as inhibitors of NEDD8-activating enzyme. *Biochimie* **2014**, *102*, 211–215. [CrossRef]
78. Lyne, P.D. Structure-based virtual screening: An overview. *Drug Discov. Today* **2002**, *7*, 1047–1055. [CrossRef]
79. Smadbeck, J.; Peterson, M.B.; Zee, B.M.; Garapaty, S.; Mago, A.; Lee, C.; Giannis, A.; Trojer, P.; Garcia, B.A.; Floudas, C.A. De novo peptide design and experimental validation of histone methyltransferase inhibitors. *PLoS ONE* **2014**, *9*, e90095. [CrossRef]
80. Woolfson, D.N.; Bartlett, G.J.; Burton, A.J.; Heal, J.W.; Niitsu, A.; Thomson, A.R.; Wood, C.W. De novo protein design: How do we expand into the universe of possible protein structures? *Curr. Opin. Struct. Biol.* **2015**, *33*, 16–26. [CrossRef]
81. Li, Q.; Quan, L.; Lyu, J.; He, Z.; Wang, X.; Meng, J.; Zhao, Z.; Zhu, L.; Liu, X.; Li, H. Discovery of peptide inhibitors targeting human programmed death 1 (PD-1) receptor. *Oncotarget* **2016**, *7*, 64967. [CrossRef]
82. Ruiz-Gómez, G.; Hawkins, J.C.; Philipp, J.; Künze, G.; Wodtke, R.; Löser, R.; Fahmy, K.; Pisabarro, M.T. Rational structure-based rescaffolding approach to De Novo design of interleukin 10 (IL-10) receptor-1 mimetics. *PLoS ONE* **2016**, *11*, e0154046. [CrossRef] [PubMed]
83. Schulz, M.N.; Hubbard, R.E. Recent progress in fragment-based lead discovery. *Curr. Opin. Pharm.* **2009**, *9*, 615–621. [CrossRef] [PubMed]
84. Kim, K.-H.; Kim, N.D.; Seong, B.-L. Pharmacophore-based virtual screening: A review of recent applications. *Expert Opin. Drug Discov.* **2010**, *5*, 205–222. [CrossRef] [PubMed]
85. Sun, H. Pharmacophore-based virtual screening. *Curr. Med. Chem.* **2008**, *15*, 1018–1024. [CrossRef] [PubMed]
86. Hansen, T.; Alst, T.; Havelkova, M.; Strøm, M.B. Antimicrobial activity of small β-peptidomimetics based on the pharmacophore model of short cationic antimicrobial peptides. *J. Med. Chem.* **2009**, *53*, 595–606. [CrossRef]

87. Caporuscio, F.; Tafi, A.; González, E.; Manetti, F.; Esté, J.A.; Botta, M. A dynamic target-based pharmacophoric model mapping the CD4 binding site on HIV-1 gp120 to identify new inhibitors of gp120–CD4 protein–protein interactions. *Bioorg. Med. Chem. Lett.* **2009**, *19*, 6087–6091. [CrossRef]
88. Hall, P.R.; Leitão, A.; Ye, C.; Kilpatrick, K.; Hjelle, B.; Oprea, T.I.; Larson, R.S. Small molecule inhibitors of hantavirus infection. *Bioorg. Med. Chem. Lett.* **2010**, *20*, 7085–7091. [CrossRef]
89. Atatreh, N.; Ghattas, M.A.; Bardaweel, S.K.; Al Rawashdeh, S.; Al Sorkhy, M. Identification of new inhibitors of Mdm2–p53 interaction via pharmacophore and structure-based virtual screening. *Drug Des. Dev.* **2018**, *12*, 3741. [CrossRef]
90. Taylor, P.; Blackburn, E.; Sheng, Y.; Harding, S.; Hsin, K.Y.; Kan, D.; Shave, S.; Walkinshaw, M. Ligand discovery and virtual screening using the program LIDAEUS. *Br. J. Pharm.* **2008**, *153* (Suppl. 1), S55–S67. [CrossRef]
91. Stahura, F.L.; Bajorath, J. New methodologies for ligand-based virtual screening. *Curr. Pharm. Des.* **2005**, *11*, 1189–1202. [CrossRef]
92. Neves, B.J.; Braga, R.C.; Melo-Filho, C.C.; Moreira Filho, J.T.; Muratov, E.N.; Andrade, C.H. QSAR-based virtual screening: Advances and applications in drug discovery. *Front Pharm.* **2018**, *9*, 1275. [CrossRef] [PubMed]
93. Wolber, G.; Seidel, T.; Bendix, F.; Langer, T. Molecule-pharmacophore superpositioning and pattern matching in computational drug design. *Drug Discov. Today* **2008**, *13*, 23–29. [CrossRef] [PubMed]
94. Yan, X.; Liao, C.; Liu, Z.; T Hagler, A.; Gu, Q.; Xu, J. Chemical structure similarity search for ligand-based virtual screening: Methods and computational resources. *Curr. Drug Targets* **2016**, *17*, 1580–1585. [CrossRef] [PubMed]
95. Maggiora, G.; Vogt, M.; Stumpfe, D.; Bajorath, J. Molecular similarity in medicinal chemistry: Miniperspective. *J. Med. Chem.* **2013**, *57*, 3186–3204. [CrossRef]
96. Geppert, H.; Vogt, M.; Bajorath, J. Current trends in ligand-based virtual screening: Molecular representations, data mining methods, new application areas, and performance evaluation. *J. Chem. Inf. Model.* **2010**, *50*, 205–216. [CrossRef]
97. Švajger, U.; Brus, B.; Turk, S.; Sova, M.; Hodnik, V.; Anderluh, G.; Gobec, S. Novel toll-like receptor 4 (TLR4) antagonists identified by structure-and ligand-based virtual screening. *Eur. J. Med. Chem.* **2013**, *70*, 393–399. [CrossRef]
98. Varney, K.M.; Bonvin, A.M.; Pazgier, M.; Malin, J.; Yu, W.; Ateh, E.; Oashi, T.; Lu, W.; Huang, J.; Diepeveen-de Buin, M. Turning defense into offense: Defensin mimetics as novel antibiotics targeting lipid II. *PLoS Pathog.* **2013**, *9*, e1003732. [CrossRef]
99. Ambaye, N.D.; Gunzburg, M.J.; Lim, R.C.; Price, J.T.; Wilce, M.C.; Wilce, J.A. The Discovery of Phenylbenzamide Derivatives as Grb7-Based Antitumor Agents. *ChemMedChem* **2013**, *8*, 280–288. [CrossRef]

molecules

MDPI

Review

Second-Generation Androgen Receptor Antagonists as Hormonal Therapeutics for Three Forms of Prostate Cancer

Pravien Rajaram, Alyssa Rivera, Kevin Muthima, Nicholas Olveda, Hubert Muchalski * and Qiao-Hong Chen *

Department of Chemistry, California State University, Fresno, CA 93740, USA; pravien@mail.fresnostate.edu (P.R.); alyssamrivera@mail.fresnostate.edu (A.R.); muthima@mail.fresnostate.edu (K.M.); nicolveda08@mail.fresnostate.edu (N.O.)

* Correspondence: hmuchalski@csufresno.edu (H.M.); qchen@csufresno.edu (Q.-H.C.); Tel.: +1-559-278-2711 (H.M.); +1-559-278-2394 (Q.-H.C.)

Academic Editor: Laura Cerchia
Received: 1 May 2020; Accepted: 21 May 2020; Published: 24 May 2020

Abstract: Enzalutamide is the first second-generation nonsteroidal androgen receptor (AR) antagonist with a strong binding affinity to AR. Most significantly, enzalutamide can prolong not only overall survival time and metastatic free survival time for patients with lethal castration-resistant prostate cancer (CRPC), but also castration-resistant free survival time for patients with castration-sensitive prostate cancer (CSPC). Enzalutamide has thus been approved by the US Food and Drug Administration (FDA) for the treatment of both metastatic (in 2012) and non-metastatic (in 2018) CRPC, as well as CSPC (2019). This is an inspiring drug discovery story created by an amazing interdisciplinary collaboration. Equally important, the successful clinical use of enzalutamide proves the notion that the second-generation AR antagonists can serve as hormonal therapeutics for three forms of advanced prostate cancer. This has been further verified by the recent FDA approval of the other two second-generation AR antagonists, apalutamide and darolutamide, for the treatment of prostate cancer. This review focuses on the rational design and discovery of these three second-generation AR antagonists, and then highlights their syntheses, clinical studies, and use. Strategies to overcome the resistance to the second-generation AR antagonists are also reviewed.

Keywords: androgen receptor; prostate cancer; enzalutamide; apalutamide; darolutamide

1. Introduction

1.1. Prostate Cancer

Prostate cancer continues to be a main health concern due to the highest incidence and the second highest cancer-related death rate in American men. In 2020, estimates indicate about 21% of all new cancer cases will be attributed to prostate cancer, while over 33,000 deaths caused by prostate cancer are projected to occur in the United States [1]. The critical driving force for prostate cancer is the androgen receptor (AR)-regulated gene expression that is initiated by the binding of androgen to AR [2]. Consequently, the mainstay therapy for castration-sensitive prostate cancer (CSPC) since 1941 is androgen deprivation therapy (ADT). However, after the initial response to ADT for about 18 to 24 months, most CSPC will inevitably shift to castration resistant prostate cancer (CRPC) [3]. In the CRPC stage, prostate cancer continues to grow under extremely low levels of male hormone testosterone in serum. The majority of prostate cancer deaths in the United States are caused by late state (metastatic) CRPC (mCRPC). Within the past decade, several new treatments have been approved for three forms of prostate cancer: metastatic castration-sensitive prostate cancer (mCSPC), non-metastatic castration-resistant prostate cancer (nmCRPC), and metastatic castration-resistant prostate cancer (mCRPC). Table 1 lists the current treatments that have been approved by the US Food & Drug Administration (FDA) since 2004, according to the information published on the official website of the US FDA. Current treatments for prostate cancer can be classified into taxane-based chemotherapeutics, hormonal therapy, immunotherapy, and radiotherapy. As illustrated in Table 1, far more hormonal therapies than other categories have recently been approved by the US FDA for prostate cancer.

Table 1. Current Treatments with Survival Benefit for Patients with Prostate Cancer.

Brand Name	Generic Name	Approval Date	Treatments	Category
Taxotere	Docetaxel in combination with prednisone	19 May 2004	mCRPC	Chemotherapy
Jevtana	Cabazitaxel in combination with prednisone	17 June 2010	mCRPC after docetaxel	Chemotherapy
Xofigo	radium-223	15 May 2013	mCRPC	Radiotherapy
Provenge	Sipuleucel-T	29 April 2010	Asymptomatic or minimally symptomatic mCRPC	Immunotherapy
Zytiga	Abiraterone acetate in combination with prednisone	28 April 2011	mCRPC after docetaxel	Hormonal therapy
Zytiga	Abiraterone acetate in combination with prednisone	10 December 2012	mCRPC before chemotherapy	Hormonal therapy
Zytiga	Abiraterone acetate in combination with prednisone	7 February 2018	mCSPC	Hormonal therapy
Erleada	Apalutamide	14 February 2018	nmCRPC	Hormonal therapy
Erleada	Apalutamide	17 September 2019	mCSPC	Hormonal therapy
XTANDI	Enzalutamide	31 August 2012	mCRPC after docetaxel	Hormonal therapy
XTANDI	Enzalutamide	13 July 2018	nmCRPC	Hormonal therapy
NUBEQA	Darolutamide	30 July 2019	nmCRPC	Hormonal therapy
XTANDI	Enzalutamide	16 December 2019	mCSPC	Hormonal therapy

nmCRPC: non-metastatic castration-resistant prostate cancer. mCRPC: metastatic castration-resistant prostate cancer mCSPC: metastatic castration-sensitive prostate cancer.

1.2. Hormonal Therapeutics

The timeline for the development of hormonal therapeutics for prostate cancer is illustrated in Figure 1. The pioneering hormonal therapeutic for prostate cancer is the well-known androgen deprivation therapy originally reported by Huggins and Hodges in 1941 [4]. At that point, orchiectomy (surgical castration) and administration of high dose of estrogen (non-surgical castration) were established to be two strategies to cut down the circulating testosterone to castrate (or near castrate) levels, resulting in appreciable biochemical response in a cohort of eight patients with metastatic prostate cancer. It was recognized by the Veterans Administration Cooperative Urological Research Group in 1970s that treatment of patients with advanced prostate cancer with high dose of estrogen led to good efficacy, but accompanying with enhanced mortality rate associated with cardiovascular complications [5]. The serious undesired effect of estrogen urged the scientists to search for a safer non-surgical castration strategy in 1980s. Encouraged by the finding that testicular production of testosterone can be indirectly controlled by long-lasting elevation of gonadotropin-releasing hormone (GnRH), GnRH agonists were designed and found to possess potential in suppressing prostate tumor growth in vivo and in clinical settings [6,7]. Synthetic GnRH agonists, e.g., goserelin (Zoladex) [8] and leuprolide (Lupron) [9], were developed as a replacement for estrogen as a better non-surgical castration strategy by the mid-1980s and have served as the centerpiece of ADT for CSPC since then. To conquer the testosterone surge as well as other side effects caused by GnRH agonists, the US FDA has approved degarelix (a GnRH antagonist) as an alternative medical castration for patients with advanced CSPC in 2008. As compared with GnRH agonists, degarelix can provide rapid suppression of prostate specific antigen (PSA) and testosterone so as to better control testosterone and prolong PSA progression-free survival [10]. Degarelix is, thus, a better non-surgical castration therapy for those CSPC patients at more advanced stages and with more apparent symptoms.

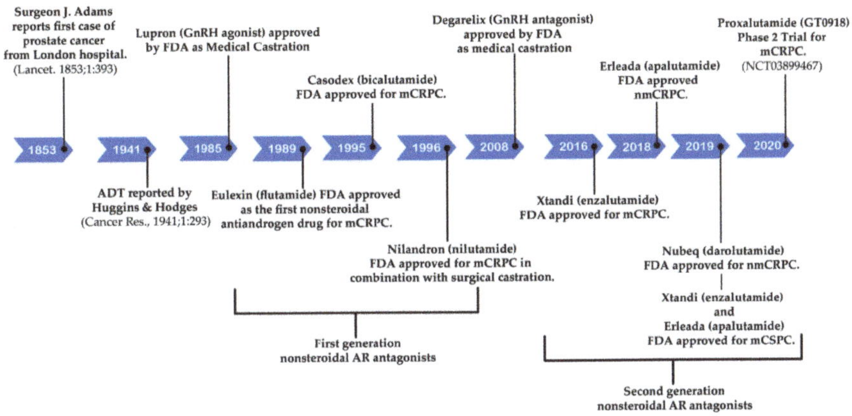

Figure 1. Timeline for the development of hormonal therapeutics for prostate cancer.

On the other hand, examination of antiandrogen compounds as another alternative to estrogen castration was initiated in the late 1960s and early 1970s, leading to the development of three first generation nonsteroidal androgen antagonists, flutamide (**1**), nilutamide, (**2**) and bicalutamide (**3**), shown in Figure 2 [11]. These antiandrogen agents were revealed to competitively bind to the ligand-binding domain on androgen receptors. Monotherapy of bicalutamide (the one with the most extensive investigation) cannot offer better clinical benefit to patients with CSPC than ADT. The combination therapy of bicalutamide with ADT is widely used by CSPC patients owing to the greater safety profile than ADT alone, even though it does not grant significant overall survival benefit [12].

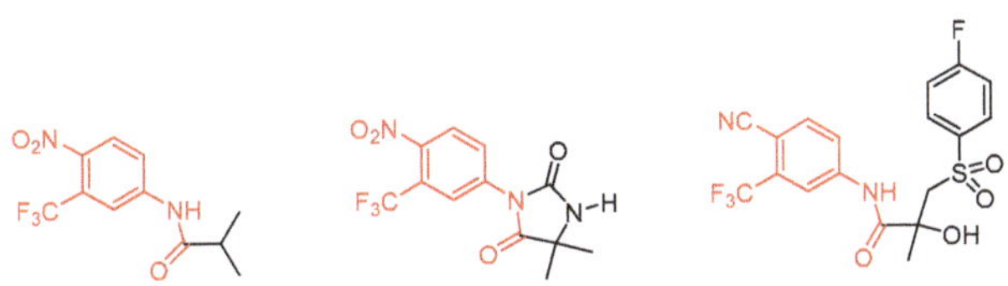

Flutamide (**1**) Nilutamide (**2**) Bicalutamide (**3**)

Figure 2. First generation of nonsteroidal AR antagonists.

The clearer understanding of the structure and function of the androgen receptor revealed that the androgen receptor plays a pivotal role for not only CSPC but also CRPC [13]. This notation stimulated the successful design and discovery of three US FDA-approved second-generation androgen receptor antagonists, enzalutamide (**4**) [14], apalutamide (**5**) [15], and darolutamide (**6**) [16] (Figure 3). As illustrated in Table 2, enzalutamide (**4**) is now the first FDA-approved antiandrogen to treat three forms of advanced prostate cancer after the US FDA approval of enzalutamide (**4**) on 16 December 2019 for the treatment of metastatic castration-sensitive prostate cancer (mCSPC). The intriguing discovery stories of these three successful second-generation nonsteroidal AR antagonists are reviewed in this article. Their syntheses, clinical studies, and clinical use are highlighted as well. Current strategies to overcome the resistance to these AR antagonists are also summarized.

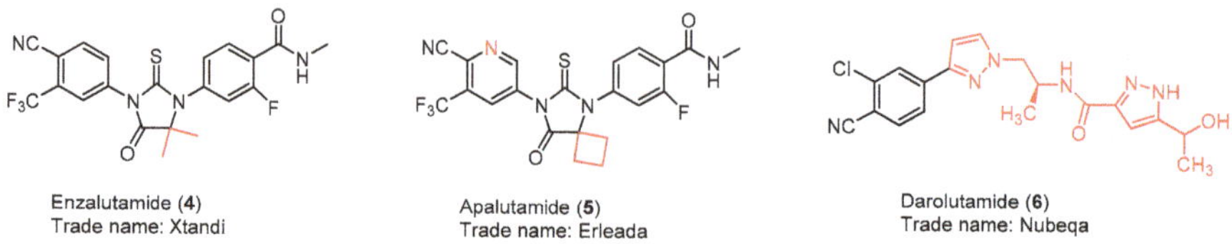

Figure 3. Second generation of nonsteroidal AR antagonists.

Table 2. FDA-approved second-generation AR antagonists for prostate cancer.

Brand Name	Generic Name	mCRPC	nmCRPC	mCSPC
XTANDI	enzalutamide	yes	yes	yes
Erleada	apalutamide	no	yes	yes
NUBEQA	darolutamide	no	yes	no

nmCRPC: non-metastatic castration-resistant prostate cancer. mCRPC: metastatic castration-resistant prostate cancer. mCSPC: metastatic castration-sensitive prostate cancer.

2. Discovery and Preclinical Studies

2.1. Enzalutamide (**4**) *and Apalutamide* (**5**)

Enzalutamide (**4**) and apalutamide (**5**) were discovered by the interdisciplinary collaboration of Sawyers/Jung groups, which was motivated by the notion that "growth of castration-resistant prostate cancer appears to depend upon continued androgen receptor signaling," facilitated by the in vitro AR-overexpressing prostate cancer cell models, and benefited from a complementary collaboration [17]. As illustrated in Figure 4, RU59063 (**7**) was selected as the original lead compound because it is a potent and selective nonsteroidal AR agonist with high affinity for AR [18,19]. Enzalutamide (**4**) and apalutamide (**5**) were eventually identified as two lead candidates for preclinical development on the grounds of in vitro evaluation of their capability of agonistic and antagonistic activity of AR signaling in a castration-resistant LNCaP/AR prostate cancer cell model [20]. The in vitro relative luciferase activity and relative PSA level were measured using bicalutamide as positive control.

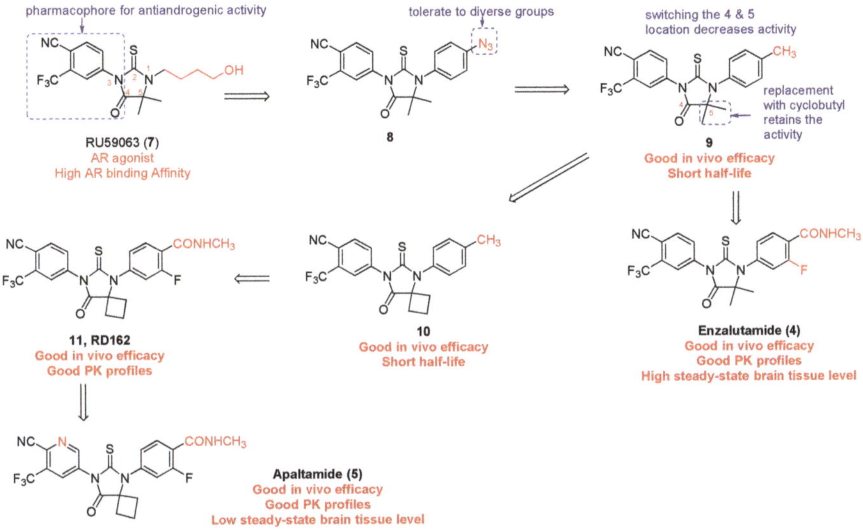

Figure 4. Discovery of enzalutamide and apalutamide.

The structural modification started with substituting the ω-hydroxybutyl at *N*1 with azidoalkyl and azidoaryl groups in the light of the hypothesis that the small polar azido group might function as a bioisostere of the hydroxyl in RU59063 (**7**). The eastern side of RU59063 (**7**) was the first focus of the chemical manipulation probably due to the fact that the electron-deficient aromatic ring on the western side is a well-established pharmacophore for anti-androgenic activity [21]. Among the first set of analogues, compound **8** was identified as the optimal derivative that had higher binding affinity than bicalutamide. Further modification on compound **8** indicated that the 4-position of the *N*1-phenyl ring can accommodate several different groups without losing the desired activity. Compound **9** with a 4-methyl on the *N*1-phenyl ring was chosen for further structure-activity relationship studies, indicating that the location for the C-4 and C-5 on the thiohydantoin ring cannot be switched and that the geminal dimethyl group on the thiohydantoin ring can be substituted by the cyclobutyl ring in compound **10**. On the basis of abovementioned promising in vitro bioassay data, compounds **9** and **10** were moved forward for in vivo evaluation in a castrate mice model with LAPC4/AR or LNCaP/AR xenografts. Both compounds are more effective than bicalutamide in suppressing PSA secretion, but with a short half-life due to rapid clearance. Considering that electron-rich *N*1-phenyl ring and hydroxylation of the benzylic methyl, directly appending electron-withdrawing groups to the *N*1-phenyl ring led to the discovery of 3-fluoroamide analogues **11** (also called RD162) and enzalutamide (also called MDV3100). Both enzalutamide and RD162 (**11**) have greater (5–8 times) AR binding affinity relative to bicalutamide in the LNCaP/AR cell line with high level expression of wild-type AR. More importantly, their binding is specific to AR because only little or no binding to other nuclear receptors was observed [14].

Both enzalutamide and RD162 (**11**) possess not only excellent in vivo anti-tumor efficacy in the castrate mice model but also superb pharmacokinetic profile [14]. The in vivo pharmacokinetic properties of RD162 (**11**) were first evaluated in mice. The results showed that, after a 24-h oral treatment with a single 20 mg/kg dose, the plasma concentration (~23 μM) of RD162 (**11**) exceeds the concentration (~1–10 μM) necessary to block AR activity. The in vivo pharmacodynamic experiments suggest that RD162 (**11**) can significantly reduce AR transcriptional function and suppress LNCaP/AR tumor cell proliferation. The excellent in vivo efficacy of RD162 (**11**) in castration-resistant prostate tumor models was confirmed to be associated with AR suppression. This is because the effective dose for antitumor efficacy in the LNCaP/AR model is closely correlated with that for AR transcriptional activity as measured by luciferase imaging experiments. The fact that enzalutamide instead of RD162 (**11**) was chosen, at that moment, as the drug candidate for further preclinical studies is simply because enzalutamide can be prepared from an inexpensive starting material. Enzalutamide was successfully approved by FDA, but was found to be associated with seizure side effect caused by antagonizing $GABA_A$ receptor in the central nervous system [22]. With the hope to find out a second-generation nonsteroidal AR antagonist with a high therapeutic index, apalutamide was later chosen for further preclinical investigation because of its lower steady-state brain tissue level in mice.

As shown in Figure 4, apalutamide (**5**, also named ARN-509) has very similar chemical structure to RD-162 (**11**) with only difference being the replacement of the *N*3-phenyl ring in RD162 (**11**) with a *N*3-pyridyl ring in apalutamide. Apalutamide possesses comparable in vitro activity to enzalutamide, but with greater anti-tumor efficacy in CRPC xenograft models and lower potential in causing seizure as an adverse effect in the central nervous system [14,23]. Specifically, enzalutamide (**4**) and apalutamide (**5**) were demonstrated to retain full antagonist activity in an AR overexpression setting and have a higher binding affinity of up to 10-fold for AR when compared to bicalutamide (**3**). Both of them compete with bicalutamide (**3**) for the same ligand-binding domain of AR. The selective binding of apalutamide (**5**) for AR over other nuclear hormone receptors was observed. Unlike the first-generation AR antagonists, both enzalutamide (**4**) and apalutamide (**5**) can interrupt multiple steps of the AR-signaling pathway, including the androgen binding to AR, nuclear translocation of AR, DNA binding, and coactivator recruitment. Good in vivo pharmacokinetic profiles, including good oral availability, long plasma half-life, and low systemic clearance, were found for both enzalutamide and apalutamide in mouse and dog models. However, apalutamide (**5**) has less chance than enzalutamide (**4**) to bind to plasma proteins, and 2-fold higher concentration of free apalutamide (**5**) was detected in mouse and human plasma. The in vivo pharmacodynamics studies of enzalutamide (**4**) and apalutamide (**5**) were carried out in a CRPC animal model with LNCaP/AR-luc xenograft tumors. Both of them have potent in vivo anti-tumor efficacy because they can significantly decrease androgen driven luciferase reporter-gene activity and reduce tumor volume compared to vehicle. However, apalutamide (**5**) only needs 10 to 30 mg/kg/d to reach maximum efficacy in the castrate mouse model with the LNCaP/AR xenografts, while enzalutamide (**4**) requires 30 to 100 mg/kg/d. Additionally, apalutamide exhibits antitumor activity in a CSPC xenograft model. The above-mentioned data provide preclinical proofs for further clinical development of apalutamide and enzalutamide for patients with CSPC and CRPC [14,23].

2.2. *Darolutamide* (**6**)

An AR transactivation screening of a group of nonsteroidal pyrazole-carboxamide and imidazole-carboxamide derivatives in an AR-HEK293 cell model in combination with a lead optimization process led to the discovery of darolutamide (**6**, also named ODM-201) [24]. Similar to enzalutamide (**4**) and apalutamide (**5**), darolutamide (**6**) is a full antagonist that has high affinity for AR in the AR overexpressing setting and suppresses nuclear translocation of AR. In contrast to enzalutamide (**4**) and apalutamide (**5**), darolutamide (**6**) possesses the following features [24]: (i) a different chemical scaffold that may bypass the side effects caused by enzalutamide (**4**) and apalutamide (**5**); (ii) antagonistic effects towards AR mutants AR(F876L), AR(W741L), and AR(T877A) that facilitate resistance to the first- and second-generation nonsteroidal AR antagonists; (iii) an inability to cross over the brain–blood barrier, suggesting a lower seizure risk than observed with enzalutamide; (iv) not increasing the concentration of serum testosterone in a mouse model; (v) having higher in vivo antitumor efficacy in the mouse model, and (vi) a shorter half-life (1.6 h vs 18.3 h for enzalutamide). Taken together, these promising preclinical results imply that darolutamide (**6**) is complementary to enzalutamide (**4**) and apalutamide (**5**) and that darolutamide (**6**) is an excellent addition to the family of the second generation of AR antagonists. However, higher dose and more frequent administration are recommended for darolutamide (**6**) due to its shorter half-life.

3. Syntheses

A detailed review of the development of synthetic approaches to enzalutamide, apalutamide, and darolutamide was recently published [25].

3.1. Synthetic Approaches to Enzalutamide (**4**) *and Apalutamide* (**5**)

Structures of enzalutamide (**4**) and apalutamide (**5**) are highly functionalized and offer multiple disconnection approaches to their synthesis. Each strategy is based on a key transformation of advanced intermediates and the bulk of the synthetic effort is spent on synthesizing those intermediates. The synthesis of the core structure of enzalutamide (**4**) and apalutamide (**5**) has been accomplished using three main strategies, which are presented in Scheme 1. Strategy 1 and Strategy 2 construct the thiohydantoin core toward the end of the synthesis, whereas Strategy 3 begins with the formation of thiohydantoin and the aromatic rings are added later. Regardless of the strategy, the assembly of the final drug begins from similar advanced aryl intermediates. Thus, the majority of process development was focused on preparation of aniline derivatives **D** and **E**, and aryl halides **H** and **I**.

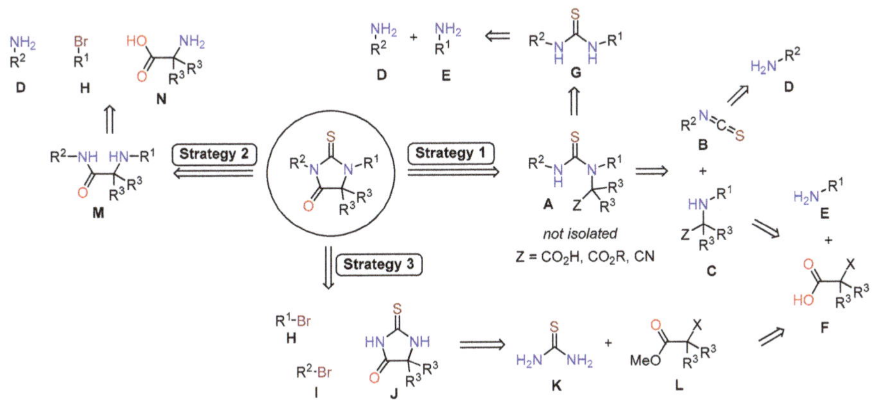

Scheme 1. Overview of synthetic approaches to hydantoin-based enzalutamide and apalutamide.

3.1.1. Strategy 1: Cyclization of Isothiocyanate

The first strategy is based on tandem condensation–cyclization cascade initiated by addition of isothiocyanate **B** to the α-amino acid derivative **C**, which delivers the thiourea intermediate **A** (Scheme 1). The compound **A** is not isolated, the nitrogen and the pendant carboxylic acid derivative (Z = CO_2H, CO_2R, or CN) react to form the thiohydantoin core. Thus, the key intermediates in this approach are isothiocyanate **B** and carboxylic acid intermediate **C**.

Sawyers and Jung disclosed the synthesis of **13** from aniline **12** and thiophosgene (Scheme 2) [17,26–28], to which alternative approaches that avoid use of thiophosgene were later developed [29–32]. The intermediate **12** needed for enzalutamide is commercially available. However, the aniline precursor of isothiocyanate fragment **18** needed for preparation of apalutamide had to be synthesized and proved to be a major challenge typical of heterocyclic amines containing both electron-rich and electron poor substituents. All published approaches to **17** vary in the order and method in which the substituents are added to 2-chloro-3-(trifluoromethyl)pyridine (**14**). The initially disclosed synthesis uses nitration–reduction sequence to install the amine functional group (Scheme 2). This strategy required uneconomical functional group interconversion (conversion **14** to hydroxypyridine **15**, then back to chloride **16** after nitration) as well as protection of the amine. The overall yield of this 7-step sequence is difficult to assess because yields for all steps were not reported. Alternately, cyanation can be accomplished prior to reduction of the nitro group and thus avoiding wasteful protection if a bromide is used instead of the chloride (steps i–k, Scheme 2) [33,34].

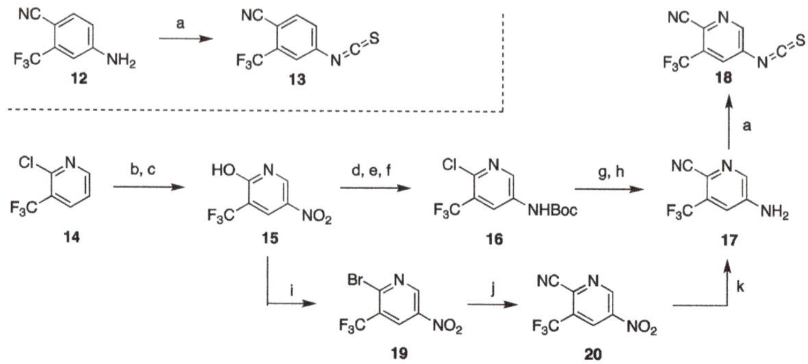

Scheme 2. Synthesis of isothiocyanate fragments of enzalutamide and apalutamide. Reaction conditions: (a) $CSCl_2$, H_2O; (b) AcOH, H_2O, reflux; (c) HNO_3, H_2SO_4, 90 °C; (d) $POCl_3$, PCl_5, 110–120 °C; H_2, (e) Raney Ni, THF; (f) Boc_2O, pyridine, DMAP, rt; (g) KCN, CuCN, phenantroline, DMA, 110 °C; (h) TFA, CH_2Cl_2; (i) $POBr_3$, PBr_3, Br_2, 90–110 °C; (j) CuCN, phenantroline, CH_3CONMe_2, 160 °C; (k) AcOH, Fe.

Highly hazardous nitration at elevated temperature can be avoided by installing the amine via C–*N* cross-coupling reaction, although functional group interconversion (Cl to OH and back to Cl) remains as part of the route (Scheme 3). Initially developed conditions for the cross-coupling delivered **23** in low yield (40%) [33,34], but the reaction conditions were later improved to reliably generate the amine **23** in 71–85% yield [35,36]. Other routes to **17** were also disclosed, but they contain serious inefficiencies are less likely to be adopted on process scale [33,34].

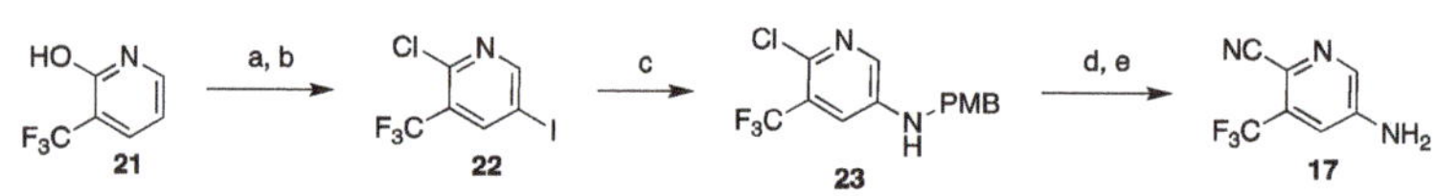

Scheme 3. Nitration-free synthesis of the substituted pyridine intermediate **17**. Reaction conditions: (a) NIS, DMF, CH_3CN, 80 °C; (b) $POCl_3$, DMF, microwave 130 °C; (c) $PMBNH_2$, $Pd(OAc)_2$, BINAP, Et_3N, $CsCO_3$, toluene; (d) $Zn(CN)_2$, $Pd_2(dba)_3$, dppf, DMF, 110 °C; (e) TFA, CH_2Cl_2.

Synthesis of the advanced intermediate **C** (R = CN, Scheme 1) can be accomplished in several ways. In their initial route to enzalutamide, Sawyers and Jung reported preparation of **26** in 52% overall yield in a 4-step sequence which begins with oxidation of 2-fluoro-4-nitrotoluene (**24**) to the corresponding carboxylic acid [17], which was converted to an *N*-methyl amide **25** via the acid chloride intermediate. Reduction of the nitro group to an amine and addition to acetone cyanohydrin furnish α-amino nitrile **26**, which upon reaction with isothiocyanate **13** under microwave heating in DMF, gave enzalutamide (**4**). In another approach, amino ester **29** was prepared in 4 steps from 4-bromo-2-fluorobenzoic acid (**27**) in 64% yield by first converting the acid to the *N*-methyl amide followed by a S_NAr reaction with 2-aminoisobutyric acid and esterification. Although this route is shorter and the overall yield is slightly higher than the synthesis of nitrile **26**, on a process scale the likely starting material would be 4-bromo-2-fluorotoluene which would add one additional step and likely reduce the overall yield (Scheme 4).

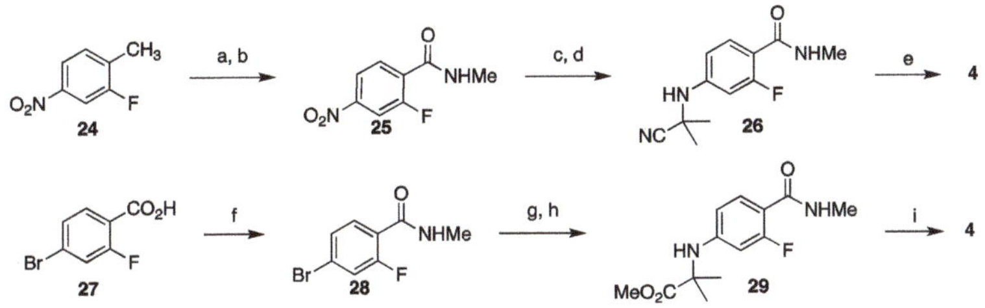

Scheme 4. Synthesis of the amino nitrile **26** (top) and amino ester **29** (bottom) for the assembly of enzalutamide. Reaction conditions: (a) CrO_3, H_5IO_6, CH_3CN, CH_2Cl_2; (b) $SOCl_2$, DMF, then $MeNH_2$; (c) Fe, AcOH, EtOAc, reflux; (d) 2-cyano-2-hydroxypropane, $MgSO_4$, EtOAc, 80 °C; (e) **13**, DFM, microwave 100 °C; (f) $SOCl_2$, DMF (cat), 2-PrOAc, 60 °C, then $MeNH_2$; (g) 2-aminoisobutyric acid, CuI, K_2CO_3, 2-acetylcyclohexanone, DMF, H_2O, 105 °C; (h) MeI, K_2CO_3, DMF, H_2O, 40 °C; **13**, DMSO, 2-PrOAc, 83–83 °C.

The amino nitrile fragment needed for assembly of apalutamide was prepared similarly in a 4-step sequence which begins with acylation of methyl amine with 2,4-difluorobenzoyl chloride (**30**) followed by S_NAr reaction with 4-methoxybenzyl amine under microwave conditions to give **31**. Acid-mediated deprotection and a Strecker reaction with cyclobutanone in the presence of sodium cyanide give amino nitrile **32** (Scheme 5, top). Although this route is relatively short, it will be difficult to implement at scale. The yield of the S_NAr reaction is low (40%) due to poor regioselectivity; the yield of the Strecker reaction was not reported. Additionally, use of cyanide at scale is challenging due to potential release of HCN. The company Hinova developed this route into a 3-step preparation (69%–82% yield) of **32** in which 2-fluoro-4-nitrobenzoic acid (**33**) was converted to a methyl amide followed by reduction of the nitro group and a Strecker reaction with cyclobutanone with TMSCN as cyanide source (Scheme 5, bottom) [37,38].

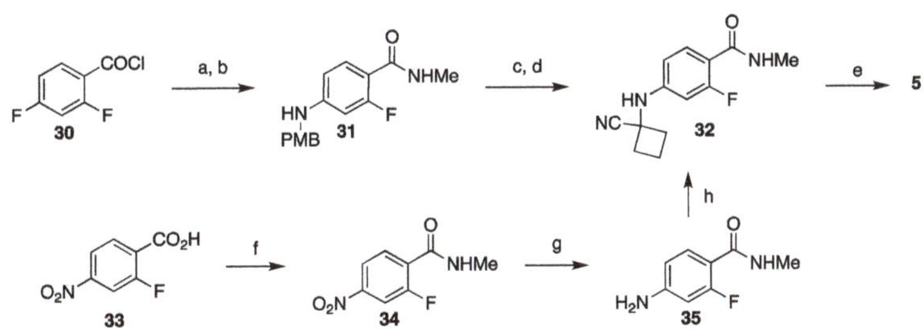

Scheme 5. Two options for synthesis of amino nitrile **32** for the assembly of apalutamide. Reaction conditions: (a) $MeNH_2$, THF; (b) $PMBNH_2$, MeCN, microwave 190 °C; (c) TFA, CH_2Cl_2; (d) cyclobutanone, NaCN; (e) **18**, $CSCl_2$, $MeCONMe_2$, 80 °C, then HCl, MeOH; (f) Me_2NH–HCl, CDI, Et_3N, CH_2Cl_2, rt; (g) Fe, AcOH, EtOAc, reflux; (h) cyclobutanone, TMSCN, AcOH, 80 °C.

Several companies subsequently explored other carboxylic acid derivatives, with the most successful one being ester-based route shown in Scheme 6. Coupling between aryl bromide **36** and cyclobutane amino acid **37** gives amino acid derivative **38** (step a, Scheme 6) [39,40]; alternatively, acid **38** can be prepared from amine **40** and α-bromo acid **41** (step b, Scheme 6) [41]. Alkylation of the carboxylic acid **38** followed by a reaction with isothiocyanide **18** delivered apalutamide in 47% yield from **38**. It is important to note that condensation/cyclization cascade of esters and isothiocyanate delivers thiohydantoin in higher yield than the same reaction with the nitrile, but the higher yield comes with trade-offs. First, one additional step will be needed to convert the ester to amide ($MeNH_2$, heat). Second, the cyclization reaction of isothiocyanate with esters produces alcohol by-product, which is reactive toward the isothiocyanate present in the reaction mixture. Therefore, excess of isothiocyanate has to be used in this step and at least one equivalent is ultimately lost to alcoholysis.

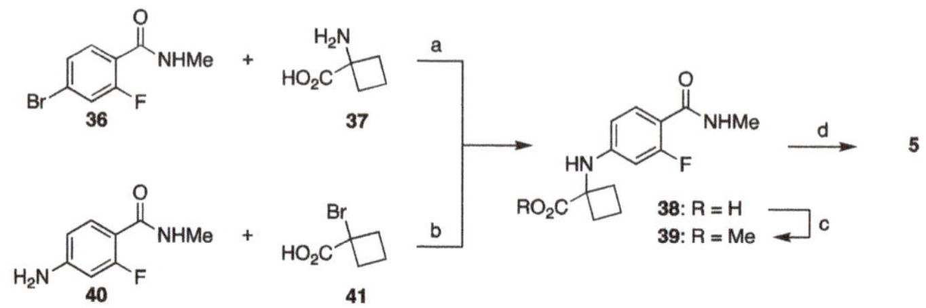

Scheme 6. Cyclobutanecarboxylic acid-based approaches to the advanced intermediate **39** needed for assembly of apalutamide. Reaction conditions: (a) DMF, K_2CO_3, CuCl, H_2O, 100–105 °C; (b) i-Pr_2Net, Et_3N, CH_2Cl_2, reflux; (c) MeI, DMF, K_2CO_3, rt; (d) **18**, DMSO, 2-PrOAc, 90 °C.

Other iterations of Strategy 1 were also used in synthesis of apalutamide where the thiohydantoin core was constructed prior to installation of the methyl benzamide (Scheme 7) [42,43]. Halogenated aniline **42** was subjected to a Strecker reaction with cyclobutanone and the resulting amino nitrile **43** was reacted with isothiocyanate **13** formed in-situ from aniline **17** and 1,1′-thiocarbonylbis(pyridine-2(1*H*)-one (vide infra). Appending the methyl amide functional group can then be accomplished in several ways (Scheme 7, step c): (i) Grignard synthesis of carboxylic acid followed by CDI coupling with methyl amine; (ii) direct Pd-catalyzed amide formation with methylamine and carbon monoxide; or (iii) Pd-catalyzed carbonylative esterification followed by a conversion of the ester to the amide.

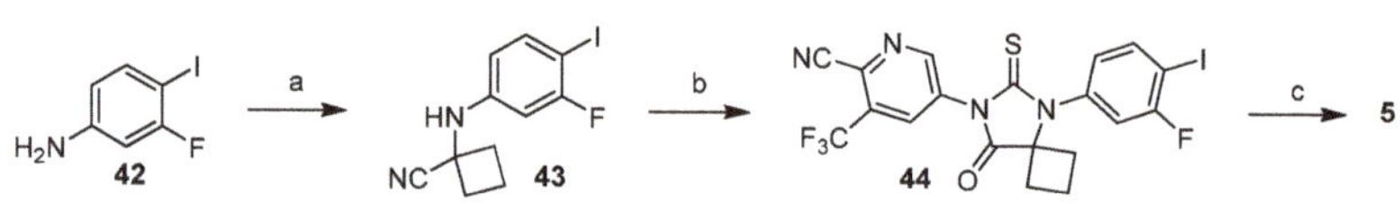

Scheme 7. Synthesis of thiohydantoin core of apalutamide and late-stage amide formation. Reaction conditions: (a) cyclobutanone, NaCN, AcOH; (b) **17**, 1,1′-thiocarbonylbis (pyridine-2(1*H*)-one, toluene, 100 °C then HCl, EtOH, DMA, 70 °C; (c) n-C_5H_{11}MgBr, THF, CO_2, then CDI, $MeNH_2$, THF; or Pd(t-$Bu_3P)_2$, CO (5 bar), i-Pr_2Net, $MeNH_2$, THF, 60 °C; or Pd$(OAc)_2$, dppf, i-Pr_2NH, CO, MeOH, 60 °C, then $MeNH_2$, MeOH.

3.1.2. Strategy 2: Late Stage Cyclization of Amino Amide

The second strategy focuses on the late stage formation of thiohydantoin core through cyclization of the amino amide **M** with thiophosgene or its surrogate (Scheme 1, Strategy 2). Depending on the chosen disconnection, the amino amide **M** can be constructed by condensation of amine **D** with amino acid **N**, or aryl-aryl cross-coupling of the amine **D** with bromide **H**. An application of this strategy was reported by Meng and co-workers in their approach to enzalutamide, which started with a carbodiimide coupling of aniline **12** and protected amino acid **45**, affording amino amide **46** after deprotection (Scheme 8). Copper-catalyzed aryl amination with methyl 4-bromo-2-fluorobenzoate (**47**) affords amino amide **49**, which undergoes the cyclization reaction with thiophosgene in the presence of 8-fold excess of DMAP to provide ester **49** in 28% overall yield [44].

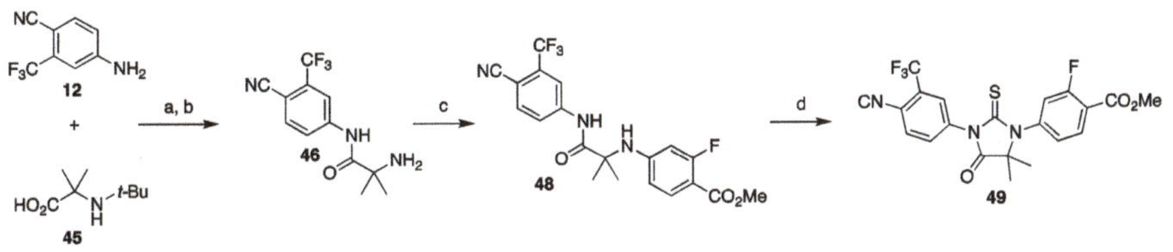

Scheme 8. Synthesis of advanced intermediate ester **49** via late-stage formation of thiohydantoin. Reaction conditions: (a) CDI, DBU, *i*-Pr_2NEt, THF, 55–65 °C; (b) HCl, 2-PrOH; (c) methyl 4-bromo-2-fluorobenzoate (**47**), acetylacetone, CuI, K_2CO_3, DMF, 120–130 °C; $CSCl_2$, DMAP, THF, 40–50 °C.

As illustrated in Scheme 9, a modified version of this strategy was used in the synthesis of apalutamide. The key differences include more streamlined synthesis of the starting aniline **12**, use of Boc as protecting group for the amino acid **50**, and use of 1,1′-thiocarbonylbis(pyridine-2(1*H*)-one (or phenylthionochloroformate) as thiophosgene alternative for the formation of thiohydantoin core [45]. This route is a highly developed process that achieves synthesis of apalutamide in seven linear steps with only three purifications. Accounting for two-step synthesis of hydroxypyridine **15** (see Scheme 2), this route achieves preparation of apalutamide in nine linear steps.

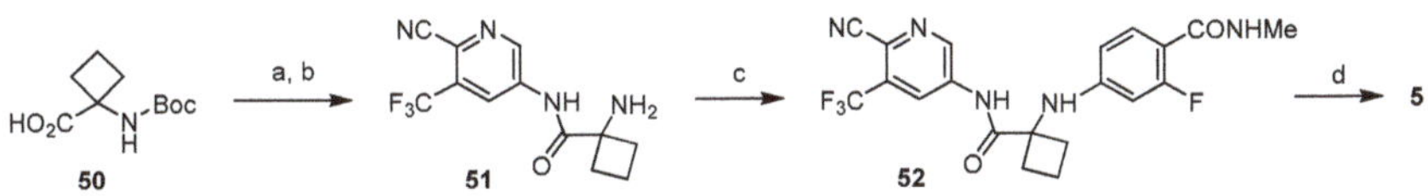

Scheme 9. Synthesis of apalutamide via late-stage, thiophosgene-free cyclization. Reaction conditions: (a) **12**, CDI, DBU, *i*-Pr_2NEt, THF, 60 °C; (b) HCl, 2-PrOH, 70 °C; (c) **28**, DMA, KOAc, CuBr, TMEDA, 120 °C; (d) 1,1′-thiocarbonylbis(pyridine2(1*H*)-one, DMAP, DMA, 90 °C.

3.1.3. Strategy 3: Functionalization of Thiohydantoin

The third strategy focuses on the formation of thiohydanotin core first and then functionalization the nitrogens (Strategy 3, Scheme 1). In comparison to the two strategies outlined above, this one is relatively less developed. Nevertheless, it holds the most promise for large-scale synthesis of enzalutamide because it is still highly divergent and, even more importantly, avoids use of thiophosgene. The reported synthesis of enzalutamide using this approach begins with a reaction of methyl 2-chloroisobutyrate (**53**) with thiourea in the presence of triethylamine to give thiohydantoin **54**. Compound **54** then undergoes two S_NAr reactions. Deprotonation with NaH in DMF followed by addition of 4-bromo-3-(trifluoromethyl)benzonitrile (**55**) furnished compound **56**, which is deprotonated again and reacted with aryl bromide **28** to provide enzalutamide (Scheme 10) [32]. It should be noted that, at the time of this writing, methyl 2-chloroisobutyrate is not widely available from commercial sources and will have to be synthesized [46].

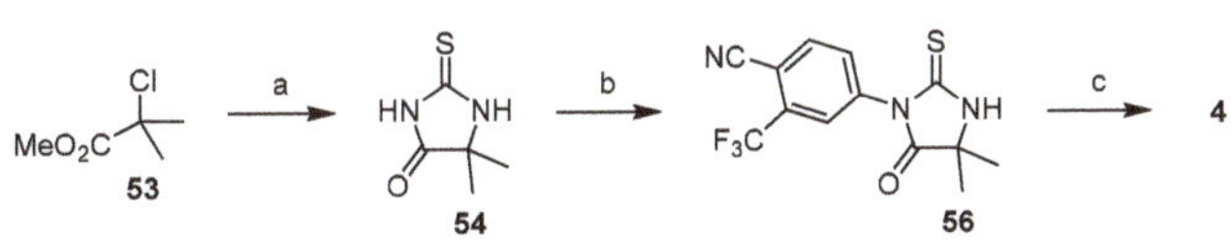

Scheme 10. Synthesis of enzalutamide via functionalization of thiohydantoin. Reaction conditions: (a) thiourea, Et_3N, DMF, 80–90 °C; (b) 4-bromo-3-(trifluoromethyl)- benzonitrile (**55**), NaH, DMF, rt; (c) **28**, NaH, DMF.

A hybrid variant of this strategy and Strategy 1 were also used in synthesis of apalutamide [47]. The ester **57** was first reacted with potassium isothiocyanate to give thiohydantoin **58**, which was then coupled with aryl bromide **59** to give apalutamide. Both **57** and **58** can be purified by crystallization, which is a significant advantage for process development (Scheme 11).

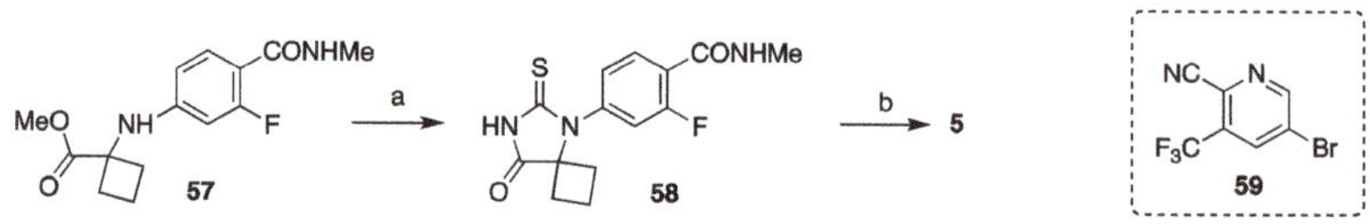

Scheme 11. Synthesis of apalutamide using atom-economical formation of isothiohydantoin core. Reaction conditions: (a) KSCN, *i*-Pr_2NEt, $MeOH/H_2O$, reflux; (b) **59**, K_2CO_3, CuI, DMF, 100–110 °C.

3.2. *Synthesis of Darolutamide*

The development of synthesis of darolutamide was mostly focused on process improvements, such as isolation via crystallization, elimination of expensive and hazardous reagents, and the general strategy remained unchanged since the original disclosure (Scheme 12) [48–51]. The synthesis relies on cross-coupling and substitution chemistry with some protection/deprotection and functional group interconversions. First, a pinacol boronic ester is installed on the THP-protected pyrazole **60** by treatment with *n*-BuLi, then with triisopropylborane, and finally with pinacol. Palladium(II) acetate-catalyzed Suzuki cross-coupling of **61** with aryl bromide **62** delivers intermediate **63**. The nitrogen was deprotected with aqueous acid and reacted with *N*-protected (*S*)-(+)-2-amino-1-propanol (**64**) under Mitsunobu conditions followed by deprotection at low pH to give intermediate **65**. The synthesis of darolutamide diastereomers was completed by amide coupling of **65** with carboxylic acid **66** followed by reduction of the methyl ketone with $NaBH_4$ in ethanol.

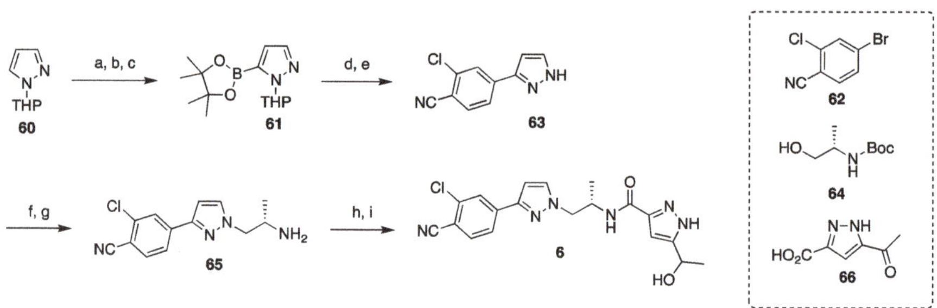

Scheme 12. Synthesis of darolutamide. Reaction conditions: (a) n-BuLi, THF, toluene; (b) $(i\text{-PrO})_3B$; (c) pinacol, AcOH; (d) **62**, $Pd(OAc)_2$, K_2CO_3, CH_3CN/H_2O, 70 °C; (e) aq HCl, MeOH, 10 °C; (f) **64**, PPh_3, DIAD, EtOAc; (g) aq HCl, 45 °C; (h) **66**, T3P, EtOAc, i-Pr_2NEt, 10 °C; (i) $NaBH_4$, EtOH.

4. Clinical Studies and Use of Second Generation Nonsteroidal AR Antagonists

Only those clinical studies directly associated with the US FDA approval of enzalutamide, apalutamide, and darolutamide were highlighted in this review.

4.1. *Enzalutamide*

Enzalutamide (also named MDV3100; trade name: Xtandi) has been approved by the FDA in 2012, 2018, and 2019, respectively, for the treatment of mCRPC, nmCRPC, and mCSPC. Enzalutamide possesses a generally good safety profile and is now widely used as a standard-of-care for the treatment of three forms of prostate cancer. The clinical use of enzalutamide not only helps to better manage prostate cancer but also verifies that androgen receptor signaling continues to be one of critical driving forces for CRPC. Enzalutamide can be sequentially used with other therapeutic methods.

The earlier clinical trials of enzalutamide were initiated by its promising efficacy and drug-like properties collected from the preclinical CRPC models. The competitive AR binding capability and clinically effective antitumor activity, together with tolerable safety profile of enzalutamide, were verified in human by a phase I/II study that enrolled 140 patients with CRPC in both pre- and post-chemotherapy settings [52]. The maximal tolerated dose for enzalutamide was determined to be 240 mg/day and the recommended dose for the advanced clinical trials was identified to be 160 mg/day. In view of these inspiring early-stage clinical results, the first phase III trial of enzalutamide, named AFFIRM, has been started to scrutinize enzalutamide versus placebo in patients with mCRPC in a post-chemotherapy setting.

4.1.1. Enzalutamide for mCRPC

With overall survival as its primary end point, AFFIRM aimed to assess whether enzalutamide can prolong the survival time of patients with mCRPC in a post-chemotherapy setting [53]. The clinical benefits derived from AFFIRM as demonstrated by the primary end points and the secondary end points were summarized in Table 3. The primary outcome from this phase III trials established enzalutamide as the first nonsteroidal AR antagonist with significant increase in patient's overall survival time. The secondary outcome suggested that enzalutamide can appreciably slow cancer progression, reduce PSA response, and improve patient's quality of life when compared to placebo. The major adverse effects of enzalutamide observed from AFFIRM are seizures, with 0.6% (five patients out of 800) of patients from the enzalutamide treatment group being reported to have a seizure. This study verified that AR and AR signaling continue to play a pivotal role for the progression of CRPC. Enzalutamide was thus quickly approved by the US FDA on 31 August 2012, for the treatment of late-stage mCRPC due to its capability of prolonging patient's life.

Table 3. Major therapeutic benefits brought by enzalutamide based on AFFIRM.

Enzalutamide AFFIRM Phase III Trial (NCT00974311)			
End Points	**Enzalutamide (n = 800)**	**Placebo (n = 399)**	**Hazard Ratio (95% CI)**
Primary End Points			
Median OS (mo)	18.4	13.6	0.63
Secondary End Points			
Median time to rPFS (mo)	8.3	2.9	0.4
Median time to first SRE (mo)	16.7	13.3	0.69
Median time to PSA progression (mo)	8.3	3	0.25
*** PSA response (%) of no.**			
decline ≥90% from baseline	25 (731)	1 (3300	
decline ≥50% from baseline	54 (731)	1 (330)	
Serious AEs (%)	39.9	38.8	

OS: Overall Survival; rPFS: Radiographic Progression-free Survival; SRE: Skeletal-related Event; PSA: Prostate-specific Antigen; AEs: Adverse Events. * Does not include patients who discontinued or died during the trial.

Inspired by the positive results from AFFIRM and the greater benefit observed in chemotherapy-naïve patients in the phase I-II clinical trial [52], another phase III trial (named PREVAIL, ClinicalTrials.gov number, NCT01212991) of enzalutamide was designed to explore the possibility of extending the application of enzalutamide to patients with mCRPC before chemotherapy [54]. A total of 1717 patients with chemotherapy-naïve mCRPC were enrolled in this trial and randomized into enzalutamide treatment (872; 160 mg daily) group and placebo group (845). Radiographic progression-free survival and overall survival were used as the two primary end points. The clinical benefits brought by enzalutamide treatment in this study with respect to all primary and secondary end points are illustrated in Table 4. It can be concluded from these data that treatment with enzalutamide resulted in a noticeable decrease in risk of radiographic progression and death, as well as a marked delay in the need of chemotherapy. Due to the promising results from PREVAIL phase III trial, the clinical use of enzalutamide was therefore extended by the US FDA to chemotherapy-naïve patients with mCRPC on 10 September 2014.

Table 4. Major therapeutic benefits brought by enzalutamide based on PREVAIL.

Enzalutamide PREVAIL Phase III Trial (NCT01212991)			
End Points	**Enzalutamide (n = 872)**	**Placebo (n = 845)**	**Hazard Ratio (95% CI)**
Primary end point			
Median OS (mo)	18.4	13.6	0.63
Median time to rPFS (mo)		3.9	0.19
Secondary end points			
Median time to first SRE (mo)	16.7	13.3	0.69
Median CC initiation time (mo)	28	10.8	0.35
Median time to PSA progression (mo)	11.2	2.8	0.17
*** PSA response (%) of no.**			
decline ≥ 90% from baseline	47 (854)	1 (777)	
decline ≥ 50% from baseline	78 (854)	3 (777)	
* Serious AEs (%) of no.	44.1 (871)	3.5 (844)	

OS: Overall Survival; rPFS: Radiographic Progression-free Survival; SRE: Skeletal-related Event; CC: Cytotoxic Chemotherapy; PSA: Prostate-specific Antigen; AEs: Adverse Events. * Does not include patients who discontinued or died during the trial.

4.1.2. Enzalutamide for nmCRPC

The patients with nmCRPC are refractory to ADT treatment and at the onset of metastasis. It has therefore been recognized that new treatment strategies are urgently needed to reduce the risk for metastasis in men with nmCRPC in accompany with a short PSA doubling time. PROSPER phase III trial was designed to investigate whether enzalutamide can meet this need [55]. This study enrolled a total of 1401 patients with nmCRPC and a PSA doubling time no more than 10 months. A total of 933 patients received enzalutamide treatment (160 mg daily) in combination with ADT; while the remaining 468 patients were assigned to the placebo group with continued ADT. Metastasis-free survival was set as the primary end point. As illustrated in Table 5, enzalutamide treatment is superior to placebo with regards to the primary end point and most of the secondary end points. The clinical results from the PROSPER trial highlighted that the risk of progression to mCRPC or death in the enzalutamide treatment group has been lowered by 71% as compared with the placebo group. Because of the promising results from the PROSPER phase III trial, enzalutamide was approved by the US FDA, after Priority Review designation, on 13 July 2018, for the treatment of patients with nmCRPC. This approval extends the enzalutamide treatment to patients with nmCRPC, and makes enzalutamide the first FDA-approved oral medicine for both mCRPC and nmCRPC.

Table 5. Major therapeutic benefits brought by enzalutamide based on PROSPER.

Enzalutamide PROSPER Phase III Trial (NCT02003924)			
End Points	**Enzalutamide (n = 933)**	**Placebo (n = 468)**	**Hazard Ratio (95% CI)**
Primary end point			
Median MFS (mo)	36.6	14.7	0.29
Median time to rPFS (mo)		3.9	0.19
Secondary end points			
Median OS (mo)			
Median time to C-FS (mo)	38.1	34	
Median first time use of CC (mo)		39.7	0.38
Median time to PP (mo)	18.5	18.4	0.96
Median time to PSA progression (mo)	37.2	3.9	0.07
*** PSA response (%)**			
decline ≥ 90% from baseline	55.9	0.4	
decline ≥ 50% from baseline	76.3	2.4	
decline to undetectable level	9.6	0	
* Serious AEs (%) of no.	24.3 (930)	18.9 (465)	

MFS: Metastasis Free Survival; rPFS: Radiographic Progression-free Survival; OS: Overall Survival; C-FS: Chemotherapy-Free Survival; PP: Pain Progression; CC: Cytotoxic Chemotherapy; PSA: Prostate-specific Antigen; AEs: Adverse Events; * Does not include patients who discontinued or died during the trial.

4.1.3. Enzalutamide for mCSPC

Patients with mCSPC is defined as those who have metastatic prostate cancer that still responds to ADT. Up to 5% of annual prostate cancer incidences belong to mCSPC in the United States [56]. With ADT as the original standard of care, most of the patients with mCSPC inevitably progress to high-risk mCRPC in 1–3 years. To help meet the needs of this big group of patients, the ARCHES Phase III trial (ClinicalTrials.gov identifier: NCT02677896) [57] aimed to investigated whether enzalutamide in combination with ADT can prolong radiographic progression-free survival using ADT alone as control. The clinical outcomes from this trial pertaining to the primary end point (radiographic progression-free survival) and key secondary end points are summarized in Table 6. A conclusion can be drawn from these data that enzalutamide, plus ADT, demonstrate clinically significant improvement in efficacy by prolonging the radiographic progression-free survival while maintaining the safety level, as compared with ADT alone. The favorable results encouraged the US FDA to grant an extension of enzalutamide for the treatment of mCSPC on 16 December 2019.

Table 6. Major therapeutic benefits brought by enzalutamide based on ARCHES.

Enzalutamide ARCHES Phase III Trial (NCT02677896)			
End Points	**Enzalutamide + ADT (n = 574)**	**Placebo + ADT (n = 576)**	**Hazard Ratio (95% CI)**
Primary End Point			
‡ Median time to rPFS based on ICR via PCWG2 (mo)		19.4	0.39
† Median time to rPFS based on ICR via PAC (mo)		19.0	0.39
Secondary End Points			
Median OS (mo)			0.19
Time to NAT	30.2		0.28
Median time to CR (mo)		13.9	0.28
PSA undetctable rate (%) of no.	68.1 (511)	17.6 (506)	
* Serious AEs (%) of no.	18.2 (572)	19.5 (574)	

rPFS: Radiographic Progression-free Survival; OS: Overall Survival; NAT: New Antineoplastic Therapy; CR: Castration resistance; PSA: Prostate-specific Antigen; AEs: Adverse Events; ‡ Radiographic Progression-Free Survival (rPFS) Based on Independent Central Review (ICR) of Bone Scan According to Prostate Cancer Clinical Trials Working Group 2 (PCWG2) Criteria; † rPFS Based on ICR of Bone Scan According to Protocol Assessment Criteria; * Does not include patients who discontinued or died during the trial.

4.2. *Apalutamide*

The promising preclinical data of apalutamide were well-mirrored by its phase I clinical trial [23,58]. Thirty men with mCRPC were enrolled in its first-in-human study. Apalutamide displayed AR inhibitory ability as evidenced by the 47% PSA response (defined as ≥50% reduction from baseline) at 12 weeks at all tested doses from 30 to 480 mg. The pharmacokinetic profile of oral-administrated apalutamide is linear and dose-dependent in the range of 30–480 mg. The rapid absorption was demonstrated by the fact that it can be measured in the plasma at 30 min after oral intake and that it can reach peak concentrations after 2–3 h. A half-life of 3–4 days was observed in the systematic circulation and most enrolled patients reached a steady-state concentration after 3 weeks of non-interrupted administration of apalutamide. A good safety profile observed from this clinical study further confirmed the high therapeutic index evaluated from the preclinical models. A daily dose of 240 mg was recommended for the follow-up clinical studies of apalutamide considering its dose to maximize the tumor regression in preclinical models, along with peak plasma concentration, safety profile, and efficacy in the phase I clinical study.

4.2.1. Apalutamide for nmCRPC

The SPARTAN trial is a randomized, double blind and multicenter phase III study that evaluated the efficacy of apalutamide in nmCRPC. There were 1207 enrolled men with nmCRPC on ADT with a PSA doubling time of over 10 months randomized to 2:1 to receive apalutamide with ADT or placebo with ADT [59].

The first interim analysis, which concluded in May 2017, determined that there was statistical significance in metastasis free survival (MFS), progression free survival (PFS), time to metastasis and time to symptomatic progression (Table 7). Due to the compelling evidence shown, the safety monitoring committee recommended that the placebo group be allowed to receive the treatment in July 2017. The second interim analysis continued to 2019 to better characterize the effect of apalutamide. It was determined that the median MFS was 40.5 months for the treatment group and 16.2 months in the placebo group with a 95% confidence interval. The four-year survival rate of apalutamide was found to be 72% compared to 65% of the placebo group. When considering the patients that crossed over from placebo to treatment, the four-year survival rate remained at 72% for apalutamide [59].

Table 7. Major therapeutic benefits brought by apalutamide based on SPARTAN.

Apalutamide SPARTAN Phase III Trial (NCT01946204)			
End Points	**Apalutamide (n = 806)**	**Placebo (n = 401)**	**Hazard Ratio (95% CI)**
Primary End Points			
Median MFS (mo)	40.5	16.2	0.28
Secondary End Points			
Median time to metastasis (mo)	40.5	16.6	0.28
Median time to PFS (mo)	40.5	14.7	0.29
Median OS (mo)		39.0	
Median time to CC (mo)			
* Serious AEs (%) of no.	24.8 (803)	23.1 (398)	

MFS: Metastasis Free Survival; PFS: Progression Free Survival; OS: Overall Survival; CC: Cytotoxic Chemotherapy; AEs: Adverse Events; * Does not include patients who discontinued or died during the trial.

Disease progression was the most frequent indicator for treatment discontinuation. Only 28% of the treatment group compared to 37% of control experienced cancer progression for discontinuation. Apalutamide treatment led to the extension of the second PFS rate by approximately 11.8 months versus placebo. The four-year second PFS rate for the treatment had a 19% difference when compared to the control [59]. Adverse effects were reported in 97% of patients in the treatment group and 94% of patents in the control group [59,60]. Median overall survival (OS) was not reached in either the treatment or placebo group, as the threshold of 427 deaths have not yet been reached as specified in the O'Brien-Fleming boundary [59].

Overall, apalutamide showed a quarter reduction for risk of death when compared to placebo as well as a higher subsequent life-prolongation, despite crossover. The resulting data for SPARTAN included statistical significance in improving MFS and time to symptomatic progression compared to placebo. The observations that apalutamide delays progression and death when combined with ongoing ADT suggests that the drug may be advantageous to high-risk nmCRPC patients. FDA immediately approved apalutamide for high-risk nmCRPC patients on 14 February 2018 [59].

4.2.2. Apalutamide for mCSPC

Apalutamide was approved by the US FDA, after a priority review, on 17 September 2019, to extend its treatment from patients with nmCRPC to those with mCSPC based on the efficacy demonstrated by its TITAN (NCT02489318) phase III trial. This clinical trial was designed as a randomized, double blind and multicenter phase III study and aimed to assess the clinical efficacy of apalutamide in combination with ADT (surgical or medical castration) in patients with mCSPC. A study of 1052 men with mCSPC were randomized 1:1 to treatment and control groups. This involved patients regardless of disease volume and with a history of docetaxel treatment and treatment for localized prostate cancer. At the conclusion of the first interim analysis in November 2018, it was found that 68.2% of patients in the apalutamide and ADT group had a 24-month radiographic progression-free survival compared to 47.5% of the placebo group (Table 8). The overall survival, measured after 200 deaths, for 24-months is 82% for apalutamide group and 73% for the placebo group. The average time for second progression-free survival was also longer in the treatment group compared to that of the placebo group. Analysis of adverse effects between apalutamide and placebo did not differ significantly [61]. In summary, the TITAN trial revealed that apalutamide in combination with ADT resulted in life-prolongation and radiographic progression-free survival relative to placebo with ADT while also preserving quality of life for men with mCSPC [61].

Table 8. Major therapeutic benefits brought by apalutamide based on TITAN.

Apalutamide TITAN Phase III Trial (NCT02489318)			
End Points	**Apalutamide + ADT (n = 525)**	**Placebo + ADT (n = 527)**	**Hazard Ratio (95% CI)**
Primary End Points			
OS (% alive)	82..4	73.5	0.67
rPFS (%)	68.2	47.5	0.48
Secondary End Points			
Median time to PSA progression (mo)		12.9	0.26
* Serious AEs (%) of no.	19.2 (574)	20.3 (527)	

OS: Overall Survival; rPFS: Radiographic Progression-free Survival; PSA: Prostate-specific Antigen; AEs: Adverse Events; * Does not include patients who discontinued or died during the trial.

4.2.3. Indirect Comparison with Enzalutamide

In the lack of direct comparative studies, Chowdhury et al. conducted a matching-adjusted indirect comparison (MAIC) of the efficacy and quality of life of apalutamide to that of enzalutamide in nmCRPC using data collected from SPARTAN and PROSPER trials [62]. A total of 1171 patients were matched from the SPARTAN trial (n = 1207) to the PROSPER trial (n = 1401). Relative to enzalutamide, apalutamide was better tolerated based on adverse events with an overall decrease in fatigue, low appetite, hypertension, and nausea occurrences. It was also associated with a better health-related qualify of life based on the Functional Assessment of Cancer Therapy-Prostate score [63]. Additionally, the calculated hazard ratios for apalutamide versus enzalutamide were 0.77 for OS and 0.91 for MFS [62]. Based on these MAIC results, apalutamide demonstrates slightly better overall tolerability and is associated with slightly higher efficacy in nmCRPC patients.

4.3. *Darolutamide*

It has recently been recognized that early and effective suppression of AR signaling may serve as a good strategy to manage nmCRPC [64], which has been firmly supported by the obvious metastasis-free survival benefits reported in the PROPER trial for enzalutamide and the SPARTAN trial for apalutamide. The clinical phases I and II studies [65,66] suggest that darolutamide provides not only meaningful antitumor efficacy but also a favorable safety profile in clinical settings. ARAMIS phase III trial was thus conducted to further assess the treatment benefits and the possible adverse events of darolutamide in men with nmCRPC. A total of 1509 men with nmCRPC and a PSA doubling time no more than 10 months were enrolled in this trial and were randomized in a 2:1 ratio to receive darolutamide (600 mg twice daily) plus ADT or ADT alone. Metastasis free survival was employed as the primary end point, and the appearance of metastasis was judged by blinded and independent central imaging review. The therapeutic benefits of darolutamide were consistently and affirmatively judged by the primary end point and the entire secondary end points (Table 9). Darolutamide in combination with ADT was demonstrated to prolong metastasis-free survival by 22 months and to reduce the risk of metastasis or death by 59% when compared with ADT alone. The therapeutic benefits brought by darolutamide, enzalutamide, or apalutamide are generally similar in patients with nmCRPC. However, darolutamide exhibited a good safety profile in this phase III trial with approximately similar incidence of adverse events in the darolutamide treatment and placebo groups. The fact that darolutamide has less common adverse effects in the phase III trial relative to enzalutamide and apalutamide is associated with its low penetration of the blood-brain barrier as evidenced in preclinical studies. Darolutamide was approved by the US FDA on 30 July 2019, for the treatment of nmCRPC in line with ARAMIS phase III trial [16].

Table 9. Major therapeutic benefits brought by darolutamide based on ARAMIS.

Darolutamide ARMIS Phase III Trial (NCT02200614)			
End Points	**Darolutamide (n = 955)**	**Placebo (n = 554)**	**Hazard Ratio (95% CI)**
Primary End Point			
Median MFS (mo)	40.4	18.4	0.41
Secondary End Points			
Median OS (mo)			0.71
Median first time use of CC (mo)		38.2	0.43
Median time to PP (mo)	40.3	25.36	0.65
Median time to SSE (mo)			0.43
* Serious AEs (%) of no.	24.8 (954)	10.5 (554)	

MFS: Metastasis Free Survival; OS: Overall Survival; PP: Pain Progression; SSE: Symptomatic Skeletal Event; AEs: Adverse Events; * Does not include patients who discontinued or died during the trial.

5. Mechanism of Action of the Second-Generation AR Antagonists

The AR is a nuclear receptor and a ligand-dependent transcription factor that regulates the expression of certain specific genes, including PSA. Its most potent native ligand is 5α-dihydrotestosterone (DHT) that is generated by intracellular metabolism of testosterone, an endogenous androgen synthesized primarily in the testes. The DHT-AR binding drives the AR translocation from cytoplasm to cell nucleus where the AR forms dimer and binds to the androgen response elements in DNA. Co-activators (coregulatory proteins) are then recruited to boost transcription, leading to prostate cancer cell proliferation and survival [2,3]. As shown in Figure 5, castration therapies (both surgical or medical) and abiraterone acetate block the androgen production, while AR antagonists restrain the AR function through competitively binding to the androgen binding site of AR in cell cytoplasm. Intriguingly, enzalutamide, apalutamide, and darolutamide mechanistically distinguish themselves from the first generation nonsteroidal AR antagonists by interfering several stages in the AR signaling pathway [14,23,24]. In addition to competitively suppressing androgen-AR binding, these second-generation nonsteroidal AR antagonists also inhibit the AR translocation from cytoplasm to cell nucleus, the coactivator recruitment, and the AR-DNA binding.

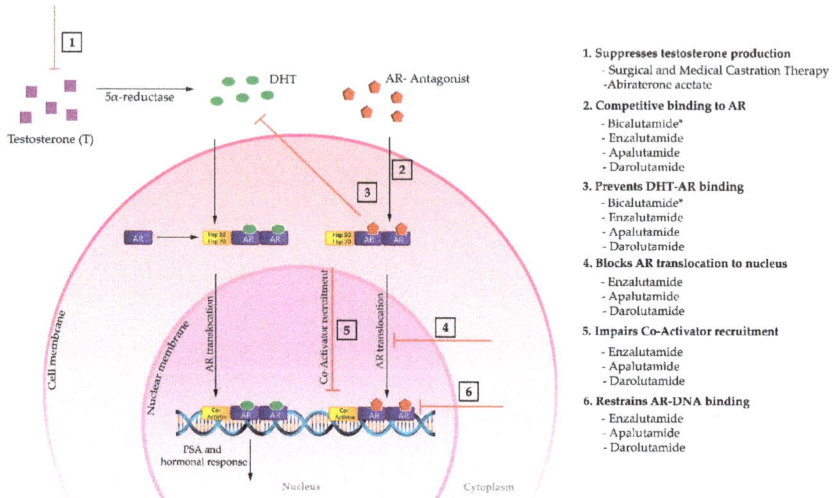

*First generation nonsteroidal AR antagonist

Figure 5. Mechanism of action of different hormonal therapies in AR signaling pathway. * First generation nonsteroidal AR antagonist.

6. Strategies to Overcome the Resistance to the Second-Generation AR Antagonists

In spite of the above-mentioned therapeutic benefits of three second-generation AR antagonists in patients with mCRPC, nmCRPC, or mCSPC, a considerable portion of patients are primarily resistant to the treatment. As summarized in Table 10, 63% of the patients with mCRPC after treating with enzalutamide are still at risk of death; 28%–41% of the patients with nmCRPC under the treatment of enzalutamide, apalutamide, or darolutamide, in combination with ADT, are on the line of progression to metastasis or death; 31%–48% of patients of mCSPC under the treatment of enzalutamide or apalutamide are exposed to radiographic progression or death. Additionally, acquired resistance emerges with the time of treatment.

Table 10. Hazard Ratios for the primary end points in the phase III trials of three AR antagonists.

Trial Name	AR Antagonist	Primary End Point	Hazard Ratio (95% CI)	Patients
AFFIRM	enzalutamide	Median overall survival	0.63	mCRPC
PROPSER	enzalutamide	Median metastasis-free survival	0.29	nmCRPC
SPARTAN	apalutamide	Median metastasis-free survival	0.28	nmCRPC
ARAMIS	darolutamide	Median metastasis-free survival	0.41	nmCRPC
ARCHES	enzalutamide	Median rPFS	0.31	mCSPC
TITAN	apalutamide	Median rPFS	0.48	mCSPC

6.1. Mechanisms of the Resistance to the Second-Generation AR Antagonists

The accurate mechanisms of the resistance to the second-generation AR antagonists are still not very clear. Several proposed mechanisms underlying the resistance to the second-generation AR antagonists are summarized in Figure 6. These mechanisms can be classified into two categories: reactivating androgen receptor signaling and bypassing androgen receptor signaling [67]. The reactivation of AR signaling can be achieved by AR amplification and AR overexpression, AR gain-of-function mutations, spliced AR variants (e.g., AR-V7), and intramolecular generation of androgens. The resistance can also be gained through bypassing AR signaling pathway including glucocorticoid receptor takeover, epithelial-mesenchymal transition, neuroendocrine transformation, autophagy, and immune system activation. More details about these proposed mechanisms have been comprehensively reviewed in the literature [67–70].

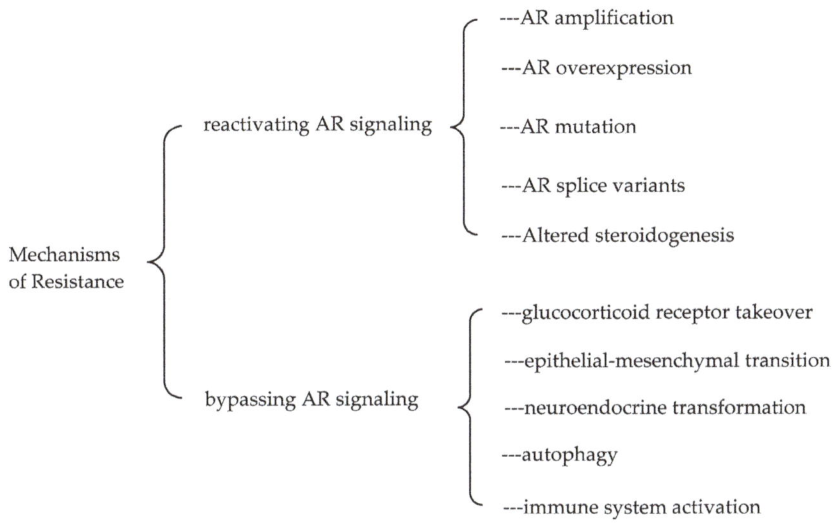

Figure 6. Mechanisms of resistance to the second-generation AR antagonists.

6.2. Strategies to Overcome the Resistance to the Second-Generation AR Antagonists

6.2.1. Combination Therapy

Combination therapy through targeting multiple complementary mechanisms of action has been recognized in recent years to be a promising strategy to overcome drug resistance [71]. Taking advantage of currently available therapies for CRPC, development of their optimal combinations as multifaceted therapies emerges as one of research hotspots in the field. Additionally, numerous of enzalutamide-based combinations are currently under clinical investigation at different phases, most of which have been tabulated by Tucci et al. in their review article [67]. With the goal to sensitize enzalutamide, these combinations were designed based on the current proposed mechanisms of resistance to the second-generation AR antagonists, as listed in Figure 6. For example, the CORT125281 (glucocorticoid receptor antagonist, NCT03437941), metformin (induces epithelial-mesenchymal transition via suppression of transforming growth factor beta 1/signal transducer and activator of transcription 3 (TGF-β1/STAT3) pathway, NCT02339168 and NCT02640534), galunisertib (TGF-*β* inhibitor, NCT02452008), AZD5363 (protein kinase B (AKT) inhibitor, NCT0331054), pembrolizumab (an anti-PD-1 checkpoint, NCT02861573 & NCT02787005), and AZD5069 (chemokine receptor antagonist, NCT03177187) are currently in clinical studies in combination with enzalutamide.

6.2.2. Target AR with Other Strategies

AR is a nuclear steroid receptor that comprises three functional domains including the ligand-binding domain (LBD, *C*-terminal end), the DNA-binding domain (DBD, central portion), and the transactivation domain (NTD or TAD, *N*-terminal end) [3]. Enzalutamide, apalutamide, and darolutamide competitively bind to the ligand-binding pocket of the LBD and inhibit the agonistic action of intrinsic ligands. The compounds that still target AR but can overcome the resistance of the second-generation AR antagonists include new LBD-targeted AR antagonists with novel chemical scaffolds, TAD (or NTD)-targeted AR antagonists, DBD-targeted AR antagonists, and AR degraders.

New AR antagonists that still bind to the LBD but with distinct chemical structures can overcome the resistance due to the point mutations, which has been exemplified by the successful story of darolutamide [72]. As abovementioned, darolutamide was developed targeting enzalutamide-resistant prostate cancer. It was revealed to suppress the transcriptional activity of some AR mutants including T878G that was responsible of converting enzalutamide into a partial AR agonist. Recently, halogen-substituted anthranilic acid derivatives have been established as a new chemical scaffold that inhibits the transactivation of both wild-type AR and AR mutants that render treatment resistance to the first-generation and second-generation nonsteroidal AR antagonists [73].

Several compounds that target the TAD or DBD of the AR have been demonstrated to possess potential in treating CRPC, which have been comprehensively summarized in an excellent review article [3]. The EPI compounds that were first isolated from marine sponges and derived from bisphenol A represent the most well-established inhibitors of AR-TAD. This group of compounds down-regulates the expression of full length AR and truncated AR variants (e.g., AR-V7) through suppressing tau-1 (transcriptional activation unit 1) and tau-5 of the TAD [74]. They inhibited AR-positive prostate cancer cell proliferation in both in vitro and in vivo experiments and suppressed the growth of AR-positive prostate cancer cell-derived tumors. The most developed EPI compound, EPI-506, has advanced to a Phase I/II clinical trial (NCT02606123) in patients with mCRPC after enzalutamide and/or abiraterone treatment.

Hairpin polyamide was developed as an AR antagonist that directly inhibits AR binding to DNA and blocks the transcription processes mediated by AR [75]. Hairpin polyamide compounds may be a good strategy to overcome the resistant to the second-generation AR antagonists because they target the transcription driven by both AR and glucocorticoid receptor. Moreover, overexpression of glucocorticoid receptor has been proposed to be one of the critical pathways leading to the resistance of the second-generation AR antagonists.

A new strategy to combat the resistance of the second-generation AR antagonists is to target AR protein for degradation, which is a completely different mechanism compared with those for AR antagonists. Additionally, AR degradation has been reported to be a likely prerequisite for prostate cancer tumor shrinkage based on an in vivo experiment [76]. AR degradation via proteolysis-targeting chimeras (PROTACs) is currently the most intriguing development in this field because this technology replaces the occupancy-driven mechanism for AR antagonist with an event-driven mechanism [77,78]. AR-PROTACs are bifunctional chimeras that can bring AR protein and the E3 ubiquitin ligase in close proximity, resulting in AR ubiquitination and subsequent degradation. AR-PROTACs have been verified in vitro and in vivo to be a better therapeutic strategy than AR antagonists for targeting AR signaling [79]. ARV-110 is the first AR-PROTAC to enter a phase I clinical trial (NCT03888612) in 2019. This clinical study aims to evaluate the pharmacokinetics, safety, and tolerability of ARV-110 in patients with mCRPC who have received more than two systemic therapies.

Additionally, the association between metformin (an antidiabetic drug) and reduced prostate cancer risk in patients with type 2 diabetics prompted a plethora of investigations on the therapeutic effects of metformin. Metformin is undergoing several clinical trials for prostate cancer, which has been summarized in the literature [80]. The mechanism of action underlying its anti-prostate cancer activity has been extensively explored [80], with the crosstalk between adenosine monophosphate-activated protein kinase (AMPK) activation and AR degradation as the most attractive one [81]. It may therefore be a new strategy, especially for prostate cancer patients with diabetics, to use AMPK activators to overcome the resistance to second-generation nonsteroidal AR antagonists. In addition, cyclin-dependent protein kinase 9 (CDK9) is a druggable target for prostate cancer because CDK9 can not only phosphorylate AR and activate AR transcriptional activity but also target anti-apoptotic proteins [82]. Therefore, CDK9 inhibitors may serve as a better therapeutic strategy over the second-generation nonsteroidal AR antagonists for the patients with CRPC.

7. Conclusions

In conclusion, an interdisciplinary collaboration led the discovery of enzalutamide as the first second-generation nonsteroidal androgen receptor (AR) antagonist with a strong binding affinity to AR. Enzalutamide can significantly prolong not only overall survival time and metastatic free survival time for patients with lethal CRPC, but also castration resistant free survival time for patients with CSPC. Enzalutamide has thus been approved by the US Food and Drug Administration (FDA) for the treatment of both metastatic (in 2012) and non-metastatic (in 2018) CRPC, as well as CSPC (2019) on the basis of the therapeutic benefits observed from AFFIRM, PREVAIL, PROSPER, and ARCHES Phase III clinical trials. Encouraged by the positive clinical results of enzalutamide, two other second-generation AR antagonists, apalutamide, and darolutamide have recently been approved by the FDA for the treatment of prostate cancer. These three second-generation AR antagonists not only offer patients with different stages of prostate cancer with alternative therapeutics, but also verified that AR signaling pathway plays a pivotal role in the progression of both CSPC and CRPC. Several approaches have been developed for the syntheses of these three second-generation AR antagonists, with three main strategies for the syntheses of the core structure of enzalutamide and apalutamide. The drawback of these AR antagonists as therapeutics for prostate cancer is the drug resistance, which can be developed by reactivating or bypassing androgen receptor signaling pathway. Combination therapies taking advantage of multiple complementary mechanisms of action and targeting AR with other mechanisms may serve as good strategies to overcome the resistance.

Author Contributions: Q.-H.C. and H.M. conceptualized this review. P.R., H.M., and Q.-H.C. performed the literature search. P.R., A.R., K.M., N.O., H.M., and Q.-H.C. interpreted and summarized the original data from the references. P.R., A.R., H.M., and Q.-H.C. drafted the manuscript. H.M. and Q.-H.C. revised and finalized the manuscript. All authors have read and agreed to the published version of the manuscript.

Funding: This research was funded by the National Institutes of Health (National Institute of General Medical Sciences) under Award Number SC2GM121185 (Q. Chen). K. Muthima was supported by the Fresno State NIH Bridges to Doctorate Program; the funding for this program is provided by the National Institutes of Health under Grant Number R25GM115293. N. Olveda was supported by the Fresno State NIH RISE Program; the funding for this program is provided by the National Institutes of Health under Grant Number R25GM131956. The APC was funded in part by the Henry Madden Library at California State University Fresno.

Acknowledgments: We thank the Department of Chemistry and College of Science and Mathematics at the California State University Fresno for all administrative support.

Conflicts of Interest: The authors declare no conflict of interest. The funders had no role in the design of the study; in the collection, analyses, or interpretation of data; in the writing of the manuscript, or in the decision to publish the results.

References

1. Siegel, R.L.; Miller Kimberly, D.; Jemal, A. Cancer statistics, 2020. *CA Cancer J. Clin.* **2020**, *70*, 7–30. [CrossRef] [PubMed]
2. Tan, E.; Li, J.; Xu, H.E.; Melcher, K.; Yong, E.-L. Androgen receptor: Structure, role in prostate cancer and drug discovery. *Acta Pharmacol. Sin.* **2014**, *36*, 3–23. [CrossRef] [PubMed]
3. Elshan, N.G.R.D.; Rettig, M.; Jung, M.E. Molecules targeting the androgen receptor (AR) signaling axis beyond the AR-Ligand binding domain. *Med. Res. Rev.* **2018**, *39*, 910–960. [CrossRef] [PubMed]
4. Huggins, C.; Hodges, C.V. Prostatic cancer. I. The effect of castration, of estrogen and of androgen injection on serum phosphatases in metastatic carcinoma of the prostate. *Cancer Res.* **1941**, *1*, 293–297.
5. Blackard, C.E. The Veterans' Administration Cooperative Urological Research Group studies of carcinoma of the prostate: A review. *Cancer Chemother. Rep.* **1975**, *59*, 225–227. [PubMed]
6. Redding, T.W.; Schally, A.V. Inhibition of prostate tumor growth in two rat models by chronic administration of D-Trp6 analog of luteinizing hormone-releasing hormone. *Proc. Natl. Acad. Sci. USA* **1981**, *78*, 6509–6512. [CrossRef] [PubMed]
7. Jacobi, G.H.; Wenderoth, U.K. Gonadotropin-releasing hormone analogs for prostate cancer: Untoward side effects of high-dose regimens acquire a therapeutical dimension. *Eur. Urol.* **1982**, *8*, 129–134. [CrossRef]

8. Walker, K.; Turkes, A.; Turkes, A.; Zwink, R.; Beacock, C.; Buck, A.; Peeling, W.; Griffiths, K. Treatment of patients with advanced cancer of the prostate using a slow-release (depot) formulation of the lhrh agonist ici 118630 (zoladex®). *J. Endocrinol.* **1984**. [CrossRef]
9. The Leuprolide Study Group Leuprolide versus Diethylstilbestrol for Metastatic Prostate Cancer. *N. Engl. J. Med.* **1984**, *311*, 1281–1286. [CrossRef]
10. Schröder, F.H.; Crawford, E.; Axcrona, K.; Payne, H.; Keane, T. Androgen deprivation therapy: Past, present and future. *BJU Int.* **2012**, *109*, 1–12. [CrossRef]
11. Anderson, J. The role of antiandrogen monotherapy in the treatment of prostate cancer. *BJU Int.* **2003**, *91*, 455–461. [CrossRef] [PubMed]
12. Schellhammer, P.F.; Sharifi, R.; Block, N.L.; Soloway, M.S.; Venner, P.M.; Patterson, A.L.; Sarosdy, M.F.; Vogelzang, N.J.; Schellenger, J.J.; Kolvenbag, G.J. Clinical benefits of bicalutamide compared with flutamide in combined androgen blockade for patients with advanced prostatic carcinoma: Final report of a double-blind, randomized, multicenter trial. Casodex Combination Study Group. *Urology* **1997**, *50*, 330–336. [CrossRef]
13. Chen, C.D.; Welsbie, D.S.; Tran, C.; Baek, S.H.; Chen, R.; Vessella, R.; Rosenfeld, M.G.; Sawyers, C.L. Molecular determinants of resistance to antiandrogen therapy. *Nat. Med.* **2003**, *10*, 33–39. [CrossRef] [PubMed]
14. Tran, C.; Ouk, S.; Clegg, N.J.; Chen, Y.; Watson, P.A.; Arora, V.; Wongvipat, J.; Smith-Jones, P.M.; Yoo, N.; Kwon, A.; et al. Development of a Second-Generation Antiandrogen for Treatment of Advanced Prostate Cancer. *Science* **2009**, *324*, 787–790. [CrossRef]
15. Smith, M.R.; Saad, F.; Chowdhury, S.; Oudard, S.; Hadaschik, B.; Graff, J.N.; Olmos, D.; Mainwaring, P.N.; Lee, J.Y.; Uemura, H.; et al. Apalutamide Treatment and Metastasis-free Survival in Prostate Cancer. *N. Engl. J. Med.* **2018**, *378*, 1408–1418. [CrossRef] [PubMed]
16. Fizazi, K.; Shore, N.; Tammela, T.L.; Ulys, A.; Vjaters, E.; Polyakov, S.; Jievaltas, M.; Luz, M.; Alekseev, B.; Kuss, I.; et al. Darolutamide in nonmetastatic, castration-resistant prostate cancer. *Yearb. Paediatr. Endocrinol.* **2019**, *380*, 1235–1346. [CrossRef]
17. Jung, M.E.; Ouk, S.; Yoo, N.; Sawyers, C.L.; Chen, C.; Tran, C.; Wongvipat, J. Structure−Activity Relationship for Thiohydantoin Androgen Receptor Antagonists for Castration-Resistant Prostate Cancer (CRPC). *J. Med. Chem.* **2010**, *53*, 2779–2796. [CrossRef]
18. Teutsch, G.; Goubet, F.; Battmann, T.; Bonfils, A.; Bouchoux, F.; Cerede, E.; Gofflo, D.; Gaillard-Kelly, M.; Philibert, D. Non-steroidal antiandrogens: Synthesis and biological profile of high-affinity ligands for the androgen receptor. *J. Steroid Biochem. Mol. Biol.* **1994**, *48*, 111–119. [CrossRef]
19. Van Dort, M.E.; Robins, D.M.; Wayburn, B. Design, synthesis, and pharmacological characterization of 4-[4,4-dimethyl-3-(4-hydroxybutyl)-5-oxo-2-thioxo-1-imidazolidinyl]-2-iodobenzonitrile as a high-affinity nonsteroidal androgen receptor ligand. *J. Med. Chem.* **2000**, *43*, 3344–3347. [CrossRef]
20. Scher, H.I.; Sawyers, C.L. Biology of Progressive, Castration-Resistant Prostate Cancer: Directed Therapies Targeting the Androgen-Receptor Signaling Axis. *J. Clin. Oncol.* **2005**, *23*, 8253–8261. [CrossRef]
21. Tucker, H.; Crook, J.W.; Chesterson, G.J. Nonsteroidal antiandrogens. Synthesis and structure-activity relationships of 3-substituted derivatives of 2-hydroxypropionanilides. *J. Med. Chem.* **1988**, *31*, 954–959. [CrossRef] [PubMed]
22. Foster, W.; Car, B.D.; Shi, H.; Levesque, P.C.; Obermeier, M.T.; Gan, J.; Arezzo, J.C.; Powlin, S.S.; Dinchuk, J.E.; Balog, A.; et al. Drug safety is a barrier to the discovery and development of new androgen receptor antagonists. *Prostate* **2010**, *71*, 480–488. [CrossRef] [PubMed]
23. Clegg, N.J.; Wongvipat, J.; Joseph, J.D.; Tran, C.; Ouk, S.; Dilhas, A.; Chen, Y.; Grillot, K.; Bischoff, E.D.; Cai, L.; et al. ARN-509: A novel antiandrogen for prostate cancer treatment. *Cancer Res.* **2012**, *72*, 1494–1503. [CrossRef] [PubMed]
24. Moilanen, A.-M.; Riikonen, R.; Oksala, R.; Ravanti, L.; Aho, E.; Wohlfahrt, G.; Nykänen, P.S.; Törmäkangas, O.P.; Palvimo, J.J.; Kallio, P.J. Discovery of ODM-201, a new-generation androgen receptor inhibitor targeting resistance mechanisms to androgen signaling-directed prostate cancer therapies. *Sci. Rep.* **2015**, *5*. [CrossRef] [PubMed]
25. Huges, D.L. Review of synthetic routes and crystalline forms of the antiandrogen oncology drugs enzalutamide, apalutamide, and darolutamide. *Org. Process Res. Dev.* **2020**, *24*, 347–362. [CrossRef]
26. Sawyers, C.L.; Jung, M.E.; Chen, C.D.; Ouk, S.; Welsbie, D.; Tran, C.; Wongvipat, J.; Yoo, D. Diarylhydantoin Compounds. PCT Int. Patent Appl. WO2006124118, 23 November 2006.

27. Sawyers, C.L.; Jung, M.E.; Chen, C.D.; Ouk, S.; Welsbie, D.; Tran, C.; Wongvipat, J.; Yoo, D. Diarylhydantoin Compounds. U.S. Patent 7709517B2, 4 May 2010.
28. Jung, M.E.; Yoo, D.; Sawyers, C.L.; Tran, C.; Wongvipat, J. Diarylhydantoin Compounds. U.S. Patent 8110594B2, 7 February 2012.
29. Chivukula, K.R.; Karuturi, V.V.R.; Benda, S.; Anke, R.; Gajula, D.; Moturu, V.R.K.M.; Indukuri, V.S.; Gorantla, S.R.A.; Chava, S. Process for the Preparation of Enzalutamide. U.S. Patent 10131636B2, 20 November 2018.
30. Suzuki, Y.; Nakagawa, S.; Kitamura, T. Process for Producing Enzalutamide Crystal Form. Int. Patent Appl. WO 2016/194813, 27 May 2016.
31. Song, L.J.; Wang, Y.; Lu, X.F.; Li, Z.Y. Synthesis of androgen receptor antagonist MDV3100. *Fine Chem. Intermed.* **2012**, *42*, 34.
32. Fu, Q.; Yue, L.; Lin, Q.; Liao, X.; Zhao, M.; Qin, Y. Method for Synthesizing Enzalutamide. Chinese Patent Appl. CN 104844520, 5 September 2017.
33. Jung, M.E.; Sawyers, C.L.; Ouk, S.; Tran, C.; Wongvipat, J. Androgen Receptor Modulator for the Treatment of Prostate Cancer and Androgen Receptor-Associated Diseases. Int. Patent Appl. WO2007126765A2, 8 November 2007.
34. Jung, M.E.; Sawyers, C.L.; Ouk, S.; Tran, C.; Wongvipat, J. Androgen Receptor Modulator for the Treatment of Prostate Cancer and Androgen Receptor-Associated Diseases. U.S. Patent 8445507B2, 21 May 2013.
35. Ouerfelli, O.; Dilhas, A.; Yang, G.; Zhao, H. Synthesis of Thiohydantoins. Int. Patent Appl. WO2008/119015A2, 2 October 2008.
36. Ouerfelli, O.; Dilhas, A.; Yang, G.; Zhao, H. Synthesis of Thiohydantoins. U.S. Patent Appl. 2010/0190991A1, 29 July 2010.
37. Pang, X.; Wang, Y.; Chen, Y. Design, synthesis, and biological evaluation of deuterated apalutamide with improved pharmacokinetic profiles. *Bioorg. Med. Chem. Lett.* **2017**, *27*, 2803–2806. [CrossRef]
38. Chen, Y.; Gong, Y. Imidazole Diketone Compound and Use Thereof. Int. Patent Appl. WO2014/190895, 4 December 2014.
39. Muthusamy, A.R.; Kanniah, S.L.; Arote, N.D.; Bhagwat, O.V.; Sonar, J.K.; Poundkar, V.B.; Wagh, Y.D. Solid State Forms of Apalutamide. Int. Patent Appl. WO 2018/112001, 21 June 2018.
40. Muthusamy, A.R.; Kanniah, S.L.; Arote, N.D.; Bhagwat, O.V.; Sonar, J.K.; Poundkar, V.B.; Wagh, Y.D. Solid State Forms of Apalutamide. U.S. Patent Appl. 2019/0322640A1, 24 October 2019.
41. Bodhuri, P.; Ceccarelli, A.P.; Emmett, M.R.; Karadeolian, A.; Souza, F.E.S.; Weeratunga, G.; Gorin, B. Processes for the Preparation of Apalutamide and Intermediates Thereof. U.S. Patent Appl. 2019/ 0276424, 12 September 2019.
42. Haim, C.B.; Horvath, A.; Weerts, E.; Albaneze-Walker, J. Processes for the Preparation of a Diarylthiohydantoin Compound. U.S. Patent Appl. 2019/0135775A9, 9 May 2019.
43. Haim, C.B.; Horvath, A.; Weerts, E.; Albaneze-Walker, J. Processes for the Preparation of a Diarylthiohydantoin Compound. U.S. Patent Appl. 2018/0002309A1, 4 January 2018.
44. Meng, X.; Shao, L.; Huang, G.; Wu, K.; Tian, P.; Xu, C.; Jiang, Z.; Xiong, L. Preparation Method of Enzalutamide of Formula (VIII). Chinese Patent Appl. CN 109651256, 4 April 2019.
45. Haim, C.B.; Horvath, A.; Edmond, J.E. Processes for the Preparation of a Diarylthiohydantoin Compound. U.S. Patent Appl. 2016/0176845A1, 23 June 2016.
46. Koyama, M.; Kawakami, T.; Okazoe, T.; Nozaki, K. Cyanide-Free One-Pot Synthesis of Methacrylic Esters from Acetone. *Chem. - A Eur. J.* **2019**, *25*, 10913–10917. [CrossRef]
47. Zheng, X.; Zhang, Y. Method for Synthesizing Apalutamide and Intermediate Thereof. Chinese Patent Appl. CN 108383749, 10 August 2018.
48. Laitinen, I.; Karjalainen, O. Process for the Preparation of Androgen Receptor Antagonists and Intermediates Thereof. U.S. Patent 10189789B2, 29 January 2016.
49. Wohlfahrt, G.; Törmäkangas, O.; Salo, H.; Höglung, L.; Karjalainen, A.; Knuuttila, P.; Holm, P. Androgen Receptor Modulating Compounds. Int. Patent Appl. WO 2011/051540A1, 5 May 2011.
50. Törmäkangas, O.; Wohlfahrt, G.; Salo, H.; Ramasubramanian, R.D.; Patra, P.K.; Martin, A.E.; Heikkinen, T.; Vesalainen, A.; Moilanen, A.; Karjalainen, A. Androgen Receptor Modulating Carboxamides. Int. Patent Appl. WO 2012/143599A1, 26 October 2012.

51. Wohlfahrt, G.; Törmäkangas, O.; Salo, H.; Höglung, L.; Karjalainen, A.; Koivikko, P.; Holm, P.; Rasku, S.; Vesalainen, A. Androgen Receptor Modulating Compounds. U.S. Patent 9657003 B2, 23 May 2017.
52. Scher, H.I.; Beer, T.M.; Higano, C.S.; Anand, A.; Taplin, M.-E.; Efstathiou, E.; Rathkopf, D.E.; Shelkey, J.; Yu, E.Y.; Alumkal, J.; et al. Antitumour activity of MDV3100 in castration-resistant prostate cancer: A phase 1–2 study. *Lancet* **2010**, *375*, 1437–1446. [CrossRef]
53. Scher, H.I.; Fizazi, K.; Saad, F.; Taplin, M.-E.; Sternberg, C.N.; Miller, K.; De Wit, R.; Mülders, P.; Hadaschik, B.; Shore, N.D.; et al. Increased Survival with Enzalutamide in Prostate Cancer after Chemotherapy. *N. Engl. J. Med.* **2012**, *367*, 1187–1197. [CrossRef]
54. Beer, T.M.; Armstrong, A.J.; Rathkopf, D.E.; Loriot, Y.; Sternberg, C.N.; Higano, C.S.; Iversen, P.; Bhattacharya, S.; Carles, J.; Chowdhury, S.; et al. Enzalutamide in Metastatic Prostate Cancer before Chemotherapy. *N. Engl. J. Med.* **2014**, *371*, 424–433. [CrossRef] [PubMed]
55. Hussain, M.; Fizazi, K.; Saad, F.; Rathenborg, P.; Shore, N.; Ferreira, U.; Ivashchenko, P.; Demirhan, E.; Modelska, K.; Phung, D.; et al. Enzalutamide in Men with Nonmetastatic, Castration-Resistant Prostate Cancer. *N. Engl. J. Med.* **2018**, *378*, 2465–2474. [CrossRef]
56. Scher, H.I.; Solo, K.; Valant, J.; Todd, M.B.; Mehra, M. Prevalence of Prostate Cancer Clinical States and Mortality in the United States: Estimates Using a Dynamic Progression Model. *PLoS ONE* **2015**, *10*, e0139440. [CrossRef] [PubMed]
57. Armstrong, A.J.; Szmulewitz, R.Z.; Petrylak, D.P.; Holzbeierlein, J.; Villers, A.; Azad, A.; Alcaraz, A.; Alekseev, B.; Iguchi, T.; Shore, N.D.; et al. ARCHES: A Randomized, Phase III Study of Androgen Deprivation Therapy With Enzalutamide or Placebo in Men With Metastatic Hormone-Sensitive Prostate Cancer. *J. Clin. Oncol.* **2019**, *37*, 2974–2986. [CrossRef]
58. Rathkopf, D.E.; Morris, M.J.; Fox, J.J.; Danila, D.C.; Slovin, S.F.; Hager, J.H.; Rix, P.J.; Maneval, E.C.; Chen, I.; Gönen, M.; et al. Phase I Study of ARN-509, a Novel Antiandrogen, in the Treatment of Castration-Resistant Prostate Cancer. *J. Clin. Oncol.* **2013**, *31*, 3525–3530. [CrossRef] [PubMed]
59. Small, E.; Saad, F.; Chowdhury, S.; Oudard, S.; Hadaschik, B.; Graff, J.; Olmos, D.; Mainwaring, P.; Lee, J.; Uemura, H.; et al. Apalutamide and overall survival in non-metastatic castration-resistant prostate cancer. *Ann. Oncol.* **2019**, *30*, 1813–1820. [CrossRef]
60. Saad, F.; Cella, D.; Basch, E.; Hadaschik, B.; Mainwaring, P.N.; Oudard, S.; Graff, J.N.; McQuarrie, K.; Li, S.; Hudgens, S.; et al. Effect of apalutamide on health-related quality of life in patients with non-metastatic castration-resistant prostate cancer: An analysis of the SPARTAN randomised, placebo-controlled, phase 3 trial. *Lancet Oncol.* **2018**, *19*, 1404–1416. [CrossRef]
61. Kwon Daniel, H.-M.; Friedlander, T.; Kwon Daniel, H.-M.; Friedlander, T. A TITAN step forward: Apalutamide for metastatic castration-sensitive prostate cancer. *Ann. Transl. Med.* **2019**, *7* (Suppl. 8), S364.
62. Chowdhury, S.; Oudard, S.; Uemura, H.; Joniau, S.; Pilon, D.; Ladouceur, M.; Behl, A.S.; Liu, J.; Dearden, L.; Sermon, J.; et al. Matching-Adjusted Indirect Comparison of the Efficacy of Apalutamide and Enzalutamide with ADT in the Treatment of Non-Metastatic Castration-Resistant Prostate Cancer. *Adv. Ther.* **2019**, *37*, 501–511. [CrossRef]
63. Chowdhury, S.; Oudard, S.; Uemura, H.; Joniau, S.; Pilon, D.; Lefebvre, P.; McQuarrie, K.; Liu, J.; Dearden, L.; Sermon, J.; et al. Matching-Adjusted Indirect Comparison of Health-Related Quality of Life and Adverse Events of Apalutamide Versus Enzalutamide in Non-Metastatic Castration-Resistant Prostate Cancer. *Adv. Ther.* **2019**, *37*, 512–526. [CrossRef]
64. Mateo, J.; Fizazi, K.; Gillessen, S.; Heidenreich, A.; Perez-Lopez, R.; Oyen, W.; Shore, N.; Smith, M.; Sweeney, C.; Tombal, B.; et al. Managing Nonmetastatic Castration-resistant Prostate Cancer. *Eur. Urol.* **2019**, *75*, 285–293. [CrossRef] [PubMed]
65. Fizazi, K.; Massard, C.; Bono, P.; Jones, R.; Kataja, V.; James, N.; A Garcia, J.; Protheroe, A.; Tammela, T.L.; Elliott, T.; et al. Activity and safety of ODM-201 in patients with progressive metastatic castration-resistant prostate cancer (ARADES): An open-label phase 1 dose-escalation and randomised phase 2 dose expansion trial. *Lancet Oncol.* **2014**, *15*, 975–985. [CrossRef]
66. Shore, N.D.; Tammela, T.L.; Massard, C.; Bono, P.; Aspegren, J.; Mustonen, M.; Fizazi, K. Safety and Antitumour Activity of ODM-201 (BAY-1841788) in Chemotherapy-naïve and CYP17 Inhibitor-naïve Patients: Follow-up from the ARADES and ARAFOR Trials. *Eur. Urol. Focus* **2018**, *4*, 547–553. [CrossRef] [PubMed]

67. Tucci, M.; Zichi, C.; Buttigliero, C.; Vignani, F.; Scagliotti, G.V.; Di Maio, M. Enzalutamide-resistant castration-resistant prostate cancer: Challenges and solutions. *OncoTargets Ther.* **2018**, *11*, 7353–7368. [CrossRef]
68. Prekovic, S.; Broeck, T.V.D.; Linder, S.; Van Royen, M.E.; Houtsmuller, A.B.; Handle, F.; Joniau, S.; Zwart, W.; Claessens, F. Molecular underpinnings of enzalutamide resistance. *Endocr.-Relat. Cancer* **2018**, *25*, R545–R557. [CrossRef]
69. Claessens, F.; Helsen, C.; Prekovic, S.; Broeck, T.V.D.; Spans, L.; Van Poppel, H.; Joniau, S. Emerging mechanisms of enzalutamide resistance in prostate cancer. *Nat. Rev. Urol.* **2014**, *11*, 712–716. [CrossRef]
70. Centenera, M.; Selth, L.A.; Ebrahimie, E.; Butler, L.M.; Tilley, W.D. New Opportunities for Targeting the Androgen Receptor in Prostate Cancer. *Cold Spring Harb. Perspect. Med.* **2018**, *8*. [CrossRef]
71. Qiu, Y.; Xu, J. Current opinion and mechanistic interpretation of combination therapy for castration-resistant prostate cancer. *Asian J. Androl.* **2019**, *21*, 270–278. [CrossRef]
72. Borgmann, H.; Lallous, N.; Ozistanbullu, D.; Beraldi, E.; Paul, N.; Dalal, K.; Fazli, L.; Haferkamp, A.; Lejeune, P.; Cherkasov, A.; et al. Moving Towards Precision Urologic Oncology: Targeting Enzalutamide-resistant Prostate Cancer and Mutated Forms of the Androgen Receptor Using the Novel Inhibitor Darolutamide (ODM-201). *Eur. Urol.* **2018**, *73*, 4–8. [CrossRef]
73. Roell, D.; Rösler, T.W.; Hessenkemper, W.; Kraft, F.; Hauschild, M.; Bartsch, S.; Abraham, T.E.; Houtsmuller, A.B.; Matusch, R.; Van Royen, M.E.; et al. Halogen-substituted anthranilic acid derivatives provide a novel chemical platform for androgen receptor antagonists. *J. Steroid Biochem. Mol. Biol.* **2019**, *188*, 59–70. [CrossRef]
74. Yang, Y.C.; Banuelos, C.A.; Mawji, N.R.; Wang, J.; Kato, M.; Haile, S.R.; McEwan, I.J.; Plymate, S.; Sadar, M.D. Targeting Androgen Receptor Activation Function-1 with EPI to Overcome Resistance Mechanisms in Castration-Resistant Prostate Cancer. *Clin. Cancer Res.* **2016**, *22*, 4466–4477. [CrossRef] [PubMed]
75. Nickols, N.G.; Dervan, P.B. Suppression of androgen receptor-mediated gene expression by a sequence-specific DNA-binding polyamide. *Proc. Natl. Acad. Sci.* **2007**, *104*, 10418–10423. [CrossRef] [PubMed]
76. Ponnusamy, S.; He, Y.; Hwang, D.-J.; Thiyagarajan, T.; Houtman, R.; Bocharova, V.; Sumpter, B.G.; Fernandez, E.; Johnson, D.L.; Du, Z.; et al. Orally Bioavailable Androgen Receptor Degrader, Potential Next-Generation Therapeutic for Enzalutamide-Resistant Prostate Cancer. *Clin. Cancer Res.* **2019**, *25*, 6764–6780. [CrossRef] [PubMed]
77. Pettersson, M.; Crews, C.M. PROteolysis TArgeting Chimeras (PROTACs)—Past, present and future. *Drug Discov. Today: Technol.* **2019**, *31*, 15–27. [CrossRef]
78. Ottis, P.; Crews, C.M. Proteolysis-Targeting Chimeras: Induced Protein Degradation as a Therapeutic Strategy. *ACS Chem. Boil.* **2017**, *12*, 892–898. [CrossRef]
79. Han, X.; Wang, C.; Qin, C.; Xiang, W.; Fernandez-Salas, E.; Yang, C.-Y.; Wang, M.; Zhao, L.; Xu, T.; Chinnaswamy, K.; et al. Discovery of ARD-69 as a Highly Potent Proteolysis Targeting Chimera (PROTAC) Degrader of Androgen Receptor (AR) for the Treatment of Prostate Cancer. *J. Med. Chem.* **2019**, *62*, 941–964. [CrossRef]
80. Zaidi, S.; Gandhi, J.; Joshi, G.; Smith, N.L.; Khan, S.A. The anticancer potential of metformin on prostate cancer. *Prostate Cancer Prostatic Dis.* **2019**, *22*, 351–361. [CrossRef]
81. Shen, M.; Zhang, Z.; Ratnam, M.; Dou, Q.P. The interplay of AMP-activated protein kinase and androgen receptor in prostate cancer cells. *J. Cell. Physiol.* **2014**, *229*, 688–695. [CrossRef]
82. Rahaman, M.H.; Kumarasiri, M.; Mekonnen, L.B.; Yu, M.; Diab, S.A.H.; Albrecht, H.; Milne, R.; Wang, S. Targeting CDK9: A promising therapeutic opportunity in prostate cancer. *Endocr.-Relat. Cancer* **2016**, *23*. [CrossRef]

molecules

MDPI

Article

Design, Synthesis, and Biological Evaluation of Proteolysis Targeting Chimeras (PROTACs) for the Dual Degradation of IGF-1R and Src

Sudhakar Manda [1,†], Na Keum Lee [1,†], Dong-Chan Oh [2] and Jeeyeon Lee [1,*]

[1] College of Pharmacy, Research Institute of Pharmaceutical sciences, Seoul National University, 1 Gwanak-ro, Gwanak-gu, Seoul 08826, Korea; sudhakariiim@gmail.com (S.M.); nklee12@snu.ac.kr (N.K.L.)

[2] Natural Products Research Institute, College of Pharmacy, Seoul National University, Seoul 08826, Korea; dongchanoh@snu.ac.kr

[*] Correspondence: jyleeut@snu.ac.kr; Tel.: +82-02-880-2471

[†] These authors contributed equally to this work.

Academic Editor: Qiao-Hong Chen
Received: 30 March 2020; Accepted: 20 April 2020; Published: 23 April 2020

Abstract: A focused PROTAC library was developed to degrade both IGF-1R and Src proteins, which are associated with various cancers. PROTACs with IGF-1R and Src degradation potentials were synthesized by tethering different inhibitor warhead units and the E3 ligase (CRBN) recruiting-pomalidomide with various linkers. The designed PROTACs 12a–b inhibited the proliferation and migration of MCF7 and A549 cancer cells with low micromolar potency (1–5 μM) in various cellular assays.

Keywords: PROTACs; anticancer activity; protein degradation; IGF-1R; Src

1. Introduction

For the past two decades, targeted protein degradation strategies have been explored widely to develop treatments for various diseases, particularly for cancers [1–4]. Proteolysis targeting chimeras (PROTACs) have emerged as a novel therapeutic strategy in drug discovery for targeted protein degradation [4–6]. PROTACs are heterobifunctional molecules that possess one warhead ligand that binds to the target protein of interest (POI), and a second ligand that recruits an E3 ligase system, which is connected by a chemical linker. The recruitment of the E3 ligase to the target protein results in ubiquitination and the subsequent degradation of the target protein by the proteasome, which is a distinct mechanism from the occupancy-driven modulation of enzyme function by conventional small-molecule inhibitors. Initially described by Crews and Deshaies in 2001, PROTACs have been successfully applied to numerous target proteins [7–12]. As opposed to the stoichiometric binding of drugs that prevent the enzymatic activity of target proteins, PROTACs need to transiently bind to their targets for degradation; this is promising for the potential to address therapeutic challenges in targeting intractable proteins in the current drug discovery [13]. In addition, they can impede the feedback-mediated increased expression of the target proteins that often result in pharmacological inefficacy by small-molecule inhibitors [14,15].

Several E3 ligases have been used in PROTAC technology to degrade recruited target proteins, which include β-TRCP, MDM2 and cIAP [7–9]. In addition, von Hippel-Lindau (VHL) and cereblon (CRBN) have been extensively studied in relation to PROTAC-mediated protein degradation [2,16–18]. Cereblon (CRBN), which is a part of a cullin-RING ubiquitin ligase complex, was identified as the target of thalidomide and its derivatives [19]. These phthalimide immunomodulatory drugs (IMiDs), including lenalidomide, pomalidomide, and thalidomide, play a pivotal role in the treatment of multiple myeloma and now serve as potent binders of the CRBN. To date, PROTACs have been successfully applied to various target proteins with different cellular locations, including estrogen and androgen receptors, BET proteins, tau protein, FKBP12, and kinases [2,11,12,17,20,21]. In particular, PROTACs, which hijack various cellular kinases, have resulted in effective target degradations [22–26]. Furthermore, the enhanced selectivity of kinase degraders, as compared to their parental kinase inhibitors, were implicated as having potential applications for clinical study [23,27]. Currently, many efforts are underway in medicinal chemistry to convert previously ineffective inhibitors to selective PROTACs for a next-generation drug platform.

The insulin-like growth factor 1 receptor (IGF-1R) is a membrane receptor tyrosine kinase that is implicated in several cancers, including prostate, breast, and lung cancers [28–30]. IGF-1R plays a key role in the proliferation, transformation and survival of various cancer cells. Frequently, its anti-apoptotic properties result in resistance to cytotoxic chemotherapeutic drugs or radiotherapy. For these reasons, the IGF-1R signaling pathway has been a major target for the development of anticancer agents [31,32]. Src, known as proto-oncogene tyrosine-protein kinase, is also associated with cancer cell survival and resistance to targeted anticancer therapies [33]. In particular, Src activation is related to the resistance of many anti-IGF-1R therapeutics. Indeed, a combined inhibition of IGF-1R and the Src family kinases have been shown to enhance antitumor effects in various cancers by decreasing the activated survival pathways [34,35]. We have also shown that the dual inhibition of IGF-1R and Src could be a viable approach to develop effective anticancer therapies to overcome resistance [36].

In this study, we report the design and synthesis of IGF-1R/Src dual degraders using the PROTAC strategy (Figure 1). The (5-cyclopropyl-1*H*-pyrazol-3-yl)pyrimidine-2,4-diamine (A) is known as a potent c-Src inhibitor with an IC_{50} value of 720 nM from the enzyme inhibition assay [37,38]. RBx10080307 (B) is known as an IGF-1R inhibitor with a cell free IC_{50} value of 277 nM [39,40]. A common structure, N^2-phenyl-N^4-(1*H*-pyrazol-3-yl)pyrimidine-2,4-diamine (C), was derived and was connected with the pomalidomide as a ligand for cereblon for dual IGF-1R/Src degradation. We reasoned that a common chemical structure would target both IGF-1R and Src, bringing both proteins close to the E3 ligase for degradation in PROTACs. We also adopted previously reported 2,4-bis-arylamino-1,3-pyrimidine (D) as an IGF-1R warhead [41], and the aminopyrazolo [3,4-*d*]pyrimidine module (E) as a Src warhead for the PROTAC approach [42,43], and compared their efficacy to those of 12 with the newly designed inhibitor units. Through extensive optimization of the linker region, we have synthesized a series of dual IGF-1R/Src degraders. Among these, PROTACs 12a and 12b were capable of inducing the degradation of both IGF-1R and Src proteins at 1–5 μM in the MCF7 (human breast cancer) and A549 (human lung cancer) cells.

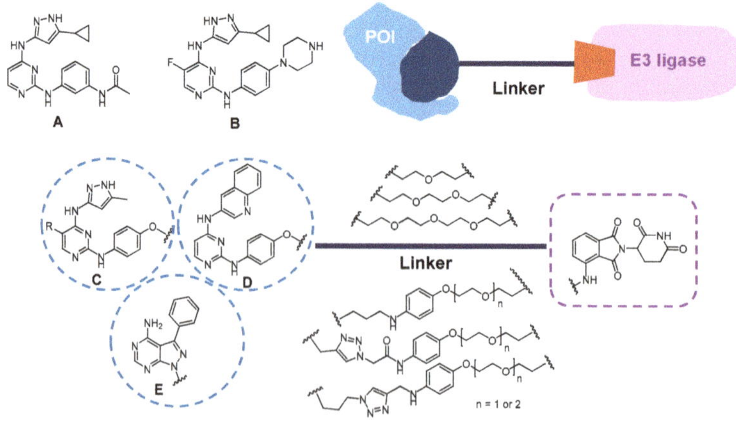

Figure 1. Chemical structures of representative Src inhibitor **A**, IGF-1R inhibitors **B**, and a schematic diagram of PROTACs for IGF-1R and Src.

2. Results

2.1. Design and Synthesis

We developed a convergent synthetic route to prepare the designed dual IGF-1R/Src PROTAC degraders and their control compounds (Scheme 1). We prepared 4a–b in two steps. An azidation was first carried out from 2-chloropolyethoxy ethanols 1a-b to provide 2a–b [44], which were coupled with 4-flouronitrobenzene 3 to give 4a–b, respectively [45]. 4c was synthesized according to the previous reports, as depicted in the supplementary information [46]. The reduction of azides 4a–c, in the presence of triphenylphosphine, leads to the amine intermediates 5a–c, which were subsequently attached with thalidomide derivative 6 to obtain 7a–c, followed by a reduction with Fe/NH_4Cl to provide 8a–c. PROTACs 10a–c were synthesized by coupling 8a–c with 2-chloro-4-arylamino-1,3-pyrimidines 9 in DMSO. The key intermediates 8a–b were also treated with their corresponding reagents 11a or 11b, to produce PROTACs 12a–d (Scheme 1) [36,47].

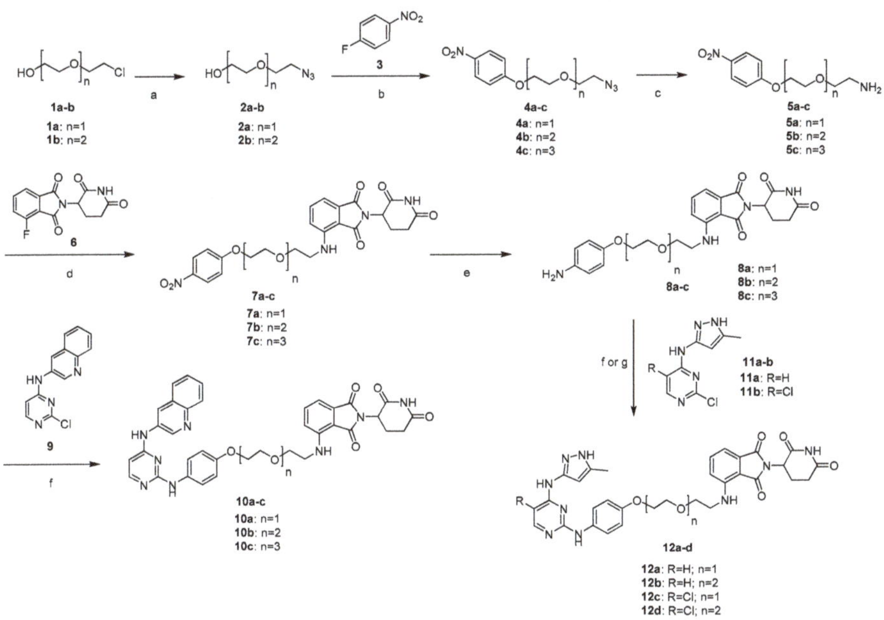

Scheme 1. Reagents and conditions: (a) NaN_3, H_2O, 80 °C, 16 h, 69–82%; (b) K_2CO_3, DMSO, 80 °C, 4 h, 53–61%; (c) Ph_3P, THF-H_2O, RT, 14 h, 61–85%; (d) DIPEA, DMF, 90 °C, 16 h; (e) Fe (powder), NH_4Cl, EtOH-H_2O, 80 °C, 2 h (42–44% over 2 steps); (f) DMSO, 100 °C, 4 h (10a–c, 12a–b; 21–57%); (g) p-TsOH, butanol, 100 °C, 4 h (12c–d; 22–32%).

The thalidomide-attached linkers 8a–b were also coupled with azidoacetic acid 13 in the presence of EDC·HCl to provide 14a–b, which were further treated with *N*-substituted 4-aminopyrazolo[3–*d*]pyrimidines intermediate (15) in the presence of copper sulfate and sodium ascorbate in THF/H_2O/tBuOH to obtain the click products 16a–b via a copper (I)-catalyzed alkyne azide 1,3-dipolar cycloaddition (CuAAC) reaction (Scheme 2). 8a-b reacted with the bromopropyl group-attached pyrazolo[3,4-*d*]pyrimidin-4-amine (17) under the basic condition yielded PROTACs 18a-b. Next, *N*-propagylation of 8a–b under the basic condition afforded 20a-b, which were coupled with azido intermediate (19) via the CuAAC reaction to obtain the desired triazole products 21a–b [36].

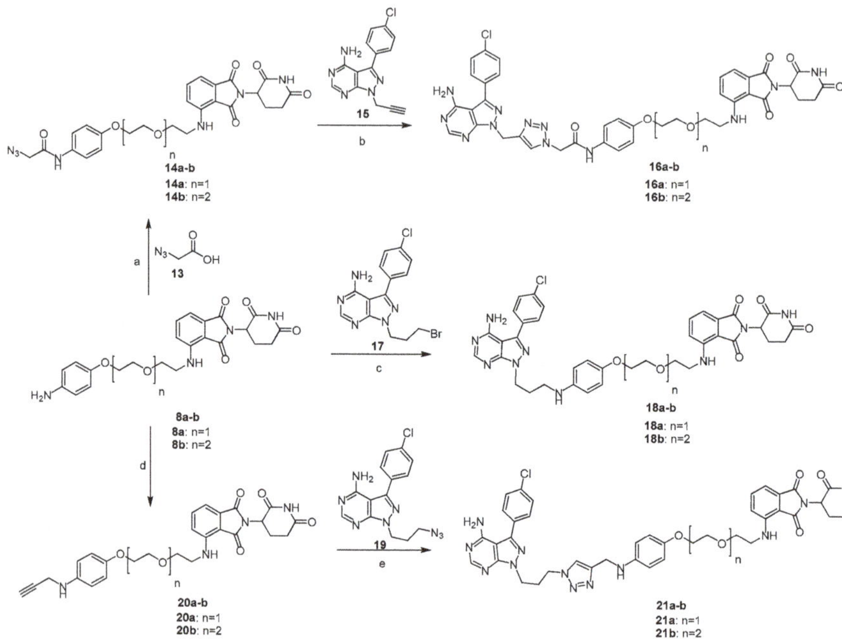

Scheme 2. Reagents and conditions: (a) EDC·HCl, DIPEA, DMF, RT, 16 h, 40–62%; (b) $CuSO_4 \cdot 5H_2O$, sodium ascorbate, THF, t-Butanol-H_2O, RT, 6 h, 26–27%; (c) K_2CO_3, DMF, 16 h, 50.5–50.8%; (d) Propargyl bromide, K_2CO_3, DMF, 16 h, 52–55%; (e) $CuSO_4 \cdot 5H_2O$, sodium ascorbate, THF, t-Butanol/H_2O, RT, 6 h, 38–40%.

2.2. *CPR3 (12a) and CPR4 (12b), Synthesized PROTAC Compounds, Inhibited Cancer Cell Proliferation*

Next, we investigated the cell cytotoxicity of the synthesized PROTAC compounds 10a–c, 12a–d, 16a–d, 18a–b and 21a–b in both MCF7 (human breast cancer) and A549 (human lung cancer) cells. As the cell permeability is more crucial for PROTAC compounds with higher molecular weights than for conventional small-molecule inhibitors, we first screened the synthesized compounds via the MTT assay. Cell growth inhibition was measured at the concentrations of 1 or 10 μM PROTAC compounds, and the measured absorbance values were normalized to DMSO-treated cells. In Figure 2, CPR3 and CPR4 inhibited cell growth dose-dependently in both MCF7 (Figure 2a) and A549 (Figure 2b) cells. Compounds CPR3 and CPR4, with a methyl-1*H*-pyrazole group, showed significant growth inhibitions. In contrast, other compounds did not show significant dose-dependent growth inhibitions. IC_{50} values were further determined through the growth inhibition curve by varying the concentrations from 0.5 to 80 μM. The IC_{50} values of CPR3 and CPR4 were measured to be 3.3 and 2.7 μM in MCF7 cells (Figure 2c), whereas they were 4.2 and 7.6 μM in A549 cells (Figure 2d), respectively. Taken together, CPR3 and CPR4 showed anti-cancer potency by effectively inhibiting cancer cell growth.

2.3. *CPR3 and CPR4 Degraded Both Src and IGF-1R Proteins*

Cell growth inhibition is closely related to the post translational regulation of gene expression [48]. Therefore, we examined whether CPR3 and CPR4 reduce the expression level of the IGF-1R or Src proteins, serving as a dual degrader. 2-Chloro-*N*-(5-methyl-1*H*-pyrazol-3-yl)pyrimidin-4-amine (NC) was used as a negative control. In MCF7 cells, NC did not degrade Src or the IGF-1R protein, whereas CPR3 and CPR4 all degraded Src and IGF-1R at 5 μM of concentration (Figure 3a). Similarly, CPR3 and CPR4 also degraded Src and IGF-1R in A549 cells (Figure 3b). These results indicated that CPR3 and CPR4 play a key role as a dual degrader for both IGF-1R and Src proteins.

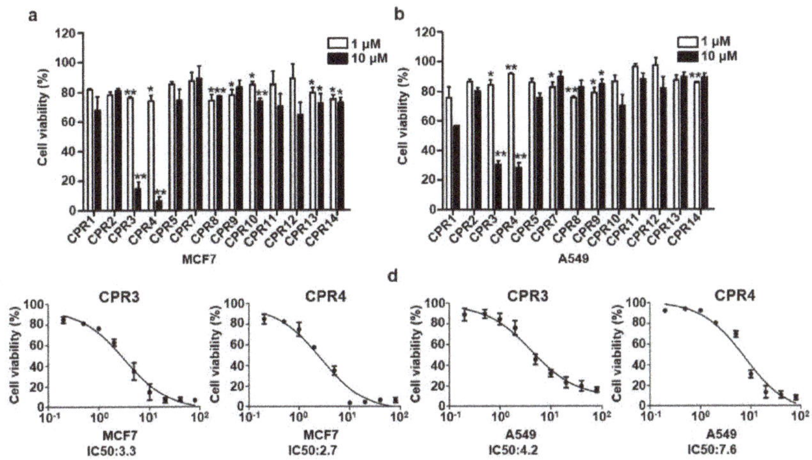

Figure 2. Inhibitory effect of PROTAC compounds on the viability of two different cancer cell lines, MCF7 (**a**) and A549 (**b**). PROTAC compounds were treated at 1 or 10 µM of concentration for 3 days in a complete RPMI-1640 medium. At various concentrations of CPR3 (**c**) or CPR4 (**d**), the IC_{50} value was calculated through the growth curve in both cell lines. Cell viability was determined by the changes in absorbance at 570 nm. * $P \leq 0.05$ and ** $P \leq 0.01$, as determined by Student's t-test.

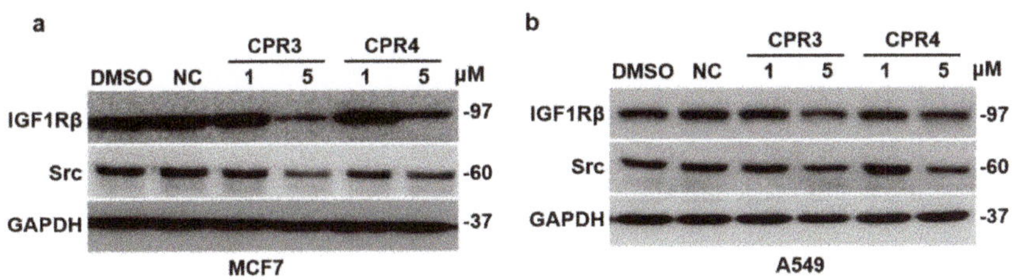

Figure 3. Immunoblotting for IGF-1R and Src in both MCF7 (**a**) and A549 (**b**) cells. The cells were treated with CPR3 or CPR4 at 1 and 5 µM of concentration for 24 h. NC was used as a negative control (5 µM). For detection of the protein expression, extracted lysate was incubated with IGF-1R or Src antibody for 1 h.

2.4. Invasion and Migration Ability Were Suppressed by CPR3 and CPR4 Treatment in Both MCF7 and A549 Cells

IGF-1R or Src mediated cancer cells were correlated with proliferation, differentiation, survival and metastasis, promoting cell-cell signal transduction. The characteristics of cancer cells have resistance to chemotherapy by processing the pathway related to the epithelial to mesenchymal transition (EMT) [49]. Therefore, we tested cell migration and invasiveness through the treatment of CPR3 and CPR4, which can block IGF-1R or Src in both MCF7 and A549 cells. In both cells, CPR3 and CPR4 significantly delayed the ratio of wound closure in a dose dependent manner, 1 or 5 µM (Figure 4), suggesting a reduction of migration by interrupting the pathway of IGF-1R or Src. In addition, Figure 4 shows a decreased invasiveness of CPR3 and CPR4 in both MCF7 (Figure 5a) and A549 (Figure 5b) cells. Cells with the ability to penetrate into the matrix were stained and counted on a bright field microscopy. The number of cells was significantly reduced at 5 µM of concentration of CPR3 and CPR4, as compared to DMSO (Figure 5). These results indicated that CPR3 and CPR4 can block the IGF-1R/Src regulated cancer cell progressions, including migration and invasion.

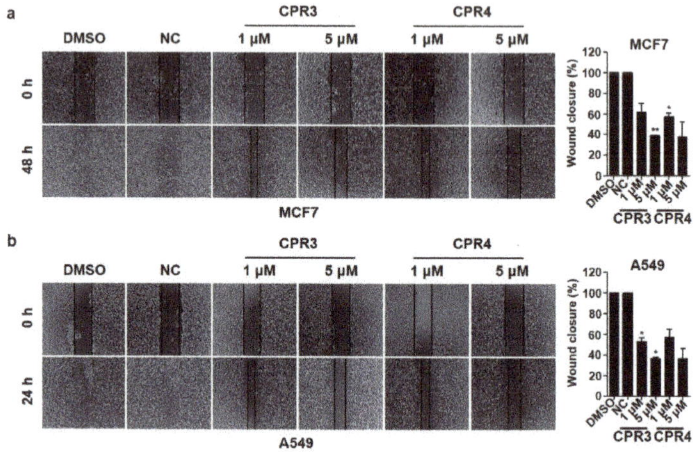

Figure 4. Wound healing images of MCF7 (**a**) and A549 (**b**) cells treated with CPR3 or CPR4 for 24 h. The PROTAC compound-treated cells were scratched with micropipette tip at 0 h. After 24 h, the migration status was monitored by bright optical microscopy. * $P \leq 0.05$ and ** $P \leq 0.01$, as determined by Student's t-test.

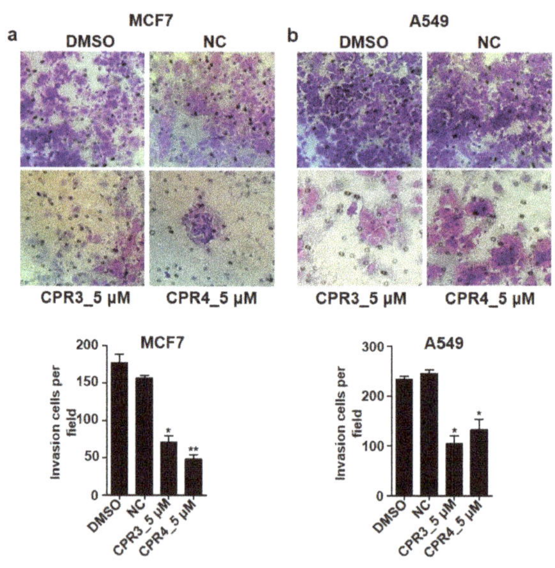

Figure 5. Invasiveness images of MCF7 (**a**) and A549 (**b**) cells treated with CPR3 or CPR4 for 24 h. The cells, resuspended in RPMI-1640 without serum, were reseeded on matrigel-coated insert transwell for 24 h. After 24 h, the cells that migrated to the membrane of the transwell were stained with 0.1% crystal violet and were counted with bright optical microscopy. * $P \leq 0.05$ and ** $P \leq 0.01$, as determined by Student's t-test.

2.5. PROTAC Compounds Inhibited the Cell Growth of Both MCF7 and A549 Cells in the Soft Agar Colony Formation Assay

Next, we examined tumorigenesis by treatment with PROTAC compounds in both MCF7 and A549 cells. It is well known that cancer cells differentiate rapidly and proliferate infinitely. In addition, the capability of single cells to form into a colony is a hallmark of cancer cell survival and proliferation.

To test cellular anchorage-independent growth in vitro, we performed the soft agar colony formation assay after treatment with PROTAC compounds. In Figure 6, the number of colonies was significantly increased in DMSO or NC in both MCF7 (Figure 6a) and A549 (Figure 6b) cells. In contrast to the control group, the colony forming ability sharply declined with a 5 μM concentration of PROTAC compounds. Moreover, the sizes of the colonies formed from a single cell were much smaller in PROTAC compounds than in DMSO or NC. These results indicated that PROTAC compounds, with the dual degradation of IGF-1R and Src, affected cell survival.

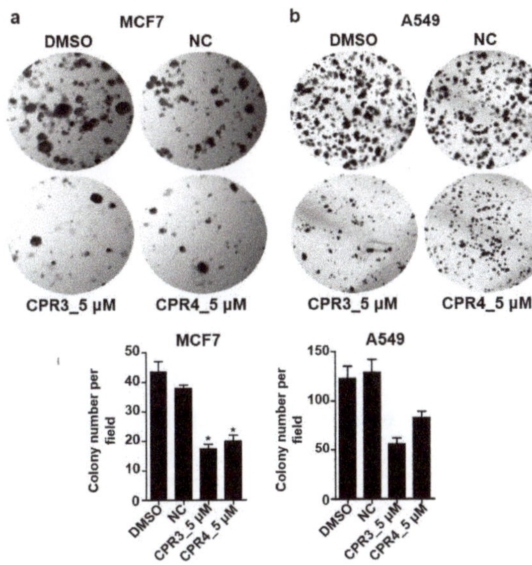

Figure 6. Soft agar colony formation images after treatment with CPR3 or CPR4 in both MCF7 (**a**) and A549 (**b**) cells. CPR3 or CPR4 was treated at 5 μM of concentration, followed by an incubation period of 2 weeks. The formed colonies were stained with 0.1% crystal violet and were detected on a bright field microscopy. * $P \leq 0.05$, as determined by Student's t-test.

3. Discussion

In this study, we rapidly synthesized and screened PROTACs for dual degradation of IGF-1R and Src by employing different warhead ligands and varied linker lengths and compositions, which brought target proteins and E3 ligases into proximity for ubiquitination. Our work demonstrated that efficient PROTAC molecules (12a–b), which had single warhead ligands that degraded two target proteins, exhibited low micromolar anticancer activity, measured by different cellular assays, including cancer cell proliferation, immunoblotting, wound healing assay, and soft agar colony formation assays.

Interestingly, the potency of the synthesized compounds obviously varied, depending on the warhead units. Our data revealed that the previously reported Src or IGF-1R modules (D and E) were not sufficient, as individual warheads, for dual PROTACs, whereas the N^2-phenyl-N^4-(1*H*-pyrazol-3-yl)pyrimidine-2,4-diamine (C) exhibited better potency for dual degradation. The induced degradation of the protein was found to be intrinsic to target proteins, which are affected by numerous factors, including the linker length and composition, E3 ligase ligand, spatial orientation of the formed ternary complex and their stability, cell permeability, and ubiquitination efficiency. One important factor for PROTACs is a drug-like property with cell permeability, for which atom numbers need to be minimized in the design of the chemical structure. Indeed, the linker size with 7-10 atoms, between the warhead ligand and the E3 ligase ligand in PROTACs 12a–b, appears to be sufficient for proximity-induced ubiquitination of Src or IGF-1R with the E3 ligase.

The possibility of off-target degradation is still likely to happen with small-warhead ligands, due to their promiscuity. However, recent advancements in PROTACs with promiscuous kinase inhibitors have shown that efficiency is not directly correlated with the binding affinity of the ligands [27]. Rather, it is more closely related to the geometry of the ternary complex of the target protein-PROTAC-E3 ligases, as well as to the efficiency of the proximity-induced enzymatic ubiquitin transfer. Further optimization needs to be followed in regard to the optimal CRBN ligand orientation, nano to pico molar potency, etc. However, our work demonstrated a facile preparation of efficient dual degraders, which enrich our knowledge in establishing dual degradation as an alternative therapeutic strategy in cancers.

4. Materials and Methods

4.1. Chemistry

4.1.1. General Information

All reagents and solvents were obtained from commercial suppliers and used as received unless otherwise specified. All reactions were performed under nitrogen atmosphere using oven-dried glassware and monitored by thin-layer chromatography (TLC) on a silica-coated plate (60 F254, Merck, Darmstadt, Germany). Separated compounds on the TLC plate were visualized under UV light at 254 nm and 365 nm (VL-4.LC, Vilber Lourmat, Eberhardzell, Germany). Column chromatography was carried out using a silica gel 230-400 mesh (ZEOprep, Zeochem, Lake Zurich, Switzerland) with *n*-hexane, EtOAc, CH_2Cl_2 and MeOH as eluents. ^{1}H NMR (400 MHz) and ^{13}C NMR (125 MHz) spectra were recorded using a FT-NMR Avance III HD (Bruker, Billerica, MA, USA) at ambient temperature. Chemical shifts were reported in ppm (parts per million) relative to tetramethylsilane and coupling constants (J) were expressed in hertz (Hz). The following abbreviations are used for multiplicities: s = singlet; brs = broad singlet; d = doublet; t = triplet; q = quartet; m = multiplet; dd = doublet of doublets. Mass-to-charge ratio (m/z) values were obtained by using high-resolution mass spectrometry (HRMS) under fast atom bombardment (FAB) conditions with a JMS-700 MStation (JEOL, Tokyo, Japan).

4.1.2. Synthesis of 10a–c, 12a–d, 16a–b, 18a–b and 21a–b

General procedure for synthesis of 8a–c: A reaction mixture of 7a–c (11.036 mmol, 1.0 eq), iron powder (10.363 mmol, 10 eq) and ammonium chloride (10.363 mmol, 10 eq) in ethanol-water (8:2) was stirred for 2 h under N_2 atmosphere at 80 °C. The reaction mixture was cooled down to room temperature, filtered through celite bed, which was washed twice with ethyl acetate. Solvent was removed under reduced pressure and the obtained residue was dissolved in ethyl acetate and washed with water and brine solution. Organic layer was dried over anhydrous sodium sulfate. Upon concentration under reduced pressure, the residue was purified by column chromatography on silica gel to give 8a–c in 42–44% yield.

*4-((2-(2-(4-aminophenoxy)ethoxy)ethyl)amino)-2-(2,6-dioxopiperidin-3-yl)isoindoline-1,3-dione (**8a**)*: Yellow solid; yield 42.1%; R_f = 0.50 (methanol/dichloromethane = 0.5:9.5); ^{1}H-NMR (400 MHz, $CDCl_3$) δ 8.57 (s, 1H), 7.43 (t, J = 8.8 Hz, 1H), 7.06 (d, J = 7.2 Hz, 1H), 6.89 (d, J = 8.4 Hz, 1H), 6.71 (d, J = 9.2 Hz, 2H), 6.58 (d, J = 9.2 Hz, 2H), 6.49 (t, J = 5.6 Hz, 1H), 4.87 (dd, J = 5.6, 12.0 Hz, 1H), 4.03 (t, J = 4.8 Hz, 2H), 3.80–3.74 (m, 4H), 3.45 (dd, J = 5.6, 11.2 Hz, 2H), 2.84–2.65 (m, 3H), 2.08–2.02 (m, 1H); ^{13}C-NMR (125 MHz, $CDCl_3$) δ 171.39, 169.18, 168.53, 167.59, 151.80, 146.77, 140.14, 135.95, 132.42, 116.75, 116.31 (2C), 115.87 (2C), 111.57, 110.24, 69.89, 69.63, 68.21, 48.78, 42.36, 31.32, 22.67; HR-MS (FAB$^+$) calcd for $C_{23}H_{25}N_4O_6$ [M + H]$^+$ 453.1774, found 453.1777.

*4-((2-(2-(2-(4-aminophenoxy)ethoxy)ethoxy)ethyl)amino)-2-(2,6-dioxopiperidin-3-yl)isoindoli ne-1,3-dione (**8b**)*: Yellow solid; yield 44.7%; R_f = 0.50 (methanol/dichloromethane = 1:9); ^{1}H-NMR (400 MHz, $CDCl_3$) δ 8.54 (s, 1H), 7.44 (t, J = 7.2 Hz, 1H), 7.05 (d, J = 7.2 Hz, 1H), 6.88 (d, J = 8.4 Hz, 1H), 6.71 (d, J = 8.8 Hz, 2H), 6.58 (d, J = 8.8 Hz, 2H), 6.47 (t, J = 5.6 Hz, 1H), 4.84 (dd, J = 5.2, 12.0 Hz, 1H), 4.02 (t,

J = 4.8 Hz, 2H), 3.79 (t, J = 5.2 Hz, 2H), 3.71–3.65 (m, 6H), 3.43 (dd, J = 5.6, 11.2 Hz, 3H), 2.77–2.64 (m, 3H), 2.04-2.00 (m, 1H); ^{13}C-NMR (125 MHz, $CDCl_3$) δ 171.29, 169.18, 168.46, 167.59, 151.85, 146.77, 140.11, 135.95, 132.42, 116.73, 116.30 (2C), 115.79 (2C), 111.53, 110.19, 70.70, 70.66, 69.92, 69.44, 68.07, 48.78, 42.32, 31.31, 22.65; HR-MS (FAB$^+$) calcd for $C_{25}H_{29}N_4O_7$ [M + H]$^+$ 497.2036, found 497.2029.

*4-((2-(2-(2-(2-(4-aminophenoxy)ethoxy)ethoxy)ethoxy)ethyl)amino)-2-(2,6-dioxopiperidin-3-yl)isoindoline -1,3-dione (**8c**):* Yellow solid; yield 42.9%; R_f = 0.50 (methanol/dichloromethane = 1:9); ^{1}H-NMR (400 MHz, $CDCl_3$) δ 8.46 (s, 1H), 8.13 (d, J = 9.2 Hz, 2H), 7.44 (t, J = 8.4 Hz, 1H), 7.05 (d, J = 6.8 Hz, 1H), 6.93 (d, J = 9.2 Hz, 2H), 6.87 (d, J = 8.4 Hz, 1H), 6.44 (t, J = 5.6 Hz, 1H), 4.88 (dd, J = 6.0, 12.4 Hz, 1H), 4.17 (t, J = 4.4 Hz, 2H), 3.85 (t, J = 4.8 Hz, 2H), 3.70–3.64 (m, 10H), 3.42 (dd, J = 5.6, 11.1 Hz, 2H), 2.85–2.68 (m, 3H), 2.10–2.02 (m, 1H); ^{13}C-NMR (125 MHz, $CDCl_3$) δ 171.36, 169.18, 168.54, 167.49, 163.75, 146.68, 141.42, 135.92, 132.35, 125.73 (2C), 116.67, 114.48 (2C), 111.50, 110.10, 70.75, 70.54, 70.50, 69.40, 69.22, 68.10, 48.75, 42.26, 31.28, 22.63; HR-MS (FAB$^+$) calcd for $C_{27}H_{33}N_4O_8$ [M + H]$^+$ 541.2298, found 541.2299.

General procedure for synthesis of 10a–c and 12a–b: A reaction mixture of 8a–c (0.044 mmol, 1.0 eq) and corresponding pyrimidines 9 or 11a–b (0.044 mmol, 1.0 eq) were dissolved in DMSO (1.0 mL), and the resulting mixture was stirred for 16 h under N_2 atmosphere at 90 °C. The progress of the reaction was monitored by TLC. After completion of the reaction, 50 mL of cold water was added and extracted with ethyl acetate (3 × 50 mL). The combined organic layer was dried over anhydrous sodium sulfate. Upon concentration under reduced pressure, the residue was purified by column chromatography on silica gel to give 10a–c and 12a–b, respectively. 21–57% yields.

*2-(2,6-dioxopiperidin-3-yl)-4-((2-(2-(4-((4-(quinoline-3-ylamino)pyrimidin-2-yl)amino)pheno xy)ethoxy) ethyl)amino)isoindoline-1,3-dione (**10a**, CPR-2)*: Yellow solid; yield 52.0%; R_f = 0.45 (methanol/dichloromethane = 1:9); mp 160.2–161.8 °C; ^{1}H-NMR (400 MHz, MeOD + $CDCl_3$) δ 8.81 (s, 1H), 8.70 (s, 1H), 7.90 (d, J = 5.6 Hz, 1H), 7.85–7.83 (m, 1H), 7.53–7.42 (m, 4H), 7.35 (d, J = 9.2 Hz, 2H), 6.98-6.95 (m, 2H), 6.87 (d, J = 9.2 Hz, 2H), 6.19 (d, J = 6.0 Hz, 1H), 4.85 (dd, J = 5.6, 12.4 Hz, 1H), 4.14 (t, J = 4.4 Hz, 2H), 3.87 (t, J = 4.8 Hz, 2H), 3.79 (t, J = 5.6 Hz, 2H), 3.48 (t, J = 5.2 Hz, 2H), 2.68–2.53 (m, 3H), 1.99–1.87 (m, 1H); ^{13}C-NMR (125 MHz, MeOD + $CDCl_3$) δ 174.08, 170.92, 170.46, 169.29, 162.30, 161.34, 156.69, 156.32, 147.99, 145.73, 144.42, 137.28, 134.97, 133.92, 133.60, 129.87, 128.86, 128.83 (2C), 128.26, 124.99, 124.87, 118.17, 116.25 (2C), 112,67, 111.33, 99.83, 71.05, 70.95, 69.10, 50.06, 43.45, 32.49, 23.85; HRMS (FAB$^+$) calcd for $C_{36}H_{33}N_8O_6$ [M + H]$^+$ 673.2523, found 673.2532.

*2-(2,6-dioxopiperidin-3-yl)-4-((2-(2-(2-(4-((4-(quinolin-3-ylamino)pyrimidin-2-yl)amino)phen oxy)ethoxy) ethoxy)ethyl)amino)isoindoline-1,3-dione (**10b**, CPR-5)*: Yellow solid; yield 57.7%; R_f = 0.45 (methanol/dichloromethane = 1:9); mp 185.3–186.4 °C; ^{1}H-NMR (400 MHz, DMSO-d_6) δ 11.06 (s, 1H), 9.82 (s, 1H), 9.10 (s, 1H), 8.85 (s, 2H), 8.02 (d, J = 5.6 Hz, 1H), 7.86 (d, J = 9.2 Hz, 1H), 7.69 (brs, 1H), 7.54–7.49 (m, 5H), 7.08 (d, J = 8.8 Hz, 1H), 6.97 (d, J = 6.8 Hz, 1H), 6.83 (d, J = 9.2 Hz, 2H), 6.57 (t, J = 6.0 Hz, 1H), 6.25 (d, J = 5.6 Hz, 1H), 4.99 (dd, J = 5.6, 12.8 Hz, 1H), 4.01 (t, J = 4.4 Hz, 2H), 3.72 (t, J = 4.8 Hz, 2H), 3.60–3.56 (m, 6H), 3.46–3.40 (m, 2H), 2.85–2.76 (m, 1H), 2.53–2.48 (m, 2H), 1.96–1.91 (m, 1H); ^{13}C-NMR (125 MHz, MeOD + $CDCl_3$) δ 173.69, 170.58, 170.29, 169.04, 162.05, 161.17, 156.78, 156.05, 147.74, 145.64, 144.31, 137.07, 134.69, 133.73, 133.39, 129.66, 128.84, 128.64, 128.61, 128.09, 124.68, 124.61 (2C), 117.91, 115.97 (2C), 112.52, 111.07, 99.53, 71.82, 71.67, 70.91, 70.53, 68.82, 49.88, 43.21. 32.35, 23.68; HRMS (FAB$^+$) calcd for $C_{38}H_{37}N_8O_7$ [M + H]$^+$ 717.2785, found 717.2770.

*2-(2,6-dioxopiperidin-3-yl)-4-((2-(2-(2-(2-(4-((4-(quinolin-3-ylamino)pyrimidin-2-yl)amino)phenoxy) ethoxy)ethoxy)ethoxy)ethyl)amino)isoindoline-1,3-dione (**10c**, CPR-1)*: Yellow solid; yield 21.0%; R_f = 0.45 (methanol/dichloromethane = 1:9); mp 151.8–152.9 °C; ^{1}H-NMR (400 MHz, DMSO-d_6) δ 11.05 (s, 1H), 9.77 (s, 1H), 9.05 (s, 1H), 8.88 (brs, 1H), 8.86 (s, 1H), 8.03 (d, J = 5.6 Hz, 1H), 7.87 (d, J = 9.6 Hz, 1H), 7.70 (brs, 1H), 7.55–7.48 (m, 5H), 7.07 (d, J = 8.4 Hz, 1H), 6.97 (d, J = 6.8 Hz, 1H), 6.84 (d, J = 9.2 Hz, 2H), 6.55 (t, J = 5.6 Hz, 1H), 6.25 (d, J = 5.6 Hz, 1H), 5.01 (dd, J = 5.0, 12.8 Hz, 1H), 4.01 (t, J = 4.4 Hz, 2H), 3.70 (t, J = 4.4 Hz, 2H), 3.58–3.52 (m, 10H), 3.40 (dd, J = 5.2, 10.8 Hz, 2H), 2.87–2.78 (m, 1H), 2.55–2.49 (m, 2H), 1.99–1.94 (m, 1H); ^{13}C-NMR (125 MHz, $CDCl_3$) δ 172.76, 170.03, 169.22, 167.68, 160.78, 159.85, 156.15, 154.50, 146.63, 145.50, 144.23, 135.89, 132.88, 132.86, 132.32, 128.72, 128.26, 127.63, 127.36, 126.94,

123.82, 122.48 (2C), 116.67, 114.82 (2C), 111.51, 110.08, 97.51, 70.78, 70.68, 70.60 (2C), 69.74, 69.34, 67.72, 48.83, 42.28, 31.44, 22.79; HR-MS (FAB$^+$) calcd for $C_{40}H_{41}N_8O_8$ $[M + H]^+$ 761.3047, found 761.3039.

*2-(2,6-dioxopiperidin-3-yl)-4-((2-(2-(4-((4-((5-methyl-1H-pyrazol-3-yl)amino)pyrimidin-2-yl) amino) phenoxy)ethoxy)ethyl)amino)isoindoline-1,3-dione (**12a**, CPR-3)*: Yellow solid; yield 32.6%; R_f = 0.45 (methanol/dichloromethane = 1:9); mp 158.1–159.3 °C; ^{1}H-NMR (400 MHz, MeOD + $CDCl_3$) δ 7.84 (d, *J* = 6.0 Hz, 1H), 7.42 (dd, *J* = 7.2, 8.4 Hz, 1H), 7.34 (d, *J* = 9.2 Hz, 2H), 7.00 (d, *J* = 6.8 Hz, 1H), 6.90 (d, *J* = 8.8 Hz, 1H), 6.83 (d, *J* = 8.8 Hz, 2H), 6.13 (s, 1H), 5.87 (s, 1H), 4.85 (dd, *J* = 5.6, 12.4 Hz, 1H), 4.08 (t, *J* = 4.4 Hz, 2H), 3.80 (t, *J* = 4.8 Hz, 2H), 3.73 (t, *J* = 5.2 Hz, 2H), 3.44 (t, *J* = 5.2 Hz, 2H), 2.77–2.58 (m, 3H), 2.16 (s, 3H), 2.04–1.99 (m, 1H); ^{13}C-NMR (125 MHz, DMSO-d_6) δ 172.84, 170.11, 168.94, 167.31, 160.75, 159.39, 157.14, 150.01, 147.37, 146.40, 141.86, 138.84, 136.21, 132.11, 117.41, 115.46 (2C), 115.24 (2C), 110.70, 109.31, 104.99, 95.52, 69.09, 68.93, 67.64, 48.58, 41.71, 31.01, 22.16, 10.63; HR-MS (FAB$^+$) calcd for $C_{31}H_{32}N_9O_6$ $[M + H]^+$ 626.2476, found 626.2477.

*2-(2,6-dioxopiperidin-3-yl)-4-((2-(2-(2-(4-((4-((5-methyl-1H-pyrazol-3-yl)amino)pyrimidin-2-yl)amino) phenoxy)ethoxy)ethoxy)ethyl)amino)isoindoline-1,3-dione (**12b**, CPR-4)*: Yellow solid; yield 44.5%; R_f = 0.45 (methanol/dichloromethane = 1:9); mp 176.2–177.5 °C; ^{1}H-NMR (400 MHz, MeOD + $CDCl_3$) δ 7.75 (d, *J* = 6.4 Hz, 1H), 7.43 (dd, *J* = 7.2, 8.4 Hz, 1H), 7.32 (d, *J* = 8.8 Hz, 2H), 7.00 (d, *J* = 7.2 Hz, 1H), 6.91 (d, *J* = 8.8 Hz, 1H), 6.86 (d, *J* = 9.2 Hz, 2H), 6.23 (s, 1H), 5.96 (s, 1H), 4.85 (dd, *J* = 5.2, 11.2 Hz, 1H), 4.08 (t, *J* = 4.4 Hz, 2H), 3.83 (t, *J* = 4.8 Hz, 2H), 3.71–3.65 (m, 6H), 3.42 (t, *J* = 5.2 Hz, 2H), 2.75–2.65 (m, 3H), 2.18 (s, 3H), 2.06–1.98 (m, 1H); ^{13}C-NMR (125 MHz, DMSO-d_6) δ 172.80, 170.08, 168.94, 167.29, 160.72, 159.36, 157.06, 150.84, 147.35, 146.40, 140.13, 138.85, 136.20, 132.08, 117.44, 116.17 (2C), 115.31 (2C), 110.66, 109.24, 105.01, 95.47, 69.90, 69.79, 69.19, 68.91, 67.53, 48.55, 41.68, 30.98, 22.14, 10.62; HRMS (FAB$^+$) calcd for $C_{33}H_{36}N_9O_7$ $[M + H]^+$ 670.2738, found 670.2745.

*4-((2-(2-(4-((5-chloro-4-((5-methyl-1H-pyrazol-3-yl)amino)pyrimidin-2-yl)amino)phenoxy) ethoxy)ethyl) amino)-2-(2,6-dioxopiperidin-3-yl)isoindoline-1,3-dion(**12c**, CPR-10)*: To the solution of 8a (30 mg, 0.066 mmol) in n-butanol (4.0 mL) were added 11b (16 mg, 0.066 mmol) and p-toluenesulfonic acid monohydrate (13.5 mg, 0.066 mmol). The resulting mixture was stirred for 4 h under N_2 atmosphere at 100 °C. The progress of reaction was monitored by TLC. After completion of the reaction, the reaction mixture was cooled down to room temperature, saturated $NaHCO_3$ solution was added to adjust pH to 7, then extracted with ethyl acetate (3 x 20 mL). The combined organic layer was dried over anhydrous sodium sulfate. After concentration of the reaction mixture under reduced pressure, the residue was purified by column chromatography on silica gel to give 12c (13.19 mg, 32.5%) as a yellow solid. R_f = 0.45 (methanol/dichloromethane = 1:9); mp 196.2–197.8 °C; ^{1}H-NMR (400 MHz, MeOD + $CDCl_3$) δ 7.90 (s, 1H), 7.46 (t, *J* = 8.4 Hz, 1H), 7.32 (d, *J* = 8.8 Hz, 2H), 6.98 (dd, *J* = 7.2, 10.4 Hz, 2H), 6.85 (d, *J* = 8.8 Hz, 2H), 6.20 (s, 1H), 4.92 (dd, *J* = 6.0, 12.4 Hz, 1H), 4.11 (t, *J* = 4.4 Hz, 2H), 3.83 (t, *J* = 4.4 Hz, 2H), 3.76 (t, *J* = 5.2 Hz, 2H), 3.47 (t, *J* = 5.2 Hz, 2H), 2.74–2.63 (m, 3H), 2.20 (s, 3H), 2.04–1.96 (m, 1H); ^{13}C-NMR (125 MHz, DMSO-d_6) δ 172.80, 170.07, 168.91, 167.28, 157.04, 156.78, 155.09, 149.72, 146.38, 145.70, 142.45, 138.74, 136.19, 132.09, 117.40, 115.44 (2C), 114.91 (2C), 113.15, 110.67, 109.28, 98.02, 69.08, 68.92, 67.63, 48.56, 41.70, 30.98, 22.14, 10.73; HR-MS (FAB$^+$) calcd for $C_{31}H_{31}ClN_9O_6$ $[M + H]^+$ 660.2086, found 660.2077.

*4-((2-(2-(2-(4-((5-chloro-4-((5-methyl-1H-pyrazol-3-yl)amino)pyrimidin-2-yl)amino)phenoxy) ethoxy) ethoxy)ethyl)amino)-2-(2,6-dioxopiperidin-3-yl)isoindoline-1,3-dione (**12d**, CPR-12)*: 12d was synthesized according to the procedure for 12c. Yellow solid; yield 22.6%; R_f = 0.55 (EtOAc); mp 180.9–182.1 °C; ^{1}H-NMR (400 MHz, $CDCl_3$) δ 8.00 (brs, 1H), 7.94 (s, 1H), 7.60 (brs, 1H), 7.42 (t, *J* = 7.2 Hz, 1H), 7.30 (d, *J* = 9.2 Hz, 2H), 7.01 (d, *J* = 7.2 Hz, 1H), 6.87 (d, *J* = 8.4 Hz, 1H), 6.78–6.71 (m, 2H), 6.63 (brs, 1H), 6.42 (t, *J* = 5.6 Hz, 1H), 6.03 (s, 1H), 4.85 (dd, *J* = 5.6, 12.4 Hz, 1H), 4.11–4.08 (m, 2H), 3.84 (t, *J* = 4.8 Hz, 2H), 3.75–3.69 (m, 6H), 3.46–3.42 (m, 2H), 2.81–2.59 (m, 3H), 2.24 (s, 3H), 2.05–2.02 (m, 1H); ^{13}C-NMR (125 MHz, DMSO-d_6) δ 172.79, 170.07, 168.93, 167.28, 157.04, 156.78, 155.10, 149.74, 146.40, 145.69, 142.41, 138.74, 136.19, 132.08, 117.42, 115.30 (2C), 114.92 (2C), 113.16, 110.65, 109.24, 98.01, 69.90, 69.79, 69.24, 68.91, 67.54, 48.56, 41.69, 30.98, 22.14, 10.73; HR-MS (FAB$^+$) calcd for $C_{33}H_{35}ClN_9O_7$ $[M + H]^+$ 704.2348, found 704.2340.

General procedure for synthesis of 14a–b: Dried round bottom flask with stir bar was charged with azidoacetic acid 13 (0.06 mmol, 1.0 eq) and *N*-ethyl-*N*′-(3-dimethylaminopropyl)carbodiimide hydrochloride (EDC·HCl) (0.120 mmol, 2.0 eq) followed by slow addition of dry DMF (3 mL). Then substituted alkyl amine 8a–b (0.06 mmol, 1.0 eq) was added, followed by addition of diisopropyl ethylamine (0.018 mmol, 3.0 eq). The resulting mixture was stirred for 16 h at room temperature. After completion of the reaction, cooled water was added to the reaction mixture, which was extracted with ethyl acetate twice. Separated organic layer was dried with anhydrous sodium sulfate and solvent was evaporated under reduced pressure. Crude product was purified by column chromatography on silica gel using EtOAc: Hexane as mobile phase to get desired product 14a–b in 40–63% yields.

*2-azido-N-(4-(2-(2-((2-(2,6-dioxopiperidin-3-yl)-1,3-dioxoisoindolin-4-yl)amino)ethoxy)ethox y)phenyl) acetamide (**14a**):* Yellow solid; yield 40.6%; R_f = 0.50 (methanol/dichloromethane = 1:9); ^{1}H-NMR (400 MHz, $CDCl_3$) δ 8.23 (s, 1H), 7.97 (s, 1H), 7.46 (t, *J* = 7.2 Hz, 1H), 7.38 (d, *J* = 9.2 Hz, 2H), 7.07 (d, *J* = 7.2 Hz, 1H), 6.88 (t, *J* = 8.8 Hz, 3H), 6.53 (brs, 1H), 4.88 (dd, *J* = 5.2 Hz, *J* = 12.0 Hz 1H), 4.14-4.10 (m, 4H), 3.84 (t, *J* = 4.8 Hz, 2H), 3.78 (t, *J* = 5.2 Hz, 2H), 3.46 (t, *J* = 5.2 Hz, 2H), 2.87–2.70 (m, 3H), 2.11–2.08 (m, 1H); ^{13}C-NMR (125 MHz, $CDCl_3$) δ 171.08, 169.17, 168.41, 167.59, 164.47, 156.01, 146.79, 136.02, 132.46, 130.08, 121.77 (2C), 116.74, 115.19 (2C), 111.69, 110.33, 69.80, 69.72, 67.88, 52.96, 48.84, 42.41, 31.40, 22.76; HR-MS (FAB$^+$) calcd for $C_{25}H_{26}N_7O_7$ $[M + H]^+$ 536.1894, found 536.1894.

*2-azido-N-(4-(2-(2-(2-((2-(2,6-dioxopiperidin-3-yl)-1,3-dioxoisoindolin-4-yl)amino)ethoxy) ethoxy)ethoxy) phenyl)acetamide (**14b**):* Yellow solid; yield 62.8%; R_f = 0.70 (ethyl acetate); ^{1}H-NMR (400 MHz, $CDCl_3$) δ 8.08 (s, 1H), 7.93 (s, 1H), 7.46 (t, *J* = 8.0 Hz, 1H), 7.38 (d, *J* = 8.8 Hz, 2H), 7.07 (d, *J* = 7.2 Hz, 1H), 6.90–6.84 (m, 3H), 6.46 (t, *J* = 6.4 Hz, 1H), 4.83 (dd, *J* = 6.8, 13.2 Hz, 1H), 4.12-4.07 (m, 4H), 3.84 (t, *J* = 4.8 Hz, 2H), 3.73–3.68 (m, 6H), 3.44 (dd, *J* = 5.6 Hz, 2H), 2.84–2.65 (m, 3H), 2.08–2.03 (m, 1H); ^{13}C-NMR (125 MHz, $CDCl_3$) δ 170.93, 169.20, 168.28, 167.60, 164.42, 156.09, 146.82, 136.04, 132.49, 129.99, 121.83 (2C), 116.76, 115.01 (2C), 111.63, 110.24, 70.86, 70.76, 69.76, 69.49, 67.71, 52.96, 48.84, 42.41, 31.39, 22.71; HR-MS (FAB$^+$) calcd for $C_{27}H_{30}N_7O_8$ $[M + H]^+$ 580.2156, found 580.2156.

3-(4-chlorophenyl)-1-(prop-2-yn-1-yl)-1H-pyrazolo[3,4-d]pyrimidin-4-amine (**15**): Compound 15 was synthesized according to the reported procedure [36,50].

*2-(4-((4-amino-3-(4-chlorophenyl)-1H-pyrazol[3,4-d]pyrimidin-1-yl)methyl)-1H-1,2,3-triazol -1-yl)-N-(4-(2-(2-((2-(2,6-dioxopiperidin-3-yl)-1,3-dioxoisoindolin-4-yl)amino)ethoxy)ethoxy)phen yl)acetamide (**16a**, CPR-7)*: To a reaction mixture of 8a (12 mg, 0.022 mmol) and 15 (6.3 mg, 0.022 mmol) dissolved in THF (1.0 mL) was added t-butanol (0.5 mL). Then $CuSO_4 \cdot 5H_2O$ (1.1 mg, 0.004 mmol) dissolved in 0.2 mL of water was added to it, followed by the addition of sodium ascorbate (3.55 mg, 0.017 mmol) dissolved in 0.2 mL of water. The reaction mixture was stirred at room temperature for 6 h. The progress of reaction was monitored by TLC. After completion of the reaction, solvent was evaporated, and the residue was extracted with ethyl acetate (3 x 20 mL). The combined organic layer was dried over anhydrous sodium sulfate. Upon concentration under reduced pressure, the residue was purified by column chromatography on silica gel to give 16a (5 mg, 27.2%) as a yellow solid. R_f = 0.15 (methanol/ethyl acetate = 1:9); mp 186.3–187.6 °C; ^{1}H-NMR (400 MHz, MeOD + $CDCl_3$) δ 8.28 (s, 1H), 7.98 (s, 1H), 7.59 (d, *J* = 8.4 Hz, 2H), 7.48-7.41 (m, 3H), 7.32 (d, *J* = 9.2 Hz, 2H), 6.99 (d, *J* = 6.8 Hz, 1H), 6.93 (d, *J* = 8.4 Hz, 1H), 6.79 (d, *J* = 9.2 Hz, 2H), 5.71 (s, 2H), 5.15 (s, 2H), 4.87 (dd, *J* = 6.0, 12.4 Hz, 1H), 4.07 (t, *J* = 4.4 Hz, 2H), 3.80 (t, *J* = 4.8 Hz, 2H), 3.74 (t, *J* = 5.2 Hz, 2H), 3.44 (t, *J* = 5.2 Hz, 2H), 2.73–2.63 (m, 3H), 2.05–1.96 (m, 1H); ^{13}C-NMR (125 MHz, MeOD + $CDCl_3$) δ 173.62, 170.49, 170.22, 169.03, 164.18, 157.27, 156.78, 154.71, 147.73, 145.77, 143.70, 137.07, 136.73, 133.37, 131.74 (2C), 131.65 (2C), 130.76, 130.61, 126.08, 124.26, 122.55 (2C), 117.90, 115.99 (2C), 112.55, 112.16, 111.12, 70.73, 70.68, 68.78, 53.81, 43.45, 43.22, 32.33, 30.61, 23.68; HR-MS (FAB$^+$) calcd for $C_{39}H_{36}ClN_{12}O_7$ $[M + H]^+$ 819.2518, found 819.2532.

*2-(4-((4-amino-3-(4-chlorophenyl)-1H-pyrazolo[3,4-d]pyrimidin-1-yl)methyl)-1H-1,2,3-triazol-1-yl)-N-(4-(2-(2-(2-((2-(2,6-dioxopiperidin-3-yl)-1,3-dioxoisoindolin-4-yl)amino)ethoxy) ethoxy)ethoxy)phenyl)acetamide (**16b**, CPR-9)*: 16b was synthesized according to the procedure for 16a. Yellow solid; yield 26.8%; R_f = 0.20 (ethyl acetate); mp 192.8–194.1 °C; ^{1}H-NMR (400 MHz, MeOD) δ 8.28 (s, 1H), 7.92 (s, 1H), 7.55 (d,

J = 6.4 Hz, 2H), 7.46-7.38 (m, 4H), 7.31 (d, J = 9.2 Hz, 2H), 6.99 (d, J = 6.8 Hz, 1H), 6.86 (d, J = 8.4 Hz, 1H), 6.76 (d, J = 9.2 Hz, 2H), 5.69 (s, 2H), 5.09 (s, 2H), 4.77 (dd, J = 5.2, 12.4 Hz, 1H), 3.78 (t, J = 4.8 Hz, 2H), 3.68-3.58 (m, 6H), 3.39 (t, J = 5.2 Hz, 2H), 3.29-3.27 (m, 2H), 2.73-2.59 (m, 3H), 2.00–1.94 (m, 1H); ^{13}C-NMR (125 MHz, MeOD + $CDCl_3$) δ 173.69, 170.51, 170.29, 169.19, 169.12, 164.28, 157.73, 156.85, 147.78, 137.14, 136.81, 136.43, 133.42, 131.81 (2C), 131.64 (2C), 130.82, 130.67, 129.34, 126.22, 122.61 (2C), 119.64, 117.97, 117.61, 115.87 (2C), 112.53, 111.08, 71.75, 71.65, 70.79, 70.49, 68.66, 53.80, 43.50, 43.23, 32.36, 30.67, 23.70; HR-MS (FAB$^+$) calcd for $C_{41}H_{40}ClN_{12}O_8$ [M + H]$^+$ 863.2781, found 863.2768.

1-(3-bromopropyl)-3-(4-chlorophenyl)-1H-pyrazolo[3,4-d]pyrimidin-4-amine (**17**): To a reaction mixture of 22 (400 mg, 1.628 mmol) and 1,3-dibromo propane (394 mg, 1.953 mmol) dissolved in DMF (4.0 mL) was added K_2CO_3 (562 mg, 4.070 mmol). The resulting mixture was stirred at room temperature for 16 h. The progress of the reaction was monitored by TLC. After completion of the reaction, cold water was added and extracted with ethyl acetate (3 x 20 mL). The combined organic layer was dried over anhydrous sodium sulfate. Upon concentration under reduced pressure, the residue was purified by column chromatography on silica gel to give 17 (388 mg, 65.0%) as a white solid. R_f = 0.80 (methanol/dichloromethane = 1:9); ^{1}H-NMR (400 MHz, $CDCl_3$) δ 8.35 (s, 1H), 7.62 (d, J = 8.8 Hz, 2H), 7.50 (d, J = 8.8 Hz, 2H), 5.90 (brs, 2H), 4.57 (t, J = 6.8 Hz, 2H), 3.42 (t, J = 6.8 Hz, 2H), 2.54–2.47 (m, 2H); ^{13}C-NMR (125 MHz, $CDCl_3$) δ 157.84, 155.94, 154.66, 143.32, 135.36, 131.55, 129.68 (2C), 129.60 (2C), 98.38, 45.55, 32.52, 29.79; HR-MS (FAB$^+$) calcd for $C_{14}H_{14}BrClN_5$ [M + H]$^+$ 366.0121, found 366.0121.

*4-((2-(2-(4-((3-(4-amino-3-(4-chlorophenyl)-1H-pyrazolo[3,4-d]pyrimidin-1-yl)propyl)amino) phenoxy)ethoxy)ethyl)amino)-2-(2,6-dioxopiperidin-3-yl)isoindoline-1,3-dione(**18a**, CPR-8)*: To the solution of 8a (20 mg, 0.044 mmol) in DMF (3.0 mL) were added potassium carbonate (12.21 mg, 0.066 mmol) and 17 (16.2 mg, 0.044 mmol). The reaction mixture was stirred for 16 h under N_2 atmosphere at room temperature. The progress of reaction was monitored by TLC. After completion of the reaction, cold water (20 mL) was added and extracted with ethyl acetate (3 x 20 mL). The combined organic layer was dried over anhydrous sodium sulfate. Upon concentration under reduced pressure, the residue was purified by column chromatography on silica gel to give 18a (16.5 mg, 50.6%) as a yellow solid. R_f = 0.50 (methanol/dichloromethane = 1:9); mp 146.3–147.6 °C; ^{1}H-NMR (400 MHz, $CDCl_3$) δ 8.35 (s, 1H), 7.63 (d, J = 8.4 Hz, 2H), 7.48–7.42 (m, 3H), 7.05 (d, J = 6.8 Hz, 1H), 6.89 (d, J = 8.4 Hz, 1H), 6.71 (d, J = 8.8 Hz, 2H), 6.58 (d, J = 8.8 Hz, 2H), 6.46 (t, J = 6.0 Hz, 1H), 5.53 (brs, 2H), 4.84 (dd, J = 5.2, 12.4 Hz, 1H), 4.45 (td, J = 7.2, 2.8 Hz, 2H), 4.03 (t, J = 4.4 Hz, 2H), 3.91 (td, J = 6.8, 2.4 Hz, 2H), 3.78 (p, 2H), 3.74 (t, J = 5.2 Hz, 2H), 3.46 (dd, J = 5.6, 11.2 Hz, 2H), 2.88 (dd, J = 12.8, 2.8 Hz, 1H), 2.72–2.66 (m, 2H), 2.23 (p, 2H), 2.04–1.99 (m, 1H); ^{13}C-NMR (125 MHz, $CDCl_3$) δ 170.94, 169.29, 168.75, 167.69, 157.69, 155.86, 154.51, 151.75, 146.77, 142.98, 140.30, 135.93, 135.13, 132.49, 131.75, 129.79 (2C), 129.49 (2C), 116.69, 116.23 (2C), 115.91 (2C), 111.57, 110.37, 98.40, 69.94, 69.71, 68.21, 49.56, 44.84, 42.42, 38.29, 31.96, 27.73, 22.06; HR-MS (FAB$^+$) calcd for $C_{37}H_{37}ClN_9O_6$ [M + H]$^+$ 738.2555, found 738.2544.

*4-((2-(2-(2-(4-((3-(4-amino-3-(4-chlorophenyl)-1H-pyrazolo[3,4-d]pyrimidin-1-yl)propyl)amin o)phenoxy) ethoxy)ethoxy)ethyl)amino)-2-(2,6-dioxopiperidin-3-yl)isoindoline-1,3-dione (**18b**, CPR-11)*: 18b was synthesized according to the procedure for 18a. Yellow solid; yield 50.8%; R_f = 0.45 (methanol/dichloromethane = 1:9); mp 148.2–149.9 °C; ^{1}H-NMR (400 MHz, $CDCl_3$) δ 8.35 (s, 1H), 7.63 (d, J = 8.4 Hz, 2H), 7.49–7.42 (m, 3H), 7.05 (d, J = 6.8 Hz, 1H), 6.88 (d, J = 8.8 Hz, 1H), 6.70 (d, J = 8.8 Hz, 2H), 6.57 (d, J = 8.8 Hz, 2H), 6.44 (t, J = 5.6 Hz, 1H), 4.82 (dd, J = 4.8, 12.0 Hz, 1H), 4.49-4.20 (m, 2H), 4.01 (t, J = 4.8 Hz, 2H), 3.93–3.87 (m, 2H), 3.78 (t, J = 5.2 Hz, 2H), 3.70–3.63 (m, 6H), 3.43 (dd, J = 5.2, 10.8 Hz, 2H), 2.88–2.82 (m, 1H), 2.74–2.62 (m, 2H), 2.23 (p, 2H), 2.06–1.97 (m, 1H); ^{13}C-NMR (125 MHz, $CDCl_3$) δ 170.94, 169.29, 168.75, 167.70, 157.65, 155.80, 154.49, 151.86, 146.77, 143.01, 140.19, 135.93, 135.14, 132.49, 131.74, 129.79 (2C), 129.50 (2C), 116.68, 116.25 (2C), 115.80 (2C), 111.52, 110.31, 98.39, 70.76, 70.71, 69.97, 69.53, 68.08, 49.55, 44.84, 42.37, 38.26, 31.94, 27.74, 22.04; HR-MS (FAB$^+$) calcd for $C_{39}H_{41}ClN_9O_7$ [M + H]$^+$ 782.2817, found 782.2834.

1-(3-azidopropyl)-3-(4-chlorophenyl)-1H-pyrazolo[3,4-d]pyrimidin-4-amine (**19**): To the solution of 17 (200 mg, 0.545 mmol) in DMF (2.0 mL) was added sodium azide (46.10 mg, 0.709 mmol) at room temperature. The reaction mixture was stirred for 16 h under N_2 atmosphere at room temperature.

The progress of reaction was monitored by TLC. After completion of the reaction, cold water (50 mL) was added and extracted with ethyl acetate (3 x 20 mL). The combined organic layer was dried over anhydrous sodium sulfate. Upon concentration under reduced pressure, the residue was purified by column chromatography on silica gel to give 19 (119 mg, 66.1%) as a white solid. R_f = 0.50 (EtOAc/n-Hexane = 1:1); ^{1}H-NMR (400 MHz, $CDCl_3$) δ 8.36 (s, 1H), 7.62 (d, *J* = 8.0 Hz, 2H), 7.50 (d, *J* = 8.4 Hz, 2H), 5.90 (brs, 2H), 4.52 (t, *J* = 6.4 Hz, 2H), 3.36 (t, *J* = 6.4 Hz, 2H), 2.23–2.17 (m, 2H); ^{13}C-NMR (125 MHz, $CDCl_3$) δ 157.84, 155.96, 154.63, 143.31, 135.36, 131.55, 129.67 (2C), 129.60 (2C), 98.34, 48.71, 44.26, 28.93; HR-MS (FAB$^+$) calcd for $C_{14}H_{14}ClN_8$ [M + H]$^+$ 329.1030, found 329.1033.

*2-(2,6-dioxopiperidin-3-yl)-4-((2-(2-(4-(prop-2-yn-1-ylamino)phenoxy)ethoxy)ethyl)amino)iso indoline -1,3-dione (**20a**)*: To the solution of 8a (50 mg, 0.110 mmol) in DMF (3.0 mL) were added potassium carbonate (22.9 mg, 0.165 mmol) and propargyl bromide (14.5 mg, 0.110 mmol) at room temperature. The reaction mixture was stirred for 16 h under N_2 atmosphere at room temperature. The progress of reaction was monitored by TLC. After completion of the reaction, cold water (20 mL) was added and extracted with ethyl acetate (3 x 20 mL). The combined organic layer was dried over anhydrous sodium sulfate. Upon concentration under reduced pressure, the residue was purified by column chromatography on silica gel to give 20a (30 mg, 55.4%) as a yellow solid. R_f = 0.60 (ethyl acetate = 100%); ^{1}H-NMR (400 MHz, $CDCl_3$) δ 7.45 (t, *J* = 8.4 Hz, 1H), 7.07 (d, *J* = 7.2 Hz, 1H), 6.91 (d, *J* = 8.4 Hz, 1H), 6.73 (d, *J* = 8.8 Hz, 2H), 6.59 (d, *J* = 8.8 Hz, 2H), 6.49 (t, *J* = 5.6 Hz, 1H), 4.92 (dd, *J* = 7.6, 12.4 Hz, 1H), 4.55 (d, *J* = 2.4 Hz, 2H), 4.04 (t, *J* = 4.4 Hz, 2H), 3.81–3.74 (m, 4H), 3.47 (dd, *J* = 5.2, 10.8 Hz, 2H), 3.00–2.93 (m, 1H), 2.81–2.72 (m, 2H), 2.14 (s, 1H), 2.08–2.04 (m, 1H); ^{13}C-NMR (125 MHz, $CDCl_3$) δ 170.11, 169.23, 167.96, 167.63, 151.77, 146.81, 140.30, 135.97, 132.46, 116.75, 116.23 (2C), 115.92 (2C), 111.61, 110.33, 77.94, 70.76, 69.94, 69.70, 68.22, 49.52, 42.42, 31.87, 29.62, 21.92; HR-MS (FAB$^+$) calcd for $C_{26}H_{27}N_4O_6$ [M + H]$^+$ 491.1931, found 491.1938.

*2-(2,6-dioxopiperidin-3-yl)-4-((2-(2-(2-(4-(prop-2-yn-1-ylamino)phenoxy)ethoxy)ethoxy)ethyl) amino) isoindoline-1,3-dione (**20b**)*: 20b was synthesized according to the procedure for 20a. White solid; yield 52.5%; R_f = 0.60 (EtOAc/n-Hexane = 1:1); ^{1}H-NMR (400 MHz, $CDCl_3$) δ 7.45 (t, *J* = 8.4 Hz, 1H), 7.07 (d, *J* = 6.8 Hz, 1H), 6.90 (d, *J* = 8.4 Hz, 1H), 6.72 (d, *J* = 8.8 Hz, 2H), 6.59 (d, *J* = 8.8 Hz, 2H), 6.47 (t, *J* = 5.6 Hz, 1H), 4.87 (dd, *J* = 4.8, 7.2 Hz, 1H), 4.55 (d, *J* = 2.4 Hz, 2H), 4.03 (t, *J* = 4.8 Hz, 2H), 3.81 (t, *J* = 5.2 Hz, 2H), 3.72–3.66 (m, 6H), 3.44 (dd, *J* = 5.6, 11.2 Hz, 2H), 2.97–2.86 (m, 1H), 2.76–2.67 (m, 2H), 2.15 (s, 1H), 2.08–2.01 (m, 1H); ^{13}C-NMR (125 MHz, $CDCl_3$) δ 170.10, 169.23, 167.95, 167.66, 151.90, 146.81, 140.20, 135.98, 132.48, 116.74, 116.26 (2C), 115.82 (2C), 111.58, 110.30, 77.97, 70.77, 70.74, 69.99, 69.57, 69.51, 68.11, 49.51, 42.39, 31.85, 29.63, 21.93; HR-MS (FAB$^+$) calcd for $C_{28}H_{31}N_4O_7$ [M + H]$^+$ 535.2193, found 535.2200.

*4-((2-(2-(4-(((1-(3-(4-amino-3-(4-chlorophenyl)-1H-pyrazolo[3,4-d]pyrimidin-1-yl)propyl)-1H-1,2,3-triazol -4-yl)methyl)amino)phenoxy)ethoxy)ethyl)amino)-2-(2,6-dioxopiperidin-3-yl)isoindol ine-1,3-dione (**21a**, CPR-13)*: 21a was synthesized according to the procedure for 16a. Yellow solid; yield 40.1%; R_f = 0.45 (methanol/dichloromethane = 1:9); mp 159.1–160.6 °C; ^{1}H-NMR (400 MHz, $CDCl_3$) δ 8.35 (s, 1H), 7.69 (s, 1H), 7.61 (d, *J* = 8.4 Hz, 2H), 7.48 (d, *J* = 8.4 Hz, 2H), 7.42 (t, *J* = 7.2 Hz, 1H), 7.01 (d, *J* = 7.2 Hz, 1H), 6.88 (d, *J* = 8.4 Hz, 1H), 6.70 (d, *J* = 8.8 Hz, 2H), 6.57 (d, *J* = 8.8 Hz, 2H), 6.47 (t, *J* = 5.6 Hz, 1H), 5.13-5.04 (m, H), 4.92 (dd, *J* = 5.2, 12.4 Hz, 1H), 4.47 (t, *J* = 7.2 Hz, 2H), 4.34 (t, *J* = 6.8 Hz, 2H), 4.03 (t, *J* = 4.8 Hz, 2H), 3.78 (t, *J* = 4.8 Hz, 2H), 3.74 (t, *J* = 5.6 Hz, 2H), 3.44 (dd, *J* = 4.4, 10.0 Hz, 2H), 2.97–2.90 (m, 1H), 2.79–2.68 (m, 2H), 2.53 (p, 2H), 2.07-2.00 (m, 1H); ^{13}C-NMR (125 MHz, $CDCl_3$) δ 170.52, 169.25, 168.70, 167.80, 167.68, 159.35, 157.61, 155.89, 154.58, 146.79, 146.73, 143.55, 143.07, 135.94, 135.40, 132.46, 131.37, 129.69 (2C), 129.62 (2C), 123.83, 116.74, 116.44 (2C), 115.90 (2C), 111.56, 110.33, 69.92, 69.68, 68.23, 49.54, 47.58, 44.12, 42.39, 35.62, 31.91, 29.98, 22.04; HR-MS (FAB$^+$) calcd for $C_{40}H_{40}ClN_{12}O_6$ [M + H]$^+$ 819.2882, found 819.2887.

*4-((2-(2-(2-(4-(((1-(3-(4-amino-3-(4-chlorophenyl)-1H-pyrazolo[3,4-d]pyrimidin-1-yl)propyl)-1H-1,2,3-triazol-4-yl)methyl)amino)phenoxy)ethoxy)ethoxy)ethyl)amino)-2-(2,6-dioxopiperidin-3-yl)isoindoline-1,3-dione (**21b**, CPR-14)*: 21b was synthesized according to the procedure for 16a. Yellow solid; yield 38.3%; R_f = 0.250 (methanol/dichloromethane = 1:9); mp 164.5–165.9 °C; ^{1}H-NMR (400 MHz, $CDCl_3$) δ 8.35 (s, 1H),

7.69 (s, 1H), 7.61 (d, J = 8.0 Hz, 2H), 7.48 (d, J = 8.4 Hz, 2H), 7.41 (t, J = 7.6 Hz, 1H), 6.99 (d, J = 7.2 Hz, 1H), 6.87 (d, J = 8.8 Hz, 1H), 6.69 (d, J = 8.4 Hz, 2H), 6.57 (d, J = 8.4 Hz, 2H), 6.45 (t, J = 6.0 Hz, 1H), 5.12–5.03 (m, 2H), 4.88 (dd, J = 5.2, 11.6 Hz, 1H), 4.47 (t, J = 6.0 Hz, 2H), 4.36 (t, J = 7.2 Hz, 2H), 4.01 (t, J = 5.2 Hz, 2H), 3.79 (t, J = 5.2 Hz, 2H), 3.71-3.65 (m, 6H), 3.44–3.40 (m, 2H), 2.93–2.87 (m, 1H), 2.75–2.64 (m, 2H), 2.55 (p, 2H), 2.04–1.98 (m, 1H); ^{13}C-NMR (125 MHz, MeOD+$CDCl_3$) 170.75, 169.10, 168.74, 167.77, 155.58, 154.17, 146.67, 146.60, 135.90, 135.39, 135.15, 133.28, 132.35, 132.27, 131.00, 130.89, 129.57 (2C), 129.51 (2C), 128.92, 128.67, 116.72 (2C), 111.40 (2C), 109.99, 109.50, 70.58, 70.52, 69.82, 69.37, 68.01, 47.62, 44.02, 42.09, 35.33, 31.62, 29.80, 29.54, 21.90; HR-MS (FAB$^+$) calcd for $C_{42}H_{44}ClN_{12}O_7$ $[M + H]^+$ 863.3144, found 863.3149.

4.2. *Anticancer Activity*

4.2.1. MTT Assay

MCF7 (human breast cancer) and A549 (human lung cancer) cells were obtained from the Korean Cell Line Bank (KCLB, Seoul, Korea) and incubated in 5% CO_2 at 37 °C. The cells were plated in 96-well culture plates (SPL Life Science Co., Gyeonggi-do, Republic of Korea) for 24 h. For cell viability test, the synthesized PROTACs were treated at the various concentrations from 0 to 80 μM for 3 days. After that, 100 μL of 20 mM MTT (3-(4,5-Dimethylthiazol-2-yl)-2,5-Diphenyltetrazolium Bromide) (Thermo Fisher Scientific, Rockford, IL, USA) (5 mg/mL) dissolved in RPMI-1640 medium was added to the incubated well for 3 h. The supernatant was discarded and 100 μL of DMSO was reacted with viable cells. The product of reaction was measured by absorbance at 570 nm using Mithras2 plate reader (Berthold Technologies, Bad Wildbad, Germany).

4.2.2. Western Blot Assay

The PROTAC-treated MCF7 (human breast cancer) and A549 (human lung cancer) cells were lysed with 1X lysis buffer containing protease inhibitor. Extracted protein lysate (20 μg) were loaded on 12% SDS-polyacrylamide gel electrophoresis and transferred to a polyvinylidene difluoride membrane (ATTO, Tokyo, Japan). The membrane was blocked with 3% Bovine Serum Albumin (BSA) in tris-phosphate buffer containing 0.1% Twin 20, and incubated with primary antibodies for 1 h at room temperature. The following antibodies were IGF1Rβ (1:200, Santa Cruz Biotechnology, Santa Cruz, CA, USA) and Src (1:000, Cell Signaling Technology, Beverly, MA, USA) and GAPDH (1:200, Santa Cruz Biotechnology) as internal control. The signal was reacted with ECL solution (GenDEPOT, Barker, TX, USA) and detected on an Image Quant LAS 4000 biomolecular imager (GE Healthcare, Chicago, IL, USA).

4.2.3. Wound Healing and Invasion Assay

MCF7 (human breast cancer) and A549 (human lung cancer) cells were treated with 1 or 5 μM of PROTAC compounds for 24 h. After 24 h, the treated cells were collected and re-implanted (3×10^5) on 24-well culture plates for 24 h. When cells reached confluence, wound healing assay was performed by scratching with pipette tips. For invasion assay, matrigel (BD Biosciences, San Diego, CA, USA) coated transwell (BD Biosciences, San Diego, CA, USA, 353097, 8 μm pore size) was used to mimic extra cellular matrix in vitro. The PROTAC-treated cells (1×10^5) suspended in RPMI-1640 without FBS were seeded into transwell and each of the insert wells was put in 24-well culture plates containing RPMI-1640 with FBS. After incubation, the membrane of insert transwell was stained with 0.1% crystal violet (Sigma Aldrich, St. Louis, USA). The wound closure or invasive images were analyzed based on bright field microscopy.

4.2.4. Soft Agar Colony Formation Assay

To investigate growth ability on solid surface in vitro, a colony forming assay was performed by using top and bottom agarose method. The base of layer was poured with 1.5 mL of 0.5% agarose

(BD Biosciences, San Diego, CA, USA) containing RPMI-1640 with FBS and solidified. 1 mL of PROTAC-treated cells (3×10^5) resuspended in complete medium with 0.3% agarose (BD Biosciences, San Diego, CA, USA) was covered on the base of layer. The plates were incubated for approximately 2 weeks in 5% CO_2 at 37 °C. Formed colony was counted on bright field microscopy.

5. Conclusions

We developed dual degrader PROTACs to target both IGF-1R and Src, which are associated with various cancer cells. We evaluated the degradation potentials of the synthesized PROTAC compounds by different cellular assays. Interestingly, PROTACs with a dual IGF-1R/Src inhibitor warhead (**C**), which possess a common structure from the reported IGF-1R and Src inhibitors, showed significant degradation potency, whereas previously reported individual modules, with similar sizes for Src or IGF-1R, were not active in PROTACs. Our data support the notion that the binding affinities of warhead ligands are not the sole determinant of PROTAC efficiency. Off-target effects, with promiscuous ligands, may be counteracted with other factors, including the formation of a stable ternary complex with target protein-E3 ligase, as well as efficient ubiquitination. Our dual degrader PROTACs, along with various cell-based assays, indicated that the PROTACs developed in this study serve as valuable tools to understand the mechanism and process of induced degradation of target proteins, which will result in next-generation anticancer therapeutics.

Supplementary Materials: The following are available online: Experimental details, synthesis of intermediates (7a–c, 9, 11a–b, 15, 17 and 19), ^1H and ^{13}C-NMR spectra of the synthesized compounds.

Author Contributions: Conceptualization, J.L.; methodology, S.M. and N.L.; validation, N.L.; formal analysis, S.M. and N.L.; investigation, J.L.; writing—original draft preparation, S.M. and N.L.; writing—review and editing, J.L.; review and editing, D.O.; supervision, J.L.; funding acquisition, J.L. and D.O. All authors have read and agreed to the published version of the manuscript.

Funding: This research was funded by the National Research Foundation of Korea (NRF) grants (NRF-2018R1A2B2005535 and 2018R1A4A1021703) funded by the Korean government (MSIT).

Conflicts of Interest: The authors declare no conflict of interest.

References

1. Salami, J.; Crews, C.M. Waste disposal-An attractive strategy for cancer therapy. *Science* **2017**, *355*, 1163–1167. [CrossRef] [PubMed]
2. Winter, G.E.; Buckley, D.L.; Paulk, J.; Roberts, J.M.; Souza, A.; Dhe-Paganon, S.; Bradner, J.E. Drug Development. Phthalimide conjugation as a strategy for in vivo target protein degradation. *Science* **2015**, *348*, 1376–1381. [CrossRef]
3. Mullard, A. First targeted protein degrader hits the clinic. *Nat. Rev. Drug Discov.* **2019**. [CrossRef] [PubMed]
4. Chamberlain, P.P.; Hamann, L.G. Development of targeted protein degradation therapeutics. *Nat. Chem. Biol.* **2019**, *15*, 937–944. [CrossRef] [PubMed]
5. Toure, M.; Crews, C.M. Small-Molecule PROTACS: New Approaches to Protein Degradation. *Angew. Chem. Int. Ed. Engl.* **2016**, *55*, 1966–1973. [CrossRef] [PubMed]
6. Lai, A.C.; Crews, C.M. Induced protein degradation: An emerging drug discovery paradigm. *Nat. Rev. Drug Discov.* **2017**, *16*, 101–114. [CrossRef] [PubMed]
7. Sakamoto, K.M.; Kim, K.B.; Kumagai, A.; Mercurio, F.; Crews, C.M.; Deshaies, R.J. Protacs: Chimeric molecules that target proteins to the Skp1-Cullin-F box complex for ubiquitination and degradation. *Proc. Natl. Acad. Sci. USA* **2001**, *98*, 8554–8559. [CrossRef]
8. Schneekloth, A.R.; Pucheault, M.; Tae, H.S.; Crews, C.M. Targeted intracellular protein degradation induced by a small molecule: En route to chemical proteomics. *Bioorg. Med. Chem. Lett.* **2008**, *18*, 5904–5908. [CrossRef]
9. Itoh, Y.; Ishikawa, M.; Naito, M.; Hashimoto, Y. Protein knockdown using methyl bestatin-ligand hybrid molecules: Design and synthesis of inducers of ubiquitination-mediated degradation of cellular retinoic acid-binding proteins. *J. Am. Chem. Soc.* **2010**, *132*, 5820–5826. [CrossRef]

10. Zhou, B.; Hu, J.; Xu, F.; Chen, Z.; Bai, L.; Fernandez-Salas, E.; Lin, M.; Liu, L.; Yang, C.Y.; Zhao, Y.; et al. Discovery of a Small-Molecule Degrader of Bromodomain and Extra-Terminal (BET) Proteins with Picomolar Cellular Potencies and Capable of Achieving Tumor Regression. *J. Med. Chem.* **2018**, *61*, 462–481. [CrossRef]
11. Zengerle, M.; Chan, K.H.; Ciulli, A. Selective Small Molecule Induced Degradation of the BET Bromodomain Protein BRD4. *ACS Chem. Biol.* **2015**, *10*, 1770–1777. [CrossRef] [PubMed]
12. Chu, T.T.; Gao, N.; Li, Q.Q.; Chen, P.G.; Yang, X.F.; Chen, Y.X.; Zhao, Y.F.; Li, Y.M. Specific Knockdown of Endogenous Tau Protein by Peptide-Directed Ubiquitin-Proteasome Degradation. *Cell Chem. Biol.* **2016**, *23*, 453–461. [CrossRef] [PubMed]
13. Lazo, J.S.; Sharlow, E.R. Drugging Undruggable Molecular Cancer Targets. *Annu. Rev. Pharm. Toxicol.* **2016**, *56*, 23–40. [CrossRef] [PubMed]
14. Duncan, J.S.; Whittle, M.C.; Nakamura, K.; Abell, A.N.; Midland, A.A.; Zawistowski, J.S.; Johnson, N.L.; Granger, D.A.; Jordan, N.V.; Darr, D.B.; et al. Dynamic reprogramming of the kinome in response to targeted MEK inhibition in triple-negative breast cancer. *Cell* **2012**, *149*, 307–321. [CrossRef]
15. Visakorpi, T.; Hyytinen, E.; Koivisto, P.; Tanner, M.; Keinänen, R.; Palmberg, C.; Palotie, A.; Tammela, T.; Isola, J.; Kallioniemi, O.P. In vivo amplification of the androgen receptor gene and progression of human prostate cancer. *Nat. Genet.* **1995**, *9*, 401–406. [CrossRef]
16. Hon, W.C.; Wilson, M.I.; Harlos, K.; Claridge, T.D.; Schofield, C.J.; Pugh, C.W.; Maxwell, P.H.; Ratcliffe, P.J.; Stuart, D.I.; Jones, E.Y. Structural basis for the recognition of hydroxyproline in HIF-1 alpha by pVHL. *Nature* **2002**, *417*, 975–978. [CrossRef]
17. Schneekloth, J.S., Jr.; Fonseca, F.N.; Koldobskiy, M.; Mandal, A.; Deshaies, R.; Sakamoto, K.; Crews, C.M. Chemical genetic control of protein levels: Selective in vivo targeted degradation. *J. Am. Chem. Soc.* **2004**, *126*, 3748–3754. [CrossRef]
18. Gadd, M.S.; Testa, A.; Lucas, X.; Chan, K.H.; Chen, W.Z.; Lamont, D.J.; Zengerle, M.; Ciulli, A. Structural basis of PROTAC cooperative recognition for selective protein degradation. *Nat. Chem. Biol.* **2017**, *13*, 514. [CrossRef]
19. Ito, T.; Ando, H.; Suzuki, T.; Ogura, T.; Hotta, K.; Imamura, Y.; Yamaguchi, Y.; Handa, H. Identification of a primary target of thalidomide teratogenicity. *Science* **2010**, *327*, 1345–1350. [CrossRef]
20. Raina, K.; Lu, J.; Qian, Y.M.; Altieri, M.; Gordon, D.; Rossi, A.M.K.; Wang, J.; Chen, X.; Dong, H.Q.; Siu, K.; et al. PROTAC-induced BET protein degradation as a therapy for castration-resistant prostate cancer. *Proc. Natl. Acad. Sci. USA* **2016**, *113*, 7124–7129. [CrossRef]
21. Bondeson, D.P.; Mares, A.; Smith, I.E.D.; Ko, E.; Campos, S.; Miah, A.H.; Mulholland, K.E.; Routly, N.; Buckley, D.L.; Gustafson, J.L.; et al. Catalytic in vivo protein knockdown by small-molecule PROTACs. *Nat. Chem. Biol.* **2015**, *11*, 611. [CrossRef] [PubMed]
22. Lai, A.C.; Toure, M.; Hellerschmied, D.; Salami, J.; Jaime-Figueroa, S.; Ko, E.; Hines, J.; Crews, C.M. Modular PROTAC Design for the Degradation of Oncogenic BCR-ABL. *Angew. Chem. Int. Ed. Engl.* **2016**, *55*, 807–810. [CrossRef] [PubMed]
23. Olson, C.M.; Jiang, B.S.; Erb, M.A.; Liang, Y.K.; Doctor, Z.M.; Zhang, Z.N.; Zhang, T.H.; Kwiatkowski, N.; Boukhali, M.; Green, J.L.; et al. Pharmacological perturbation of CDK9 using selective CDK9 inhibition or degradation. *Nat. Chem. Biol.* **2018**, *14*, 163. [CrossRef] [PubMed]
24. Jiang, B.; Wang, E.S.; Donovan, K.A.; Liang, Y.; Fischer, E.S.; Zhang, T.; Gray, N.S. Development of Dual and Selective Degraders of Cyclin-Dependent Kinases 4 and 6. *Angew. Chem. Int. Ed. Engl.* **2019**, *58*, 6321–6326. [CrossRef] [PubMed]
25. Su, S.; Yang, Z.; Gao, H.; Yang, H.; Zhu, S.; An, Z.; Wang, J.; Li, Q.; Chandarlapaty, S.; Deng, H.; et al. Potent and Preferential Degradation of CDK6 via Proteolysis Targeting Chimera Degraders. *J. Med. Chem.* **2019**, *62*, 7575–7582. [CrossRef]
26. Smith, B.E.; Wang, S.L.; Jaime-Figueroa, S.; Harbin, A.; Wang, J.; Hamman, B.D.; Crews, C.M. Differential PROTAC substrate specificity dictated by orientation of recruited E3 ligase. *Nat. Commun.* **2019**, *10*, 131. [CrossRef]
27. Bondeson, D.P.; Smith, B.E.; Burslem, G.M.; Buhimschi, A.D.; Hines, J.; Jaime-Figueroa, S.; Wang, J.; Hamman, B.D.; Ishchenko, A.; Crews, C.M. Lessons in PROTAC Design from Selective Degradation with a Promiscuous Warhead. *Cell Chem. Biol.* **2018**, *25*, 78–87. [CrossRef]
28. Li, R.; Pourpak, A.; Morris, S.W. Inhibition of the Insulin-like Growth Factor-1 Receptor (IGF1R) Tyrosine Kinase as a Novel Cancer Therapy Approach. *J. Med. Chem.* **2009**, *52*, 4981–5004. [CrossRef]

29. Wu, J.; Li, W.; Craddock, B.P.; Foreman, K.W.; Mulvihill, M.J.; Ji, Q.S.; Miller, W.T.; Hubbard, S.R. Small-molecule inhibition and activation-loop trans-phosphorylation of the IGF1 receptor. *EMBO J.* **2008**, *27*, 1985–1994. [CrossRef]
30. Pollak, M.N.; Schernhammer, E.S.; Hankinson, S.E. Insulin-like growth factors and neoplasia. *Nat. Rev. Cancer* **2004**, *4*, 505–518. [CrossRef]
31. Min, H.Y.; Yun, H.J.; Lee, J.S.; Lee, H.J.; Cho, J.; Jang, H.J.; Park, S.H.; Liu, D.; Oh, S.H.; Lee, J.J.; et al. Targeting the insulin-like growth factor receptor and Src signaling network for the treatment of non-small cell lung cancer. *Mol. Cancer* **2015**, *14*, 113. [CrossRef] [PubMed]
32. Dziadziuszko, R.; Camidge, D.R.; Hirsch, F.R. The insulin-like growth factor pathway in lung cancer. *J. Thorac. Oncol. Off. Publ. Int. Assoc. Study Lung Cancer* **2008**, *3*, 815–818. [CrossRef] [PubMed]
33. Yeatman, T.J. A renaissance for SRC. *Nat. Rev. Cancer* **2004**, *4*, 470–480. [CrossRef]
34. Dayyani, F.; Parikh, N.U.; Varkaris, A.S.; Song, J.H.; Moorthy, S.; Chatterji, T.; Maity, S.N.; Wolfe, A.R.; Carboni, J.M.; Gottardis, M.M.; et al. Combined Inhibition of IGF-1R/IR and Src family kinases enhances antitumor effects in prostate cancer by decreasing activated survival pathways. *PLoS ONE* **2012**, *7*, e51189. [CrossRef] [PubMed]
35. Shin, D.H.; Lee, H.J.; Min, H.Y.; Choi, S.P.; Lee, M.S.; Lee, J.W.; Johnson, F.M.; Mehta, K.; Lippman, S.M.; Glisson, B.S.; et al. Combating resistance to anti-IGFR antibody by targeting the integrin beta3-Src pathway. *J. Natl. Cancer Inst.* **2013**, *105*, 1558–1570. [CrossRef]
36. Lee, H.J.; Pham, P.C.; Hyun, S.Y.; Baek, B.; Kim, B.; Kim, Y.; Min, H.Y.; Lee, J.; Lee, H.Y. Development of a 4-aminopyrazolo[3,4-d]pyrimidine-based dual IGF1R/Src inhibitor as a novel anticancer agent with minimal toxicity. *Mol. Cancer* **2018**, *17*, 50. [CrossRef]
37. Kwarcinski, F.E.; Steffey, M.E.; Fox, C.C.; Soellner, M.B. Discovery of Bivalent Kinase Inhibitors via Enzyme-Templated Fragment Elaboration. *ACS Med. Chem. Lett.* **2015**, *6*, 898–901. [CrossRef]
38. Kwarcinski, F.E.; Fox, C.C.; Steffey, M.E.; Soellner, M.B. Irreversible inhibitors of c-Src kinase that target a nonconserved cysteine. *ACS Chem. Biol.* **2012**, *7*, 1910–1917. [CrossRef]
39. Tandon, R.; Senthil, V.; Nithya, D.; Pamidiboina, V.; Kumar, A.; Malik, S.; Chaira, T.; Diwan, M.; Gupta, P.; Venkataramanan, R.; et al. RBx10080307, a dual EGFR/IGF-1R inhibitor for anticancer therapy. *Eur. J. Pharmacol.* **2013**, *711*, 19–26. [CrossRef]
40. Tandon, R.; Kapoor, S.; Vali, S.; Senthil, V.; Nithya, D.; Venkataramanan, R.; Sharma, A.; Talwadkar, A.; Ray, A.; Bhatnagar, P.K.; et al. Dual epidermal growth factor receptor (EGFR)/insulin-like growth factor-1 receptor (IGF-1R) inhibitor: A novel approach for overcoming resistance in anticancer treatment. *Eur. J. Pharmacol.* **2011**, *667*, 56–65. [CrossRef]
41. Buchanan, J.L.; Newcomb, J.R.; Carney, D.P.; Chaffee, S.C.; Chai, L.; Cupples, R.; Epstein, L.F.; Gallant, P.; Gu, Y.; Harmange, J.C.; et al. Discovery of 2,4-bis-arylamino-1,3-pyrimidines as insulin-like growth factor-1 receptor (IGF-1R) inhibitors. *Bioorg. Med. Chem. Lett.* **2011**, *21*, 2394–2399. [CrossRef] [PubMed]
42. Schenone, S.; Radi, M.; Musumeci, F.; Brullo, C.; Botta, M. Biologically driven synthesis of pyrazolo[3,4-d]pyrimidines as protein kinase inhibitors: An old scaffold as a new tool for medicinal chemistry and chemical biology studies. *Chem. Rev.* **2014**, *114*, 7189–7238. [CrossRef] [PubMed]
43. Kumar, A.; Ahmad, I.; Chhikara, B.S.; Tiwari, R.; Mandal, D.; Parang, K. Synthesis of 3-phenylpyrazolopyrimidine-1,2,3-triazole conjugates and evaluation of their Src kinase inhibitory and anticancer activities. *Bioorg. Med. Chem. Lett.* **2011**, *21*, 1342–1346. [CrossRef] [PubMed]
44. Abellan-Flos, M.; Tanc, M.; Supuran, C.T.; Vincent, S.P. Exploring carbonic anhydrase inhibition with multimeric coumarins displayed on a fullerene scaffold. *Org. Biomol. Chem.* **2015**, *13*, 7445–7451. [CrossRef]
45. Song, Z.; Jin, Y.; Ge, Y.; Wang, C.; Zhang, J.; Tang, Z.; Peng, J.; Liu, K.; Li, Y.; Ma, X. Synthesis and biological evaluation of azole-diphenylpyrimidine derivatives (AzDPPYs) as potent T790M mutant form of epidermal growth factor receptor inhibitors. *Bioorg. Med. Chem.* **2016**, *24*, 5505–5512. [CrossRef]
46. Lu, J.; Qian, Y.; Altieri, M.; Dong, H.; Wang, J.; Raina, K.; Hines, J.; Winkler, J.D.; Crew, A.P.; Coleman, K.; et al. Hijacking the E3 Ubiquitin Ligase Cereblon to Efficiently Target BRD4. *Chem. Biol.* **2015**, *22*, 755–763. [CrossRef]
47. Degorce, S.L.; Boyd, S.; Curwen, J.O.; Ducray, R.; Halsall, C.T.; Jones, C.D.; Lach, F.; Lenz, E.M.; Pass, M.; Pass, S.; et al. Discovery of a Potent, Selective, Orally Bioavailable, and Efficacious Novel 2-(Pyrazol-4-ylamino)-pyrimidine Inhibitor of the Insulin-like Growth Factor-1 Receptor (IGF-1R). *J. Med. Chem.* **2016**, *59*, 4859–4866. [CrossRef]

48. Wang, Z.; Liu, G.; Mao, J.; Xie, M.; Zhao, M.; Guo, X.; Liang, S.; Li, H.; Li, X.; Wang, R. IGF-1R Inhibition Suppresses Cell Proliferation and Increases Radiosensitivity in Nasopharyngeal Carcinoma Cells. *Mediat. Inflamm.* **2019**, 5497467. [CrossRef]
49. Cox, O.T.; O'Shea, S.; Tresse, E.; Bustamante-Garrido, M.; Kiran-Deevi, R.; O'Connor, R. IGF-1 Receptor and Adhesion Signaling: An Important Axis in Determining Cancer Cell Phenotype and Therapy Resistance. *Front. Endocrinol.* **2015**, *6*, 106. [CrossRef]
50. Kumar, A.; Wang, Y.; Lin, X.; Sun, G.; Parang, K. Synthesis and evaluation of 3-phenylpyrazolo[3,4-d]pyrimidine-peptide conjugates as Src kinase inhibitors. *ChemMedChem* **2007**, *2*, 1346–1360. [CrossRef]

Sample Availability: Samples of the compounds are not available from the authors.

molecules

MDPI

Article

Phenylpyrazalopyrimidines as Tyrosine Kinase Inhibitors: Synthesis, Antiproliferative Activity, and Molecular Simulations

Bhupender S. Chhikara [1,2], Sajda Ashraf [3], Saghar Mozaffari [4], Nicole St. Jeans [2], Dindyal Mandal [2,4], Rakesh Kumar Tiwari [2,4], Zaheer Ul-Haq [3,*] and Keykavous Parang [2,4,*]

1. Department of Chemistry, Aditi Mahavidyalaya, University of Delhi, Bawana, Delhi 110039, India; bschhikara@gmail.com
2. Department of Biomedical and Pharmaceutical Sciences, College of Pharmacy, University of Rhode Island, Rhode Island, Kingston, RI 02881, USA; nicolestjean@ymail.com (N.S.J.); mandal@chapman.edu (D.M.); tiwari@chapman.edu (R.K.T.)
3. Dr. Panjwani Center for Molecular Medicine and Drug Research, ICCBS, University of Karachi, Karachi 75210, Pakistan; sajda.ashraf@yahoo.com
4. Center For Targeted Drug Delivery, Department of Biomedical and Pharmaceutical Sciences, Chapman University School of Pharmacy, Harry and Diane Rinker Health Science Campus, California, Irvine, CA 92618, USA; mozaf100@mail.chapman.edu

* Correspondence: zaheer.qasmi@iccs.edu (Z.U.-H.); parang@chapman.edu (K.P.); Tel.: +92-321-9255-322 (Z.U.-H.); +1-714-516-5489 (K.P.); Fax: +92-21-99261713 (Z.U.-H.); +1-714-516-5481 (K.P.)

Academic Editor: Qiao-Hong Chen
Received: 15 April 2020; Accepted: 29 April 2020; Published: 2 May 2020

Abstract: *N*1-(α,β-Alkene)-substituted phenylpyrazolopyrimidine derivatives with acetyl and functionalized phenyl groups at α- and β-positions, respectively, were synthesized by the reaction of 3-phenylpyrazolopyrimidine (PhPP) with bromoacetone, followed by a chalcone reaction with differently substituted aromatic aldehydes. The Src kinase enzyme assay revealed modest inhibitory activity (half maximal inhibitory concentration, IC_{50} = 21.7–192.1 μM) by a number of PhPP derivatives. Antiproliferative activity of the compounds was evaluated on human leukemia (CCRF-CEM), human ovarian adenocarcinoma (SK-OV-3), breast carcinoma (MDA-MB-231), and colon adenocarcinoma (HT-29) cells in vitro. 4-Chlorophenyl carbo-enyl substituted 3-phenylpyrazolopyrimidine (**10**) inhibited the cell proliferation of HT-29 and SK-OV-3 by 90% and 79%, respectively, at a concentration of 50 μM after 96 h incubation. The compound showed modest inhibitory activity against c-Src (IC_{50} = 60.4 μM), Btk (IC_{50} = 90.5 μM), and Lck (IC_{50} = 110 μM), while it showed no activity against Abl1, Akt1, Alk, Braf, Cdk2, and PKCa. In combination with target selection and kinase profiling assay, extensive theoretical studies were carried out to explore the selectivity behavior of compound **10**. Specific interactions were also explored by examining the changing trends of interactions of tyrosine kinases with the phenylpyrazolopyrimidine derivative. The results showed good agreement with the experimental selectivity pattern among c-Src, Btk, and Lck.

Keywords: protein kinase; phenylpyrazolopyrimidine; antiproliferative activity; enzyme inhibition; molecular simulation

1. Introduction

Cancer cells show the overexpression of different protein tyrosine kinases (PTKs). These enzymes catalyze the phosphorylation of many protein substrates by the transfer of the γ-phosphate group from ATP to specific tyrosine residues. PTKs have critical roles in signal transduction pathways.

Src family kinases (SFKs) have nine different PTKs, including c-Src, c-Yes, Fyn, Lck, Lyn, Hck, Frk, Blk, and c-Fgr of which Src is the prototype [1]. SFKs have essential roles in the regulation of a wide variety of normal cellular signal transduction pathways, such as cell division, differentiation, growth factor signaling, survival, adhesion, migration, and invasion [2]. Src tyrosine kinase expression is frequently elevated in several tumors, including breast, colon, prostate, lung, ovary, and pancreas, when it is compared with the adjacent healthy tissues. Src kinase was shown to be the critical modulator of cancer cell metastasis and invasion [3].

In recent years, a number of small cell-permeable inhibitors of protein kinases were investigated for the treatment of different cancers [4]. Different small molecules that were actively investigated as kinase inhibitor include quinazolines [5], quinolinecarbonitriles [6], pyrazolopyrimidines [7,8], imidazo [1,5-a]pyrazines [9], Calixarene [10], benzotriazines [11,12], indoles [13], and ATP- phosphopeptide conjugates [14]. The research effort led to the generation of small molecules for the treatment of different malignancies. Imatinib, a 2-phenylaminopyrimidine, was approved for the treatment of chronic myelogenous leukemia (CML) and gastrointestinal stromal tumors (GISTs) [15]. Dasatinib (BMS-354825), a pyrimidinylthiazole derivative, was approved to use in patients with CML after imatinib treatment [16], and bosutinib (SKI-606), a 3-quinolinecarbonitrile analogue, is known to suppress migration and invasion of human breast cancer cells [17]. Ibrutinib (Figure 1) is a pyrazolopyrimidine-based [18] small-molecule kinase inhibitor that was approved for the treatment of B-cell cancers like mantle cell lymphoma, chronic lymphocytic leukemia, and Waldenström's macroglobulinemia [19,20].

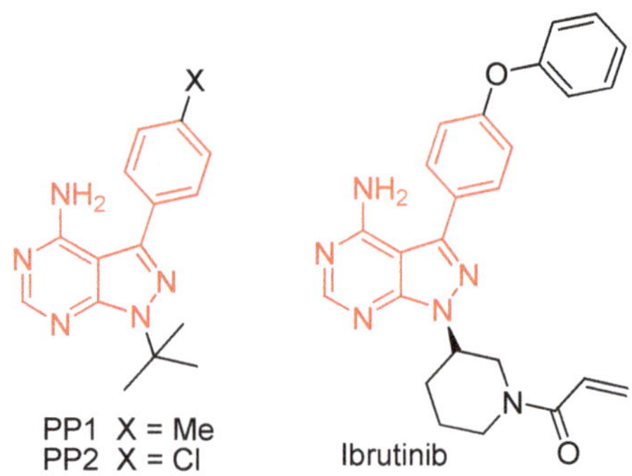

Figure 1. Chemical structures of 3-phenylpyrazolopyrimidine (PhPP) derivatives (PP1 and PP2) and Ibrutinib.

A number of crystallographic studies showed that adenosine 5′-(β,γ-imido)triphosphate (AMP-PNP), an ATP mimic, binds to the ATP-binding site of c-Src (Protein Data Bank (PDB) 2SRC) [21]. Furthermore, complexes of 3-phenylpyrazolopyrimidine (PhPP) derivatives (PP1 and PP2) (Figure 1) act as ATP-binding site inhibitors of Hck (PDB 1QCF) and Lck (PDB 1QPE) [22]. Indeed, the pyrazolopyrimidine core of PP1 and PP2 (Figure 1) mimics the adenine base of ATP in binding to the nucleotide-binding site. In another study [8], we showed that the 3-phenyl group interacts with a large hydrophobic pocket in the ATP-binding site, contributing significantly to Src kinase inhibitory activity. There is also another cavity formed from side chains of helix αC and helix αD that is normally occupied by a carbohydrate moiety followed by a triphosphate group of ATP. This cavity is mostly unfilled by the tert-butyl of 3-phenylpyrazolopyrimidines (PP1 and PP2). Furthermore, we investigated the variation of *N*1 substitution in 3-phenylpyrazolopyrimidines with different 1,2,3-triazoles containing hydrophobic residues to interact with amino acids of this cavity and contribute to the enhancement of Src kinase inhibitory potency [8]. The cysteine residue present in the cavity could be a potential target to bind with PhPP molecules irreversibly, leading to a potential increase in kinase inhibition.

Here, we describe the synthesis and evaluation of kinase inhibitory activity of *N*1-substituted PhPP with α-acetyl-β-phenyl-alkene groups (Figure 2). We hypothesized that this substitution at the *N*1 position of PhPP could contribute significantly to the kinase inhibition through generating specific interactions. We further extended our study to investigate the selectivity profile of one of the active compounds (**10**) with a panel of nine different kinases by applying MD and MMGBSA calculations. This study helped to reveal the inhibitory mechanism of PhPP derivatives based on their distinct structural characteristics required for its interaction with a specific kinase.

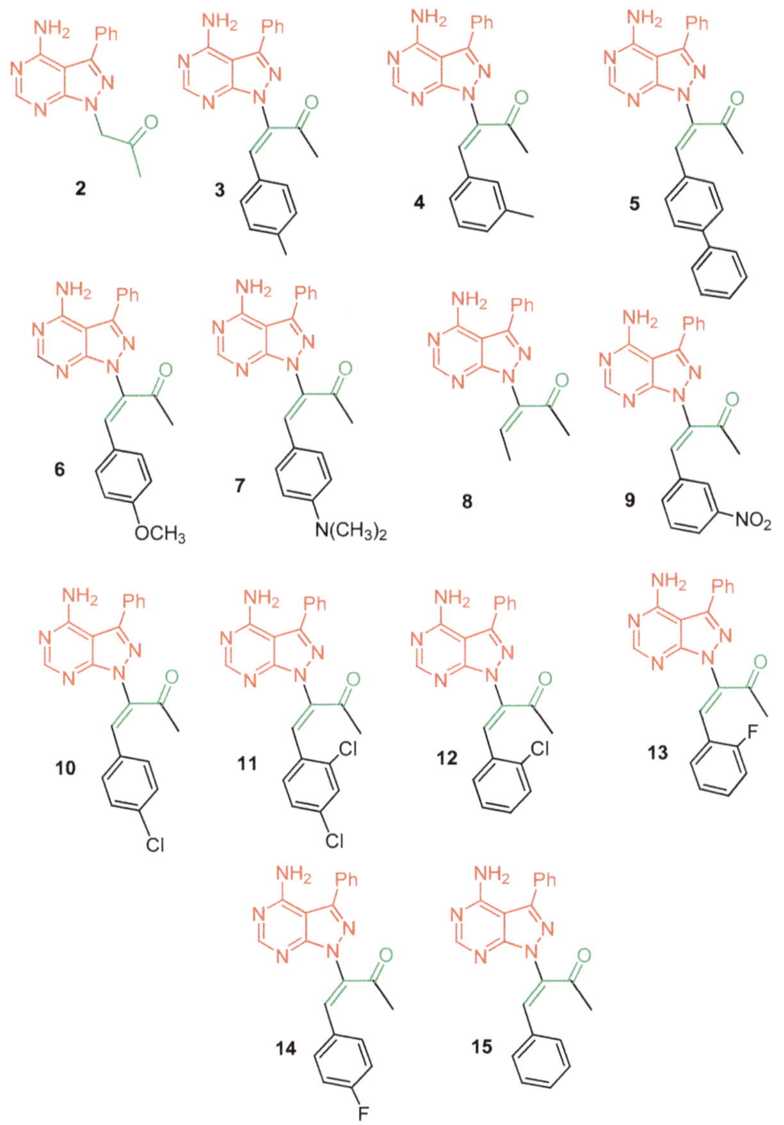

Figure 2. Chemical structures of *N*1-substituted PhPP with α-acetyl-β-phenyl-alkene groups (*E* and *Z* isomers).

2. Results and Discussion

2.1. Chemical Synthesis

The products were synthesized by following the chemical pathway shown in Scheme 1. The PhPP (**1**) was synthesized according to a reported procedure [23]. The N1 of **1** was substituted with bromoacetone in the presence of potassium carbonate as a base. Product **2** was confirmed by NMR, which showed the disappearance of the proton peak of NH at 8.07 ppm of **1** and appearance of the peak at 5.24 ppm and 2.21 ppm for CH_2 and CH_3, respectively, in ^1H NMR. Furthermore, ^{13}C NMR showed peaks at 201.34 ppm, 56.15 ppm, and 27.14 ppm representing the carbonyl group, CH_2, and CH_3, respectively, in product **2**.

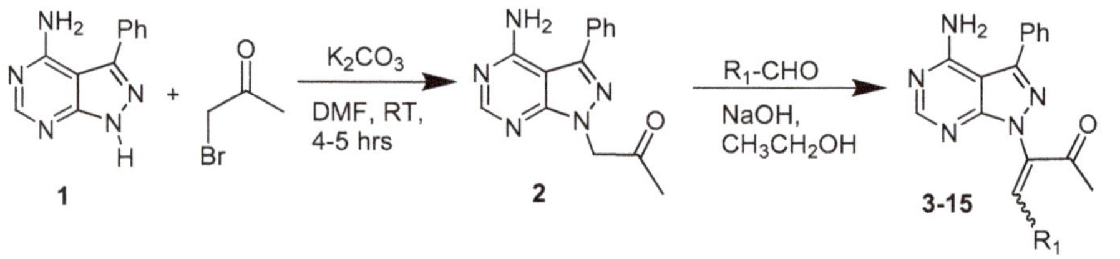

R₁	
3 *p*-(CH_3)Ph-	**10** *p*-(Cl)Ph-
4 *m*-(CH_3)Ph-	**11** 2,4-diCl-Ph-
5 4-(Ph)-Ph-	**12** *o*-(Cl)Ph
6 4- (OCH_3)Ph-	**13** *o*-(F)Ph-
7 *p*-($N(CH_3)_2$Ph-	**14** p-(F)Ph-
8 -CH_3	**15** Ph-
9 *m*-(NO_2)Ph-	

Scheme 1. Chemical synthesis of PhPP derivatives.

Next, the double bond group was introduced by the chalcone reaction. The anion of **2** generated by sodium hydroxide was reacted with different benzaldehydes at room temperature to give product **3**. The ratio of starting material and amount of solvent defined the formation of product and side products. A higher concentration (i.e., less amount of solvent ethanol) and the presence of higher equivalents of **2** than the aldehyde lead to a second internal Michael reaction where the anion of **2** reacts with product **3**, leading to the formation of side product as indicated by Electrospray Ionization Mass Spectrometry (ESI-MS) at 659 Da (data not shown). In an optimum condition, the aldehyde and reactant **2** should be present in more than 1.4:1 equivalent, and solvent ethanol should be present in approximately 20 mL for 26 mg (0.1 mmol) of **2**. Out of two possible products after the conjugation of **2** with 4-methylbenzaldehyde, only product **3** was observed, suggesting the reaction of the carbanion of methylene (CH_2) group between the carbonyl and nitrogen rather than that of methyl (CH_3). The formation of product **3** was confirmed by ESI-MS by the presence of a mass peak at 370 Da $[M + H]^+$. This was confirmed by ^1H NMR, which showed the absence of a peak at 5.24 ppm for CH_2 of **2**, while the three protons for CH_3 were present at 2.31 ppm. Correspondingly, in ^{13}C NMR, the peak at 56.15 ppm (assigned to CH_2) was absent in **3** while the peak at 26.13 ppm (assigned to CH_3 with slight upfield shift) was present. Furthermore, out of EZ possible isomers for the double bond, both the isomers were present as indicated by NOE NMR spectra, possibly by rotation introduced due to keto-enol tautomerism.

In the case of product **8**, the chalcone reaction was carried with precaution to avoid the formation of side products due to the presence of α-hydrogen in acetaldehyde. The anion of **2** was generated first with 1.1 equivalent of sodium hydroxide over extended time and added to the solution of acetaldehyde (1.2 equivalents). The reaction was quenched with acetic acid after 30 min. The product was confirmed by ESI-MS and NMR. The products were purified by HPLC and showed a purity of 95–99%.

2.2. *Src-Kinase Assay*

In vitro Src kinase assay for some of the compounds was conducted, as presented in Table 1. As results indicated, the compounds were moderately active against the Src kinase. Among all the tested compounds, compounds **6** and **4** were found to be the most potent with IC_{50} values of 21.7 and 24.7 μM, respectively. Compounds **3** and **7** exhibited IC_{50} values of 32.9 μM and 36.8, respectively. Compound **5** showed the lowest activity with an IC_{50} of 192.1 μM. Since the compounds showed only moderate Src kinase inhibitory activity, they were evaluated for antiproliferative activity first to find the lead compound for further kinase inhibitory assays.

Table 1. In vitro Src kinase inhibition assay for the selected compounds.

Compound No.	IC_{50} (μM) [a]
3	32.9
4	24.7
5	192.1
6	21.7
7	36.9
Staurosporine	0.6
PP2	0.5

[a] All experiments were repeated in triplicate. All the standard deviations were in the range of 6–13%.

2.3. *Antiproliferative Activities*

The effect of compounds on the cell proliferation of cancer cells was evaluated in vitro in a human leukemia cell line (CCRF-CEM) according to the previously reported procedures [24,25], breast adenocarcinoma (MDA-MB-231), ovarian adenocarcinoma (SK-OV-3), and colon adenocarcinoma (HT-29) cell lines up to 72 h. Doxorubicin (Dox) was used as a positive control as shown previously [26–29]. These cell lines were selected to determine the antiproliferative activity against diverse cancer cells. Compounds **10** and **11** consistently inhibited the cell proliferation 72–96 h in all cell lines. The percentage of cell proliferation was significantly reduced in HT-29 cells in the presence of **10** and **11** when compared with Dox and other compounds. Compound **10** was more effective in the order of HT-29 (90%) > CCRF-CEM, SK-OV-3 (79%) > MDA-MB-231 (60%), while Dox showed HT-29 (75%) > CCRF-CEM, SK-OV-3 (73%) > MDM-MB-231 (64%) after 96 h. Compounds **2**, **7**, **9**, and **12** were found to be inactive in reducing the cell proliferation in all the cell lines after 24–96 h while other compounds **3** and **13–15** exhibited comparable or slightly less antiproliferative activity (Figure 3A–D) than compounds **10** and **11** after 96 h. These data indicate that the presence of the chlorine group at the para position in compounds **10** and **11** were effective in improving the antiproliferative activities. However, the absence of phenyl and/or double bonds in compounds **2** and **8** significantly reduced the antiproliferative activities versus **10** and **11**. The presence of *p*-dimethylamino, *m*-nitro, and *o*-chlorine in **7**, **9**, and **12** were not productive while *o*-fluorine (**13**), *p*-fluorine (**14**), unsubstituted phenyl (**15**), and *p*-Cl (**10** and **11**) enhanced the antiproliferative activity. Compounds **5** and **6** with *p*-ph and *p*-methoxy exhibited antiproliferative activity against some of the cell lines, with **5** being more active in HT-29 and **6** in CCRF-CEM and SK-OV3 cells. However, their activity was generally less than compounds **3**, **10**, **11**, **13**, and **14**. Compounds **10** and **11** exhibited IC_{50} values of 25.5 μM and 34.3 μM, respectively, after 72 h incubation against SK-OV-3 cells (Figure 4).

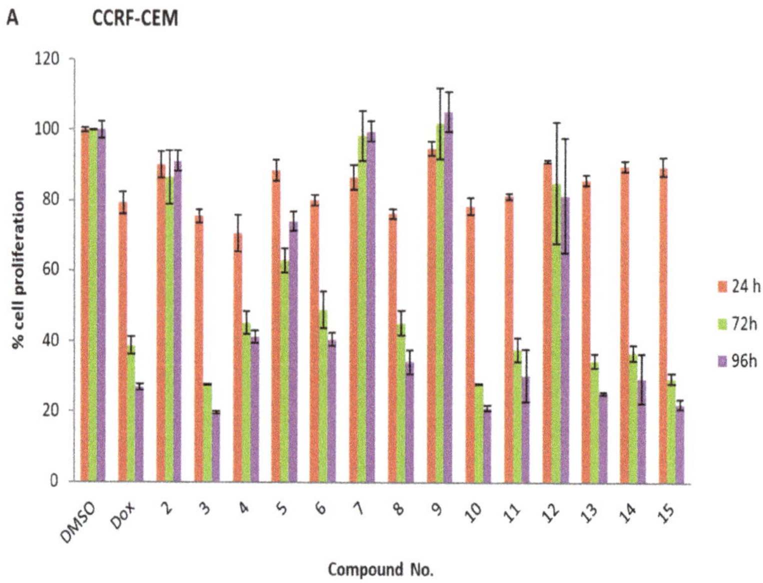

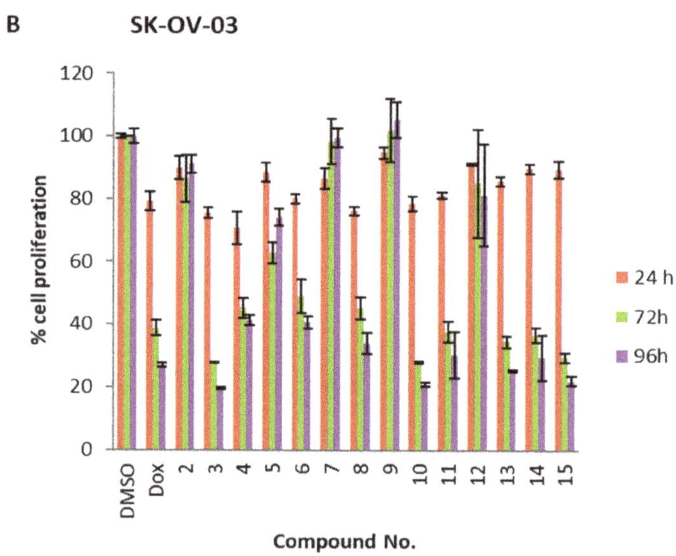

Figure 3. *Cont.*

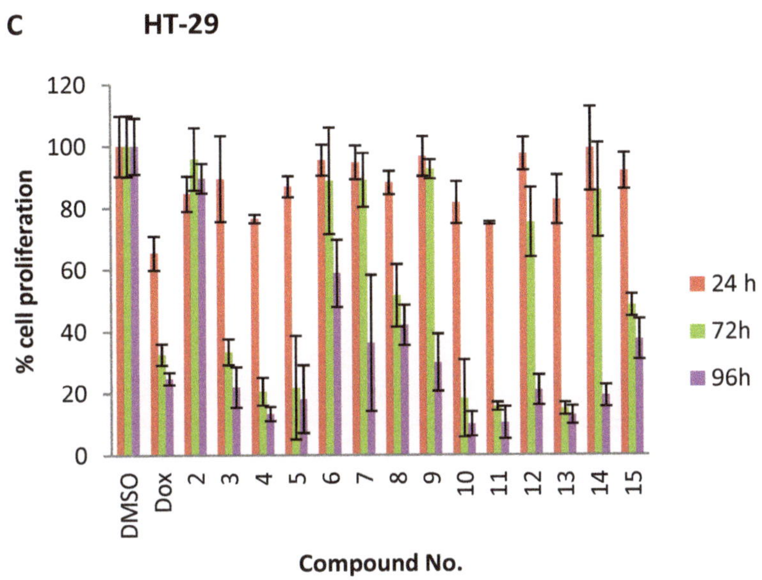

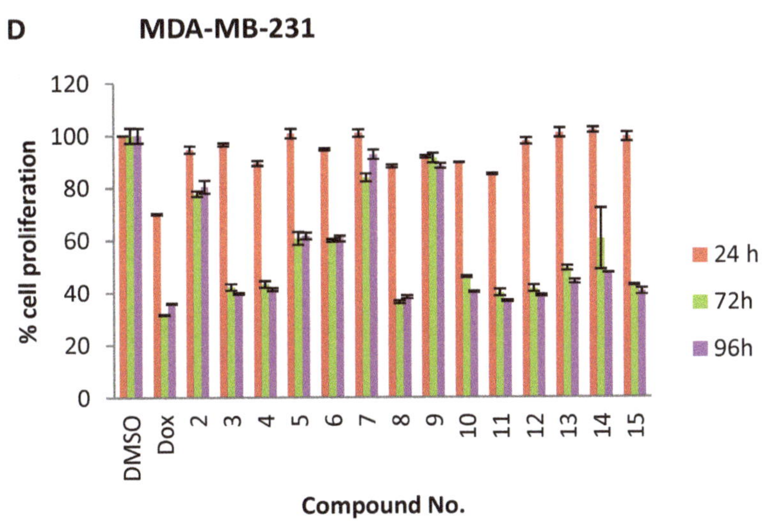

Figure 3. Antiproliferative activity of PhPP derivatives (50 μM) and doxorubicin (Dox) (1 μM) against CCRF-CEM (**A**), SK-OV-3 (**B**), HT-29 (**C**), and MDA-MB-231 (**D**) cell lines. All experiments were repeated in triplicate.

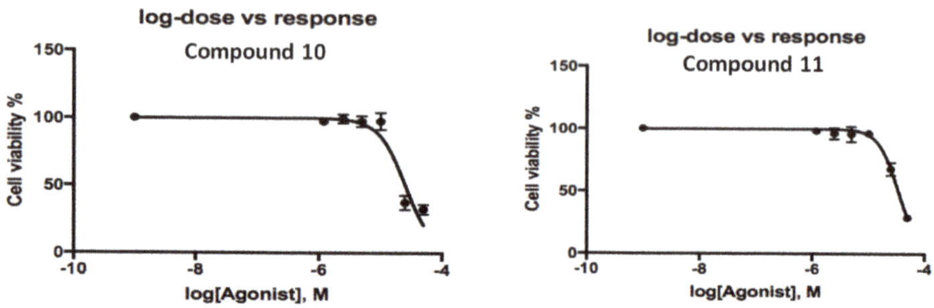

Figure 4. Dose-response curves of **10** (**left**) and **11** (**right**) after 72 h incubation against SK-OV-3 cells.

Compound **10** was selected for further evaluation against a panel of kinases to determine the mechanism of activity. The results are shown in Table 2 against Abl1, Akt1, Alk, Braf, Btk, Cdk2, cSrc, Lck, and PKCa enzymes. The data indicate modest activity against Btk, c-Src, and Lck while the compound was inactive or showed very low inhibition activity against other kinases.

Table 2. The activity of compound **10** against a panel of protein kinases.

Kinase	Compound 10 IC_{50} (μM)	Control Compound IC_{50} (μM)
Abl1	NA [a]	0.85 [b]
Akt1	>150	0.012 [b]
Alk	NA	0.01 [b]
Braf	NA	0.018 [c]
Btk	95.4	0.067 [b]
Cdk2/Cyclin A1	NA	0.0039 [b]
c-Src	64.1	0.0085 [b]
Lck	110	0.011 [b]
PKCa	NA	0.0016 [b]

[a] Not active (NA) indicates no inhibition or compound activity that could not be fit to an IC_{50} curve; [b] Staurosporine; [c] GW5074.

2.4. Molecular Modeling

To rationalize the activity of compound **10**, KEGG pathway and molecular dynamics simulation studies were utilized to explore the specific behavior of the *Z* configuration compound **10** against multiple kinases.

2.4.1. Target Identification

Conventional identification of drug targets is an expensive, time-consuming, and difficult process; only a few drug targets can be identified. In contrast, the computational method permits a great deal of analysis within a short period and brings a large number of potential drug targets from a pool of information [30]. In the present study, an integrated in silico approach was used to identify potential targets [31] for the active compound **10**. Initially, the disease search tool in the KEGG database was used against breast, ovarian, and colorectal cancer to extract the targets that may be involved in these diseases (Figures 5–7) [32]. KEGG uses the knowledge of gene function and linking this information with advanced order functional information by using systematic analysis. The schematic presentation of the KEGG pathway shows genes marked as light-blue color as a drug target and genes marked as pink as associated with the disease, whereas when the gene is linked with both a disease and a drug target, its color is split into light blue and pink. There were several target proteins involved in one pathway; therefore, protein-drug association servers Similarity Ensemble Approach (SEA, http://sea.bkslab.org/) [33], Search Tool for the Retrieval of Interacting Genes (STRING, http://string-db.org) [34], and Search Tool for Interacting Chemicals (STITCH, http://stitch.embl.de/) [35] were used. The STRING database was used to explain the molecular function, biological processes, cellular components, and pathways of the target proteins. The SEA relates target proteins based on set-wise chemical similarity among their compounds. A total of 14 potential targets (Btk, Itk, c-Src, EGFR, Akt1, Fyn, Lyn, Lck, PKC, Abl1, Hck, Cdk2, Braf, and Her2) were selected based on the data obtained from these servers that further proved the reliability of text mining and molecular docking.

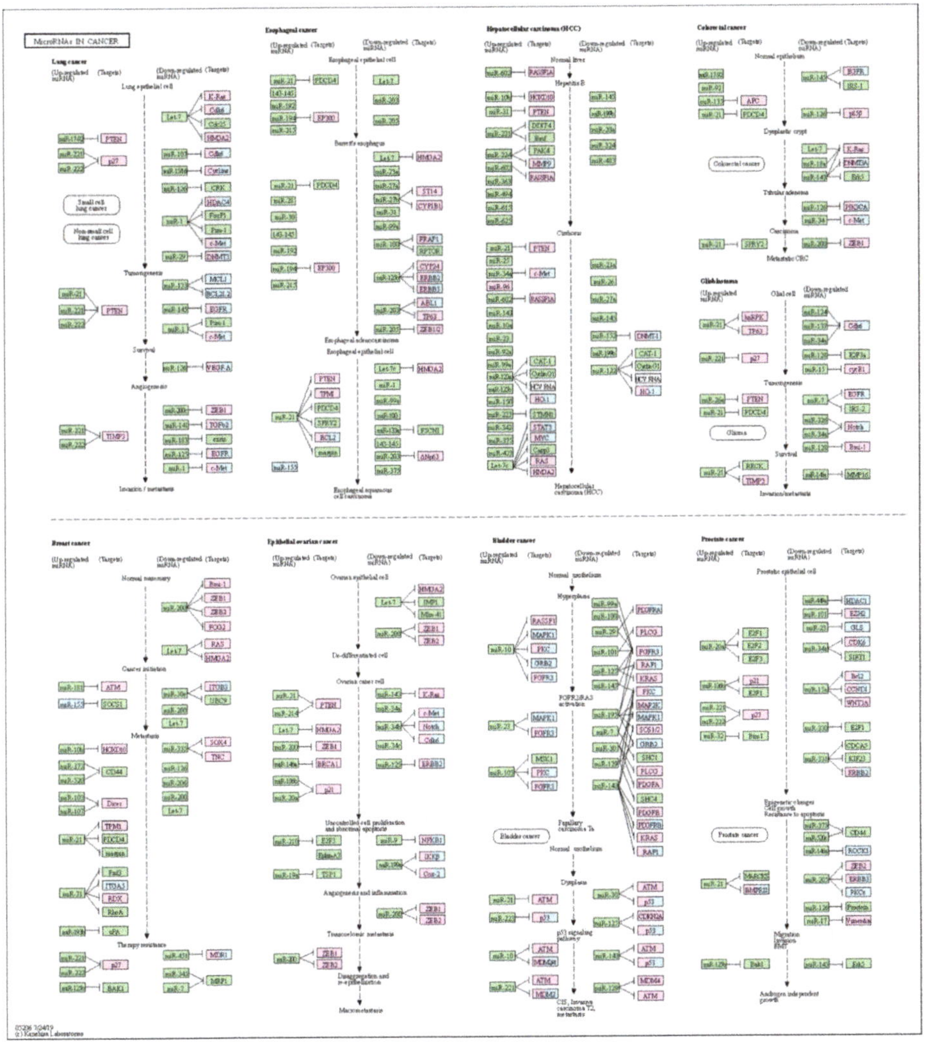

Figure 5. The KEGG pathway for ovarian cancer.

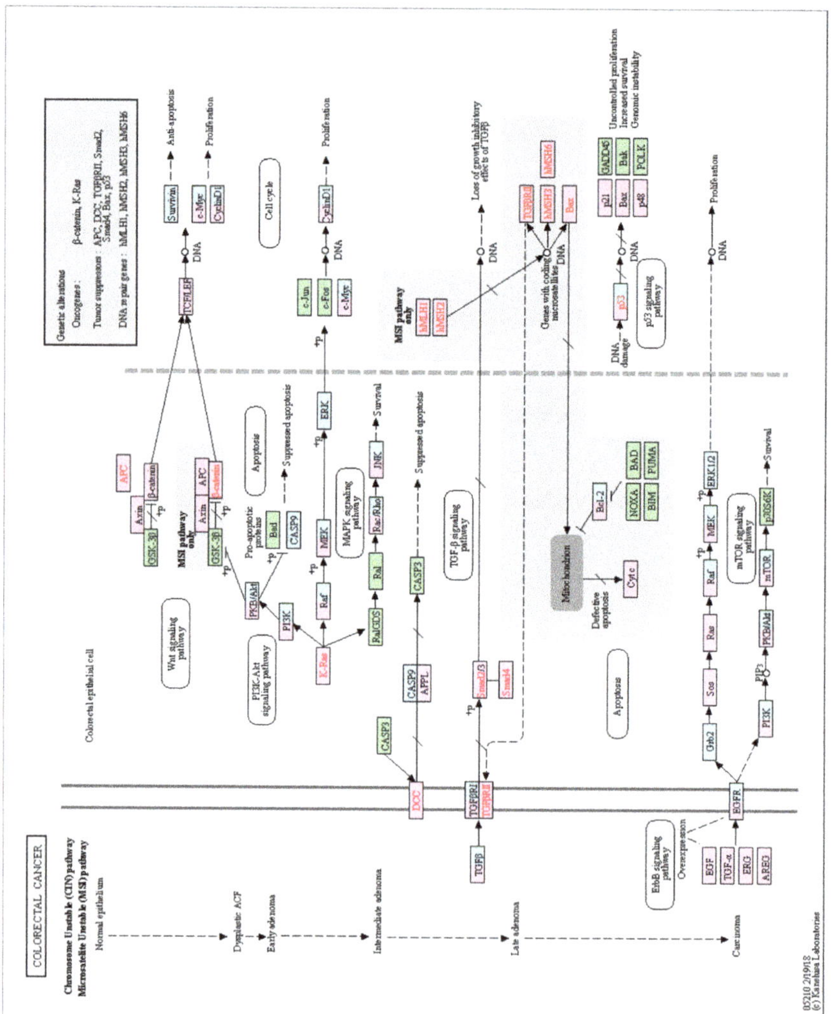

Figure 6. The KEGG pathway for colorectal cancer.

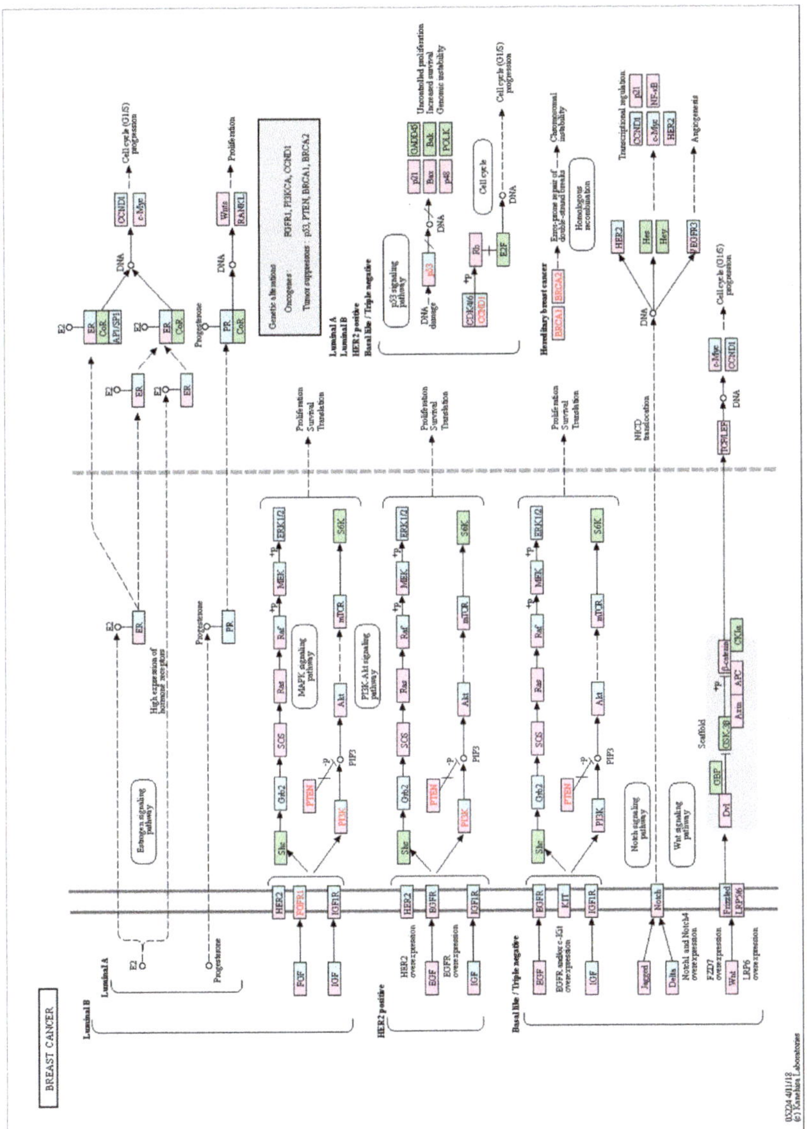

Figure 7. The KEGG pathway for breast cancer.

2.4.2. Docking Studies

The known compounds that were already reported as inhibitors of the target proteins, as well as nature and crucial active site residues, were specified in their accessible complexes, used as a positive control. Prior to docking, validation of the software and docking conditions was performed by retrieving the control compounds from their crystal complexes and then redocking by MOE against their relevant targets. The redocking results are presented in Table 3. After validation, docking of compound **10** was performed with all 14 targets, and their docking scores were compared with the control in order to select a target with the highest docking score. We observed that compound **10** presented good scores against Btk, Itk, c-Src, EGFR, Akt1, Fyn, Lyn, Lck, PKC, and Abl1 kinase as compared to Hck, Cdk2, Braf, and Her2. The docking scores of compound **10** are presented in Table 4.

Table 3. Predicted binding affinity (docking scores in kcal/mol) and root-mean-square deviation (RMSD) of control inhibitors against related proteins.

Target Proteins	Docking Score of Comp. 10	RMSD (Å)
c-Src	−8.3240	1.5
Btk	−7.6201	0.75
Itk	−8.1748	1.4
EGFR	−7.7890	1.56
Fyn	−7.5002	1.32
Lyn	−5.9252	1.23
Hck	−5.1107	0.9
Her2	−8.7522	0.54
Lck	−7.7834	0.45
PKC	−6.4224	0.82
Braf	−6.8762	1.52
Abl1	−6.7421	0.85
Akt1	−7.8654	0.74
Cdk2	−5.2409	0.95

Table 4. MM/PBSA derived binding free energies of complexes computed from the MD simulations.

	c-Src	PKC	Akt	Alk	Btk	CDK2	Lck	Abl1	Braf
VDWAALS	−40.343	−46.197	−35.635	−35.533	−46.946	−50.067	−34.248	−40.962	−31.802
EEL	−13.296	−19.577	−15.181	−3.935	−13.128	−29.554	−15.558	−18.300	−10.603
EPB/EGB	32.183	39.385	33.442	23.836	36.678	54.064	32.371	39.952	26.077
ESURF/ECAVITY/ ENPOLAR	−5.024	−5.873	−3.961	−4.54	−5.820	−6.421	−4.623	−5.313	−4.283
DELTA G binding (PB)	−20.633	−21.653	−15.645	−5.210	−15.683	−6.893	−18.093	−9.629	−20.433

2.4.3. Structure Architecture of Kinases

The structure of all protein kinase domains is composed of a small, typically β-stranded *N*-lobe linked with a small hinge region to a bigger α-helical C-lobe. In protein kinases, ATP binds to the cavity that lies between *N*- and C-terminal lobes creating the kinase activation site, where the adenine moiety of ATP is packed like a sandwich between hydrophobic residues, while it is associated with the hinge region by hydrophilic contact. Typical kinase elements include the G-loop (glycine-rich residues forming the active site roof), A-loop, or activation loop crucial for kinase activation and deactivation, C-helix responsible for the selectivity of the active site, and the hinge region that plays a vital role in inhibitor binding. The ATP-binding site categorized into five distinct regions: adenine region where the adenine moiety of ATP forms a hydrogen bond with the hinge, hydrophobic region-I corresponds to the entrance pocket, hydrophobic region-II also known as the selectivity pocket is determined by an extremely conserved DFG (aspartate-phenylalanine-glycine) motif, a hydrophilic region where the ATP sugar binds, and a solvent-exposed region for phosphate binding.

2.4.4. Molecular Dynamic Simulation

Although X-ray crystallography and molecular docking are powerful techniques for biological macromolecules, they are unable to examine the protein's flexibility and they provide a momentary binding mode. Therefore, MD simulation was used to investigate the ligand-protein interactions [36] and the conformational changes which occur in the structure of kinases with respect to motions. Based on the docking results, nine complexes were selected for further MD simulation to understand the binding mechanism of compound **10** and its stability against multiple kinases.

c-Src

The stereo view of the binding mode of Src (PDB ID: 2SRC) is depicted in Figure 8A. It was found that, initially, compound **10** was bound to the active site of Src kinase similar to a cognate ligand by making a hydrogen bond with the NH group of Met341 and CO group of Glu339, while these bonds were observed to undergo destabilization during the simulation. Comparatively, three new hydrogen bonds were formed, involving the side chain amino group of Lys295 (solvent accessible area) and the hydroxyl group of Ser345, which interact with the pyrazolopyrimidine scaffold located in the adenine region of Src kinase. The spatial position of the compound was found to be different from the observed dock pose because of major conformational changes during simulation.

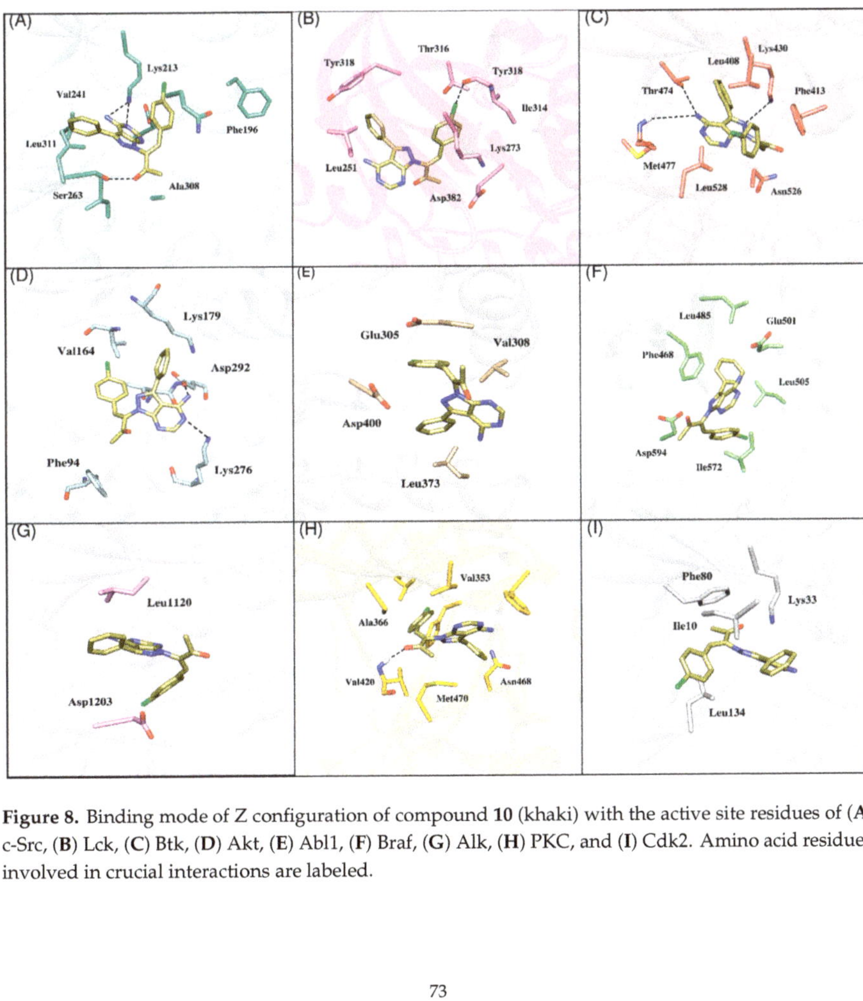

Figure 8. Binding mode of Z configuration of compound **10** (khaki) with the active site residues of **(A)** c-Src, **(B)** Lck, **(C)** Btk, **(D)** Akt, **(E)** Abl1, **(F)** Braf, **(G)** Alk, **(H)** PKC, and **(I)** Cdk2. Amino acid residues involved in crucial interactions are labeled.

The activation loop in the DFG-in conformation provides enough space to accommodate the ring of compound **10**, which may cause a collision with Phe405 of the DFG-out conformation. Moreover, distinct hydrophobic interactions were also observed with Leu273, and Val281 (hydrophobic region I) that maintain the binding mode of complexes. The MD results suggest that the non-flexible part of the compound might be the reason for its moderate activity as compared to the reference compound.

Lck

The binding elements responsible for the modest activity of Lck kinase are depicted in Figure 8B. Consistent with the results from other reported studies, compound **10** is well accommodated in the ATP site of Lck by forming multiple hydrophobic, π-stacking, π-cation, and Van der Waals interactions with Leu251, Ala271, Lys273, Thr316, Lys318, and Asp382. Due to the different conformation of the DFG motif, compound **10** slightly moves toward the adenine region with its core pyrimidine ring in the adenine region by forming a hydrophilic interaction with Met319. In the meantime, Phe385 of the DFG motif is involved in a weak hydrophobic interaction due to the far distance. The chloro-benzene ring engages the gatekeeper residue Thr316 via hydrophobic interaction, while the non-substituted benzene ring occupies the extended hydrophobic pocket, forming π-stacking and Van der Waals interactions with Leu251, Ala271, and Tyr318. The complex was further stabilized by the formation of a halogen bond between the backbone of the carbonyl oxygen of Ile314 and the fluorine of the compound **10**. In summary, a marked similarity of interaction was observed with the reference compound except for the hydrophilic interaction responsible for the inhibitory activity of Lck kinase.

Btk

The docked complex of BTK presented a number of hydrophilic and hydrophobic interactions with the active site residues Leu408, Val416, Lys430, Thr474, Glu475, Met477, Leu528, Asp539, and Phe540. The compound occupied the same position consistent with the reference compound. Molecular dynamics studies revealed that compound **10** binding to BTK, is stable and it was found to involve in hydrogen bond interactions with key residues of the glycine-rich P-loop like Leu408, Gly409, and Asp539. Transient hydrogen bond interactions were also detected with crucial active site residues Glu475 and Met477 of the hinge region, catalytic residue Lys430, and the DFG motif that is crucial for kinase activity, indicating that compound **10** probably has the appropriate interaction profile with BTK (Figure 8C).

Akt

According to the binding mode of the Akt complex [37], compound **10** adopts a Y-shape conformation, where the presence of residues Phe469 and Phe472 that are essential for the regulatory control of Akt1, make the pocket hydrophobic. Initially, the pyrimidine ring occupies the adenosine portion of the binding site, forming hydrogen bonding to the hinge region of the kinase through Ala230 (Figure 8D). During the simulation, this hydrogen bond is replaced by hydrophobic interactions, while the phenyl substituent presents a parallel aromatic interaction with Phe438. Moreover, residues Lys179, Leu181, and Val164 also stabilize the compound by making hydrophobic contact. In general, theoretical studies indicate that compound **10** stabilizes Akt via hydrophobic interactions; however, after losing its interactions with the hinge region, the gatekeeper residue and the DFG motif lead to its low kinase inhibitory properties.

Abl

The binding mode of the Abl1 complex (Figure 8E) showed that the compound is accommodated in the lipophilic channel slightly away from the hinge region. The bent conformation of the molecule does not allow its tight binding to the ATP site. This resultant compound is unable to mimic interaction with the adenine moiety of ATP. Only a few hydrophobic interactions were observed with Glu305, Val308, Leu473, and Asp400, but these interactions were also not found to be persistent throughout the md simulation. It is hypothesized that the absence of specific interactions of compound **10** with the residues of the hinge region and DFG motif could be the reason for its inactivity.

Braf

According to the docking calculations, compound **10** is involved in a number of hydrophilic and hydrophobic interactions with Braf kinase. However, after a short 50 ns production run, the simulated binding mode provided a different picture to understand the selectivity trend. During the simulation, these non-bonded interactions were weakened due to loop flipping of the motif from the DGF-in to the DGF-out conformation. However, in order to accommodate the core pyrimidine ring, the benzene ring was required to tilt out of the plane due to restricted space. As a result of this movement, intermolecular interactions broke, which penalized the binding affinity of compound **10** for Braf (Figure 8F).

Alk

The binding interactions of the Alk with compound **10** are depicted in Figure 8G. The complex obtained after simulation indicates that the compound partially aligned on the reference compound ceritinib, and it was unable to form any hydrophilic interaction with the active site residues, especially with the hinge region. A similar type of binding mode was observed in the case of PKC (Figure 8H) and Cdk2 (Figure 8I).

2.4.5. Binding Free Energy Calculations

MM/PBSA is considered as the best choice for predicting the binding affinities of a protein-ligand complex with implicit solvent at a low computational cost. It has the potential to recognize the true binding structure of the complex from docking. In the present study, MM/PBSA was used to re-rank the nine complexes after a short production run of 50 ns. The calculated binding free energy of all complexes is presented in Table 4 [38]. The binding position and atomic interaction between protein kinases and ligand are the main factors that play a role in measuring the binding affinity. The predicted binding poses of compound **10** significantly overlaid with the reported inhibitors of c-Src, Lck, Btk, and Akt, but partially aligned in the case of Braf and Alk. According to Table 4, the binding free energy computed for c-Src, Lck, and Akt complexes was −20.63, −15.64, and −18.09, respectively, which were more stable than ALK, CDK2, and Abl1 kinases, agreeing with the selectivity profile observed experimentally. In order to comprehend the effect of the individual energy term in the binding process, total binding free energy was decomposed into the Eele, Evdw, EGB, and ESURF energy components. The values of these components indicated that van der Waals (ΔGvdw) energy contributed significantly to the total binding free energy. The superior contribution of Van der Waals interaction (Table 4) was in agreement with the fact that compound **10** mainly stabilizes via hydrophobic interactions with the kinases.

3. Experimental Protocols

3.1. Materials and Methods

Bromoacetone was purchased from ChemService Inc. (West Chester, PA, USA). Anhydrous dichloromethane, anhydrous pyridine, *N,N*-dimethylformamide (DMF), and other chemicals and reagents were purchased from Sigma-Aldrich Chemical Co. (Milwaukee, WI, USA). The chemical structures of final products were characterized by nuclear magnetic resonance spectra (^{1}H NMR, ^{13}C NMR) determined on a Bruker (Billerica, MA, USA) NMR spectrometer (400 MHz) or a Varian (Silicon Valley, CA, USA) NMR spectrometer (500 MHz). ^{13}C NMR spectra were fully decoupled. Chemical shifts were reported in parts per millions (ppm) using deuterated solvent peak as the standard. The chemical structures of final products were confirmed by a high-resolution Biosystems QStar Elite (QStar Technologies, Denver, CO, USA) time-of-flight electrospray mass spectrometer. Details of procedures and spectroscopic data of the respective compounds are presented below. Final compounds were purified on a Phenomenex (Torrance, CA, USA) Prodigy 10 μm ODS reverse-phase column (2.1 cm × 25 cm) with a Hitachi (Tokyo, Japan) HPLC system using a gradient system of acetonitrile or methanol and water ($CH_3CN/CH_3OH/H_2O$, 0–100%, pH 7.0, 60 min). The purity of final products (>99%) was confirmed by analytical HPLC. The analytical HPLC was performed on the Hitachi analytical HPLC system using a C18 Shimadzu (Kyoto, Japan) Premier 3 μm column (150 cm × 4.6 mm) using two different isocratic systems, and a flow rate of 1 mL/min with UV detection at 265 nm.

3.2. Synthesis

3-Phenyl-1*H*-pyrazolo[3,4-*d*]pyrimidin-4-amine (**1**): Compound **1** was synthesized according to a previously reported procedure [23].

1-(4-Amino-3-phenyl-1*H*-pyrazolo[3,4-*d*]pyrimidin-1-yl)propan-2-one (**2**): Compound **1** (156 mg, 0.73 mmol) and potassium carbonate (200 mg, 1.4 mmol) were taken in dry DMF (10 mL). Bromoacetone (100 mg, 0.72 mmol) was diluted with dry DMF (5 mL) and was added dropwise to the reaction mixture at room temperature. The reaction mixture was stirred for 4 h at room temperature. After completion of the reaction, the solvent was removed under reduced pressure, added water (50 mL) and extracted with dichloromethane. The organic layer was filtered through filter paper and dried over Na_2SO_4 (anhydrous). The crude product was further purified on silica gel flash chromatography using dichloromethane and methanol (0–20%) as eluents. 160 mg, 81% yield. ^{1}H-NMR ($CDCl_3$, 500 MHz, δ ppm): 8.3 (s, 1H), 7.7 (d, *J* = 11 Hz, 2H), 7.5–7.5 (m, 3H), 5.2 (s, 2H), 2.2 (s, 3H).^{13}C NMR ($CDCl_3$, 125 MHz, δ ppm): 201.3, 158.1, 156.2, 155.2, 145.4, 132.8, 129.4, 129.3, 128.4, 98.4, 56.1, 27.1. HR-MS (ESI-TOF) (*m/z*): calculated for $C_{14}H_{13}N_5O + H^+$: 268.1193; found, 268.0852 $[M + H]^+$.

General Procedure for the Synthesis of Pyrazolopyrimidine Chalcones:

Compound **2** (26 mg, 0.1 mmol) was dissolved in ethanol (5 mL). Sodium hydroxide (5 mg, 20 μL of 250 mg/mL NaOH solution in water) was added to the compound **2** solution. The reaction mixture solution was stirred for 15 min. Then, a solution of *p*-methylbenzaldehyde (24 mg, 0.2 mmol) in ethanol (15 mL) was added to the reaction mixture. The reaction mixture was allowed to stir at room temperature for 5 h. On completion of the reaction, the reaction mixture was neutralized with dilute acetic acid in ethanol and purified over reverse phase HPLC using water and methanol as eluents to obtain pure product **3** (22 mg, 61% yield). A similar procedure was adopted for the synthesis of other pyrazolopyrimidine derivatives.

3-(4-Amino-3-phenyl-1*H*-pyrazolo[3,4-*d*]pyrimidin-1-yl)-4-*p*-tolylbut-3-en-2-one (**3**). (Yield: 61%). ^{1}H-NMR ($CDCl_3$, 500 MHz, δ ppm): 8.3 (s, 1H), 7.7 (s, 1H), 7.7 (d, *J* = 7 Hz, 2H), 7.6–7.5 (m, 3H), 7.0 (d, *J* = 8.2 Hz, 2H), 6.9 (d, *J* = 8.2 Hz, 2H), 2.3 (s, 3H), 2.9 (s, 3H). ^{13}C NMR ($CDCl_3$, 125 MHz, δ ppm): 194.3, 157.9, 156.9, 155.8, 146.8, 141.8, 140.5, 132.7, 131.8, 130.7, 129.6, 129.5, 129.4, 128.5, 26.1, 21.5. HR-MS (ESI-TOF) (*m/z*): calculated for $C_{22}H_{19}N_5O + H^+$: 370.1662; found, 370.1534 $[M + H]^+$.

3-(4-Amino-3-phenyl-1*H*-pyrazolo[3,4-d]pyrimidin-1-yl)-4-*m*-tolylbut-3-en-2-one (**4**). (Yield: 64%). ^{1}H-NMR ($CDCl_3$, 500 MHz, δ ppm): 8.3 (s, 1H), 7.9 (s, 1H), 7.7 (d, *J* = 7 Hz, 2H), 7.6–7.5 (m, 3H), 7.1–7.0 (m, 2H), 6.8 (s, 1H), 6.7 (d, *J* = 10 Hz, 1H), 2.3 (s, 3H), 2.2 (s, 3H). ^{13}C NMR ($CDCl_3$, 125 MHz, δ ppm): 194.3, 157.8, 155.1, 154.9, 146.8, 140.6, 133.9, 131.7, 131.5, 130.2, 129.5, 129.4,128.6, 128.4, 26.2, 21.3. HR-MS (ESI-TOF) (*m/z*): calculated for $C_{22}H_{19}N_5O + H^+$: 370.1662; found, 370.1454 $[M + H]^+$.

3-(4-Amino-3-phenyl-1*H*-pyrazolo[3,4-d]pyrimidin-1-yl)-4-*p*-biphenylbut-3-en-2-one (**5**). (Yield: 59%). ^{1}H-NMR ($CDCl_3$, 500 MHz, δ ppm): 8.0 (s, 1H), 7.9 (s, 1H), 7.7 (d, *J* = 8.2 Hz, 2H), 7.6–7.6 (m, 3H), 7.6–7.4 (m, 9H), 2.3 (s, 3H). ^{13}C NMR ($CDCl_3$, 125 MHz, δ ppm): 191.9, 147.2, 135.2, 131.1, 130.3, 129.9, 129.9, 129.8, 129.4, 129.0, 128.7, 128.5, 128.5, 127.7, 127.3, 127.3, 127.2, 127.1, 127.0, 126.1, 22.5. HR-MS (ESI-TOF) (*m/z*): calculated for $C_{27}H_{21}N_5O + H^+$: 432.1819; found, 432.1616 $[M + H]^+$.

3-(4-Amino-3-phenyl-1*H*-pyrazolo[3,4-d]pyrimidin-1-yl)-4-(4-methoxyphenyl)but-3-en-2-one (**6**). (Yield: 63%). ^{1}H-NMR ($CDCl_3$, 500 MHz, δ ppm): 8.3 (s, 1H), 7.9 (s, 1H), 7.7 (d, *J* = 7 Hz, 2H), 7.6–7.5 (m, 3H),

6.9 (d, J = 8.9 Hz, 2H), 6.7 (d, J = 8.9 Hz, 2H), 3.7 (s, 3H), 2.3 (s, 3H). ^{13}C NMR ($CDCl_3$, 125 MHz, δ ppm): 194.2, 161.9, 158.0, 156.9, 155.7, 146.9, 140.2, 132.8, 132.7, 130.6, 129.5, 129.4, 128.5, 124.3, 114.4, 98.9, 55.3, 26.0. HR-MS (ESI-TOF) (*m/z*): calculated for $C_{22}H_{19}N_5O_2 + H^+$: 386.1612; found, 386.1573 $[M + H]^+$.

3-(4-Amino-3-phenyl-1*H*-pyrazolo[3,4-d]pyrimidin-1-yl)-4-(4-(dimethylamino)phenyl)but-3-en-2-one (**7**). (Yield: 66%). ^{1}H-NMR ($CDCl_3$, 500 MHz, δ ppm): 8.3 (s, 1H), 7.9 (s, 1H), 7.7 (d, J = 8 Hz, 2H), 7.6–7.5 (m, 3H), 6.8 (d, J = 9.1 Hz, 2H), 6.4 (d, J = 9.1 Hz, 2H), 2.9 (s, 6H), 2.3 (s, 3H). ^{13}C NMR ($CDCl_3$, 125 MHz, δ ppm): 194.4, 162.1, 158.2, 157.1, 155.9, 147.1, 140.4, 133.0, 132.9, 130.8, 129.7, 129.6, 128.7, 124.5, 114.6, 99.0, 41.4, 26.3. HR-MS (ESI-TOF) (*m/z*): calculated for $C_{23}H_{22}N_6O + H^+$: 399.1928; found, 399.1981 $[M + H]^+$.

3-(4-Amino-3-phenyl-1*H*-pyrazolo[3,4-d]pyrimidin-1-yl)-pent-3-en-2-one (**8**). (Yield: 60%). ^{1}H-NMR ($CDCl_3$, 500 MHz, δ ppm): 8.37 (s, 1H), 7.8–7.7 (m, 2H), 7.6–7.5 (m, 3H), 7.4 (q, J = 7.1 Hz, 1H), 2.3 (s, 3H), 1.8 (d, J = 7 Hz, 3H). ^{13}C NMR ($CDCl_3$, 100 MHz, δ ppm): 157.9, 156.3, 154.8, 141.7, 132.6, 129.6, 129.5, 129.5, 128.5. 128.4, 98.3, 56.2, 26.1, 14.6. HR-MS (ESI-TOF) (*m/z*): calcd for $C_{16}H_{15}N_5O + H^+$: 294.1349; found, 294.099 $[M + H]^+$.

3-(4-Amino-3-phenyl-1*H*-pyrazolo[3,4-d]pyrimidin-1-yl)-4-(3-nitrophenyl)but-3-en-2-one (**9**). (Yield: 44%). ^{1}H-NMR ($CDCl_3$, 500 MHz, δ ppm): 8.3 (s, 1H), 7.9 (s, 1H), 7.7 (d, J = 7 Hz, 2H), 7.5–7.5 (m, 3H), 6.9 (d, J = 8.9 Hz, 2H), 6.7 (d, J = 8.9 Hz, 1H), 2.3 (s, 3H). ^{13}C NMR ($CDCl_3$, 125 MHz, δ ppm): 194.2, 161.9, 158.0, 156.9, 155.7, 146.9, 140.2, 132.8, 132.7, 130.6, 129.5, 129.4, 128.5, 124.3, 114.4, 98.9, 55.3, 26.0. HR-MS (ESI-TOF) (*m/z*): calculated for $C_{21}H_{16}N_6O_3 + H^+$: 401.1357; found, 401.0957 $[M + H]^+$, 801.1652 $[2M + H]^+$.

3-(4-Amino-3-phenyl-1*H*-pyrazolo[3,4-d]pyrimidin-1-yl)-4-(4-chlorophenyl)but-3-en-2-one (**10**). (Yield: 57%). ^{1}H-NMR ($CDCl_3$, 500 MHz, δ ppm): 8.1 (s, 1H), 7.9 (s, 1H), 7.6 (m, 2H), 7.5–7.5 (m, 3H), 7.2 (d, J = 8.6 Hz, 2H), 6.9 (d, J = 8.6 Hz, 2H), 2.4 (s, 3H). ^{13}C NMR ($CDCl_3$, 125 MHz, δ ppm): 192.4, 153.7, 153.5, 149.5, 147.2, 140.6, 137.9, 132.5, 131.5, 131.3, 130.9, 130.4, 130.1, 129.5, 128.1, 97.6, 55.3, 25.8. HR-MS (ESI-TOF) (*m/z*): calculated for $C_{21}H_{16}ClN_5O + H^+$: 390.1116; found, 390.0951 $[M + 1]^+$.

3-(4-Amino-3-phenyl-1*H*-pyrazolo[3,4-d]pyrimidin-1-yl)-4-(2,4-dichlorophenyl)but-3-en-2-one (**11**). (Yield: 58%). ^{1}H-NMR ($CDCl_3$, 500 MHz, δ ppm): 8.3 (s, 1H), 7.9 (s, 1H), 7.7 (d, J = 7 Hz, 2H), 7.5–7.5 (m, 3H), 6.9 (s, 1H), 6.7 (d, J = 8.6 Hz, 2H), 2.6 (s, 3H). ^{13}C NMR ($CDCl_3$, 125 MHz, δ ppm): 192.2, 153.7, 136.9, 136.2, 130.9, 130.2, 130.1, 129.8, 129.0, 128.2, 128.1, 127.5, 127.5, 97.6, 66.4, 53.4, 25.9. HR-MS (ESI-TOF) (*m/z*): calculated for $C_{21}H_{15}Cl_2N_5O + H^+$: 424.0726; found, 424.1220 $[M + H]^+$.

3-(4-Amino-3-phenyl-1*H*-pyrazolo[3,4-d]pyrimidin-1-yl)-4-(2-chlorophenyl)but-3-en-2-one (**12**). (Yield: 57%). ^{1}H-NMR ($CDCl_3$, 500 MHz, δ ppm): 8.3 (s, 1H), 8.2 (s, 1H), 7.6–7.5 (m, 5H), 7.3–7.2 (m, 4H), 2.6 (s, 3H). ^{13}C-NMR ($CDCl_3$, 125 MHz, δ ppm): 153.6, 153.3, 149.1, 146.5, 138.2, 132.0, 130.8, 130.2, 130.1, 129.3, 128.9, 128.1, 126.9, 52.5, 25.9. HR-MS (ESI-TOF) (*m/z*): calcd for $C_{21}H_{16}ClN_5O + H^+$: 390.1116; found, 390.1427 $[M + H]^+$.

3-(4-Amino-3-phenyl-1*H*-pyrazolo[3,4-d]pyrimidin-1-yl)-4-(2-fluorophenyl)but-3-en-2-one (**13**). (Yield: 62%). ^{1}H-NMR ($CDCl_3$, 500 MHz, δ ppm): 8.3 (s, 1H), 7.9 (s, 1H), 7.7 (d, J = 7 Hz, 2H), 7.6–7.5 (m, 3H), 7.2–6.9 (m, 4H), 2.3 (s, 3H). ^{13}C NMR ($CDCl_3$, 125 MHz, δ ppm): 193.8, 158.1, 155.6, 147.4, 132.8, 132.7, 130.3, 131.7, 129.7, 129.5, 129.5, 129.3, 129.2, 128.4, 128.4, 128.4, 98.7, 26.2. HR-MS (ESI-TOF) (*m/z*): calculated for $C_{21}H_{16}FN_5O + H^+$: 374.1412; found, 374.1526 $[M + H]^+$.

3-(4-Amino-3-phenyl-1*H*-pyrazolo[3,4-d]pyrimidin-1-yl)-4-(4-fluorophenyl)but-3-en-2-one (**14**). (Yield: 64%). ^{1}H-NMR ($CDCl_3$, 500 MHz, δ ppm): 8.1 (s, 1H), 7.8 (s, 1H), 7.5–7.4 (m, 5H), 6.9 (dd, J = 14 Hz, J = 5.6 Hz, 2H), 6.8 (t, J = 7.6 Hz, 2H), 2.4 (s, 3H). ^{13}C NMR ($CDCl_3$, 125 MHz, δ ppm): 192.5, 153.7, 153.5, 147.2, 140.7, 132.5, 132.4, 130.9, 130.1, 130.0, 128.1, 128.1, 116.7, 116.5, 25.7. HR-MS (ESI-TOF) (*m/z*): calculated for $C_{21}H_{16}FN_5O + H^+$: 374.1412; found, 374.1679 $[M + H]^+$.

3-(4-Amino-3-phenyl-1*H*-pyrazolo[3,4-d]pyrimidin-1-yl)-4-phenyl but-3-en-2-one (**15**). (Yield: 59%). ^{1}H-NMR ($CDCl_3$, 500 MHz, δ ppm): 8.2 (s, 1H), 8.0 (s, 1H), 7.7–7.6 (m, 5H), 7.4–6.9 (m, 5H), 2.5 (s, 3H). ^{13}C-NMR ($CDCl_3$, 125 MHz, δ ppm): 192.5, 153.7, 153.5, 147.2, 140.7, 132.5, 132.4, 130.9, 130.1, 130.0, 128.1, 128.1, 116.7, 116.5, 25.7. HR-MS (ESI-TOF) (*m*/*z*): calculated for $C_{21}H_{17}N_5O + H^+$: 356.1506; found, 356.1703 $[M + H]^+$.

3.3. *Kinase Enzyme Assay*

3.3.1. c-Src Kinase Activity Assay

The effect of compounds on the activity of *c*-Src kinase was assessed using a Transcreener® ADP [2,8] fluorescence intensity (FI) Assay, from Bell Brook Labs, Madison, WI, USA, (catalog no. 3013-1K) according to the manufacturer's protocol. A 384-well low-volume black non-binding surface round-bottom microplate was purchased from Corning Inc. (Corning, NY, USA) (#3676). In summary, the kinase reaction was started in the 384-well low volume black microplate with the incubation of 2.5 µL of the reaction cocktail (0.7 nM of His_6-Src kinase domain in kinase buffer) with 2.5 µL of prediluted compounds (dissolved in 10% DMSO, 4× target concentration) for 10 min at room temperature using microplate shaker. The reaction cocktail was made using the kinase buffer HEPES (200 mM, pH 7.5), $MgCl_2$ (16 mM), EGTA (8 mM), DMSO (4%), Brij-35 (0.04%), and 2-mercaptoethanol (43 mM). The kinase reaction was started by adding 5 µL of ATP/substrate (40 µM/600 µM) cocktail and incubated for 30 min at room temperature on a microplate shaker. Src optimal peptide (AEEEIYGEFEAKKKK) was used as the substrate for the kinase reaction. The kinase reaction was stopped by adding 10 µL of the 1× ADP Detection Mixture to the enzyme reaction mixture and mixed using a plate shaker. The mixture was incubated at room temperature for 1 h, and the fluorescence intensity was measured. The 1× ADP Detection Mixture was prepared by adding ADP^2 Antibody-IRDyeR QC-1 (10 µg/mL) and ADP Alexa594 Tracer (8 nM) to Stop and Detect Buffer B(1×). The fluorescence Intensity measurements were performed using a fluorescence intensity optical module using the excitation of 580 nm and emission of 630 nm with bandwidths of 10 nm by Optima, BMG Labtech microplate reader (BMG Labtech, Ortenberg, Germany). The IC_{50} values of the compounds were calculated using ORIGIN 6.0 (Origin Lab, Microcal Software, Inc. Northhampton, MA, USA) software. IC_{50} is the concentration of the compound that inhibited enzyme activity by 50%. All the experiments were carried out in triplicate.

3.3.2. Evaluation of Compound **10** Against a Panel of Kinases (Abl1, Akt1, Alk, Braf, Btk, Cdk2, cSrc, Lck, and PKCa)

Compound **10** was evaluated for inhibitory activity against Abl1, Akt1, Alk, Braf, Btk, Cdk2, cSrc, Lck, and PKCa, in duplicate by Reaction Biology Corporation. Compounds were tested in a five-dose IC_{50} mode with four-fold serial dilution starting at 20 µM. Control compounds Staurosporine and GW5074 were tested in a 10-dose IC_{50} starting at 20 µM with a four-fold or three-fold serial dilution, respectively. All kinase reactions were performed at 200 µM ATP. The compounds were pre-incubated with the enzyme and substrate mixture about 20 min, and then ATP was added to start the reaction. The reaction was 2 h at room temperature. Curve fits were performed when the activities at the highest concentration of compounds were less than 65%. The detailed experimental procedure is provided here. An IC_{50} value of less than 0.04 nM or higher than 1 µM is estimated based on the best curve fitting available. The substrates for kinases are shown in Table 5.

Table 5. Substrates used for kinases.

Kinases	Kinase (Invitrogen) Cat#	Kinase Conc. in Reaction (nM)	Substrate	Substrate Conc. in Reaction
Abl1	PR4348B	0.25	ABLtide	20 μM
c-Src	P3044	0.6	pEY	0.2 mg/mL
Akt1	PR3878D	8	Crosstide	20 μM
Alk	PV3867	1.5	pEY	0.2 mg/mL
Cdk2/Cyclin A1	C29-10BG	15	Histone H1	20 μM
PKCa	PR1455C	0.5	Histone H1 + Lipid Activator	20 μM
Braf	PR6995A	30	MEK1 (K97R)	5 μM
Lck	P3043	8	pEY + Manganese	0.2 mg/mL
Btk	PV3363	8	pEY	0.2 mg/mL

Base Reaction buffer was prepared from 20 mM Hepes (pH 7.5), 10 mM $MgCl_2$, 1 mM EGTA, 0.02% Brij35, 0.02 mg/mL BSA, 0.1 mM Na_3VO_4, 2 mM DTT, and 1% DMSO. Required cofactors were added individually to each kinase reaction. Testing compounds were dissolved in 100% DMSO to a specific concentration. The serial dilution was conducted by Integra Viaflo Assist in DMSO. The substrate was prepared in a freshly prepared reaction buffer. The required cofactors for each kinase were added to the substrate solution. The kinase was added into the substrate solution, and the solution was gently mixed. The compounds in 100% DMSO were added into the kinase reaction mixture by Acoustic technology (Echo550; nanoliter range) and incubated for 20 min at room temperature. P-ATP (Specific activity 10 μCi/μl) was added into the reaction mixture to initiate the reaction. The mixture was incubated for 2 h at room temperature. The radioactivity was detected using the filter-binding method. The kinase activity data were expressed as the percentage remaining kinase activity in test samples compared to vehicle (dimethyl sulfoxide) reactions. IC_{50} values, and curve fits were obtained using GraphPad Prism software (version 7, Informer Technologies, Inc., Los Angeles, CA, USA).

3.4. Cell Culture and Cell Proliferation Assay

3.4.1. Cell Culture

Human leukemia cell line CCRF-CEM (ATCC no. CCL-119), human ovarian adenocarcinoma cell line SK-OV-3 (ATCC no. HTB-77), human breast carcinoma cell line MDA-MB-231 (ATCC no.HTB-26), and human colon adenocarcinoma cell line HT-29 (ATCC no. HTB-38) were obtained from American Type Culture Collection. Cells were grown on 75 cm^2 cell culture flasks with RPMI-16 medium (for leukemia cells) and EMEM (Eagle's minimum essential medium) (for SK-OV-3, HT-29, MDA-MB-231 cells), supplemented with 10% fetal bovine serum (FBS), and 1% penicillin-streptomycin solution (10,000 units of penicillin and 10 mg of streptomycin in 0.9% NaCl) in a humidified atmosphere of 5% CO_2, 95% air at 37 °C.

3.4.2. Cell Proliferation Assay

The cell proliferation assay was carried out using a CellTiter 96 aqueous one-solution cell proliferation assay kit (Promega, Madison, WI, USA). Briefly, upon reaching about 75–80% confluence, 5000 cells/well were plated in 96-well microplate in 100 μL of the medium. After seeding for 24 h, the cells were treated with 50 μM compound in triplicate. Doxorubicin (10 μM) was used as a positive control. At the end of the sample exposure period (72 h), 20 μL of CellTiter 96 aqueous solution was added. The plate was returned to the incubator for 1 h in a humidified atmosphere at 37 °C. The absorbance of the formazan product was measured at 490 nm using a microplate reader. The blank control was recorded by measuring the absorbance at 490 nm with wells containing medium mixed with CellTiter 96 aqueous solution but no cells. The percentage of cell survival was calculated as the OD value of cells treated with test compound − OD value of culture medium/(OD value of control cells

– OD value of culture medium) × 100%. The same strategy was used for generating a dose-response graph for compound **10**.

3.5. Molecular Modeling

3.5.1. Target Fishing

Potential targets were identified against the phenylpyrazolopyrimidine scaffold using a combination of information integration, chemometric methods, and data mining approaches. Initially, targets involved in breast, ovarian, and colorectal cancer pathways were extracted from the database of KEGG. In the next step, protein network association servers STRING, STITCH, and SEA were used to characterize the protein-ligand interactions. Similarly, the PhPP scaffold was also searched using different search engines to understand protein-ligand interactions. Based on the above-mentioned information, we selected fourteen different targets, including Btk, Itk, c-Src, EGFR [39], Braf, Fyn, Lyn, Hck, Cdk2/4, Alk, Akt1 Lck, PKC, and Abl1 kinase. To understand the binding mechanism of active compound **10** against all selected targets, molecular docking and MD simulations were performed.

3.5.2. Preparation of Complexes

Crystal structures of the Anaplastic lymphoma kinase [PDB ID: 4MKC], ABL1 kinase [PDB ID: 6HD4], Protein kinase B also known as AKT [PDB ID: 4GV1], bruton tyrosine kinase [PDB ID: 6DIS], BRAF [PDB ID: 6B8U], c-Src kinase [PDB ID: 2SRC], CDK2 [PDB ID: 4KD1], LCK [PDB ID: 2OFU], ITK [PDB ID: 4HUC], EGFR [PDB ID: 4HJO], FYN [PDB ID: 2DQ7], LYN [PDB ID: 2ZV9], HCK [PDB ID: 1QCF], and PKCa [PDB ID: 3IW4] were retrieved from RCSB Protein Databank. The missing part of the starting structures was constructed using MOE software (Molecular Operating Environment, v2016.08, 2016). Compound partial charges were derived with the MMFF94x force field. All stabilizing agents, water molecules, and ions present in the crystal structures were removed. The protonate 3D module in MOE was used for assigning the protonation state to every titratable residue at physiological conditions within the complexes. MOE docking suite was employed for docking studies. The standard default settings were used with the London dG scoring function as a fitness function in all calculations.

3.5.3. MD Simulations

After analysis of docking results, nine complexes were subjected to all-atom MD simulation using the graphics processing unit (GPU) version of the PMEMD.cuda engine provided with Amber18 [40]. The gaff [41] and ff14SB force field [42] were implemented to ligand and protein in all simulations, respectively. Each complex was neutralized by adding counter ions, and the systems were solvated by a cubic box of the TIP3P water model with a 10 Å box size from the solute. Systems were relaxed by adjusting hydrogen position, while 1000 cycles of steepest descent, and 5000 cycles of the conjugate gradient with restraints of 100 kcal·mol^{-1} were applied on heavy atoms. Finally, another minimization of 5000 steps was performed to relax the system without any restraint. It was followed by equilibration of each system by gradual heating from 0 K to 300 K in the NVT ensemble. Systems were further equilibrated under the NPT ensemble (Pressure = 1 atm). The production run of 50 ns was performed for each system using the isothermal-isobaric (NPT) ensemble at constant temperature and pressure with periodic boundary conditions. The Particle Mesh Ewald Method (PMEM) [43] was used to calculate long-range electrostatic interactions with cut off value of 8 Å for the non-bonded (electrostatics and Van der Waals) interactions. An integration time step of 2 fs was set to integrate Newton's equations of motion. The SHAKE algorithm [44] was employed to restrain the bonds involving hydrogen atoms. The trajectories were analyzed using CPPTRAJ module incorporated in AMBER suite. All visualization was performed using Chimera and VMD.

3.5.4. MM/PBSA Calculations

The binding free energy calculation for each complex was performed using the MM(GB/PB)SA method based on 1000 frames extracted from the 50 ns trajectory. The equations associated with binding free energy calculation were as follows:

$$\Delta G = G_{complex} - (G_{receptor} + G_{compound}) \quad (1)$$

$$G = H - TS \quad (2)$$

$$H = E_{vdw} + E_{ele} + E_{int} + G_{gb} + G_{surf} \quad (3)$$

The total binding free energy is ΔG, whereas the free energies for the complex, receptor, and compound are represented as $G_{complex}$, $G_{receptor}$, and $G_{compound}$, respectively. The terms H and TΔS were used for the contribution of enthalpy and entropy. The binding free energy further decomposed into electrostatic (E_{ele}), Van der Waals interaction (E_{vdw}), internal energy (E_{int}), and polar (G_{gb}) and non-polar desolvation energy (G_{surf}). The value of the dielectric constant was set to 1, and the external was set to 80 for solute protein (εin). The Generalized Born (GB) model established by Onufriev (GBOBC1) with modified Bondi radii (mbondi2) and igb = 2 implemented in AMBER18 was used to calculate the electrostatic contribution to the solvation free energy. The non-polar surface area was calculated using the LCPO model. The offset (β) and surface tension (γ) values were set to 0.92 kcal/mol and 0.00542 kcal/(mol·Å2), respectively.

4. Conclusions

A number of novel *N*1-(α,β-alkene) substituted phenylpyrazolopyrimidine (PhPP) derivatives with acetyl and functionalized phenyl groups at α- and β-positions were synthesized, and they showed modest inhibitory activity (IC_{50} = 21.7–192.1 μM) against c-Src kinases. A number of para-chlorophenyl substituted compounds, **10** and **11,** consistently inhibited the cell proliferation 72–96 h in all cell lines and were more effective against HT-29 cells. Compound **10** was also found to be modestly active against c-Src, Lck, and Btk. The target-based study of these compounds was performed by text mining, similarity search, and ligand-protein interaction pattern to identify potential targets. Further MD simulation and binding free energy calculations were carried out to discriminate the selectivity of the investigated compound with a panel of different kinases and provide more in-depth structural insight into the interaction pattern involved in the inhibition process. The structural and energetic features highlighted in this study can provide a theoretical basis for further research on selective protein kinase inhibitors.

Author Contributions: Methodology: B.S.C., N.S.J., S.A., S.M., and R.K.T.; writing—original draft preparation: B.S.C., Z.U.-H, and K.P.; supervision: Z.U.-H. and K.P.; funding acquisition: K.P.; performed the synthesis: B.S.C. and N.S.J.; conducted the antiproliferative assays: S.M. and D.M.; performed the kinase assays: R.K.T.; performed molecular modeling: S.A.; supervised, wrote, and edited the manuscript: Z.U.-H. and K.P. All authors contributed to writing the manuscript, editing, and reviewing of the manuscript. All authors read and agreed to the published version of the manuscript.

Funding: This research was funded by the American Cancer Society Grant # RSG-07-290-01-CDD.

Acknowledgments: We acknowledge the financial support from the American Cancer Society Grant # RSG-07-290-01-CDD and Chapman University School of Pharmacy.

Conflicts of Interest: The authors declare no conflicts of interest.

References

1. Yeatman, T.J. A renaissance for SRC. *Nat. Rev. Cancer* **2004**, *4*, 470–480. [CrossRef] [PubMed]
2. Summy JM, G.G. Src family kinases in tumor progression and metastasis. *Cancer Metastasis Rev.* **2003**, *22*, 337–358. [CrossRef] [PubMed]

3. Irby, R.B.; Yeatman, T.J. Role of Src expression and activation in human cancer. *Oncogene* **2000**, *19*, 5636–5642. [CrossRef] [PubMed]
4. Jiao, Q.; Bi, L.; Ren, Y.; Song, S.; Wang, Q.; Wang, Y.S. Advances in studies of tyrosine kinase inhibitors and their acquired resistance. *Mol. Cancer* **2018**, *17*, 36. [CrossRef] [PubMed]
5. Wagner, J.; Von Matt, P.; Sedrani, R.; Albert, R.; Cooke, N.; Ehrhardt, C.; Geiser, M.; Rummel, G.; Stark, W.; Strauss, A.; et al. Discovery of 3-(1*H*-indol-3-yl)-4-[2-(4-methylpiperazin-1-yl)quinazolin-4-yl]-pyrrole-2,5-dione (AEB071), a potent and selective inhibitor of protein kinase C isotypes. *J. Med. Chem.* **2009**, *52*, 6193–6196. [CrossRef]
6. Tsou, H.R.; Overbeek-Klumpers, E.G.; Hallett, W.A.; Reich, M.F.; Floyd, M.B.; Johnson, B.D.; Michalak, R.S.; Nilakantan, R.; Discafani, C.; Golas, J.; et al. Optimization of 6,7-disubstituted-4-(arylamino)quinoline-3-carbonitriles as orally active, irreversible inhibitors of human epidermal growth factor receptor-2 kinase activity. *J. Med. Chem.* **2005**, *48*, 1107–1131. [CrossRef] [PubMed]
7. Schenone, S.; Radi, M.; Musumeci, F.; Brullo, C.; Botta, M. Biologically driven synthesis of pyrazolo [3, 4-d] pyrimidines as protein kinase inhibitors: An old scaffold as a new tool for medicinal chemistry and chemical biology studies. *Chem. Rev.* **2014**, *114*, 7189–7238. [CrossRef]
8. Kumar, A.; Ahmad, I.; Chhikara, B.S.; Tiwari, R.; Mandal, D.; Parang, K. Synthesis of 3-phenylpyrazolopyrimidine-1,2,3-triazole conjugates and evaluation of their Src kinase inhibitory and anticancer activities. *Bioorg. Med. Chem. Lett.* **2011**, *21*, 1342–1346. [CrossRef]
9. Mukaiyama, H.; Nishimura, T.; Kobayashi, S.; Ozawa, T.; Kamada, N.; Komatsu, Y.; Kikuchi, S.; Oonota, H.; Kusama, H. Synthesis and c-Src inhibitory activity of imidazo[1,5-a]pyrazine derivatives as an agent for treatment of acute ischemic stroke. *Bioorg. Med. Chem.* **2007**, *15*, 868–885. [CrossRef]
10. Trush, V.; Cherenok, S.; Tanchuk, V.; Kalchenko, V.; Vovk, A. Evaluation of inhibition of protein tyrosine phosphatase 1B by calixarene-based α-ketophosphonic acids. *Chem. Biol. Lett.* **2015**, *2*, 1–5.
11. Rao, V.K.; Chhikara, B.S.; Tiwari, R.; Shirazi, A.N.; Parang, K.; Kumar, A. One-pot regioselective synthesis of tetrahydroindazolones and evaluation of their antiproliferative and Src kinase inhibitory activities. *Bioorg. Med. Chem. Lett.* **2012**, *22*, 410–414. [CrossRef] [PubMed]
12. Rao, M.S.; Chhikara, B.S.; Tiwari, R.; Shirazi, A.N.; Parang, K.; Kumar, A. Microwave-assisted and scandium triflate catalyzed synthesis of tetrahydrobenzo[a]xanthen-11-ones. *Monatshefte fur Chemie* **2012**, *143*, 263–268. [CrossRef]
13. Rao, V.K.; Chhikara, B.S.; Shirazi, A.N.; Tiwari, R.; Parang, K.; Kumar, A. 3-substitued indoles: One-pot synthesis and evaluation of anticancer and Src kinase inhibitory activities. *Bioorg. Med. Chem. Lett.* **2011**, *21*, 3511–3514. [CrossRef] [PubMed]
14. Nam, N.H.; Lee, S.; Ye, G.; Sun, G.; Parang, K. ATP-phosphopeptide conjugates as inhibitors of Src tyrosine kinases. *Bioorg. Med. Chem.* **2004**, *12*, 5753–5766. [CrossRef]
15. Deininger, M.; Buchdunger, E.; Druker, B.J. The development of imatinib as a therapeutic agent for chronic myeloid leukemia. *Blood* **2005**, *105*, 2640–2653. [CrossRef]
16. Shah, N.P.; Tran, C.; Lee, F.Y.; Chen, P.; Norris, D.; Sawyers, C.L. Overriding imatinib resistance with a novel ABL kinase inhibitor. *Science* **2004**, *305*, 399–401. [CrossRef]
17. Vultur, A.; Buettner, R.; Kowolik, C.; Liang, W.; Smith, D.; Boschelli, F.; Jove, R. SKI-606 (bosutinib), a novel Src kinase inhibitor, suppresses migration and invasion of human breast cancer cells. *Mol. Cancer Ther.* **2008**, *7*, 1185–1194. [CrossRef]
18. Martina Ferrari, S.; La Motta, C.; Sartini, S.; Baldini, E.; Materazzi, G.; Politti, U.; Ruffilli, I.; Ulisse, S.; Miccoli, P.; Antonelli, A. Pyrazolopyrimidine derivatives as antineoplastic agents: With a special focus on thyroid cancer. *Mini Rev. Med. Chem.* **2016**, *16*, 86–93. [CrossRef]
19. Crisci, S.; Di Francia, R.; Amitrano, F.; Saggese, M.; Mele, S.; Ronga, G.; De Filippi, R.; Berretta, M.; Rossi, P.; Pinto, A. Overview of Targeted Drugs for Mature B-Cell Non-hodgkin Lymphomas. *Front. Oncol.* **2019**, *9*, 443. [CrossRef]
20. Akinleye, A.; Chen, Y.; Mukhi, N.; Song, Y.; Liu, D. Ibrutinib and novel BTK inhibitors in clinical development. *J. Hematol. Oncol.* **2013**, *6*, 59. [CrossRef]
21. Xu, W.; Doshi, A.; Lei, M.; Eck, M.J.; Harrison, S.C. Crystal Structures of c-Src Reveal Features of Its Autoinhibitory Mechanism. *Mol. Cell* **1999**, *3*, 629–638. [CrossRef]

22. Zhu, X.; Kim, J.L.; Newcomb, J.R.; Rose, P.E.; Stover, D.R.; Toledo, L.M.; Zhao, H.; Morgenstern, K.A. Structural analysis of the lymphocyte-specific kinase Lck in complex with non-selective and Src family selective kinase inhibitors. *Structure* **1999**, *7*, 651–661. [CrossRef]
23. Bookser, B.C.; Ugarkar, B.G.; Matelich, M.C.; Lemus, R.H.; Allan, M.; Tsuchiya, M.; Nakane, M.; Nagahisa, A.; Wiesner, J.B.; Erion, M.D. Adenosine Kinase Inhibitors. 6. Synthesis, Water Solubility, and Antinociceptive Activity of 5-Phenyl-7-(5-deoxy-β-d-ribofuranosyl)pyrrolo[2,3-d]pyrimidines Substituted at C4 with Glycinamides and Related Compounds. *J. Med. Chem.* **2005**, *48*, 7808–7820. [CrossRef] [PubMed]
24. Chhikara, B.S.; Parang, K. Development of cytarabine prodrugs and delivery systems for leukemia treatment. *Expert Opin. Drug Deliv.* **2010**, *7*, 1399–1414. [CrossRef] [PubMed]
25. Chhikara, B.S.; Mandal, D.; Parang, K. Synthesis and evaluation of fatty acyl ester derivatives of cytarabine as anti-leukemia agents. *Eur. J. Med. Chem.* **2010**, *45*, 4601–4608. [CrossRef]
26. Chhikara, B.S.; Rathi, B.; Parang, K. Critical evaluation of pharmaceutical rational design of nano-delivery systems for doxorubicin in cancer therapy. *J. Mater. Nanosci.* **2019**, *6*, 47–66.
27. Nasrolahi Shirazi, A.; Tiwari, R.; Chhikara, B.S.; Mandal, D.; Parang, K. Design and biological evaluation of cell-penetrating peptide-doxorubicin conjugates as prodrugs. *Mol. Pharm.* **2013**, *10*, 488–499. [CrossRef]
28. Chhikara, B.S.; St. Jean, N.; Mandal, D.; Kumar, A.; Parang, K. Fatty acyl amide derivatives of doxorubicin: Synthesis and in vitro anticancer activities. *Eur. J. Med. Chem.* **2011**, *46*, 2037–2042. [CrossRef]
29. Chhikara, B.S.; Mandal, D.; Parang, K. Synthesis, anticancer activities, and cellular uptake studies of lipophilic derivatives of doxorubicin succinate. *J. Med. Chem.* **2012**, *55*, 1500–1510. [CrossRef]
30. Behera, D.K.; Behera, P.M.; Acharya, L.; Dixit, A. Development and validation of pharmacophore and QSAR models for influenza PB2 inhibitors. *Chem. Biol. Lett.* **2017**, *4*, 1–8.
31. Sharma, D.; Pathak, M.; Sharma, R.; Sharma, N.; Tyagi, P.; Chawla, R.; Basu, M.; Ojha, H. Homology modeling and docking studies of VP24 protein of Ebola virus with an antiviral drug and its derivatives. *Chem. Biol. Lett.* **2017**, *4*, 27–32.
32. Kanehisa, M.; Shlomi, T.; Ruppin, E.; Koonin, E.; Snoddy, J.; Gerstein, M.; Sheffer, M.; Alon, U. KEGG: Kyoto Encyclopedia of Genes and Genomes. *Nucl. Acid. Res.* **2000**, *28*, 27–30. [CrossRef] [PubMed]
33. Wang, Z.; Liang, L.; Yin, Z.; Lin, J. Improving chemical similarity ensemble approach in target prediction. *J. Cheminform.* **2016**, *8*, 20. [CrossRef] [PubMed]
34. Roth, A.; Franceschini, A.; Szklarczyk, D.; Heller, D.; Simonovic, M.; Wyder, S.; von Mering, C.; Huerta-Cepas, J.; Forslund, K.; Bork, P.; et al. STRING v10: Protein–protein interaction networks, integrated over the tree of life. *Nucl. Acid. Res.* **2014**, *43*, D447–D452.
35. Szklarczyk, D.; Santos, A.; Von Mering, C.; Jensen, L.J.; Bork, P.; Kuhn, M. STITCH 5: Augmenting protein-chemical interaction networks with tissue and affinity data. *Nucl. Acid. Res.* **2016**, *44*, D380–D384. [CrossRef] [PubMed]
36. Chandel, V.; Raj, S.; Rathi, B.; Kumar, D. In silico identification of potent FDA approved drugs against Coronavirus COVID-19 main protease: A drug repurposing approach. *Chem. Biol. Lett.* **2020**, *7*, 166–175.
37. Wencheng, X.; Zhang, L.; Yin, Y.; Yang, D.; Zhao, G. 3D-QSAR and molecular docking studies of ATP-competitive Akt inhibitors with the scaffold 4-(piperazin-1-yl)pyrimidine. *Chem. Biol. Lett.* **2014**, *1*, 44–54.
38. Kollman, P.A.; Massova, I.; Reyes, C.; Kuhn, B.; Huo, S.; Chong, L.; Lee, M.; Lee, T.; Duan, Y.; Wang, W.; et al. Calculating structures and free energies of complex molecules: Combining molecular mechanics and continuum models. *Acc. Chem. Res.* **2000**, *33*, 889–897. [CrossRef]
39. Chandel, V.; Srivastava, M.; Srivastava, A.; Asthana, S.; Kumar, D. In-silico interactions of active Phytochemicals with c-MYC EGFR and ERBB2 oncoproteins. *Chem. Biol. Lett.* **2020**, *7*, 47–54.
40. Case, D.A.; Cheatham, T.E.; Darden, T.; Gohlke, H.; Luo, R.; Merz, K.M.; Onufriev, A.; Simmerling, C.; Wang, B.; Woods, R.J. The Amber biomolecular simulation programs. *J. Comput. Chem.* **2005**, *26*, 1668–1688. [CrossRef]
41. Wang, J.; Wolf, R.M.; Caldwell, J.W.; Kollman, P.A.; Case, D.A. Development and testing of a general Amber force field. *J. Comput. Chem.* **2004**, *25*, 1157–1174. [CrossRef] [PubMed]
42. Maier, J.A.; Martinez, C.; Kasavajhala, K.; Wickstrom, L.; Hauser, K.E.; Simmerling, C. ff14SB: Improving the Accuracy of Protein Side Chain and Backbone Parameters from ff99SB. *J. Chem. Theor. Comput.* **2015**, *11*, 3696–3713. [CrossRef] [PubMed]

43. Darden, T.; York, D.; Pedersen, L. Particle mesh Ewald: An N·log(N) method for Ewald sums in large systems. *J. Chem. Phys.* **1993**, *98*, 10089–10092. [CrossRef]
44. Ryckaert, J.C.; Ciccotti, G.; Berendsen, H.J.C. Numerical Integration of the Cartesian Equations of Motion of a System with Constraints. *J. Comp. Phys.* **1977**, *23*, 327–341. [CrossRef]

Sample Availability: Samples of the limited number the compounds are available from the authors upon request.

molecules

MDPI

Article

Synthesis, Docking Studies and Biological Activity of New Benzimidazole- Triazolothiadiazine Derivatives as Aromatase Inhibitor

Ulviye Acar Çevik [1,2], Betül Kaya Çavuşoğlu [3], Begüm Nurpelin Sağlık [1,2], Derya Osmaniye [1,2], Serkan Levent [1,2], Sinem Ilgın [4], Yusuf Özkay [1,2,*] and Zafer Asım Kaplancıklı [1]

1 Department of Pharmaceutical Chemistry, Faculty of Pharmacy, Anadolu University, Eskisehir 26470, Turkey; uacar@anadolu.edu.tr (U.A.Ç.); bnsaglik@anadolu.edu.tr (B.N.S.); dosmaniye@anadolu.edu.tr (D.O.); serkanlevent@anadolu.edu.tr (S.L.); zakaplan@anadolu.edu.tr (Z.A.K.)

2 Doping and Narcotic Compounds Analysis Laboratory, Faculty of Pharmacy, Anadolu University, Eskisehir 26470, Turkey

3 Department of Pharmaceutical Chemistry, Faculty of Pharmacy, Bülent Ecevit University, Zonguldak 67100, Turkey; betulkaya@anadolu.edu.tr

4 Department of Pharmaceutical Toxicology, Faculty of Pharmacy, Anadolu University, Eskisehir 26470, Turkey; silgin@anadolu.edu.tr

* Correspondence: yozkay@anadolu.edu.tr; Tel.: +90-222-335-0580 (ext. 3603)

Academic Editor: Filippo Minutolo

Received: 3 March 2020; Accepted: 1 April 2020; Published: 2 April 2020

Abstract: In the last step of estrogen biosynthesis, aromatase enzyme catalyzes the conversion of androgens to estrogens. Aromatase inhibition is an important way to control estrogen-related diseases and estrogen levels. In this study, sixteen of benzimidazole-triazolothiadiazine derivatives have been synthesized and studied as potent aromatase inhibitors. First, these compounds were tested for their anti-cancer properties against human breast cancer cell line (MCF-7). The most active compounds **5c**, **5e**, **5k**, and **5m** on MCF-7 cell line were subject to further in vitro aromatase enzyme inhibition assays to determine the possible mechanisms of action underlying their activity. Compound **5e** showed slight less potent aromatase inhibitory activity than that of letrozole with IC_{50} = 0.032 ± 0.042 μM, compared to IC_{50} = 0.024 ± 0.001 μM for letrozole. Furthermore, compound **5e** and reference drug letrozole were docked into human placental aromatase enzyme to predict their possible binding modes with the enzyme. Finally, ADME parameters (absorption, distribution, metabolism, and excretion) of synthesized compounds (**5a–5p**) were calculated by QikProp 4.8 software.

Keywords: aromatase; MCF-7; NIH3T3; benzimidazole; triazolothiadiazine; docking; ADME

1. Introduction

Aromatase is a member of the cytochrome P450 enzyme that catalyzes the biosynthesis of estrogens from androgens [1,2]. Estrogen levels have been shown to be higher in breast cancer cells. Inhibition of aromatase is one of the effective current therapeutic strategies for controlling estrogen-dependent breast cancer. Therefore, one of the commonly used classes of drugs for the management of estrogen-dependent cancer is aromatase inhibitors (AIs) [1,3,4].

Aromatase inhibitors that have been used clinically can be categorized as first-, second-, and third generations based on their evolution time or steroidal or steroidal or non-steroidal aromatase inhibitors (NSAIs) based on their structural similarity with steroids [5,6].

Aminoglutethimide is the prototype nonsteroidal inhibitor of aromatase. Problems with the side effects and selectivity of aminoglutethimide led to the development of the second-generation of nonsteroidal aromatase inhibitor (Fadrazole bearing imidazole structure) [7]. However, this compound still has some nonselective inhibitory activity with respect to progesterone, corticosterone, and aldosterone biosynthesis. Competitive nonsteroidal inhibitors can also be constructed with a triazole ring, which is found in the third generation of aromatase inhibitors [8–10]. Most of the nonsteroidal aromatase inhibitors of therapeutic importance act covalently bind to the substrate-binding site of aromatase by coordinate the heme iron [11–13]. Especially, the heterocyclic nitrogen atom of triazole and imidazole plays an important role by coordinating with the heme iron of the aromatase enzyme [12,13]. Some studies have shown that imidazole and triazole derivatives have promising aromatase inhibition [14–17].

Recent clinical studies have shown that aromatase inhibitors, especially the third-generation, are more effective than fulvestrant and tamoxifen because of their lower side effects and higher clinical efficacy. Nevertheless, the development of acquired resistance after prolonged AIs therapy, undesirable side effects (bone loss, cardiac events, increased rash, insomnia, headaches, and arthralgia) limits their use in clinical practice. Thus, the search for new potent molecules that impair cancer growth, strongly inhibit aromatase enzyme, and present fewer side effects is of major importance [18–21].

In the previous study, 3-[4-(5-methyl-1*H*-benzo[*d*]imidazol-2-yl)phenyl]-6- (substituted phenyl) -7H-[1,2,4] triazolo [3,4-b] [1,3,4]thiadiazines derivatives have been synthesized and promising compounds have been obtained that need further development as a new class of aromatase inhibitors [22]. In this study, new benzimidazole-triazolothiadiazine derivatives were synthesized and structure of these compounds was characterized by spectroscopic data. Their antiproliferative activities against MCF-7 were evaluated. To identify the possible modes of action, aromatase inhibition experiments were performed for the most active compounds against the MCF-7 cell line. Finally, in silico prediction of pharmacokinetic profiles (ADME) were calculated for physicochemical properties of these drug candidates.

2. Results and Discussion

2.1. Chemistry

Synthesis of the target compounds was accomplished according to the steps illustrated in Scheme 1. Substituents of the synthesized compounds (**5a–5p**) were shown in Table 1. The starting intermediated compound (**1a**,**1b**) was prepared by the reaction of 1,2-phenylenediamine and sodium metabisulfite with 4-formylbenzoic acid methyl ester as described in a previous study [23]. The ester derivative (**1a**,**1b**) reacted with hydrazine hydrate producing compounds **2a**, **2b** in a microwave synthesis reactor. Then, the compounds-(5-substitüe-1*H*-benzimidazol-2-yl)benzoic acid hydrazide derivatives (**2a**,**2b**) were treated with carbon disulfide in NaOH solution affording, after acidic treatment, compounds **3a**, **3b**. The reaction of compound **3a**, **3b** with hydrazine hydrate in the presence of ethanol produced compounds **4a**, **4b**. Then cyclization of compounds **4a**, **4b** with appropriate phenacyl bromide in the presence of anhydrous ethanol provided the desired final products (**5a–5p**). The characterization of these new derivatives was done by their spectroscopic (^{1}H NMR, ^{13}C NMR and Mass) data. ^{1}H NMR and ^{13}C NMR spectra of the synthesized compounds were observed at the expected region. Mass spectra (HRMS) of all the synthesized compounds showed that the molecular ion $[M + H]^+$ peak is in agreement with their molecular formula (see Supplementary Materials).

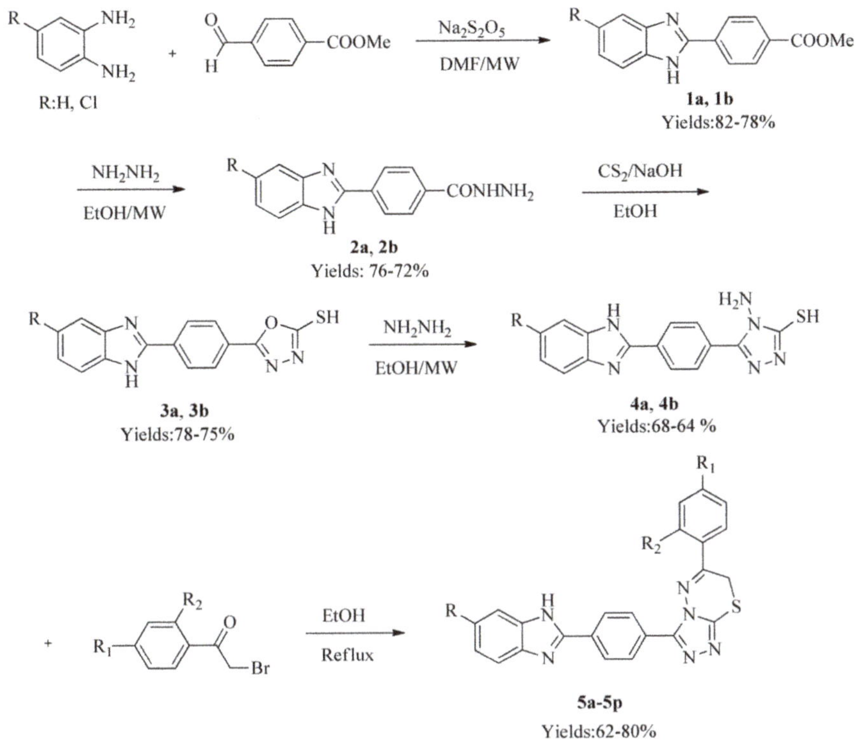

Scheme 1. The reaction sequence for the synthesis of the compounds (**5a–5p**).

Table 1. The synthesized compounds (**5a–5p**).

Comp.	R	R^1	R^2
5a	-H	-H	-H
5b	-H	-Cl	-H
5c	-H	-F	-H
5d	-H	$-CH_3$	-H
5e	-H	-CN	-H
5f	-H	-Br	-H
5g	-H	-F	-F
5h	-H	-Cl	-Cl
5i	-Cl	-H	-H
5j	-Cl	-Cl	-H
5k	-Cl	-F	-H
5l	-Cl	$-CH_3$	-H
5m	-Cl	-CN	-H
5n	-Cl	-Br	-H
5o	-Cl	-F	-F
5p	-Cl	-Cl	-Cl

2.2. Cytotoxicity Assay

The newly synthesized compounds were evaluated for their in vitro anticancer potential against MCF-7 breast cancer cell lines by MTT assay [24] using cisplatin as a reference standard. The 50% inhibitory concentration (IC_{50}) values were determined for these compounds. In addition, the cytotoxic activities of compounds **5c**, **5e**, **5k**, and **5m** were assessed against healthy NIH3T3 [25] cells, in order to express the selectivity toward carcinogenic cells. The IC_{50} values of test compounds were determined as the mean IC_{50} of 4 independent experiments. Results are presented in Table 2, as IC_{50} values are in μM and revealed that some of the tested compounds were remarkably more cytotoxic than the cisplatin against MCF-7 cell lines. Concerning MCF-7 cell line, the most potent compounds were the 4-cyano derivatives **5e** and **5m** with IC_{50} = 0.016 ± 0.001 and 0.018 ± 0.001 μM, respectively compared to IC_{50} = 0.020 ± 0.009 μM for the reference drug cisplatin. Furthermore, the most promising activity was observed for the compounds **5c** and **5k** bearing 4-fluorophenyl derivatives with IC_{50}= 0.119 ± 0.005 and 0.110 ± 0.005 μM, respectively compared to IC_{50} = 0.020 ± 0.009 μM for the reference drug cisplatin.

Table 2. IC_{50} (μM) values of compounds (**5a–5p**) (n = 4).

Comp.	MCF-7	NIH3T3
5a	0.142 ± 0.007	-
5b	0.0414 ± 0.001	-
5c	**0.119 ± 0.005**	**81.8 ± 2.4**
5d	0.194 ± 0.006	-
5e	**0.016 ± 0.001**	**≥1000**
5f	0.318 ± 0.019	-
5g	0.245 ± 0.004	-
5h	0.342 ± 0.017	-
5ı	0.205 ± 0.005	-
5j	0.258 ± 0.011	-
5k	**0.110 ± 0.005**	**77.6 ± 2.1**
5l	0.352 ± 0.019	-
5m	**0.018 ± 0.001**	**≥1000**
5n	0.264 ± 0.011	-
5o	0.373 ± 0.011	-
5p	0.147 ± 0.001	-
Cisplatin	**0.020 ± 0.009**	**≥1000**

Benzimidazole-triazolothiadiazine derivatives led to a promising increase in the anti-proliferative activity. The synthesized compounds can be divided into two groups as nonsubstituted benzimidazole and 5-chlorobenzimidazole. Test compounds showed variable activities against MCF-7. In particular, compounds **5e** and **5m** displayed the highest cytotoxic activity against MCF-7 cell line. The most active compounds **5e** and **5m** carried a 4-cyanophenyl substituent. The chlorine substituent in the fifth position (**5m**) of the benzimidazole ring did not significantly affect the activity. Compounds **5c** and **5k** carrying fluorine substituents in the fourth position of the phenyl ring showed lower activity than compounds **5e** and **5m** bearing cyano group in the fourth position of the phenyl ring.

2.3. Aromatase Inhibition Assay

The in vitro anti-aromatase activity of the most active compounds **5c**, **5e**, **5k,** and **5m** was valued using commercial fluorometric assay kit (Aromatase-CYP19A Inhibitor Screening kit, Bio Vision) with letrozole as the reference drug. Results are presented in Table 3. The IC_{50} values of compounds were in the sub-micromolar range (2.276 ± 0.106–0.03 2 ± 0.001 μM). The best value was shown by compound **5e** with IC_{50} value (0.032 ± 0.001 μM).

Table 3. IC_{50} (μM) values of compounds **5c**, **5e**, **5k**, **5m,** and letrozole.

Comp.	Aromatase Inhibition
5c	1.716 ± 0.042
5e	**0.032 ± 0.001**
5k	2.276 ± 0.106
5m	1.562 ± 0.064
Letrozole	**0.024 ± 0.001**

2.4. Molecular Docking

After the most active derivative was selected as compound **5e** according to in vitro aromatase enzyme inhibition assay and letrozole, molecular docking studies were performed to explain its binding modes with human aromatase enzyme active site. For this purpose, the crystal structure of human aromatase enzyme (PDB ID: 3EQM) [26] was retrieved from the Protein Data Bank server (www.pdb.org). The 2D and 3D docking poses of compound 5e are presented in Figures 1 and 2. The docking poses of letrozole are presented in Figures 3 and 4.

According to docking poses, it is understood that compound 5e displays compatible settlement with the enzyme active region. The benzimidazole ring in the structure forms two π–π interactions with Arg115 and Phe134. Also, it can be seen from 2D docking pose, this compound is in interaction with Hem molecules and Cys437 via its nitrogen atoms of triazolothiadiazine ring by salt bridge. There is another π–π interaction between 4-cyanophenyl ring and HEM molecule. The nitrogen atom of cyano group at C-4 position of phenyl ring interacts with hydroxyl of Ser314 doing hydrogen bonding. It is thought that this interaction is important for compound **5e** in terms of explaining its inhibitory activity. It is seen that the presence of an electron withdrawing group such as cyano at this position is a positive contribution to the activity.

As seen in the docking poses, letrozole is settled down in the enzyme active site properly. For letrozole, it is seen that benzonitrile ring creates π–π interaction with HEM molecule. Another π–π interaction is observed between 1,2,4-triazole ring and Arg115. Also, this 1,2,4-triazole ring forms two hydrogen bonds via its second and fourth nitrogen atoms with amino groups of Ala438 and Arg115, respectively.

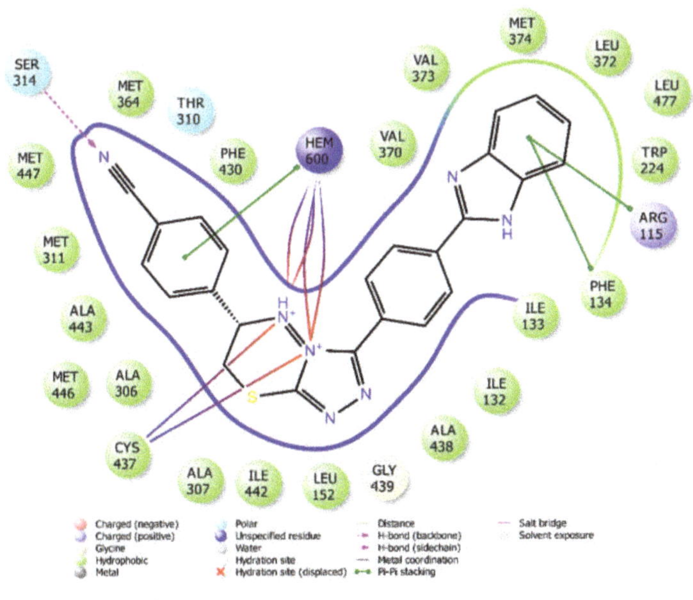

Figure 1. Two-dimensional interaction mode of compound **5e** in the enzyme active site (Human aromatase PDB Code: 3EQM).

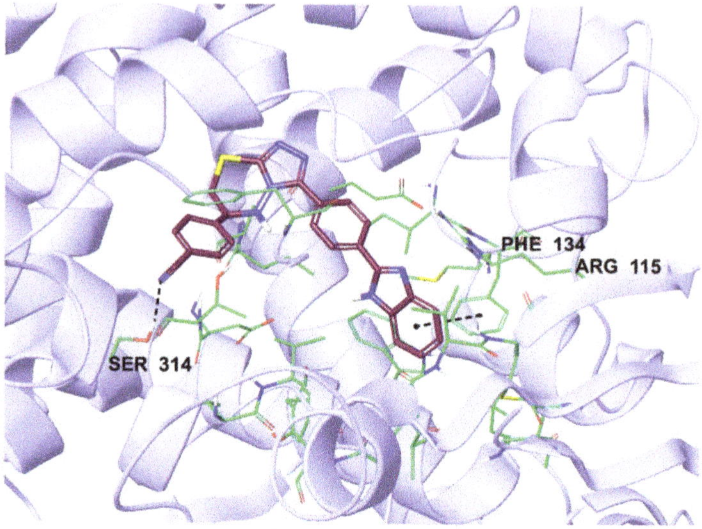

Figure 2. The interacting mode of compound **5e** in the active region of human aromatase. The inhibitor, colored with maroon, and the important residues, colored with purple, in the active site of the enzyme are presented by tube model.

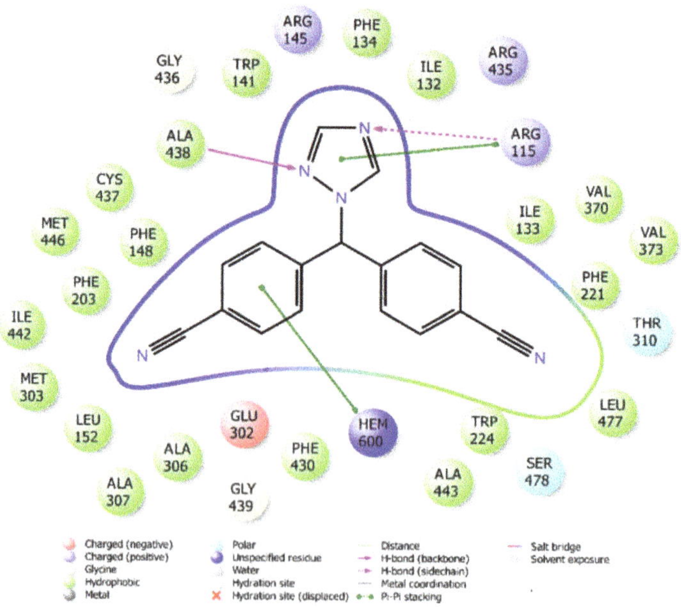

Figure 3. Two-dimensional interaction mode of letrozole in the enzyme active site (Human aromatase PDB Code: 3EQM).

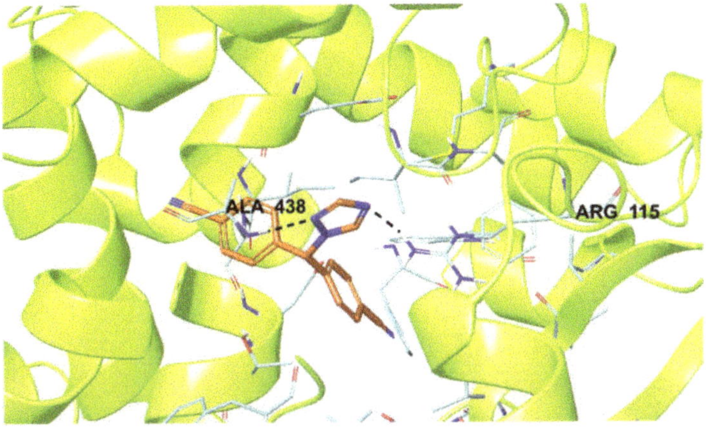

Figure 4. The interacting mode of letrozole in the active region of human aromatase. The inhibitor, colored with orange, and the important residues, colored with turquoise, in the active site of the enzyme are presented by tube model.

2.5. Theoretical Determination of ADME Properties

QikProp allows to provide acceptable ranges for comparing the predicted properties of compounds with those of 95% of known drugs and estimate drug-likeness properties. The drug-likeness of a compound was assessed according to Jorgensen's rule of three [27], which regards PCaco (>22 nm/s), logS (>−5.7), primary metabolites (PM) (<7), and Lipinski's rule of five [28], which considers number of hydrogen bond acceptors (≤10) and donors (≤5), molecular weight (<500 Da), and octanol/water partition coefficient (≤5).

Table 4. presents the predicted ADME properties of all compounds. According to Lipinski's rule of five and Jorgensen's rule of three, all compounds (**5a–5p**) are in accordance with the rule by causing no more than one violation. Consequently, according to predictions of ADME properties, it can be suggested that the active compounds may have a good pharmacokinetic profile.

Table 4. Calculated ADME parameters.

Comp.	MW	RB	DM	MV	DHB	AHB	PSA	logP	logS	PCaco	logBB	PMDCK	PM	CNS	%HOA	VRF	VRT
5a	408.48	0	13.539	1230.58	1	4.5	66.81	5.226	−7.577	1145.907	−0.361	1066.282	2	0	100	1	1
5b	442.925	0	11.536	1274.691	1	4.5	66.813	5.722	−8.323	1145.871	−0.207	2630.568	2	0	100	1	1
5c	426.47	0	11.294	1246.689	1	4.5	66.815	5.463	−7.944	1145.883	−0.255	1928.038	2	0	100	1	1
5d	422.506	0	14.175	1289.517	1	4.5	66.81	5.533	−8.145	1145.907	−0.388	1066.282	3	0	100	1	1
5e	433.489	1	7.968	1297.278	1	6	92.606	4.468	−8.534	236.976	−1.255	194.119	2	−2	95.607	0	1
5f	487.376	0	11.913	1283.596	1	4.5	66.813	5.799	−8.439	1145.858	−0.198	2828.358	2	0	100	1	1
5g	444.461	0	12.598	1251.337	1	4.5	65.595	5.544	−8.02	1167.271	−0.2	2431.401	2	0	100	1	1
5h	477.37	0	12.709	1287.743	1	4.5	64.6	5.897	−8.422	1199.257	−0.099	3927.141	2	0	100	1	1
5i	442.925	0	12.609	1274.528	1	4.5	66.806	5.721	−8.321	1145.207	−0.208	2625.13	2	0	100	1	1
5j	477.37	0	10.697	1318.639	1	4.5	66.809	6.217	−9.068	1145.171	−0.054	6476.318	2	0	100	1	1
5k	460.915	0	10.455	1290.637	1	4.5	66.811	5.957	−8.688	1145.183	−0.101	4746.726	2	0	100	1	1
5l	456.951	0	13.229	1333.465	1	4.5	66.806	6.028	−8.891	1145.207	−0.235	2625.13	3	0	100	1	1
5m	467.934	1	7.409	1341.226	1	6	92.602	4.96	−9.274	236.832	−1.117	477.911	2	−2	100	0	1
5n	521.821	0	11.046	1327.544	1	4.5	66.809	6.294	−9.184	1145.158	−0.044	6963.267	2	0	92.631	2	1
5o	478.906	0	11.99	1295.266	1	4.5	65.591	6.038	−8.764	1166.535	−0.046	5985.589	2	0	100	1	1
5p	511.815	0	12.056	1331.676	1	4.5	64.597	6.391	−9.166	1198.487	0.055	9667.877	2	1	93.553	2	1

MW: Molecular weight **RB:** Number of rotatable bonds (recommended value: 0-15) **DM:** Computed dipole moment (recommended value: 1-12.5) **MV:** Total solvent-accessible volume (recommended value: 500-2000) **DHB:** Estimated number of hydrogen bond donors (recommended value: 0-6) **AHB:** Estimated number of hydrogen bond acceptors (recommended value: 2-20) **PSA:** Van der Waals surface area of polar nitrogen and oxygen atoms and carbonyl carbon atoms (recommended value: 7-200) **logP:** Predicted octanol/water partition coefficient (recommended value: -2-6.5) **logS:** Predicted aqueous solubility (recommended value: -6.5-0.5) **PCaco:** Predicted apparent Caco-2 cell permeability (recommended value: <25 poor, >500 great) **logBB:** Predicted brain/blood partition coefficient (recommended value: -3-1.2) **PMDCK:** Predicted apparent MDCK cell permeability (recommended value: <25 poor, >500 great) **PM:** Number of likely metabolic reactions (recommended value: 1-8) **CNS:** Predicted central nervous system activity (recommended value: −2 (inactive), +2 (active)) **%HOA:** Predicted human oral absorption percent (recommended value: >80% is high, <25% is poor) **VRF:** Number of violations of Lipinski's rule of five. The rules are: MW < 500, logP < 5, DHB ≤ 5, AHB≤ 10, Positive PSA value. **VRT:** Number of violations of Jorgensen's rule of three. The three rules are: logS > -5.7, PCaco > 22 nm/s, PM < 7.

3. Materials and Methods

3.1. Chemistry

Whole chemicals employed in the synthetic procedure were purchased from Sigma-Aldrich Chemicals (Sigma-Aldrich Corp., St. Louis, MO, USA) or Merck Chemicals (Merck KGaA, Darmstadt, Germany). Melting points of the obtained compounds were determined by MP90 digital melting point apparatus (Mettler Toledo, OH, USA) and were uncorrected. Microwave syntheses were realized by using a Monowave 300 high-performance microwave reactor (Anton-Paar, Austria). ^{1}H NMR and ^{13}C NMR spectra of the synthesized compounds were registered by a Bruker 300 MHz and 75 MHz digital FT-NMR spectrometer (Bruker Bioscience, Billerica, MA, USA) in DMSO-d_6, respectively. Splitting patterns were designated as follows: s: singlet; d: doublet; t: triplet; m: multiplet in the NMR spectra. Coupling constants (*J*) were reported as Hertz. M+1 peaks were determined by Shimadzu LC/MS ITTOF system (Shimadzu, Tokyo, Japan). All reactions were monitored by thin-layer chromatography (TLC) using Silica Gel 60 F254 TLC plates (Merck KGaA, Darmstadt, Germany).

3.1.1. Synthesis of 4-(5-substitüe-1H-benz[d]imidazol-2-yl)benzoic Acid Methyl Ester (**1a**,**1b**)

Yields: 82–78%. 4-(5-substitüe-1*H*-benz[*d*]imidazol-2-yl)benzoic acid hydrazide derivatives (**2a**,**2b**) (yields: 76–72%) and 5-[4-(5(6)-substituted-1*H*-benz[*d*]imidazol-2-yl)phenyl]-1,3,4-oxadiazole-2-thiol derivatives (**3a**,**3b**) (yields: 78–7 %) were prepared following the reported procedures [23].

3.1.2. 4-Amino-5-(4-(5-substitüe-1H-benzo[d]imidazol-2-yl)phenyl)-4H-1,2,4-triazole-3-thiol (**4a**,**4b**)

Compound **3a** or **3b** (0.02 mol) was dissolved in ethanol. Hydrazine hydrate (5 mL) was added to the mixture. The reaction mixture was heated at 240 °C and 10 bar for 10 min under microwave synthesis reactor (Anton-Paar Monowave 300). After the reaction ended, the product was washed with water, dried, and crystallized using ethanol (96%) [22]. Yields: 68–64%.

3.1.3. 3-(4-(5-substitüe-1H-benzo[d]imidazol-2-yl)phenyl)-6-(substitüephenyl)-7H-[1,2,4]triazole [3,4-b][1,3,4]thiadiazine (**5a**–**5p**)

Compound **4a** or **4b** (0.003 mol) and appropriate phenacyl bromide (0.003 mol) in ethanol was heated under reflux for 8 h. After the reaction ended, the product was filtered and dried [22].

3-(4-(1H-benzo[d]imidazol-2-yl)phenyl)-6-phenyl-7H-[1,2,4]triazole[3,4-b][1,3,4] thiadiazine (5a): Yields: 77%. Mp 230.7–232.9 °C. ^{1}H-NMR (300 MHz, DMSO-d_6): δ = 4.52 (2H, s, -CH_2-), 7.52-7.55 (2H, m, aromatic CH), 7.59–7.67 (3H, m, Aromatic CH), 7.83–7.86 (2H, m, aromatic CH), 8.06–8.09 (2H, m, aromatic CH), 8.34 (2H, d, *J*=8.67 Hz, 1,4-disubstitutedbenzene), 8.43 (2H, d, *J*=8.64 Hz, 1,4-disubstitutedbenzene). ^{13}C-NMR (75 MHz, DMSO-d6): δ = 23.31, 114.89, 125.84, 126.55, 128.13, 128.50, 129.13, 129.65, 132.64, 133.78, 134.17, 143.96, 149.21, 151.22, 156.82, 163.07. HRMS (*m*/*z*): $[M + H]^+$ calcd for $C_{23}H_{16}N_6S$: 409.1224; found: 409.1230.

3-(4-(1H-benzo[d]imidazol-2-yl)phenyl)-6-(4-chlorophenyl)-7H-[1,2,4]triazole[3,4-b][1,3,4] thiadiazine (**5b**): Yields: 72%. Mp 190.9–192.6 °C. ^{1}H-NMR (300 MHz, DMSO-d_6): δ = 4.50 (2H, s, -CH_2-), 7.56–7.59 (2H, m, aromatic CH), 7.65–7.70 (3H, m, aromatic CH), 7.86–7.89 (2H, m, aromatic CH), 8.06–8.09 (2H, m, aromatic CH), 8.31 (2H, d, *J*=8.61 Hz, 1,4-disubstitutedbenzene), 8.57 (2H, d, *J*=8.61 Hz, 1,4-Disubstitutedbenzene). ^{13}C-NMR (75 MHz, DMSO-d_6): δ=23.27, 114.67, 125.49, 126.35, 128.87, 129.11, 129.32, 129.45, 129.73, 129.92, 130.11, 130.71, 132.62, 133.01, 137.50, 144.01, 148.52, 151.17, 156.87. HRMS (*m*/*z*): $[M + H]^+$ calcd for $C_{23}H_{15}N_6SCl$: 443.0843; found: 443.0840.

3-(4-(1*H*-benzo[*d*]imidazol-2-yl)phenyl)-6-(4-fluorophenyl)-7H-[1,2,4]triazole[3,4-b][1,3,4] thiadiazine (**5c**): Yields: 69%. Mp 274.2–277.1 °C. ^{1}H-NMR (300 MHz, DMSO-d_6): δ = 4.50 (2H, s, -CH_2-), 7.12 (1H, s, aromatic CH), 7.29 (1H, s, aromatic CH), 7.46–7.52 (4H, m, aromatic CH), 7.81–7.84 (2H, m, aromatic CH), 8.33 (2H, d, *J* = 8.64 Hz, 1,4-disubstitutedbenzene), 8.51 (2H, d, J=8.76 Hz, 1,4-disubstitutedbenzene).

^{13}C-NMR (75 MHz, DMSO-d_6): δ = 23.27, 114.32, 114.90, 116.76 (d, J = 21.98 Hz), 126.40, 127.68, 127.96, 128.43, 128.56, 128.69, 128.87, 128.95, 130.32 (d, J = 2.77 Hz), 130.78 (d, J = 8.43 Hz), 134.60, 143.66, 151.30, 155.71, 166.36 (d, J = 249.53 Hz). HRMS (m/z): $[M + H]^+$ calcd for $C_{23}H_{15}N_6FS$: 427.1137; found: 427.1136.

3-(4-(1H-benzo[d]imidazol-2-yl)phenyl)-6-(4-methylphenyl)-7H-[1,2,4]triazole[3,4-b][1,3,4] thiadiazine (**5d**): Yields: 70%. Mp 207.5–209.1 °C. ^{1}H-NMR (300 MHz, DMSO-d_6): δ = 2.41 (3H, s, CH_3), 4.49 (2H, s, -CH_2-), 7.41 (2H, d, J = 8.13 Hz, 1,4-disubstitutedbenzene), 7.52–7.55 (2H, m, benzimidazole CH), 7.83–7.86 (2H, m, benzimidazole CH), 7.97 (2H, d, J = 8.25 Hz, 1,4-disubstitutedbenzene), 8.33 (2H, d, J = 8.58 Hz, 1,4-disubstitutedbenzene), 8.43 (2H, d, J = 8.61 Hz, 1,4-disubstitutedbenzene). ^{13}C-NMR (75 MHz, DMSO-d_6): δ=21.55, 23.18, 114.86, 125.84, 126.42, 128.08, 128.24, 128.47, 129.02, 129.22, 129.71, 130.20, 130.90, 134.11, 142.96, 144.00, 147.35, 149.13, 151.07, 156.69. HRMS (m/z): $[M + H]^+$ calcd for $C_{24}H_{18}N_6S$: 423.1381; found: 423.1386.

3-(4-(1H-benzo[d]imidazol-2-yl)phenyl)-6-(4-cyanophenyl)-7H-[1,2,4]triazole[3,4-b][1,3,4] thiadiazine (**5e**): Yields: 68%. Mp 259.3–263.1 °C. ^{1}H-NMR (300 MHz, DMSO-d_6): δ = 4.53 (2H, s, -CH_2-), 7.56–7.58 (2H, m, benzimidazole CH), 7.85–7.88 (2H, m, benzimidazole CH), 8.06 (2H, d, J = 8.37 Hz, 1,4-disubstitutedbenzene), 8.21 (2H, d, J = 8.46 Hz, 1,4-disubstitutedbenzene), 8.30 (2H, d, J = 8.49 Hz, 1,4-disubstitutedbenzene), 8.42 (2H, d, J = 8.49 Hz, 1,4-disubstitutedbenzene). ^{13}C-NMR (75 MHz, DMSO-d_6): δ = 23.35, 114.58, 114.71, 118.68, 125.51, 126.39, 127.20, 128.48, 128.74, 128.87, 129.19, 129.43, 129.84, 133.03, 133.44, 137.97, 143.97, 148.72, 151.25, 155.45. HRMS (m/z): $[M + H]^+$ calcd for $C_{24}H_{15}N_7S$: 434.1186; found: 434.1182.

3-(4-(1H-benzo[d]imidazol-2-yl)phenyl)-6-(4-bromophenyl)-7H-[1,2,4]triazole[3,4-b][1,3,4] thiadiazine (**5f**): Yields: 74%. Mp 284.8–286.2 °C. ^{1}H-NMR (300 MHz, DMSO-d_6): δ = 4.50 (2H, s, -CH_2-), 7.53–7.56 (3H, m, aromatic CH), 7.81–7.85 (3H, m, aromatic CH), 7.99–8.02 (2H, m, aromatic CH), 8.32 (2H, d, J = 8.64 Hz, 1,4-disubstitutedbenzene), 8.42 (2H, d, J = 8.70 Hz, 1,4-disubstitutedbenzene). ^{13}C-NMR (75 MHz, DMSO-d_6): δ = 23.20, 114.91, 125.04, 125.96, 126.50, 127.03, 128.56, 129.19, 130.09, 130.90, 132.37, 132.67, 133.00, 142.94, 143.96, 147.34, 149.17, 151.22, 155.95. HRMS (m/z): $[M + H]^+$ calcd for $C_{23}H_{15}N_6SBr$: 487.0311; found: 487.0335.

3-(4-(1H-benzo[d]imidazol-2-yl)phenyl)-6-(2,4-difluorohenyl)-7H-[1,2,4]triazole [3,4-b][1,3,4] thiadiazine (**5g**): Yields: 72%. Mp 208.5–210.7 °C. ^{1}H-NMR (300 MHz, DMSO-d_6): δ = 4.42 (2H, s, -CH_2-), 7.46–7.49 (4H, m, aromatic CH), 7.79–7.82 (3H, m, aromatic CH), 7.29–7.35 (2H, m, aromatic CH), 8.45–8.51 (2H, m, aromatic CH). ^{13}C-NMR (75 MHz, DMSO-d_6): δ = 25.37, 113.01 (dd, J_1 = 3.08 Hz, J_2 = 21.45 Hz), 106.08 (d, J = 26.01 Hz), 114.05, 114.45, 119.72 (dd, J_1 = 3.02 Hz, J_2 = 11.51 Hz), 126.56, 127.17, 128.25, 128.75, 129.15, 132.37, 132.67 (dd, J_1 = 3.12 Hz, J_2 = 10.36 Hz), 134.23, 135.55, 143.74, 148.22, 151.06, 153.70, 164.66 (d, J = 251.18 Hz), 164.83 (d, J = 250.91 Hz). HRMS (m/z): $[M + H]^+$ calcd for $C_{23}H_{14}N_6SF_2$: 445.1053; found: 445.1041.

3-(4-(1H-benzo[d]imidazol-2-yl)phenyl)-6-(2,4-dichlorophenyl)-7H-[1,2,4]triazole[3,4-b] [1,3,4] thiadiazine (**5h**): Yields: 77%. Mp 190.7–193.4 °C. ^{1}H-NMR (300 MHz, DMSO-d_6): δ = 4.36 (2H, s, -CH_2-), 7.34–7.37 (3H, m, aromatic CH), 7.65 (1H, dd, J_1 = 2.04 Hz, J_2 = 8.34 Hz, aromatic CH), 7.70–7.73 (2H, m, aromatic CH), 7.78–7.81 (1H, m, aromatic CH), 8.20 (2H, d, J = 8.64 Hz, 1,4-disubstitutedbenzene), 8.40 (2H, d, J = 8.61 Hz, 1,4-disubstitutedbenzene). ^{13}C-NMR (75 MHz, DMSO-d_6): δ = 26.23, 115.05, 115.32, 124.22, 124.72, 126.99, 127.78, 128.08, 128.29, 128.57, 128.96, 129.59, 130.38, 132.93, 133.05, 133.74, 136.86, 143.65, 149.92, 151.62, 156.53. HRMS (m/z): $[M + H]^+$ calcd for $C_{23}H_{14}N_6SCl_2$: 477.0457; found: 477.0450.

3-(4-(5-chloro-1H-benzo[d]imidazol-2-yl)phenyl)-6-phenyl-7H-[1,2,4]triazole[3,4-b][1,3,4] thiadiazine (**5i**): Yields: 80%. Mp: 247.3–249.6 °C. ^{1}H-NMR (300 MHz, DMSO-d_6): δ = 4.50 (2H, s, -CH_2-), 7.49 (1H, dd, J_1 = 1.89 Hz, J_2=8.67 Hz, aromatic CH), 7.59–7.62 (3H, m, aromatic CH), 7.78–7.84 (2H, m, aromatic

CH), 8.03–8.06 (2H, m, aromatic CH), 8.27 (2H, d, *J* = 8.64 Hz, 1,4-disubstitutedbenzene), 8.37 (2H, d, *J* = 8.64 Hz, 1,4-disubstitutedbenzene). ^{13}C-NMR (75 MHz, DMSO-d_6): δ = 23.32, 114.60, 116.29, 125.95, 126.40, 128.11, 128.47, 128.97, 129.20, 129.63, 129.94, 132.62, 133.27, 133.71, 135.39, 143.97, 150.42, 151.04, 156.76. HRMS (*m/z*): [M + H]$^+$ calcd for $C_{23}H_{15}N_6SCl$: 443.0826; found: 443.0840.

3-(4-(5-chloro-1*H*-benzo[*d*]imidazol-2-yl)phenyl)-6-(4-chlorophenyl)-7H-[1,2,4]triazole [3,4-b][1,3,4] thiadiazine (**5j**): Yields: 70%. Mp: 226.0–228.9 °C. ^{1}H-NMR (300 MHz, DMSO-d_6): δ = 4.46 (2H, s, -CH_2-), 7.33–7.37 (1H, m, benzimidazole CH), 7.63 (2H, d, *J* = 8.61 Hz, 1,4-disubstitutedbenzene), 7.68–7.73 (2H, m, benzimidazole CH), 8.04 (2H, d, *J* = 8.61 Hz, 1,4-disubstitutedbenzene), 8.19 (2H, d, *J* = 8.46 Hz, 1,4-disubstitutedbenzene), 8.39 (2H, d, *J* = 8.43 Hz, 1,4-disubstitutedbenzene). ^{13}C-NMR (75 MHz, DMSO-d_6): δ = 23.13, 115.14, 116.51, 124.18, 127.79, 128.20, 128.33, 128.83, 128.98, 129.19, 129.68, 129.87, 130.51, 131.57, 132.60, 137.42, 143.58, 151.40, 155.59. HRMS (*m/z*): [M + H]$^+$ calcd for $C_{23}H_{14}N_6SCl_2$: 477.0427; found: 477.0450.

3-(4-(5-chloro-1*H*-benzo[*d*]imidazol-2-yl)phenyl)-6-(4-fluorophenyl)-7H-[1,2,4]triazole [3,4-b][1,3,4] thiadiazine (**5k**): Yields: 71%. Mp: 249.1–250.9 °C. ^{1}H-NMR (300 MHz, DMSO-d_6): δ = 4.48 (2H, s, -CH_2-), 7.38 (1H, dd, J_1 = 1.98 Hz, J_2 = 8.58 Hz, aromatic CH), 7.46–7.48 (2H, m, aromatic CH), 7.71–7.74 (1H, m, aromatic CH), 7.77 (1H, s, aromatic CH), 8.12–8.14 (2H, m, aromatic CH), 8.25 (2H, d, *J* = 8.64 Hz, 1,4-disubstitutedbenzene), 8.40 (2H, d, *J* = 8.61 Hz, 1,4-disubstitutedbenzene). ^{13}C-NMR (75 MHz, DMSO-d_6): δ = 23.45, 114.95, 116.45, 116.77 (d, *J* = 22.09 Hz), 124.83, 128.07, 128.21, 128.39, 128.84, 128.89, 130.30 (d, *J* = 2.99 Hz), 130.85 (d, *J* = 8.93 Hz), 135.26, 137.58, 143.69, 150.99, 151.27, 155.73, 164.82 (d, *J* = 249.42 Hz). HRMS (*m/z*): [M + H]$^+$ calcd for $C_{23}H_{14}N_6FSCl$: 461.0741; found: 461.0746.

3-(4-(5-chloro-1*H*-benzo[*d*]imidazol-2-yl)phenyl)-6-(4-methylphenyl)-7H-[1,2,4]triazole [3,4-b][1,3,4] thiadiazine (**5l**): Yields: 65%. Mp: 250.7–252.3 °C. ^{1}H-NMR (300 MHz, DMSO-d_6): δ = 4.46 (2H, s, -CH2-), 7.40 (2H, d, *J* = 8.07 Hz, 1,4-disubstitutedbenzene), 7.45 (1H, dd, J_1 = 1.95 Hz, J_2 = 8.67 Hz, benzimidazole CH), 7.76–7.79 (1H, m, benzimidazole CH), 7.82–7.83 (1H, m, benzimidazole CH), 7.95 (2H, d, *J* = 8.31 Hz, 1,4-disubstitutedbenzene), 8.28 (2H, d, *J* = 8.67 Hz, 1,4-disubstitutedbenzene), 8.37 (2H, d, *J* = 8.67 Hz, 1,4-disubstitutedbenzene). ^{13}C-NMR (75 MHz, DMSO-d_6): δ = 21.54, 23.15, 114.88, 116.44, 125.26, 127.74, 128.08, 128.21, 128.95, 129.24, 129.72, 130.21, 130.90, 134.62, 136.89, 142.95, 143.90, 150.99, 151.15, 156.66. HRMS (*m/z*): [M + H]$^+$ calcd for $C_{24}H_{17}N_6SCl$: 457.0994; found: 457.0997.

3-(4-(5-chloro-1*H*-benzo[*d*]imidazol-2-yl)phenyl)-6-(4-cyanophenyl)-7H-[1,2,4]triazole [3,4-b][1,3,4] thiadiazine (**5m**): Yields: 62%. Mp: 254.0–255.7 °C. ^{1}H-NMR (300 MHz, DMSO-d_6): δ = 4.53 (2H, s, -CH_2-), 7.50 (1H, dd, J_1 = 1.95 Hz, J_2 = 8.70 Hz, benzimidazole CH), 7.85–7.86 (1H, m, aromatic CH), 8.06–8.08 (3H, m, aromatic CH), 8.21 (2H, d, *J* = 8.61 Hz, 1,4-disubstitutedbenzene), 8.26 (2H, d, *J* = 8.64 Hz, 1,4-disubstitutedbenzene), 8.38 (2H, d, *J* = 8.64 Hz, 1,4-disubstitutedbenzene). ^{13}C-NMR (75 MHz, DMSO-d_6): δ = 23.30, 114.57, 114.71, 118.70, 125.83, 126.85, 128.48, 128.86, 129.11, 129.37, 129.81, 133.46, 133.58, 135.73, 137.98, 143.88, 150.56, 151.33, 155.41. HRMS (*m/z*): [M + H]$^+$ calcd for $C_{24}H_{14}N_7SCl$: 468.0782; found: 468.0793.

3-(4-(5-chloro-1*H*-benzo[*d*]imidazol-2-yl)phenyl)-6-(4-bromophenyl)-7H-[1,2,4]triazole [3,4-b][1,3,4] thiadiazine (**5n**): Yields: 76%. Mp: 243.4–247.3 °C. ^{1}H-NMR (300 MHz, DMSO-d_6): δ = 4.48 (2H, s, -CH_2-), 7.43 (1H, dd, J_1 = 1.98 Hz, J_2 = 8.67 Hz, benzimidazole CH), 7.75 (1H, s, aromatic CH), 7.80–7.82 (3H, m, aromatic CH), 7.99 (2H, d, *J* = 8.70 Hz, 1,4-disubstitutedbenzene), 8.26 (2H, d, *J* = 8.58 Hz, 1,4-disubstitutedbenzene), 8.37 (2H, d, *J* = 8.64 Hz, 1,4-disubstitutedbenzene). ^{13}C-NMR (75 MHz, DMSO-d_6): δ=23.14, 115.01, 116.52, 124.92, 126.45, 128.10, 129.05, 130.07, 131.76, 132.00, 132.15, 132.67, 133.00, 141.45, 143.77, 148.89, 149.69, 151.39, 155.91. HRMS (*m/z*): [M + H]$^+$ calcd for $C_{23}H_{14}N_6SClBr$: 520.9930; found: 520.9945.

3-(4-(5-chloro-1*H*-benzo[*d*]imidazol-2-yl)phenyl)-6-(2,4-difluorohenyl)-7H-[1,2,4]triazole [3,4-b][1,3,4] thiadiazine (**5o**): Yields: 66%. Mp: 182.2–185.0 °C. ^{1}H-NMR (300 MHz, DMSO-d_6): δ = 4.39 (2H, s,

-CH_2-), 7.28–7.34 (1H, m, aromatic CH), 7.42–7.48 (1H, m, aromatic CH), 7.48–7.52 (2H, m, aromatic CH), 7.77–7.83 (2H, m, aromatic CH), 7.93–8.01 (1H, m, aromatic CH), 8.25 (2H, d, J = 8.64 Hz, 1,4-disubstitutedbenzene), 8.44 (2H, d, J = 8.58 Hz, 1,4-disubstitutedbenzene). ^{13}C-NMR (75 MHz, DMSO-d_6): δ = 25.31, 105.76 (d, J = 26.01 Hz), 106.28, 113.19 (dd, J_1 = 2.63 Hz, J_2 = 20.86 Hz), 114.74, 116.39, 119.76 (dd, J_1 = 3.73 Hz, J_2 = 7.83 Hz), 125.45, 127.49, 128.32, 128.94, 129.14, 129.40, 132.71 (dd, J_1 = 3.21 Hz, J_2 = 9.80 Hz), 134.22, 143.80, 151.60, 151.26, 153.78, 161.28 (d, J = 252.62 Hz), 164.46 (d, J = 256.22 Hz). HRMS (m/z): $[M + H]^+$ calcd for $C_{23}H_{13}N_6F_2SCl$: 479.0632; found: 479.0652.

3-(4-(5-chloro-1*H*-benzo[*d*]imidazol-2-yl)phenyl)-6-(2,4-dichlorophenyl)-7H-[1,2,4]triazole [3,4-b][1,3,4] thiadiazine (**5p**): Yields: 68%. Mp: 114.4–116.5 °C. ^{1}H-NMR (300 MHz, DMSO-d_6): δ = 4.35 (2H, s, -CH_2-), 7.25 (1H, dd, J_1 = 1.74 Hz, J_2 = 8.52 Hz, aromatic CH), 7.65 (2H, dd, J_1 = 2.07 Hz, J_2 = 8.34 Hz, aromatic CH), 7.88 (2H, d, J = 8.34 Hz, aromatic CH), 7.90 (1H, m, aromatic CH), 8.16 (2H, d, J = 8.61 Hz, 1,4-disubstitutedbenzene), 8.32 (2H, d, J = 8.58 Hz, 1,4-disubstitutedbenzene). ^{13}C-NMR (75 MHz, DMSO-d_6): δ = 26.33, 106.76, 125.55, 127.29, 127.35, 128.58, 128.90, 129.64, 130.37, 131.63, 132.35, 132.96, 133.06, 133.44, 133.77, 136.56, 136.84, 143.51, 149.25, 151.77, 156.48. HRMS (m/z): $[M + H]^+$ calcd for $C_{23}H_{13}N_6SCl_3$: 511.0037; found: 511.0061.

3.2. Cytotoxicity Assay

The anticancer activity of compounds **5a–5p** were screened according to the MTT assays. The MTT assays were performed as previously described [24,25]. Cisplatin was used as the reference drug for the MCF7 cell line in the MTT assays.

3.3. Aromatase Inhibition Assay

This method was carried out according to the kit procedure (Bio Vision, Aromatase (CYP19A) Inhibitor Screening Kit (Fluorometric)). The compounds were dissolved in dimethyl sulfoxide (DMSO) and added to the assay in at least seven concentrations ranging from 10^{-3}–10^{-9} M. The recombinant human aromatase stock was prepared by reconstituting with 1 mL of aromatase assay buffer. The contents were mixed thoroughly by vortexing to obtain a homogeneous solution and the solution was transferred to a 15-mL conical tube. The volume was brought to 2450 µL with the aromatase assay buffer and 50 µl of NADPH production system (100X) was added for a final total volume of 2.5 mL. Letrozole was used as a positive inhibition control. For solvent control, a small aliquot of aromatase assay buffer containing the organic solvent was used to dissolve the test compounds that were prepared. Reaction wells containing test compounds and the corresponding no inhibitor controls (which may also serve as a solvent control), as well as a background control (containing no fluorogenic Aromatase Substrate) were prepared. The plate was incubated for at least 10 min at 37 °C to allow test ligands to interact with the aromatase. After incubation, 30 µl of the aromatase substrate/NADP+ mixture was added to each well. Immediately (within 1 min), the fluorescence at Ex/Em = 488/527 nm was measured.

3.4. Molecular Docking

A structure-based in silico procedure was applied to discover the binding modes of compound 5e to human aromatase enzyme active site. The crystal structures of human aromatase (PDB ID: 3EQM) [26] was retrieved from the Protein Data Bank server (www.pdb.org).

The structures of ligands were built using the Schrödinger Maestro [29] interface and then were submitted to the Protein Preparation Wizard protocol of the Schrödinger Suite 2016 Update 2 [30]. The ligands were prepared by the LigPrep 3.8 [31] to assign the protonation states at pH 7.4 ± 1.0 and the atom types, correctly. Bond orders were assigned, and hydrogen atoms were added to the structures. The grid generation was formed using Glide 7.1 [32]. Flexible docking runs were performed with single precision docking mode (SP).

3.5. Theoretical Determination of ADME Properties

Physicochemical parameters of obtained compounds (**5a–5p**) were evaluated by using QikProp 4.8 [33].

4. Conclusions

Inhibition of aromatase has proved to be an effective approach for the treatment of hormone-dependent breast cancer in the postmenopausal women. Imidazole and triazole groups are important rings for the development new potent aromatase inhibitors with high affinity for the enzyme. A series of benzimidazole-triazolothiadiazine derivatives have been synthesized with different substituents at benzimidazole and phenyl rings. The newly synthesized compounds were tested for their anti-cancer properties against human breast cancer cell line (MCF-7). The synthesized compounds were then tested in in vitro aromatase assay and two compounds (**5e** and **5m**) exhibited activity similar to letrozole.

Supplementary Materials: The following are available online.

Author Contributions: Z.A.K., Y.Ö., conceived and designed the experiments; D.O., U.A.Ç. performed the synthesis; S.L. performed analysis studies; B.N.S., U.A.Ç., and S.I. performed activity tests; D.O., U.A.Ç., B.N.S., B.K.Ç. wrote the paper. All authors have read and agreed to the published version of the manuscript.

Acknowledgments: This study was financially supported by Anadolu University Scientific Projects Fund, Project No: 1905S032.

Conflicts of Interest: The authors declare no conflict of interest.

References

1. Chamduang, C.; Pingaew, R.; Prachayasittikul, V.; Prachayasittikul, S.; Ruchirawat, S.; Prachayasittikul, V. Novel triazole-tetrahydroisoquinoline hybrids as human aromatase inhibitors. *Bioorg. Chem.* **2019**, *93*, 103327. [CrossRef] [PubMed]
2. Doiron, J.; Richard, R.; Touré, M.M.; Picot, N.; Richard, R.; Čuperlović-Culf, M.; Robichaud, G.A.; Touaibia, M. Synthesis and structure–activity relationship of 1-and 2-substituted-1, 2, 3-triazole letrozole-based analogues as aromatase inhibitors. *Eur. J. Med. Chem.* **2011**, *46*, 4010–4024. [CrossRef] [PubMed]
3. Henneberta, O.; Montes, M.; Favre-Reguillon, A.; Chermetted, H.; Ferroudc, C.; Mortin, R. Epimerase activity of the human 11β-hydroxysteroid dehydrogenase type 1 on 7-hydroxylated C19-steroids. *J. Steroid Biochem. Mol. Biol.* **2009**, *114*, 57–63. [CrossRef] [PubMed]
4. Leechaisit, R.; Pingaew, R.; Prachayasittikul, V.; Worachartcheewan, A.; Prachayasittikul, S.; Ruchirawat, S.; Prachayasittikul, V. Synthesis, molecular docking, and QSAR study of bis-sulfonamide derivatives as potential aromatase inhibitors. *Bioorg. Med. Chem.* **2019**, *27*, 115040. [CrossRef]
5. Brueggemeier, R.W.; Hackett, J.C.; Diaz-Cruz, E.S. Aromatase inhibitors in the treatment of breast cancer. *Endocr. Rev.* **2005**, *26*, 331–345. [CrossRef]
6. Cepa, M.M.; da Silva, E.J.T.; Correia-da-Silva, G.; Roleira, F.M.; Teixeira, N.A. Synthesis and biochemical studies of 17-substituted androst-3-enes and 3,4-epoxyandrostanes as aromatase inhibitors. *Steroids* **2008**, *73*, 1409–1415. [CrossRef]
7. Bonfield, K.; Amato, E.; Bankemper, T.; Agard, H.; Steller, J.; Keeler, J.M.; Roy, D.; McCallum, A.; Paula, S.; Ma, L. Development of a new class of aromatase inhibitors: Design, synthesis and inhibitory activity of 3-phenylchroman-4-one (isoflavanone) derivatives. *Bioorg. Med. Chem.* **2012**, *20*, 2603–2613. [CrossRef]
8. Rampogu, S.; Baek, A.; Bavi, R.S.; Son, M.; Cao, G.P.; Kumar, R.; Park, C.; Zeb, A.; Rana, R.M.; Park, S.J.; et al. Identification of Novel Scaffolds with Dual Role as Antiepileptic and Anti-Breast Cancer. *IEEE/ACM Trans. Comput. Biol. Bioinform.* **2018**, *16*, 1663–1674. [CrossRef]
9. Trunet, P.F.; Vreeland, F.; Royce, C.; Chaudri, H.A.; Cooper, J.; Bhatnagar, A.S. Clinical use of aromatase inhibitors in the treatment of advanced breast cancer. *J. Steroid. Biochem. Mol. Biol.* **1997**, *61*, 241–245. [CrossRef]

10. Steele, R.E.; Mellor, L.B.; Sawyer, W.K.; Wasvary, J.M.; Browne, L.J. In vitro and in vivo studies demonstrating potent and selective estrogen inhibition with the nonsteroidal aromatase inhibitor CGS 16949A. *Steroids* **1987**, *50*, 147161. [CrossRef]
11. Kato, S.; Endoh, H.; Masuhiro, Y.; Kitamoto, T.; Uchiyama, S.; Sasaki, H.; Masushige, S.; Gotoh, Y.; Nishida, E.; Kawashima, H.; et al. Activation of the estrogen receptor through phosphorylation by mitogen-activated protein kinase. *Science* **1995**, *270*, 1491–1494. [CrossRef] [PubMed]
12. Sable, P.M.; Potey, L.C. Synthesis and antiproliferative activity of imidazole and triazole derivatives of flavonoids. *Pharm. Chem. J.* **2018**, *52*, 438–443. [CrossRef]
13. Gilardi, G.; Di Nardo, G. Heme iron centers in cytochrome P450: Structure and catalytic activity. *Rend. Lincei* **2017**, *28*, 159–167. [CrossRef]
14. Asadi, P.; Khodarahmi, G.; Farrokhpour, H.; Hassanzadeh, F.; Saghaei, L. Quantum mechanical/molecular mechanical and docking study of the novel analogues based on hybridization of common pharmacophores as potential anti-breast cancer agents. *Res. Pharm. Sci.* **2017**, *12*, 233.
15. Mojaddami, A.; Sakhteman, A.; Fereidoonnezhad, M.; Faghih, Z.; Najdian, A.; Khabnadideh, S.; Rezaei, Z. Binding mode of triazole derivatives as aromatase inhibitors based on docking, protein ligand interaction fingerprinting, and molecular dynamics simulation studies. *Res. Pharm. Sci.* **2017**, *12*, 21. [CrossRef]
16. Song, Z.; Liu, Y.; Dai, Z.; Liu, W.; Zhao, K.; Zhang, T.; Dai, Y. Synthesis and aromatase inhibitory evaluation of 4-N-nitrophenyl substituted amino-4H-1,2,4-triazole derivatives. *Bioorg. Med. Chem.* **2016**, *24*, 4723–4730. [CrossRef]
17. Adhikari, N.; Amin, S.A.; Jha, T.; Gayen, S. Integrating regression and classification-based QSARs with molecular docking analyses to explore the structure-antiaromatase activity relationships of letrozole-based analogs. *Can. J. Chem.* **2017**, *95*, 1285–1295. [CrossRef]
18. Prachayasittikul, V.; Pingaew, R.; Worachartcheewan, A.; Sitthimonchai, S.; Nantasenamat, C.; Prachayasittikul, S.; Ruchirawat, S.; Prachayasittikul, V. Aromatase inhibitory activity of 1, 4-naphthoquinone derivatives and QSAR study. *EXCLI J.* **2017**, *16*, 714.
19. Augusto, T.V.; Amaral, C.; Varela, C.L.; Bernardo, F.; da Silva, E.T.; Roleira, F.F.; Costa, S.; Teixeria, N.; Correia-da-Silva, G. Effects of new C6-substituted steroidal aromatase inhibitors in hormone-sensitive breast cancer cells: Cell death mechanisms and modulation of estrogen and androgen receptors. *J. Steroid. Biochem. Mol. Biol.* **2019**, *195*, 105486. [CrossRef]
20. Shoombuatong, W.; Schaduangrat, N.; Nantasenamat, C. Towards understanding aromatase inhibitory activity via QSAR modeling. *EXCLI J.* **2018**, *17*, 688.
21. Prior, A.M.; Yu, X.; Park, E.J.; Kondratyuk, T.P.; Lin, Y.; Pezzuto, J.M.; Sun, D. Structure-activity relationships and docking studies of synthetic 2-arylindole derivatives determined with aromatase and quinone reductase 1. *Bioorg. Med. Chem. Lett.* **2017**, *27*, 5393–5399. [CrossRef] [PubMed]
22. Acar Çevik, U.; Sağlık, B.N.; Osmaniye, D.; Levent, S.; Kaya Çavuşoğlu, B.; Karaduman, A.B.; Ozkay, Y.; Kaplancıklı, Z.A. Synthesis and docking study of benzimidazole–triazolothiadiazine hybrids as aromatase inhibitors. *Arch. Pharm.* **2020**, e2000008. [CrossRef] [PubMed]
23. Çevik, U.A.; Osmaniye, D.; Çavuşoğlu, B.K.; Sağlik, B.N.; Levent, S.; Ilgin, S.; Ozkay, Y.; Kaplancikli, Z.A. Synthesis of novel benzimidazole–oxadiazole derivatives as potent anticancer activity. *Med. Chem. Res.* **2019**, *28*, 2252–2261. [CrossRef]
24. Evren, A.E.; Yurttaş, L.; Eksellı, B.; Akalın-Cıftcı, G. Novel tri-substituted thiazoles bearing piperazine ring: Synthesis and evaluation of their anticancer activity. *Lett. Drug Des. Discov.* **2019**, *16*, 547–555. [CrossRef]
25. Çevik, U.A.; Sağlık, B.N.; Ardıç, C.M.; Özkay, Y.; Atlı, Ö. Synthesis and evaluation of new benzimidazole derivatives with hydrazone moiety as anticancer agents. *Turk. J. Biochem.* **2018**, *43*, 151–158. [CrossRef]
26. Ghosh, D.; Griswold, J.; Erman, M.; Pangborn, W. Structural basis for androgen specificity and oestrogen synthesis in human aromatase. *Nature* **2009**, *457*, 219. [CrossRef]
27. Jorgensen, W.L.; Duffy, E.M. Prediction of drug solubility from structure. *Adv. Drug Deliv. Rev.* **2002**, *54*, 355–366. [CrossRef]
28. Lipinski, C.A.; Lombardo, F.; Dominy, B.W.; Feeney, P.J. Experimental and computational approaches to estimate solubility and permeability in drug discovery and development settings. *Adv. Drug Deliv. Rev.* **1997**, *23*, 3–25. [CrossRef]
29. *Maestro*, version 10.6; Schrödinger, LLC: New York, NY, USA, 2016.
30. *The Schrödinger Suite 2016 Update 2*; Schrödinger, LLC: New York, NY, USA, 2016.

31. *LigPrep*, version 3.8; Schrödinger, LLC: New York, NY, USA, 2016.
32. *Glide*, version 7.1; Schrödinger, LLC: New York, NY, USA, 2016.
33. *QikProp*, version 4.8; Schrödinger, LLC: New York, NY, USA, 2016.

Sample Availability: Samples of the compounds **5a–5p** are available from the authors.

molecules

MDPI

Article

Synthesis, Characterization and Biological Evaluation of Novel Dihydropyranoindoles Improving the Anticancer Effects of HDAC Inhibitors

Murat Bingul [1,2,3], Greg M. Arndt [2,4], Glenn M. Marshall [2,5], Belamy B. Cheung [2,6,*], Naresh Kumar [1,*] and David StC. Black [1,*]

1 School of Chemistry, UNSW Sydney, Sydney, NSW 2052, Australia; muratbingul1983@gmail.com
2 Children's Cancer Institute, Lowy Cancer Research Centre, UNSW Sydney, Sydney, NSW 2052, Australia; garndt@ccia.unsw.edu.au (G.M.A.); gmarshall@ccia.unsw.edu.au (G.M.M.)
3 School of Pharmacy, Dicle University, 21280 Diyarbakır, Turkey
4 ACRF Drug Discovery Centre for Childhood Cancer, Children's Cancer Institute, Lowy Cancer Research Centre, UNSW Sydney, Sydney, NSW 2052, Australia
5 Kids Cancer Centre, Sydney Children's Hospital, Randwick, NSW 2031, Australia
6 School of Women's and Children's Health, UNSW Sydney, Sydney, NSW 2052, Australia
* Correspondence: bcheung@ccia.unsw.edu.au (B.B.C.); n.kumar@unsw.edu.au (N.K.); d.black@unsw.edu.au (D.S.B.); Tel.: +61-2-9385-2450 (B.B.C.); +61-2-9385-4698 (N.K.); +61-2-9385-4657 (D.S.B.)

Academic Editor: Qiao-Hong Chen
Received: 28 February 2020; Accepted: 16 March 2020; Published: 18 March 2020

Abstract: The dihydropyranoindole scaffold was identified as a promising target for improving the anti-cancer activity of HDAC inhibitors from the preliminary screening of a library of compounds. A suitable methodology has been developed for the preparation of novel dihydropyranoindoles via the Hemetsberger indole synthesis using azido-phenylacrylates, derived from the reaction of corresponding alkynyl-benzaldehydes with methyl azidoacetate, followed by thermal cyclization in high boiling solvents. Anti-cancer activity of all the newly synthesized compounds was evaluated against the SH-SY5Y and Kelly neuroblastoma cells as well as the MDA-MB-231 and MCF-7 breast adenocarcinoma cell lines. Biological studies showed that the tetracyclic systems had significant cytotoxic activity at higher concentration against the neuroblastoma cancer cells. More importantly, these systems, at the lower concentration, considerably enhanced the SAHA toxicity. In addition to that, the toxicity of designated systems on the healthy human cells was found to be significantly less than the cancer cells.

Keywords: dihydropyranoindole; anticancer; HDAC inhibitors; neuroblastoma; breast cancer

1. Introduction

Chemotherapy is one of the most widely used treatments for high-risk cancer patients [1,2]. A range of well-known agents, namely Doxorubicin, Cyclophosphamide, Etoposide have been used to combat various cancers in modern chemotherapeutic therapy [3,4]. However, a major problem faced in chemotherapy is resistance to commonly-used anti-cancer drugs [5]. Therefore, development of novel anti-cancer chemotherapeutic agents is of utmost importance in the area of drug discovery and development.

The histone deacetylase (HDAC) inhibitors are a class of chemotherapeutic agents that hold promise in cancer therapy [6,7]. HDAC inhibitors have been reported to suppress cell proliferation and angiogenesis, induce cell differentiation and promote apoptosis in a number of cancer cell types [8,9]. Suberoylanilide hydroxamic acid (SAHA) is the first HDAC inhibitor to obtain meet FDA approval [10], and has been considered to be a highly promising anticancer therapeutic agent due to its potent cytotoxic effect on a number of tumor cell types as well as low toxicity towards healthy normal cells [11–13]. However, single agent treatment with SAHA has been found to be ineffective against several cancers [14,15]. On the other hand, the combination of SAHA with other chemotherapeutic agents with different mechanisms of action has been considered to be more promising as the drug resistance caused by single agent therapies may be overcome [14,16]. Due to the significant cytotoxic effects observed during clinical trials of SAHA in combination with a variety of chemotherapeutic agents, many synthetic compounds have been produced and screened to identify molecules capable of enhancing the cytotoxic activity of SAHA, while producing fewer side effects.

In order to provide a basis for this study, a subset (10,560 compounds) of the Walter & Eliza Hall Institute (WEHI) compound library was screened to identify molecules that can act synergistically with a clinical dose of SAHA to overcome drug resistance in SAHA-resistant MDA-MB-231 breast cancer cell lines [17]. The compounds that reduced viability to <40% in the presence of SAHA but to >70% in the absence of SAHA, with a difference of at least 55% between the two conditions have been identified as hit molecules for their SAHA enhancing capability [17]. A structural analysis of the hit molecules demonstrated that the main structural feature to be the presence of 5- or 6-membered fused heterocyclic systems, most commonly containing one or more nitrogen atoms. Furthermore, these fused systems typically involved 3 or 4 conjoined rings. Due to the ongoing experiments regarding the hit molecules, the structures of these compounds are not discussed in this manuscript.

Identification of New Target Molecules

The starting point of the current work was the selection of a range of compounds exhibiting structural similarity to the hits from compound library in order to expand the structural diversity of the screening set. The six related monomeric dihydropyranoindoles **1–3** and dimeric furoquinolines **4–6** were selected in order to understand the effect of the indole and quinoline structures, as well as the fused dihydropyran and furan rings, on biological activities (Figure 1). The molecules were tested against SH-SY5Y neuroblastoma and MDA-MB-231 breast cancer cell lines, using the Alamar blue (Resazurin) assay [18] to measure the cell viability. The same screening conditions were used with WEHI screening. Briefly, the designated cells were exposed to 1 μM SAHA, 10 μM compound and the combination of SAHA and compound for 72 h.

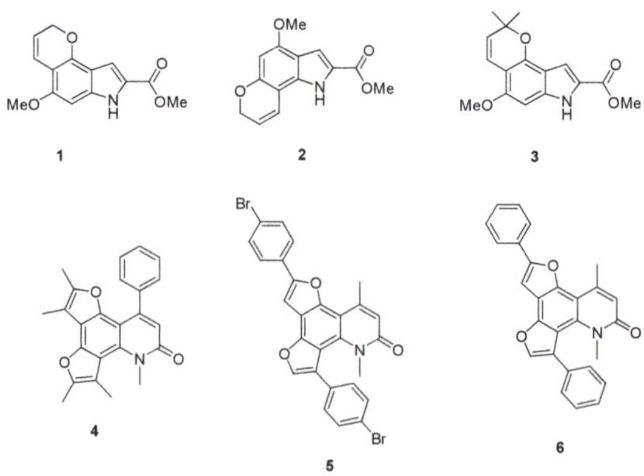

Figure 1. Six compounds from the NK library.

The in vitro assays revealed that the MDA-MB-231 were the more resistant cell lines than the SH-SY5Y cell lines for the single and combination treatments of all compounds. The compounds **5** and **6**, analogues of quinolines, displayed the lowest reduction on SH-SY5Y cell viability and also no SAHA enhancement was found by the combination with SAHA (Figure S1A, see Supplementary

Materials). In the case of compound **6**, the single and combination treatments showed no inhibition of MDA-MB-231 cell viability, while the 20% and 5% of inhibitions were obtained with the treatment of compound **5** alone and combination with 1 μM SAHA (Figure S1B, see Supplementary Materials). The compound **4** was the most active ligand among the quinoline candidates, with 30% inhibition of SH-SY5Y cell viability in the absence of SAHA and 20% additional cytotoxic effect in the presence of SAHA (Figure S1A, see Supplementary Materials). The designated compound displayed 25% reduction on MDA-MB-231 cells, while no SAHA enhancement effect was obtained against the same cell line (Figure S1B, see Supplementary Materials).

Overall, **1**, **3** and **4** were determined as the most promising compounds as SAHA enhancer and it was concluded that the indole heterocyclic systems **1** and **3** were found to be a potential target for the SAHA enhancement with the higher differential values between in the absence and presence of SAHA In order to further validate these compounds **1**, **3** and **4** as viable lead structures, it was essential to determine their toxicity towards normal and non-malignant cells. The most effective ligands were screened against the MRC-5 normal human lung fibroblast cells, as described for cytotoxic assay. This screen showed that the toxicity of **3** was found to be greater than **1** and **4** proposing that specificity of **3** against the normal and cancer cells was not different (Figure S2, see Supplementary Materials). The single treatment of compound **3** showed the cytotoxic activity with the values of 33% and 28% reduction against the SH-SY5Y and MDA-MB-231 cells respectively, while the toxicity of this compound against the MRC-5 cells was 26% and 30% greater than the SH-SY5Y and MDA-MB-231 cancer cells. However, compounds **1** and **4** displayed non-toxic behavior on the MRC-5 healthy human cells with values of 103% and 98% viable cells.

Based on the results of screening against the cancer cells and toxicity study on normal cells, the indole heterocyclic system **1** was identified as promising leads for further development on the enhancement of SAHA activity and compound **1** was also determined to be non-toxic across the healthy human cells. The main work described in this manuscript focused on the synthesis, characterization and in vitro biological evaluation of a series of targeted compounds based on tricyclic and tetracyclic dihydropyrano derivatives. The effectiveness of the novel compounds as single agents and in combination with a clinical dose of SAHA was determined against neuroblastoma and breast cancer cells.

2. Results and Discussion

The preparation of dihydropyranoindole systems was achieved by two synthetic methods, and the generality of these pathways were discussed in this paper. 3,4-Dihydroxybenzaldehyde **7** has been given as an example for the representation of two possible methods which could be used for the preparation of the desired pyranoindole methyl 5,10-dihydro-7*H*-dipyrano [3,2-*e*:2′,3′-*g*]indole-6-carboxylate **10** (Figure 2). The first method was to prepare the compound **10** via methyl hydroxyindole-2-carboxylate **8** which could be prepared by the Hemetsberger indole synthesis [19]. Methyl hydroxyindole-2-carboxylate **8** on reacting with haloalkynes would give the alkyne indole-ether **9** which upon Claisen cyclization would afford the desired dihydropyranoindole **10**. As an alternative pathway, aryl ether benzaldehyde **11** would be prepared via simple alkylation of phenol **7** with haloalkynes and the Hemetsberger indole synthesis would then be applied to build the indole moiety. It is anticipated that thermal cyclization would yield the desired compound **10** in one step.

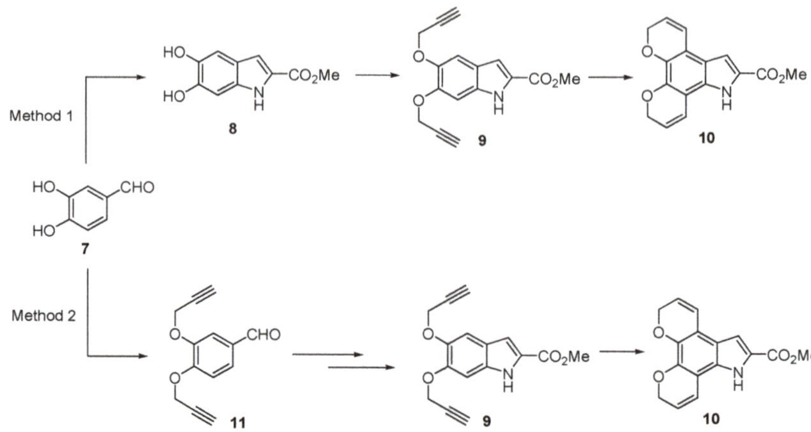

Figure 2. Two methods for the preparation of pyranoindole systems.

2.1. Preparation of Tetracyclic Dihydropyranoindole 10 Via (Method 1)

In the first synthetic method, methyl 5,6-dihydroxyindole-2-carboxylate **8** was generated via the Hemetsberger indole synthesis by benzyl-protected benzaldehydes and the subsequent deprotection afforded the corresponding hydroxyindoles. The 3,4-dihydroxybenzaldehyde **7** was reacted with benzyl bromide in the presence of potassium carbonate in acetone to afford the protected carbaldehydes **12** [20] in 88% yield (Scheme 1). Treatment of 3,4-dibenzyloxy benzaldehyde **12** with methyl azidoacetate in methanol, in the presence of strong basic environment (sodium methoxide) gave the vinyl azido intermediate **13** in 59% yield. Thermal decomposition of the arylazido **13** was performed by heating at reflux in xylene, generating the methyl 5,6-dibenzyloxyindole-2-carboxylate **14** in 71% yield. Hydrogenolysis of the benzyl group was carried out by treating the compound **14** with 5% *w/w* palladium on carbon under hydrogen atmosphere at room temperature for 2 h, to yield the desired methyl 5,6-dihydroxyindole-2-carboxylate **8** [21] in 77% yield. The dihydroxyindole **8** was reacted with propargyl bromide in the presence of potassium carbonate in acetone (Scheme 1). The desired dipropargyloxyindole intermediate **9** was prepared in 61% yield. The Claisen cyclization of **9** was explored in xylene, 1,2-dichlorobenzene and toluene. It was found that heating at reflux in chlorobenzene gave the optimum result in terms of the completion of the reaction as well as the yield and purity of the product. Using this approach, the desired tetracyclic dihydropyranoindole **10** was isolated in 51% yield.

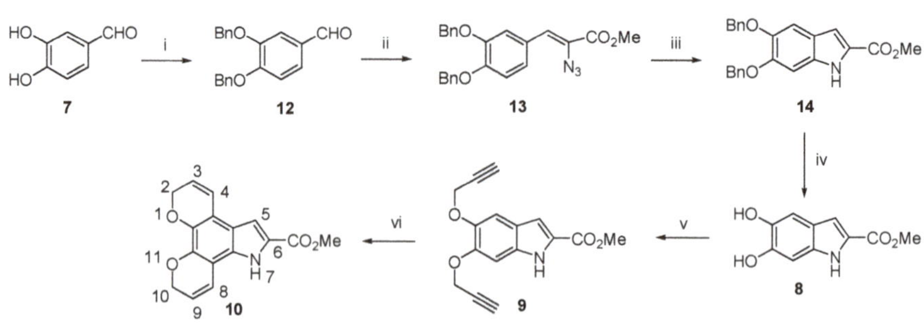

Scheme 1. Reagents and conditions: (i) Benzyl bromide, K_2CO_3, DMF, reflux, overnight; (ii) Methyl azidoacetate, NaOMe, anhyd. MeOH, <−10 °C, 4 h; (iii) Xylene, reflux, 2 h, (iv) 5% Pd/C, H_2, MeOH/THF, 2h, rt, (v) Propargyl bromide, K_2CO_3, acetone, reflux, 4 h, 61%, (vi) Chlorobenzene, reflux 2 h, 52%.

The possible reaction mechanism could be explained as in Figure 3. Methyl 5,6-bis(prop-2-yn-1-yloxy)-1*H*-indole-2-carboxylate **9** undergoes an initial Claisen rearrangement to generate intermediate **A**, which subsequently enolizes to produce 5,6-dihydroxyindole derivative (intermediate **B**). A double hydride shift in intermediate **B** gives the keto intermediate **C**, which undergoes an electrocyclic ring closing reaction to form methyl 5,10-dihydro-2*H*-dipyrano[3,2-*e*:2′,3′-*g*]indole-6-carboxylate **10**.

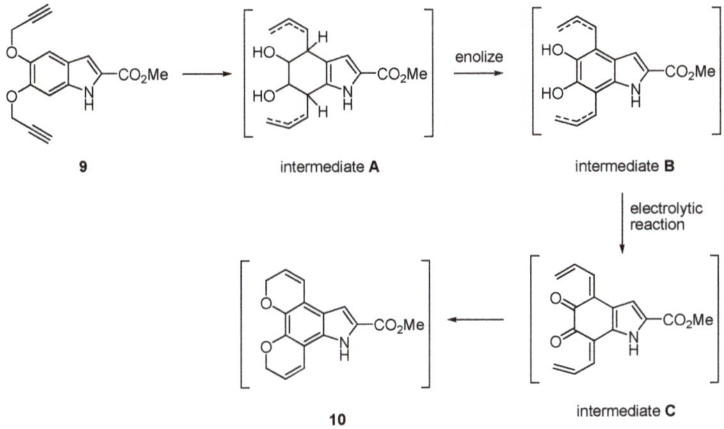

Figure 3. Possible reaction mechanism.

The ^{1}H-NMR spectrum of compound **10** in $CDCl_3$ showed a singlet at 3.96 ppm corresponding to the methyl ester protons, and two doublets of doublets at 4.91 and 4.96 ppm assigned to the two CH_2 groups. A multiplet at 5.87–5.97 ppm corresponded to H3 and H9, while another multiplet at 6.72–6.80 ppm corresponded to H4 and H8. Furthermore, H3 appeared as a doublet at 7.19 ppm and the NH proton appeared as a broad singlet at δ 8.85 ppm. The DEPT 135 spectrum of compound **10** confirmed the structure of the molecule, displaying the loss of two CH carbon signals as a result of cyclization of the alkyne group as well as the appearance of two negative signals at 64.68 and 64.72 ppm corresponding to the methylene carbon atoms in the product.

2.2. *Alternative Pathway for the Preparation of Tetracyclic Dihydropyranoindole 10 (Method 2)*

The alternative approach began with the reaction of 3,4-dihydroxybenzaldehyde **7** with propargyl bromide under basic conditions (potassium carbonate), which afforded the propargyloxy benzaldehyde **11** [22] in 87% yield. At this point, two synthetic strategies using benzaldehyde **11** as a key intermediate were envisioned (Scheme 2). The first route involved Claisen cyclization to build the dihydropyrano rings **15**, followed by the application of the Hemetsberger indole synthesis to construct the indole scaffold via the unsaturated azido intermediate **16** (Route 1). The cyclization of the aryl ether intermediate **11** was attempted by refluxing in high-boiling solvents such as xylene, toluene, 1,2-dichlorobenzene and chlorobenzene (Scheme 2). In all cases, the novel compound **15** was afforded in low yields, with unreacted starting material being recovered as the major product. The highest yield (35%) was obtained by the use of chlorobenzene. In order to synthesize the desired tetracyclic dihydropyranoindole **10**, the standard Hemetsberger indole synthesis was applied to new intermediate **15**. The condensation of benzaldehyde **15** with methyl azidoacetate was carried out at low temperature (ice-salt bath) in the presence of sodium methoxide. The addition of a small amount of crushed ice to the reaction mixture resulted in the isolation of azido ester **16** as an oily compound which was found to be unstable at room temperature, and was hence used in the next step without further purification. It was postulated that the presence of the dihydropyran ring caused the generation of an unstable azido ester intermediate.

Thermal cyclization of the azido ester **16** was performed by heating at reflux in xylene, which afforded the desired dihydropyranoindole **10** in 62% yield.

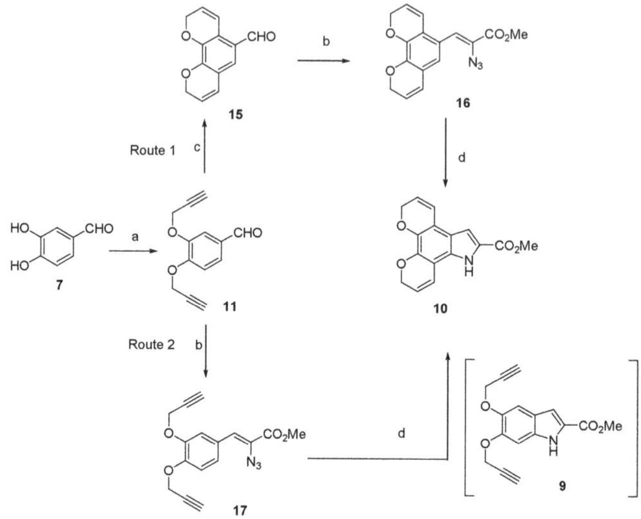

Scheme 2. Reagents and conditions: (a) Propargyl bromide, K_2CO_3, acetone, reflux, 4 h, (b) Methyl azidoacetate, metallic Na, anhyd. MeOH, <−10 °C, 2 h (c) Chlorobenzene, reflux, 2 h, (d) Xylene, reflux, 4 h.

In the second route, it was anticipated that the indole heterocyclic system could be constructed first, followed by the installation of dihydropyrano rings onto the indole moiety. Since the cyclization of both aryl ether and unsaturated azide ester moieties require refluxing conditions in a high-boiling solvent, it was predicted that the indole and dihydropyran rings could be prepared in one step from the key azide intermediate **17** (Route 2). The benzaldehyde **11** was condensed with methyl azidoacetate under strongly basic conditions at low temperature to generate the novel unsaturated stable azide intermediate **17** in 63% yield (Scheme 2). Since xylene was the common solvent for the generation of the indole moiety from the azido ester intermediate, the cyclization reaction was first carried out in refluxing xylene. As anticipated, the thermal cyclization of intermediate **17** resulted in both the decomposition of the azidocinnamate moiety and formation of the indole heterocyclic system, as well as the cyclization of the propargyloxy moiety to furnish the fused pyran ring in a single step. Hence, the desired tetracyclic dihydropyranoindole **10** was obtained in a yield of 72%.

Taken altogether, it was concluded that the first method is a less favorable synthetic pathway consisting of six steps to prepare the desired dihydropyranoindole and also generating the lowest of yield (51%) at the final step. In the case of the second method, route 1 was also found to be an unfavorable synthetic method for further synthesis due to the low-yielding cyclization step to generate the new tricyclic aldehyde **15**, the formation of the unstable azido intermediate **16** from the Hemestberger indole synthesis and the four step pathway for the desired dihydropyranoindole **10**. On the other hand, route 2 of the second strategy was deemed to be the most favorable synthetic route towards dihydropyranoindoles, as it contained three steps to afford the desired dihydropyranoindole and gave the highest yield of 72%. Thus, route 2 of the second method was chosen for further studies in this study.

2.3. The Preparation of Monomeric Hydropyrano System

The synthetic strategy (Route 2) was extended to the synthesis of indole systems containing a single fused dihydropyran ring. Hence, 4-hydroxy-3-methoxy benzaldehyde **18** was reacted with propargyl bromide in the presence of potassium carbonate to give aryl ether **19a** [23] in 84% yield, which was then reacted with methyl azidoacetate under basic conditions to give azidocinnamate **20a** in 76% yield (Scheme 3). Interestingly, thermal cyclization of the **20a** in xylene afforded the corresponding propargyloxy indole **21a** in the yield of 68% instead of the expected dihydropyranoindole system **22a**. Further heating of indole **21a** in refluxing chlorobenzene afforded the desired dihydropyranoindole **22a** in 77% yield.

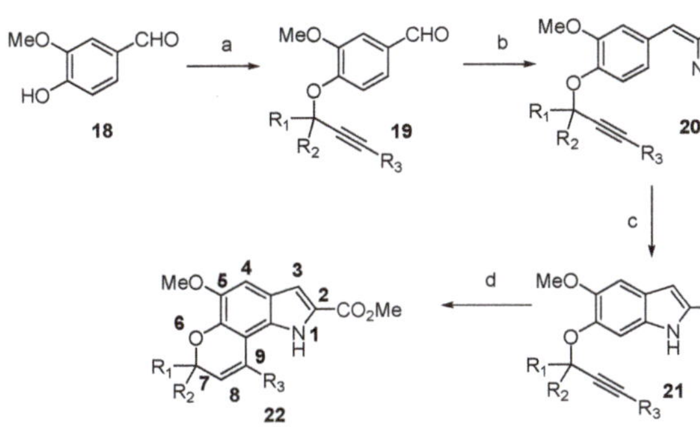

Compound	R_1	R_2	R_3
22a	H	H	H
22b	H	H	Me
22c	Me	Me	H

Scheme 3. Reagents and conditions: (a) Propargyl bromide or 3-chloro-3-methylbut-1-yne or 1-bromobut-2-yne, K_2CO_3, acetone, reflux, 4 h, (b) Methyl azidoacetate, metallic Na, anhyd. MeOH, <−10 °C, 2 h (c) Xylene, reflux, 4 h, (d) Chlorobenzene, reflux, 2 h.

The ^{1}H-NMR spectrum of compound **22a** in $CDCl_3$ showed the presence of two singlets at 3.94 ppm and 3.96 ppm corresponding to the methoxy and methyl ester protons, and doublets of doublets at 4.96 ppm corresponding to the CH_2 protons. Protons H8 and H9 appeared as multiplets in a range of 5.89–5.95 ppm and 6.73–6.79 ppm respectively. Furthermore, H4 appeared as a singlet at 7.02 ppm, while H3 was appeared as a doublet at 7.13 ppm (J = 2.1 Hz) due to its coupling with the NH proton, which resonated as a broad singlet at 8.94 ppm. The DEPT 135 spectrum showed the presence of a negative peak at 65.79 ppm corresponding to a methylene carbon atom. Furthermore, the spectrum revealed the absence of the alkyne CH signal due to cyclization of the alkyne moiety in indole **21a**.

The synthesis of tricyclic dihydropyranoindole systems containing methyl substituents on the fused dihydropyran ring at different positions was also investigated. To achieve this, 4-hydroxy-3-methoxybenzaldehyde **18** was reacted with 1-bromobut-2-yne and 3-chloro-3-methylbut-1-yne in the presence of potassium carbonate to give the aryl ether aldehydes **19b** [24] and **19c** [25] in 92% and 84% yields, respectively (Scheme 3). The aldehydes **19b** and **19c** were treated with methyl azidoacetate in the presence of sodium methoxide to give azidocinnamates **20b** and **20c** in yields of 61% and 62%. Finally, the thermal cyclization of the unsaturated azide **20b** and **20c** in refluxing xylene generated the desired product **22c** in 74% yields, while the indole ether **21b** was isolated in 67% yield. The desired dihydropyranoindole **22b** was obtained in 49% yield, by the further cyclization of **21b** in refluxing chlorobenzene.

In the ^{1}H-NMR spectrum of methyl 5-methoxy-7,7-dimethyl-1,7-dihydropyrano[2,3-*g*]indole-2-carboxylate **22c**,the two methyl groups appeared as a singlet at 1.55 ppm, while H8 and H9 appeared as doublet signals at 5.71 and 6.66 ppm (J = 9.7 Hz). Furthermore, H4 appeared as a singlet at 7.01 ppm and H3 appeared as a doublet at 7.13 ppm (J = 2.1 Hz), confirming that cyclization occurred at C7. In the ^{1}H-NMR spectrum of the cyclization product **22b**, the olefinic proton on the dihydropyran ring appeared as multiplet signals in the ranges of 5.65–5.68 ppm, due to coupling with the neighboring

CH_2 and CH_3 groups. For compound **22b**, the O-CH_2 protons resonated as a multiplet at 4.77 ppm and the methyl protons of the dihydropyran ring appeared as a quartet at 1.71 ppm.

The same synthetic route was applied to 3-hydroxy-4-methoxy benzaldehyde **23** in order to generate an analogue with the dihydropyran ring fused at a different position. Thus, hydroxybenzaldehyde **23** was reacted with propargyl bromide in the presence of potassium carbonate to generate the intermediate ether **24a** [26] in 87% yield, which upon reaction with methyl azidoacetate in strongly basic conditions gave the azidocinnamate **25a** in 72% yield (Scheme 4). Heating the azidocinnamate **25a** in refluxing xylene gave the propargyloxy indole **26a** in 73% yield, which was then cyclized in chlorobenzene to afford the desired dihydropyranoindole **27a** in 74% yield.

The ^{1}H-NMR spectrum of compound **27a** in $CDCl_3$ showed two singlet signals at 3.92 and 3.93 ppm corresponding to the methoxy and methyl ester protons, and doublets of doublets at 4.90 ppm corresponding to the CH_2 protons. H8 and H9 appeared as multiplets at 5.89–5.95 and 6.76–6.79 ppm respectively. The H4 appeared as a singlet at 6.77 ppm, while H1 appeared as a doublet at 7.17 ppm (J = 2.1 Hz). Moreover, the NH proton resonated as a broad singlet at δ 8.96 ppm. The formation of the desired dihydropyranoindole was further confirmed by DEPT 135 spectroscopy which revealed the presence of a negative peak at 65.71 ppm corresponding to the CH_2 group accompanied by the disappearance of the signal corresponding to the CH group of the starting alkyne **26a**.

3-Hydroxy-4-methoxybenzaldehyde **23** was further treated with 1-bromobut-2-yne and 3-chloro-3-methylbut-1-yne under basic conditions to generate the corresponding intermediates **24b** [24] and **24c** [27] 89% and 82% yields, respectively (Scheme 4). The aryl ethers **24b** and **24c** were condensed with methyl azidoacetate in the presence of sodium methoxide to generate the azidoacrylates **25b** and **25c** in 64% and 62% yields respectively. Thermal decomposition of the unsaturated azides **25b** gave the indole ethers **26b** in 71%, while the desired hydropyrano compound **27c** was directly isolated in 68% yield. The desired dihydropyranoindoles **27b** was obtained in 54% yields respectively, by the cyclization of **26b** and in refluxing chlorobenzene. It was also of interest to construct new dihydropyranoindole systems containing substituents other than a methyl group on a pyran ring. The haloalkyne, 3-phenylprop-2-yn-1-ol, was treated with 3-hydroxy-4-methoxybenzaldehyde **23** in the presence of potassium carbonate to produce the alkylated carbaldehyde **24d** in 92% yield (Scheme 4). The reaction between the aryl ether **24d** with methyl azidoacetate afforded the unsaturated azido ester **25d** in 64% yield. Finally, heating compound **25d** in refluxing xylene afforded the corresponding indole ether **26d** in 74% yield, which further underwent thermal cyclization in chlorobenzene to furnish the desired dihydropyranoindole **27d** in 81% yield.

In the ^{1}H-NMR spectrum of methyl 5-methoxy-7,7-dimethyl-3,7-dihydropyrano[3,2-*e*]indole-2-carboxylate **27c**, the two methyl groups appeared as a sharp singlet at 1.53 ppm. The H8 and H9 of the dihydropyran ring appeared as two doublets at 5.73 and 6.68 ppm that coupled to each other with a coupling constant of 9.7 Hz. H1 appeared as a doublet (J = 2.1 Hz) at 7.20 ppm while H4 was assigned as a singlet at 6.79 ppm. In the ^{1}H-NMR spectrum of the cyclization product **27b** the olefinic protons on the dihydropyran ring appeared as multiplet signals in range of 5.69–5.72, due to coupling with the neighboring CH_2 and CH_3 groups. The characteristic O-CH_2 protons resonated as a multiplet at 4.77 ppm, while the methyl group of the dihydropyran ring appeared at as a quartet 1.63 ppm. The ^{1}H-NMR spectrum of compound **27d** displayed the O-CH_2 protons as a doublet at 4.85 ppm with a coupling constant of 4.4 Hz, and the olefinic proton as a multiplet at 5.94–5.97 ppm. The aromatic protons of phenyl ring appeared as multiplet in the range of 7.34–7.44 ppm. The H4 and H1 appeared as two singlets at 5.98 and 6.88 ppm.

Similar attempts were made to the prepare methyl substituted tetracyclic dihydropyranoindole compounds from the 3,4-dihydroxybenzaldehyde **7**, 1-bromobut-2-yne and 3-chloro-3-methylbut-1-yne. The benzaldehyde **7** was alkylated with 2 equivalents of 1-bromobut-2-yne in the presence of potassium carbonate to generate the novel aryl ether **29** in 87% yield (Scheme 5). The benzaldehyde **29** was then treated with methyl azidoacetate under strongly basic conditions to generate the azido compound **30** in 63% yield, which subsequently underwent thermal decomposition in refluxing xylene to afford the indole ether **31** in 65% yield. However, the cyclization of **31** could not be achieved in a number of solvents, including chlorobenzene, toluene, xylene and 1,2-dichlorobenzene which resulted in the formation of decomposed reaction mixture. The reaction between 3,4-dihydroxybenzaldehyde **7** and 3-chloro-3-methylbut-1-yne was investigated in an attempt to produce the dipropargyloxybenzaldehyde intermediate **28** (Scheme 5). However, this reaction resulted in a black reaction mixture, presumably due to decomposition.

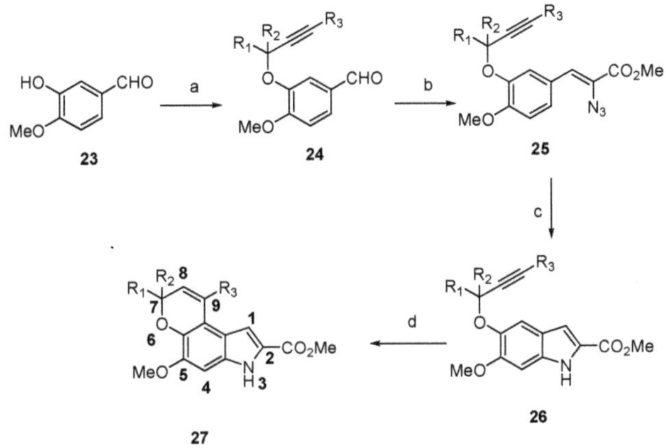

Compound	R_1	R_2	R_3
27a	H	H	H
27b	H	H	Me
27c	Me	Me	H
27d	H	H	Ph

Scheme 4. Reagents and conditions: (a) Propargyl bromide or 3-chloro-3-methylbut-1-yne or1-bromobut-2-yne or 3-phenylprop-2-yn-1-ol, K_2CO_3, acetone, reflux, 4 h, (b) Methyl azidoacetate, metallic Na, anhyd. MeOH, <−10 °C, 2 h (c) Xylene, reflux, 4 h, (d) Chlorobenzene, reflux, 2 h.

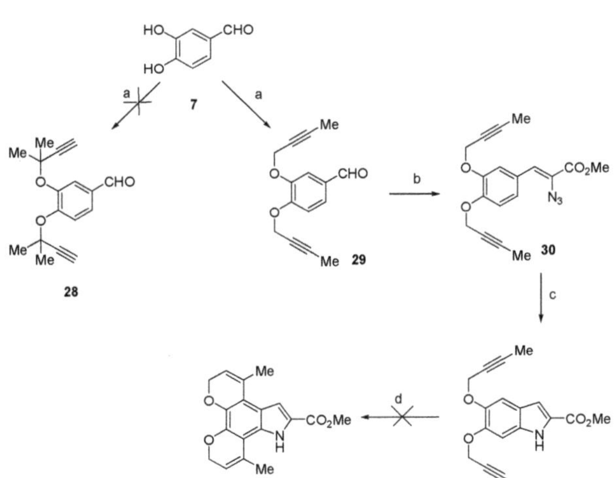

Scheme 5. Reagents and conditions: (a) 1-Bromobut-2-yne or 3-Chloro-3-methyl-1-butyne, K_2CO_3, acetone, reflux, 4 h, (b) methyl azidoacetate, metallic Na, anhydrous MeOH, −10 °C, 2 h (c) Xylene, reflux, 2 h, (d) Xylene, chlorobenzene, toluene, 1,2-dichlorobenzene reflux, overnight.

2.4. Biological Study

2.4.1. Preliminary Biological Screening of Dihydropyranoindoles for SAHA Enhancement Activity

Novel dihydropyranoindole analogues were screened to determine the levels of SAHA enhancement activity as well as their own cytotoxic profile against the SH-SY5Y and Kelly neuroblastoma cells and the MDA-MB-231 and MCF-7 breast adenocarcinoma cell lines using the Alamar blue (Resazurin) assay [18]. Briefly, the cells were allowed to attach for 24 h in a 96-well culture plate before being exposed to the ligands at a concentration of 10 μM in DMSO for 72 h, either in the presence or absence of SAHA. Comparative values for cell viability in each well were determined by a Wallac 1420 Victor III spectrophotometer, which measured light absorbance in each well at 570 nm. The mean and standard deviation (SD) values for each compound were calculated from at least three replicate experiments. The anticancer activity of the compounds was evaluated by comparison to a negative (DMSO) control. Figure 4 shows the tested novel dihydropyranoindoles synthesized in this study and the compound **33** was selected from the NK library. In this assay, the cell lines were exposed to SAHA, 10 μM of the compounds as well as the combination of SAHA with the compounds for 72 h.

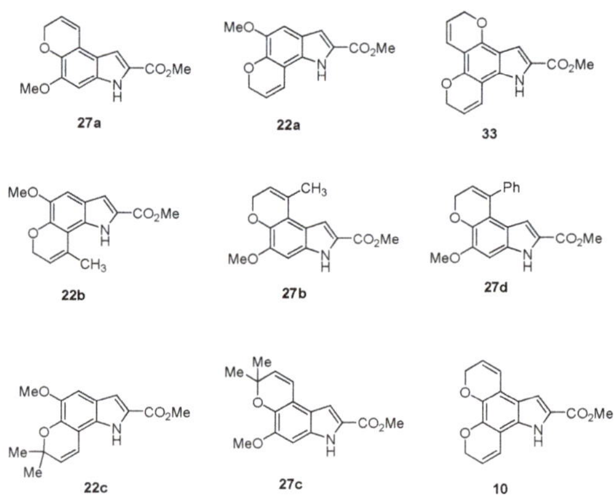

Figure 4. Synthesized and selected compounds.

According to the results from the screening, the neuroblastoma cells were found to be the more sensitive cells towards the treatment of new pyranoindoles, while these compounds showed a moderate effect on the breast cancer cell lines (Figures S3A,B and S4A,B, see Supplementary Materials). MDA-MB-231 cells were determined as the most resistant cell line for the single as well as the combination treatments (Figure S3A, see Supplementary Materials). The dihydropyranoindole **27c** exhibited the greatest cell viability inhibition with the values of 34% and 35% in the absence and presence of SAHA against the MDA-MB-231 cells. The SAHA enhancement was achieved by the additional reduction value of 20% across MDA-MB-231 viability. MCF-7 cells showed an identical pattern of sensitivity. However, most of the dihydropyranoindoles were able to reduce the viability by the value of 20% (Figure S3, see Supplementary Materials).

Compound **33** displayed the highest reduction with the 35% inhibition, while compounds **27c** and **22c** generated similar reductions with the values of 20% and 22% on the same cell line. Unfortunately the combination of pyranoindoles with 1 μM SAHA had very low SAHA enhancement by the average values of 5% across the MCF-7 cell lines.

It was observed that dihydropyranoindoles had a variety of impact on the viability of neuroblastoma cells (Kelly and SH-SY5Y) with the single and combination treatments (Figure S4A,B, see Supplementary Materials). Out of all the novel ligands synthesized, ligand **33** had the strongest cytotoxic activity with the reduction value of 50% at 10 μM, while ligands **27c** and **10** showed similar inhibition behaviors by the average reduction value of 32% against Kelly cells for the single treatment. The dihydropyranoindoles **27c** and **33** displayed the enhancement of SAHA cytotoxicity with the values of 24 and 22% respectively (Figure S4A, see Supplementary Materials). The value of 40% SAHA enhancement was obtained by the combination of compound **33**. However, the ligand **33** was considered as self-toxic compound due to the reduction value for the single treatment. The levels of individual cytotoxic efficiency against the SH-SY5Y were found to be higher than those observed on the Kelly cells (Figure S4B, see Supplementary Materials). The compounds **27d** and **10** showed the greatest cytotoxic activity reducing 44% and 56% of the cells respectively. Most importantly, the enhancement of SAHA activity was achieved by the treatment of almost all of the novel dihydropyranoindole analogues showing at least 20% additional reduction to SAHA cytotoxicity. Although the highest SAHA enhancement was obtained in the case of compound **10** with the value of 55%, it was not considered as a promising enhancer since the single treatment also generated the greatest reduction (56%) on the SH-SY5Y cell. The best enhancers were assigned as compounds **22a**, **27a**, **27c** and **33** with the reduction values of 25%, 29%, 30% and 31%respectively due to the lower toxicity but the higher enhancement effects on SAHA cytotoxicity.

2.4.2. Determination of SAHA Enhancement Activity of Selected Dihydropyranoindoles at Lower Concentrations

Since the levels of SAHA enhancement were found to be promising, further investigations were carried out using five different concentrations (0.01, 0.1, 1, 10, 20 μM), using the Alamar blue (Resazurin) assay [18] to determine whether the lower concentrations would provide higher enhancement of the SAHA cytotoxicity or the cytotoxic manner would be dependent on the dose usage. The initial screening revealed that the single treatment of dihydropyranoindoles **33**, **27c** and **10** at a concentration of 10 μM showed the highest cytotoxic efficiency against the Kelly cells. The designated compounds were treated with the Kelly cells by the combinations of 0.5 μM SAHA with the five different concentrations (0.01, 0.1, 1, 10, 20 μM) and the results are shown at Figure S5A,C (see Supplementary Materials). In general, the single treatment of these compounds provided lower cytotoxic activity at the concentrations of 0.01, 0.1 and 1 μM compared with the values at 10 μM and the cell viability differentials between the absence and presence of SAHA were greater than those at 10 μM concentrations, suggesting that the designated compounds behave as suitable SAHA enhancers (Figure S5A,C, see Supplementary Materials). Similar SAHA enhancement pattern was observed at the concentrations of 0.01, 0.1 and 1 μM for all three compounds, while the combination of 1 μM compound **27c** or **10** with the 0.5 μM SAHA revealed the best SAHA enhancement with the values of 24% and 25% additional inhibition (Figure S5B,C, see Supplementary Materials).

In addition to those two compounds, compound **33** showed the greatest viability differentials with the values of 61%, 63% and 65% at the concentrations of 0.01, 0.1 and 1 μM and the desired SAHA enhancement was observed for all the concentrations. The lowest concentration of compound **33** (0.01 μM) revealed a remarkable reduction with the value of 25%, while the best combination for the highest SAHA enhancement was determined as a 10:0.5 ratio of compound and SAHA with the additional reduction value of 55% (Figure S5 A, see Supplementary Materials). It was concluded that the highest cell viability differentials was achieved by the use of nanomolar concentrations in the case of all three compounds and the best SAHA enhancer was determined as compound **33**.

Similarly, in the case of the SH-SY5Y cell line, further investigations were undertaken with **27a**, **33** and **27c** which were chosen due to their highest additional effects on the SAHA cytotoxicity with the lower toxicity behavior in the absence of SAHA. Compound **10** was also explored to determine its cytotoxic behavior as well as the SAHA enhancement potential at lower concentrations. The combinations of 1 μM SAHA with the five different concentrations (0.01, 0.1, 1, 10, 20 μM) of designated compounds were treated with the SH-SY5Y cells and the results are shown at Figure S6A–D (see Supplementary Materials).

The SAHA enhancement pattern was found to be identical on SH-SY5Y value for all cases of combinations of **27a** with SAHA. The highest viability differential was obtained in the ratio 1:10 of SAHA to compound with the reduction value of 35% (Figure S6A, see Supplementary Materials). The dose-dependent pattern of single treatments of **33** and **27c** suggested that these compounds displayed higher toxicity at 20 μM with the values of 45% and 55% reductions. Furthermore, the combinations of these compounds at the concentrations of 0.01, 0.1 and 1 μM with SAHA enhanced the SAHA cytotoxicity in a similar manner and the best combinations were found to be as the ratio 1:10 of SAHA to compound with the additional reduction values of 28% and 33% (Figure S6B,C, see Supplementary Materials). The greatest cytotoxicity was obtained at a concentration of 20 μM of **10** alone with the reduction values of 88% on SH-SY5Y cell viability and the ratio of 1:20 SAHA to compound combination provided 94% cell death (Figure S6D, see Supplementary Materials).

More importantly, at the lower concentrations (0.01, 0.1 and 1 μM) of **10**, the cytotoxicity was found to be lower with the average reduction value of 25%. Encouragingly, the biggest cell viability differential was obtained at the ratio of 1:10 SAHA to compound with the value of 44%, and the greatest SAHA enhancement was also found as 37% at the same combination. It was concluded that **10** was the most cytotoxic compound at higher concentration (20 μM, 88% reduction) and also it was found to be the best SAHA enhancer at the ratio of 1:10 SAHA to compound combination.

2.4.3. SAR Study of Selected Dihydropyranoindoles

These observations suggested an important structure-activity relationship among **27a**, **33**, **27c** and **10**. That is, the incorporation of tetracyclic dihydropyranoindoles **33** and **10** resulted in lower cell viability reductions at higher concentrations (20 μM) and also this system was found to offer the best enhancement with the ratio of 1:10 SAHA to compound combinations against both neuroblastoma cancer cells (Kelly and SH-SY5Y). The SAR analysis revealed that the location of dihydropyran ring on the benzene ring was important for the cytotoxic efficiency of tricyclic dihydropyranoindoles, The compounds **27c**, an example of dihydropyrano[3,2-*e*]indole system, was found to be more potent than the dihydropyranoindole **22c** which is a member of dihydropyrano[2,3-*g*]indole scaffold against both neuroblastoma cells (Kelly and SH-SY5Y). In comparison of two tricyclic dihydropyranoindoles **27c** and **22c** at 20 μM, it was found that the compound **27c** reduced 20% more SH-SY5Y cell with the combination of 1 μM SAHA than compound **22c**, while the 20% SAHA enhancement was achieved using the combination of compound **27c** and SAHA but no SAHA enhancement was found with the compound **22c** in the case of Kelly cells. Furthermore, the dihydropyrano[2,3-*g*]indole analogues **22a** and **22b** displayed the lowest reduction on Kelly cells in the presence and absence of SAHA. Similar results were observed in the case of SH-SY5Y cells with the exception of 21% additional reduction on SAHA enhancement obtained by the use of **22a**.

2.4.4. Toxicity Study Against Normal Cells

While selected dihydropyranoindoles showed potent SAHA enhancement activity against Kelly and SH-SY5Y neuroblastoma and MCF-7 and MDA-MB-231 breast cancer cells, they must be markedly less toxic against the healthy cells in order to be considered as potential SAHA enhancers. Thus, the dihydropyranoindoles **27a**, **33**, **27c** and **10** were also examined for their toxicity effects on the MRC-5 and WI-38 lung fibroblasts in order to determine whether these compounds exhibited selectivity for tumor cells (Figure S7A–D, see Supplementary Materials). Comparison of the cytotoxic activity and toxicity levels of the dihydropyranoindoles against cancer cells and the healthy cells revealed that the cancer cells were more sensitive to the dihydropyranoindoles compared to the normal cells. The toxicity of 1 μM of SAHA reduced the viability of MRC-5 and WI-38 cells with the value of 9% and 24% respectively, while **27a** alone displayed a similar pattern of toxicity against normal cells with values of 10% for MRC-5 and 22% for WI-38 at a concentration of 10 μM (Figure S7A, see Supplementary Materials). The viability of MRC-5 and WI-38 were reduced 21% and 16%, 3% and 26% by the use of **33** and **10** alone (Figure S7B,C, see Supplementary Materials), while the highest toxicity levels were obtained in the case of **27c** with the reduction values of 20% and 43% (Figure S7D, see Supplementary Materials). The combination treatments were found to be quite identical to the reduction values of single treatments of each compound. These observations demonstrated that **27a**, **33** and **10** were either less toxic or slightly less toxic than SAHA, while **27c** displayed more toxicity than SAHA for both normal cells.

3. Materials and Methods

3.1. General Information

Commercially available reagents were purchased from Fluka (Sydney, NSW, Australia), Aldrich (Sydney, NSW, Australia), Acros Organics (Morris Plains, NJ, USA), Alfa Aesar (Lancashire, UK) and Lancaster (Lancashire, UK) and purified if necessary. The synthetic procedures have been reported for all compounds as general methods and appropriate references have been given for known compounds. ^{1}H (300 MHz) and ^{13}C-NMR (75 MHz) spectra were obtained in the designated solvents on a DPX 300 spectrometer (Bruker, Sydney, NSW, Australia). Melting points were measured using a Mel-Temp melting point apparatus and are uncorrected. Infrared spectra were recorded on Avatar Series FT-IR spectrophotometer as KBr disks (Thermo Nicolet, Waltham, MA, USA). Ultraviolet spectra were measured using a Cary 100 spectrophotometer (Varian, Santa Clara, CA, USA) in the designated solvents and data reported as wavelength (λ) in nm and adsorption coefficient (ε) in $cm^{-1}M^{-1}$. High-resolution [ESI] mass spectra were recorded by the UNSW Bioanalytical Mass Spectrometry Facility, on an Orbitrap LTQ XL (Thermo Scientific, Waltham, MA, USA) ion trap mass spectrometer using a nanospray (nano-electrospray) ionization source.

3.1.1. GP-1: General Procedure for the Benzylation of Dihydroxybenzaldehydes

A solution of hydroxybenzaldehyde (1 equiv.), anhydrous potassium carbonate (per hydroxyl group, 1 equiv.) and benzyl bromide (per hydroxyl group, 1 equiv.) in anhydrous DMF (100 mL) was heated at reflux until TLC analysis showed consumption of the starting aldehyde (9 h). Upon cooling to room temperature, the reaction mixture was diluted with water (300 mL) and the resulting precipitate was collected via filtration and washed with water (2 × 250 mL). Upon drying, the residue was recrystallized from dichloromethane and *n*-hexane to give the title compound.

3.1.2. GP-2: General Procedure for the Preparation of Vinyl-Azido Intermediates

A solution of sodium methoxide was prepared via the portion-wise addition of metallic sodium (17 equiv.) to anhydrous methanol (30 mL) with stirring under nitrogen. A dropping funnel was attached to the reaction flask and charged with the corresponding aldehyde (1 equiv.) and methyl azidoacetate (10 equiv.) in methanol (15 mL). The contents of the funnel were added dropwise to the sodium methoxide solution over 1.5 h under a nitrogen atmosphere. Once the addition was completed, the reaction mixture was warmed to 5 °C, where it remained for 4 h. The heterogeneous mixture was poured into crushed ice. The resulting precipitate was filtered, washed with water and dried to give the title compound. The crude product was used in the next step without further purification.

3.1.3. GP-3: General Procedure for the Preparation of Methyl Benzyloxyindole-2-carboxylates

The vinyl azido intermediate (6.66 mmol) was dissolved in xylene (50 mL) and the reaction mixture was heated under reflux for 6 h. After refluxing, the solvent was evaporated under reduced pressure and the remaining residue was extracted with boiling hexane. Upon cooling, the resulting solid was filtered to give crude product which was recrystallized from dichloromethane and *n*-hexane to give the title compound.

3.1.4. GP-4: General Procedure for the Hydrogenolysis of Methyl Dibenzyloxyindole-2-carboxylate

After vacuum/H_2 cycles to remove air from the reaction flask, a stirred mixture of benzyloxyindole (1 mmol) and 5% Pd/C (10% *w/w*) in THF/MeOH (1:1, 15 mL) was exposed to a hydrogen atmosphere (1 atm) and stirred at room temperature for 2 h. The reaction mixture was filtered through a pad of Celite® and the filtrate was then concentrated under reduced pressure. The crude product was purified by flash column chromatography (SiO_2), eluted with dichloromethane to give the title compounds.

3.1.5. GP-5: General Procedure for the Synthesis of Propargyloxybenzaldehydes:

Propargyl bromide (per hydroxyl group, 1.2 equiv.) was added to a mixture of potassium carbonate (per hydroxyl group, 1 equiv.) and hydroxybenzaldehyde (1 equiv.) in acetone. The reaction mixture was heated under reflux with stirring until no more starting material remained (~30 h). The reaction mixture was cooled to room temperature and Et_2O (100 mL) was added. The ethereal solution was washed with NaOH (1 N, 3 × 50 mL). The organic layer was dried over $MgSO_4$, concentrated under reduced pressure and recrystallized from dichloromethane/*n*-hexane to give the compound.

3.1.6. GP-6 General Procedure for the Synthesis of Dihydropyranoindoles:

A solution of alkyne indole ethers (1.04 mmol) in chlorobenzene (20 mL) was heated under reflux until TLC analysis showed consumption of the starting indole (12 h). The heating was discontinued and the solvent was evaporated under reduced pressure. The crude product was purified using flash column chromatography (SiO_2), eluted with 30% dichloromethane/*n*-hexane, to give the dihydropyranoindole.

Methyl 2-azido-3-(3,4-dibenzyloxyphenyl)-propenoate (**13**) The *title* compound was prepared as described in GP-2 from 3,4-dibenzyloxybenzaldehyde (**12**) (2.95 g, 9.3 mmol) and methyl azidoacetate (10.69 g, 93 mmol) in anhydrous methanol (30 mL) to give the product (2.27 g, 59%) as a pale yellow granular solid; m.p. 114–116 °C; IR (KBr): υ_{max} 2917, 2119, 1701, 1683, 1590, 1508, 1432, 1379, 1233, 1201, 1130, 999, 802, 728 cm^{-1}; UV-vis (CH_3CN): λ_{max}325 (24,500); ^{1}H-NMR: (300 MHz, $CDCl_3$): δ 3.91 (s, 3H, CO_2Me), 5.25 (s, 4H, 2 × O-CH_2), 6.83 (s, 1H, CH=C), 7.35–7.52 (m, 12H, ArH), 7.64 (d, *J* = 2.2 Hz, 1H, H2′); ^{13}C-NMR: (75.6 MHz, $CDCl_3$): δ 52.7 ($CO_2\underline{Me}$), 70.9 (CH_2), 71.3 (CH_2), 113.8 (C2′), 116.6 (C5′), 123.3 ($\underline{C}$H=C), 125.4 (C6′), 125.7 (ArC), 126.6 (ArC), 127.1 (2 × ArC), 127.2 (2 × ArC), 127.8 (ArC), 127.9 (ArC), 128.5 (2 × ArC), 128.6 (2 × ArC), 136.8 (C1′), 137.1 (CH=$\underline{C}$), 148.3 (C4′), 150.1 (C3′), 164.1 ($\underline{C}O_2Me$); HRMS (+ESI): Found *m/z* 438.1439 $[M + Na]^+$, $C_{24}H_{21}N_3O_4Na$ requires 438.1439.

Methyl 5,6-dibenzyloxyindole-2-carboxylate (**14**) The *title* compound was prepared as described in GP-3 from methyl 2-azido-3-(3′,4′-dibenzyloxyphenyl)propenoate (**13**) (2.76 g, 6.66 mmol) in xylene (50 mL) to give the product (1.84 g, 71%) as a yellow granular solid; m.p. 148–150 °C; IR (KBr): υ_{max} 3309, 2942, 2871, 2113, 1680, 1627, 1519, 1488, 1452, 1353, 1288, 1246, 1208, 1144, 1000, 918, 905, 839, 794 cm^{-1}; UV-vis (CH_3CN): λ_{max} 208 nm (ε 72,400 cm^{-1} M^{-1}), 320 (31,700); ^{1}H-NMR (300 MHz, $CDCl_3$): δ 3.93 (s, 3H, CO_2Me), 5.21 (s, 2H, O-CH_2), 5.24 (s, 2H, O-CH_2), 7.00 (s, 1H, H4), 7.01 (s, 1H, H7), 7.23 (d, *J* = 2.1 Hz, 1H, H3), 7.33–7.51 (m, 10H, ArH), 8.73 (bs, 1H, NH); ^{13}C-NMR (75.6 MHz, $CDCl_3$): 51.8 ($CO_2\underline{Me}$), 71.3 (CH_2), 72.0 (CH_2), 97.0 (C7), 107.0 (C4), 108.8 (C3), 121.0 (ArC), 126.0 (C2), 127.0 (ArC), 127.2 (2 × ArC), 127.3 (ArC), 127.7 (2 × ArC), 127.8 (ArC), 128.4 (ArC), 128.5 (ArC), 132.4 (ArC), 137.0 (ArC), 137.4 (2 × ArC), 145.8 (C5), 149.9 (C6), 162.1 ($\underline{C}O_2Me$); HRMS (+ESI): Found *m/z* 410.1364 $[M + Na]^+$, $C_{24}H_{21}NO_4Na$ requires 410.1363.

Methyl 5,6-dihydroxyindole-2-carboxylate (**8**) The *title* compound was prepared as described in GP-4 from methyl 5,6-dibenzyloxyindole-2-carboxylate (**14**) (0.387 g, 1.0 mmol) and 5% Pd/C catalyst (40 mg) in methanol/THF mixture (15 mL) to give the product (159 mg, 77%) as yellow solid; m.p. 256–258 °C; IR (KBr): υ_{max} 3437, 3315, 2953, 2107, 1653, 1632, 1531, 1506, 1437, 1311, 1283, 1230, 1198, 1139, 992, 937, 849, 825, 767 cm^{-1}; UV-vis (CH_3CN): λ_{max} 203 nm (ε 42,100 cm^{-1} M^{-1}), 318 (27,000);^{1}H-NMR (300MHz, d_6-DMSO): δ 3.82 (s, 3H, CO_2Me), 6.79 (d, *J* = 0.8 Hz, 1H, H4), 6.88 (s, 1H, H3), 6.90 (d, *J* = 0.8 Hz, 1H, H7), 8.84 and 9.17 (bs, each 1H, OH), 11.28 (bs, 1H, NH); ^{13}C-NMR (75.6 MHz, $CDCl_3$): 52.0

(CO_2Me), 97.3 (C7), 105.4 (C4), 108.4 (C3), 120.3 (ArC), 125.0 (C2), 133.2 (ArC), 142.3 (C5), 146.7 (C6), 162.5 (CO_2Me); HRMS (+ESI): Found *m/z* 230.0423 $[M + Na]^+$, $C_{10}H_9NO_4Na$ requires 230.0424.

Methyl 5,6-bis(prop-2-yn-1-yloxy)-1H-indole-2-carboxylate (**9**) The *title* compound was prepared as described in GP-5 from methyl 5,6-dihydroxyindole-2-carboxylate (**8**) (993 mg, 4.8 mmol), potassium carbonate (1.32 g, 9.6 mmol) and propargyl bromide (1.36 g, 10.6 mmol) in acetone to give the product (828 mg, 61%) as a yellow solid;m.p. 170–172 °C; IR (KBr): ν_{max} 3332, 3285, 2939, 2925, 2865, 2292, 2108, 1720, 1684, 1625, 1520, 1480, 1435, 1380, 1365, 1280, 1247, 1203, 1150 1024, 986, 892, 819, 805, 759, 720, 672 cm^{-1}; UV-vis (CH_3CN): λ_{max} 209 nm (ε 28,300 cm^{-1} M^{-1}), 313 (18,000); ^{1}H-NMR (300 MHz, $CDCl_3$): δ 2.55 (t, J = 1.6 Hz, 1H, CH≡C), 2.57 (t, J = 1.6 Hz, 1H, CH≡C), 3.95 (s, 3H, CO_2Me), 4.82 (d, J = 2.4 Hz, 2H, O-CH_2), 4.85 (d, J = 2.4 Hz, 2H, O-CH_2), 7.10 (d, J = 0.7 Hz, 1H, H7), 7.16 (q, J = 0.9 Hz, 1H, H3), 7.31 (s, 1H, H4), 8.86 (bs, 1H, NH), ^{13}C-NMR (75.6 MHz, $CDCl_3$): δ51.8 (CO_2Me), 57.0 (O-CH_2), 57.5 (O-CH_2), 75.7 (C≡CH), 75.7 (C≡CH), 78.6 (C≡CH), 79.1 (C≡CH), 97.2 (C7), 107.2 (C4), 108.9 (C3), 121.3 (aryl C), 126.4 (C2), 132.4 (aryl C), 144.2 (C4), 148.2 (C5), 162.1 (CO_2Me); HRMS (+ESI): Found *m/z* 306.0736 $[M + Na]^+$, $C_{16}H_{13}NO_4Na$ requires 306.0737.

2,9-Dihydropyrano[3,2-h]chromene-5-carbaldehyde (**15**) The *title* compound was prepared as described in GP-6 from 3,4-bis(prop-2-yn-1-yloxy)benzaldehyde (**11**) (214 mg, 1.04 mmol) in chlorobenzene (20 mL) to give the product (77 mg, 35%) as a white solid; m.p. 102–104 °C; IR (KBr): ν_{max} 1680, 1570, 1490, 1440, 1340, 1301, 1205, 1102, 995, 945, 900, 898, 861, 745 cm^{-1}; UV-vis (CH_3CN): λ_{max} 225 nm (ε 27,400 cm^{-1} M^{-1}), 268 (18,800), 305 (17,500); ^{1}H-NMR (300 MHz, $CDCl_3$): δ 4.40 (dd, J = 3.0, 1.4 Hz, 2H, O-CH_2), 4.79 (dd, J = 3.0, 1.4 Hz, 2H, O-CH_2), 6.97 (d, J = 8.7 Hz, 2H, H4 and H7), 7.37 (s, 1H, H6), 7.40–7.42 (m, 2H, H3 and H8), 9.80 (s, 1H, CHO); ^{13}C-NMR (75.6 MHz, $CDCl_3$): δ71.3 (O-CH_2), 71.5 (O-CH_2), 119.6 (C6), 120.6 (aryl C), 121.6 (C4), 121.8 (C7), 125.3 (aryl C), 126.5 (C3), 126.9 (C8), 127.1 (C5), 147.9 (aryl C), 154.3 (aryl C), 190.7 (CHO); HRMS (+ESI): Found *m/z* 237.0533 $[M + Na]^+$, $C_{13}H_{10}O_3Na$ requires 237.0528.

3,4-Bis(but-2-yn-1-yloxy)benzaldehyde (**29**) The *title* compound was prepared as described in GP-5 from 3,4-dihydroxybenzaldehyde (7) (660 mg, 4.8 mmol), potassium carbonate (1.32 g, 9.6 mmol) and 1-bromobut-2-yne (1.40 g, 10.6 mmol) in acetone to give the product (1.01 g, 87%) as a white solid; m.p. 86–88 °C; IR (KBr): ν_{max} 1688, 1582, 1499, 1431, 1375, 1248, 1201, 1125, 987, 920, 857, 797, 729 cm^{-1}; UV-vis (CH_3CN): λ_{max} 228 nm (ε 31,500 cm^{-1} M^{-1}), 272 (22,200), 303 (14,800); ^{1}H-NMR (300 MHz, $CDCl_3$): δ 1.85–1.87 (m, 6H, 2 × C-CH_3), 4.79 (q, J = 2.3 Hz, 2H, O-CH2), 4.82 (q, J = 2.3 Hz, 2H, O-CH2), 7.17 (d, J = 8.2 Hz, 1H, H5), 7.52 (dd, J = 8.2, 1.9 Hz, 1H, H6), 7.57 (d, J = 1.9 Hz, 1H, H2), 9.89 (s, 1H, CHO); ^{13}C-NMR (75.6 MHz, $CDCl_3$): δ 3.6 (C-CH_3), 3.7 (C-CH_3), 57.2 (2 × O-CH_2), 73.1 (C-CH_3), 73.3 (C-CH_3), 84.6 (C≡C(CH_3)), 84.9 (C≡C(CH_3)), 112.0 (C5), 112.7 (C2), 126.4 (C6), 130.3 (aryl C), 147.9 (C4′), 152.9 (C3′), 190.8 (CHO); HRMS (+ESI): Found *m/z* 265.0840 $[M + Na]^+$, $C_{15}H_{14}O_3Na$ requires 265.0835.

4-Methoxy-3-((3-phenylprop-2-yn-1-yl)oxy)benzaldehyde (**24d**) The *title* compound was prepared as described in GP-5 from 3-hydroxy-4-methoxybenzaldehyde **23** (730 mg, 4.8 mmol), potassium carbonate (662 mg, 4.8 mmol) and 3-phenylprop-2-yn-1-yl-4-methylbenzenesulfonate (1.66 g, 5.8 mmol) in acetone to give the product (1.17 g, 92%) as a white solid; m.p. 112–114 °C; IR (KBr): ν_{max} 1673, 1579, 1506, 1430, 1378, 1256, 1221, 1165, 1130, 1012, 931, 874, 810, 754, 686 cm^{-1}; UV-vis (CH_3CN): λ_{max} 232 nm (ε 45,500 cm^{-1} M^{-1}), 272 (21,500), 302 (14,800); ^{1}H-NMR (300 MHz, $CDCl_3$): δ 4.00 (s, 3H, OMe), 5.08 (s, 2H, O-CH2), 7.03 (d, J = 8.2 Hz, 1H, H5), 7.30–7.33 (m, 3H, ArH), 7.34–7.45 (m, 2H, ArH), 7.54 (dd, J = 8.2, 1.9 Hz, 1H, H6), 7.68 (d, J = 1.9 Hz, 1H, H2), 9.90 (s, 1H, CHO); ^{13}C-NMR (75.6 MHz, $CDCl_3$): δ 56.2 (OMe), 57.5 (O-CH_2), 83.0 (C≡C(Ph)), 88.0 (C-Ph), 110.9 (C5), 112.1 (C2), 122.1 (aryl C), 127.1 (2 × aryl CH), 127.8 (aryl CH), 128.8 (C6), 130.0 (aryl C), 131.9 (2 × aryl CH), 147.5 (C4), 155.0 (C3), 190.7 (CHO); HRMS (+ESI): Found *m/z* 289.0837 $[M + Na]^+$, $C_{17}H_{14}O_3Na$ requires 289.0835.

Methyl (Z)-2-azido-3-(3,4-bis(prop-2-yn-1-yloxy)phenyl) acrylate (**17**) The *title* compound was prepared as described in GP-2 from 3,4-bis(prop-2-yn-1-yloxy)benzaldehyde (**11**) (558 mg, 2.6 mmol) and methyl azidoacetate (2.99 g, 26.0 mmol) in anhydrous methanol (30 mL) to give the product (582 mg, 63%) as a pale yellow granular solid; m.p. 114–116 °C; IR (KBr): ν_{max} 2954, 2123, 1709, 1594, 1506, 1433, 1378, 1239, 1133, 1081, 1009, 793, 745, 683 cm^{-1}; UV-vis (CH_3CN): λ_{max} 327 nm (ε 19,100 cm^{-1} M^{-1}); ^{1}H-NMR (300 MHz,$CDCl_3$): δ 2.57 (t, *J* = 2.4 Hz, 1H, CH≡C), 2.59 (t, *J* = 2.4 Hz, 1H, CH≡C), 3.92 (s, 3H, CO_2Me), 4.83 (d, *J* = 2.4 Hz, 4H, 2 × O-CH2), 6.91 (s, 1H, CH=C), 7.09 (d, *J* = 8.5 Hz, 1H, H5′), 7.44 (dd, *J* = 8.5, 2.0 Hz, 1H, H6′), 7.77 (d, *J* = 2.0 Hz, 1H, H2′), ^{13}C-NMR (75.6 MHz, $CDCl_3$): δ 52.8 ($CO_2\underline{Me}$), 56.6 (OMe), 57.0 (2 × O-CH_2), 76.1 (C≡$\underline{C}$H), 76.2 (C≡$\underline{C}$H), 77.2 ($\underline{C}$≡CH), 77.4 ($\underline{C}$≡CH), 113.8 (C5′), 116.6 (C2′), 123.9 ($\underline{C}$H=C), 125.3 (C6′), 125.6 (aryl C), 146.9 (aryl C), 148.5 (aryl C), 164.1 ($\underline{C}O_2Me$); HRMS could not be determined due to the unstable properties of the compound

Methyl (Z)-2-azido-3-(4-methoxy-3-(prop-2-yn-1-yloxy)phenyl)acrylate (**25a**) The *title* compound was prepared as described in GP-2 from 4-methoxy-3-(prop-2-yn-1-yloxy)benzaldehyde (24a) (494 mg, 2.6 mmol) and methyl azidoacetate (2.99 g, 26.0 mmol) in anhydrous methanol (30 mL) to give the product (537 mg, 72%) as a pale yellow granular solid; m.p. 116–118 °C; IR (KBr): ν_{max} 2951, 2101, 1698, 1592, 1507, 1432, 1379, 1254, 1214, 1139, 1084, 1016, 809, 745 cm^{-1}; UV-vis (CH_3CN): λ_{max} 235 nm (ε 16,600 cm^{-1} M^{-1}), 330 (27,100); ^{1}H-NMR (300 MHz, $CDCl_3$): δ 2.58 (t, *J* = 2.4 Hz, 1H, CH≡C), 3.94 (s, 3H, OMe), 3.94 (s, 3H, CO_2Me), 4.83 (d, *J* = 2.4 Hz, 2H, O-CH2), 6.90 (s, 1H, CH=C), 6.93 (d, *J* = 8.5 Hz, 1H, H5′), 7.43 (dd, *J* = 8.5, 2.0 Hz, 1H, H6′), 7.76 (d, *J* = 2.0 Hz, 1H, H2′); ^{13}C-NMR (75.6 MHz, $CDCl_3$): δ 52.8 ($CO_2\underline{Me}$), 55.9 (OMe), 56.8 (O-CH_2), 76.0 (C≡$\underline{C}$H), 77.4 ($\underline{C}$≡CH), 111.2 (C5′), 116.1 (C2′), 123.4 ($\underline{C}$H=C), 125.6 (C6′), 125.0 (aryl C), 126.1 (CH=$\underline{C}$), 146.3 (C4′), 150.8 (C3′), 164.1 ($\underline{C}O_2Me$); HRMS (+ESI): Found *m/z* 310.0800 [M + Na]$^+$, $C_{14}H_{13}N_3O_4Na$ requires 310.0798.

Methyl (Z)-2-azido-3-(3-methoxy-4-(prop-2-yn-1-yloxy) phenyl)acrylate (**20a**) The *title* compound was prepared as described in GP-2 from 3-methoxy-4-(prop-2-yn-1-yloxy)benzaldehyde (**19a**) (494 mg, 2.6 mmol) and methyl azidoacetate (2.99 g, 26.0 mmol) in anhydrous methanol (30 mL) to give the product (567 mg, 76%) as a pale yellow granular solid; m.p. 120–122 °C; IR (KBr): ν_{max} 2920, 2122, 1704, 1592, 1509, 1450, 1345, 1243, 1206, 1141, 1008, 922, 804, 764 cm^{-1}; UV-vis (CH_3CN): λ_{max} 323 nm (ε 17,500 cm^{-1} M^{-1}); ^{1}H-NMR (300 MHz, $CDCl_3$): δ 2.56 (t, *J* = 2.4 Hz, 1H, CH≡C), 3.94 (s, 3H, OMe), 3.95 (s, 3H, CO_2Me), 4.83 (d, *J* = 2.4 Hz, 2H, O-CH2), 6.91 (s, 1H, CH=C), 7.06 (d, *J* = 8.5 Hz, 1H, H5′), 7.43 (dd, *J* = 8.5, 1.9 Hz, 1H, H6′), 7.56 (d, *J* = 1.9 Hz, 1H, H2′); ^{13}C-NMR (75.6 MHz, $CDCl_3$): δ 52.8 ($CO_2\underline{Me}$), 55.9 (OMe), 56.5 (O-CH_2), 76.2 (C≡$\underline{C}$H), 77.4 ($\underline{C}$≡CH), 113.3 (C5′), 113.5 (C2′), 123.7 ($\underline{C}$H=C), 124.4 (C6′), 125.5 (aryl C), 127.3 (CH=$\underline{C}$), 147.9 (C3′), 149.1 (C4′), 164.1 ($\underline{C}O_2Me$); HRMS could not be determined due to the unstable properties of the compound.

Methyl (Z)-2-azido-3-(3,4-bis(but-2-yn-1-yl)oxy)phenyl) acrylate (**30**) The *title* compound was prepared as described in GP-2 from 3,4-bis(but-2-yn-1-yloxy)benzaldehyde (**29**) (629 mg, 2.6 mmol) and methyl azidoacetate (2.99 g, 26.0 mmol) in anhydrous methanol (30 mL) to give the product (555 mg, 63%) as a pale yellow granular solid; m.p. 124–126 °C; IR (KBr): ν_{max} 2918, 2119, 1712, 1687, 1590, 1506, 1432, 1373, 1314, 1243, 1128, 992, 804, 745 cm^{-1}; UV-vis (CH_3CN): λ_{max} 307 nm (ε 14,500 cm^{-1} M^{-1}); ^{1}H-NMR (300 MHz, $CDCl_3$): δ 1.87 (t, *J* = 2.3 Hz, 6H, 2 × C-CH_3), 3.93 (s, 3H, $CO_2\underline{Me}$), 4.79 (q, *J* = 2.3 Hz, 2H, O-CH_2), 4.82 (q, *J* = 2.3 Hz, 2H, O-CH_2), 6.91 (s, 1H CH=C), 7.05 (d, *J* = 8.5 Hz, 1H, H5′), 7.44 (dd, *J* = 8.5, 1.8 Hz, 1H, H6′), 7.73 (d, *J* = 2.0 Hz, 1H, H2′); ^{13}C-NMR (75.6 MHz, $CDCl_3$): δ 3.7 (2×C-$\underline{C}H_3$), 52.8 ($CO_2\underline{Me}$), 57.1 (OMe), 57.2 (O-CH_2), 57.5 (O-CH_2), 73.9 (2×$\underline{C}$-CH_3), 84.2 ($\underline{C}$≡C(CH_3)), 84.9 ($\underline{C}$≡C(CH_3)), 113.2 (C5′), 116.0 (C2′), 125.3 ($\underline{C}$H=C), 125.8 (C6′), 126.5 (aryl C), 126.6 (CH=$\underline{C}$), 147.9 (C4′), 148.8 (C3), 164.2 ($\underline{C}O_2Me$); HRMS could not be determined due to the unstable properties of the compound.

Methyl (Z)-2-azido-3-(3-(but-2-yn-1-yloxy)-4-methoxyphenyl) acrylate (**25b**) The *title* compound was prepared as described in GP-2 from 3-(but-2-yn-1-yloxy)-4-methoxybenzaldehyde (**24b**) (530 mg, 2.6 mmol) and methyl azidoacetate (2.9 g, 26.0 mmol) in anhydrous methanol (30 mL) to give the product (500 mg, 64%) as a pale yellow granular solid; m.p. 96–98 °C; IR (KBr): ν_{max} 2951, 2101, 1698, 1592,

1507, 1431, 1379, 1254, 1139, 1016, 810, 745 cm^{-1}; UV-vis (CH_3CN): λ_{max} 327 nm (ε 25,700 cm^{-1} M^{-1}); ^{1}H-NMR (300 MHz, $CDCl_3$): δ 1.89 (t, *J* = 2.3 Hz, 3H, CH_3), 3.93 (s, 3H, OMe), 3.94 (s, 3H, CO_2Me), 4.78 (q, *J* = 2.3 Hz, 2H, O-CH_2), 6.91 (d, *J* = 8.5 Hz, 1H, H5′), 6.92 (s, 1H, CH=C), 7.41 (dd, *J* = 8.5, 2.0 Hz, 1H, H6′), 7.73 (d, *J* = 2.0 Hz, 1H, H2′); ^{13}C-NMR (75.6 MHz, $CDCl_3$): δ 3.7 (C-$\underline{C}H_3$), 52.8 ($CO_2\underline{Me}$), 55.9 (OMe), 57.4 (O-CH_2), 73.7 ($\underline{C}$-CH_3), 84.3 ($\underline{C}$≡C(CH_3)), 111.0 (C5′), 115.6 (C2′), 123.3 ($\underline{C}$H=C), 125.6 (C6′), 125.9 (aryl C), 126.0 (CH=$\underline{C}$), 146.7 (C4′), 150.7 (C3′), 164.2 ($\underline{C}O_2$Me); HRMS (+ESI): Found *m/z* 324.0944 [M + Na]$^+$, $C_{15}H_{15}N_3O_4Na$ requires 324.0955.

Methyl (Z)-2-azido-3-(4-(but-2-yn-1-yloxy)-3-methoxyphenyl)acrylate (**20b**) The *title* compound was prepared as described in GP-2 from 4-(but-2-yn-1-yloxy)-3-methoxybenzaldehyde (19b)(530 mg, 2.6 mmol) and methyl azidoacetate (2.99 g, 26.0 mmol) in anhydrous methanol (30 mL) to give the product (477 mg, 61%) as a pale yellow granular solid; m.p. 94–96 °C; IR (KBr): ν_{max} 2920, 2120, 1702, 1592, 1509, 1434, 1377, 1244, 1140, 1011, 801, 763 cm^{-1}; UV-vis (CH_3CN): λ_{max} 324 nm (ε 14,900 cm^{-1} M^{-1}); ^{1}H-NMR (300 MHz, $CDCl_3$): δ 1.87 (t, *J* = 2.3 Hz, 3H, CH_3), 3.94 (s, 3H, OMe), 3.94 (s, 3H, $CO_2\underline{Me}$), 4.77 (q, *J* = 2.3 Hz, 2H, O-CH2), 6.90 (s, 1H, CH=C), 7.05 (d, *J* = 8.5 Hz, 1H, H5′), 7.38 (dd, *J* = 8.5, 1.8, Hz, 1H, H6′), 7.53 (d, *J* = 1.8 Hz, 1H, H2′); ^{13}CNMR (75.6 MHz, $CDCl_3$): δ 3.7 (C-$\underline{C}H_3$), 52.8 ($CO_2\underline{Me}$), 55.9 (OMe), 57.1 (O-CH_2), 73.5 ($\underline{C}$-CH_3), 84.4 ($\underline{C}$≡C(CH_3)), 112.9 (C5′), 113.3 (C2′), 123.4 (aryl C), 124.5 ($\underline{C}$H=C), 125.8 (C6′), 126.8 (CH=$\underline{C}$), 14.34 (C3′), 149.0 (C4′), 164.2 ($\underline{C}O_2$Me); HRMS (+ESI): Found *m/z* 324.0955 [M + Na]$^+$, $C_{15}H_{15}N_3O_4Na$ requires 324.0955.

Methyl (Z)-2-azido-3-(4-methoxy-3-((3-phenylprop-2-yn-1-yl) oxy)phenyl)acrylate (**25d**) The *title* compound was prepared as described in GP-2 from 4-methoxy-3-((3-phenylprop-2-yn-1-yl)oxy)benzaldehyde (**24d**) (692 mg, 2.6 mmol) and methyl azidoacetate (2.99 g, 26.0 mmol) in anhydrous methanol (30 mL) to give the product (632 mg, 67%) as a pale yellow granular solid; m.p. 118–120 °C; IR (KBr): ν_{max} 2921, 2827, 2119, 1674, 1612, 1580, 1506, 1431, 1378, 1275, 1232, 1129, 1008, 966. 873, 809, 753, 686 cm^{-1}; UV-vis (CH_3CN): λ_{max} 234 nm (ε 57,700 cm^{-1} M^{-1}), 272 (22,600), 306 (21,800); ^{1}H-NMR (300 MHz, $CDCl_3$): δ 3.93 (s, 3H, OMe), 3.96 (s, 3H, CO_2Me), 5.04 (d, *J* = 6.0 Hz, 2H, O-CH2), 6.91 (s, 1H, CH≡C), 6.92 (d, *J* = 8.0 Hz, 1H, H5′), 7.09 (dd, *J* = 8.0, 1.8 Hz, 1H, H6′), 7.27–7.33 (m, 3H, ArH), 7.43–7.46 (m, 2H, ArH), 7.85 (d, *J* = 1.8 Hz, 1H, H2′); ^{13}C-NMR (75.6 MHz, $CDCl_3$): δ 52.6 ($CO_2\underline{Me}$), 55.9 (OMe), 57.5 (O-CH_2), 83.9 ($\underline{C}$-Ph), 87.5 ($\underline{C}$≡C(Ph)), 111.1 (C5′), 116.0 (C2′), 120.4 (aryl C), 125.7 ($\underline{C}$H=C), 126.0 (C6′), 126.1 (aryl C), 128.3 (2×aryl CH), 128.6 (CH=$\underline{C}$), 130.6 (aryl CH), 131.9 (2×aryl CH), 146.7 (C4′), 150.9 (C3′), 164.2 ($\underline{C}O_2$Me); HRMS (+ESI): Found *m/z* 386.1099 [M + Na]$^+$, $C_{20}H_{17}N_3O_4Na$ requires 386.1117.

Methyl (Z)-2-azido-3-(4-methoxy-3-((2-methylbut-3-yn-2-yl) oxy)phenyl)acrylate (**25c**) The *title* compound was prepared as described in GP-2 from 4-methoxy-3-((2-methylbut-3-yn-2-yl)oxy)benzaldehyde (**24c**) (567 mg, 2.6 mmol) and methyl azidoacetate (2.99 g, 26.0 mmol) in anhydrous methanol (30 mL) to give the product (507 mg, 62%) as a pale yellow granular solid; m.p. 122–124 °C; IR (KBr): ν_{max} 2988, 2835, 2094, 1691, 1619, 1565, 1506, 1425, 1374, 1253, 1138, 1084, 1027, 962. 891, 799, 756, 687 cm^{-1}; UV-vis (CH_3CN): λ_{max} 238 nm (ε 16,800 cm^{-1} M^{-1}), 328 (35,400); ^{1}H-NMR (300 MHz, $CDCl_3$): δ 1.70 (s, 6H, 2 × C-CH_3), 2.59 (d, *J* = 0.9 Hz, 1H, CH≡C), 3.87 (s, 3H, OMe), 3.92 (s, 3H, CO_2Me), 6.91 (s, 1H, CH=C), 6.90 (d, *J* = 8.5 Hz, 1H, H5′), 7.45 (dd, *J* = 1.9, 8.5 Hz, 1H, H6′), 8.16 (d, *J* = 2.0 Hz, 1H, H2′);^{13}C-NMR (75.6 MHz, $CDCl_3$): δ 29.3 (2×C-$\underline{C}H_3$), 52.7 ($CO_2\underline{Me}$), 55.7 (OMe), 73.6 (C≡$\underline{C}$H), 74.1 ($\underline{C}$-(CH_3)$_2$), 86.1 ($\underline{C}$≡CH), 111.5 (C5′), 123.2 (C2′), 124.8 ($\underline{C}$H=C), 125.7 (C6′), 125.9 (aryl C), 127.4 (CH=$\underline{C}$), 144.2 (C4′), 153.9 (C3′), 164.2 ($\underline{C}O_2$Me); HRMS (+ESI): Found *m/z* 338.1099 [M + Na]$^+$, $C_{16}H_{17}N_3O_4Na$ requires 338.1117.

Methyl (Z)-2-azido-3-(3-methoxy-4-((2-methylbut-3-yn-2-yl)oxy)phenyl)acrylate (**20c**) The *title* compound was prepared as described in GP-2 from 3-methoxy-4-((2-methylbut-3-yn-2-yl)oxy)benzaldehyde (**19c**) (567 mg, 2.6 mmol) and methyl azidoacetate (2.1 g, 26. mmol) in anhydrous methanol (30 mL) to give the product (524 mg, 62%) as a pale yellow granular solid; m.p. 116–118 °C; IR (KBr): ν_{max} 2975, 2802, 2112, 1703, 1635, 1565, 1512, 1400, 1387, 1212, 1100, 1052, 998, 957, 888, 765, 745, 677 cm^{-1}; UV-vis (CH_3CN): λ_{max} 328 nm (ε 17,100 cm^{-1} M^{-1}); ^{1}H-NMR (300 MHz, $CDCl_3$): δ 1.72 (s, 6H, 2 × C-CH_3),

2.60 (d, *J* = 0.9 Hz, 1H, CH≡C), 3.89 (s, 3H, OMe), 3.93 (s, 3H, CO_2Me), 6.91 (s, 1H, CH=C), 7.33 (dd, *J* = 8.5, 1.9 Hz, 1H, H6′), 7.45 (d, *J* = 8.5 Hz, 1H, H5′), 7.52 (d, *J* = 1.9 Hz, 1H, H2′); ^{13}C-NMR (75.6 MHz, $CDCl_3$): δ 29.4 (2 × C-$\underline{C}H_3$), 52.8 ($CO_2\underline{Me}$), 55.9 (OMe), 73.9 (C≡$\underline{C}$H), 73.9 ($\underline{C}$-$(CH_3)_2$) 85.8 ($\underline{C}$≡CH), 113.9 (C5′), 121.5 (C2′), 123.8 ($\underline{C}$H=C), 123.9 (C6′), 125.7 (aryl C), 128.5 (CH=$\underline{C}$), 146.1 (C3′), 152.0 (C4′), 164.1 ($\underline{C}O_2Me$); HRMS (+ESI): Found *m/z* 338.1104 $[M + Na]^+$, $C_{16}H_{17}N_3O_4Na$ requires 338.1117.

Methyl 6-methoxy-5-(prop-2-yn-1-yloxy)-1H-indole-2-carboxylate (**26a**) The *title* compound was prepared as described in GP-3 from methyl (Z)-2-azido-3-(3-(but-2-yn-1-yloxy)-4-methoxyphenyl)acrylate (**25a**) (596 mg, 2.08 mmol) in xylene (20 mL) to give the product (196 mg, 73%) as a yellow solid; m.p. 164–166 °C; IR (KBr): ν_{max} 3325, 3259, 2953, 2925, 2123, 1671, 1624, 1520, 1480, 1440, 1367, 1320, 1249, 1208, 1185, 1146, 1005, 890, 833, 766, 694 cm^{-1}; UV-vis (CH_3CN): λ_{max} 208 nm (ε 40,600 cm^{-1} M^{-1}), 318 (28,700); ^{1}H-NMR (300 MHz, $CDCl_3$): δ 2.55 (t, *J* = 2.4 Hz, 1H, CH≡C), 3.95 (s, 3H, OMe), 3.96 (s, 3H, CO_2Me), 4.82 (d, *J* = 2.4 Hz, 2H, O-CH_2), 6.90 (d, *J* = 0.8 Hz, 1H, H4), 7.16 (q, *J* = 0.9 Hz, 1H, H3), 7.28 (s, 1H, H7), 8.91 (bs, 1H, NH), ^{13}C-NMR (75.6 MHz, $CDCl_3$): δ 51.8 ($CO_2\underline{Me}$), 56.0 (OMe), 57.3 (O-CH_2), 75.7 (C≡$\underline{C}$H), 78.7 ($\underline{C}$≡CH), 94.0 (C7), 106.6 (C4), 109.0 (C3), 120.2 (aryl C), 125.9 (C2), 132.9 (aryl C), 143.7 (C6), 150.6 (C5), 162.3 ($\underline{C}O_2Me$); HRMS (+ESI): Found *m/z* 282.0725 $[M + Na]^+$, $C_{14}H_{13}NO_3Na$ requires 282.0742.

Methyl 5-methoxy-6-(prop-2-yn-1-yloxy)-1H-indole-2-carboxylate (**21a**) The *title* compound was prepared as described in GP-3 from methyl (Z)-2-azido-3-(4-(but-2-yn-1-yloxy)-3-methoxyphenyl)acrylate (**20a**) (596 mg, 2.08 mmol) in xylene (20 mL) to give the product (183 mg, 68%) as a yellow solid; m.p. 152–154 °C; IR (KBr): ν_{max} 3325, 3241, 2999, 2937, 2113, 1681, 1638, 1522, 1475, 1452, 1360, 1280, 1237, 1211, 1195, 1143, 1003, 924, 843, 819, 761, 675 cm^{-1}; UV-vis (CH_3CN): λ_{max} 209 nm (ε 35,800 cm^{-1} M^{-1}), 308 (21,400); ^{1}H-NMR (300 MHz, $CDCl_3$): δ 2.57 (t, *J* = 2.4 Hz, 1H, CH≡C), 3.95 (s, 3H, OMe), 3.96 (s, 3H, CO_2Me), 4.85 (d, *J* = 2.4 Hz, 2H, O-CH_2), 7.08 (d, *J* = 0.8 Hz, 1H, H4), 7.11 (s, 1H, H7), 7.15 (q, *J* = 0.9 Hz, 1H, H3), 8.87 (bs, 1H, NH); ^{13}C-NMR (75.6 MHz, $CDCl_3$): δ 51.8 ($CO_2\underline{Me}$), 56.2 (OMe), 56.9 (O-CH_2), 76.1 (C≡$\underline{C}$H), 77.4 ($\underline{C}$≡CH), 96.8 (C7), 103.0 (C4), 108.7 (C3), 121.4 (aryl C), 126.1 (C2), 131.6 (aryl C), 146.6 (C5), 147.6 (C6), 162.2 ($\underline{C}O_2Me$); HRMS (+ESI): Found *m/z* 282.0726 $[M + Na]^+$, $C_{14}H_{13}NO_3Na$ requires 282.0742.

Methyl 5,6-bis(but-2-yn-1-yloxy)-1H-indole-2-carboxylate (**31**) The *title* compound was prepared as described in GP-3 from methyl (Z)-2-azido-3-(3,4-bis(but-2-yn-1-yloxy)phenyl)acrylate (**30**) (704 mg, 2.08 mmol) in xylene (20 mL) to give the product 210 mg, 65%) as a yellow solid; m.p. 146–148 °C; IR (KBr): ν_{max} 3332, 2912, 2294, 2120, 1682, 1644, 1519, 1434, 1379, 1244, 1204, 1145, 984, 891, 819, 765 cm^{-1}; UV-vis (CH_3CN): λ_{max} 210 nm (ε 39,600 cm^{-1} M^{-1}), 317 (24,900); ^{1}H-NMR (300 MHz, $CDCl_3$): δ 1.87 (q, *J* = 2.4 Hz, 6H, 2 × C-CH_3), 3.96 (s, 3H, CO_2Me), 4.76 (q, *J* = 2.4 Hz, 2H, O-CH2), 4.79 (q, *J* = 2.4 Hz, 2H, O-CH2), 7.08 (d, *J* = 0.7 Hz, 1H, H4), 7.16 (q, *J* = 0.9 Hz, 1H, H3), 7.25 (s, 1H, H7), 9.03 (bs, 1H, NH); ^{13}C-NMR (75.6 MHz, $CDCl_3$): δ 3.7 (2 × C-$\underline{C}H_3$), 51.8 ($CO_2\underline{Me}$), 57.4 and 57.8 (O-CH_2), 73.9 ($\underline{C}$-CH_3), 74.2 ($\underline{C}$-CH_3), 83.8 ($\underline{C}$≡C(CH_3)), 84.2 ($\underline{C}$≡C(CH_3)), 96.5 (C7), 106.1 (C4), 108.9 (C3), 120.9 (aryl C), 126.0 (C2), 132.5 (aryl C), 144.4 (C5), 148.5 (C6), 162.3 ($\underline{C}O_2Me$); HRMS (+ESI): Found *m/z* 334.1046 $[M + Na]^+$, $C_{18}H_{17}NO_4Na$ requires 334.1050.

Methyl 5-(but-2-yn-1-yloxy)-6-methoxy-1H-indole-2-carboxylate (**26b**) The *title* compound was prepared as described in GP-3 from methyl (Z)-2-azido-3-(3-(but-2-yn-1-yloxy)-4-methoxyphenyl)acrylate (**25b**) (626 mg, 2.08 mmol) in xylene (20 mL) to give the product (201 mg, 71%) as a yellow solid; m.p. 160–162 °C; IR (KBr): ν_{max} 3324, 3258, 3009, 2918, 2795, 2123, 2108, 1672, 1600, 1520, 1490, 1425, 1400, 1385, 1346, 1249, 1208, 1185, 1146, 1005, 980, 890, 833, 766 cm^{-1}; UV-vis (CH_3CN): λ_{max} 208 nm (ε 27,700 cm^{-1} M^{-1}), 319 (18,900);^{1}H-NMR (300 MHz, $CDCl_3$): δ 1.88 (q, *J* = 2.4 Hz, 3H, C-CH_3), 3.95 (s, 3H, OMe), 3.96 (s, 3H, CO_2Me), 4.77 (q, *J* = 2.4 Hz, 2H, O-CH_2), 6.88 (d, *J* = 0.7 Hz, 1H, H4), 7.16 (q, *J* = 0.9 Hz, 1H, H3), 7.23 (s, 1H, H7), 8.82 (bs, 1H, NH); ^{13}C-NMR (75.6 MHz, $CDCl_3$): δ 5.2 (C-$\underline{C}H_3$), 53.2 ($CO_2\underline{Me}$), 57.4 (OMe), 59.1 (O-CH_2), 75.5 ($\underline{C}$-CH_3), 85.3 ($\underline{C}$≡C), 95.2 (C7), 107.1 (C4), 110.4 (C3), 121.7 (aryl C),

127.1 (C2), 134.0 (aryl C), 145.5 (C6), 151.9 (C5), 163.7 (C̲O$_2$Me); HRMS (+ESI): Found *m/z* 296.0884 [M + Na]$^+$, $C_{15}H_{15}NO_4Na$ requires 296.0899.

Methyl 6-(but-2-yn-1-yloxy)-5-methoxy-1H-indole-2-carboxylate (**21b**) The *title* compound was prepared as described in GP-3 from methyl (Z)-2-azido-3-(4-(but-2-yn-1-yloxy)-3-methoxyphenyl)acrylate (**20b**) (626 mg, 2.08 mmol) in xylene (20 mL) to give the product (190 mg, 67%) as a yellow solid; m.p. 164–166 °C; IR (KBr): ν_{max} 3324, 3224, 3005, 2936, 2835, 2215, 2108, 1680, 1584, 1495, 1455, 1433, 1362, 1285, 1243, 1228, 1146, 1045, 988, 946, 846, 819, 760, 672 cm^{-1}; UV-vis (CH_3CN): λ_{max} 210 nm (ε 37,100 cm^{-1} M^{-1}), 319 (22,300); ^{1}H-NMR (300 MHz, $CDCl_3$): δ 1.87 (q, *J* = 2.4 Hz, 3H, C-CH$_3$), 3.94 (s, 3H, OMe), 3.96 (s, 3H, CO$_2$Me), 4.80 (q, *J* = 2.4 Hz, 2H, O-CH2), 7.06 (d, *J* = 0.7 Hz, 1H, H4), 7.08 (s, 1H, H7), 7.14 (q, *J* = 0.9 Hz, 1H, H3), 9.01 (bs, 1H, NH); ^{13}C-NMR (75.6 MHz, $CDCl_3$): δ 3.7 (C-C̲H$_3$), 51.8 (CO$_2$M̲e̲), 56.1 (OMe), 57.4 (O-CH$_2$), 73.8 (C̲-CH$_3$), 84.3 (C̲≡C(CH$_3$)), 96.2 (C7), 102.7 (C4), 108.7 (C3), 121.0 (aryl C), 125.8 (C2), 131.8 (aryl C), 146.1 (C5), 148.0 (C6), 162.3 (C̲O$_2$Me); HRMS (+ESI): Found *m/z* 296.0883 [M + Na]$^+$, $C_{15}H_{15}NO_4Na$ requires 296.0889.

Methyl 6-methoxy-5-((3-phenylprop-2-yn-1-yl)oxy)-1H-indole-2-carboxylate (**26d**) The *title* compound was prepared as described in GP-3 from methyl (Z)-2-azido-3-(4-methoxy-3-((3-phenylprop-2-yn-1-yl)oxy)phenyl)acrylate (**25d**) (754 mg, 2.08 mmol) in xylene (20 mL) to give the product (257 mg, 74%) as a yellow solid; m.p. 138–140 °C; IR (KBr): ν_{max} 3326, 2984, 2924, 2740, 2113, 1675, 1645, 1520, 1480, 1439, 1381, 1247, 1195, 1145, 996, 845, 823, 761, 672 cm^{-1}; UV-vis (CH_3CN): λ_{max} 203 nm (ε 58,900 cm^{-1} M^{-1}), 318 (22,200); ^{1}H-NMR (300 MHz, $CDCl_3$): δ 3.95 (s, 3H, OMe), 3.98 (s, 3H, CO$_2$Me), 5.04 (s, 2H, O-CH2), 6.90 (s, 1H, H4), 7.17 (q, *J* = 0.9 Hz, 1H, H3), 7.31 (s, 1H, H7), 7.32–7.36 (m, 3H, ArCH), 7.44–7.47 (m, 2H, ArCH), 8.84 (bs, 1H, NH); ^{13}C-NMR (75.6 MHz, $CDCl_3$): δ 51.8 (CO$_2$M̲e̲), 56.0 (OMe), 58.2 (O-CH$_2$), 84.1 (C̲≡C(Ph)), 87.4 (C̲-Ph), 93.9 (C7), 106.6 (C4), 109.0 (C3), 120.3 (aryl C), 122.4 (aryl C), 125.8 (C2), 128.2 (2 × aryl CH), 128.5 (aryl CH), 131.8 (2 × aryl CH), 132.8 (aryl C), 144.0 (C6), 150.7 (C5), 162.2 (C̲O$_2$Me); HRMS (+ESI): Found *m/z* 336.1221 [M + H]$^+$, $C_{20}H_{18}NO_4$ requires 336.1236.

Methyl 5,10-dihydro-7H-dipyrano[3,2-e:2′,3′-g]indole-6-carboxylate (**10**) *Method 2: Route 2* The title compound was prepared as described in GP-3 from methyl (Z)-2-azido-3-(3,4-bis(prop-2-yn-1-yloxy)phenyl) acrylate (**9**) (646 mg, 2.08 mmol) in xylene (20 mL) to give the product (61.4 mg, 72%) as a yellow solid; m.p. 168–170 °C; IR (KBr): ν_{max} 3415, 3328, 2947, 2831, 2341, 2116, 1674, 1640, 1575, 1524, 1486, 1441, 1400, 1274, 1213, 1158, 1135, 1025, 1000, 920, 813, 755 cm^{-1}; UV-vis (CH_3CN): λ_{max} 225 nm (ε 24,100 cm^{-1} M^{-1}), 269 (13,800), 360 (13,000); ^{1}H-NMR (300 MHz, $CDCl_3$): δ 3.96 (s, 3H, CO$_2$Me), 4.91 (dd, J = 3.8, 1.8 Hz, 2H, O-CH$_2$), 4.94 (dd, *J* = 3.8, 1.8 Hz, 2H, O-CH$_2$), 5.87–5.97 (m, 2H, H3 and H9), 6.72–6.80 (m, 2H, H4 and H8), 7.19 (d, *J* = 2.1 Hz, 1H, H5), 8.85 (s, 1H, NH); ^{13}C-NMR (75.6 MHz, $CDCl_3$): δ52.0 (CO$_2$M̲e̲), 65.7 (O-CH$_2$), 65.8 (O-CH$_2$), 106.5 (C5), 107.0 (aryl C), 115.3 (aryl C), 118.8 (C4), 119.3 (C8), 120.8 (aryl C), 121.8 (C3), 121.9 (C9), 126.5 (C6), 128.8 (aryl C), 138.1 (aryl C), 141.7 (aryl C), 162.3 (C̲O$_2$Me); HRMS (+ESI): Found *m/z* 306.0736 [M + Na]$^+$, $C_{16}H_{13}NO_4Na$ requires 306.0737.

This compound was also prepared by the methods described below. Method 1: The title compound was prepared as described in GP-6 from methyl 5,6-bis(prop-2-yn-1-yloxy)-1*H*-indole-2-carboxylate (**16**) (118 mg, 0.42 mmol) in chlorobenzene (30 mL) to give the product (43.5 mg, 51%) as a yellow solid.

Method 2: Route 1 The title compound was prepared as described in GP-6 from methyl (Z)-2-azido-3-(2*H*,10*H*-pyrano[4,3-h]chromen-5-yl)acrylate (**17**) (646 mg, 2.08 mmol) in xylene (20 mL) to give the product (52.9 mg, 62%) as a yellow solid.

Methyl 5-methoxy-3,7-dihydropyrano[3,2-e]indole-2-carboxylate (**27a**) The title compound was prepared as described in GP-6 from methyl 6-methoxy-5-(prop-2-yn-1-yloxy)-1H-indole-2-carboxylate (**26a**) (108 mg, 0.42 mmol) in chlorobenzene (30 mL) to give the product (80 mg, 74%) as a yellow solid; m.p. 166–168 °C; IR (KBr): ν_{max} 3325, 2948, 2839, 2340, 2110, 1677, 1637, 1515, 1439, 1271, 1193, 1143, 1098,

998, 931, 883, 808, 752 cm^{-1}; UV-vis (CH_3CN): λ_{max} 212 nm (ε 37,400 cm^{-1} M^{-1}), 271 (13,300), 322 (30,600); ^{1}H-NMR (300 MHz, $CDCl_3$): δ 3.92 (s, 3H, OMe), 3.93 (s, 3H, CO_2Me), 4.90 (dd, *J* = 3.7, 1.7 Hz, 2H, O-CH2), 5.89–5.95 (m, 1H, H8), 6.76–6.79 (m, 1H, H9), 6.79 (s, 1H, H4), 7.17 (d, *J* = 2.1 Hz, 1H, H1), 8.96 (s, 1H, NH); ^{13}C-NMR (75.6 MHz, $CDCl_3$): δ 51.8 ($CO_2\underline{Me}$), 56.0 (OMe), 65.7 (O-CH_2), 93.8 (C4), 106.1 (C1), 114.9 (aryl C), 118.3 (aryl C), 121.6 (C9), 121.8 (C8), 126.0 (C2), 132.2 (aryl C), 139.3 (aryl C), 148.8 (C5), 162.2 ($\underline{C}O_2Me$); HRMS (+ESI): Found *m/z* 282.0731 [M + Na]$^+$, $C_{14}H_{13}NO_4Na$ requires 282.0737.

Methyl 5-methoxy-1,7-dihydropyrano[2,3-g]indole-2-carboxylate (**22a**) The *title* compound was prepared as described in GP-6 from methyl 5-methoxy-6-(prop-2-yn-1-yloxy)-1*H*-indole-2-carboxylate (**21a**) (108 mg, 0.42 mmol) in chlorobenzene (30 mL) to give the product (83 mg, 77%) as a yellow solid; m.p. 188–190 °C; IR (KBr): ν_{max} 3327, 2944, 2827, 2366, 2106, 1677, 1528, 1444, 1306, 1221, 1148, 1101, 989, 955, 831, 755 cm^{-1}; UV-vis (CH_3CN): λ_{max} 226 nm (ε 28,100 cm^{-1} M^{-1}), 290 (16,700), 339 (18,400); ^{1}H-NMR (300 MHz, $CDCl_3$): δ 3.94 (s, 3H, OMe), 3.96 (s, 3H, CO_2Me), 4.96 (dd, *J* = 3.8, 1.8 Hz, 2H, O CH_2), 5.89–5.95 (m, 1H, H8), 6.75–6.79 (m, 1H, H9), 7.02 (s, 1H, H4), 7.13 (d, *J* = 2.1 Hz, 1H, H3), 8.94 (s, 1H NH); ^{13}C-NMR (75.6 MHz, $CDCl_3$): δ51.9 ($CO_2\underline{Me}$), 56.2 (OMe), 65.7 (O-CH_2), 103.1 (C4), 107.1 (aryl C), 109.2 (C3), 119.3 (aryl C), 120.8 (C8), 121.0 (C9), 126.0 (C2), 128.7 (aryl C), 137.6 (aryl C), 145.2 (C5), 162.3 ($\underline{C}O_2Me$); HRMS (+ESI): Found *m/z* 282.0738 [M + Na]$^+$, $C_{14}H_{13}NO_4Na$ requires 282.0737.

Methyl 5-methoxy-9-methyl-3,7-dihydropyrano[3,2-e]indole-2-carboxylate (**27b**) The *title* compound was prepared as described in GP-6 from methyl 5-(but-2-yn-1-yloxy)-6-methoxy-1*H*-indole-2-carboxylate (**26b**) (114 mg, 0.42 mmol) in chlorobenzene (30 mL) to give the product (62 mg, 54%) as a yellow solid; m.p. 196–198 °C; IR (KBr): ν_{max} 3310, 2948, 2925, 2833, 2106, 1675, 1640, 1517, 1495, 1439, 1366, 1274, 1265, 1194, 1146, 1080, 1004, 960, 880, 815, 765, 672 cm^{-1}; UV-vis (CH_3CN): λ_{max} 213 nm (ε 28,900 cm^{-1} M^{-1}), 267 (9,500), 322 (24,200); ^{1}H-NMR (300 MHz, $CDCl_3$): δ 1.63 (s, 3H, C-CH_3), 3.94 (s, 3H, OMe), 3.95 (s, 3H, CO_2Me), 4.77 (q, *J* = 2.4 Hz, 2H, O-CH_2), 5.69–5.72 (m, 1H, H8), 6.87 (s, 1H, H1), 7.23 (s, 1H, H4), 8.82 (bs, 1H, NH); ^{13}C-NMR (75.6 MHz, $CDCl_3$): δ 22.6 (C-$\underline{C}H_3$), 51.8 ($CO_2\underline{Me}$), 56.1 (OMe), 65.2 (O-CH_2), 93.8 (C4), 109.3 (C1), 117.4 (aryl C), 117.9 (aryl C), 118.3 (C8), 126.5 (C2), 132.0 ($\underline{C}$-CH_3), 132.9 (aryl C), 140.4 (aryl C), 149.0 (C5), 162.2 ($\underline{C}O_2Me$); HRMS (+ESI): Found *m/z* 296.0887 [M + Na]$^+$, $C_{15}H_{15}NO_4Na$ requires 296.0893.

Methyl 5-methoxy-9-methyl-1,7-dihydropyrano[2,3-g]indole-2-carboxylate (**22b**) The *title* compound was prepared as described in GP-6 from methyl 6-(but-2-yn-1-yloxy)-5-methoxy-1*H*-indole-2-carboxylate (**21b**) (114 mg, 0.42 mmol) in chlorobenzene (30 mL) to give the product (56 mg, 49%) as a yellow solid; m.p. 176–178 °C; IR (KBr): ν_{max} 3410, 2980, 2930, 2845, 1695, 1645, 1606, 1534, 1445, 1430, 1385, 1375, 1232, 1189, 1139, 1096, 1040, 998, 981, 927, 857, 744, 712cm^{-1}; UV-vis (CH_3CN): λ_{max} 224 nm (ε 32,500 cm^{-1} M^{-1}), 286 (22,200), 337 (23,500); ^{1}H-NMR (300 MHz, $CDCl_3$): δ 1.71 (s, 3H, C-CH_3), 3.94 (s, 3H, OMe), 3.96 (s, 3H, CO_2Me), 4.77 (q, *J* = 1.6 Hz, 2H, O-CH_2), 5.65–5.68 (m, 1H, H8), 7.05 (s, 1H, H4), 7.14 (d, *J* = 2.1 Hz, 1H, H3), 8.81 (bs, 1H, NH), ^{13}C-NMR (75.6 MHz, $CDCl_3$): δ 20.8 (C-$\underline{C}H_3$), 51.8 ($CO_2\underline{Me}$), 56.2 (OMe), 65.4 (O-CH_2), 103.2 (C4), 108.9 (C3), 109.9 (aryl C), 117.7 (C8), 121.9 (aryl C), 126.0 (C2), 128.7 ($\underline{C}$-CH_3), 129.3 (aryl C), 144.2 (aryl C), 145.4 (C5), 162.1 ($\underline{C}O_2Me$); HRMS (+ESI): Found *m/z* 296.0886 [M + Na]$^+$, $C_{15}H_{15}NO_4Na$ requires 296.0893.

Methyl 5-methoxy-9-phenyl-3,7-dihydropyrano[3,2-e]indole-2-carboxylate (**27d**) The *title* compound was prepared as described in GP-6 from methyl 6-methoxy-5-((3-phenylprop-2-yn-1-yl)oxy)-1*H*-indole-2-carboxylate (**26d**) (140 mg, 0.42 mmol) in chlorobenzene (30 mL) to give the product (113 mg, 81%) as a yellow solid; m.p. 188–190 °C; IR (KBr): ν_{max} 3311, 2949, 2816, 2114, 1684, 1639, 1598, 1515, 1500, 1438, 1400, 1360, 1260, 1241, 1193, 1141, 1042, 1011, 995, 920, 823, 759, 703 cm^{-1}; UV-vis (CH_3CN): λ_{max} 274 nm (ε 11,600 cm^{-1} M^{-1}), 326 (26,400); ^{1}H-NMR (300 MHz, $CDCl_3$): δ 3.82 (s, 3H, OMe), 4.00 (s, 3H, CO_2Me), 4.85 (d, *J* = 4.4 Hz, 2H, O-CH_2), 5.94–5.97 (m, 1H, H8), 5.98 (s, 1H, H4), 6.88 (s, 1H, H1), 7.30–7.34 (m, 2H, ArH), 7.41–7.44 (m, 3H, ArH), 8.76 (bs, 1H, NH), ^{13}C-NMR (75.6 MHz, $CDCl_3$): δ 51.7 ($CO_2\underline{Me}$), 58.1 (OMe), 65.1 (O-CH_2), 94.2 (C4),

109.4 (C1), 117.0 (aryl C), 117.5 (aryl C), 125.0 (C2), 120.4 (C8), 127.9 (aryl CH), 128.3 (2 × arylCH), 128.5 (2 × aryl CH), 132.8 (aryl C), 139.4 (C-Ph), 139.4 (aryl C), 141.1 (aryl C), 149.0 (C5), 162.1 ($\underline{C}O_2Me$); HRMS (+ESI): Found *m/z* 358.1057 $[M + Na]^+$, $C_{20}H_{17}NO_4Na$ requires 358.1055.

Methyl 5-methoxy-7,7-dimethyl-3,7-dihydropyrano[3,2-e] indole-2-carboxylate (**27c**)
The title compound was prepared as described in GP-3 from methyl (Z)-2-azido-3-(4-methoxy-3-((2-methylbut-3-yn-2-yl)oxy)phenyl)acrylate (**25c**) (654 mg, 2.08 mmol) in xylene (20 mL) to give the product (220 mg, 68%) as a yellow solid; m.p. 144–146 °C; IR (KBr): ν_{max} 3316, 2962, 2975, 2111, 1681, 1625, 1600, 1510, 1439, 1400, 1366, 1270, 1230, 1192, 1131, 1075, 999, 934, 887, 818, 754, 728 cm^{-1}; UV-vis (CH_3CN): λ_{max} 219 nm (ε 40,000 cm^{-1} M^{-1}), 271 (13,500), 323 (31,100); ^{1}H-NMR (300 MHz, $CDCl_3$): δ 1.53 (s, 6H, 2 × CH_3), 3.92 (s, 3H, OMe), 3.95 (s, 3H, CO_2Me), 5.73 (d, *J* = 9.7 Hz, 1H, H8), 6.68 (d, *J* = 9.7 Hz, 1H, H9), 6.79 (s, 1H, H4), 7.19 (d, *J* = 2.1 Hz, 1H, H1), 9.00 (bs, 1H, NH); ^{13}C-NMR (75.6 MHz, $CDCl_3$): δ 27.3 (2 × C-$\underline{C}H_3$), 51.7 ($CO_2\underline{Me}$), 58.1 (OMe), 76.2 ($\underline{C}$-$(CH_3)_2$), 93.1 (C4), 106.1 (C1), 113.4 (aryl C), 118.2 (aryl C), 119.3 (C9), 125.7 (C2), 130.6 (C8), 132.0 (aryl C), 138.1 (aryl C), 149.5 (C5), 162.3 ($\underline{C}O_2Me$); HRMS (+ESI): Found *m/z* 310.1044 $[M + Na]^+$, $C_{16}H_{17}NO_4Na$ requires 310.1050.

Methyl 5-methoxy-7,7-dimethyl-1,7-dihydropyrano[2,3-g] indole-2-carboxylate (**22c**)
The title compound was prepared as described in GP-3 from methyl (Z)-2-azido-3-(3-methoxy-4-((2-methylbut-3-yn-2-yl)oxy)phenyl)acrylate (**20c**) (654 mg, 2.08 mmol) in xylene (20 mL) to give the product (203 mg, 74%) as a yellow solid; m.p. 158–160 °C; IR (KBr): ν_{max} 3338, 2955, 2919, 2845, 2111, 1676, 1640, 1595, 1534, 1444, 1370, 1350, 1310, 1265, 1217, 1195, 1134, 1099, 1050, 985, 960, 880, 826, 760, 714 cm^{-1}; UV-vis (CH_3CN): λ_{max} 226 nm (ε 29,600 cm^{-1} M^{-1}), 262 (15,200), 341 (19,000); ^{1}H-NMR (300 MHz, $CDCl_3$): δ 1.55 (s, 6H, 2 × CH_3), 3.93 (s, 3H, OMe), 3.96 (s, 3H, CO_2Me), 5.71 (d, *J* = 9.7 Hz, 1H, H8), 6.66 (d, *J* = 9.7 Hz, 1H, H9), 7.02 (s, 1H, H4), 7.13 (d, *J* = 2.1 Hz, 1H, H3), 8.95 (bs, 1H, NH); ^{13}C-NMR (75.6 MHz, $CDCl_3$): δ 27.4 (2 × C-$\underline{C}H_3$), 51.8 ($CO_2\underline{Me}$), 56.5 (OMe), 76.6 ($\underline{C}$-$(CH_3)_2$), 103.3 (C4), 105.8 (aryl C), 109.3 (C3), 116.8 (C9), 120.6 (aryl C), 125.7 (C2), 128.9 (aryl C), 129.8 (C8), 142.3 (aryl C), 149.9 (C5), 162.4 ($\underline{C}O_2Me$); HRMS (+ESI): Found *m/z* 288.1228 $[M + H]^+$, $C_{16}H_{18}NO_4$ requires 288.1236.

3.2. Cell Biology Techniques

The SH-SY5Y and Kelly human neuroblastoma cell lines were generously donated by Dr. J. Biedler (Memorial Sloan-Kettering Cancer Center, New York, NY, USA). The MDA-MB-231 and MCF-7 breast cancer cell lines were purchased from the American Type Culture Collection. All cell lines were cultured under standard conditions at 37 °C in 5% CO_2 as an adherent monolayer in Dulbecco's modified Eagle's medium supplemented with L-glutamine (DMEM) (Invitrogen, Waltham, MA, USA) and 10% fetal calf serum (FCS) (Thermo Fisher Scientific, Waltham, MA, USA).

Method for Cell Viability Assays

Cell viability was measured by the standard Alamar blue assay, as previously described [18]. Briefly, cells were allowed to attach for 24 h in 96-well culture plates. The cells were then continuously exposed to serial dilutions of the hydrazide-hydrazone derivatives for 72 h, either in the presence or absence of SAHA (0.5 or 1 μM), with five replicate wells for each determination. Cell viability was determined by the addition of 22 μL of Alamar blue reagent, recorded at comparative 0 h and 5 h values, using a Wallac 1420 Victor III spectrophotometer (GMI, Ramsey, MN, USA), which measured light absorbance in each well at 570 nm. The cell viability of each plate was calculated as a percentage compared to matched DMSO controls (0.5%). The mean (+/'SEM) is shown for three independent experiments.

3.3. Statistical Analysis

Results of the cell viability studies were statistically analyzed using the two-tailed, unpaired Student's t-test. Results are expressed as mean values with 95% confidence intervals.

4. Conclusions

The studies presented in this study have contributed to the investigation of the potential of dihydropyranoindoles to act as SAHA enhancers for the treatment of neuroblastoma and breast cancer cells. To the best of our knowledge, this is the first study which was carried out on the combination of SAHA with dihydropyranoindoles. The desired tricyclic and tetracyclic dihydropyranoindoles was achieved by the reaction of corresponding hydroxybenzaldehydes with haloalkynes followed by the application of the Hemetsberger indole synthesis to yield the related indoles. Claisen cyclization in the presence of chlorobenzene afforded the desired compounds in good yields. Some of the dihydropyranoindoles were successfully synthesized from the corresponding azido intermediates in one step by the thermal decomposition step of the Hemetsberger indole synthesis. The biological studies revealed that the breast cancer cells displayed significant resistance towards the combination treatments of the dihydropyranoindoles compared to the neurobalstoma cells. It was also found that tetracyclic analogues of dihydropyranoindoles **33** and **10** were found to be more favorable for the enhancement of SAHA activity, while only dihydropyrano[3,2-*e*]indole tricyclic systems **27a** and **27c** resulted in the additional reduction of the SAHA cytotoxicity against the neuroblastoma cell lines. Taken altogether, the tetracyclic dihydropyranoindole **10** was determined as the most cytotoxic compound at the concentration 20 μM, while the lower concentration of the designated compound displayed the best enhancement on SAHA activity with the value of 44% additional reduction at the ratio of 1:10 SAHA to compound.

Supplementary Materials: The following figures are available online: **Figure S1** Cell viability of A) SH-SY5Y, B) MDA-MB-231 cancer cells treated with the selected six compounds **1–6** (10 μM) over 72 h. Error bars represent mean values (±S.D.) for three independent determinations. **Figure S2**. Comparative toxicity of compounds **1, 3** and **4** (10 μM) against SH-SY5Y, MDA-MB-231 and MRC-5 cell lines after 72 h exposure. Error bars represent mean values (±S.D.) for three independent determinations. **Figure S3**. Cell viability of A) MCF-7 $p < 0.01$ B) MDA-MB-231 $p < 0.05$ breast cancer cells treated with 10 μM compounds over 72 h, in the presence or absence of 1 μM of SAHA. Error bars represent mean values (±S.D.) for three independent determinations **Figure S4**. Cell viability of A) Kelly $p \geq 0.05$ (ns) B) SH-SY5Y $p < 0.0005$ neuroblastoma cancer cellstreated with 10 μM compounds over 72 h, in the presence or absence of 1 μM of SAHA. Error bars represent mean values (±S.D.) for three independent determinations. **Figure S5**. Cell viability of KELLY neuroblastoma cancer cells treated with compounds A) **33** $p < 0.01$ B) **27c** $p < 0.05$ and C) **10** $p < 0.05$ at different concentrations (0.01, 0.1, 1, 10, 20 μM) over 72 h in the absence and presence of SAHA. Error bars represent mean values (±S.D.) for three independent determinations. **Figure S6**. Cell viability of SH-SY5Y neuroblastoma cancer cells treated with compounds A) **27a**, $p < 0.0005$ B) **33**, $p < 0.0005$ C) **10**, $p < 0.01$ and D) **27c**, $p < 0.01$ at different concentrations (0.01, 0.1, 1, 10, 20 μM) over 72 h in the absence and presence of SAHA. Error bars represent mean values (±S.D.) for three independent determinations. **Figure S7**. Comparative toxicity of compounds A) **27a**, $p < 0.05$ B) **33**, $p < 0.05$ C) **10**, $p < 0.05$ and D) **27c**, $p < 0.0005$ (10 μM) against cancer cells (Kelly, SH-SY5Y, MCF-7 and MDA-MB-231) and human lung fibroblasts (WI-38 and MRC-5) cell lines after 72 h exposure. Error bars represent mean values (±S.D.) for three independent determinations.

Author Contributions: N.K., D.S.B., G.M.M. and B.B.C. conceived and designed the experiments, G.M.A. provided the data from library screening, M.B. performed the experiments, analyzed, interpreted the data and wrote the paper, N.K. and G.M.M. supported financially. All authors have read and agree to the published version of the manuscript.

Funding: This research was funded by Australian Research Council Discovery Project, grant number DP180100845.

Acknowledgments: We thank the University of New South Wales, and the Australian Research Council (ARC) for funding to N.K. and D.S.B. Mass spectrometric analysis for this work was carried out at the Bioanalytical Mass Spectrometry Facility, UNSW and was supported in part by infrastructure funding from the New South Wales Government as part of its co-investment in the National Collaborative Research Infrastructure Strategy. This research was supported by Australian Postgraduate Research Scholarships, University of NSW, Program Grants from the NHMRC Australia, Cancer Institute NSW Australia and Cancer Council NSW Australia. The Children's Cancer Institute Australia for Medical Research is affiliated with the University of NSW and Sydney Children's Hospital.

Conflicts of Interest: The authors declare no conflict of interest.

References

1. Matthay, K.K.; Yanik, G.; Messina, J.; Quach, A.; Huberty, J.; Cheng, S.C.; Veatch, J.; Goldsby, R.; Brophy, P.; Kersun, L.S.; et al. Phase II study on the effect of disease sites, age, and prior therapy on response to iodine-131-metaiodobenzylguanidine therapy in refractory neuroblastoma. *J. Clin. Oncol.* **2007**, *25*, 1054–1060. [CrossRef]
2. DuBois, S.G.; Kalika, Y.; Lukens, J.N.; Brodeur, G.M.; Seeger, R.C.; Atkinson, J.B.; Haase, G.M.; Black, C.T.; Perez, C.; Shimada, H.; et al. Metastatic sites in stage IV and IVS neuroblastoma correlate with age, tumor biology, and survival. *J. Pediat Hematol Onc.* **1999**, *21*, 181–189. [CrossRef] [PubMed]
3. Matthay, K.K.; Reynolds, C.P.; Seeger, R.C.; Shimada, H.; Adkins, E.S.; Haas-Kogan, D.; Gerbing, R.B.; London, W.B.; Villablanca, J.G. Iodine-131- metaiodobenzylguanidine double infusion with autologous stem-cellrescue for neuroblastoma: A new approaches to neuroblastoma therapyphase I study. *J. Clin Oncol.* **2009**, *27*, 1020–1025. [CrossRef] [PubMed]
4. Smith, M.A.; Seibel, N.L.; Altekruse, S.F.; Ries, L.A.G.; Melbert, D.L.; O'Leary, M.; Smith, F.O.; Reaman, G.H. Outcomes for children and adolescents with cancer: Challenges for the twenty-first century. *J. Clin. Oncol.* **2010**, *28*, 2625–2634. [CrossRef]
5. Lautz, T.B.; Jie, C.; Clark, S.; Naiditch, J.A.; Jafari, N.; Qiu, Y.Y.; Zheng, X.; Chu, F.; Madonna, M.B. The effect of vorinostat on the development of resistance to doxorubicin in neuroblastoma. *PLoS ONE* **2012**, *7*, 40816. [CrossRef] [PubMed]
6. Huang, J.M.; Sheard, M.A.; Ji, L.Y.; Sposto, R.; Keshelava, N. Combination of Vorinostat and Flavopiridol Is Selectively Cytotoxic to Multidrug-Resistant Neuroblastoma Cell Lines with Mutant *TP53*. *Mol. Cancer Ther.* **2010**, *9*, 3289–3301. [CrossRef]
7. Ozaki, K.; Kishikawa, F.; Tanaka, M.; Sakamoto, T.; Tanimura, S.; Kohno, M. Histone deacetylase inhibitors enhance the chemosensitivity of tumor cells with cross-resistance to a wide range of DNA-damaging drugs. *Cancer Sci.* **2008**, *99*, 376–384. [CrossRef] [PubMed]
8. Basu, H.S.; Mahlum, A.; Mehraein-Ghomi, F.; Kegel, S.J.; Guo, S.; Peters, N.R.; Wilding, G. Pre-treatment with anti-oxidants sensitizes oxidatively stressed human cancer cells to growth inhibitory effect of suberoylanilide hydroxamic acid (SAHA). *Cancer Chemoth. Pharm.* **2011**, *67*, 705–715. [CrossRef]
9. Richon, V.M. Cancer biology: Mechanism of antitumour action of vorinostat (suberoylanilide hydroxamic acid), a novel histone deacetylase inhibitor. *Brit. J. Cancer* **2006**, *95*, 2–6. [CrossRef]
10. Duvic, M.; Zhang, C. Clinical and laboratory experience of vorinostat (suberoylanilide hydroxamic acid) in the treatment of cutaneous T-cell lymphoma. *Brit. J. Cancer.* **2006**, *95*, 13–19. [CrossRef]
11. Mann, B.S.; Johnson, J.R.; He, K.; Sridhara, R.; Abraham, S.; Booth, B.P.; Verbois, L.; Morse, D.E.; Jee, J.M.; Pope, S.; et al. Vorinostat for treatment of cutaneous manifestations of advanced primary cutaneous T-cell lymphoma. *Clin. Cancer Res.* **2007**, *13*, 2318–2322. [CrossRef] [PubMed]
12. Kelly, W.K.; O'Connor, O.A.; Krug, L.M.; Chiao, J.H.; Heaney, M.; Curley, T.; MacGregore-Cortelli, B.; Tong, W.; Secrist, J.P.; Schwartz, L.; et al. Phase I study of an oral histone deacetylase inhibitor, suberoylanilide hydroxamic acid, in patients with advanced cancer. *J. Clin. Oncol.* **2005**, *23*, 3923–3931. [CrossRef] [PubMed]
13. Krug, L.M.; Curley, T.; Schwartz, L.; Richardson, S.; Marks, P.; Chiao, J.; Kelly, W.K. Potential role of histone deacetylase inhibitors in mesothelioma: Clinical experience with suberoylanilide hydroxamic acid. *Clin. Lung. Cancer* **2006**, *7*, 257–261. [CrossRef] [PubMed]
14. Rundall, B.K.; Denlinger, C.E.; Jones, D.R. Suberoylanilide hydroxamic acid combined with gemcitabine enhances apoptosis in non-small cell lung cancer. *Surgery.* **2005**, *138*, 360–367. [CrossRef] [PubMed]
15. Sonnemann, J.; Gange, J.; Kumar, K.S.; Muller, C.; Bader, P.; Beck, J.F. Histone deacetylase inhibitors interact synergistically with tumor necrosis factor-related apoptosis-inducing ligand (TRAIL) to induce apoptosis in carcinoma cell lines. *Investig. New Drug.* **2005**, *23*, 99–109. [CrossRef] [PubMed]
16. Denlinger, C.E.; Rundall, B.K.; Jones, D.R. Proteasome inhibition sensitizes non-small cell lung cancer to histone deacetylase inhibitor-induced apoptosis through the generation of reactive oxygen species. *J. Thorac Cardiov Sur.* **2004**, *128*, 740–748. [CrossRef]
17. Arndt, G.; Children's Cancer Institute, Sydney, Australia. Personal Communication, 2009.
18. Marks, P. Discovery and development of SAHA as an anticancer agent. *Oncogene.* **2007**, *26*, 1351–1356. [CrossRef]

19. Hemetsberger, H.; Knittel, D.; Weidmann, H. Synthese und Thermolyse von α-Azidoacrylestern. *Monatsh. Chem.* **1972**, *103*, 149. [CrossRef]
20. McElhanon, J.R.; Wu, M.J.; Escobar, M.; Chaudhry, U.; Hu, C.L.; McGrath, D.V. Asymmetric Synthesis of a Series of Chiral AB2 Monomers for Dendrimer Construction. *J. Org. Chem.* **1997**, *62*, 908–915. [CrossRef]
21. Büchi, G.; Kamikawa, T. An alternative synthesis of 5,6-dihydroxy-2,3-hydroindole-2-carboxylates (Cyclodopa). *J. Org. Chem.* **1977**, *42*, 4153–4154. [CrossRef]
22. Li, J.; Zhang, D.M.; Zhu, X.; He, Z.J.; Liu, S.; Li, M.F.; Pang, J.Y.; Lin, Y.C. Studies on synthesis and structure-activity relationship (SAR) of derivatives of a new natural product from marine fungi as inhibitors of influenza virus neuraminidase. *Mar. Drugs.* **2011**, *9*, 1887–1901. [CrossRef] [PubMed]
23. Guantai, E.M.; Ncokazi, K.; Egan, T.J.; Gut, J.; Rosenthal, P.J.; Smith, P.J.; Chibale, K. Design, synthesis and in vitro antimalarial evaluation of triazole-linked chalcone and dienone hybrid compounds. *Bioorg. Med. Chem.* **2010**, *18*, 8243–8256. [CrossRef] [PubMed]
24. Elomri, A.; Michel, S.; Tillequin, F.; Koch, M. A novel synthesis of 6-demethoxyacronycine. *Heterocycles* **1992**, *34*, 799–806.
25. Suresh, T.; Kumar, R.N.; Mohan, P.S. A Facile approach to dibenzo [bf| [1,6] naphthyridines using Vilsmeier Conditions. *Heterocycl Commun.* **2003**, *9*, 83–88. [CrossRef]
26. Zammit, S.C.; Cox, A.J.; Gow, R.M.; Zhang, Y.; Gilbert, R.E.; Krum, H.; Kelly, D.J.; Williams, S.J. Evaluation and optimization of antifibrotic activity of cinnamoyl anthranilates. *Bioorg. Med. Chem. Lett.* **2009**, *19*, 7003–7006. [CrossRef]
27. Crombie, L.; Jamieson, S.V. Dihydrostilbenes of cannabis. Synthesis of canniprene. *J. Chem. Soc. Perkin Trans. 1* **1982**, 1467–1475. [CrossRef]

Sample Availability: Samples of the compound are not available from the authors.

molecules

MDPI

Article

Design, Synthesis, and In Vitro Evaluation of the Photoactivatable Prodrug of the PARP Inhibitor Talazoparib

Jiaguo Li [1,2], Dian Xiao [2], Lianqi Liu [2], Fei Xie [2], Wei Li [2], Wei Sun [1,*], Xiaohong Yang [1,*] and Xinbo Zhou [2,*]

1 School of Pharmaceutical Sciences, Jilin University, Changchun 130021, China; li_jiaguo@126.com

2 National Engineering Research Center for the Emergency Drug, Beijing Institute of Pharmacology and Toxicology, Beijing 100850, China; be_xiaodian@163.com (D.X.); llianqi@126.com (L.L.); xiefei0058@163.com (F.X.); a_moon1096@163.com (W.L.)

* Correspondence: wsun@jlu.edu.cn (W.S.); xiaohongyang88@126.com (X.Y.); zhouxinbo@bmi.ac.cn (X.Z.); Tel.: +86-010-6693-0674 (X.Z.)

Academic Editor: Qiao-Hong Chen

Received: 26 November 2019; Accepted: 16 January 2020; Published: 18 January 2020

Abstract: In this article, we report the design, synthesis, photodynamic properties, and in vitro evaluation of photoactivatable prodrug for the poly (ADP-ribose) polymerase 1 (PARP-1) inhibitor Talazoparib. In order to yield a photoactivatable, inactive prodrug, photoactivatable protecting groups (PPGs) were employed to mask the key pharmacophore of Talazoparib. Our study confirmed the good stability and photolytic effect of prodrugs. A PARP-1 enzyme inhibition assay and PARylation experiment showed that the inhibitory activity of the prodrug was reduced 380 times and more than 658 times, respectively, which proved that the prodrug's expected activity was lost after PPG protection. In *BRCA1*- and *BRCA2*-deficient cell lines, the inhibitory activity of the compound was significantly restored after ultraviolet (UV) irradiation. The results indicate that the photoactivatable prodrug strategy is an interesting approach for studying PARP inhibitors. Meanwhile, the described photoactivatable prodrug also provided a new biological tool for the mechanism research of PARP.

Keywords: Talazoparib; PARP inhibitor; prodrug; o-nitro-benzyl; photoactivatable protecting groups

1. Introduction

DNA repair in normal cells mainly relies on the base excision repair (BER) pathway for single-strand DNA breaks and the homologous recombination (HR) pathway for double-strand DNA breaks [1]. Poly (ADP-ribose) polymerase (PARP) plays a key role in the repair of single-strand DNA breaks, through its ability to bind to DNA gaps and recruit other DNA repair enzymes in the BER pathway [1–4]. The tumor suppressor proteins encoded by the breast cancer genes *BRCA1* and *BRCA2* participate in the HR of double-strand DNA breaks [5]. Usually, in tumor cells with *BRCA1* and *BRCA2* mutations or defects, the inhibition of the PARP enzyme can lead to the accumulation of single-strand DNA breaks, owing to the HR repair pathway being blocked, which causes further double-strand DNA breaks and finally results in the death of tumor cells [6–8]. Currently, PARP inhibitors have been a hot topic in the tumor research area. Among them, Olaparib, Rucaparib, Niraparib, and Talazoparib have been approved for the treatment of *BRCA*-deficient breast, ovarian, fallopian tube, and primary peritoneal cancers [9]. In addition, PARP inhibitors are also used in combination with some kinase inhibitors, and show significant synergistic antitumor effects on prostate cancer, pancreatic cancer, gastric cancer, acute leukemia, and non-small-cell lung cancer [10–13]. The number of diseases illustrate the huge potential for therapeutic agents and for biological probes in PARP research.

Talazoparib (trade name: Talzenna), an oral PARP inhibitor developed by Pfizer, was approved by the U.S. Food and Drug Administration (FDA) on 16 October 2018 [14,15]. It is currently the most active compound among the PARP inhibitors, with an IC_{50} of 0.57 nM, which is 4–10 times lower than that of the other PARP inhibitors [16]. The clinical dose of Talazoparib is only 1 mg (once a day). In contrast, to achieve similar effects as Talazoparib, the dosage of Olaparib [17] and Niraparib [18] are 400 mg (twice a day) and 300 mg (once a day), respectively. In addition, while Talazoparib is highly effective in killing tumor cells, there may still be serious side effects, such as myelodysplastic syndrome or acute myeloid leukemia [14,19]. In light of the immense significance of PARP inhibitors, we aimed to develop a relevant, photoactivatable Talazoparib prodrug.

Photoactivatable prodrugs are usually designed by blocking a key pharmacophore moiety of the inhibitor using photoactivatable protecting groups (PPGs), which have been widely used in biology and medicine in recent years as a non-invasive approach [20–22]. This method can provide temporal and spatial control for the release of bioactive substance by UV irradiation. Thus, highly active inhibitors can be generated in irradiated areas of interest at defined points in time. The photoactivatable prodrugs can serve as a novel biological tool for kinetic or mechanistic studies. Moreover, blocked inhibitors may minimize the systemic side effects of Talazoparib, in order to enable a higher dosage of inactive prodrugs.

The o-nitrobenzyl system and its derivatives are one of the most commonly used PPGs [23–26]. The photolysis mechanism is intramolecular rearrangement. As shown in Figure 1, under 365 nm UV irradiation, carbonyl compounds containing o-nitrobenzyl can form a highly active bi-radical, which will undergo hydrogen abstraction on the carbon atom at the γ position and release the parent drugs [26–29]. The advantages of such PPG technology are a high release speed and easy chemical synthesis. At the same time, the UV release wavelength of 365 nm involves less DNA damage than wavelengths shorter than 300 nm, and is harmless to tissues and cells at low doses [29,30]. This method has potential clinical application value [25,26]. For example, irradiation can be temporarily applied to the lesion site during or after surgery to release active substances for killing residual cancer cells, thereby preventing postoperative recurrence. Optical fibres and endoscopic probes can also be used to transmit the required light to the action site to treat some superficial tumors.

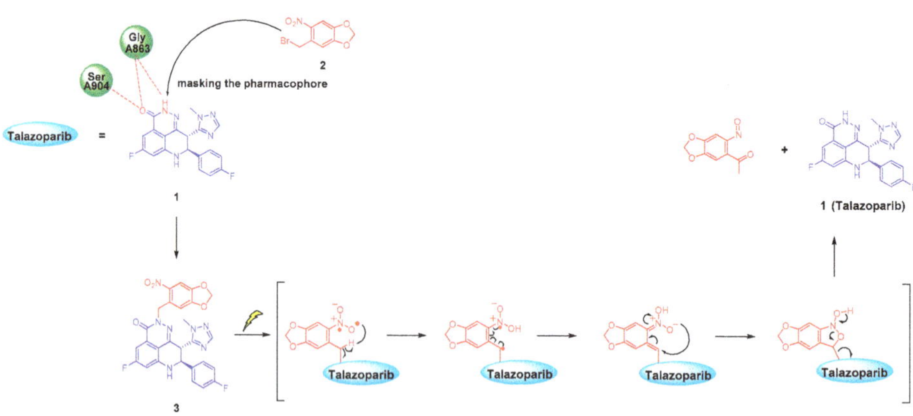

Figure 1. Photolysis mechanism of o-nitrobenzyl upon 365 nm UV irradiation and the inferred drug release process of the Talazoparib prodrug.

In this study, we report the design, synthesis, photodynamic properties, and in vitro evaluation of a photoactivatable prodrug for the PARP-1 inhibitor Talazoparib. We used the concept of PPGs to covalently bond o-nitrobenzyl derivatives (herein designated as compound **2**) to the lactam pharmacophore of Talazoparib, under the guidance of molecular docking; this disrupts its key hydrogen bonding interaction with the PARP protein residue to yield an inactive photoactivatable prodrug, i.e., compound **3**. Our research proved that newly designed prodrug **3** showed good stability and could be rapidly deprotected after UV radiation. A PARP-1 enzyme inhibition assay and PARylation experiment showed that inhibitory activity of the PPG-protected prodrug was greatly reduced by 380 and more than 658 times, respectively. In addition, in *BRCA1*- and *BRCA2*-deficient cell lines, the inhibitory activity of the prodrug **3** was significantly restored after transitory UV irradiation, and the data implies that inhibitory activity could increase with prolonged irradiation time. The results of this preliminary study indicate that the photoactivatable prodrug strategy was an interesting approach for studying PARP inhibitors. Meanwhile, the described photoactivatable prodrugs also provide a novel biological tool for the signal transduction research.

2. Results and Discussion

2.1. Molecular Modelling

Molecular docking of the Tazaloparib into the catalytic domain of PARP-1 (catPARP-1) revealed that its lactam moiety was the key pharmacodynamic group (PDB ID 4PJT). N and O atoms on the lactam moiety could form hydrogen bonds with the Gly863 and Ser904 residues of PARP-1, respectively (Figure 2A) [31,32]. To block its pharmacophoric features, we linked PPGs (namely, compound **2**) to the lactam moiety to form compound **3**, and simulated the action mode of this compound in the same activity pocket. Consistent with our hypothesis, no proper binding of compound **3** to the enzyme active sites were found during the docking; that is, the PPGs blocked the interaction of the lactam moiety with the Gly863 and Ser904 residues (Figure 2B). In addition, the introduction of PPGs led to spatial conflict, which rendered compound **3** unable to maintain the same binding mode as Talazoparib, and the whole molecule was turned over by a certain angle degree (Figure 2C). Inspired by this docking result, we synthesised compound **3** and carried out the following series of photochemical characterisations and biological evaluations.

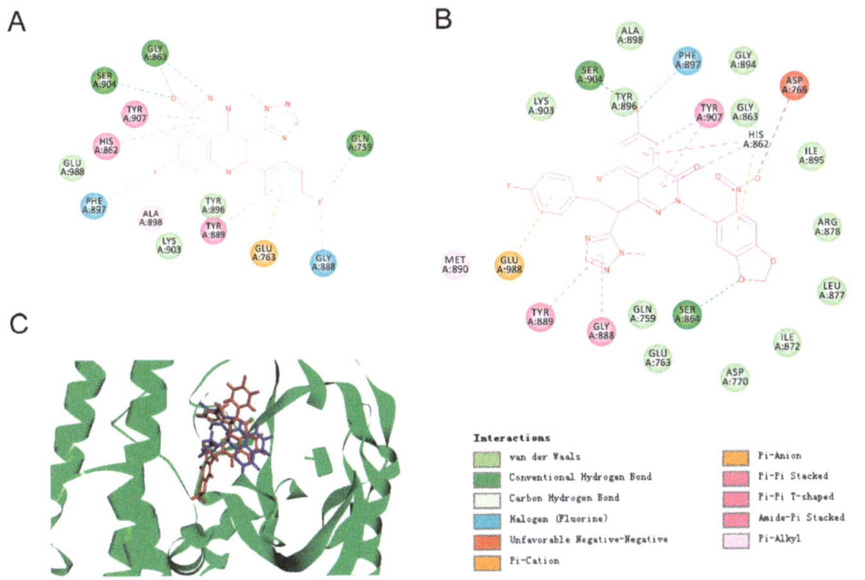

Figure 2. Predicted ligand binding models relative to the catalytic domain of poly (ADP-ribose) polymerase 1 (catPARP-1). (**A**) The co-crystallized binding modes of Talazoparib and the catPARP-1 protein were taken from PDB ID 4PJT. (**B**) Predicted co-crystallized binding poses of compound **3** in a complex with catPARP-1. (**C**) Superimposition of the binding models of Tazaloparib (blue) and compound **3** (red) with catPARP-1 protein (green).

2.2. *Chemistry*

As shown in Scheme 1, Talazoparib could generate the intermediate compound **4** under the action of n-Butyllithium. Compound **4** subsequently underwent a nucleophilic substitution reaction with compound **2** to generate the photoactivatable target compound **3**.

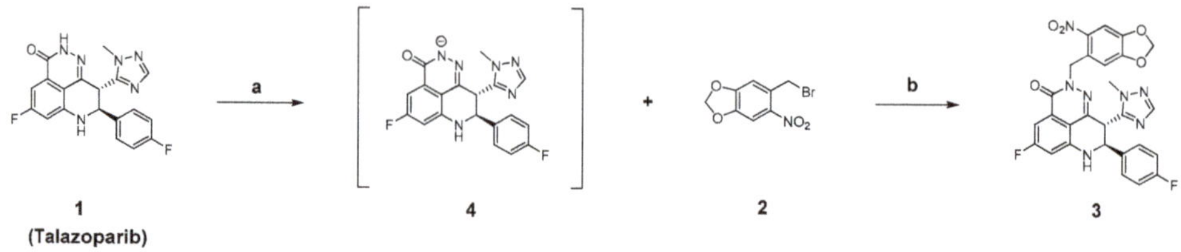

Scheme 1. Synthesis of compound **3**. Reagents: (a) n-BuLi, tetrahydrofuran (THF), N_2, −80 °C, 10 min; (b) THF, N_2, 0 °C, 1 h.

2.3. *Stability Assays and UV Cleavage Test In Vitro*

2.3.1. UV Stability of Talazoparib

Talazoparib should have sufficient stability at the light radiation wavelength used; otherwise, it will be degraded immediately after release or even before the breaking of the PPG covalent bond. Therefore, we first evaluated the UV stability of Talazoparib at a wavelength of 365 nm. To this end, we used a UV cross-linker with an emission wavelength of 365 nm (4.1 mWs/cm^2) to irradiate 2.63 mM Talazoparib in methanol, and took aliquots of the sample at different times for high-performance liquid chromatography (HPLC) analysis. The result indicated that there was no significant loss of Talazoparib in the peak area within 10 min, showing good UV stability (Figure 3A). In addition, the UV/vis absorption spectra of Talazoparib and compound **3** was shown in supplementary materials (See Figure S1).

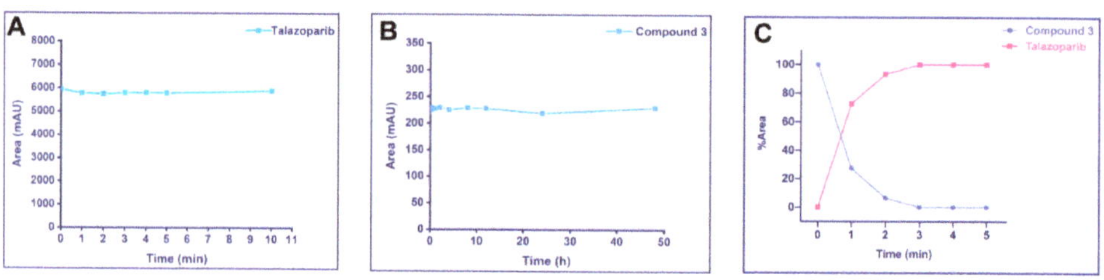

Figure 3. Stability assays and UV cleavage test in vitro. Compounds were irradiated at 365 nm (4.1 mW/cm^2). Samples were determined on a C18 column using a water/acetonitrile (ACN) gradient. The detection wavelength for high-performance liquid chromatography (HPLC) analysis was 220 nm. The peak area or peak area percentage was plotted against the irradiation time. (**A**) UV stability of Talazoparib: 2.63 mM Talazoparib in methanol were irradiated up to 10 min, and aliquot samples at different time points were analyzed by HPLC. Talazoparib was stable under the described UV irradiation. (**B**) Phosphate-buffered saline (PBS) stability of the photoactivatable prodrug: 20 µM compound **3** in pH = 7.4 PBS (containing 10% DMSO) were incubated at 37 °C for 48 h and analyzed by HPLC. The peak area of compound **3** did not show significant changes. (**C**) UV cleavage test on compound **3**: 20 µM of the compound in methanol was irradiated at 365 nm for 5 min and analyzed by HPLC. By progressing irradiation, compound **3** was converted into Talazoparib.

2.3.2. Stability of the Photoactivatable Prodrug in Phosphate-Buffered Saline

The synthesised photoactivatable prodrug should be sufficiently stable. If a high dose of inactive prodrugs were converted to the parent drug in advance, this might produce some undesirable toxic and side effects. Therefore, we tested the stability of compound **3** in phosphate-buffered saline (PBS) with the same pH as blood. Then 20 μM of compound **3** were added to pH = 7.4 PBS containing 10% dimethyl sulfoxide, which was incubated in a 37 °C thermostatic incubator for 48 h under normal brightness, during which samples of equal concentration were taken at different time points for HPLC analysis. The results were plotted according to the sampling time points and the peak areas of the compound (Figure 3B). The peak area of compound **3** did not show significant changes within 48 h, indicating that the compound **3** had good stability in PBS.

2.3.3. UV Release of the Photoactivatable Prodrug

A photoactivatable prodrug needs to not only have good stability, but also be rapidly and effectively released at the irradiated site. Therefore, we tested the photolysis of compound **3**. Figure 3C shows the release situation of compound **3** (20 μM in methanol) after UV irradiation. Under the current experimental conditions, compound **3** could rapidly and completely release Talazoparib in 3 min. In addition, the release experiment also provided a reference for the irradiation duration to be used for the subsequent cell experiments.

2.4. Enzymatic Experiments In Vitro

2.4.1. Inhibition of the PARP-1 Enzyme

According to the guidance of molecular docking, after the PPG was introduced at the lactam pharmacophore of Talazoparib, the prodrug **3** should have had a reduced inhibitory effect on the PARP-1 enzyme. Therefore, we evaluated the inhibitory activities of Talazoparib and compound **3** on PARP-1. As shown in the dose-dependent curve in Figure 4A, the inhibitory activity of the PPG-inactivated compound **3** was significantly lower than that of Talazoparib. The IC_{50} values of Talazoparib and compound **3** were 0.005 and 1.919 μM, respectively, indicating that the inhibitory activity was reduced by 380 times (Table 2). This was consistent with the prediction from the molecular docking. The test results strongly proved that the interaction between the inhibitor and PARP-1 enzyme could be significantly blocked after introducing PPG to the lactam pharmacophore of Talazoparib.

Table 1. Inhibitory activity of Talazoparib and compound **3** on poly (ADP-ribose) (PAR) polymerization.

Test Compound	Inhibit Polymerization of PAR
	IC_{50} (μM)
Talazoparib	<0.0005
3	0.329

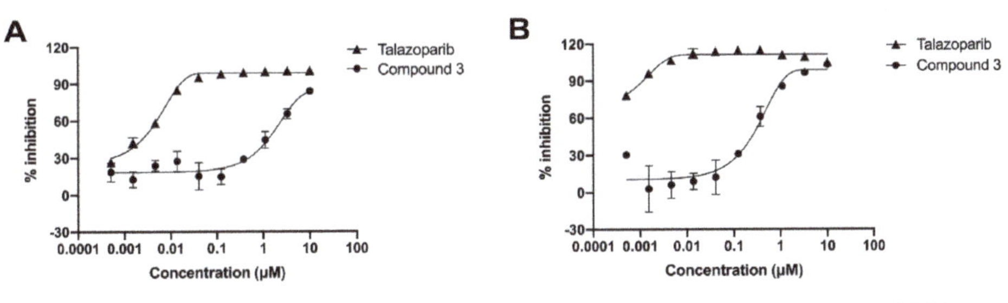

Figure 4. (**A**) Dose–response curve of Talazoparib and compound **3** on PARP-1 enzyme inhibition. Compound **3** showed a significant decrease in the inhibitory activity compared to the active Talazoparib to PARP-1 enzyme. Error bars represent standard deviation from duplicate determinations, and results are shown as mean ± standard deviation (SD). The IC_{50} value is presented in Table 2. (**B**) Dose–response curve of Talazoparib and compound **3** on PARylation assay. The ability of compound **3** to inhibit the

polymerization of PAR significant decreased compared to the active Talazoparib in Hela cells. Error bars represented standard deviation from duplicate determinations, and results are shown as mean ± SD. The IC_{50} value is presented in Table 1.

Table 2. Poly (ADP-ribose) polymerase 1 (PARP-1) enzyme inhibitory activity of Talazoparib and compound **3**.

Test Compound	Inhibition of PARP-1 Enzyme
	IC_{50} (μM)
Talazoparib	0.005
3	1.919

2.4.2. PARylation Assay

The inhibitory activity of compounds on the PARP-1 enzyme could also be evaluated at the cellular level by using a hydrogen peroxide solution to damage the DNA of cells. Under normal circumstances, PARP-1 would be activated immediately, and the poly (ADP-ribose) polymer would be synthesised with NAD+ as the substrate. In the presence of a PARP-1 inhibitor, however, the biological function of PARP-1 would be inhibited. Therefore, the inhibitory activity on PARP-1 can be determined by detecting the level of poly (ADP-ribose) [16,33]. From the data in Figure 4B and Table 1, it can be seen that Talazoparib showed a strong inhibitory effect on poly ADP-ribosylation in HeLa cells, with an IC_{50} value of less than 0.0005 μM, whereas compound **3** showed a weak inhibitory effect, with an IC_{50} value of 0.329 μM, a decrease of 658 times at least.

2.5. Compound's Cytotoxicity Assay in the Absence and Presence of UV Irradiation

After confirming that the introduction of PPG could block the inhibitory activity of Talazoparib on PARP-1, we speculated that compound **3** should also have less cytotoxicity than Talazoparib. To verify this idea, cell proliferation inhibition experiments were conducted. As Talazoparib should only be applied to *BRCA1* or BRCA2-defective cell lines, the principle is simultaneous inhibition of the BER pathway and HR repair pathway of DNA to produce a synthetic lethality effect and consequently, the apoptosis of the tumour cells. Therefore, we selected the well-recognized *BRCA1*- and *BRCA2*-defective cell lines MX-1 and Capan-1 for the following tests. The results indicate that Talazoparib exhibited effective cytotoxicity in the MX-1 and Capan-1 cell lines (IC_{50} values: 0.015 μM and 0.003 μM, respectively). In contrast, the PPG-inactivated compound **3** showed no significant cytotoxicity, with IC_{50} values of 1.873 μM and 0.863 μM, respectively (Figure 5 and Table 3).

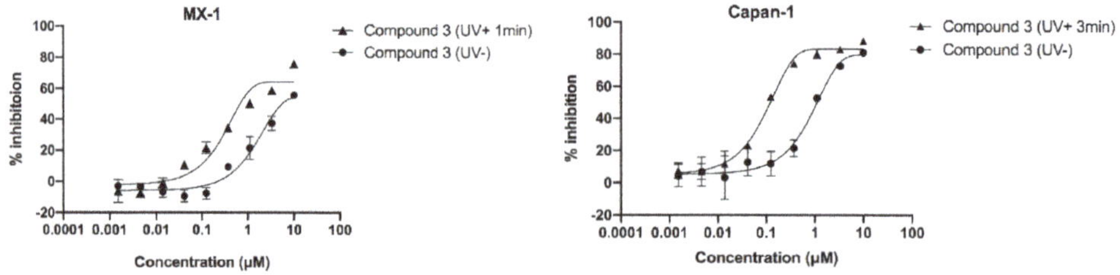

Figure 5. Dose–response curves of compound **3** in the absence and presence of ultraviolet irradiation. Cells were incubated for 1 h with the compounds and were then irradiated at 365 nm (4.1 mW/cm^2). Cell growth was determined 10 days after incubation with the compounds. Irradiated compounds showed left-shifted dose–response curve compared to that of the unirradiated compounds. Error bars represent the standard deviation from duplicate determinations, and results are shown as mean ± SD. The IC_{50} value is presented in Table 3.

Table 3. Capan-1 and MX-1 cell inhibitory activities of Talazoparib and compound **3** in the absence and presence ultraviolet radiation.

Test Compound	MX-1 Cell (UV + 1 min) IC_{50} (μM)	Capan-1 Cell (UV + 3 min IC_{50} (μM)
Talazoparib (UV-)	0.015	0.003
3 (UV-)	1.873	0.863
3 (UV+)	0.577	0.092

Next, we tested whether the inhibitory activity of compound **3** could be restored after UV irradiation. In order to negate the influence of UV irradiation on cells, to avoid interfering with the experiment results, we first measured the maximum tolerance of cells to UV light. As shown in Figure 6, the MX-1 cell line was relatively sensitive to UV irradiation, and could tolerate an irradiation duration of 1 min, whereas further extension of the duration would affect cell proliferation. In contrast, the Capan-1 cell line could tolerate UV irradiation for a relatively long time, and approximately 85% of the cells were still alive after irradiation for 5 min. On the basis of the principle of maximising drug release, while ensuring normal cell proliferation as much as possible, we determined the UV irradiation durations for the MX-1 and Capan-1 cells to be 1 min and 3 min, respectively.

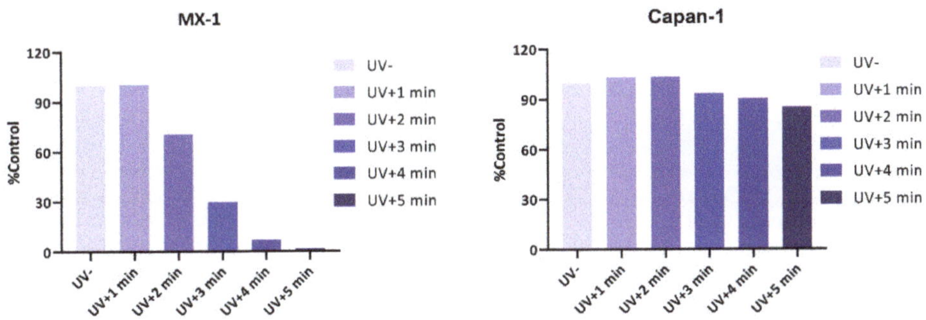

Figure 6. Cellular ultraviolet light tolerance test. Cells were irradiated at 365 nm (4.1 mW/cm^2) for indicated periods of time, and cell growth was determined after 10 days. The MX-1 cell line was relatively sensitive to UV irradiation. Radiation over 1 min affected cell proliferation. In contrast, the Capan-1 cell line tolerated UV irradiation for a relatively long time.

As shown in Table 3, the inhibitory activity of compound **3** on MX-1 cells after UV irradiation was approximately three times higher than that on the non-irradiated group (IC_{50} values: 1.873 μM vs. 0.577 μM, respectively). However, it did not reach the same level of inhibition as the parent drug Talazoparib, likely because the irradiation duration of 1 min was not enough to allow the release of all the compound **3**. Therefore, we tested the Capan-1 cells that could tolerate a longer UV irradiation duration. To our delight, the IC_{50} value of compound **3** for Capan-1 cells was 0.092 μM after 3 min of irradiation, which was nine times higher than that of the non-irradiated group (IC_{50} value: 0.863 μM). Further analysis was needed to determine the reason why the inhibitory activity of compound **3** still did not reach the same level as Talazoparib after UV irradiation. We simulated the same cytotoxicity experimental conditions to evaluate the photolysis of 10 μM compound **3** (10 μM is the starting concentration of compound **3** in cytotoxicity experiments) in a 96-well plate. The results showed that compound **3** was not released completely after 3 min UV irradiation (see Figure S2).

The above cytotoxicity experiment data indicated that compound **3** could significantly restore the effective activity of Talazoparib after being irradiated by UV light, and the data from both cells imply that inhibitory activity could increase with prolonged irradiation time. However, owing to the limited types of *BRCA*-deficient cells that could be selected for study and their restrictive UV light tolerance, compound **3** did not reach the same level of inhibitory activity as Talazoparib. The experimental results could provide inspiration for future research.

2.6. Verification of the Toxicity of Leaving Photoactivatable Protecting Groups

Subsequently, the leaving PPG after irradiation was also evaluated for its cytotoxicity. Compound **3** was obviously not suitable for verifying this, since it released active Talazoparib after its photocleavage. Therefore, we used an indirect test method by synthesising compound **6** via the nucleophilic substitution reaction between the non-cytotoxic Boc-protected amino acid L-alanine (Boc-Ala), as reported in the literature, and compound **2** under the catalysis of potassium carbonate (Scheme 2), and examined compound **6'**s effect on cell proliferation before and after irradiation [25,26].

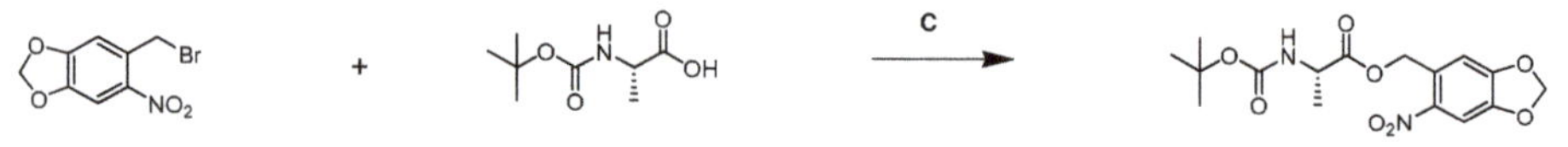

3 **5** **6**

Scheme 2. Synthesis of compound **6**. Reagents: (c) K_2CO_3, reflux, 5 h.

We first evaluated the photolysis of compound **6**, and the experimental results showed that 20 μM of compound **6** in methanol solution were almost completely released within 20 min (see Figure S3). Next, we used the same initial concentration as that of compound **3** for the measurement. To fully release the drug, we UV-irradiated compound **6** at different concentrations for 20 min, and then added each sample to cells for co-culture. As a result, compound **6** showed no significant cytotoxicity in MX-1 and Capan-1 cells both before and after irradiation (Figure 7 and Table 4). Since the Boc–Ala released after irradiation was not cytotoxic, the results verified that the leaving PPG at the indicated concentrations did not cause any cytotoxicity. This therefore proved that the cytotoxicity of compound **3** after irradiation could be attributed entirely to the released Talazoparib.

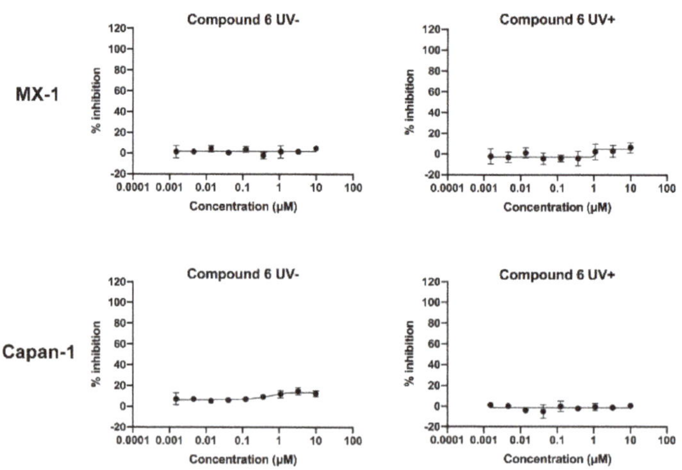

Figure 7. Dose–response curves of compound **6** in the absence and presence of ultraviolet radiation in the MX-1 and Capan-1 cells. After 20 min of irradiation at 365 nm (4.1 mW/cm^2), the compounds were transferred to 96-well plates and incubated with the cells. Cell growth was determined 10 days after incubation with the compounds. Irradiated compounds showed similar dose–response curves as that of unirradiated compounds. Error bars represent standard deviation from duplicate determinations, and results are shown as mean ± SD. The IC_{50} value is presented in Table 4.

Table 4. MX-1 and Capan-1 cell inhibitory activities of compound **6** in the absence and presence ultraviolet radiation.

Test Compound	MX-1 Cell IC_{50} (μM)	Capan-1 Cell IC_{50} (μM)
6 (UV-)	>10	>10
6 (UV+)	>10	>10

3. Materials and Methods

3.1. Molecular Docking

The catPARP-1 crystal structure (PDB ID 4PJT) was downloaded from the Protein Data Bank. Molecular docking was carried out using Gold (The Cambridge Crystallographic Data Centre). Before docking calculations, water molecules of the crystal structure were deleted, and hydrogen atoms were added. The whole 4PJT was defined as a receptor, and the site sphere was selected based on the active site of 4PJT. Compound **3** was placed during the molecular docking procedure. After the end of molecular modelling, types of interactions of the docked protein with ligand were analyzed.

3.2. Chemistry

All of the reagents and solvents were purchased from Innochem (Beijing, China), Aladdin (Shanghai, China), Energy Chemical (Shanghai, China), TCI (Tokyo, Japan), Ark Pharm (Libertyville, IL, USA), and used without additional purification. Anhydrous solvents were stored in sure-seal bottles under dry nitrogen. Analytical thin-layer chromatography was conducted on pre-coated silica gel plates (Yantai Dexin Biotechnology Co., Ltd., Yantai, China). Visualization was accomplished with 254 nm and 365 nm UV light. Column chromatography was performed using silica gel (200–300 mesh; Qingdao Ocean Chemical Engineering Co., Ltd., Qingdao, China).

Nuclear magnetic resonance (NMR) spectra were obtained on a JNM-ECA-400 400 MHz spectrometer (JEOL Ltd., Tokyo, Japan). Chemical shifts were reported in ppm and TMS was used as the internal standard. Coupling constants (*J*) are given in Hertz. Spin multiplicities were reported as the following abbreviations: s (singulet), d (doublet), dd (doublet doublet), t (triplet), q (quadruplet), m (multiplet). The mass spectrometry (MS) systems were the API 3000 triple-quadrupole mass spectrometer equipped with a Turbo Ion Spray electrospray ionization (ESI) source (AB Sciex, Concord, ON, Canada). HPLC analysis was performed using an Agilent 1260 Series (California, CA, USA).

3.2.1. Synthesis of (8*S*,9*R*)-5-Fluoro-8-(4-fluorophenyl)-9-(1-methyl-1*H*-1,2,4-triazol-5-yl)-2-((6-nitrobenzo[d][1,3]dioxol-5-yl)methyl)-2,7,8,9-tetrahydro-3*H* pyrido[4,3,2-de]phthalazin-3-one (**3**)

To a solution of Talazoparib (70 mg, 0.18 mmol) in anhydrous tetrahydrofuran (THF) (30 mL) was added to a 100 mL, two-necked flask with a magnetic stir bar. The flask was evacuated and backfilled with argon three times. Then 2.5 M n-Butyllithium (108 μL, 0.27 mmol) in hexanes were added the reaction solution, and the mixture was cooled at −80 °C. After stirring for 10 min, a solution of 5-(bromomethyl)-6-nitrobenzo[d][1,3] dioxole (93.9 mg, 0.27 mmol) in anhydrous THF was slowly added to the mixture, was warmed to 0 °C, and stirred overnight. When the reaction was completed, the mixture was carefully quenched by ammonium chloride saturated solution, and was extracted with ethyl acetate (50 mL × 3). The combined organic layers were washed with brine, dried over anhydrous sodium sulfate, and concentrated. The crude product was purified by column chromatography (dichloromethane/methanol = 50:1) to give compound **3** (46 mg, yield 45.7%) as a light yellow solid; ^{1}H NMR (400 MHz, DMSO-d_6) δ 7.79 (s, 1H); 7.73 (s, 1H); 7.63 (s, 1H); 7.53–7.45 (m, 2H); 7.20–7.13 (m, 2H); 7.10 (dd, *J* = 9.0, 2.4 Hz, 1H); 6.93 (dd, *J* = 11.1, 2.5 Hz, 1H); 6.61 (s, 1H); 6.22–6.21 (m, 2H); 5.40–5.29 (m, 2H); 5.08–5.00 (m, 2H); 3.56 (s, 3H). ESI m/z (M + H)$^+$ calculated for $C_{27}H_{20}F_2N_7O_5{}^+$ 560.15 found 560.15.

3.2.2. (6-Nitrobenzo[d][1,3]dioxol-5-yl)methyl (tert-butoxycarbonyl)-L-alaninate (**6**)

To a solution of (tert-butoxycarbonyl)-L-alanine (190 mg, 1.0 mmol) in acetone, potassium carbonate (207.31 mg, 1.50 mmol) and compound **3** were added. Then the mixture was stirred and heated at reflux for 5 h. After the reaction completed, the mixture was cooled to room temperature and removed under reduced pressure. The residue was dissolved in water and then the aqueous solution was extracted with dichloromethane (50 mL × 3). The combined organic layers were washed with brine, dried over anhydrous sodium sulfate, and concentrated to give the crude product, which was purified by column chromatography (ethyl acetate/petroleum ether = 5:1) to give compound **6** (264 mg, yield 71.4%) as a light yellow solid; ^{1}H NMR (400 MHz, DMSO-d_6) δ 7.74 (s, 1H); 7.46 (d, J = 7.3 Hz, 1H); 7.22 (s, 1H), 6.26 (s, 2H); 5.43–5.32 (m, 2H); 4.15–4.08 (m, 1H); 1.38 (s, 9H); 1.27 (d, J = 7.4 Hz, 3H). ESI m/z $(M + Na)^+$ calculated for $C_{16}H_{20}N_2NaO_8{}^+$ 391.11 found 391.11.

3.3. *Talazoparib UV Stability Assays*

Talazoparib was dissolved in methanol (2.63 mM), and the solution was divided into six equal portions for UV irradiation at 365 nm by using an UV crosslinker (CL-1000L UVP Crosslinker, 5 × 8 W; Analytikjena, IL, USA). The irradiation times were 1 min, 2 min, 3 min, 4 min, 5 min, and 10 min. The irradiated solution was transferred to a volumetric flask and diluted to the same volume with methanol. Then HPLC analysis was performed to detect the compound peak area. Samples were determined on an Agilent Eclipse Plus C18 column (4.6 × 150 mm, 5 μm particle size; California, CA, USA) using a mobile phase A (water) and mobile phase B (acetonitrile (ACN)) to elute. The gradient changed from 70% A to 30% A in 10 min, then continuing to elute with 30% A for 5 min. The flow rate was 1 mL/min, and the detection wavelength was 220 nm.

3.4. *Phosphate-Buffered Saline Stability of the Photoactivatable Prodrug*

Twenty μM of the test compound in pH = 7.4 PBS, containing 10% DMSO, were transferred to 13 1 mL volumetric flasks in equal volumes, incubated at 37 °C. The volumetric flasks were taken out at 0 min, 5 min, 10 min, 15 min, 30 min, 1 h, 2 h, 4 h, 8 h, 12 h, 24 h, 48 h, and 7 days, and were frozen at −80 °C. The samples were thawed in sequence and diluted to the same volume with methanol. Then HPLC analysis was performed to detect the compound peak area. Samples were determined on an Agilent Eclipse Plus C18 column (4.6 × 150 mm, 5 μm particle size; California, CA, USA) using a mobile phase A (water) and mobile phase B (ACN) to elute. The gradient changed from 70% A to 30% A in 10 min, continuing to elute with 30% A for 5 min. The flow rate was 1 mL/min, and the detection wavelength was 220 nm.

3.5. *UV Cleavage Test for Photoactivatable Prodrug*

The compound was dissolved in methanol (20 μM), and the solution were irradiated at 365 nm by using an UV crosslinker. Every minute from 0 to 10 min, aliquot samples (200 μL) were determined on an Agilent Eclipse Plus C18 column (4.6 × 150 mm, 5 μm particle size) using mobile phase A (water) and mobile phase B (ACN) to elute. The gradient changed from 70% A to 30% A in 10 min, continuing to elute with 30% A for 5 min. The flow rate was 1 mL/min and the detection wavelength was 220 nm. The peak areas percentage of the compounds at each time point were plotted against the sampling time.

3.6. *PARP-1 Enzyme Inhibition Assay*

A PARP-1 Chemiluminescent Assay Kit (Cat# 80569, BPS, San Diego, CA, USA) was used to detect the ability of compounds to inhibit PARP-1 enzyme activity. All experimental steps followed the operating manual. Firstly, each well was precoated with 25 μL 1× histone mixture that was diluted in PBS by incubation at 4 °C overnight. The wells were blocked by adding 100 μL of blocking buffer, then incubated at room temperature for 90 min. Then 12.5 μL of the prepared 1× PARP assay mixture and 1× activated DNA in 1× PARP buffer were added into each well of the assay plate, and 2.5 μL of compound or solvent control were added at varying concentrations. The reaction was initiated by the addition of 10 μL 1 ng/μL PARP-1 enzyme in 1× PARP buffer at room temperature for 60 min. Next, the reaction solution was added with 25 μL of diluted Streptavidin-HRP (1:50 in blocking buffer) to each well at room temperature for an additional 30 min. Finally, 25 μL of Horseradish Peroxidase (HRP) chemiluminescent substrate A and 25 μL of HRP chemiluminescent substrate B were mixed on ice, and the mixture was added by 50 μL per well. The luminescent signal was measured using a multi-function microplate reader, and IC_{50} values were calculated using GraphPad Prism 8.0 software.

3.7. PARylation Assay

The cellular PARylation assay evaluated the ability of test compounds to inhibit polymerization of PAR. Hela cells were seeded in 96-well plates (10,000 cells/well) in 200 μL of cell complete medium, and were allowed to adhere for 4 h at 37 °C in a humidified atmosphere of 5% CO_2. The medium was then removed from the plates, and the cells were treated with varying concentrations of test compounds for 18 h. 100 μL serum-free medium with 500 μM H_2O_2 solution was added, and the plate was kept at 37 °C for 5 min. Next, cells were fixed for 20 min with prechilled methanol at −20 °C and were incubated with 60 μL Poly(ADP-ribose) monoclonal antibody (1:2000) (prepared at 1x PBS containing 0.05% Tween-20 with 1% bovine serum albumin) at 37 °C for 2 h, followed by incubation with 60 μL IRDye 800CW goat anti-mouse IgG (diluted to 1:5000) and DNA stain DRAQ5 (1:5000) (prepared at 1× PBS containing 0.05% Tween-20 with 1% bovine serum albumin) at 37 °C for 2 h. The fluorescent signal was normalized with the DRAQ5 signal, and IC_{50} values were calculated using GraphPad Prism 8.0 software.

3.8. Cell Proliferation Assay

To assess the cytotoxicity of test compounds on *BRCA*-deficient cells using a CellTiter-Glo assay. MX-1 cells (*BRCA1*-deficient) and Capan-1 cells (*BRCA2*-deficient) were seeded in 96-well plates at densities that allowed linear growth for 10 days, and adhered overnight at 37 °C in a humidified atmosphere of 5% CO_2. Cells were treated in their recommended growth medium containing varying concentrations of test compounds. When the cells were incubated with the test compounds for 1 h, the cell culture plates were irradiated to the corresponding time with an ultraviolet crosslinker (for compounds that did not require UV irradiation, this step could be omitted). After 10 days of incubation, CellTiter-Glo Reagent (Promega, Madison, WI, USA) was added to the plates, which continued to be incubated for 30 min at room temperature. Chemiluminescence values were recorded by a multiplate reader, and IC_{50} values were calculated using GraphPad Prism 8.0 software.

4. Conclusions

In summary, this paper reports, for the first time, a photoactivatable Talazoparib prodrug. During the research process, we blocked the key lactam pharmacophore of Talazoparib with PPGs under the guidance of computer molecular docking. The in vitro enzyme inhibition assay and PARylation experiment proved that the inhibitory activity of the PPG-inactivated compound was greatly reduced (by 380 and more than 658 times, respectively). In *BRCA1*- and *BRCA2*- deficient cell lines, the prodrug could significantly restore the effective activity of Talazoparib after being irradiated by UV light, and the data imply that inhibitory activity could increase with prolonged irradiation time. However, because of the limitations of the relatively few types of *BRCA*-deficient cells that could be selected for study, as well as their restricted tolerance to UV light, we could not obtain the same level of inhibitory activity from the irradiated prodrug as from the parent drug. Further structural optimisation of the compound and appropriate cell selection would be helpful for further research on this photoactivatable Talazoparib prodrug strategy.

In conclusion, the results of this preliminary study prove that the photoactivatable prodrug strategy was an interesting approach for studying PARP inhibitors. On the one hand, the described photoactivatable prodrug could provide a new biological tool for the mechanism research of PARP.

On the other hand, photoactivatable prodrug also create new possibilities for therapeutic applications. However, this requires profound research on the prodrug' stability, toxicity, and bioavailability, and further cell and animal studies will be planned to address these questions.

Supplementary Materials: The following are available online at http://www.mdpi.com/1420-3049/25/2/407/s1, Figure S1: UV/Vis absorption spectra of compound 3 and Talazoparib in methanol solution, Figure S2: UV-cleavage test on the compound 3 in culture medium DMEM, Figure S3: UV-cleavage test on the compound 6, Figure S4 and S6: The ^{1}H-NMR spectrometry of compound 3 and 6, Figure S5 and S7: Mass spectrometry of compound 3 and 6.

Author Contributions: Conceptualization, J.L.; methodology, J.L.; software, L.L.; validation, W.S., X.Y. and X.Z.; formal analysis, D.X. and F.X.; investigation, D.X. and W.L.; resources, X.Z.; data curation, J.L. and L.L.; writing—original draft preparation, J.L.; writing—review and editing, W.S., X.Y., and X.Z.; supervision, X.Y. and X.Z.; project administration, X.Z.; funding acquisition, X.Z. All authors have read and agreed to the published version of the manuscript.

Funding: This research was funded by the National Science and Technology Major Project for Major New Drugs Innovation and Development, under grant no. 2018ZX09711003-009, and the Chinese National Natural Science Foundation, under grant no. 81872736.

Acknowledgments: The authors gratefully acknowledge research support from the Dan Jiang laboratory for structural confirmation.

Conflicts of Interest: The authors declare no conflict of interest.

References

1. Sulai, N.H.; Tan, A.R. Development of poly(ADP-ribose) polymerase inhibitors in the treatment of BRCA-mutated breast cancer. *Clin. Adv. Hematol. Oncol.* **2018**, *16*, 491–501.
2. Althaus, F.R.; Richter, C. ADP-ribosylation of proteins. Enzymology and biological significance. *Mol. Biol. Biochem. Biophys.* **1987**, *37*, 1–237. [PubMed]
3. Chambon, P.; Weill, J.D.; Mandel, P. Nicotinamide mononucleotide activation of new DNA-dependent polyadenylic acid synthesizing nuclear enzyme. *Biochem. Biophys. Res. Commun.* **1963**, *11*, 39–43. [CrossRef]
4. Virag, L.; Szabo, C. The therapeutic potential of poly(ADP-ribose) polymerase inhibitors. *Pharmacol. Rev.* **2002**, *54*, 375–429. [CrossRef] [PubMed]
5. Turk, A.A.; Wisinski, K.B. PARP inhibitors in breast cancer: Bringing synthetic lethality to the bedside. *Cancer* **2018**, *124*, 2498–2506. [CrossRef]
6. Bryant, H.E.; Schultz, N.; Thomas, H.D.; Parker, K.M.; Flower, D.; Lopez, E.; Kyle, S.; Meuth, M.; Curtin, N.J.; Helleday, T. Specific killing of BRCA2-deficient tumours with inhibitors of poly(ADP-ribose) polymerase. *Nature* **2005**, *434*, 913–917. [CrossRef]
7. Farmer, H.; McCabe, N.; Lord, C.J.; Tutt, A.N.J.; Johnson, D.A.; Richardson, T.B.; Santarosa, M.; Dillon, K.J.; Hickson, I.; Knights, C.; et al. Targeting the DNA repair defect in BRCA mutant cells as a therapeutic strategy. *Nature* **2005**, *434*, 917–921. [CrossRef]
8. Rhee, H.K.; Lim, S.Y.; Jung, M.J.; Kwon, Y.; Kim, M.H.; Choo, H.Y. Synthesis of isoquinolinone-based tetracycles as poly (ADP-ribose) polymerase-1 (PARP-1) inhibitors. *Bioorg. Med. Chem.* **2009**, *17*, 7537–7541. [CrossRef]
9. Liu, J.F.; Tolaney, S.M.; Birrer, M.; Fleming, G.F.; Buss, M.K.; Dahlberg, S.E.; Lee, H.; Whalen, C.; Tyburski, K.; Winer, E.; et al. A Phase 1 trial of the poly(ADP-ribose) polymerase inhibitor olaparib (AZD2281) in combination with the anti-angiogenic cediranib (AZD2171) in recurrent epithelial ovarian or triple-negative breast cancer. *Eur. J. Cancer* **2013**, *49*, 2972–2978. [CrossRef]
10. Parsels, L.A.; Karnak, D.; Parsels, J.D.; Zhang, Q.; Vélez-Padilla, J.; Reichert, Z.R.; Wahl, D.R.; Maybaum, J.; O'Connor, M.J.; Lawrence, T.S.; et al. PARP1 Trapping and DNA Replication Stress Enhance Radiosensitization with Combined WEE1 and PARP Inhibitors. *Mol. Cancer Res.* **2018**, *16*, 222–232. [CrossRef]
11. Garcia, T.B.; Snedeker, J.C.; Baturin, D.; Gardner, L.; Fosmire, S.P.; Zhou, C.; Jordan, C.T.; Venkataraman, S.; Vibhakar, R.; Porter, C.C. A Small-Molecule Inhibitor of WEE1, AZD1775, Synergizes with Olaparib by Impairing Homologous Recombination and Enhancing DNA Damage and Apoptosis in Acute Leukemia. *Mol. Cancer Ther.* **2017**, *16*, 2058–2068. [CrossRef] [PubMed]

12. Karnak, D.; Engelke, C.G.; Parsels, L.A.; Kausar, T.; Wei, D.; Robertson, J.R.; Marsh, K.B.; Davis, M.A.; Zhao, L.; Maybaum, J.; et al. Combined inhibition of Wee1 and PARP1/2 for radiosensitization in pancreatic cancer. *Clin. Cancer Res. Off. J. Am. Assoc. Cancer Res.* **2014**, *20*, 5085–5096. [CrossRef] [PubMed]
13. Bang, Y.J.; Im, S.A.; Lee, K.W.; Cho, J.Y.; Song, E.K.; Lee, K.H.; Kim, Y.H.; Park, J.O.; Chun, H.G.; Zang, D.Y.; et al. Randomized, Double-Blind Phase II Trial With Prospective Classification by ATM Protein Level to Evaluate the Efficacy and Tolerability of Olaparib Plus Paclitaxel in Patients With Recurrent or Metastatic Gastric Cancer. *J. Clin. Oncol. Off. J. Am. Soc. Clin. Oncol.* **2015**, *33*, 3858–3865. [CrossRef] [PubMed]
14. Pfizer Inc. TALZENNATM (Talazoparib) Capsules, for Oral Use: US Prescribing Information. Available online: http://www.fda.gov/ (accessed on 18 October 2018).
15. US FDA. FDA Approves Talazoparib for gBRCAm HER2-Negative Locally Advanced or Metastatic Breast Cancer [Media Release]. Available online: http://www.fda.gov/ (accessed on 16 October 2018).
16. Shen, Y.; Rehman, F.L.; Feng, Y.; Boshuizen, J.; Bajrami, I.; Elliott, R.; Wang, B.; Lord, C.J.; Post, L.E.; Ashworth, A. BMN 673, a novel and highly potent PARP1/2 inhibitor for the treatment of human cancers with DNA repair deficiency. *Clin. Cancer Res. Off. J. Am. Assoc. Cancer Res.* **2013**, *19*, 5003–5015. [CrossRef] [PubMed]
17. Fong, P.C.; Boss, D.S.; Yap, T.A.; Tutt, A.; Wu, P.; Mergui-Roelvink, M.; Mortimer, P.; Swaisland, H.; Lau, A.; O'Connor, M.J.; et al. Inhibition of poly(ADP-ribose) polymerase in tumors from BRCA mutation carriers. *N. Engl. J. Med.* **2009**, *361*, 123–134. [CrossRef] [PubMed]
18. Sandhu, S.K.; Schelman, W.R.; Wilding, G.; Moreno, V.; Baird, R.D.; Miranda, S.; Hylands, L.; Riisnaes, R.; Forster, M.; Omlin, A.; et al. The poly(ADP-ribose) polymerase inhibitor niraparib (MK4827) in BRCA mutation carriers and patients with sporadic cancer: A phase 1 dose-escalation trial. *Lancet Oncol.* **2013**, *14*, 882–892. [CrossRef]
19. Hoy, S.M. Talazoparib: First Global Approval. *Drugs* **2018**, *78*, 1939–1946. [CrossRef]
20. Pelliccioli, A.P.; Wirz, J. Photoremovable protecting groups: Reaction mechanisms and applications. *Photochem. Photobiol. Sci.* **2002**, *1*, 441–458. [CrossRef]
21. Mayer, G.; Heckel, A. Biologically active molecules with a "light switch". *Angew. Chem. Int. Ed.* **2006**, *45*, 4900–4921. [CrossRef]
22. Ellis-Davies, G.C. Caged compounds: Photorelease technology for control of cellular chemistry and physiology. *Nat. Methods* **2007**, *4*, 619–628. [CrossRef]
23. Kaplan, J.H.; Forbush, B.; Hoffman, J.F. Rapid photolytic release of adenosine 5′-triphosphate from a protected analog: Utilization by the sodium:potassium pump of human red blood cell ghosts. *Biochemistry* **1978**, *17*, 1929–1935. [CrossRef] [PubMed]
24. Engels, J.; Schlaeger, E.J. Synthesis, structure, and reactivity of adenosine cyclic 3′,5′-phosphate benzyl triesters. *J. Med. Chem.* **1977**, *20*, 907–911. [CrossRef] [PubMed]
25. Pinchuk, B.; Horbert, R.; Döbber, A.; Kuhl, L.; Peifer, C. Photoactivatable Caged Prodrugs of VEGFR-2 Kinase Inhibitors. *Molecules* **2016**, *21*, 570. [CrossRef] [PubMed]
26. Horbert, R.; Pinchuk, B.; Davies, P.; Alessi, D.; Peifer, C. Photoactivatable Prodrugs of Antimelanoma Agent Vemurafenib. *ACS Chem. Biol.* **2015**, *10*, 2099–2107. [CrossRef]
27. Shin, W.S.; Han, J.; Kumar, R.; Lee, G.G.; Sessler, J.L.; Kim, J.-H.; Kim, J.S. Programmed activation of cancer cell apoptosis: A tumor-targeted phototherapeutic topoisomerase I inhibitor. *Sci. Rep.* **2016**, *6*, 29018. [CrossRef]
28. Ibsen, S.; Zahavy, E.; Wrasdilo, W.; Berns, M.; Chan, M.; Esener, S. A Novel Doxorubicin Prodrug with Controllable Photolysis Activation for Cancer Chemotherapy. *Pharm. Res.* **2010**, *27*, 1848–1860. [CrossRef]
29. Matsumura, Y.; Ananthaswamy, H.N. Toxic effects of ultraviolet radiation on the skin. *Toxicol. Appl. Pharmacol.* **2004**, *195*, 298–308. [CrossRef]
30. Bliman, D.; Nilsson, J.R.; Kettunen, P.; Andréasson, J.; Grøtli, M. A Caged Ret Kinase Inhibitor and its Effect on Motoneuron Development in Zebrafish Embryos. *Sci. Rep.* **2015**, *5*, 13109. [CrossRef]
31. Aoyagi-Scharber, M.; Gardberg, A.S.; Yip, B.K.; Wang, B.; Shen, Y.; Fitzpatrick, P.A. Structural basis for the inhibition of poly(ADP-ribose) polymerases 1 and 2 by BMN 673, a potent inhibitor derived from dihydropyridophthalazinone. *Acta Crystallogr. Sect. F Struct. Biol. Commun.* **2014**, *70*, 1143–1149. [CrossRef]

32. Wang, B.; Chu, D.; Feng, Y.; Shen, Y.; Aoyagi-Scharber, M.; Post, L.E. Discovery and Characterization of (8S,9R)-5-Fluoro-8-(4-fluorophenyl)-9-(1-methyl-1H-1,2,4-triazol-5-yl)-2,7,8,9-tetrahydro-3H-pyrido[4,3,2-de]phthalazin-3-one (BMN 673, Talazoparib), a Novel, Highly Potent, and Orally Efficacious Poly(ADP-ribose) Polymerase-1/2 Inhibitor, as an Anticancer Agent. *J. Med. Chem.* **2016**, *59*, 335–357.
33. Jones, P.; Altamura, S.; Boueres, J.; Ferrigno, F.; Fonsi, M.; Giomini, C.; Lamartina, S.; Monteagudo, E.; Ontoria, J.M.; Orsale, M.V.; et al. Discovery of 2-{4-[(3S)-piperidin-3-yl]phenyl}-2H-indazole-7-carboxamide (MK-4827): A novel oral poly(ADP-ribose)polymerase (PARP) inhibitor efficacious in BRCA-1 and -2 mutant tumors. *J. Med. Chem.* **2009**, *52*, 7170–7185. [CrossRef] [PubMed]

Sample Availability: Samples of the compounds are not available from the authors.

molecules

MDPI

Article

P-MAPA and Interleukin-12 Reduce Cell Migration/Invasion and Attenuate the Toll-Like Receptor-Mediated Inflammatory Response in Ovarian Cancer SKOV-3 Cells: A Preliminary Study

Luiz Antonio Lupi [1], Flávia Karina Delella [2], Maira Smaniotto Cucielo [1], Graziela Gorete Romagnoli [3], Ramon Kaneno [3], Iseu da Silva Nunes [4], Raquel Fantin Domeniconi [1], Marcelo Martinez [5], Francisco Eduardo Martinez [1], Wagner José Fávaro [6] and Luiz Gustavo de Almeida Chuffa [1,*]

1. Department of Anatomy, UNESP-São Paulo State University, Institute of Biosciences, Botucatu, 18618-689 São Paulo, Brazil; luiz.lupi@unesp.br (L.A.L.); maira.cucielo@gmail.com (M.S.C.); raquel.domeniconi@unesp.br (R.F.D.); fe.martinez@unesp.br (F.E.M.)
2. Department of Morphology, UNESP-São Paulo State University, Institute of Biosciences, Botucatu, 18618-689 São Paulo, Brazil; flavia.delella@unesp.br
3. Department of Microbiology and Immunology, UNESP-São Paulo State University, Institute of Biosciences, Botucatu, 18618-689 São Paulo, Brazil; graziela.romagnoli@unesp.br (G.G.R.); rskaneno@yahoo.com.br (R.K.)
4. Farmabrasilis R&D Division, Campinas, 13279-020 SP, Brazil; iseununes@gmail.com
5. Department of Morphology and Pathology, Federal University of São Carlos, 13565-905 São Paulo, Brazil; martinez@ufscar.br
6. Department of Structural and Functional Biology, UNICAMP-University of Campinas, Campinas, 13083-970 São Paulo, Brazil; favarowj@unicamp.br

* Correspondence: guchuffa@yahoo.com.br; Tel.: +55-(14)-3880-0027

Academic Editor: Qiao-Hong Chen
Received: 16 October 2019; Accepted: 9 December 2019; Published: 18 December 2019

Abstract: Immunotherapies have emerged as promising complementary treatments for ovarian cancer (OC), but its effective and direct role on OC cells is unclear. This study examined the combinatory effects of the protein aggregate magnesium–ammonium phospholinoleate–palmitoleate anhydride, known as P-MAPA, and the human recombinant interleukin-12 (hrIL-12) on cell migration/invasion, apoptosis, toll-like receptor (TLR)-mediated inflammation, and cytokine/chemokine profile in human OC cell line SKOV-3. P-MAPA and IL-12 showed cancer cell toxicity under low doses after 48 h. Although apoptosis/necrosis and the cell cycle were unchanged by the treatments, P-MAPA enhanced the sensitivity to paclitaxel (PTX) and P-MAPA associated with IL-12 significantly reduced the migratory potential and invasion capacity of SKOV-3 cells. P-MAPA therapy reduced TLR2 immunostaining and the myeloid differentiation factor 88 (MyD88), but not the TLR4 levels. Moreover, the combination of P-MAPA with IL-12 attenuated the levels of MyD88, interferon regulatory factor 3 (IRF3) and nuclear factor kappa B (NF-kB p65). The IL-12 levels were increased and P-MAPA stimulated the secretion of cytokines IL-3, IL-9, IL-10, and chemokines MDC/CCL22 and, regulated on activation, normal T cells expressed and secreted (RANTES)/CCL5. Conversely, combination therapy reduced the levels of IL-3, IL-9, IL-10, MDC/CCL22, and RANTES/CCL5. Collectively, P-MAPA and IL-12 reduce cell dynamics and effectively target the TLR-related downstream molecules, eliciting a protective effect against chemoresistance. P-MAPA also stimulates the secretion of anti-inflammatory molecules, possibly having an immune response in the OC microenvironment.

Keywords: ovarian cancer; P-MAPA; IL-12; TLR signaling; inflammation; chemoresistance

1. Introduction

Ovarian cancer (OC) is the fifth largest cause of cancer-related death in the United States and is the most lethal of all gynecological malignancies [1]. OC originates from the ovarian surface epithelium, fallopian tube (fimbriae region) or endometriosis-related tissue, and often exhibits a late diagnosis due to the lack of clear signs or symptoms in the early stages of development [2–5]. Unfortunately, there is no screening method for achieving the best curative result, and traditional chemotherapy and surgery are limited for patients with advanced OC [6]. After cisplatin and paclitaxel (PTX) resistance, several patients become susceptible to developing recurrent OC and metastasis [7]. Therefore, new therapeutic options that overcome chemoresistance and enhance drug sensitivity are promising for the treatment of OC.

Immunotherapies have demonstrated great efficiency by activating host immune responses into the OC microenvironment [8]; however, what is happening with the cancer cells as a direct result of immunostimulation requires further investigation. We recently reported the effect of the immunomodulatory agent termed protein aggregate magnesium-ammonium phospholinoleate-palmitoleate anhydride (P-MAPA), a natural biopolymer extracted from the *Aspergillus oryzae*, which exhibits a number of antitumor responses in different experimental models of cancer [9–11]. In association with cisplatin, P-MAPA showed a greater survival rate and a reduced OC volume in addition to the increased expression of proteins involved in toll-like receptor (TLR)-mediated inflammatory response (canonical and non-canonical pathways) in OC-bearing animals [11]. Recent studies also supported the immunological mechanism of action of P-MAPA through the activation of TLR2 and TLR4 signaling in both cancer and infections, in addition to regulating the activity of T cells (especially CD4+T and CD8+T cells) and natural killer (NK) cells [9,10]. Importantly, P-MAPA did not show toxicity in preclinical in vitro (V-79 Chinese hamster cell line) and in vivo models (Swiss mice, Wistar rats, and monkeys) nor in human clinical trial phase I [9]; its effects in cancer treatment have been tested in non-muscle invasive urinary bladder cancer [9,10] and in OC [11]. The directive role of P-MAPA on human OC cells, considering its feasibility, sensibility, resistance, and toxicity, has not been explored yet.

TLRs are transmembrane molecules that signal via myeloid differentiation factor 88 (MyD88) or TLR-associated activator of interferon (TRIF) to induce cell proliferation, chemoresistance, and cytokine/chemokine production [12]. Most importantly, TLRs can trigger a different response depending on the cell type (e.g., cancer cell or immune cell), and particularly, TLR4 has been reported to be a precursor of the immune escape of OC cells [13,14]. The crosstalk between the immunoadjuvant and the OC cells targeting the TLR signaling and related cytokine secretion has never been proposed as to their impact and specific response.

Interleukin-12 (IL-12) is a cytokine related to innate and adaptive immunity, being mainly produced by the antigen-presenting cells (APCs), such as B lymphocytes, dendritic cells (DCs), and others [15,16]. It acts on T and NK cells stimulating a cytotoxic CD8+ response and inducing cytokine production, especially interferon-γ (IFN-γ) [15,17]; IL-12 is involved in the differentiation of naïve T cells into a polarized T helper 1 (Th1) immune response. Patients with recurrent OC who underwent IL-12 treatment, in a well-established dosage regimen, showed significant tumor regression [18]; the major challenge involving the treatment with IL-12 is related to the adverse effects due to its high diffusion and toxicity (e.g., lymphopenia and irreversible elevation of transaminases at 600 ng/kg and neutropenia, fatigue, and headache at 300 ng/kg) [19], and a more precise and direct administration may limit their undesirable effects. Notably, a phase II study involving intraperitoneal infusions of recombinant IL-12 in patients with residual disease $\leq$1 cm showed to be well-tolerated after fist-line therapy for OC-related peritoneal carcinomatosis [19]. Recently, Cohen et al. [16] studied the relationship between membrane-bound IL-12 in tumor cells and the potential to disrupt protumorigenic signaling and tumor outgrowth within peritoneal cavities; IL-12 significantly led to a tumor refractory state, thereby delaying the onset of metastatic disease.

Because P-MAPA is thought to increase IFN-γ levels, which may potentiate the Thelper (Th1)-mediated immune response, and adjuvant therapies with IL-12 have long been proposed as beneficial for patients with OC, this study investigates the effects of P-MAPA and IL-12, alone or in combination, on cancer cell activities with focus to the TLR-mediated inflammatory process and cytokines/chemokines profiling in human SKOV-3 cell line.

2. Results

2.1. P-MAPA and IL-12 Reduce Cell Viability and Induce Apoptosis in the Presence of PTX in SKOV-3 Cells

An MTT assay was carried out using three biological and technical replicates to unravel the most suitable dose and period of treatment. Based on previous results, the SKOV-3 cells were challenged with P-MAPA at doses of 25 μg/mL, 50 μg/mL, and 100 μg/mL, and rhIL-12 at doses of 0.5 ng/mL, 1 ng/mL, and 2 ng/mL for 24 h, 48 h, and 72 h. Then, we tested three different cell concentrations to achieve the better treatment response (1×10^3 cells, 1×10^4 cells, and 5×10^4 cells; Supplementary Figure S1). The SKOV-3 cell viability was efficiently reduced after the low-dose P-MAPA treatment (25 μg/mL for 48 h; viability was reduced by ~27%), and then started to increase after 72 h exposure (Figure 1A). Treatment with rhIL-12 also showed reduction in cell viability at an intermediate dose of 1 ng/mL mainly after 48-h exposure (Figure 1B; viability reduction by ~25% after 48 h). Combinatory therapy with P-MAPA and IL-12 also reduced the cell viability by about 33% (Figure 1C), and the treatment doses were set at 25 μg/mL of P-MAPA and 1 ng/mL of IL-12. Annexin V- fluorescein isothiocyanate (FITC)/Propidium iodide (PI) staining was used to effectively determine the apoptosis/necrosis rate induced by P-MAPA and rhIL-12 immunotherapies. In this study, we set early apoptosis (Annexin V-FITC+/PI−) as apoptosis and late apoptosis (Annexin V+/PI+) and necrosis (Annexin V−/PI+) as necrosis. The apoptosis index was not influenced by P-MAPA, IL-12, or P-MAPA+IL-12 (Figure 1D,E), which pointed out that these agents are unable to induce cell death at this concentration. We also observed that P-MAPA and IL-12 did not alter the cell cycle significantly (Figure 1F,G). These data indicate that these immunotherapeutic agents do not have a direct and high toxic effect to the cell, which is, in fact, expected from immunotherapies. Because the treatments did not promote cell death or cell proliferation, the reduction of cell viability might have been a result of decreased cell metabolism, because the MTT test indirectly reflects the mitochondrial activity.

To better understand whether P-MAPA and IL-12 therapies potentially increase the effect of standard chemotherapy, they were tested in association with PTX (Figure 2A,B). After 48 h, P-MAPA decreased cell viability in association with different doses of PTX compared with cells treated with PTX only (~30% reduction with 5 μM PTX; ~30% reduction with 2.5 μM PTX; ~24% reduction with 1.25 μM PTX and ~34% reduction with 0.625 μM PTX). Because IL-12 had no effect on cell viability when associated with PTX, the decreased cell viability observed after combining P-MAPA with IL-12 in association with doses of PTX is probably due to the P-MAPA effect (~19% reduction with 5 μM PTX, ~30% reduction with 2.5 μM PTX, ~30% reduction with 1.25 μM PTX, and ~38% reduction with 0.625 μM PTX). To confirm these effects on SKOV-3 cell death, an Annexin V-FITC/PI assay was performed using the lowest dose of PTX (0.625 μM). Concordantly, with the MTT results, P-MAPA and P-MAPA+IL-12 increased cell death in association with PTX at dose of 0.625 μM. The apoptosis/necrosis ratio of PTX was 0.64 and became higher when associated with P-MAPA (1.18) or P-MAPA+IL-12 (0.88), thus enhancing the P-MAPA effect as apoptotic inductor. Finally, PTX significantly increased the number of cells in G0/G1 and decreased cells in G2/M phase of the cell cycle, thus inducing cell cycle arrest. In this case, the addition of P-MAPA and IL-12 did not potentiate the PTX effects in cell cycle (Figure 2D,E).

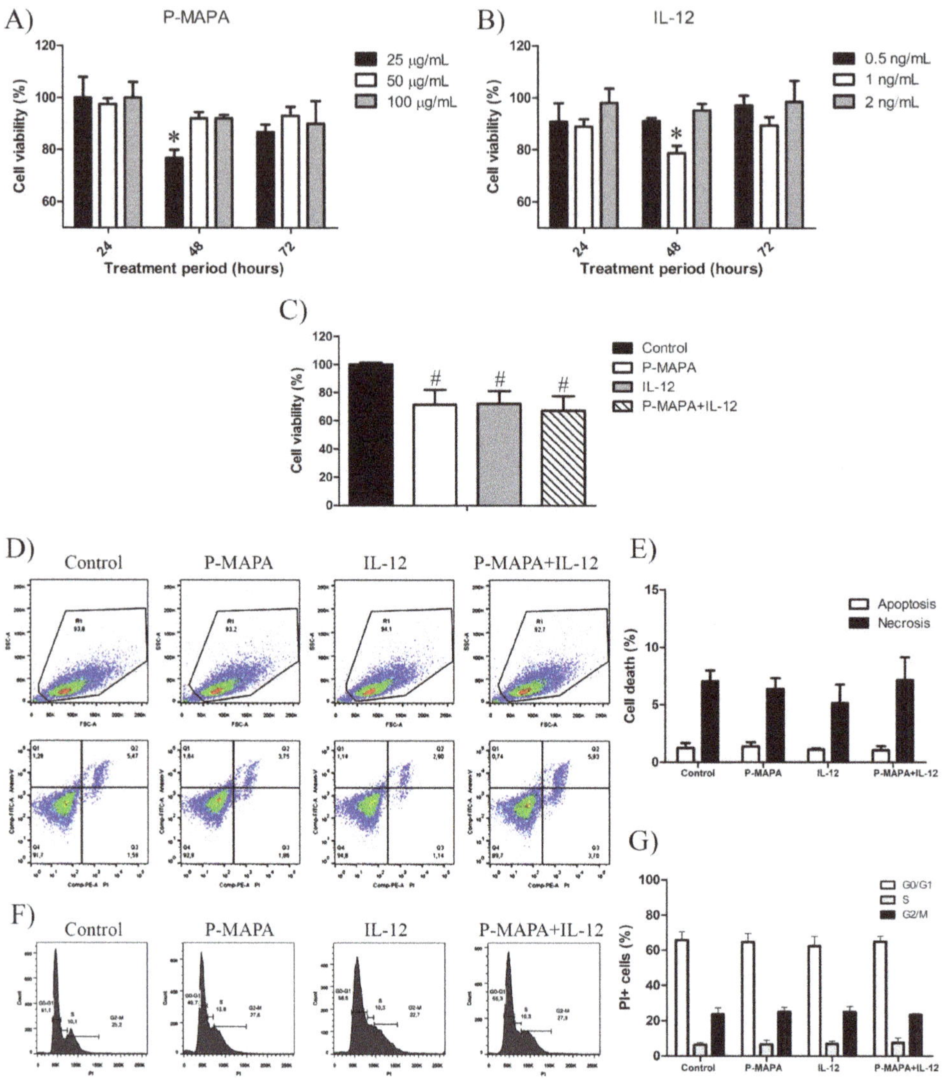

Figure 1. Protein aggregate magnesium–ammonium phospholinoleate–palmitoleate anhydride (P-MAPA) and interleukin-12 (IL-12) suppress cell viability without changing the apoptosis rate and cell cycle. SKOV-3 cells were treated with various concentrations of P-MAPA (**A**) and IL-12 (**B**) for 24, 48, and 72 h, and the cytotoxicity (expressed as percentage) was assayed by MTT; (**C**) Cell viability (%) after standardization of treatments (25 µg P-MAPA and 1 ng IL-12) after 48 h exposure; 1×10^3 SKOV-3 cells showed the best reproducibility. (**D**) Representative apoptotic index in SKOV-3 cells treated with P-MAPA and IL-12 for 48 h detected by annexin V/PI flow cytometry. (**E**) Percentage of cells in apoptosis and necrosis. (**F**) Representative cell cycle analysis in SKOV-3 cells treated with P-MAPA and IL-12 for 48 h detected by PI and RNAase flow cytometry. (**G**) Percentage of PI+ cells in G0/G1, S, and G2/M phases. The samples were assayed in three technical and biological replicates. Results are expressed as the mean ± SD and described as column chart. * $p < 0.05$ vs. different doses at 48 h; # $p < 0.05$ vs. control group.

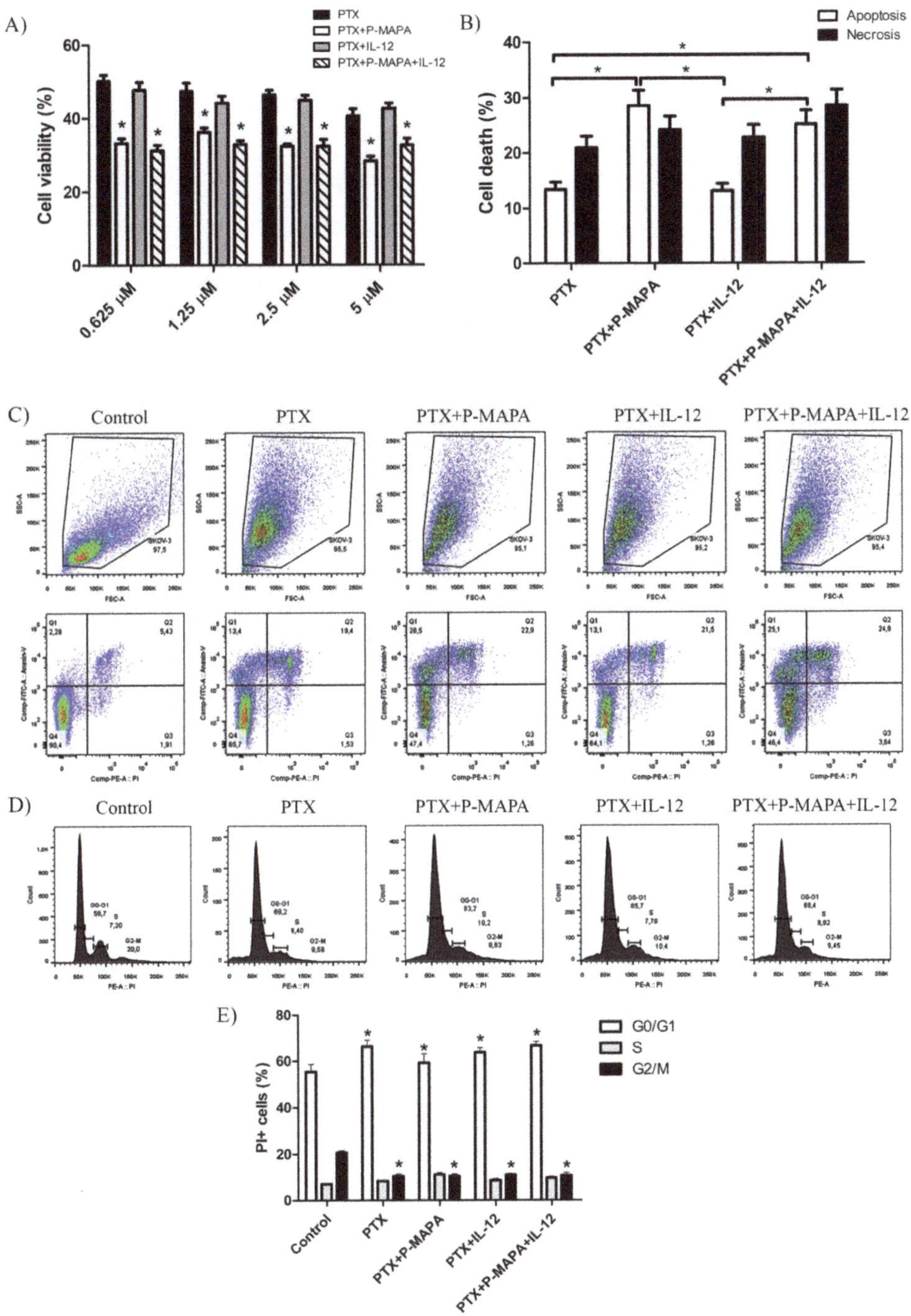
A)
PTX
PTX+P-MAPA
PTX+IL-12
PTX+P-MAPA+IL-12
Cell viability (%)
0.625 μM
1.25 μM
2.5 μM
5 μM
B)
Apoptosis
Necrosis
Cell death (%)
PTX
PTX+P-MAPA
PTX+IL-12
PTX+P-MAPA+IL-12
C)
Control
PTX
PTX+P-MAPA
PTX+IL-12
PTX+P-MAPA+IL-12
D)
Control
PTX
PTX+P-MAPA
PTX+IL-12
PTX+P-MAPA+IL-12
E)
PI+ cells (%)
G0/G1
S
G2/M
Control
PTX
PTX+P-MAPA
PTX+IL-12
PTX+P-MAPA+IL-12

Figure 2. P-MAPA and P-MAPA+IL-12 reduce cell viability and apoptosis/necrosis rate in the presence of PTX. (**A**) Cell viability was assessed by an MTT assay; SKOV-3 cells were treated with various concentrations of PTX alone or in association with P-MAPA and IL-12 for 48 h. * $p < 0.05$ vs. PTX and PTX+IL-12 groups. (**B**) Percentage of cells in apoptosis and necrosis after exposure to 0.625 μM PTX plus P-MAPA, IL-12, or P-MAPA+IL-12. * $p < 0.05$. (**C**) Representative apoptotic index in SKOV-3 cells detected by Annexin V/PI flow cytometry. (**D**) Representative cell cycle analysis in SKOV-3 cells treated with PTX, P-MAPA and IL-12 for 48 h detected by PI and RNase flow cytometry. (**E**) Percentage of PI+ cells in the G0/G1, S, and G2/M phases. The samples were assayed in three technical and biological replicates.* $p < 0.05$ vs. control group. Results are expressed as the mean ± SD.

2.2. Combination of P-MAPA with IL-12 Is Essential to Reduce Cell Migration Whereas P-MAPA Alone Decreased The Invasive Potential of SKOV-3 Cells

To investigate the inhibitory effect of P-MAPA and IL-12 as a single or combinatory treatment on SKOV-3 cells, a wound-healing assay was performed in different periods. Although the treatment with IL-12 showed a reduced migration rate (~ 17%) after 36 h and 48 h exposure, cells treated with P-MAPA migrated significantly less (~ 13%) only at 48 h exposure (Figure 3A,B). Combination of P-MAPA and IL-12 reduced the migratory potential of cells after 36 h and 48 h treatment (>20%), being the most efficient after 36 h (Figure 3A,B); this overall analysis suggests that IL-12 was more effective than P-MAPA in delaying wound closure. SKOV-3 cells that were treated with 0.9% saline solution (control group) had an accelerated growth and migration rate when compared with all the treatments. Because the wound-healing assay might be biased by cell proliferation, transwell migration and invasion assays were performed and effectively showed that P-MAPA reduced cell migration when administered alone or in association with IL-12 (Figure 4A). When Geltrex® was added to the chambers, the number of invasive cells was reduced after P-MAPA treatment in comparison to IL-12 treatment or its association (Figure 4B).

2.3. Immunotherapy with P-MAPA and IL-12 Significantly Reduced the TLR-Mediated Downstream Molecules Involved in the Inflammatory Process of SKOV-3 Cells

One of the most important factors responsible for the acquisition of malignant phenotypes of OC cells is associated with chemoresistance to treatments and uncovering new agents that downregulate the inflammatory pathway(s) may be of significant interest. To evaluate whether P-MAPA or IL-12 play a role on OC-related inflammation, TLR2- and TLR4-mediated pathways were evaluated through canonical and non-canonical signaling. Although the expressions of TLR2 and TLR4 did not vary significantly, the downstream target molecules were affected by the treatments (Figure 5A,B). P-MAPA and IL-12 alone or in combination led to a profound reduction in the MyD88 levels (0.53-, 0.48-, and 0.61-fold reduction, respectively vs. the control group; Figure 5A,B). We also evaluated the NF-kB p65 expression in the extracts of SKOV-3 cells, and notably, IL-12 alone or combined with P-MAPA induced a significant reduction in the p65 levels (0.66- and 0.63-fold reduction, respectively vs. control group; Figure 5A,B). To explore the non-canonical pathway, the TRIF and IRF3 levels were measured. Although the TRIF levels were unchanged after the treatments ($p > 0.05$), P-MAPA, IL-12, and the combination of P-MAPA with IL-12 induced a significant decrease in the IRF3 levels (0.70-, 0.43-, and 0.71-fold reduction, respectively vs. the control group; Figure 5A,B). These findings provide evidence that P-MAPA and IL-12 potentially act on MyD88-dependent and MyD88-independent pathways, which also encourages the possibility that these immunomodulatory agents could even increase the chemosensitivity of other therapeutics.

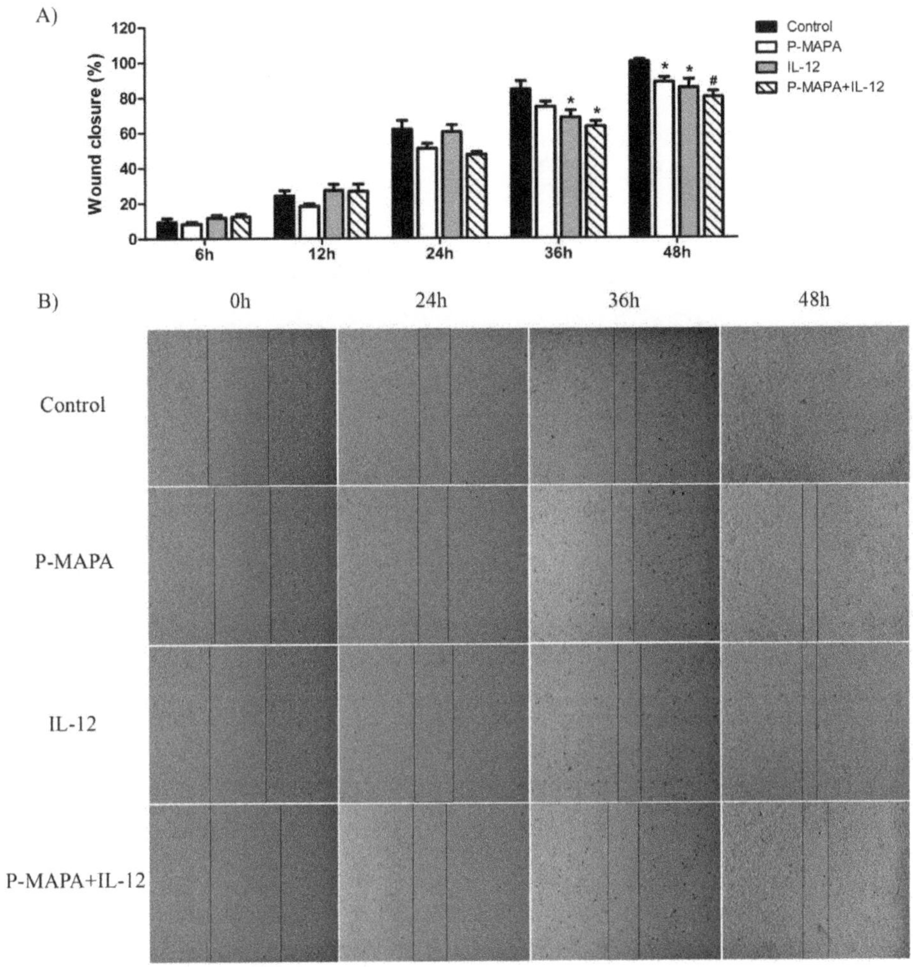

Figure 3. Migratory potential of SKOV-3 cells determined by wound-healing assay. (**A**) Percentage of wound closure after 0, 6, 12, 24, 36, and 48 h. * $p < 0.05$, # $p < 0.01$ vs. control group. (**B**) Photographs of each wound-healing analysis at 0, 24, 36, and 48 h which were representative for specific closing area; vertical black bars were used to show the incision edges (10× magnification). The samples were assayed in three technical and biological replicates.

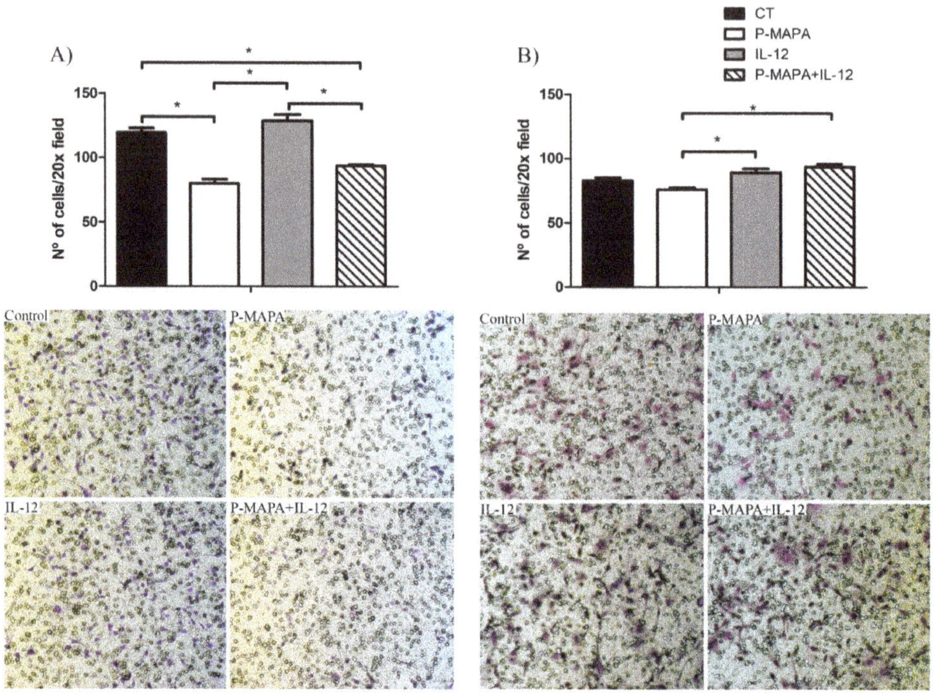

Figure 4. Effects of P-MAPA and IL-12 alone or in combination on the migration and invasion capacity of SKOV-3 cells. (**A**) Cell migration was measured by the amount of cells located in the lower part of the insert. (**B**) Cell invasion was determined by the amount of cells located in the lower part of the insert previously covered by Geltrex®. Representative images of the assay were obtained at 20× magnification. The samples were assayed in three technical and biological replicates. Results are expressed as the mean ± SD; * $p < 0.05$; CT, control group.

To further investigate and elucidate the location and the relative expression levels of the TLR2 and TLR4 receptors, an immunofluorescence assay was performed on SKOV-3 cells. As evidenced by the cellular fluorescence level, the P-MAPA treatment significantly decreased the expression level of cytoplasmic and nuclear TLR2 (48% fluorescence reduced vs. the control group; Figure 5C). On the contrary, IL-12 and the combination of P-MAPA and IL-12 promoted the highest TLR2 immunofluorescence intensity (135% and 151% fluorescence level, respectively vs. P-MAPA; Figure 5C), which suggests that IL-12 is responsible for restoring TLR2 activation after P-MAPA therapy in SKOV-3 cells. Lastly, the relative immunofluorescence of the TLR4 was unchanged after the treatments (Figure 5D).

2.4. P-MAPA Stimulates the Secretion of Pro- and Anti-Inflammatory Molecules, Whereas Its Association with IL-12 Induced the Synthesis of Inflammatory Cytokines in SKOV-3 Cells

To determine which cytokines/chemokines are secreted by the SKOV-3 cells and how P-MAPA and IL-12 act to regulate its production, a wide range of these molecules were evaluated in both supernatants (Figure 6A) and cellular extracts (Figure 6B). As expected, the IL-12 levels were higher in the cells treated with IL-12 and P-MAPA+IL-12 (244% and 243% fold-increased, respectively vs. the control group, and 154% and 155% fold-increased, respectively vs. the P-MAPA group; Figure 6A); IL-12 was slightly elevated with P-MAPA, even at low concentrations.

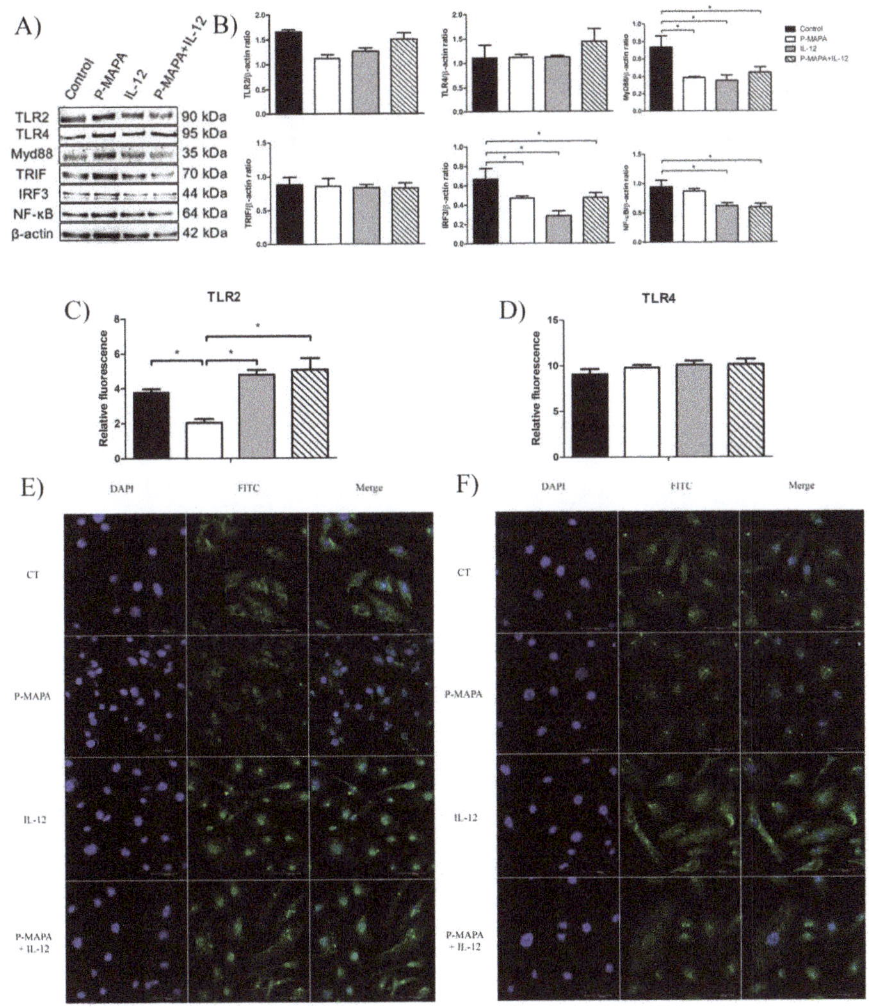

Figure 5. TLR2- and TLR4-mediated signaling pathways are involved with inflammatory process and chemoresistance in human OC. (**A**) Representative protein profiles of TLR2, TLR4, MyD88, TRIF, IRF3, and NF-kB; fractions containing 50 μg protein were pooled from 5 samples per group. (**B**) Individual blots were used for densitometric analysis of the TLR2 and TLR4 levels and related downstream molecules (MyD88, TRIF, IRF3, and NF-kB) after normalization to the β-actin. Data are expressed as the mean ± SD. * $p < 0.05$ vs. control group. Relative fluorescence intensity of TLR2 (**C**) and TLR4 (**D**) receptors. The values are expressed as the mean ± SD. The samples were assayed in three technical and biological replicates. * $p < 0.05$. Confocal imaging of TLR2 (**E**) and TLR4 (**F**) immunostaining using fluorescein isothiocyanate (FITC)-conjugated antibodies anti-TLR2 and anti-TLR4 was obtained in SKOV-3 cells (Alexafluor®488, bar = 50 μm). DAPI was used for nuclear staining and merged images were performed using Image J software. Negative controls were used. CT, control; DAPI, 4′,6-diamidino-2-phenylindole; FITC, fluorescein isothiocyanate.

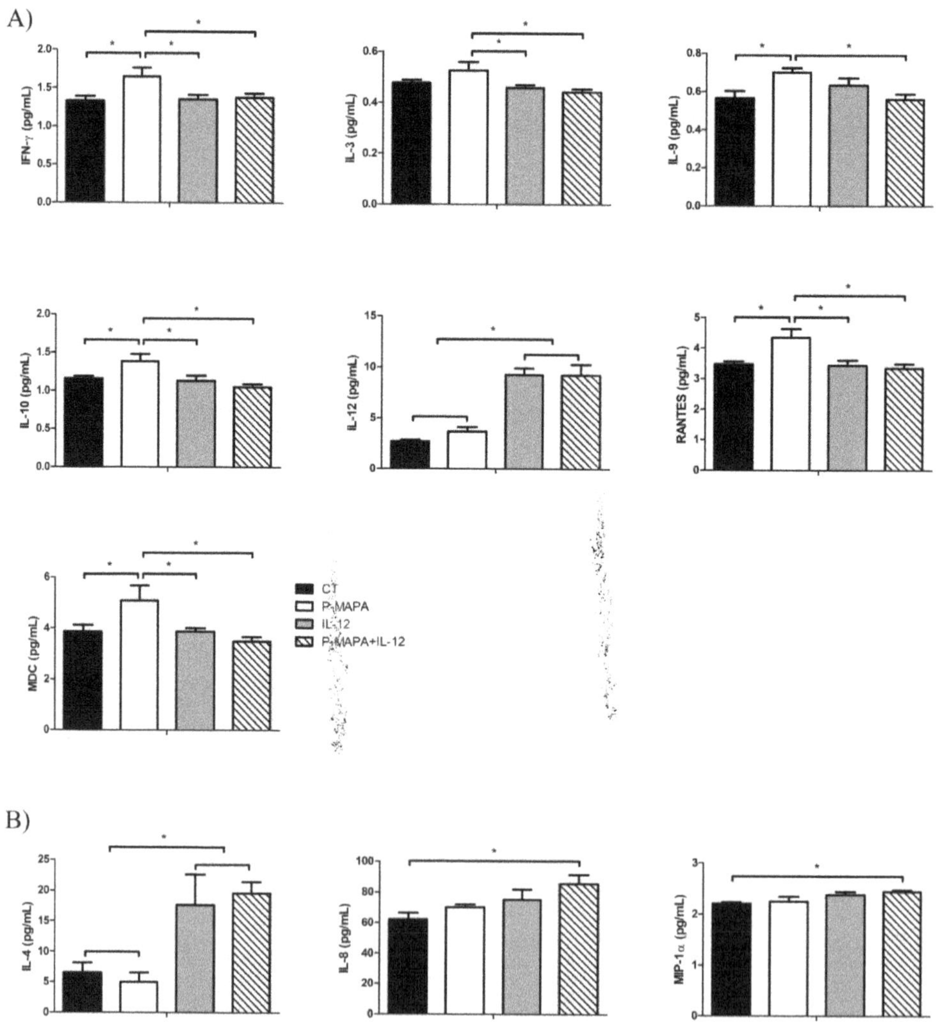

Figure 6. Multiplex analysis of cytokines and chemokines produced by SKOV-3 cells in response to P-MAPA and IL-12 treatments. (**A**) Concentrations of IFN-γ, IL-3, IL-9, IL-10, IL-12, RANTES, and MDC were altered in the supernatants of cell culture. (**B**) Levels of IL-4, IL-8, and MIP-1α were altered in SKOV-3 cell extracts. All data are expressed as the mean ± SD. * $p < 0.05$ as compared with the corresponding group; One-way ANOVA complemented by the Tukey test. The samples were assayed in three technical and biological replicates. CT, control; IFN-γ, interferon gamma; RANTES, regulated on activation, normal T cell expressed and secreted; MDC, macrophage-derived chemokine; MIP-1α, macrophage inflammatory protein 1-alpha.

Comparing the treatments, P-MAPA significantly stimulated the secretion of IFN-γ (24% vs. the control, IL-12 and P-MAPA+IL-12 groups; Figure 6A), which is probably related to the activation of the Th1 response. P-MAPA also stimulated IL-10 (21% vs. control, 23% vs. IL-12 and 32% vs. P-MAPA+IL-12 groups), MDC/CCL22 (31% vs. control and IL-12 groups, and 45% vs. P-MAPA+IL-12), and, regulated on activation, normal T cells expressed and secreted (RANTES)/CCL5 (25% vs. the control, 27% vs. the IL-12, and 30% vs. the P-MAPA+IL-12 groups). Furthermore, P-MAPA increased IL-3 and treatment with IL-12 or P-MAPA+IL-12 promoted a reduction in its levels (13% and 17% reduction, respectively vs. P-MAPA; Figure 6A). Treatment with P-MAPA also increased the IL-9 levels (25% increased vs. the control and P-MAPA+IL-12 groups; Figure 6A). A part of these results suggests the secretion of molecules involved in the Th2 response (e.g., IL-10, CCL22), but their regulatory signaling combined with other molecules released by immune cells into the OC microenvironment could not be proved to have a favorable or unfavorable effect. The IL-4 levels were internally elevated in SKOV-3 cells (Figure 6B) after therapies with IL-12 alone or combined with P-MAPA (169% and 254% increased vs. the control group and 198% and 293% increased vs. the P-MAPA group, respectively). Interestingly, the association of P-MAPA with IL-12 induced the highest production of intracellular IL-8 (37% vs. the control group) and MIP-1α (11% vs. control group; Figure 6B). In brief, cytokines that were not significantly influenced by P-MAPA and IL-12 included IL-1β, IL-2, IL-6, IL-7, IL-13, IL-15, IL-17, IP-10, MCP-1, and MIP-1β (Supplementary Tables S1 and S2).

3. Discussion

We reported that lower doses of P-MAPA efficiently reduce cell invasion, whereas P-MAPA in combination with IL-12 reduces cell migration in addition to attenuating the TLR-mediated inflammatory response in human SKOV-3 cells (Figure 7). Although these compounds have individually showed important effects in reducing OC volume and mass while enhancing overall survival and immunostimulation in animals and humans [11,16], this study is the first to describe a therapeutic rationale against human OC, thus revealing the mechanisms underlying cancer cell-related inflammatory aspects rather than those of immune cells.

P-MAPA and IL-12 elicited a decrease in cell metabolism, but no effect on cell apoptosis/necrosis and cell cycle was observed. Although an MTT assay is largely used as the viability/toxicity assay, it could be biased by decreased metabolism activity. This utilizes mitochondrial machinery to convert a colorless tetrazolium salt solution into purple formazan crystals [20]. Once we had pursued a treatment dose with low cell toxicity but considerable modulatory potential, we believed that either P-MAPA or IL-12 may be changing OC cell metabolism to a reduced activity (metabolomics could be of significant value to find the targets more precisely). The impact of this reduction was indeed confirmed by the migration and invasion assays. P-MAPA was able to reduce the migration and invasion capacity, and the delayed wound closure in IL-12-treated cells may be likely due to its decreased metabolic activity. Given that lower doses of P-MAPA and IL-12 are recommended to be well-tolerated, OC cell apoptosis could be prevented by the low-level toxicity of chemicals; conversely, these concentrations are safely used to activate immune responses and modulate cell metabolism. When associated with PTX, P-MAPA was able to increase cell death and apoptosis/necrosis ratio without potentiating the PTX effects on cell cycle. In accordance with a previous study in which approximately 50% of SKOV-3 cells died after 48 h exposure to 5 μM of PTX [21], we observed that P-MAPA not only was effective to increase cell death in the presence of PTX but also to maintain cell toxicity even after considerably lower levels of PTX. This increase in cell death might be a result of apoptosis induction, since the apoptosis/necrosis ratio was significantly higher in animals treated with the combination of P-MAPA and PTX. Because apoptosis lead to the release of the damage-associated molecular pattern (DAMP), this higher ratio may facilitate immunogenic cell death (ICD) [22].

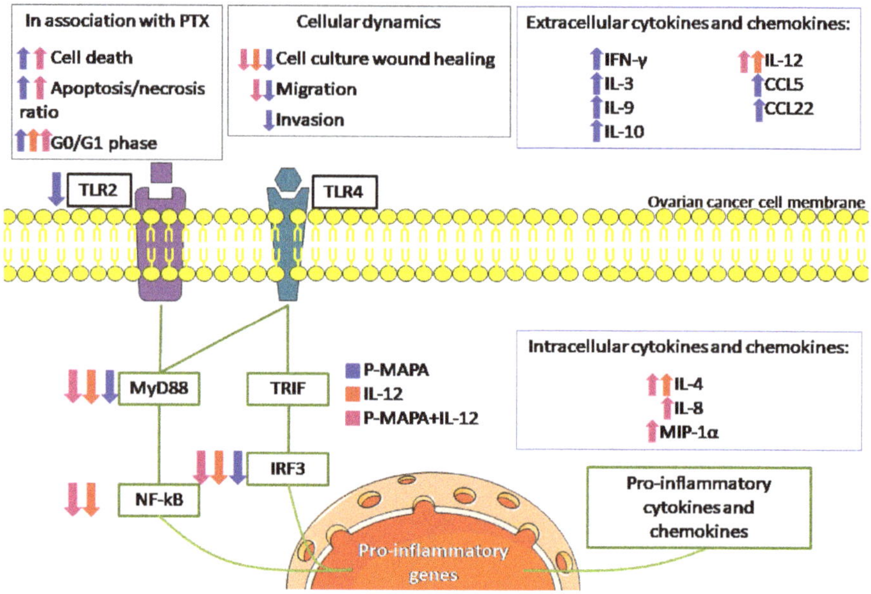

Figure 7. Schematic view of the effects of P-MAPA and IL-12 on human SKOV-3 cells. The effect of each treatment is shown by its representative color. Up and down arrows indicate whether the treatment increased or decreased, respectively, such as cellular function or molecule at these levels. The treatments reduced the downstream molecules (MyD88, NF-kB, and IRF3, with the exception of P-MAPA in reducing NF-kB) of both canonical and non-canonical toll-like receptor (TLR) signaling pathways, and only P-MAPA significantly downregulated the TLR2 levels. The intracellular cytokine/chemokine levels were increased after treatment with IL-12 (IL-4) or P-MAPA+IL-12 (IL-4, IL-8 and MIP-1α); P-MAPA was more effective in increasing the secretion of the following cytokines/chemokines: IFN-γ, IL-3, IL-9, IL-10, RANTES/CCL5, MDC/CCL22). As expected, IL-12 was used to treat SKOV-3 cells and appeared increased after IL-12 and P-MAPA+IL-12 treatments. Although IL-12 only reduced the SKOV-3 cells' wound closure, P-MAPA efficiently regulated the cellular dynamics by reducing the wound closure, cell migration and invasion. The combination of P-MAPA with IL-12 decreased the period of wound closure and cell migration rate. MyD88, myeloid differentiation primary response 88; NF-kB, nuclear factor kappa B; TRIF, TIR-domain-containing adapter-inducing interferon-β; IRF-3, interferon regulatory factor 3; TLR2, toll-like receptor 2; TLR4, toll-like receptor 4; P-MAPA, protein aggregate magnesium-ammonium phospholinoleate-palmitoleate anhydride; IL, interleukin; MIP-1α, macrophage inflammatory protein 1α; IFN-γ, interferon gamma; RANTES, regulated on activation, normal T cell expressed and secreted; MDC, macrophage-derived chemokine; CCL, C-C motif chemokine ligand.

The pro-inflammatory actions of TLR signaling in cancer cells and immune cells may severely affect tumor progression [23], and, particularly, the immunosuppressive OC microenvironment needs to be continuously immunostimulated [23,24]. Although TLR4 was unchanged by the treatments, P-MAPA induces a reduction in the TLR2 levels together with downstream molecules in SKOV-3 cells. Additionally, we found TLR2 nuclear expression in SKOV-3 cells treated with P-MAPA. Although we are not the first to observe nuclear staining of TLR2 and TLR4 [25], the effect of the switch of cytoplasmic to nuclear expression in SKOV-3 cells remains unclear. Based on our results, this nuclear expression seems not to have any negative effect favoring cancer development. Although the TLR2-induced MyD88-dependent pathway is related to an increase in IL-12 secretion [26], the immunoregulatory mechanisms whereby IL-12 restores TLR2 to levels close to control remain to be elucidated. In immune cells, P-MAPA has reportedly been described as a TLR4 agonist [9–11], thereby enhancing the synthesis of cytokines and activating a Th1-polarized response. Our data evidenced the protective effect of P-MAPA in attenuating TLR2-mediated signaling in OC cells. The activation of TLR, especially via MyD88, is associated with increased tumor growth, chemoresistance, and the early recurrence of ovarian epithelial tumors [7,27]. In addition, OC expressing high levels of MyD88 presents a higher proliferative index and increased production of pro-inflammatory cytokines and chemokines [7,28,29]. Importantly, the association of P-MAPA and IL-12 decreased the levels of MyD88 in SKOV-3 cells compared with their respective control; because P-MAPA and P-MAPA + IL-12 also significantly decreased the migratory and invasive potential of the cells, it can be suggested that the MyD88-dependent signaling pathway may be one of the mechanisms by which SKOV-3 cells promote migration and invasion. It has also been reported that increased expression of MyD88 is related to a decreased sensitivity to chemotherapy (e.g., PTX) in the MyD88-negative OC A2780 cell line [30]; moreover, the activation of MyD88 and NF-kB in MyD88-positive SKOV-3 cells promoted cell proliferation and tumor growth, likely due to the increased secretion of pro-inflammatory cytokines, thus rendering the cells PTX resistant [13]. In this line, the downregulation of MyD88 and NF-kB may be a possible mechanism by which P-MAPA improves the chemosensitivity of PTX in SKOV-3 cells.

The activation of TLR4/MyD88/NF-kB signaling by ligands is strongly related to an inflammatory microenvironment, thereby contributing to a more aggressive OC phenotype and poorer clinical outcomes in women [31]. In SKOV-3 cells, silencing the membrane-associated RING-CH (MARCH), an ubiquitin ligase that downregulates MHC class II expression, resulted in reduced cell migration and invasion in addition to inhibition of NF-kB signaling [32], thus reinforcing that NF-kB may play a role in the regulation of numerous cellular dynamics. Taken together, the combination of P-MAPA and IL-12 was efficient to induce the downregulation of both MyD88 and NF-kB, which can be of great value to enhance the overall survival of patients while attenuating OC progression and metastasis.

TRIF activation is responsible for triggering the TLR non-canonical pathway, thus activating several transcriptional factors, such as NF-kB, IRF3 and AP-1, and resulting in cytokines and type I IFN production [33,34]. Although few studies have explored the role of TRIF/IRF3 in OC cells, they seem to be critical for therapy [35]. Recently, Chuffa et al. [23] reported the downregulation of TRIF and IRF3 in OC-induced rats, whereby the immunomodulatory agent dramatically reduced the volume and mass of ovarian tumors. Importantly, P-MAPA and IL-12, either alone or in association, significantly downregulated IRF3 levels, evidencing the potential of immunotherapies to act by both canonical and non-canonical TLR pathways.

Immunostimulatory and immunosuppressive molecules can contribute to either inhibiting or enhancing anti-tumor immune activity of such a response by immunotherapy. We screened a number of molecules displaying important effects in OC, but most of them displayed no changes in SKOV-3 cells after P-MAPA and IL-12 treatments. Treatment of SKOV-3 with rhIL-12 showed its availability in both IL-12 and P-MAPA+IL-12 groups, thus proving that the agent was present in the supernatants; whether IL-12 therapy was still capable of stimulating more IL-12 production by the cells is uncertain. IL-3 levels are stimulated by P-MAPA therapy, and this increase might be protective for patients during OC chemotherapy; administration of rhIL-3 to patients with platelet count < 75,000/mm^3 is effective to fight thrombocytopenia and neutropenia after chemotherapy [36]. Moreover, IL-3 is able to intensify the dose of carboplatin for primary advanced OC [37]. P-MAPA also enhanced IL-9 secretion by SKOV-3 cells, and this effect seems to have a dual impact on the immune system. IL-9 was initially recognized as a T-cell growth factor with oncogenic potential. However, Th9 cell-secreted IL-9 has been revisited for the immunity of some tumors [38]. IL-9 activates innate immune cells like mast cells, contributing to tumor growth prevention [38], and in addition to Th9 cell-derived IL-3, induction of adaptive anti-cancer responses that favor DCs survival has been reported in various cancers [39].

Regulatory T (Treg) cells can infiltrate into solid OC or ascitic fluid, contributing to an immunosuppressive microenvironment by secreting IL-10 and TGFB-1 while reducing the IFN-γ levels [40]. Because these cytokines participate either in stimulating or inhibiting the activities of other immune cells, P-MAPA seems to work as a double-edge sword regarding the SKOV-3 cells. Although mechanistically unclear, P-MAPA contributes partially to reducing the immunosuppression, likely due to the increased levels of IFN-γ rather than IL-10. In fact, high IFN-γ secretion meets our proposal by enhancing OC-cell immunogenicity through the recruitment of CD8+T and natural killer (NK) cells, in addition to increasing the anti-tumor activity of macrophages; we recently found that P-MAPA reduces Treg cells and stimulates CD8+T effector cells in OC-bearing animals (unpublished data). Recently, the expression of programmed death-ligand 1 (PD-L1) on tumor cells represents an important pathway by which malignant cells evade the immune system. In SKOV-3 cells, PD-L1 was variably found in the surface and cytoplasm [41], and its expression was correlated with high levels of TNF-α, IL-10, and IL-6 released from tumor-associated macrophages (TAMs). Because P-MAPA and IL-12 attenuated the downstream mediators of the TLR signaling, the altered expression of some cytokines may be independent of TLR-mediated inflammatory response.

A complex network represented by chemokines and its receptors, growth factors, inflammatory products, and other molecules (e.g., NF-kB), is responsible for tumor progression or rejection. Chemokines signal not only for tumor cells but may control tumor development through activation of specific receptors expressed in a variety of cells, thereby regulating the traffic of infiltrating macrophages, lymphocytes, DCs, and neutrophils [42]. The secretion of CCL5, which binds to the CCR4 receptor, is strongly associated with the presence of tumor-infiltrating CD8+T cells; the upregulation of its receptor in activated vaccine-primed T cells improved tumor homing in OC [43]. In SKOV-3 cells, the levels of CCL22/MDC and CCL5/RANTES were higher after P-MAPA therapy. Although these chemokines appear to be associated with a poor prognosis when released by immune cells, the functional meaning of their production by OC cells as to their significance in the OC microenvironment remains to be investigated. CCL22 is secreted by DCs and macrophages and acts on target cells by interacting with the CCR4 receptor located in the cell surface [44]. CCL22 is correlated to the chemoattraction of Treg cells in advanced stages of OC, and its expression was increased in response to IFN-γ signaling [45]. This finding partially corroborates our results in which both CCL22 and IFN-γ were higher in SKOV-3 cells after P-MAPA therapy; in contrast, P-MAPA does not promote elevation in the number of Treg cells (data not shown). A previous study by Giuntoli et al. [46] showed that ascites specimens originating from patients with malignant OC were accomplished by elevated levels of IL-6, IL-8, IL-10, IL-15, IP-10, MCP-1, MIP-1β, and VEGF, in contrast to significantly reduced levels of IL-2, IL-5, IL-7, IL-17, and CCL5/RANTES. Although controversial, IL-8 production by human OC cells plays a role in controlling tumor growth [47], and MIP-1α is involved in the recruitment of Th1 and cytotoxic effector T cells [48]. We found a higher secretion IL-8 and MIP-1α after combinatory treatment of P-MAPA and IL-12. Partially supporting our results, IL-8 levels have already been reported to be augmented in OC, even after the downregulation of NF-kB [49]; however, the alternative mechanism involved with this production remains unclear. Additionally, we observed increased levels of RANTES after P-MAPA treatment. RANTES is responsible for recruiting T cells, macrophages, eosinophils, and basophils into the inflammatory sites. In addition to IL-2 and IFN-γ, RANTES is thought to induce the activation and proliferation of NK cells while enhancing the anti-tumor response in animal models [46]. In addition to the overexpression of VEGF and MCP-1, a reduction in RANTES levels is associated with activating pathways for tumor growth. Normally, OCs produce large amounts of RANTES, and this production is correlated with the infiltration of TAMs, CD8+T cells, and tumor progression [50,51]; these chemokines are further related to the acquisition of polarized immune responses (Th1 versus Th2). Although some negative effects are associated with the efficacy of chemotherapy related to RANTES, therapy with P-MAPA may be helpful against tumor expansion.

4. Materials and Methods

4.1. Cell Line and Cell Culture

The human OC cell line SKOV-3 was purchased from the American Type Culture Collection (ATCC, Rockville, MD, USA). The SKOV-3 cells were routinely incubated in RPMI 1640 (Life Technologies, Grand Island, NY, USA) supplemented with 10% Fetal Bovine Serum (FBS) and 1% anti-anti solution (100 mg/mL penicillin G, and 100 μg/mL streptomycin (Merck, Darmstadt, Germany). The culture medium was changed every 2 to 3 days. All cells were maintained at 37 °C in a humidified atmosphere of 5% CO_2.

4.2. Treatments with P-MAPA and IL-12

To evaluate the in vitro effect of the treatments, different doses of P-MAPA (25 μg/mL, 50 μg/mL, and 100 μg/mL) were tested in accordance with Favaro et al. [9]. Initially, 5 mg P-MAPA was diluted in 1 mL of saline solution to achieve the desired stock solution of 5 mg/mL, which were then diluted in the cell culture medium to obtain the testing doses. For the treatment with recombinant (rh)IL-12, concentrations of 0.5 ng/mL, 1 ng/mL, and 2 ng/mL were diluted in the culture medium based on the previous report by Su et al. [52]. For the combination of P-MAPA and IL-12, the most effective dose and incubation period were determined after performing an MTT assay. The saline solution was used as a solvent vehicle control and prepared in the same volume and dilution for both treatments. All experiments were performed at 0, 24, 48, and 72 h time exposure and assayed in three technical and biological replicates.

4.3. Cell Cytotoxicity (MTT Assay)

The SKOV-3 cells were seeded in a 96-well plate at a density of 1×10^3 cells/well. The cellular activity and/or toxicity were evaluated in different concentrations of P-MAPA and IL-12 and periods (0, 24, and 48 h) to define the best treatment protocol. For this experiment, the choice of dose and period of treatment was the combination of high cellular viability with low toxicity and efficient signaling regulation. Thereafter, different doses of PTX were associated with P-MAPA and IL-12 to verify the sensitivity effects. An MTT solution (5 mg/mL) was added to the wells for 4 h, and the crystals were diluted with DMSO under agitation. The concentration was determined by an Epoch microplate reader (BioTek Instruments, Highland Park, PO, USA) at 540 nm, being the reference curve fixed at 650 nm. The percentage of crystal formation was calculated by fixing the control group crystal formation as 100%.

4.4. Apoptosis Rate by Annexin V-FITC/PI Staining

During the apoptosis process, cells normally externalize the phospholipid phosphatidylserine (PS), which binds with high affinity to Annexin V in the presence of calcium. Herein, we used the Annexin V assay with the BD Pharmingen^{TM} Annexin V-FITC Apoptosis Detection Kit (ApoAlert Annexin V, Clontech, CA, USA). The SKOV-3 cells (1×10^5 cells) were placed in a 6-well plate and left for 6 h to attach. The cells were then treated with 25 µg/mL of P-MAPA, 1 ng/mL of rhIL-12 or their association for 48 h. In addition, P-MAPA and IL-12 were added to the lowest dose of PTX (0.625 µM) to confirm chemosensitivity. After the treatment period, cells were trypsinized and centrifuged (Centrifuge 5804 R, Eppendorf, Hamburg, Germany)) for 10 min at 1200 rpm for culture medium removal. The cell pellet was washed twice with phosphate-buffered saline (PBS) and centrifuged at 10,000 rpm for 30 s, followed by resuspension with 100 µL Annexin V binding buffer and incubation with Annexin V and propidium iodide (PI) for 15 min in the dark at room temperature. After the incubation, the prepared cells were then analyzed by flow cytometry in a FACSCantoTMII with FACSDiva (BD Biosciences, Clontech, CA, USA) software. The flow cytometric results were analyzed by the FlowJo software (vX.10.6 version, Tree Stars Inc., Ashland, OR, USA).

4.5. Cell Cycle Determination by PI Staining

The cell cycle stages (G0/G1, S, and G2/M) were performed by flow cytometry analysis through the DNA content measurement of nuclei stained with PI dye. After all the treatments, the SKOV-3 cells (1×10^5) were trypsinized, washed with PBS, and centrifuged for 5 min at 1500 rpm. After the cells were fixed in 70% cold ethanol at 4 °C for 1 h, they were incubated with PI staining solution of 50 µg/mL PI and 10 mg/mL RNase A for 1 h at room temperature in a dark room. Flow cytometry was performed in a FACSCantoTMII with FACSDiva (BD Biosciences, Clontech, CA, USA) software to analyze DNA content. The relative ratios of cells in the G0/G1, S, and G2/M phases were calculated using FlowJo software (vX.10.6 version, Tree Stars Inc.).

4.6. Wound-Healing Assay

The wound-healing method was performed to verify the effects of P-MAPA and rhIL-12 alone or in combination on cell migration capacity. Briefly, 3×10^5 SKOV-3 cells were placed in 6-well plates with a serum-free culture medium for cell starvation. When the cells reached high confluence, a wound was created through the confluent cell monolayer using an angled tip at 45°, and the SKOV-3 cells were then immediately treated with the pre-determined doses of P-MAPA, rhIL-12, or both, diluted in 2 mL of complete RPMI 1640 medium. Images were obtained at 0 h, 6 h, 12 h, 24 h, 36 h, and 48 h until the wound closure. Migration area (%) was measured using Image-J software. All experiments were analyzed in biological and technical triplicate.

4.7. Cell Migration Using Transwell Insert

To evaluate the migratory potential of the cells, 1×10^4 SKOV-3 cells were seeded in triplicates into the upper chambers of 24-well ThinCert™ cell culture inserts (GBO, Americana, SP, Brazil) with PVDF filters (8.0 µm pore size) containing the corresponding treatment diluted in serum free RPMI 1640 medium. In the lower chamber, RPMI supplemented with 10% FBS was added as a chemotactic factor. After the plates were incubated at 37 °C and 5% CO_2 for 24 h, the cells in the upper chamber were gently removed with a cotton swab. The cells that had migrated to the lower surface of the insert through the 8.0 µm pore were fixed in methanol for 8 min and stained with hematoxylin for 45 s. The migrated cells were photographed with 20× objectives under an inverted microscope (ZeissAxiovert®, Germany). Four non-overlapped images were randomly analyzed for each well and the migrated cells were counted using Image J software.

4.8. Invasion Assay

The invasion assay was performed using a 24-well ThinCert™ cell culture insert (GBO, Americana, SP, Brazil) with PVDF filters (8.0 μm pore size). Briefly, 24-well plates were previously coated with Geltrex® (ThermoFisher, Waltham, MA, USA), which mimics the biological basement membrane matrix, and 1×10^4 cells were placed in the upper chamber with a serum-free culture medium containing the treatments. After 24 h, the invasive potential was determined by the amount of cells capable of crossing the barrier when chemotactically attracted by the RPMI 1640 medium supplemented with 10% FBS in the lower chamber. The protocol of cell fixing and staining was the same described for cell migration. Finally, four non-overlapped images were randomly analyzed per well and the invasive cells were counted using Image J software.

4.9. Immunofluorescence Assay

After the SKOV-3 cells were seeded in coverslips and treated with P-MAPA, rhIL-12, or their association for 48 h, they were fixed in methanol for 8 min at room temperature and then washed in sterile ice-cold PBS. To avoid nonspecific bindings, a blocking solution containing 3% (*v*/*v*) bovine serum albumin (BSA) was added for 1 h. Then, cells were incubated overnight with rabbit polyclonal anti-TLR2 and anti-TLR4 antibodies diluted 1:200 (Abcam, Cambridge, MA) for 4 h, followed by post incubation with secondary polyclonal anti-IgG conjugated to FITC (1:200 dilution in 1% BSA, Santa Cruz Biotechnology, Inc., CA) for 1 h. After the reactions, 4,6-diamidino-2-phenylindole (DAPI; Sigma, St Louis, MO) was used for nuclei staining. Positive staining was analyzed using a confocal fluorescence microscope Zeiss Axiophot II (Carl Zeiss, Oberköchen, Germany) at different magnification (excitation filter 590 nm, emission filter 650 nm) and for DAPI staining (excitation filter 365 nm, emission filter 485 nm). The relative fluorescence in FITC images was calculated using Image J software.

4.10. Western Blot Analysis

After the treatments, five replicates of each experiment were used. After being washed with cold PBS, 1×10^6 SKOV-3 cells were added to radioimmunoprecipitation assay buffer (RIPA) lysis buffer containing protease inhibitors and rapidly frozen for 24 h. Under constant agitation for 30 min at 4 °C, the cells were resuspended and transferred to 1.5 mL tubes and centrifuged for 20 min at 12,000 rpm. Protein quantification was performed using a Bradford assay, and the same amount of protein (40 μg) was solubilized in 1.5×Laemmli buffer and then used for 4–20% SDS-PAGE (Bio-Rad Laboratories, Hercules, CA, USA). After electrophoresis was carried out on tris-glycine running buffer system (120 V for 2 h), the proteins were electro-transferred (350 mA) to nitrocellulose membranes, and then blocked with 3% BSA in tris-buffered saline plus tween 20 (TBS-T) solution for 1 h. Afterward, the proteins were incubated with respective primary antibodies (1:500; Abcam, Cambridge, UK) at 4 °C overnight: anti-TLR2, anti-TLR4, anti-MyD88, anti-NF-kB p65, anti-TRIF, anti-IRF3. Subsequently, the membranes were washed three times and then incubated for 90 min with specific secondary antibodies (Sigma-Aldrich, St. Louis, MO, USA) diluted 1:20,000 in 1% BSA. After sequential washes, positive reactions were performed using ECL kit (Thermo Fisher Scientific, MA). All of the blots were calculated using individual samples obtained from three replicates/group and were represented as the mean optical density (band intensity/housekeeping protein). β-actin was used as the endogenous control.

4.11. Cytokine and Chemokine Assay

Levels of different cytokines and chemokines were determined in both supernatants and cell homogenates using a MilliPlex® Map Kit (EMD Millipore, Darmstadt, Germany) with a standard 20-plex detection kit according to the manufacturer's protocols. The human cytokine/chemokine Panel I kit (cat. no. HCYTOMAG-60K) included the following analytes: interferon-gamma (IFN-γ), interleukin (IL)-1β, IL-2, IL-3, IL-4, IL-6, IL-7, IL-8, IL-9, IL- 10, IL-12, IL-13, IL-15, IL-17, IP-10, macrophage-derived chemokine (MDC/CCL22), monocyte chemotactic protein-1 (MCP-1), macrophage inflammatory protein-1 (MIP)-1α, MIP-1β, and regulated upon activation normal T cell expressed and secreted (RANTES/CCL5). The concentrations were ranged between 0 and the lowest detectable level in each assay before log transformation. The analyses combined fluorescent cytometry and ELISA technology, so that each magnetic bead was added to a specific anti-cytokine to achieve a specific binding. For this experiment, the levels of analytes varied from 0.4 to 3500 pg/mL and the intra-assay CV was < 10%, inter-assay CV < 15%. No cross-reactivity was observed among cytokines and other molecules. The fluorescence intensity was measured using the MAGPIX system (Luminex Corporation, Austin, TX, USA).

4.12. Statistical Analysis

All data were evaluated using the analysis of variance (ANOVA) and presented as the mean ± standard deviation (SD). Significant results were then compared by Tukey or Newman-Keuls *post hoc* tests, and statistical significance was set at $p < 0.05$ for all analyses. Data were analyzed and constructed using GraphPad Prism 5.0 scientific graphing software (GraphPad Software, San Diego, CA, USA).

5. Conclusions

In summary, we demonstrated that P-MAPA in association with IL-12, both considered potent immunomodulatory agents, exhibited anti-cancer activities on human SKOV-3 cells. Although P-MAPA combined with IL-12 promotes a reduction in cell viability and cell migration, P-MAPA alone reduces the invasion capacity and enhances apoptosis in the presence of PTX. Similarly to either P-MAPA or IL-12 alone, the combinatory therapy induced the downregulation of TLR-downstream molecules involved with inflammation, which may result in protection against chemoresistance; these effects seem to be associated with TLR2 suppression rather than TLR4 signaling. P-MAPA alone stimulated the secretion of pro- and anti-inflammatory mediators, and its association with IL-12 increased the production of IL-4, -8, and MIP-1α by the SKOV-3 cells; this may promote changes in the immune responsiveness of the OC microenvironment. In addition to the effect on OC-infiltrated immune cells, these immunotherapies might provide a sustained opportunity for a novel combined strategy against malignant OC cells.

Supplementary Materials: The following are available online. Figure S1: MTT assay was tested with different cell densities to find the most appropriate strategy for cell counting. SKOV-3 cells at density of 1×10^3 were representative to determine cell viability; Table S1: Multiplex assay of the cytokines and chemokines (pg/mL) in the supernatant of cell culture; Table S2: Multiplex assay of the cytokines and chemokines (pg/mL) in the SKOV-3 cells.

Author Contributions: L.A.L., L.G.d.A.C., F.K.D.: conceived the hypothesis of the study, collected and analyzed the data, and drafted the manuscript. W.J.F., F.E.M., M.M., G.G.R., R.K., M.S.C., R.F.D., I.d.S.N.: participated in its design, intellectual conception of the study, and in the acquisition of data. All authors have read and agreed to the published version of the manuscript.

Funding: We would like to give a special thanks to Farmabrasilis-Brazil, FAPESP (*Fundação de Amparo à Pesquisa do Estado de São Paulo*, grant numbers: 2019/00906-6 and 2016/03993-9), CAPES (grant number: 0708/2018), and CNPq (grant number: 401040/2016-0) by providing financial support.

Acknowledgments: We are grateful to HélioKushima and Valeria Sandrim from Department of Pharmacology, IBB/UNESP, Botucatu, SP, Brazil, for excellent technical assistance and support.

Conflicts of Interest: The authors declare no conflict of interest.

Abbreviations

BSA	Bovine serum albumin
CEEA	Ethical Committee of the Institute of Bioscience/UNESP
CEMIB	Multidisciplinary Center for Biological Investigation
DAB	Diaminobenzidine
DAPI	6-diamidino-2-phenylindole
DCs	Dendritic cells
FITC	Fluorescein Isothiocyanate
HRP-conjugated	Horseradish peroxidase-conjugated
H	Hematoxylin
IFN	Interferon
IFN-γ	Interferon gamma
IL-6	Interleukin 6
IL-8	Interleukin 8
IRF3	Interferon regulatory factor 3
MyD88	Myeloid differentiation factor 88
NF-kB p65	Nuclear factor kappa B subunit p65
NK	natural killer cells
OC	ovarian cancer
PBS	phosphate-buffered saline
P-MAPA	Protein aggregate magnesium-ammonium phospholinoleate-palmitoleate anhydride
PTX	paclitaxel
RIPA	Radioimmunoprecipitation assay buffer
SDS-PAGE	Sodium dodecyl sulphate-polyacrylamide gel electrophoresis
TBS-T	Tris-Buffered Saline plus Tween 20
CD4 + T	CD4-positive T cells
CD8 + T	CD8-positive T cells
Th1	T helper 1
TLR (s)	Toll-like receptor (s)
TLR2	Toll-like receptor 2
TLR4	Toll-like receptor 4
TRIF	TIR domain-containing adaptor inducing interferon-beta

References

1. Siegel, R.L.; Miller, K.D.; Jemal, A. Cancer statistics, 2018. *CA Cancer J. Clin.* **2018**, *68*, 7–30. [CrossRef] [PubMed]
2. Fallows, S.; Price, J.; Atkinson, R.J.; Johnston, P.G.; Hickey, I.; Russell, S.E. P53 mutation does not affect prognosis in ovarian epithelial malignancies. *J. Pathol.* **2001**, *194*, 68–75. [CrossRef] [PubMed]
3. Cannistra, S.A. Cancer of the ovary. *N. Engl. J. Med.* **2004**, *351*, 2519–2565. [CrossRef] [PubMed]
4. Chuffa, L.G.; Fioruci-Fontanelli, B.A.; Mendes, L.O.; Fávaro, W.J.; Pinheiro, P.F.; Martinez, M.; Martinez, F.E. Characterization of chemically induced ovarian carcinomas in an ethanol-preferring rat model: Influence of long-term melatonin treatment. *PLoS ONE* **2013**, *8*, e81676. [CrossRef] [PubMed]
5. Chuffa, L.G.; Lupi-Júnior, L.A.; Costa, A.B.; Amorim, J.P.; Seiva, F.R. The role of sex hormones and steroid receptors on female reproductive cancers. *Steroids* **2017**, *118*, 93–108. [CrossRef]
6. Ebell, M.H.; Culp, M.B.; Radke, T.J. A systematic review of symptoms for the diagnosis of ovarian cancer. *Am. J. Prev. Med.* **2016**, *50*, 384–394. [CrossRef]
7. Kelly, M.G.; Alvero, A.B.; Chen, R.; Silasi, D.A.; Abrahams, V.M.; Chan, S.; Visintin, I.; Rutherford, T.; Mor, G. TLR-4 signaling promotes tumor growth and paclitaxel chemoresistance in ovarian cancer. *Cancer Res.* **2006**, *66*, 3859–3868. [CrossRef]
8. Bronte, G.; Cicero, G.; Sortino, G.; Pernice, G.; Catarella, M.T.; D'Alia, P.; Cusenza, S.; Lo Dico, S.; Bronte, E.; Sprini, D.; et al. Immunotherapy for recurrent ovarian cancer: A further piece of the puzzle or a striking strategy? *Expert Opin. Biol. Ther.* **2014**, *14*, 103–114. [CrossRef]
9. Fávaro, W.J.; Nunes, O.S.; Seiva, F.R.; Nunes, I.S.; Woolhiser, L.K.; Durán, N.; Lenaerts, A.J. Effects of P-MAPA immunomodulator on Toll-like receptors and p53: Potential therapeutic strategies for infectious diseases and cancer. *Infect. Agent. Cancer* **2012**, *7*, 1–15.
10. Garcia, P.V.; Seiva, F.R.; Carniato, A.P.; de Mello Júnior, W.; Duran, N.; Macedo, A.M.; de Oliveira, A.G.; Romih, R.; de Oliveira, A.G.; Romih, R.; et al. Increased toll-like receptors and p53 levels regulate apoptosis and angiogenesis in non-muscle invasive bladder cancer: Mechanism of action of P-MAPA biological response modifier. *BMC Cancer* **2016**, *16*, 422. [CrossRef]
11. de Almeida Chuffa, L.G.; de Moura Ferreira, G.; Lupi, L.A.; da Silva Nunes, I.; Fávaro, W.J. P-MAPA immunotherapy potentiates the effect of cisplatin on serous ovarian carcinoma through targeting TLR4 signaling. *J. Ovarian Res.* **2018**, *11*, 8. [CrossRef]
12. Chen, R.; Alvero, A.B.; Silasi, D.A.; Steffensen, K.D.; Mor, G. Cancers take their Toll–the function and regulation of Toll-like receptors in cancer cells. *Oncogene* **2008**, *27*, 225–233. [CrossRef]
13. Szajnik, M.; Szczepanski, M.J.; Czystowska, M.; Elishaev, E.; Mandapathil, M.; Nowak-Markwitz, E.; Spaczynski, M.; Whiteside, T.L. TLR4 signaling induced by lipopolysaccharide or paclitaxel regulates tumor survival and chemoresistance in ovarian cancer. *Oncogene* **2009**, *28*, 4353–4363. [CrossRef] [PubMed]
14. Wang, A.C.; Su, Q.B.; Wu, F.X.; Zhang, X.L.; Liu, P.S. Role of TLR4 for paclitaxel chemotherapy in human epithelial ovarian cancer cells. *Eur. J. Clin. Investig.* **2009**, *39*, 157–164. [CrossRef] [PubMed]
15. Trinchieri, G. Interleukin-12 and the regulation of innate resistance and adaptive immunity. *Nat. Rev. Immunol.* **2003**, *3*, 133–146. [CrossRef] [PubMed]
16. Cohen, C.A.; Shea, A.A.; Heffron, C.L.; Schmelz, E.M.; Roberts, P.C. Interleukin-12 Immunomodulation Delays the Onset of Lethal Peritoneal Disease of Ovarian Cancer. *J. Interferon Cytokine Res.* **2016**, *36*, 62–73. [CrossRef] [PubMed]
17. Colombo, M.P.; Trinchieri, G. Interleukin-12 in anti-tumor immunity and immunotherapy. *Cytokine Growth Factor Rev.* **2002**, *13*, 155–168. [CrossRef]

18. Hurteau, J.A.; Blessing, J.A.; DeCesare, S.L.; Creasman, W.T. Evaluation of recombinanthuman interleukin-12 in patients with recurrent or refractory ovarian cancer: Agynecologic oncology group study. *Gynecol. Oncol.* **2001**, *82*, 7–10. [CrossRef]
19. Lenzi, R.; Edwards, R.; June, C.; Seiden, M.V.; Garcia, M.E.; Rosenblum, M.; Freedman, R.S. Phase II study of intraperitoneal recombinant interleukin-12 (rhIL-12) in patients with peritoneal carcinomatosis (residual disease <1 cm) associated with ovarian cancer or primary peritoneal carcinoma. *J. Transl. Med.* **2007**, *5*, 66.
20. Präbst, K.; Engelhardt, H.; Ringgeler, S.; Hübner, H. Cell Viability Assays: Methods and Protocols. *Methods Mol. Biol.* **2017**, *1601*, 117.
21. Ahn, H.J.; Kim, Y.S.; Kim, J.U.; Han, S.M.; Shin, J.W.; Yang, H.O. Mechanism of taxol-inducedapoptosis in human SKOV3 ovarian carcinoma cells. *J. Cell Biochem.* **2004**, *91*, 1043–1052. [CrossRef]
22. Wang, Y.J.; Fletcher, R.; Yu, J.; Zhang, L. Immunogenic effects of chemotherapy-induced tumor cell death. *Genes Dis.* **2018**, *5*, 194–203. [CrossRef]
23. Chuffa, L.G.; Fioruci-Fontanelli, B.A.; Mendes, L.O.; Ferreira Seiva, F.R.; Martinez, M.; Fávaro, W.J.; Domeniconi, R.F.; Pinheiro, P.F.; Delazari Dos Santos, L.; Martinez, F.E. Melatonin attenuates the TLR4-mediated inflammatory response through MyD88- and TRIF-dependent signaling pathways in an in vivo model of ovarian cancer. *BMC Cancer* **2015**, *15*, 34. [CrossRef]
24. Lavoue, V.; Thedrez, A.; Leveque, J.; Foucher, F.; Henno, S.; Jauffret, V.; Belaud-Rotureau, M.A.; Catros, V.; Cabillic, F. Immunity of human epithelial ovarian carcinoma: The paradigm of immunesuppression in cancer. *J. Transl. Med.* **2013**, *11*, 1–12. [CrossRef]
25. Jouhi, L.; Koljonen, V.; Böhling, T.; Haglund, C.; Hagström, J. The expression of toll-like receptors 2, 4, 5, 7 and 9 in Merkel cell carcinoma. *Anticancer Res.* **2015**, *35*, 1843–1849.
26. Zhu, G.; Gui, Z. Effect of silkworm peptide on inducting M1 type polarization andTh1 activation via TLR2-induced MyD88-dependent pathway. *Food Sci. Nutr.* **2019**, *7*, 1251–1260. [CrossRef] [PubMed]
27. d'Adhemar, C.J.; Spillane, C.D.; Gallagher, M.F.; Bates, M.; Costello, K.M.; Barry-O'Crowley, J.; Haley, K.; Kernan, N.; Murphy, C.; Smyth, P.C.; et al. The MyD88+ phenotype is an adverse prognostic factor in epithelial ovarian cancer. *PLoS ONE* **2014**, *9*, e100816. [CrossRef]
28. Kim, K.H.; Jo, M.S.; Suh, D.S.; Yoon, M.S.; Shin, D.H.; Lee, J.H.; Choi, K.U. Expression and significance of the TLR4/MyD88 signaling pathway in ovarian epithelial cancers. *World J. Surg. Oncol.* **2012**, *10*, 193. [CrossRef] [PubMed]
29. Gaikwad, S.M.; Thakur, B.; Sakpal, A.; Singh, R.K.; Ray, P. Differential activation of NF-κB signaling is associated with platinum and taxane resistance in MyD88deficient epithelial ovarian cancer cells. *Int. J. Biochem. Cell Biol.* **2015**, *61*, 90–102. [CrossRef] [PubMed]
30. Zhan, Y.; Xiang, F.; Wu, R.; Xu, J.; Ni, Z.; Jiang, J.; Kang, X. MiRNA-149 modulates chemosensitivity of ovarian cancer A2780 cells to paclitaxel by targeting MyD88. *J. Ovarian Res.* **2015**, *8*, 48. [CrossRef] [PubMed]
31. Li, Z.; Block, M.S.; Vierkant, R.A.; Fogarty, Z.C.; Winham, S.J.; Visscher, D.W.; Kalli, K.R.; Wang, C.; Goode, E.L. The inflammatory microenvironment in epithelial ovarian cancer: A role for TLR4 and MyD88 and related proteins. *Tumour Biol.* **2016**, *37*, 13279–13286. [CrossRef] [PubMed]
32. Meng, Y.; Hu, J.; Chen, Y.; Yu, T.; Hu, L. Silencing MARCH1 suppresses proliferation, migration and invasion of ovarian cancer SKOV3 cells via downregulation of NF-κB and Wnt/β-catenin pathways. *Oncol. Rep.* **2016**, *36*, 2463–2470. [CrossRef] [PubMed]
33. Yamamoto, M.; Sato, S.; Hemmi, H.; Hoshino, K.; Kaisho, T.; Sanjo, H.; Takeuchi, O.; Sugiyama, M.; Okabe, M.; Takeda, K.; et al. Role of adaptor TRIF in the MyD88-independent toll-like receptor signaling pathway. *Science* **2003**, *301*, 640–643. [CrossRef] [PubMed]

34. Ullah, M.O.; Sweet, M.J.; Mansell, A.; Kellie, S.; Kobe, B. TRIF-dependent TLR signaling, its functions in host defense and inflammation, and its potential as a therapeutic target. *J. Leukoc. Biol.* **2016**, *100*, 27–45. [CrossRef] [PubMed]
35. Muccioli, M.; Sprague, L.; Nandigam, H.; Pate, M.; Benencia, F. Toll-like receptors as novel therapeutic targets for ovarian cancer. *ISRN Oncol.* **2012**, *2012*, 642141. [CrossRef] [PubMed]
36. Yamamoto, K.; Yajima, A.; Terashima, Y.; Nozawa, S.; Taketani, Y.; Yakushiji, M.; Noda, K. Phase II clinical study on the effects of recombinant human interleukin-3 onthrombocytopenia after chemotherapy for advanced ovarian cancer. SDZ ILE 964[IL-3] Study Group. *J. Immunother.* **1999**, *22*, 539–545. [CrossRef]
37. Veldhuis, G.J.; Willemse, P.H.; van Gameren, M.M.; Aalders, J.G.; Mulder, N.H.; Mull, B.; Biesma, B.; deVries, E.G. Recombinant human interleukin-3 to dose-intensify carboplatin and cyclophosphamide chemotherapy in epithelial ovarian cancer: A phase I trial. *J. Clin. Oncol.* **1995**, *13*, 733–740. [CrossRef]
38. Rivera-Vargas, T.; Humblin, E.; Végran, F.; Ghiringhelli, F.; Apetoh, L. Th9 cells inanti-tumor immunity. *Semin. Immunopathol.* **2017**, *39*, 39–46. [CrossRef]
39. Park, J.; Li, H.; Zhang, M.; Lu, Y.; Hong, B.; Zheng, Y.; He, J.; Yang, J.; Qian, J.; Yi, Q. Murine Th9 cells promote the survival of myeloid dendritic cells in cancerimmunotherapy. *Cancer Immunol. Immunother.* **2014**, *63*, 835–845. [CrossRef]
40. Singh, M.; Loftus, T.; Webb, E.; Benencia, F. Minireview: Regulatory T Cells and Ovarian Cancer. *Immunol. Investig.* **2016**, *45*, 712–720. [CrossRef]
41. Qu, Q.X.; Xie, F.; Huang, Q.; Zhang, X.G. Membranous and cytoplasmic expression ofPD-L1 in ovarian cancer cells. *Cell. Physiol. Biochem.* **2017**, *43*, 1893–1906. [CrossRef] [PubMed]
42. Barbieri, F.; Bajetto, A.; Florio, T. Role of chemokine network in the development and progression of ovarian cancer: A potential novel pharmacological target. *J. Oncol.* **2010**, *2010*, 426956. [CrossRef] [PubMed]
43. Zsiros, E.; Duttagupta, P.; Dangaj, D.; Li, H.; Frank, R.; Garrabrant, T.; Hagemann, I.S.; Levine, B.L.; June, C.H.; Zhang, L.; et al. The ovarian cancer chemokine landscape isconducive to homing of vaccine-primed and CD3/CD28-costimulated T cells prepared for adoptive therapy. *Clin. Cancer Res.* **2015**, *21*, 2840–2850. [CrossRef]
44. Vulcano, M.; Albanesi, C.; Stoppacciaro, A.; Bagnati, R.; D'Amico, G.; Struyf, S.; Transidico, P.; Bonecchi, R.; Del Prete, A.; Allavena, P.; et al. Dendritic cells as a major source of macrophage-derived chemokine/CCL22 in vitro and in vivo. *Eur. J. Immunol.* **2001**, *31*, 812–822. [CrossRef]
45. Fialová, A.; Partlová, S.; Sojka, L.; Hromádková, H.; Brtnický, T.; Fučíková, J.; Kocián, P.; Rob, L.; Bartůňková, J.; Spíšek, R. Dynamics of T-cell infiltration during thecourse of ovarian cancer: The gradual shift from a Th17 effector cell response toa predominant infiltration by regulatory T-cells. *Int. J. Cancer* **2013**, *132*, 1070–1079.
46. Giuntoli, R.L., 2nd; Webb, T.J.; Zoso, A.; Rogers, O.; Diaz-Montes, T.P.; Bristow, R.E.; Oelke, M. Ovarian cancer-associated ascites demonstrates altered immune environment: Implications for antitumor immunity. *Anticancer Res.* **2009**, *29*, 2875–2884.
47. Lee, L.F.; Hellendall, R.P.; Wang, Y.; Haskill, J.S.; Mukaida, N.; Matsushima, K.; Ting, J.P. IL-8 reduced tumorigenicity of human ovarian cancer in vivo due to neutrophil infiltration. *J. Immunol.* **2000**, *164*, 2769–2775. [CrossRef]
48. Colvin, E.K. Tumor-associated macrophages contribute to tumor progression in ovarian cancer. *Front. Oncol.* **2014**, *4*, 137. [CrossRef]
49. Tino, A.B.; Chitcholtan, K.; Sykes, P.H.; Garrill, A. Resveratrol and acetyl-resveratrol modulate activity of VEGF and IL-8 in ovarian cancer cell aggregates via attenuation of the NF-κB protein. *J. Ovarian Res.* **2016**, *9*, 84. [CrossRef]
50. Milliken, D.; Scotton, C.; Raju, S.; Balkwill, F.; Wilson, J. Analysis of chemokinesand chemokine receptor expression in ovarian cancer ascites. *Clin. Cancer Res.* **2002**, *8*, 1108–1114.

51. Soria, G.; Ben-Baruch, A. The inflammatory chemokines CCL2 and CCL5 in breastcancer. *Cancer Lett.* **2008**, *267*, 271–285. [CrossRef] [PubMed]
52. Su, W.; Ito, T.; Oyama, T.; Kitagawa, T.; Yamori, T.; Fujiwara, H.; Matsuda, H. The direct effect of IL-12 on tumor cells: IL-12 acts directly on tumor cells to activate NF-kB and enhance IFN-g-mediated STAT1 phosphorylation. *Biochem. Biophys. Res. Commun.* **2001**, *280*, 503–5121. [CrossRef] [PubMed]

Sample Availability: Samples of the compounds are not available from the authors.

molecules

MDPI

Article

Design, Synthesis, and Biological Evaluation of Pyridineamide Derivatives Containing a 1,2,3-Triazole Fragment as Type II c-Met Inhibitors

Hehua Xiong [†], Jianxin Cheng [†], Jianqing Zhang, Qian Zhang, Zhen Xiao, Han Zhang, Qidong Tang * and Pengwu Zheng *

School of Pharmacy, Jiangxi Science & Technology Normal University, Nanchang 330013, China; 18296154955@163.com (H.X.); cjx3159@163.com (J.C.); zhang1405474771@163.com (J.Z.); 15797966937@163.com (Q.Z.); xz950420@163.com (Z.X.); zbl1045762244@163.com (H.Z.)

* Correspondence: tangqidongcn@126.com (Q.T.); zhengpw@jxstnu.edu.cn (P.Z.); Tel.: +86-791-8380-2393 (P.Z.)

† These authors contribute equally to this work.

Academic Editor: Qiao-Hong Chen

Received: 21 November 2019; Accepted: 10 December 2019; Published: 18 December 2019

Abstract: A series of 4-(pyridin-4-yloxy)benzamide derivatives containing a 1,2,3-triazole fragment were designed, synthesized, and their inhibitory activity against A549, HeLa, and MCF-7 cancer cell lines was evaluated. Most compounds exhibited moderate to potent antitumor activity against the three cell lines. Among them, the promising compound **B26** showed stronger inhibitory activity than Golvatinib, with IC_{50} values of 3.22, 4.33, and 5.82 μM against A549, HeLa, and MCF-7 cell lines, respectively. The structure–activity relationships (SARs) demonstrated that the modification of the terminal benzene ring with a single electron-withdrawing substituent (fluorine atom) and the introduction of a pyridine amide chain with a strong hydrophilic group (morpholine) to the hinge region greatly improved the antitumor activity. Meanwhile, the optimal compound **B26** showed potent biological activity in some pharmacological experiments in vitro, such as cell morphology study, dose-dependent test, kinase activity assay, and cell cycle experiment. Finally, the molecular docking simulation was performed to further explore the binding mode of compound **B26** with c-Met.

Keywords: 4-(pyridin-4-yloxy)benzamide; 1,2,3-triazole; c-Met; inhibitor

1. Introduction

Cancer has become a serious threat to human life and health [1,2]. c-Met tyrosine kinase is a kind of type III tyrosine kinase, which is closely related to cellular activities [3] such as growth, reproduction, metastasis, etc. However, abnormal expression of c-Met kinases in cells usually triggers the occurrence, invasion, and metastasis of various cancer diseases [4]. c-Met kinase has been found overexpressed in various cancer cells and has become an attractive target for cancer treatment [5,6]. Nowadays, developing small molecule c-Met kinase inhibitors has become a hotspot in the treatment of human cancer [7].

c-Met inhibitors are classified as type I and type II inhibitors according to the binding mode of inhibitors with c-Met. Usually, c-Met inhibitors of type I are single-target inhibitors that bind to the hinge region of the ATP pocket, and c-Met inhibitors of type II are multitarget inhibitors that bind to the hinge region and an extra hydrophobic pocket [8,9]. With the development of biology and pharmacology, the intracellular mechanisms have been elucidated, and research in small molecule inhibitors has made significant progress. Type II c-Met inhibitors possess more potent inhibitory activity and better tolerance to drug resistance through binding to kinases of multiple types. Cabozantinib, a c-Met inhibitor of type II, was approved by the FDA for treatment of prostate cancer in 2012. Some representative c-Met inhibitors (type II) in the clinical trial phase are listed in Figure 1, including

Golvatinib, BMS-777607, Altriatinib, and TAS-115 [10–12]. Furthermore, according to the structure characteristics of inhibitors, the skeleton of c-Met inhibitor (type II) was summarized into blocks A, B, C, and D by our research group, as shown in Figure 1 [13].

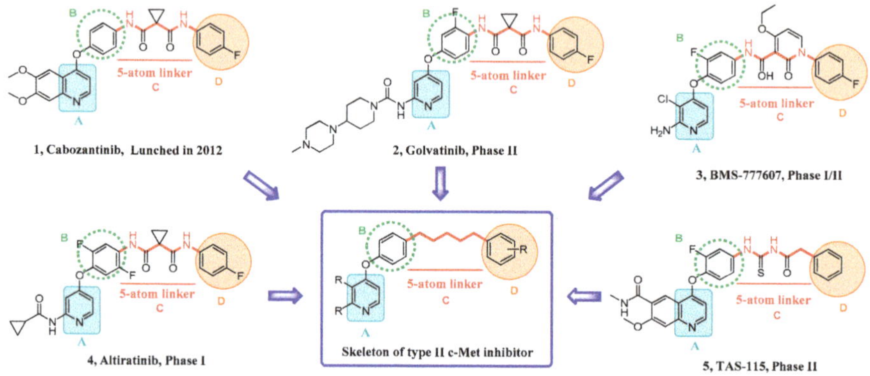

Figure 1. Some representative c-Met inhibitors of type II and the summarized skeleton.

We explored the SARs of c-Met inhibitors (type II) bearing pyridinamide structure using Golvatinib as a lead compound in this study. In order to guide our modification of the lead compound, a molecular docking simulation of Golvatinib and c-Met protein was performed, as shown in Figure 2. The docking results indicated that blocks A and C, which possessed hydrogen bonding interactions with residues Met1160, Asp1222, and Lys1110, played a key role in maintaining the inhibitory activity against c-Met. Therefore, the modification was mainly concentrated on blocks A and C. Firstly, a pyridylamide structure in block A, including hydrogen bond donor and hydrogen bond acceptor atoms, was introduced into the meta position of pyridine in order to enhance the interaction with the hinge region residues, and then some alkyl chains bearing morpholine or thiophene groups were connected to the terminal of the pyridine amide structure for better water solubility of compounds. Then, a 1,2,3-triazole fragment with good biological activity and two hydrogen bond acceptor atoms was introduced to block C for more tight combination between the compounds and c-Met. In addition, considering the steric hindrance problem [14], H/F atoms and different substituents were introduced in blocks B and D, respectively, to explore their effects on biological activity of target compounds. Finally, a series of small molecule inhibitors containing the 1,2,3-triazole fragment were designed, synthesized, and biologically evaluated.

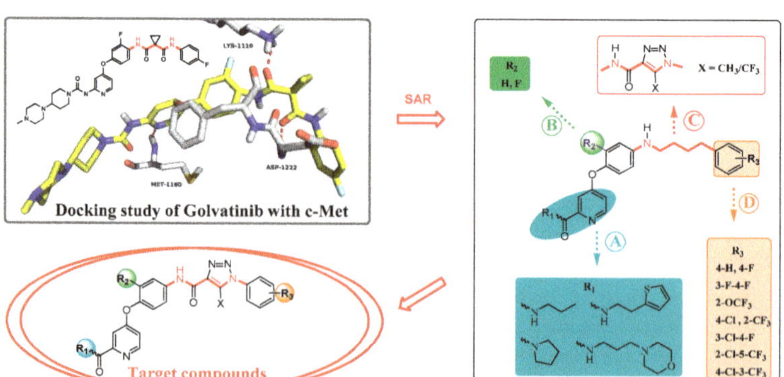

Figure 2. Design strategy of target compounds based on the molecular simulation and structure–activity relationships (SARs).

2. Results and Discussion

2.1. Chemistry

The synthesis route of target compounds **B1–B27** is shown in Scheme 1. Firstly, the commercially available pyridinecarboxylic acid **6** was reacted with $SOCl_2$ using NaBr as catalyst to yield 4-chloropicolinoyl chloride **7**, which was then converted into ethyl 4-chloropicolinate **8** with ethanol. Next, 4-chloropicolinate **8** was subjected to nucleophilic substitute with *p*-nitrophenol or 2-fluoro-4-nitrophenol using chlorobenzene as solvent to give picolinate analogues **9a–9b**, which were then dissolved in 1,4-dioxane and hydrolyzed with NaOH aqueous solution to obtain picolinic acid analogues **10a–10b**. Intermediates **10a–10b** were reacted with $SOCl_2$ to get the corresponding acyl chlorides and then connected with amines (including propan-1-amine, 2-(thiophen-2-yl)ethan-1-amine, pyrrolidine and 3-morpholinopropan-1-amine) to obtain picolinamide analogues **11a–11e**. Finally, the key intermediates **12a–12e** were produced by the reduction of **11a–11e** with hydrazine hydrate as reducing agent. Other intermediates **13a–13i**, which have been reported in our previous research [15], were combined with intermediates **12a–12e** by a nucleophilic substitute reaction to get the target compounds **B1–B27**.

The structural information of the target compounds was confirmed by ^{1}H-NMR, ^{13}C-NMR, and TOF MS (ES+), which were consistent with the structures depicted.

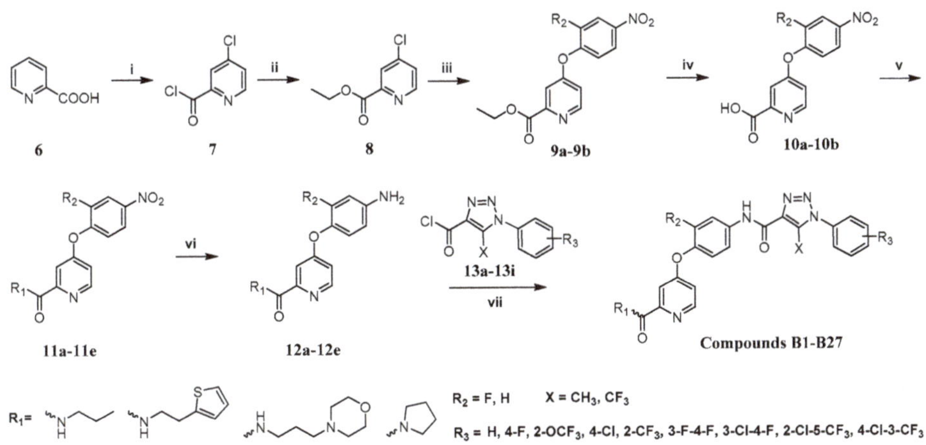

Scheme 1. The synthetic route for target compounds **B1–B27**. Reagents and conditions: (i) NaBr, $SOCl_2$, 85 °C, 18 h; (ii) triethylamine, dichloromethane (DCM), EtOH, 0 °C, 1 h; (iii) *p*-nitrophenol or 2-fluoro-4-nitrophenol, chlorobenzene, 135 °C, 4 h; (iv) 1,4-dioxane, sodium hydroxide (10%), r.t., 0.5 h; (v) $SOCl_2$, amines, Et_3N, DCM, 0–85 °C, 1 h; (vi) EtOH, activated carbon, $FeCl_3 \cdot 6H_2O$, hydrazine hydrate (80%), 90 °C, 4 h. (vii) EtOH, activated carbon, $FeCl_3 \cdot 6H_2O$, hydrazine hydrate (80%), 90 °C, 4 h; (vii) DCM, $NaHCO_3$, 0 °C, 1 h.

2.2. Antitumor Activity of Compounds *B1–B27* Against A549, HeLa, and MCF-7 Cell Lines and SAR Analysis

The antitumor activity of target compounds against A549, HeLa, and MCF-7 cell lines was evaluated to investigate their inhibitory activity against cancer cells [16]. The antitumor activities of compounds were displayed as the IC_{50} (half-inhibitory concentration) values, as shown in Tables 1 and 2. Most compounds exhibited moderate to potent antitumor activity against three cell lines. Compounds **B25–B27** possessed more potent inhibitory activity than Golvatinib, as shown in Table 2, with IC_{50} values in the range of 3.22–13.60 μM. The optimal compound **B26** showed excellent inhibitory activity against A549, HeLa, and MCF-7 cell lines with IC_{50} values of 3.22 ± 0.12, 4.33 ± 0.09, and 5.82 ± 0.09 μM, respectively, which were more efficient than Golvatinib (8.14 ± 0.45, 15.17 ± 0.17, and 16.91 ± 0.29 μM).

Table 1. Antitumor activities of the target compounds **B1–B18** against A549, HeLa, and MCF-7 cell lines.

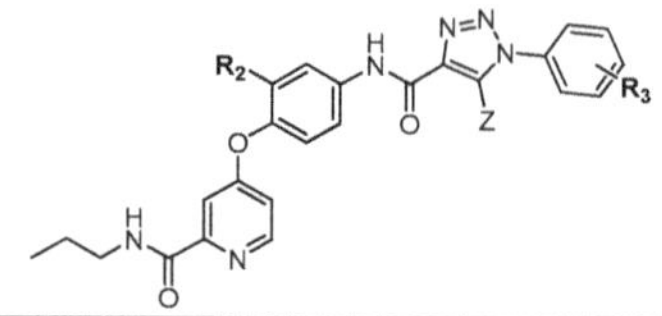

Compd.	R_2	R_3	Z	IC_{50} (μM) ± SD		
				A549	HeLa	MCF-7
B1	H	4-H	CH_3	46.55 ± 1.90	52.31 ± 5.42	63.05 ± 2.44
B2		4-F	CH_3	21.30 ± 0.66	42.06 ± 6.03	32.13 ± 0.86
B3		2-OCF_3	CH_3	32.67 ± 1.16	53.94 ± 4.23	48.71 ± 3.26
B4		4-Cl	CF_3	56.26 ± 2.26	48.23 ± 1.59	120.76 ± 1.25
B5		2-CF_3	CF_3	35.57 ± 1.03	59.55 ± 2.94	270.40 ± 12.35
B6		3-F-4-F	CF_3	256.30 ± 10.37	170.38 ± 13.69	NA [a]
B7		3-Cl-4-F	CF_3	221.98 ± 21.46	295.65 ± 15.37	NA
B8		2-Cl-5-CF_3	CF_3	238.07 ± 17.84	NA	NA
B9		4-Cl-3-CF_3	CF_3	357.24 ± 14.50	NA	NA
B10	F	4-H	CH_3	33.31 ± 1.25	41.55 ± 2.26	60.50 ± 3.99
B11		4-F	CH_3	19.70 ± 0.89	46.57 ± 1.59	29.11 ± 1.30
B12		2-OCF_3	CH_3	24.24 ± 0.71	53.04 ± 1.11	42.26 ± 1.09
B13		4-Cl	CF_3	46.13 ± 3.59	55.43 ± 2.30	82.48 ± 2.34
B14		2-CF_3	CF_3	32.94 ± 2.33	40.68 ± 1.09	84.45 ± 12.34
B15		3-F-4-F	CF_3	123.07 ± 10.23	240.60 ± 22.49	332.01 ± 20.08
B16		3-Cl-4-F	CF_3	150.58 ± 12.21	270.24 ± 13.56	NA
B17		2-Cl-5-CF_3	CF_3	223.34 ± 10.89	NA	NA
B18		4-Cl-3-CF_3	CF_3	246.70 ± 21.23	NA	NA
Golvatinib [b]				8.14 ± 0.45	15.17 ± 0.17	16.91 ± 0.29

[a] NA: Low inhibitory activity, [b] Used as the positive control.

Table 2. Antitumor activities of the target compounds **B10–B12** and **B19–B27** against A549, HeLa, and MCF-7 cell lines.

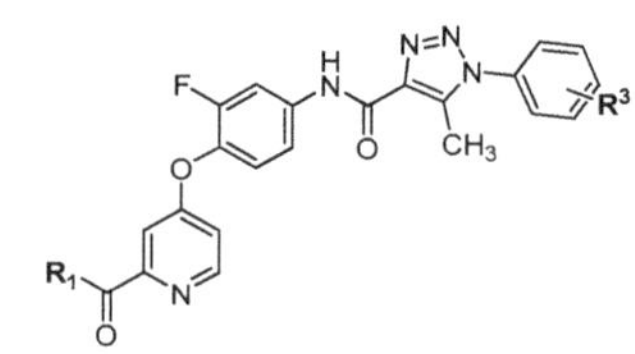

Compd.	R_1	R_3	IC_{50} (μM) ± SD		
			A549	HeLa	MCF-7
B10	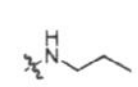	4-H	33.31 ± 1.25	41.55 ± 2.26	60.50 ± 3.99
B11		4-F	19.70 ± 0.89	46.57 ± 1.59	29.11 ± 1.30
B12		2-OCF_3	24.24 ± 0.71	53.04 ± 1.11	42.26 ± 1.09
B19	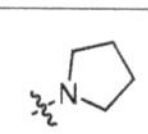	4-H	27.25 ± 0.79	32.31 ± 2.11	39.08 ± 0.97
B20		4-F	12.10 ± 0.31	21.84 ± 1.93	19.12 ± 0.21
B21		2-OCF_3	17.72 ± 0.42	29.55 ± 2.04	41.10 ± 1.21
B22	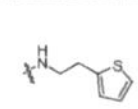	4-H	19.88 ± 0.75	45.18 ± 3.89	33.80 ± 1.11
B23		4-F	12.52 ± 0.37	15.19 ± 0.96 [a]	35.11 ± 3.05
B24		2-OCF_3	13.34 ± 0.58	19.73 ± 0.83	44.82 ± 2.96
B25	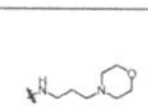	4-H	6.43 ± 0.21	10.51 ± 0.68	13.60 ± 0.86
B26		4-F	3.22 ± 0.12	4.33 ± 0.09	5.82 ± 0.09
B27		2-OCF_3	4.91 ± 0.09	5.72 ± 0.17	9.34 ± 0.52
Golvatoinib [b]			8.14 ± 0.45	15.17 ± 0.17	16.91 ± 0.29

[a] Bold values show the IC_{50} values of the target compounds lower than the values of the positive control; [b] Used as the positive control.

According to the antitumor activity of compounds **B1–B27** listed in Tables 1 and 2, the SARs were summarized as follows. Overall, the F atom on the meta-central benzene ring provided stronger inhibitory activity against cancer cells than H atom, for example, compounds **B1–B8** displayed less inhibitory activity than compounds **B9–B18**. A single substitution (such as H/F/OCF_3/Cl/CF_3) linked to the terminal benzene ring was favorable for maintaining the biological activity, such as compounds **B1–B5** and **B10–B15** that possessed moderate antitumor activity with IC_{50} values less than 60 μM against A549 and HeLa cell lines. However, the double substituents connected to the terminal benzene ring obviously impaired the inhibitory activity of compounds **B6–B9** and **B15–B18,** whose IC_{50} values were more than 120 μM against three cell lines. A possible explanation would be that the introduction of two substituents to the terminal benzene ring may create steric hindrance, which made it difficult for compounds to extend into the hydrophobic pocket and to bind tightly to c-Met kinase.

Inspired by the inhibitory activity of compounds **B1–B3** and **B10–B12**, as shown in Table 1, the F atom of the central benzene ring and the single group (H, F, or OCF_3) of the terminal benzene ring were reserved to perform a SAR study of the pyridine amide moiety. Hydrophilic groups, including morpholine or thiophene groups attached to the terminal of pyridine amide, have a great contribution to inhibitory activity of the compounds **B22–B27** (with IC_{50} values in the range of 3.22–45.18 μM).

In summary, introducing morpholino groups and F atoms to the pyridylpropyl amide and the terminal benzene ring, respectively, made significant advances in the inhibitory activity.

2.3. *Dose-Dependent Test of Compound **B26** Against A549 Cells*

To explore the relationship between concentrations and antitumor activity of compound **B26**, we carried out a dose-dependent test based on the MTT method [16], in which A549 cells were treated with seven different concentrations of compound **B26** (0.137, 0.411, 1.234, 3.704, 11.11, 33.33, and 100 μM), using Golvatinib as a positive control, as seen in Figure 3. The results revealed that compound **B26** could effectively inhibit cancer cells in a dose-dependent manner. Notably, compound **B26** inhibited A549 cells more than 50% at the concentration of 3.704 μM, while the inhibitory rate of Golvatinib was less than 40% at the same concentration.

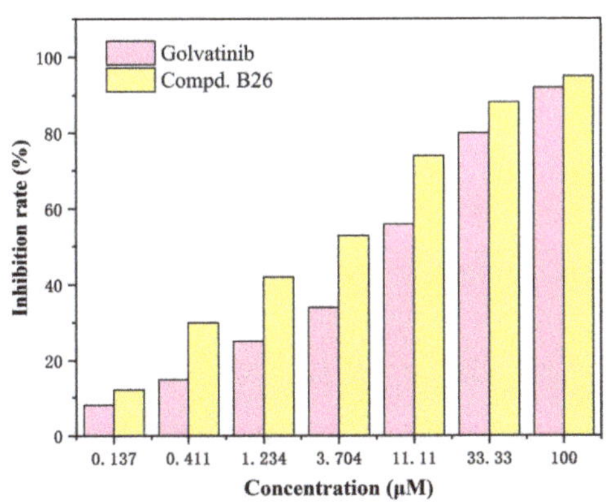

Figure 3. Relationship between concentration and inhibition rate of compound **B26** against A549 cells.

2.4. *Cell Cycle Study of A549 Cells Treated with Compound **B26***

To further investigate the inhibitory pattern of compound **B26** on the growth of cancer cells, cell cycle distribution analysis [17] was carried out on A549 cells, as shown in Figure 4. Compound **B26** at concentrations of 5, 10, and 15 μM and Golvatinib at a concentration of 5 μM were delivered to A549 cells for 24 h, as shown in Figure 4. With the increased concentration of compound **B26**, the percentage of cells blocked in G_0/G_1 phase was increased from 65.44% to 79.18%, while the percentage in the S phase decreased from 21.91% to 16.56%. There was no significant change in G_2/M phase. The result showed that compound **B26** (74.41%) and Golvatinib (74.77%) had the same inhibitory effect on A549 cells at the concentration of 5 μM, both of which could block cells in the G_0/G_1 phase.

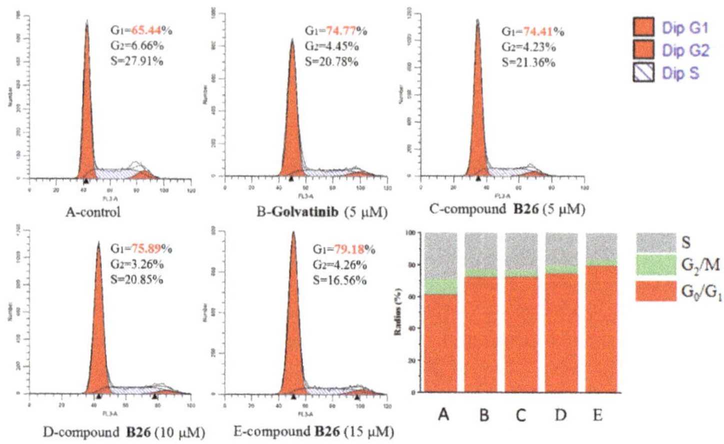

Figure 4. Cell cycle study of A549 cells treated with compound **B26** and Golvatinib.

2.5. c-Met Enzyme Assay of Compounds B25–B27 and Staurosporine

Compounds **B25**, **B26**, and **B27**, possessing potent antitumor activity against A549, HeLa, and MCF-7 cell lines, were selected to investigate their c-Met kinase assay by mobility shift assay method [18] with staurosporine as a positive control, which was used to insure the reliability of the experimental data. Compound **B26** exhibited potent inhibitory activity against c-Met with an inhibition rate of 36% at the concentration of 0.625 μM, as shown in Table 3.

Table 3. c-Met kinase activity of selected compounds **B25**, **B26**, **B27**, and staurosporine.

Compound (0.625 μM)	Rates (%)
B25	4.3
B26	36.0
B27	23.8
Staurosporine	87.3

2.6. Molecular Docking Simulation of Compounds (B26 and Golvatinib) and c-Met

Next, we further explored the binding mode of compound **B26** and Golvatinib with c-Met kinase (PDB: 3LQ8, extracted from the PDB database) through molecule docking simulation using AutoDock 4.2 software [19], as shown in Figure 5. The docking results indicated that compound **B26** and Golvatinib in an extended conformation formed strong hydrogen bonding interactions with residues Met1160, Asp1222, and Lys1110, as shown in Figure 5a–d. Interestingly, the pyridylamide structure of compound **B26** formed a bidentate hydrogen bond with residue Met1160, as shown in Figure 5a,b, which may offer a stronger ability of compound **B26** to bind with c-Met. Compound **B26** formed more hydrogen bonding interactions with Met1160 than Golvatinib, which may explain the better antitumor activity of compound **B26**.

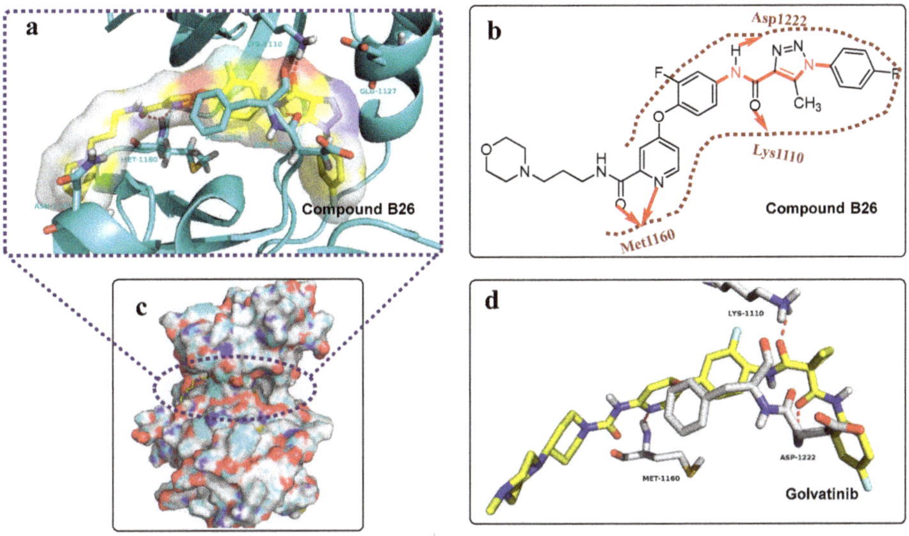

Figure 5. Figure 5a, 5b, and 5c are partial views, two-dimensional partial views, and integral cavity views of the docking results of c-Met (PDB code: 3LQ8) and compound **B26**, respectively. Figure 5d shows partial views of c-Met and Golvatinib. The c-Met protein and compounds are displayed by cartoons and sticks, respectively. Hydrogen bonding interactions between compounds and c-Met are indicated with dashed lines or arrows in red.

3. Experimental Section

3.1. Chemistry

Unless specifically required, all reagents used in the experiments were purchased as commercial analytical grade and used without further purification. Frequently used solvents (dichloromethane, ethyl acetate, tetrahydrofuran, 1,4-dioxane, methanol, ethanol, etc.) were absolutely anhydrous. Flash column chromatography was performed on silica gel (300 mesh) using a mixture of petroleum ether (PE) and ethyl acetate (EA). The reaction process was monitored by thin-layer chromatography (TLC, SH-GH254) and spots were visualized with ultraviolet analyzer (light in 254 or 365 nm). ^{1}H-NMR and ^{13}C-NMR spectra analysis of compounds was implemented in Bruker 400 MHz spectrometer (Bruker Bioscience, Billerica, MA, USA) using tetramethylsilane (TMS) as an internal standard at room temperature. Mass spectrometry (MS) of target compounds was carried out Waters High Resolution Quadrupole Time of Flight Tandem Mass Spectrometry (Waters, Xevo G2-XS Tof). The melting point of the compounds was measured by SGW X-4 micro melting point instrument. The purity of compounds was determined by an Agilent 1260 liquid chromatograph equipped with an Inertex-C18 column, and all were more than 95%.

3.1.1. Preparation of 4-Chloropicolinoyl Chloride (7)

Pyridinecarboxylic acid **6** (10.00 g, 0.081 mol), NaBr (0.10 g, 0.001 mol), and a drop of *N*,*N*-dimethylformamide (DMF) were added in thionyl chloride ($SOCl_2$, 50 mL) and stirred at 85 °C for 18 h. The reaction was monitored by TLC. After completion of the reaction, the solvent was removed under vacuum to obtain a yellow liquid, which was dissolved in DCM for further use.

3.1.2. Preparation of Ethyl 4-Chloropicolinate (8)

Dichloromethane (30 mL), ethanol (16.43 g, 0.170 mol), and triethylamine (17.17 g, 0.170 mol) were successively added to a beaker and stirred at 0 °C for 0.5 h. Subsequently, a mixture of

4-chloropicolinoyl chloride **7** (16.43 g, 0.110 mol) and DCM (5 mL) was added dropwise, stirred at 0 °C for 0.5 h, and monitored by TLC. After completion of the reaction, NaOH solution was added to the mixture to adjust the pH value 9–10. Ultimately, the organic layers were combined and dried to obtain a brown liquid.

3.1.3. Preparation of Ethyl 4-(4-Nitrophenoxy)picolinate (**9a**) and Ethyl4-(2-Fluoro-4-Nitrophenoxy) picolinate (**9b**)

Intermediate **8** (13.22 g, 0.071 mol) and *p*-nitrophenol or 2-fluoro-4-nitrophenol (0.026 mol) were dissolved in chlorobenzene (40 mL) and then stirred at 130 °C for 4 h. The completion of the reaction was monitored by TLC. After completion of the reaction, the cold petroleum ether (100 mL) was poured into the reaction solvent and stirred at room temperature for 0.5 h. Next, petroleum ether (100 mL) was poured off to give a viscous liquid, which was then dissolved in DCM (300 mL) and extracted with aqueous solution of NaOH. The organic layer was combined, dried, and concentrated under vacuum to get a pale yellow solid.

3.1.4. Preparation of 4-(4-Nitrophenoxy)picolinic Acid (**10a**) and 4-(2-Fluoro-4-Nitrophenoxy)picolinic Acid (**10b**)

Intermediates **9a–9b** (0.035 mol) were dissolved in 1,4-dioxane (50 mL) and stirred at room temperature for 0.5 h. A solution of 10% NaOH (2.28 mL, 0.057 mol) was then added dropwise to the above mixture, stirred at room temperature for 0.5 h, and monitored by TLC. After completion of the reaction, the solvent was evaporated under vacuum to give a white solid. The white solid was then dissolved in saturated NaCl solution (500 mL) and stirred at room temperature for 10 h. Subsequently, after the pH of the solution was adjusted to 2–3 by 75% hydrochloric acid (HCl), a yellow solid was precipitated, filtered, and dried.

3.1.5. Preparation of 4-(4-Nitrophenoxy)picolinamide or 4-(2-Fluoro-4-Nitrophenoxy)picolinamide Analogues (**11a–11e**)

Intermediates **10a–10b** (0.020 mol) and one drop of DMF were successively dissolved in $SOCl_2$ (50 mL) and stirred at 85 °C for 0.5 h. Then reaction solvent was concentrated in vacuum, dissolved in DCM (8 mL), and added dropwise to a mixture of DCM (50 mL), ammonia analogs (0.020 mol), and triethylamine (0.020 mol). The reaction solution was stirred at 0 °C for 0.5 h, and monitored by TLC. Finally, a gray slid was obtained by the same post-treatment method as that used for preparation of ethyl 4-chloropicolinate **8**.

3.1.6. Preparation of 4-(4-Aminophenoxy)picolinamide or 4-(2-Fluoro-4-aminophenoxy)picolinamide Analogues (**12a–12e**)

Intermediates **11a–11e** (0.016 mol), activated carbon (1.92 g, 0.160 mol), and $FeCl_3{\cdot}6H_2O$ (0.43 g, 0.016 mol) were dissolved in ethanol (30 mL) and stirred at 90 °C for 0.5 h. Then, 80% hydrazine hydrate (8.00 g, 0.128 mol) was added dropwise and stirred for 3.5 h. The reaction was monitored by TLC. After completion of the reaction, the solution was filtered, concentrated, and recrystallized to give a green solid.

3.1.7. Preparation of 5-Methyl-1-Phenyl-1H-1,2,3-Triazole-4-Carbonyl Chloride or 1-Phenyl-5-(trifluoromethyl)-1H-1,2,3-Triazole-4-Carbonyl Chloride Analogues (**13i–13e**)

The preparation of intermediates **13a–13i** was carried out according to our previous research [15].

3.1.8. Preparation of Target Compounds **B1–B27**

Intermediates **12a–12e** (0.002 mol) and sodium bicarbonate (4.20 g, 0.005 mol) were dissolved in DCM and stirred at 0 °C for 0.5 h. The solution of intermediates **13a–13i** (0.002 mol) and DCM were added dropwise to the above mixture, and stirred at 0 °C for 0.5 h. The reaction was monitored by TLC. After completion of the reaction, the solution was extracted with a mixture of DCM/NaOH (500 mL) three times and then the organic layers were combined, dried over sodium sulfate, evaporated, and purified by chromatographic column to possess a light yellow or white solid.

4-(4-(5-methyl-1-phenyl-1H-1,2,3-triazole-4-carboxamido)phenoxy)-N-propylpicolinamide (**B1**) Light yellow solid; Yield: 78.5%; m.p.: 116.8–117.1 °C; ^{1}H-NMR (400 MHz, DMSO-d_6, ppm) δ 10.75 (s, 1H), 8.82 (s, 1H), 8.52 (d, J = 5.5 Hz, 1H), 8.03 (s, 1H), 8.01 (s, 1H), 7.67 (s, 2H), 7.64 (d, J = 6.4 Hz, 2H), 7.43 (s, 1H), 7.23 (d, J = 8.4 Hz, 2H), 7.18 (d, J = 4.5 Hz, 1H), 3.22 (dd, J = 12.8, 6.3 Hz, 2H), 2.59 (s, 3H), 1.50 (dt, J = 14.1, 7.0 Hz, 2H), 0.84 (t, J = 7.2 Hz, 3H). TOF MS ES+ (m/z): $[M + H]^+$, calcd for $C_{25}H_{24}N_6O_3$: 457.1988, found, 457.1986.

4-(4-(1-(4-fluorophenyl)-5-methyl-1H-1,2,3-triazole-4-carboxamido)phenoxy)-N-propylpicolinamide (**B2**) Light yellow solid; Yield: 59.3%; m.p.: 110.4–110.8 °C; ^{1}H-NMR (400 MHz, DMSO-d_6, ppm) δ 10.64 (s, 1H), 8.71 (s, 1H), 8.40 (d, J = 5.6 Hz, 1H), 7.91 (s, 1H), 7.89 (s, 1H), 7.65 (d, J = 4.8 Hz, 1H), 7.63 (d, J = 4.6 Hz, 1H), 7.39 (t, J = 8.7 Hz, 2H), 7.31 (d, J = 2.1 Hz, 1H), 7.11 (d, J = 8.8 Hz, 2H), 7.06 (d, J = 3.1 Hz, 1H), 3.10 (dd, J = 13.3, 6.6 Hz, 2H), 2.46 (s, 3H), 1.38 (dt, J = 14.2, 7.1 Hz, 2H), 0.72 (t, J = 7.3 Hz, 3H). TOF MS ES+ (m/z): $[M + H]^+$, calcd for $C_{25}H_{23}FN_6O_3$: 475.1894, found, 475.1896.

4-(4-(5-methyl-1-(2-(trifluoromethoxy)phenyl)-1H-1,2,3-triazole-4-carboxamido)phenoxy)-N-propylpicolinamide (**B3**) White solid; Yield: 78.2%; m.p.: 97.7–98.0 °C; ^{1}H-NMR (400 MHz, DMSO-d_6, ppm) δ 10.81 (s, 1H), 8.81 (s, 1H), 8.52 (d, J = 5.3 Hz, 1H), 8.03 (s, 1H), 8.01 (s, 1H), 7.88 (d, J = 7.7 Hz, 1H), 7.84 (d, J = 7.6 Hz, 1H), 7.78 (d, J = 7.7 Hz, 1H), 7.72 (t, J = 7.2 Hz, 1H), 7.42 (s, 1H), 7.23 (d, J = 8.6 Hz, 2H), 7.18 (d, J = 0.8 Hz, 1H), 3.22 (d, J = 6.2 Hz, 2H), 2.46 (s, 3H), 1.51 (dd, J = 14.0, 7.0 Hz, 2H), 0.84 (t, J = 7.2 Hz, 3H). TOF MS ES+ (m/z): $[M + H]^+$, calcd for $C_{26}H_{23}F_3N_6O_4$: 541.1811, found, 541.1813.

4-(4-(1-(4-chlorophenyl)-5-(trifluoromethyl)-1H-1,2,3-triazole-4-carboxamido)phenoxy)-N-propylpicolinamide (**B4**) White solid; Yield: 66.4%; m.p.: 159.0–159.2 °C; ^{1}H-NMR (400 MHz, DMSO-d_6, ppm) δ 11.19 (s, 1H), 8.80 (s, 1H), 8.52 (d, J = 5.5 Hz, 1H), 7.99 (s, 1H), 7.97 (d, J = 1.2 Hz, 1H), 7.79 (d, J = 4.4 Hz, 3H), 7.75 (d, J = 8.7 Hz, 1H), 7.42 (s, 1H), 7.27 (d, J = 8.7 Hz, 2H), 7.19 (d, J = 5.5 Hz, 1H), 3.23 (dd, J = 13.2, 6.7 Hz, 2H), 1.57–1.47 (m, 2H), 0.84 (t, J = 7.4 Hz, 3H). ^{13}C-NMR (100 MHz, DMSO-d_6, ppm) δ 165.73, 163.13, 156.58, 152.54, 150.36(2,C), 149.46, 142.31, 136.19, 135.84, 134.09, 129.70(2,C), 128.22(2,C), 122.40(2,C), 121.33(2,C), 114.18(2,C), 108.95, 40.58, 22.34, 11.27. TOF MS ES+ (m/z): $[M + H]^+$, calcd for $C_{25}H_{20}ClF_3N_6O_3$: 545.1316, found, 545.1317.

N-propyl-4-(4-(5-(trifluoromethyl)-1-(2-(trifluoromethyl)phenyl)-1H-1,2,3-triazole-4-carboxamido)phenoxy) picolinamide (**B5**) White yellow solid; Yield: 69.4%; m.p.: 163.4–163.7 °C; ^{1}H-NMR (400 MHz, DMSO-d_6, ppm) δ 11.26 (s, 1H), 8.80 (s, 1H), 8.53 (d, J = 5.2 Hz, 1H), 8.15–8.09 (m, 2H), 8.05 (d, J = 7.2 Hz, 1H), 8.00 (d, J = 7.7 Hz, 3H), 7.43 (s, 1H), 7.27 (d, J = 8.5 Hz, 2H), 7.18 (d, J = 2.7 Hz, 1H), 3.23 (dd, J = 12.4, 6.0 Hz, 2H), 1.57–1.47 (m, 2H), 0.84 (t, J = 7.3 Hz, 3H). ^{13}C-NMR (100 MHz, DMSO-d_6, ppm) δ 165.72, 163.14, 156.20, 152.53, 150.36(2,C), 149.53, 141.89, 135.72, 134.28(2,C), 132.86, 132.02, 130.02(2,C), 127.71, 122.60(2,C), 121.29(2,C), 114.17(2,C), 108.96, 40.57, 22.33, 11.24. TOF MS ES+ (m/z): $[M + H]^+$, calcd for $C_{26}H_{20}F_6N_6O_3$: 579.1580, found, 579.1573.

4-(4-(1-(3,4-difluorophenyl)-5-(trifluoromethyl)-1H-1,2,3-triazole-4-carboxamido)phenoxy)-N-propylpicolinamide (**B6**) Light yellow solid; Yield: 85.0%; m.p.: 97.6–97.8 °C; ^{1}H-NMR (400 MHz, DMSO-d_6, ppm) δ 11.21 (s, 1H), 8.80 (s, 1H), 8.52 (d, J = 4.9 Hz, 1H), 8.12 (s, 1H), 7.98 (d, J = 6.9 Hz, 2H), 7.81 (d, J = 8.9 Hz, 1H), 7.74 (s, 1H), 7.41 (s, 1H), 7.27 (d, J = 6.9 Hz, 2H), 7.20 (d, J = 2.3 Hz, 1H), 3.26–3.19 (m, 2H), 1.52 (dd, J = 13.7, 6.8 Hz, 2H), 0.84 (t, J = 7.1 Hz, 3H). ^{13}C-NMR (100 MHz, DMSO-d_6, ppm) δ 165.73, 163.13, 156.48, 152.54, 150.36(2,C), 149.48, 142.09, 135.81, 131.59, 124.44, 122.46(2,C), 121.32(2,C), 118.63, 118.44, 117.06, 116.86, 114.19(2,C), 108.93, 40.58, 22.34, 11.26. TOF MS ES+ (m/z): $[M + H]^+$, calcd for $C_{25}H_{19}F_5N_6O_3$: 547.1517, found, 547.1517.

4-(4-(1-(3-chloro-4-fluorophenyl)-5-(trifluoromethyl)-1H-1,2,3-triazole-4-carboxamido)phenoxy)-N-propylpicolinamide (**B7**) White solid; Yield: 81.6%; m.p.: 153.6–153.9 °C; ^{1}H-NMR (400 MHz, DMSO-d_6, ppm) δ 11.23 (s,

1H), 8.80 (t, J = 5.9 Hz, 1H), 8.52 (d, J = 5.6 Hz, 1H), 7.99 (s, 1H), 7.97 (s, 1H), 7.79 (d, J = 4.0 Hz, 3H), 7.42 (s, 1H), 7.27 (d, J = 8.6 Hz, 2H), 7.18 (d, J = 3.8 Hz, 1H), 3.23 (dd, J = 13.3, 6.5 Hz, 2H), 1.57–1.47 (m, 2H), 0.84 (t, J = 7.3 Hz, 3H). ^{13}C-NMR (100 MHz, DMSO-d_6, ppm) δ 165.73, 163.15, 156.61, 152.52, 150.33(2,C), 149.45, 142.38, 136.20, 135.87, 134.06, 129.69(2,C), 128.18(2,C), 122.39(2,C), 121.29(2,C), 114.13(2,C), 108.99, 40.58, 22.34, 11.25. TOF MS ES+ (*m/z*): [M + H]$^+$, calcd for $C_{25}H_{19}ClF_4N_6O_3$: 563.1222, found, 563.1216.

4-(4-(1-(2-chloro-5-(trifluoromethyl)phenyl)-5-(trifluoromethyl)-1H-1,2,3-triazole-4-carboxamido)phenoxy)-N-propylpicolinamide (**B8**) White solid; Yield: 56.7%; m.p.: 143.3–143.7 °C; ^{1}H-NMR (400 MHz, DMSO-d_6, ppm) δ 11.30 (s, 1H), 8.81 (s, 1H), 8.65 (s, 1H), 8.53 (d, J = 4.9 Hz, 1H), 8.21 (d, J = 8.0 Hz, 1H), 8.15 (d, J = 7.9 Hz, 1H), 8.00 (d, J = 8.4 Hz, 2H), 7.42 (s, 1H), 7.27 (d, J = 8.5 Hz, 2H), 7.19 (d, J = 2.1 Hz, 1H), 3.22 (dd, J = 12.2, 6.0 Hz, 2H), 1.52 (dq, J = 13.9, 7.1 Hz, 2H), 0.84 (t, J = 7.1 Hz, 3H). ^{13}C-NMR (100 MHz, DMSO-d_6, ppm) δ 165.72, 163.14, 156.13, 152.54, 150.37(2,C), 149.56, 141.97, 135.71, 135.05, 133.58, 131.78(2,C), 131.49, 130.44, 127.03, 122.63(2,C), 121.28(2,C), 114.18(2,C), 108.96, 40.58, 22.33, 11.25. TOF MS ES+ (*m/z*): [M + H]$^+$, calcd for $C_{26}H_{19}ClF_6N_6O_3$: 613.1190, found, 613.1189.

4-(4-(1-(4-chloro-3-(trifluoromethyl)phenyl)-5-(trifluoromethyl)-1H-1,2,3-triazole-4-carboxamido)phenoxy)-N-propylpicolinamide (**B9**) Light yellow solid; Yield: 66.3%; m.p.: 155.5–155.8 °C; ^{1}H-NMR (400 MHz, DMSO-d_6, ppm) δ 11.21 (s, 1H), 8.81 (s, 1H), 8.53 (d, J = 5.3 Hz, 1H), 8.44 (s, 1H), 8.17 (d, J = 8.1 Hz, 1H), 8.10 (d, J = 8.4 Hz, 1H), 7.99 (d, J = 8.7 Hz, 2H), 7.41 (s, 1H), 7.27 (d, J = 8.6 Hz, 2H), 7.19 (d, J = 2.9 Hz, 1H), 3.22 (dd, J = 12.8, 6.2 Hz, 2H), 1.52 (dq, J = 14.8, 7.4 Hz, 2H), 0.84 (t, J = 7.3 Hz, 3H). TOF MS ES+ (*m/z*): [M + H]$^+$, calcd for $C_{26}H_{19}ClF_6N_6O_3$: 613.1190, found, 613.1188.

4-(2-fluoro-4-(5-methyl-1-phenyl-1H-1,2,3-triazole-4-carboxamido)phenoxy)-N-propylpicolinamide (**B10**) White solid; Yield: 76.8%; m.p.: 143.3–143.7 °C; ^{1}H-NMR (400 MHz, DMSO-d_6, ppm) δ 10.96 (s, 1H), 8.83 (s, 1H), 8.54 (d, J = 5.4 Hz, 1H), 8.11 (d, J = 13.2 Hz, 1H), 7.86 (d, J = 8.7 Hz, 1H), 7.67 (d, J = 2.6 Hz, 5H), 7.48–7.39 (m, 2H), 7.23 (d, J = 4.7 Hz, 1H), 3.23 (dd, J = 12.9, 6.3 Hz, 2H), 2.59 (s, 3H), 1.57–1.47 (m, 2H), 0.84 (t, J = 7.3 Hz, 3H). ^{13}C-NMR (100 MHz, DMSO-d_6, ppm) δ 165.66, 163.43, 160.15, 153.09, 150.87(2,C), 138.46, 138.29, 135.61, 130.48, 130.09(3,C), 125.84(3,C), 124.07, 117.64, 113.82, 109.37, 108.46, 41.02, 22.73, 11.67, 9.86. TOF MS ES+ (*m/z*): [M + H]$^+$, calcd for $C_{25}H_{23}FN_6O_3$: 475.1894, found, 475.1894.

4-(2-fluoro-4-(1-(4-fluorophenyl)-5-methyl-1H-1,2,3-triazole-4-carboxamido)phenoxy)-N-propylpicolinamide (**B11**) White solid; Yield: 65.1%; m.p.: 143.5–143.8 °C; ^{1}H-NMR (400 MHz, DMSO-d_6, ppm) δ 10.95 (s, 1H), 8.82 (s, 1H), 8.54 (d, J = 5.1 Hz, 1H), 8.10 (d, J = 12.7 Hz, 1H), 7.86 (d, J = 8.6 Hz, 1H), 7.76 (s, 2H), 7.51 (t, J = 8.4 Hz, 2H), 7.44 (d, J = 12.9 Hz, 2H), 7.22 (d, J = 2.5 Hz, 1H), 3.22 (d, J = 6.0 Hz, 2H), 2.58 (s, 3H), 1.51 (dd, J = 13.9, 6.9 Hz, 2H), 0.84 (t, J = 7.2 Hz, 3H). ^{13}C-NMR (100 MHz, DMSO-d_6, ppm) δ 165.65, 164.20, 163.42, 161.74, 160.11, 153.08, 150.88, 138.75, 138.22, 131.99, 128.44, 128.35, 124.08, 117.65, 117.18(2,C), 116.95, 113.83, 109.60, 109.38, 108.44, 41.01, 22.73, 11.67, 9.78. TOF MS ES+ (*m/z*): [M + H]$^+$, calcd for $C_{25}H_{22}F_2N_6O_3$: 493.1800, found, 493.1797.

4-(2-fluoro-4-(5-methyl-1-(2-(trifluoromethoxy)phenyl)-1H-1,2,3-triazole-4-carboxamido)phenoxy)-N-propylpicolinamide (**B12**) Light yellow solid; Yield: 63.2%; m.p.: 132.6–132.9 °C; ^{1}H-NMR (400 MHz, DMSO-d_6, ppm) δ 10.99 (s, 1H), 8.82 (s, 1H), 8.55 (d, J = 5.6 Hz, 1H), 8.10 (d, J = 13.2 Hz, 1H), 7.88 (d, J = 7.5 Hz, 1H), 7.85 (d, J = 8.0 Hz, 2H), 7.79 (d, J = 8.4 Hz, 1H), 7.73 (t, J = 7.5 Hz, 1H), 7.46 (d, J = 9.0 Hz, 1H), 7.41 (d, J = 2.5 Hz, 1H), 7.23 (dd, J = 5.5, 2.6 Hz, 1H), 3.26–3.20 (m, 2H), 2.46 (s, 3H), 1.58–1.47 (m, 2H), 0.85 (t, J = 7.4 Hz, 3H). TOF MS ES+ (*m/z*): [M + H]$^+$, calcd for $C_{26}H_{22}F_4N_6O_4$: 559.1717, found, 559.1717.

4-(4-(1-(4-chlorophenyl)-5-(trifluoromethyl)-1H-1,2,3-triazole-4-carboxamido)-2-fluorophenoxy)-N-propylpicolinamide (**B13**) Light yellow solid; Yield: 76.3%; m.p.: 176.5–176.8 °C; ^{1}H-NMR (400 MHz, DMSO-d_6, ppm) δ 11.37 (s, 1H), 8.81 (s, 1H), 8.55 (d, J = 5.3 Hz, 1H), 8.06 (d, J = 12.8 Hz, 1H), 7.79 (d, J = 7.4 Hz, 5H), 7.48 (d, J = 8.9 Hz, 1H), 7.44 (s, 1H), 7.27–7.20 (m, 1H), 3.23 (d, J = 6.1 Hz, 2H), 1.52 (dd, J = 14.1, 7.1 Hz, 2H), 0.84 (t, J = 7.3 Hz, 3H). TOF MS ES+ (*m/z*): [M + H]$^+$, calcd for $C_{25}H_{19}ClF_4N_6O_3$: 563.1222, found, 563.1216.

4-(2-fluoro-4-(5-(trifluoromethyl)-1-(2-(trifluoromethyl)phenyl)-1H-1,2,3-triazole-4-carboxamido)phenoxy)-N-propylpicolinamide (**B14**) Light yellow solid; Yield: 79.6%; m.p.: 172.8–173.1 °C; ^{1}H-NMR (400 MHz, DMSO-d_6, ppm) δ 11.43 (s, 1H), 8.82 (s, 1H), 8.55 (d, *J* = 5.3 Hz, 1H), 8.12 (s, 1H), 8.09 (d, *J* = 4.7 Hz, 1H), 8.05 (s, 1H), 8.00 (d, *J* = 9.1 Hz, 2H), 7.84 (d, *J* = 8.3 Hz, 1H), 7.49 (d, *J* = 8.9 Hz, 1H), 7.44 (s, 1H), 7.24 (d, *J* = 2.5 Hz, 1H), 3.23 (d, *J* = 5.6 Hz, 2H), 1.55–1.49 (m, 2H), 0.84 (t, *J* = 7.2 Hz, 3H). ^{13}C-NMR (100 MHz, DMSO-d_6, ppm) δ 165.15, 163.01, 156.39, 152.70, 150.48(2,C), 141.52, 134.25(2,C), 134.18, 132.86, 132.00, 129.99(2,C), 127.65, 123.86(2,C), 117.59, 113.43(2,C), 109.61, 109.39, 108.12, 40.60, 22.31, 11.21. TOF MS ES+ (*m/z*): [M + H]$^+$, calcd for $C_{26}H_{22}F_4N_6O_3$: 543.1614, found, 543.1616.

4-(4-(1-(3,4-difluorophenyl)-5-(trifluoromethyl)-1H-1,2,3-triazole-4-carboxamido)-2-fluorophenoxy)-N-propylpicolinamide (**B15**) White solid; Yield: 55.4%; m.p.: 134.4–134.8 °C; ^{1}H-NMR (400 MHz, DMSO-d_6, ppm) δ 11.40 (s, 1H), 8.83 (s, 1H), 8.55 (d, *J* = 5.4 Hz, 1H), 8.13 (d, *J* = 9.0 Hz, 1H), 8.06 (d, *J* = 13.0 Hz, 1H), 7.82 (d, *J* = 7.0 Hz, 2H), 7.74 (s, 1H), 7.48 (t, *J* = 8.8 Hz, 1H), 7.42 (s, 1H), 7.25 (d, *J* = 2.0 Hz, 1H), 3.22 (d, *J* = 6.2 Hz, 2H), 1.52 (d, *J* = 7.1 Hz, 2H), 0.84 (t, *J* = 7.1 Hz, 3H). TOF MS ES+ (*m/z*): [M + H]$^+$, calcd for $C_{26}H_{19}F_7N_6O_3$: 597.1485, found, 597.1486.

4-(4-(1-(3-chloro-4-fluorophenyl)-5-(trifluoromethyl)-1H-1,2,3-triazole-4-carboxamido)-2-fluorophenoxy)-N-propylpicolinamide (**B16**) White solid; Yield: 59.7%; m.p.: 163.3–163.5 °C; ^{1}H-NMR (400 MHz, DMSO-d_6, ppm) δ 11.39 (s, 1H), 8.82 (t, *J* = 5.8 Hz, 1H), 8.56 (d, *J* = 5.6 Hz, 1H), 8.23 (d, *J* = 4.8 Hz, 1H), 8.06 (d, *J* = 12.9 Hz, 1H), 7.88 (d, *J* = 8.5 Hz, 1H), 7.83 (d, *J* = 8.8 Hz, 1H), 7.77 (t, *J* = 8.9 Hz, 1H), 7.48 (t, *J* = 9.0 Hz, 1H), 7.42 (s, 1H), 7.25 (d, *J* = 5.4 Hz, 1H), 3.23 (dd, *J* = 13.3, 6.5 Hz, 2H), 1.53 (dt, *J* = 14.5, 7.4 Hz, 2H), 0.85 (t, *J* = 7.4 Hz, 3H). TOF MS ES+ (*m/z*): [M + H]$^+$, calcd for $C_{25}H_{18}ClF_5N_6O_3$: 581.1127, found, 581.1128.

4-(4-(1-(2-chloro-5-(trifluoromethyl)phenyl)-5-(trifluoromethyl)-1H-1,2,3-triazole-4-carboxamido)-2-fluorophenoxy)-N-propylpicolinamide (**B17**) White solid; Yield: 64.5%; m.p.: 154.1–154.4 °C; ^{1}H-NMR (400 MHz, DMSO-d$_6$, ppm) δ 11.48 (s, 1H), 8.83 (s, 1H), 8.65 (s, 1H), 8.55 (d, *J* = 5.0 Hz, 1H), 8.21 (d, *J* = 7.8 Hz, 1H), 8.15 (d, *J* = 8.2 Hz, 1H), 8.07 (d, *J* = 12.9 Hz, 1H), 7.84 (d, *J* = 8.6 Hz, 1H), 7.49 (t, *J* = 8.8 Hz, 1H), 7.43 (s, 1H), 7.25 (d, *J* = 1.4 Hz, 1H), 3.23 (d, *J* = 6.0 Hz, 2H), 1.52 (dd, *J* = 13.9, 6.9 Hz, 2H), 0.84 (t, *J* = 7.3 Hz, 3H). TOF MS ES+ (m/z): [M + H]$^+$, calcd for $C_{26}H_{18}ClF_7N_6O_3$: 631.1089, found, 631.1089.

4-(4-(1-(4-chloro-3-(trifluoromethyl)phenyl)-5-(trifluoromethyl)-1H-1,2,3-triazole-4-carboxamido)-2-fluorophenoxy)-N-propylpicolinamide (**B18**) White solid; Yield: 55.9%; m.p.: 153.4–153.7 °C; ^{1}H-NMR (400 MHz, DMSO-d$_6$, ppm) δ 11.41 (s, 1H), 8.83 (s, 1H), 8.56 (d, *J* = 5.3 Hz, 1H), 8.45 (s, 1H), 8.18 (d, *J* = 8.4 Hz, 1H), 8.12–8.01 (m, 2H), 7.84 (d, *J* = 8.4 Hz, 1H), 7.48 (t, *J* = 8.9 Hz, 1H), 7.42 (s, 1H), 7.25 (s, 1H), 3.26–3.19 (m, 2H), 1.52 (dq, *J* = 14.4, 7.0 Hz, 2H), 0.84 (t, *J* = 7.2 Hz, 3H). TOF MS ES+ (m/z): [M + H]$^+$, calcd for $C_{26}H_{18}ClF_7N_6O_3$: 631.1089, found, 631.1096.

N-(3-fluoro-4-((2-(pyrrolidine-1-carbonyl)pyridin-4-yl)oxy)phenyl)-5-methyl-1-phenyl-1H-1,2,3-triazole-4-carboxamide (**B19**) Light yellow solid; Yield: 63.2%; m.p.: 169.7–170.0 °C; ^{1}H-NMR (400 MHz, DMSO-d_6, ppm) δ 10.94 (s, 1H), 8.50 (d, *J* = 4.4 Hz, 1H), 8.09 (d, *J* = 12.9 Hz, 1H), 7.84 (d, *J* = 8.4 Hz, 1H), 7.65 (d, *J* = 14.4 Hz, 5H), 7.42 (t, *J* = 8.6 Hz, 1H), 7.13 (d, *J* = 14.2 Hz, 2H), 3.59 (s, 2H), 3.45 (s, 2H), 2.59 (s, 3H), 1.82 (s, 4H). TOF MS ES+ (*m/z*): [M + H]$^+$, calcd for $C_{26}H_{23}FN_6O_3$: 487.1897, found, 487.1902.

N-(3-fluoro-4-((2-(pyrrolidine-1-carbonyl)pyridin-4-yl)oxy)phenyl)-1-(4-fluorophenyl)-5-methyl-1H-1,2,3-triazole-4-carboxamide (**B20**) Light yellow solid; Yield: 66.4%; m.p.: 164.3–164.7 °C; ^{1}H-NMR (400 MHz, DMSO-d_6, ppm) δ 10.94 (s, 1H), 8.51 (d, *J* = 5.3 Hz, 1H), 8.09 (d, *J* = 13.2 Hz, 1H), 7.84 (d, *J* = 8.4 Hz, 1H), 7.75 (d, *J* = 3.2 Hz, 2H), 7.51 (t, *J* = 8.4 Hz, 2H), 7.42 (t, *J* = 8.9 Hz, 1H), 7.18 (s, 1H), 7.12 (d, *J* = 4.6 Hz, 1H), 3.59 (s, 2H), 3.45 (s, 2H), 2.57 (s, 3H), 1.81 (s, 4H). TOF MS ES+ (*m/z*): [M + H]$^+$, calcd for $C_{26}H_{22}F_2N_6O_3$: 505.1800, found, 505.1807.

N-(3-fluoro-4-((2-(pyrrolidine-1-carbonyl)pyridin-4-yl)oxy) phenyl)-5-methyl-1-(2-(trifluoromethoxy)phenyl)-1H-1,2,3-triazole-4-carboxamide (**B21**) White solid; Yield: 66.5%; m.p.: 176.3–176.6 °C; ^{1}H-NMR (400 MHz,

DMSO-d_6, ppm) δ 11.00 (s, 1H), 8.51 (d, J = 4.9 Hz, 1H), 8.09 (d, J = 12.8 Hz, 1H), 7.89 (d, J = 7.3 Hz, 1H), 7.85 (d, J = 8.0 Hz, 2H), 7.79 (d, J = 8.2 Hz, 1H), 7.75–7.70 (m, 1H), 7.43 (t, J = 8.6 Hz, 1H), 7.16 (s, 1H), 7.11 (d, J = 1.9 Hz, 1H), 3.60 (s, 2H), 3.46 (s, 2H), 2.46 (s, 3H), 1.82 (s, 4H). TOF MS ES+ (m/z): $[M + H]^+$, calcd for $C_{27}H_{22}F_4N_6O_4$: 571.1717, found, 571.1722.

4-(2-fluoro-4-(5-methyl-1-phenyl-1H-1,2,3-triazole-4-carboxamido)phenoxy)-N-(2-(thiophen-2-yl)ethyl)picolinamide (**B22**) Light yellow solid; Yield: 61.9%; m.p.: 124.6–125.0 °C; ^{1}H NMR (400 MHz, DMSO-d_6, ppm) δ 10.97 (s, 1H), 8.98 (t, J = 5.9 Hz, 1H), 8.55 (d, J = 5.6 Hz, 1H), 8.11 (d, J = 13.2 Hz, 1H), 7.86 (d, J = 8.8 Hz, 1H), 7.67 (d, J = 2.3 Hz, 5H), 7.48–7.41 (m, 2H), 7.32 (d, J = 4.9 Hz, 1H), 7.24 (d, J = 3.0 Hz, 1H), 6.96-6.91 (m, 1H), 6.89 (d, J = 2.6 Hz, 1H), 3.54 (dd, J = 13.4, 6.8 Hz, 2H), 3.06 (t, J = 7.1 Hz, 2H), 2.59 (s, 3H). TOF MS ES+ (*m/z*): $[M + H]^+$, calcd for $C_{28}H_{23}FN_6O_3S$: 543.1614, found, 543.1616.

4-(2-fluoro-4-(1-(4-fluorophenyl)-5-methyl-1H-1,2,3-triazole-4-carboxamido)phenoxy)-N-(2-(thiophen-2-yl) ethyl)picolinamide (**B23**) White solid; Yield: 51.7%; m.p.: 110.4–110.8 °C; ^{1}H-NMR (400 MHz, DMSO-d_6, ppm) δ 10.99 (s, 1H), 9.00 (t, J = 5.7 Hz, 1H), 8.57 (d, J = 5.6 Hz, 1H), 8.13 (d, J = 13.2 Hz, 1H), 7.88 (d, J = 8.8 Hz, 1H), 7.79 (d, J = 4.8 Hz, 1H), 7.77 (d, J = 4.8 Hz, 1H), 7.54 (t, J = 8.7 Hz, 2H), 7.47 (d, J = 9.1 Hz, 1H), 7.43 (d, J = 2.1 Hz, 1H), 7.34 (d, J = 4.6 Hz, 1H), 7.26 (d, J = 2.4 Hz, 1H), 6.98–6.94 (m, 1H), 6.91 (s, 1H), 3.55 (dd, J = 13.3, 6.8 Hz, 2H), 3.08 (t, J = 7.1 Hz, 2H), 2.60 (s, 3H). TOF MS ES+ (*m/z*): $[M + H]^+$, calcd for $C_{28}H_{22}F_2N_6O_3S$: 561.1520, found, 561.1529.

4-(2-fluoro-4-(5-methyl-1-(2-(trifluoromethoxy)phenyl)-1H-1,2,3-triazole-4-carboxamido)phenoxy)-N-(2-(thiophen-2-yl)ethyl)picolinamide (**B24**) White solid; Yield: 56.6%; m.p.: 103.4–103.7 °C; ^{1}H-NMR (400 MHz, DMSO-d_6, ppm) δ 10.98 (s, 1H), 8.94 (s, 1H), 8.55 (d, J = 5.3 Hz, 1H), 8.10 (d, J = 13.2 Hz, 1H), 7.88 (d, J = 6.4 Hz, 2H), 7.84 (d, J = 7.0 Hz, 1H), 7.78 (d, J = 8.1 Hz, 1H), 7.72 (t, J = 7.4 Hz, 1H), 7.44 (t, J = 8.8 Hz, 2H), 7.31 (d, J = 4.1 Hz, 1H), 7.23 (d, J = 2.3 Hz, 1H), 6.96–6.92 (m, 1H), 6.90 (s, 1H), 3.55 (d, J = 6.2 Hz, 2H), 3.07 (t, J = 6.9 Hz, 2H), 2.47 (s, 3H). TOF MS ES+ (m/z): $[M + H]^+$, calcd for $C_{29}H_{22}F_4N_6O_4S$: 627.1437, found, 627.1439.

4-(2-fluoro-4-(5-methyl-1-phenyl-1H-1,2,3-triazole-4-carboxamido)phenoxy)-N-(3-morpholinopropyl)picolinamide (**B25**) White solid; Yield: 42.6%; m.p.: 108.3–108.6 °C; ^{1}H-NMR (400 MHz, DMSO-d_6, ppm) δ 10.67 (s, 1H), 9.05 (s, 1H), 8.53 (s, 1H), 8.03 (d, J = 7.5 Hz, 2H), 7.67 (s, 5H), 7.45 (s, 1H), 7.23 (d, J = 7.6 Hz, 1H), 7.17 (s, 1H), 3.64 (s, 4H), 3.36 (s, 2H), 2.60 (s, 3H), 2.44 (s, 6H), 1.72 (s, 2H). ^{13}C-NMR (100 MHz, DMSO-d_6, ppm) δ 166.25, 163.53, 159.92, 152.85, 150.72, 149.29, 138.56, 138.11, 136.82, 135.67, 130.44, 130.10(2,C), 125.83(2,C), 122.70(2,C), 121.51(2,C), 114.53, 109.30, 66.25(2,C), 56.81, 53.53(2,C), 38.36, 25.59, 9.85. TOF MS ES+ (*m/z*): $[M + H]^+$, calcd for $C_{29}H_{30}FN_7O_4$: 560.2421, found, 560.2416.

4-(2-fluoro-4-(1-(4-fluorophenyl)-5-methyl-1H-1,2,3-triazole-4-carboxamido)phenoxy)-N-(3-morpholinopropyl) picolinamide (**B26**) White solid; Yield: 39.3%; m.p.: 108.5–108.9 °C; ^{1}H-NMR (400 MHz, DMSO-d_6, ppm) δ 10.73 (s, 1H), 9.10 (s, 1H), 8.52 (d, J = 3.7 Hz, 1H), 8.03 (d, J = 7.9 Hz, 2H), 7.76 (s, 2H), 7.52 (d, J = 6.9 Hz, 2H), 7.43 (s, 1H), 7.23 (d, J = 7.9 Hz, 2H), 3.61 (s, 4H), 3.35 (s, 2H), 2.59 (s, 3H), 2.34 (s, 6H), 1.68 (s, 2H). ^{13}C-NMR (100 MHz, DMSO-d_6, ppm) δ 166.25, 163.48, 159.87, 152.90, 150.69, 149.33, 138.38, 136.78, 132.06, 128.39, 128.30, 122.71(2,C), 121.46(2,C), 117.16(2,C), 116.93(2,C), 114.50, 109.32, 66.54(2,C), 57.08, 53.77(2,C), 38.55, 25.80, 9.74. TOF MS ES+ (*m/z*): $[M + H]^+$, calcd for $C_{29}H_{29}F_2N_7O_4$: 578.2327, found, 578.2347.

4-(2-fluoro-4-(5-methyl-1-(2-(trifluoromethoxy)phenyl)-1H-1,2,3-triazole-4-carboxamido)phenoxy)-N-(3-morpholinopropyl)picolinamide (**B27**) White solid; Yield: 41.0%; m.p.: 97.6–97.9 °C; ^{1}H-NMR (400 MHz, DMSO-d_6, ppm) δ 10.78 (s, 1H), 9.05 (s, 1H), 8.54 (s, 1H), 7.99 (d, J = 5.2 Hz, 2H), 7.86 (d, J = 3.8 Hz, 2H), 7.79 (s, 1H), 7.73 (s, 1H), 7.41 (s, 1H), 7.23 (d, J = 6.1 Hz, 2H), 3.91 (d, J = 8.3 Hz, 2H), 3.85 (d, J = 11.1 Hz, 2H), 3.36 (d, J = 5.0 Hz, 2H), 3.06 (s, 4H), 2.45 (s, 2H), 1.98 (s, 2H). TOF MS ES+ (m/z): $[M + H]^+$, calcd for $C_{30}H_{29}F_4N_7O_5$: 643.1059, found, 643.1094.

^{1}H-NMR spectra of representative target compounds (**B1**, **B6**, **B12**, **B13**, **B20**, **B25**, and **B26**), ^{13}C-NMR spectra of representative target compounds (**B6**, **B7**, **B10**, **B11**, **B14**, **B25**, and **B26**), and TOF-MS spectra of representative target compounds (**B13**, **B17**, **B19**, **B21**, **B22**, **B25**, and **B26**) can be seen in the Supplementary Materials.

3.2. Antitumority Assay

The antitumor activities of target compounds were determined by the MTT method using Golvatinib as a positive control. All cancer cell lines (A549, HeLa, and MCF-7) were cultured with Dulbecco Modified Eagle Medium (DMEM) or Roswell Park Memorial Institute (1640) containing 10% fetal bovine serum and 0.1% penicillin–streptomycin, under ambient conditions of 5% CO_2 and 37 °C. Cells were digested with an appropriate amount of Trypsin–EDTA solution to obtain the cell suspension, which was diluted with medium and inoculated into 96-well plates at $5*10^4$ cells per well. After cells were incubated for 24 h, the target compounds diluted by medium to suitable concentrations were added into 96-well plates, and the cells were cultured continue for 72 h. Next, the medium was removed, and then thiazolyl blue tetrazolium bromide (MTT) was added to each well to treat cells for 3.5 h. Ultimately, dimethyl sulfoxide (DMSO) was added to each well after removal of MTT and the absorbance values were measured with the ELISA (enzyme-linked immunosorbent assay) reader. All antitumor activities were tested for three times. The IC_{50} values were the average of three measurements and were calculated using the Bacus Laboratories Incorporated Slide Scanner (Bliss) software.

3.3. Dose-Dependent Test

The dose-dependent effect of compound **B26** on A549 cells was tested by the MTT method using Golvatinib as a positive control. The experimental procedure was identical to that of the cytotoxic activity, wherein the concentration of the test compound was configured to be seven and the cytotoxic activity was five. Seven different concentrations of compound **B26** treated on A549 cells to obtain the corresponding inhibition rates. Experimental data was obtained by Orange (2018 64 bit) software based on the inhibition rate.

3.4. Cell Morphology Studies

Cell morphology studies aimed to explore the morphological changes of A549 cells with and without treatment with compound **B26**, and the cell morphology was visualized by acridine orange (AO) staining. The culture environment of A549 cells was consistent with that in the antitumor activity experiments. Cells were digested with Trypsin–EDTA solution to get the cell suspension, which was diluted with 1640 medium and inoculated into a 24-well plate at $2*10^4$ cells per well. After incubating for 12 h, compound **B26** diluted to suitable concentrations by 1640 medium was added into a 24-well plate, and cell culture was continued for 12 h. Then, the 1640 medium in the well plate was removed and every well were washed three times with phosphate buffer saline (PBS). After washing with PBS three times, A549 cells were treated with AO for 15 min. A549 cells were washed three times with PBS again, and the cell morphology distribution was observed directly by a fluorescence microscope. Ultimately, the picture is exported via computer.

3.5. Cell Cycle Study

A549 cells were seeded into six-well plates at $1*10^5$ cells per well and incubated for 24 h. Then, the medium containing DMEM (control, without compound) or compound **B26** with different concentrations was added to the culture plate, and A549 cells were further cultured for 24 h. Then, A549 cells were collected into a centrifuge tube and fixed with a small amount of ice-cold 70% ethanol at 4 °C for 6–12 h. Cells washed three times with PBS were incubated with Rnase (1 mg/mL, diluted with PBS) for 30 min at room temperature. Finally, propidium iodide (PI) was added to staining without light for 30 min at room temperature, and the DNA content was measured by flow cytometry within 1 h. Experimental data was obtained by Modify software.

3.6. c-Met Kinase Assay

The kinase assay was implemented through Mobility shift assay. The Mixture the configured available Brij-35 (0.0015%) and 50 mM HEPES (pH = 7.5) to get a kinase buffer base. Then, compounds **B25**, **B26**, and **B27** were configured to five concentrations using dimethyl sulfoxide. The kinase buffer containing the compounds or dimethyl sulfoxide was added to 96-well plates and mixed on the shaker for fifteen minutes. Next, the solution was transferred in duplicate from a 96-well plate to a 384-well plate, and then an enzyme solution (c-Met kinase mixed with kinase buffer) was added to each well. After incubation of the 384-well plate for 10 min at room temperature, a 2.5*peptide solution (formed by the addition of FAM-labeled peptide and ATP to the kinase base buffer) was added to each well. After incubation at 28 °C for a certain period of time, a stop buffer was added to each well for stop the reaction. The inhibition value is obtained by converting the conversion data on the caliper. The formula is that percent inhibition = (max − conversion) / (max − min) * 100. Among them, "max" stands for DMSO control, "min" stands for low control. Finally, the IC_{50} values were obtained by fitting the inhibition rate data using the XLFit excel add-in version software.

3.7. Molecular Docking Study

All the molecular docking simulations were performed by the AutoDock 4.2 software. The crystal structure of c-Met (PDB code: 3LQ8) used in the docking was downloaded from http://www.rcsb.org/. The preparation process of the protein for docking mainly involves the addition of hydrogen atoms and charges, elimination of unrelated water molecules, immobilization of exact residues, and removal of endogenous ligands (Foretinib), etc. The preparation process of the molecules for docking mainly includes the addition of hydrogen atoms and charges. Then the prepared molecules (target compounds) were docked to the certified binding site of c-Met protein. Subsequently, the genetic algorithm was used for energy optimization. All the docking results were modified and processed by PyMOL 1.8.x software (https://pymol.org).

4. Conclusions

In conclusion, a series of 4-(pyridin-4-yloxy)benzamide derivatives bearing a triazole fragment were designed and synthesized. In addition, we evaluated them for antitumor activity against three cancer cell lines and c-Met kinase activity (only for compounds **B25–B27**) in vitro. The pharmacological results indicated that most compounds showed moderate antitumor activity against the three cancer cell lines. In particular, compound **B26** showed excellent inhibitory activity with IC_{50} values of 3.22, 4.33, and 5.82 μM against A549, HeLa, and MCF-7 cell lines, which were more potent than Golvatinib, respectively. The SARs study indicated that the introduction of a morpholino group in the hydrophilic region was more favorable than an alkane chain in terms of antitumor activity, and a single electron-withdrawing substituent (such as a fluorine atom) on the terminal phenyl ring improved the inhibitory activity of the target compounds. Further studies will be carried out in the near future.

Supplementary Materials: The Supplementary Materials are available online at http://www.mdpi.com/1420-3049/25/1/10/s1.

Author Contributions: P.Z., Q.T. and J.C. conceived and designed the experiments; H.X., J.Z., Q.Z., Z.X. and H.Z. performed the experiments and statistics analysis; J.C. and H.X. completed the molecular docking simulation and H.X. started the project and wrote the paper. All authors have read and agreed to the published version of the manuscript.

Funding: We gratefully acknowledge the generous support provided by Natural Science Foundation of National Natural Science Foundation of China (NSFC No. 81660572), Jiangxi Province (20171BAB215071, 20192ACBL21009) and Top-notch talent project of Jiangxi Science & Technology Normal University (2016QNBJRC002).

Conflicts of Interest: The authors declare no conflict of interest.

References

1. Miller, K.D.; Nogueira, L.; Mariotto, B.; Rowland, J.H.; Yabroff, K.R.; Alfano, C.M.; DVM, J.A.; Kramer, J.L.; Siegel, R.L. Cancer Treatment and Survivorship Statistics. *CA Cancer J. Clin.* **2016**, *66*, 271–289. [CrossRef] [PubMed]
2. Luo, T.; Zhang, S.G.; Zhu, L.F.; Zhang, F.X.; Li, W.; Zhao, K.; Wen, X.X.; Yu, M.; Zhan, Y.Q.; Chen, H.; et al. A Selective c-Met and Trks Inhibitor Indo5 Suppresses Hepatocellular Carcinoma Growth. *J. Exp. Clin. Canc. Res.* **2019**, *38*, 130–143. [CrossRef] [PubMed]
3. Moslehi, J.J.; Michael, D. Tyrosine Kinase Inhibitor–Associated Cardiovascular Toxicity in Chronic Myeloid Leukemia. *J. Clin. Oncol.* **2015**, *33*, 4210–4222. [CrossRef] [PubMed]
4. Bouattour, M.; Raymond, E.; Qin, S.; Cheng, A.L.; Stammberger, U.; Locatelli, G.; Faivre, S. Recent Developments of c-Met as a Therapeutic Target in Hepatocellular Carcinoma. *Hepatology* **2018**, *67*, 1132–1149. [CrossRef] [PubMed]
5. Kim, H.J.; Kang, S.K.; Kwon, W.S.; Kim, S.T.; Jeong, I.; Jeung, H.C.; Kragh, M.; Horak, I.D.; Chung, H.C.; Rha, S.Y. Forty-Nine Gastric Cancer Cell Lines with Integrative Genomic Profiling for Development of c-Met Inhibitor. *Nt. J. Cancer* **2018**, *143*, 151–159. [CrossRef] [PubMed]
6. Hong, D.S.; LoRusso, P.; Hamid, O.; Janku, F.; Kittaneh, M.; Catenacci, D.V.T.; Chan, E.; Bekaii-Saab, T.; Gadgeel, S.M.; Loberg, R.T.; et al. Phase I Study of AMG 337, a Highly Selective Small-Molecule Met Inhibitor, in Patients with Advanced Solid Tumors. *Clin. Cancer Res.* **2019**, *25*, 2403–2413. [CrossRef] [PubMed]
7. Liu, Y.; Jin, S.Y.; Peng, X.; Lu, D.; Zeng, L.M.; Sun, Y.M.; Ai, J.; Geng, M.Y.; Hu, Y.H. Pyridazinone Derivatives Displaying Highly Potent and Selective Inhibitory Activities Against c-Met Tyrosine Kinase. *Eur. J. Med. Chem.* **2016**, *108*, 322–333. [CrossRef] [PubMed]
8. Li, M.J.; Wu, G.Z.; Kaas, Q.; Jiang, T.; Yu, R.L. Development of Efficient Docking Strategies and Structure–Activity Relationship Study of the c-Met Type II Inhibitors. *J. Mol. Graph Model* **2017**, *75*, 241–249. [CrossRef] [PubMed]
9. Zhao, Y.M.; Zhang, J.K.; Zhuang, R.X.; He, R.Y.; Xi, J.J.; Pan, X.W.; Shao, Y.D.; Pan, Y.M.; Sun, J.J.; Cai, Z.B.; et al. Synthesis and Evaluation of a Series of Pyridine and Pyrimidine Derivatives as Type II c-Met Inhibitors. *Bioorgan. Med. Chem.* **2017**, *25*, 3195–3205. [CrossRef] [PubMed]
10. Nakazawa, Y.; Kawano, S.; Matsui, J.; Funahashi, Y.; Tohyama, Q.; Muto, H.; Nakagawa, T.; Matsushima, T. Multitargeting Strategy Using Lenvatinib and Golvatinib: Maximizing Anti-Angiogenesis Activity in a Preclinical Cancer Model. *Cancer Sci.* **2015**, *106*, 201–207. [CrossRef] [PubMed]
11. Parikh, P.K.; Ghate, M.D. Recent Advances in the Discovery of Small Molecule c-Met Kinase Inhibitors. *Eur. J. Med. Chem.* **2018**, *143*, 1103–1138. [CrossRef] [PubMed]
12. Darwish, H.W.; Abdelhameed, A.S.; Bakheit, A.H.; Alanazi, A.M. A New Method to Determine the New C-Met Inhibitor "Cabozantinib" in Dosage Form and Human Plasma via Micelle-Enhanced Spectrofluorimetry. *RSC Adv.* **2015**, *5*, 40484–40490. [CrossRef]
13. Tang, Q.D.; Duan, Y.L.; Wang, L.X.; O'Yang, Y.Q.; Wang, C.L.; Mei, H.; Tang, S.; Xiong, Y.H.; Zheng, P.W.; Gong, P.; et al. Synthesis and Antiproliferative Activity of Pyrrolo[2, 3-b]pyridine Derivatives Bearing the 1, 8-Naphthyridin-2-One Moiety. *Eur. J. Med. Chem.* **2018**, *143*, 266–275. [CrossRef] [PubMed]
14. Zhang, L.; Zhao, J.Y.; Zhang, B.C.; Lu, T.; Chen, Y.D. Discovery of [1, 2, 4] triazolo [3, 4-b][1, 3, 4] thiadiazole Derivatives as Novel, Potent and Selective c-Met Kinase Inhibitors: Synthesis, SAR Study, and Biological Activity. *Eur. J. Med. Chem.* **2018**, *150*, 809–816. [CrossRef] [PubMed]
15. Wang, L.X.; Xu, S.; Liu, X.B.; Chen, X.Y.; Xiong, H.H.; Hou, S.S.; Zou, W.S.; Tang, Q.D.; Zheng, P.W.; Zhu, W.F. Discovery of Thinopyrimidine-Triazole Conjugates as c-Met Targeting and Apoptosis Inducing Agents. *Bioorg. Chem.* **2018**, *77*, 370–380. [CrossRef] [PubMed]
16. Dadashpour, S.; Küçükkılınç, T.T.; Ayazgök, B.; Hosseinimehr, S.J.; Chippindale, A.M.; Foroumadi, A.; Irannejad, H. Discovery of Novel 1, 2, 4-Triazolo-1, 2, 4-Triazines with Thiomethylpyridine Hinge Binders as Potent c-Met Kinase Inhibitors. *Future Med. Chem.* **2019**, *11*, 1119–1136. [CrossRef] [PubMed]
17. Olmez, I.; Zhang, Y.; Manigat, L.; Benamar, M.; Brenneman, B.; Nakano, I.; Godlewski, J.; Bronisz, A.; Lee, J.; Abbas, T.; et al. Combined c-Met/Trk Inhibition Overcomes Resistance to CDK4/6 Inhibitors in Glioblastoma. *Cancer Res.* **2018**, *78*, 4360–4369. [CrossRef] [PubMed]

18. Liu, X.B.; Kou, J.L.; Xiao, Z.; Tian, F.J.; Hu, J.Y.; Zheng, P.W.; Zhu, W.F. Design, Synthesis and Biological Evaluation of 6, 7-Disubstituted-4-Phenoxyquinoline Derivatives Bearing Pyridazinone Moiety as c-Met Inhibitors. *Molecules* **2018**, *23*, 1543. [CrossRef] [PubMed]
19. Ahmed, E.M.; Khalil, N.A.; Taher, A.T.; Refaey, R.H.; Nissan, Y.M. Triazolopyridazine Derivatives: Synthesis, Cytotoxic Evaluation, c-Met Kinase Activity and Molecular Docking. *Bioorg. Chem.* **2019**, *92*, 103272–103281. [CrossRef] [PubMed]

Sample Availability: Samples of all target compounds are available from the authors.

molecules

MDPI

Article

Synthesis and Evaluation of Novel 2*H*-Benzo[*e*]-[1,2,4]thiadiazine 1,1-Dioxide Derivatives as PI3Kδ Inhibitors

Ya-Ping Gong †, Long-Qian Tang †, Tong-Shen Liu and Zhao-Peng Liu *

Department of Medicinal Chemistry, Key Laboratory of Chemical Biology (Ministry of Education), School of Pharmaceutical Sciences, Shandong University, Jinan 250012, China; 201614474@mail.sdu.edu.cn (Y.-P.G.); lqtang.student@sina.com (L.-Q.T.); jshrlts@163.com (T.-S.L.)

* Correspondence: liuzhaop@sdu.edu.cn; Tel.: +86-531-88382006; Fax: +86-531-88382548

† Ya-Ping Gong and Long-Qian Tang contributed equally to this work.

Academic Editor: Qiao-Hong Chen
Received: 8 November 2019; Accepted: 22 November 2019; Published: 25 November 2019

Abstract: In previous work, we applied the rotation-limiting strategy and introduced a substituent at the 3-position of the pyrazolo [3,4-*d*]pyrimidin-4-amine as the affinity element to interact with the deeper hydrophobic pocket, discovered a series of novel quinazolinones as potent PI3Kδ inhibitors. Among them, the indole derivative **3** is one of the most selective PI3Kδ inhibitors and the 3,4-dimethoxyphenyl derivative **4** is a potent and selective dual PI3Kδ/γ inhibitor. In this study, we replaced the carbonyl group in the quinazolinone core with a sulfonyl group, designed a series of novel 2*H*-benzo[*e*][1,2,4]thiadiazine 1,1-dioxide derivatives as PI3Kδ inhibitors. After the reduction of nitro group in *N*-(2,6-dimethylphenyl)-2-nitrobenzenesulfonamide **5** and *N*-(2,6-dimethylphenyl)-2-nitro-5-fluorobenzenesulfonamide **6**, the resulting 2-aminobenzenesulfonamides were reacted with trimethyl orthoacetate to give the 3-methyl-2*H*-benzo[*e*][1,2,4]thiadiazine 1,1-dioxide derivatives. After bromination of the 3-methyl group, the nucleophilic substitution with the 3-iodo-1*H*-pyrazolo[3,4-*d*]pyrimidin-4-amine provided the respective iodide derivatives, which were further reacted with a series of arylboronic acids via Suzuki coupling to furnish the 2*H*-benzo[*e*][1,2,4]thiadiazine 1,1-dioxide derivatives **15a–J** and **16a–d**. In agreement with the quinazolinone derivatives, the introduction of a 5-indolyl or 3,4-dimethoxyphenyl at the affinity pocket generated the most potent analogues **15a** and **15b** with the IC_{50} values of 217 to 266 nM, respectively. In comparison with the quinazolinone lead compounds **3** and **4**, these 2*H*-benzo[*e*][1,2,4]thiadiazine 1,1-dioxide derivatives exhibited much decreased PI3Kδ inhibitory potency, but maintained the high selectivity over other PI3K isoforms. Unlike the quinazolinone lead compound **4** that was a dual PI3Kδ/γ inhibitor, the benzthiadiazine 1,1-dioxide **15b** with the same 3,4-dimethoxyphenyl moiety was more than 21-fold selective over PI3Kγ. Moreover, the introducing of a fluorine atom at the 7-position of the 2*H*-benzo[*e*][1,2,4]thiadiazine 1,1-dioxide core, in general, was not favored for the PI3Kδ inhibitory activity. In agreement with their high PI3Kδ selectivity, **15a** and **15b** significantly inhibited the SU-DHL-6 cell proliferation.

Keywords: PI3Ks; PI3Kδ inhibitors; 2*H*-benzo[*e*][1,2,4]thiadiazine 1,1-dioxide; anticancer; anticancer agents

1. Introduction

Phosphoinositide 3-kinases (PI3Ks) are a family of lipid kinases that regulate numerous biological functions, including cell growth, proliferation, differentiation, motility, and intracellular trafficking, through the phosphorylation of the phosphatidylinositol 4,5-bisphosphate (PIP2) to generate the lipid second messenger phosphatidylinositol 3,4,5-trisphosphate (PIP3) [1–3]. There are three classes of the PI3K enzyme, of which class I PI3Ks are the mostly studied and further divided into subgroups IA (PI3Kα, PI3Kβ, and PI3Kδ) and IB (PI3Kγ) based on the signaling pathways and the regulatory proteins to which they bind [4,5]. The class IA PI3K isoforms mediate the signal transduction from receptor tyrosine kinases [6], while the IB isoform PI3Kγ is principally activated by G-protein coupled receptors [7]. PI3Kα and PI3Kβ are ubiquitously expressed, while PI3Kδ and PI3Kγ are dominantly expressed in leukocytes [8–10]. All the class I PI3K isoforms are implicated in cancer [11–16]. There are also mounting evidences that support a therapeutic role for inhibition of PI3Kα in diabetes [17,18], PI3Kβ in thrombosis [19,20], PI3Kδ and PI3Kγ in both rheumatoid arthritis and asthma [21–24], PI3Kδ in activated PI3Kδ syndrome (APDS) [25–27], and PI3Kγ in idiopathic pulmonary fibrosis [28]. Therefore, the development of PI3K isoform selective inhibitors is a promising therapeutic strategy for the treatment of these PI3Ks-related diseases. The selective PI3Kδ inhibitor idelalisib (Figure 1) is approved by FDA for follicular lymphoma (FL) and small lymphocytic lymphoma (SLL) and for chronic lymphocytic leukemia (CLL) in combination with rituximab [29,30]. The dual PI3Kδ/γ inhibitor duvelisib (Figure 1) is approved for adult patients with relapsed or refractory CLL or SLL, and relapsed or refractory FL after at least two prior systemic therapies [31]. However, in the clinical application of idelalisib, infectious and autoimmune toxicities were observed, and the unique toxicities are associated with inhibition of different isoforms of the PI3K enzyme [32]. To improve the isoform selectivity of the quinazolinone-based PI3Kδ inhibitors, in previous work, we introduced a pyrazolo [3,4-*d*]pyrimidin-4-amine moiety as the hinge region binding group, a substituent at the 3-position of the pyrazolo[3,4-*d*]pyrimidine core as the affinity element to interact with the deeper hydrophobic pocket, and a 2,6-dimethylphenyl to limit the free rotation of the 3-phenyl in idelalisib, discovered the indole derivative **3** as one of the most selective PI3Kδ inhibitors (IC_{50} = 8.6 nM) with more than 3630-fold, 390-fold and 40-fold selective for PI3Kδ over PI3Kα, β and γ, and the 3,4-dimethoxyphenyl derivative **4** as a potent and selective dual PI3Kδ/γ inhibitor (IC_{50} = 8.4 nM for PI3Kδ, IC_{50} = 62 nM for PI3Kγ) with more than 1400-fold, 820-fold selective for PI3Kδ over PI3Kα and PI3Kβ [33]. Considering the importance of sulfonamides in drug discovery [34–36], we replaced the carbonyl group in the quinazolinone core, and reported here the synthesis and preliminary evaluation of 2*H*-benzo[*e*][1,2,4]thiadiazine 1,1-dioxide derivatives as PI3Kδ inhibitors.

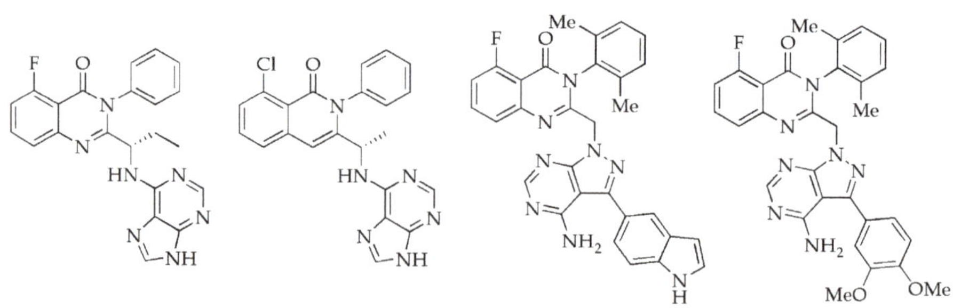

1 (Idelalisib) 2 (Duvelisib) 3 4

Figure 1. Selective PI3Kδ and dual PI3Kδ/γ inhibitors.

2. Results and Discussion

2.1. Chemistry

All the new 2*H*-benzo[*e*][1,2,4]thiadiazine 1,1-dioxide derivatives were prepared following a general synthetic route shown in Scheme 1. The 2-nitrobenzene-1-sulfonamides **5** and **6** were readily prepared according to the reported method by the reaction of 2-nitrobenzene-1-sulfonyl chloride or 5-fluoro-2-nitrobenzene-1-sulfonyl chloride with 2,6-dimethylbenzenamine in methanol and water solution in the presence of CH_3COONa under refluxing conditions [37]. Reduction of the nitro group to amine was carried out using hydrazine monohydrate in the presence of ferric chloride and activated charcoal in methanol under reflux conditions in excellent yields (95% and 99%). The resulting 2-aminobenzenesulfonamides **7** and **8** were reacted with trimethyl orthoacetate to give the corresponding 3-methyl-2*H*-benzo[*e*][1,2,4]thiadiazine 1,1-dioxide derivatives **9** and **10** in 51% and 40%, respectively. In the bromination of the allyl methyl group using *N*-bromosuccinimide (NBS), the main compounds were found to be the dibrominated products. Therefore, compounds **9** and **10** were reacted with only 0.5 equivalent of NBS in glacial acetic acid to give the monobrominated derivatives **11** and **12** in moderate yields (79% and 72% based on NBS). Nucleophilic substitution of **11** and **12** with 3-iodo-1*H*-pyrazolo[3,4-*d*]pyrimidin-4-amine, which was readily prepared from 5-amino-1*H*-pyrazole-4-carbonitrile in two steps by the known procedures [38], resulted in the iodides **13** and **14** in 86 and 58% yields, respectively. Finally, the incorporation of the affinity elements was achieved through the Suzuki coupling of **13** and **14** with the appropriate boronic acid in dioxane and water catalyzed by $Pd(PPh_3)_4$ under refluxing conditions, and the target 2*H*-benzo[*e*][1,2,4]thiadiazine 1,1-dioxide derivatives **15a–J** and **16a–d** were obtained in 34–91% and 51–84% yields. The structures of these 2*H*-benzo[*e*][1,2,4]thiadiazine 1,1-dioxide derivatives were characterized by ^{1}H-nuclear magnetic resonance (NMR) and ^{13}C-NMR (please refer to the Supplementary Materials).

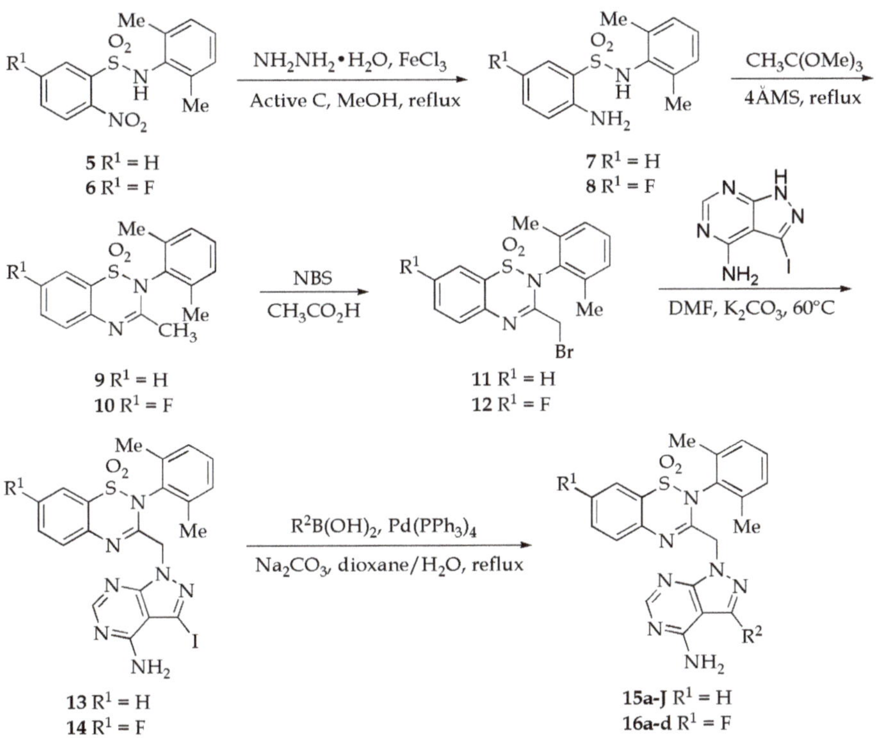

Scheme 1. Synthesis of 2*H*-benzo[*e*][1,2,4]thiadiazine 1,1-dioxide derivatives.

2.2. PI3Kδ Inhibitory Activity and Isoform Selectivity

Compounds **15a–J** were first tested for their inhibitory activity against PI3Kδ using the ADP-Glo luminescent assay [39], using a pan-PI3K inhibitor PI-103 as a positive control [40]. As shown in Table 1, the substitution at the 3-position of the pyrazolo[3,4-d]pyrimidine with 5-indolyl or 3,4-dimethoxyphenyl led to the relative potent analogues **15a** and **15b** with IC_{50} values of 217 to 266 nM, respectively. The 6-methoxypyridin-3-yl derivative **15d** exhibited moderate PI3Kδ inhibitory activity (IC_{50} = 498 nM), whereas the 3-fluoro-4-methoxyphenyl analogue **15c** only had marginal activity. In comparison with **15b**, the substitution of the 3,4-dimethoxypheny group for 2,3-dihydrobenzo[*b*][1,4]dioxin-6-yl (**15e**), benzo[*d*][1,3]dioxol-5-yl (**15f**), 4-methoxyphenyl (**15g**), 3-methoxyphenyl (**15h**), 4-(trifluoromethoxy)phenyl (**15i**), and phenyl (**15j**) was not tolerated, indicating the subtle requirements at the affinity pocket of PI3Kδ.

Table 1. PI3Kδ inhibitory activity of **15a–j** and **16a–d**.

Compd.	Structure	R	IC_{50} (nM) [a]
15a		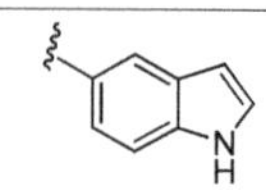	217 ± 28
15b		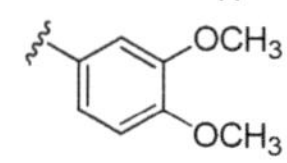	266 ± 31
15c		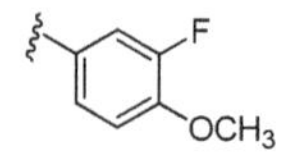	980 ± 45
15d	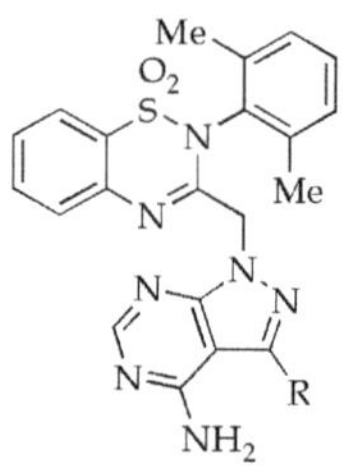	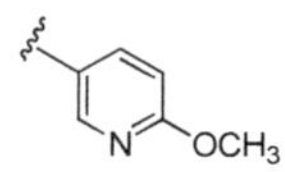	498 ± 33
15e		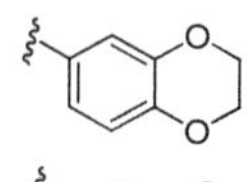	>1000
15f		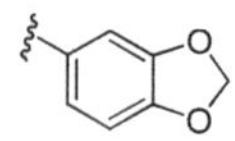	>1000
15g		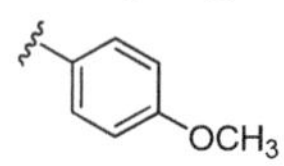	>1000
15h		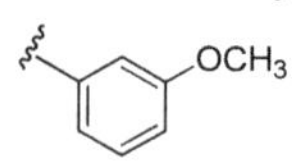	>1000
15i		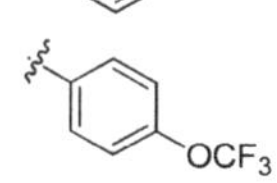	>1000
15j		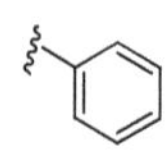	>1000
16a		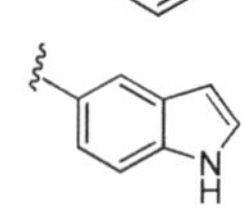	>1000
16b	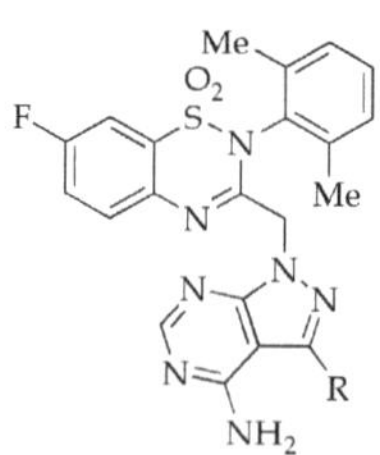	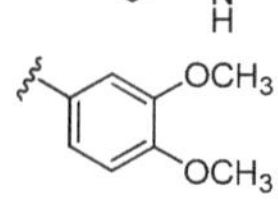	518 ± 62
16c		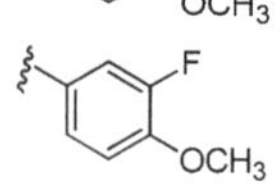	824 ± 76
16d		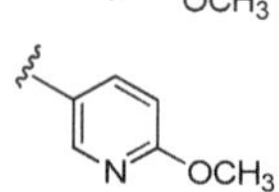	823 ± 69
	PI-103		1.6 ± 0.1

[a] The IC_{50} values are shown as the mean ± SD from two separate experiments.

In order to increase the inhibitory activity of compound **15a–d**, a fluorine atom was introduced at the 7-position of the 2*H*-benzo[*e*][1,2,4]thiadiazine 1,1-dioxide, and compounds **16a–d** were prepared and evaluated for their PI3Kδ inhibitory activity. In comparison with **15a**, the fluorinated compound **16a** lost its activity (Table 1), and compounds **16b** and **16d** showed almost 2-fold decrease in potency. In contrast, compound **16c** with a 3-fluoro-4-methoxyphenyl moiety at the affinity pocket showed a slight increase in potency.

Compared with the leading quinazolinone derivatives **3** and **4**, these 2*H*-benzo[*e*][1,2,4]-thiadiazine 1,1-dioxide derivatives **15a–j** and **16a–d** showed much decreased PI3Kδ inhibitory activity. However, the most potent derivatives **15a** and **15b** proved to be selective PI3Kδ inhibitors (Table 2). The indole derivative **15a** showed significantly lower potency against other three isoforms of class I PI3K and was more than 140-fold selective for PI3Kδ over PI3Kα, β and γ. The 3,4-dimethoxyphenyl derivative **15b** was more than 60-fold, 90-fold and 20-fold selective for PI3Kδ over PI3Kα, PI3Kβ, and PI3Kγ, respectively. In comparison with the lead **4**, **15b** was more selective over PI3Kγ (21-fold vs. 7-fold).

Table 2. The isoform selectivity and SU-DHL-6 cell growth inhibitory activity of **15a** and **15b**.

Compound	IC_{50} (nM) [a]				GI_{50} (μM) [a]
	PI3Kα	PI3Kβ	PI3Kδ	PI3Kγ	SU-DHL-6
15a	>50,000	30596 ± 875	217 ± 28	>50,000	2.13 ± 0.09
15b	16364 ± 768	24189 ± 495	266 ± 31	5838 ± 135	2.50 ± 0.11
PI-103	6.5 ± 0.7	23 ± 1.6	1.6 ± 0.1	78 ± 4.3	0.039 ± 0.011 [b]

[a] The IC_{50} or GI_{50} values are shown as the mean ± SD from two separate experiments; [b] CAL-101 was the positive control.

2.3. *SU-DHL-6 Cell Growth Inhibitory Activity*

The selective PI3Kδ inhibitors **15a** and **15b** were further evaluated for their antiproliferative activity against human B-cell SU-DHL-6. **15a** and **15b** significantly inhibited SU-DHL-6 cell proliferation with the GI_{50} of 2.13 and 2.50 μM, respectively (Table 2), which were in consistent with their PI3Kδ inhibitory potency.

2.4. *Molecular Modeling Study*

Molecular docking studies were conducted on the new discovered selective PI3Kδ inhibitors **15a** and **15b**. As shown in Figure 2, the pyrazolo[3,4-d]pyrimidine portion in both compounds **15a** and **15b** forms hydrogen bonds with Glu826 and Val828 in the hinge region.

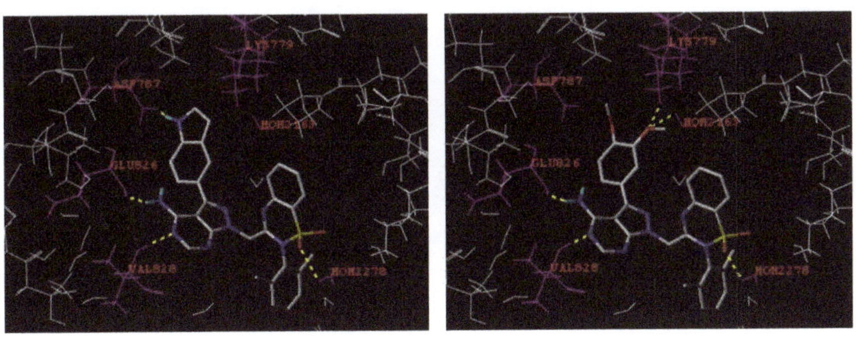

Figure 2. Molecular docking studies of **15a** (left) and **15b** (right).

Both inhibitors bind to the PI3Kδ isoform in an 'induced fit' conformation in which the 2*H*-benzo[*e*][1,2,4]thiadiazine 1,1-dioxide moiety is sandwiched between Trp760 and Met752 as these residues move apart to create the specificity pocket. The indol-5-yl (**15a**) in the specificity pocket forms an additional hydrogen bond with Asp787. Like the carbonyl oxygen in **3** and **4**, one sulfonyl oxygen in both **15a** and **15b** acts as hydrogen bond acceptor from the H_2O2278. In compound **15b**, only the 3-methoxy group forms hydrogen bonding with Lys779, while in lead **4**, the 3-methoxy interacts with Tyr813 and Asp911, the 4-methoxy interacts with Lys779 [33]. These differences may contribute its less potency against PI3Kδ than **4**. In comparison with **3** and **4**, the lack of a 8-fluorine at the 2*H*-benzo[*e*][1,2,4]thiadiazine 1,1-dioxide core in **15a** and **15b** may also be related to their lower PI3Kδ inhibitory activity.

3. Materials and Methods

3.1. General Chemical Experimental Procedures

^{1}H- and ^{13}C-NMR spectra were recorded on a Bruker-600 NMR spectrometer (Brucker Co., Ltd., Zurich, Switzerland). All spectra were recorded at room temperature for DMSO or $CDCl_3$ solutions. High resolution mass spectra (HRMS) were obtained on a 6520 QTOF instrument (Agilent Technologies Inc., Santa Clara, CA, USA by electrospray ionization (ESI). Melting points were determined on an X-6 micromelting point apparatus (Beijing Tech. Co., Ltd., Beijing, China) without corrections. Column chromatography was performed on silica gel (200–300 mesh). All reactions involving oxygen- or moisture sensitive compounds were carried out under a dry N_2 atmosphere using anhydrous solvents. Unless otherwise noted, reagents were added by syringe.

2-Amino-N-(2,6-dimethylphenyl)benzenesulfonamide (**7**)

To a stirred solution of *N*-(2,6-dimethylphenyl)-2-nitrobenzenesulfonamide (**5**, 19.4 g, 63.3 mmol) in methanol (200 mL), ferric chloride (5.1 g, 19 mmol) and activated charcoal (6.5 g) was added and refluxed for 30 min. 80% Hydrazine monohydrate (31.7 g, 633 mmol) was then added dropwise and refluxed for 5 h. After filtration, the filtrate was concentrated and the residue was dissolved in EtOAc (200 mL), washed with brine, dried over anhydrous Na_2SO_4. After filtration and evaporation, the residue was purified by silica gel chromatography (EtOAc/hexane = 1:3) to give **7** (16.5 g, 95%) as a white solid, m.p. 144–146 °C; lit. [41] m.p. 144–145 °C.

2-Amino-N-(2,6-dimethylphenyl)-5-fluorobenzenesulfonamide (**8**)

According to the procedures described for the synthesis of **7**, compound **8** were obtained as a colorless solid (16 g) in 99% yield, m.p. 185–186 °C; ^{1}H-NMR (DMSO-d_6) δ 9.44 (s, 1H, SO_2NH), 7.21 (td, *J* = 9.0, 3.0 Hz, 1H, Ar-H), 7.07 (td, *J* = 8.4, 1.5 Hz, 1H, Ar-H), 7.01 (d, *J* = 7.8 Hz, 2H, Ar-H), 6.97 (dd, *J* = 8.4, 3.0 Hz, 1H, Ar-H), 6.85 (dd, *J* = 9.0, 4.8 Hz, 1H, Ar-H), 5.85 (s, 2H, NH_2), 2.04 (s, 6H, 2,6-$(CH_3)_2$); MS (ESI) calcd. for $C_{14}H_{14}FN_2O_2S$ $[M - H]^-$: 293.1, found: 293.3.

2-(2,6-Dimethylphenyl)-3-methy-2H-benzo[e][1,2,4]thiadiazine 1,1-dioxide (**9**)

A mixture of **7** (5 g, 18.1 mmol), trimethyl orthoacetate (50 mL) and 4Ǎ molecular sieve (10 g) was refluxed for 10 h. After cooling to room temp., the mixture was concentrated and the residue was dissolved in EtOAc (200 mL), washed with brine, dried over anhydrous Na_2SO_4. After filtration and evaporation, the residue was purified by silica gel chromatography (EtOAc/hexane = 1:5) to give **9** (2.8 g, 51%) as a white solid, m.p. 162–163 °C; ^{1}H-NMR ($CDCl_3$) δ 7.89 (d, *J* = 7.8 Hz, 1H, Ar-H), 7.70 (td, *J* = 8.4, 1.2 Hz, 1H, Ar-H), 7.60 (d, *J* = 8.4 Hz, 1H, Ar-H), 7.47 (td, *J* = 7.8, 1.2 Hz, 1H, Ar-H), 7.21 (t, *J* = 7.2 Hz, 1H, Ar-H), 7.18 (d, *J* = 7.8 Hz, 2H, Ar-H), 2.22 (s, 6H, 2,6-$(CH_3)_2$), 2.11 (s, 3H, 3-CH_3); ^{13}C-NMR ($CDCl_3$) δ 154.34, 142.55, 138.58, 133.51, 132.59, 129.99, 129.27, 127.65, 127.23, 126.90, 121.01, 23.38, 18.62; MS (ESI) *m/z* calcd. for $C_{16}H_{17}N_2O_2S$ $[M + H]^+$ 301.1, found 301.0.

2-(2,6-Dimethylphenyl)-7-fluoro-3-methy-2H-benzo[e][1,2,4]thiadiazine 1,1-dioxide (**10**)

According to the procedures described for the synthesis of **9**, compound **10** were obtained as a colorless solid (6.9 g) in 40% yield, m.p. 150–151 °C; ^{1}H-NMR (DMSO-d_6) δ 7.89 (dt, *J* = 7.2, 1.5 Hz,

1H, Ar-H), 7.73 (dd, *J* = 7.2, 1.2 Hz, 2H, Ar-H), 7.36 (t, *J* = 7.2 Hz, 1H, Ar-H), 7.29 (d, *J* = 7.8 Hz, 2H, Ar-H), 2.13 (s, 6H, 2,6-$(CH_3)_2$), 2.06 (s, 3H, 3-CH_3); ^{13}C-NMR (DMSO-d_6) δ 160.28 (d, J_{C-F} = 249.2 Hz), 154.02, 139.26 (d, J_{C-F} = 3.0 Hz), 138.59, 132.62, 130.88 (d, J_{C-F} = 7.6 Hz), 130.66, 129.79, 127.96 (d, J_{C-F} = 9.1 Hz), 122.58 (d, J_{C-F} = 24.2 Hz), 107.95 (d, J_{C-F} = 27.2 Hz), 23.25, 18.47; MS (ESI) *m/z* calcd. for $C_{16}H_{16}FN_2O_2S$ $[M + H]^+$ 319.1, found 319.0.

3-Bromomethyl-2-(2,6-dimethylphenyl)-2H-benzo[e][1,2,4]thiadiazine 1,1-dioxide (**11**)

Compound **9** (1.0 g, 3.3 mmol) was dissolved in glacial acetic acid (10 mL), and then NBS (0.3 g, 1.65 mmol) was added. After the mixture was stirred at room temperature for 0.5 h, distilled water (50 mL) was added. The mixture was extracted by dichloromethane, washed with brine, dried over anhydrous Na_2SO_4. After filtration and evaporation, the residue was purified by silica gel chromatography (EtOAc/hexane = 1:10) to give **11** (0.5 g) with a conversion yield of 79% as a white solid, m.p. 150–151°C; ^{1}H-NMR ($CDCl_3$) δ 7.90 (dd, *J* = 7.8, 1.2 Hz, 1H, Ar-H), 7.75 (td, *J* = 8.4, 1.2 Hz, 1H, Ar-H), 7.69 (dd, *J* = 7.8, 0.6 Hz, 1H, Ar-H), 7.55 (td, *J* = 8.4, 1.2 Hz, 1H, Ar-H), 7.29 (t, *J* = 7.8 Hz, 1H, Ar-H), 7.19 (d, *J* = 7.8 Hz, 2H, Ar-H), 3.97 (s, 2H, CH_2Br), 2.24 (s, 6H, 2,6-$(CH_3)_2$); ^{13}C-NMR ($CDCl_3$) δ 151.86, 142.16, 138.89, 133.69, 132.14, 130.36, 129.51, 128.37, 128.25, 127.79, 121.00, 28.91, 18.95; MS (ESI) *m/z* calcd. for $C_{16}H_{16}BrN_2O_2S$ $[M + H]^+$ 379.0 and 381.0, found 381.3 and 383.4.

3-Bromomethyl-2-(2,6-dimethylphenyl)-7-fluoro-2H-benzo[e][1,2,4]thiadiazine 1,1-dioxide (**12**)

According to the procedures described for the synthesis of **11**, compound **12** were obtained as a colorless solid (0.65 g) in 72% conversion yield, m.p. 185–186 °C; ^{1}H-NMR (DMSO-d_6) δ 7.95 (dd, *J* = 8.4, 3.0 Hz, 1H, Ar-H), 7.84 (dd, *J* = 10.8, 5.4 Hz, 1H, Ar-H), 7.79 (td, *J* = 10.8, 3.0 Hz, 1H, Ar-H), 7.37 (t, *J* = 8.4 Hz, 1H, Ar-H), 7.29 (d, *J* = 9.0 Hz, 2H, Ar-H), 4.10 (s, 2H, CH_2Br), 2.14 (s, 6H, 2,6-$(CH_3)_2$); ^{13}C-NMR (DMSO-d_6) δ 161.21 (d, J_{C-F} = 250.6 Hz), 151.77, 138.82, 132.20, 131.54 (d, J_{C-F} = 9.1 Hz), 130.94, 129.97, 129.28, 128.60 (d, J_{C-F} = 9.1 Hz), 122.87 (d, J_{C-F} = 24.2 Hz), 108.32 (d, J_{C-F} = 25.7 Hz), 30.02, 18.72; MS (ESI) *m/z* calcd.for $C_{16}H_{15}BrFN_2O_2S$ $[M + H]^+$ 397.0 and 399.0, found 397.2 and 399.1.

3-((4-Amino-3-iodo-1H-pyrazolo[3,4-d]pyrimidin-1-yl)methyl)-2-(2,6-dimethylphenyl)-2H-benzo[e]-[1,2,4]thiadiazine 1,1-dioxide (**13**)

To a solution of **11** (1.1 g, 2.9 mmol) and 3-iodo-1*H*-pyrazolo[3,4-d]pyrimidin-4-amine (1.1 g, 4.4 mmol) in DMF (8 mL), K_2CO_3 (0.8 g, 5.8 mmol) was added. After stirring at 60 °C for 5 h, the mixture was poured into water (100 mL), extracted by EtOAc. The organic layer was washed with brine, dried over anhydrous Na_2SO_4. After filtration and evaporation, the residue was purified by silica gel chromatography (EtOAc/hexane = 1:10) to give **13** (1.4 g, 86%) as a white solid, m.p. 242–243 °C; ^{1}H-NMR (DMSO-d_6) δ 8.07 (s, 1H, Ar-H), 7.94 (dd, *J* = 7.8, 1.2 Hz, 1H, Ar-H), 7.80 (td, *J* = 7.8, 1.2 Hz, 1H, Ar-H), 7.65 (td, *J* = 7.8, 1.2 Hz, 1H, Ar-H), 7.43 (d, *J* = 7.8 Hz, 1H, Ar-H), 7.25 (t, *J* = 7.2 Hz, 1H, Ar-H), 7.17 (d, *J*= 7.2 Hz, 2H, Ar-H), 5.12 (s, 2H, NCH_2), 2.07 (s, 6H, 2,6-$(CH_3)_2$); ^{13}C-NMR ($CDCl_3$) δ 162.77, 161.35, 159.35, 156.17, 146.35, 143.45, 139.66, 136.44, 135.32, 134.48, 133.91, 133.26, 132.44, 108.30, 95.82, 60.13, 54.33, 23.17; MS (ESI) *m/z* calcd. for $C_{21}H_{19}IN_7O_2S$ $[M + H]^+$ 560.0, found 560.2.

3-((4-Amino-3-iodo-1H-pyrazolo[3,4-d]pyrimidin-1-yl)methyl)-2-(2,6-dimethylphenyl)-7-fluoro-2H-benzo-[e][1,2,4]thiadiazine 1,1-dioxide (**14**)

Following the procedures described for the synthesis of **13**, compound **14** were obtained as a white solid (1.6 g) in 58% yield, m.p. 243–244 °C; ^{1}H-NMR (DMSO-d_6) δ 8.08 (s, 1H, Ar-H), 7.92 (dd, *J* = 11.4, 4.2 Hz, 1H, Ar-H), 7.68 (td, *J* = 13.2, 4.2 Hz, 1H, Ar-H), 7.54 (dd, *J* = 13.2, 7.2 Hz, 1H, Ar-H), 7.26 (dd, *J* = 13.2, 10.2 Hz, 1H, Ar-H), 7.17 (d, *J* = 11.4 Hz, 2H, Ar-H), 5.13 (s, 2H, NCH_2), 2.06 (s, 6H, 2,6-$(CH_3)_2$); ^{13}C-NMR (DMSO-d_6) δ 160.89 (d, J_{C-F} = 250.7 Hz), 158.02, 156.61, 154.57, 150.89, 138.69, 131.55, 131.46 (d, J_{C-F} = 7.6 Hz), 130.64, 129.76, 128.54 (d, J_{C-F} = 7.6 Hz), 122.71 (d, J_{C-F} = 22.7 Hz), 108.28 (d, J_{C-F} = 25.7 Hz), 103.55, 91.13, 79.59, 49.55, 18.40; MS (ESI) *m/z* calcd. for $C_{21}H_{18}FIN_7O_2S$ $[M + H]^+$ 578.0, found 578.0.

3-((4-Amino-3-(1H-indol-5-yl)-1H-pyrazolo[3,4-d]pyrimidin-1-yl)methyl)-2-(2,6-dimethylphenyl)-2H-benzo[e][1,2,4]thiadiazine 1,1-dioxide (**15a**)

To a solution of **13** (180 mg, 0.30 mmol) in dioxane (4 mL) and distilled water (1.5 mL) was added 1*H*-indol-5-ylboronic acid (88 mg, 0.55 mmol), sodium carbonate anhydrous (103 mg, 0.97 mmol) and $Pd(PPh_3)_4$ (12 mg, 0.03 mmol). The mixture was degassed with N_2, and refluxed for 4 h. After cooling to room temperature, EtOAc (50 mL) and distilled water (10 mL) were added, and the organic layer was washed brine, dried over Na_2SO_4. After filtration and evaporation, the residue was purified by silica gel chromatography (EtOAc/hexane = 1:1) to give **15a** (161 mg, 91%) as a white solid, m.p. 216–217 °C; ^{1}H-NMR ($CDCl_3$) δ 11.32 (s, 1H, NH), 8.09 (s, 1H, Ar-H), 7.95 (dd, *J* = 7.8, 1.2 Hz, 1H, Ar-H), 7.81 (td, *J* = 7.8, 1.2 Hz, 2H, Ar-H), 7.65 (td, *J* = 7.8, 0.6 Hz, 1H, Ar-H), 7.57 (d, *J* = 8.4 Hz, 1H, Ar-H), 7.52 (d, *J* = 7.8 Hz, 1H, Ar-H), 7.45 (t, *J* = 3.0 Hz, 1H, Ar-H), 7.38 (dd, *J* = 8.4, 1.8 Hz, 1H, Ar-H), 7.25 (t, *J* = 7.8 Hz, 1H, Ar-H), 7.15 (d, *J* = 7.8 Hz, 2H, Ar-H), 6.55 (t, *J* = 8.4, 1.8 Hz, 1H, Ar-H), 5.20 (s, 2H, NCH_2), 2.04 (s, 6H, 2,6-$(CH_3)_2$); ^{13}C-NMR (CDCl3) δ 158.53, 156.22, 155.43, 152.04, 146.79, 141.79, 138.70, 136.53, 134.86, 131.96, 130.48, 129.70, 129.09, 128.51, 128.47, 127.83, 127.04, 123.90, 121.76, 121.20, 120.52, 112.68, 102.22, 97.86, 49.61, 18.35; HRMS (ESI) *m/z* calcd. for $C_{29}H_{25}N_8O_2S$ $[M + H]^+$ 549.1816, found 549.1829.

3-((4-Amino-3-(3,4-dimethoxyphenyl)-1H-pyrazolo[3,4-d]pyrimidin-1-yl)methyl)-2-(2,6-dimethylphenyl)-2H-benzo[e][1,2,4]thiadiazine 1,1-dioxide (**15b**)

According to the procedures described for the synthesis of **15a**, compound **15b** were obtained as a white solid (61 mg) in 75% yield, m.p. 220–222 °C; ^{1}H-NMR (DMSO-d_6) δ 8.31 (s, 1H, NH), 8.09 (s, 1H, Ar-H), 7.94 (dd, *J* = 7.8, 1.2 Hz, 1H, Ar-H), 7.81 (td, *J* = 7.8, 1.2 Hz, 1H, Ar-H), 7.65 (td, *J* = 7.2, 1.2 Hz, 1H, Ar-H), 7.50 (d, *J* = 8.4 Hz, 1H, Ar-H), 7.26 (t, *J* = 7.8 Hz, 1H, Ar-H), 7.15–7.19 (m, 4H, Ar-H), 7.12 (d, *J* = 8.4 Hz, 1H, Ar-H), 5.18 (s, 2H, NCH_2), 3.81 (s, 3H, OCH_3), 3.80 (s, 3H, OCH_3), 2.02 (s, 6H, 2,6-$(CH_3)_2$); ^{13}C-NMR (DMSO-d_6) δ 158.50, 156.26, 155.50, 151.98, 149.83, 149.51, 145.20, 141.74, 138.71, 134.86, 131.98, 130.50, 129.70, 129.13, 128.47, 127.84, 125.53, 121.19, 121.03, 112.71, 111.99, 97.70, 79.63, 56.04, 55.89, 49.64, 18.32; HRMS (ESI) *m/z* calcd. for $C_{29}H_{28}N_7O_4S$ $[M + H]^+$ 570.1918, found 570.1921.

3-((4-Amino-3-(3-fluoro-4-methoxyphenyl)-1H-pyrazolo[3,4-d]pyrimidin-1-yl)methyl)-2-(2,6-dimethyl-phenyl)-2H-benzo[e][1,2,4]thiadiazine 1,1-dioxide (**15c**)

According to the procedures described for the synthesis of **15a**, compound **15c** were obtained as a white solid (59 mg) in 66% yield, m.p. 226–227 °C; ^{1}H-NMR (DMSO-d_6) δ 8.31 (s, 1H, NH), 8.10 (s, 1H, Ar-H), 7.94 (d, *J* = 7.8 Hz, 1H, Ar-H), 7.81 (t, *J* = 7.8 Hz, 1H, Ar-H), 7.65 (t, *J* = 7.8 Hz, 1H, Ar-H), 7.49 (d, *J* = 8.4 Hz, 1H, Ar-H), 7.43–7.38 (m, 2H, Ar-H), 7.33 (t, *J* = 8.4 Hz, 1H, Ar-H), 7.25 (t, *J* = 7.8 Hz, 1H, Ar-H), 7.15 (d, *J* = 7.8 Hz, 2H, Ar-H), 5.18 (s, 2H, NCH_2), 3.90 (s, 3H, OCH_3), 2.02 (s, 6H, 2,6-$(CH_3)_2$); ^{13}C-NMR (DMSO-d_6) δ 158.50, 156.33, 155.58, 152.84, 152.03 (d, $J_{C\text{–}F}$ = 244.6 Hz), 151.85, 148.13 (d, $J_{C\text{–}F}$ = 9.1 Hz), 144.02, 141.72, 138.69, 134.86, 131.93, 130.51, 129.71, 128.82 (d, $J_{C\text{–}F}$ = 95.1 Hz), 127.82, 125.78 (d, $J_{C\text{–}F}$ = 6.0 Hz), 125.21, 121.20, 116.11 (d, $J_{C\text{–}F}$ = 19.6 Hz), 114.91, 97.67, 79.65, 56.57, 49.64, 18.32; HRMS (ESI) *m/z* calcd. for $C_{28}H_{25}FN_7O_3S$ $[M + H]^+$ 558.1718, found 558.1733.

3-((4-Amino-3-(6-methoxypyridin-3-yl)-1H-pyrazolo[3,4-d]pyrimidin-1-yl)methyl)-2-(2,6-dimethylphenyl)-2H-benzo[e][1,2,4]thiadiazine 1,1-dioxide (**15d**)

According to the procedures described for the synthesis of **15a**, compound **15d** were obtained as a white solid (41 mg) in 47% yield, m.p. 248–249 °C; ^{1}H-NMR (DMSO-d_6) δ 8.39 (d, *J* = 1.8 Hz, 1H, Ar-H), 8.31 (s, 1H, NH), 8.11 (s, 1H, Ar-H), 7.94 (dd, *J* = 7.8, 1.2 Hz, 1H, Ar-H), 7.92 (dd, *J* = 8.4, 2.4 Hz, 1H, Ar-H), 7.81 (td, *J* = 8.4, 1.2 Hz, 1H, Ar-H), 7.65 (td, *J* =7.8, 1.2 Hz, 1H, Ar-H), 7.49 (d, *J* = 7.8 Hz, 1H, Ar-H), 7.26 (t, *J* = 7.8 Hz, 1H, Ar-H), 7.16 (d, *J* = 7.8 Hz, 2H, Ar-H), 6.98 (d, *J* = 8.4 Hz, 1H, Ar-H), 5.20 (s, 2H, NCH_2), 3.92 (s, 3H, OCH_3), 2.03 (s, 6H, 2,6-$(CH_3)_2$); ^{13}C-NMR (DMSO-d_6) δ 164.14, 158.60, 156.38, 155.61, 151.81, 146.69, 142.36, 141.71, 139.29, 138.69, 134.87, 131.91, 130.51, 129.70, 129.13, 128.50, 127.80, 122.70, 121.19, 111.48, 97.92, 79.64, 53.89, 49.66, 18.33; HRMS (ESI) *m/z* calcd. for $C_{27}H_{25}N_8O_4S$ $[M + H]^+$ 541.1765, found 541.1781.

3-((4-Amino-3-(2,3-dihydrobenzo[b][1,4]dioxin-6-yl)-1H-pyrazolo[3,4-d]pyrimidin-1-yl)methyl)-2-(2,6-dimethylphenyl)-2H-benzo[e][1,2,4]thiadiazine 1,1-dioxide (**15e**)

According to the procedures described for the synthesis of **15a**, compound **15e** were obtained as a white solid (71 mg) in 64% yield, m.p. 225–226 °C; ^{1}H-NMR (DMSO-d_6) δ 8.31 (s, 1H, NH), 8.08 (s, 1H, Ar-H), 7.94 (dd, *J* = 7.8, 1.2 Hz, 1H, Ar-H), 7.82 (td, *J* = 7.8, 1.2 Hz, 1H, Ar-H), 7.65 (td, *J* = 7.8, 1.2 Hz, 1H, Ar-H), 7.51 (d, *J* = 8.4 Hz, 1H, Ar-H), 7.24 (t, *J* = 8.4 Hz, 1H, Ar-H), 7.14 (d, *J* = 7.8 Hz, 2H, Ar-H), 7.11–7.09 (m, 2H, Ar-H), 7.02 (d, *J* = 7.8 Hz, 1H, Ar-H), 5.18 (s, 2H, NCH_2), 4.30 (s, 4H, OCH_2CH_2O), 2.01 (s, 6H, 2,6-$(CH_3)_2$); ^{13}C-NMR (DMSO-d_6) δ 158.45, 156.25, 155.47, 151.92, 144.79, 144.60, 144.23, 141.74, 138.66, 134.86, 131.94, 130.47, 129.68, 129.12, 128.48, 127.83, 126.18, 121.59, 121.19, 118.30, 117.23, 97.63, 79.64, 64.67, 64.59, 49.62, 18.30; HRMS (ESI) *m/z* calcd. for $C_{29}H_{26}N_7O_4S$ $[M + H]^+$ 568.1761, found 568.1775.

3-((4-Amino-3-(benzo[d][1,3]dioxol-5-yl)-1H-pyrazolo[3,4-d]pyrimidin-1-yl)methyl)-2-(2,6-dimethyl-phenyl)-2H-benzo[e][1,2,4]thiadiazine 1,1-dioxide (**15f**)

According to the procedures described for the synthesis of **15a**, compound **15f** were obtained as a white solid (29 mg) in 34% yield, m.p. > 250 °C; ^{1}H-NMR (DMSO-d_6) δ 8.31 (s, 1H, NH), 8.08 (s, 1H, Ar-H), 7.94 (dd, *J* = 7.8, 1.2 Hz, 1H, Ar-H), 7.82 (td, *J* = 7.8, 1.2 Hz, 1H, Ar-H), 7.65 (td, *J* = 7.8, 1.2 Hz, 1H, Ar-H), 7.50 (d, *J* = 7.8 Hz, 1H, Ar-H), 7.25 (t, *J* = 7.8 Hz, 1H, Ar-H), 7.15 (d, *J* = 7.2 Hz, 2H, Ar-H), 7.12–7.09 (m, 2H, Ar-H), 7.07 (d, *J* = 8.4, 1H, Ar-H), 6.10 (s, 2H, OCH_2O), 5.17 (s, 2H, NCH_2), 2.01 (s, 6H, 2,6-$(CH_3)_2$); ^{13}C-NMR (DMSO-d_6) δ 158.44, 156.28, 155.47, 151.89, 148.36, 144.98, 141.73, 138.67, 134.87, 131.93, 130.49, 129.70, 129.14, 128.50, 127.82, 126.85, 122.65, 121.19, 109.44, 108.80, 101.89, 97.65, 79.64, 49.62, 18.30; HRMS (ESI) *m/z* calcd. for $C_{28}H_{24}N_7O_4S$ $[M + H]^+$ 554.1605, found 554.1614.

3-((4-Amino-3-(4-methoxyphenyl)-1H-pyrazolo[3,4-d]pyrimidin-1-yl)methyl)-2-(2,6-dimethylphenyl)-2H-benzo[e][1,2,4]thiadiazine 1,1-dioxide (**15g**)

According to the procedures described for the synthesis of **15a**, compound **15g** were obtained as a white solid (45 mg) in 74% yield, m.p. 248–249 °C; ^{1}H-NMR (DMSO-d_6) δ 8.32 (s, 1H, NH), 8.09 (s, 1H, Ar-H), 7.94 (dd, *J* = 7.8, 1.2 Hz, 1H, Ar-H), 7.82 (td, *J* = 7.8, 1.2 Hz, 1H, Ar-H), 7.65 (td, *J* = 7.8, 1.2 Hz, 1H, Ar-H), 7.57 (d, *J* = 8.4 Hz, 2H, Ar-H), 7.50 (d, *J* = 8.4 Hz, 1H, Ar-H), 7.25 (t, *J* = 7.8 Hz, 1H, Ar-H), 7.15 (d, *J* = 7.8 Hz, 2H, Ar-H), 7.11 (d, *J* = 8.4 Hz, 2H, Ar-H), 5.19 (s, 2H, NCH_2), 3.82 (s, 3H, OCH_3), 2.02 (s, 6H, 2,6-$(CH_3)_2$); ^{13}C-NMR (DMSO-d_6) δ160.18, 158.51, 156.26, 155.51, 151.92, 145.03, 141.75, 138.69, 134.85, 131.93, 130.48, 129.95, 129.69, 129.10, 128.49, 127.82, 125.43, 121.19, 115.12, 97.70, 79.63, 55.72, 49.60, 18.34; HRMS (ESI) *m/z* calcd. for $C_{28}H_{26}N_7O_3S$ $[M + H]^+$ 540.1812, found 540.1829.

3-((4-Amino-3-(3-methoxyphenyl)-1H-pyrazolo[3,4-d]pyrimidin-1-yl)methyl)-2-(2,6-dimethylphenyl)-2H-benzo[e][1,2,4]thiadiazine 1,1-dioxide (**15h**)

According to the procedures described for the synthesis of **15a**, compound **15h** were obtained as a white solid (46 mg) in 59% yield, m.p. 221–222 °C; ^{1}H-NMR (DMSO-d_6) δ 8.31 (s, 1H), 8.10 (s, 1H, Ar-H), 7.94 (dd, *J* = 7.8, 1.2 Hz, 1H, Ar-H), 7.82 (td, *J* = 7.8, 1.2 Hz, 1H, Ar-H), 7.63 (td, *J* = 7.8, 1.2 Hz, 1H, Ar-H), 7.50 (d, *J* = 7.8 Hz, 1H, Ar-H), 7.47 (t, *J* = 7.8 Hz, 1H, Ar-H), 7.26 (t, *J* = 7.8 Hz, 1H, Ar-H), 7.23 (d, *J* = 7.8 Hz, 1H, Ar-H), 7.20–7.11 (m, 3H, Ar-H), 7.06 (dd, *J* = 8.4, 2.4 Hz, 1H, Ar-H), 5.21 (s, 2H, NCH_2), 3.82 (s, 3H, OCH_3), 2.02 (s, 6H, 2,6-$(CH_3)_2$); ^{13}C-NMR (DMSO-d_6) δ 160.11, 158.43, 156.31, 155.56, 151.88, 145.02, 141.72, 138.70, 134.87, 134.36, 131.95, 130.86, 130.51, 129.71, 129.14, 128.48, 127.83, 121.20, 120.76, 115.19, 113.85, 97.74, 79.64, 55.63, 49.68, 18.32; HRMS (ESI) *m/z* calcd. for $C_{28}H_{26}N_7O_3S$ $[M + H]^+$ 540.1812, found 540.1825.

3-((4-Amino-3-(4-(trifluoromethoxy)phenyl)-1H-pyrazolo[3,4-d]pyrimidin-1-yl)methyl)-2-(2,6-dimethyl-phenyl)-2H-benzo[e][1,2,4]thiadiazine 1,1-dioxide (**15i**)

According to the procedures described for the synthesis of **15a**, compound **15i** were obtained as a white solid (61 mg) in 61% yield, m.p. 206–207 °C; ^{1}H-NMR (DMSO-d_6) δ 8.12 (s, 1H, Ar-H), 7.94 (dd, *J*

= 8.4, 1.2 Hz, 1H, Ar-H), 7.81 (dt, J = 8.4, 1.2 Hz, 1H, Ar-H), 7.76 (d, J =8.4 Hz, 2H, Ar-H), 7.65 (dt, J = 8.4, 0.6 Hz, 1H, Ar-H), 7.52 (d, J = 7.8 Hz, 2H, Ar-H), 7.48 (d, J = 7.8 Hz, 1H, Ar-H), 7.26 (t, J = 7.8 Hz, 1H, Ar-H), 7.16 (d, J = 7.8 Hz, 2 H, Ar-H), 5.21 (s, 2H), 2.03 (s, 6H); ^{13}C-NMR (DMSO-d_6) δ 158.52, 156.38, 155.72, 151.77, 149.08, 143.91, 141.70, 138.70, 134.87, 132.28, 131.90, 130.59, 130.53, 129.72, 129.14, 128.50, 127.80, 122.10, 121.21, 120.57 (q, $J_{C\text{–}F}$ = 256.70 Hz), 97.73, 49.68, 18.34; HRMS (ESI) *m/z* calcd. for $C_{28}H_{23}F_3N_7O_3S$ [M + H]$^+$ 594.1530, found 594.1547.

3-((4-Amino-3-phenyl-1H-pyrazolo[3,4-d]pyrimidin-1-yl)methyl)-2-(2,6-dimethylphenyl)-2H-benzo[e]-[1,2,4]thiadiazine 1,1-dioxide (**15j**)

According to the procedures described for the synthesis of **15a**, compound **15j** were obtained as a white solid (40 mg) in 73% yield, m.p. 193–194 °C; ^{1}H-NMR (DMSO-d_6) δ 8.30 (s, 1H, NH), 8.09 (s, 1H, Ar-H), 7.92 (dd, J = 7.8, 1.2 Hz, 1H, Ar-H), 7.80 (td, J = 7.8, 1.2 Hz, 1H, Ar-H), 7.66–7.62 (m, 3H, Ar-H), 7.54 (t, J = 7.8 Hz, 2H, Ar-H), 7.52–7.32 (m, 2H, Ar-H), 7.24 (t, J = 7.8 Hz, 2H, Ar-H), 7.14 (d, J = 7.8 Hz, 2H, Ar-H), 5.19 (s, 2H, NCH_2), 2.01 (s, 6H, 2,6-$(CH_3)_2$); ^{13}C-NMR (DMSO-d_6) δ 1158.46, 156.31, 155.60, 151.86, 145.16, 141.72, 138.69, 134.54, 133.53, 132.51, 131.99, 131.92, 130.51, 130.47, 129.71, 129.67, 129.27, 129.20, 128.60, 127.81, 121.20, 97.73, 79.65, 49.65, 18.34; HRMS (ESI) *m/z* calcd. for $C_{27}H_{24}N_7O_2S$ [M + H]$^+$ 510.1707, found 510.1722.

3-((4-Amino-3-(1H-indol-5-yl)-1H-pyrazolo[3,4-d]pyrimidin-1-yl)methyl)-2-(2,6-dimethylphenyl)-7-fluoro-2H-benzo[e][1,2,4]thiadiazine 1,1-dioxide (**16a**)

According to the procedures described for the synthesis of **15a**, compound **16a** were obtained as a white solid (65 mg) in 73% yield, m.p. 132–133 °C; ^{1}H-NMR (DMSO-d_6) δ 8.30 (s, 1H, NH), 8.08 (s, 1H, Ar-H), 7.91 (dd, J = 7.2, 2.4 Hz, 1H, Ar-H), 7.81 (brs, 1H, Ar-H), 7.69 (td, J = 9.6, 3.0 Hz, 1H, Ar-H), 7.61 (dd, J = 9.0, 4.8 Hz, 1H, Ar-H), 7.56 (d, J = 8.4 Hz, 1H, Ar-H), 7.44 (t, J = 3.0 Hz, 1H, Ar-H), 7.36 (dd, J = 8.4, 1.8 Hz, 1H, Ar-H), 7.25 (t, J = 7.28Hz, 1H, Ar-H), 7.16 (t, J = 7.8 Hz, 2H, Ar-H), 6.54 (s, 1H, 3-CH-indolyl), 5.20 (s, 2H, NCH_2), 2.01 (s, 6H, 2,6-$(CH_3)_2$); ^{13}C-NMR (DMSO-d_6) δ 160.08 (d, $J_{C\text{–}F}$ = 250.7 Hz), 158.52, 156.23, 155.41, 151.51, 146.84, 138.68, 138.61 (d, $J_{C\text{–}F}$ = 3.0 Hz), 136.53, 131.81, 131.44 (d, $J_{C\text{–}F}$ = 9.1 Hz), 130.55, 129.74, 128.66 (d, $J_{C\text{–}F}$ = 9.1 Hz), 128.46, 127.05, 123.87, 122.67 (d, $J_{C\text{–}F}$ = 24.2 Hz), 121.74, 120.52, 112.67, 108.19 (d, $J_{C\text{–}F}$ = 27.2 Hz), 102.21, 97.85, 79.65, 49.57, 18.32; HRMS (ESI) *m/z* calcd. for $C_{29}H_{24}FN_8O_2S$ [M + H]$^+$ 567.1721, found 567.1739.

3-((A-amino-3-(3,4-dimethoxyphenyl)-1H-pyrazolo[3,4-d]pyrimidin-1-yl)methyl)-2-(2,6-dimethylphenyl)-7-fluoro-2H-benzo[e][1,2,4]thiadiazine 1,1-dioxide (**16b**)

According to the procedures described for the synthesis of **15a**, compound **16b** were obtained as a white solid (47 mg) in 51% yield, m.p. 229–230 °C; ^{1}H-NMR (DMSO-d_6) δ 8.31 (s, 1H, NH), 8.09 (s, 1H, Ar-H), 7.91 (dd, J = 7.2, 2.4 Hz, 1H, Ar-H), 7.69 (td, J = 9.0, 2.4 Hz, 1H, Ar-H), 7.59 (dd, J = 9.0, 4.8 Hz, 1H, Ar-H), 7.26 (t, J = 7.8 Hz, 1H, Ar-H), 7.21–7.10 (m, 5H, Ar-H), 5.19 (s, 2H, NCH_2), 3.82 (s, 3H, OCH_3), 3.81 (s, 3H, OCH_3), 2.01 (s, 6H, 2,6-$(CH_3)_2$); ^{13}C-NMR (DMSO-d_6) δ 160.78 (d, $J_{C\text{–}F}$ = 250.7 Hz), 158.51, 156.27, 155.49, 151.46, 149.84, 149.52, 145.24, 138.70, 138.57 (d, $J_{C\text{–}F}$ = 3.0 Hz), 131.84, 131.41 (d, $J_{C\text{–}F}$ = 7.6 Hz), 130.57, 129.74, 128.69 (d, $J_{C\text{–}F}$ = 7.6 Hz), 125.52, 122.66 (d, $J_{C\text{–}F}$ = 24.2 Hz), 121.03, 112.72, 112.02, 108.20 (d, $J_{C\text{–}F}$ = 27.2 Hz), 97.71, 79.65, 56.04, 55.89, 49.60, 18.31; HRMS (ESI) *m/z* calcd. for $C_{29}H_{27}FN_7O_4S$ [M + H]$^+$ 588.1824, found 588.1838.

3-((4-Amino-3-(3-fluoro-4-methoxyphenyl)-1H-pyrazolo[3,4-d]pyrimidin-1-yl)methyl)-2-(2,6-dimethyl-phenyl)-7-fluoro-2H-benzo[e][1,2,4]thiadiazine 1,1-dioxide (**16c**)

According to the procedures described for the synthesis of **15a**, compound **16c** were obtained as a white solid (76 mg) in 84% yield, m.p. 201–202 °C; ^{1}H-NMR (DMSO-d_6) δ 8.31 (s, 1H, NH), 8.09 (s, 1H, Ar-H), 7.91 (dd, J = 7.2, 3.0 Hz, 1H, Ar-H), 7.69 (td, J = 7.4, 2.4 Hz, 1H, Ar-H), 7.59 (dd, J = 9.0, 4.2 Hz, 1H, Ar-H), 7.44–7.38 (m, 2H, Ar-H), 7.33 (t, J = 9.0 Hz, 1H, Ar-H), 7.26 (t, J = 7.2 Hz, 1H, Ar-H), 7.15 (d, J = 7.8 Hz, 2H, Ar-H), 5.19 (s, 2H, NCH_2), 3.90 (s, 3H, OCH_3), 2.01 (s, 6H, 2,6-$(CH_3)_2$);

^{13}C-NMR (DMSO-d_6) δ 160.89 (d, $J_{C–F}$ = 250.7 Hz), 158.50, 156.34, 155.56, 152.02 (d, $J_{C–F}$ = 246.1 Hz), 151.32, 148.14 (d, $J_{C–F}$ = 10.6 Hz), 144.06, 138.68, 138.62 (d, $J_{C–F}$ = 19.6 Hz), 131.78, 131.44 (d, $J_{C–F}$ = 7.6 Hz), 130.59, 129.74, 128.66 (d, $J_{C–F}$ = 7.6 Hz), 125.76 (d, $J_{C–F}$ = 7.6 Hz), 125.21, 122.68 (d, $J_{C–F}$ = 22.7 Hz), 116.11 (d, $J_{C–F}$ = 19.6 Hz), 114.92, 108.21 (d, $J_{C–F}$ = 25.7 Hz), 97.67, 79.63, 56.59, 49.61, 18.30; HRMS (ESI) *m/z* calcd. for $C_{28}H_{24}F_2N_7O_3S$ [M + H]$^+$ 576.1624, found 576.1637.

3-((4-Amino-3-(6-methoxypyridin-3-yl)-1H-pyrazolo[3,4-d]pyrimidin-1-yl)methyl)-2-(2,6-dimethylphenyl)-7-fluoro-2H-benzo[e][1,2,4]thiadiazine 1,1-dioxide (**16d**)

According to the procedures described for the synthesis of **15a**, compound **16d** were obtained as a white solid (51 mg) in 58% yield, m.p. 225–226 °C; ^{1}H-NMR (DMSO-d_6) δ 8.38 (s, 1H, NH), 8.31 (s, 1H, Ar-H), 8.10 (s, 1H, Ar-H), 7.90 (d, *J* = 8.4 Hz, 2H, Ar-H), 7.69 (t, *J* = 7.2 Hz, 1H, Ar-H), 7.59 (dd, *J* = 9.0, 4.2 Hz, 1H, Ar-H), 7.25 (t, *J* = 7.2 Hz, 1H, Ar-H), 7.15 (d, *J* = 8.4 Hz, 2H, Ar-H), 6.97 (d, *J* = 8.4 Hz, 1H, Ar-H), 5.20 (s, 2H, NCH_2), 3.92 (s, 3H, OCH_3), 2.01 (s, 6H, 2,6-$(CH_3)_2$); ^{13}C-NMR (DMSO-d_6) δ 164.15, 160.89 (d, $J_{C–F}$ = 250.7 Hz), 158.60, 156.39, 155.59, 151.29, 146.69, 142.41, 139.29, 138.69, 138.54 (d, $J_{C–F}$ = 3.0 Hz), 131.77, 131.45 (d, $J_{C–F}$ = 7.6 Hz), 130.59, 129.74, 128.66 (d, $J_{C–F}$ = 9.1 Hz), 122.75, 122.68, 122.67 (d, $J_{C–F}$ = 22.7 Hz), 111.48, 108.20 (d, $J_{C–F}$ = 27.2 Hz), 97.93, 79.64, 53.89, 49.63, 18.32; HRMS (ESI) *m/z* calcd. for $C_{27}H_{24}FN_8O_3S$ [M + H]$^+$ 559.1671, found 559.1678.

3.2. PI3K Kinase Assay

The ADP-Glo luminescent assay was used for PI3Kδ, PI3Kβ and PI3Kγ isoforms and the kinase-Glo luminescent assay was used for PI3Kα according to the standard protocols of Promega [40]. PI-103 was used as a positive control. The compounds were tested from 1 μM or 10 μM, 3-fold dilution, in duplicate for 10 concentrations. The kinase reaction was done in 384-well plate (Corning, Los Altos, MA, USA). Each well was loaded with test compounds (in 100% DMSO) and reaction buffer containing PI substrate. After the PI3K proteins were then added, the reaction was started by the addition of PIP2 and ATP prepared in the reaction buffer and ran for either 60 (for PI3Kα, PI3Kβ, and PI3Kγ) or 120 min (for PI3Kδ). ADP-Glo reagent was then added to terminate the reavtion. The plates were then read in a Synergy 2 reader (BioTek, Shanghai, China) for luminescence detection.

3.3. Cell Proliferation Assay

Cell proliferation was evaluated by The CellTiter-Glo luminescent cell viability assay (Promega, Shanghai, China) was used to evaluate the inhibitory activity of compounds **15a** and **15b** following the manufacturer's protocol. In brief, SU-DHL-6 (ATCC) cells were seeded in 96-well plates (Corning, Los Altos, MA, USA) at density of 1 × 10^4 cells per well, and incubated with medium alone or with the tested compounds at the indicated concentrations (50 μM in DMSO, 3-fold dilution, in duplicate for 10 concentrations). 50 μL CellTiter-Glo (Promega, Shanghai, China) reagent was added to each well to induce cell lysis, and the plate was incubated at room temperature for 10 min to stabilize luminescent signal. After 100 μL of the mixture from each well was transferred to a new 96-well black plate, the fluorescence signal was read on EnVision (Shanghai, China) and the data were analysized by XLFit 4 software (IDBS, Berlin, Germany).

3.4. Molecular Docking

X-ray cocrystal structure of PI3Kδ enzyme was downloaded from RCSB Protein Date Bank (PDB ID: 2WXH) [42]. The molecular docking of **15a** and **15b** was carried out following the same procedures as reported for compounds **3** and **4** [33].

4. Conclusions

In a continuous study to find more potent and selective PI3Kδ inhibitors based on the rotation-limiting strategy, we substituted the carbonyl in the quinazolinone core for the sulfonyl group, designed and synthesized a series of novel 2*H*-benzo[*e*][1,2,4]thiadiazine 1,1-dioxide derivatives

15a–J and **16a–d**. In agreement with the quinazolinone derivatives, the introduction of a 5-indolyl or 3,4-dimethoxyphenyl at the affinity pocket generated the most potent analogues **15a** and **15b** with the IC_{50} values of 217 to 266 nM, respectively. In comparison with the quinazolinone lead compounds **3** and **4**, the 2*H*-benzo[*e*][1,2,4]thiadiazine 1,1-dioxide derivatives exhibited much reduced PI3Kδ inhibitory activity, but maintained high selectivity over other PI3K isoforms. Unlike the quinazolinone lead compound **4** that was a dual PI3Kδ/γ inhibitor, the 2*H*-benzo[*e*][1,2,4]thiadiazine 1,1-dioxide **15b** was more than 21-fold selective over PI3Kγ. This may provide a structural base for the further design of more potent and selective PI3Kδ inhibitors. In agreement with their high PI3Kδ inhibitory activity, **15a** and **15b** exhibited high antiproliferative potency against B-cell leukemia SU-DHL-6 cells.

Supplementary Materials: Supplementary materials are available online.

Author Contributions: Conceptualization, Y.-P.G. and Z.-P.L.; methodology, Y.-P.G., L.-Q.T. and T.-S.L.; validation, Y.-P.G., L.-Q.T. and T.-S.L.; formal analysis, L.-Q.T. and Y.-P.G.; investigation, Y.-P.G., L.-Q.T. and T.-S.L.; resources, Z.-P.L.; data curation, L.-Q.T. and Y.-P.G.; writing—original draft preparation, L.-Q.T.; writing—review and editing, Z.-P.L.; visualization, Y.-P.G. and L.-Q.T.; supervision, Z.-P.L.; project administration, Z.-P.L.; funding acquisition, Z.-P.L.

Funding: This work was partially supported by the key research and development program of Shandong province (2017CXGC1401).

Conflicts of Interest: The authors declare no conflict of interest.

Abbreviations

PI3Ks	Phosphoinositide 3-kinases
PIP2	Phosphatidylinositol 4,5-bisphosphate
NBS	*N*-Bromosuccinimide
ADP	Adenosine diphosphate
ATP	Adenosine triphosphate
DMSO	Dimethyl sulfoxide
APDS	PI3Kδ syndrome
FL	Follicular lymphoma
SLL	Small lymphocytic lymphoma
CLL	Chronic lymphocytic leukemia

References

1. Toker, A.; Cantley, L.C. Signalling through the lipid products of phosphoinositide-3-OH kinase. *Nature* **1997**, *387*, 673–676. [CrossRef] [PubMed]
2. Cantley, L.C. The phosphoinositide 3-kinase pathway. *Science* **2002**, *296*, 1655–1657. [CrossRef] [PubMed]
3. Brachmann, S.M.; Yballe, C.M.; Innocenti, M.; Deane, J.A.; Fruman, D.A.; Thomas, S.M.; Cantley, L.C. Role of phosphoinositide 3-kinase regulatory isoforms in development and actin rearrangement. *Mol. Cell. Biol.* **2005**, *25*, 2593–2606. [CrossRef] [PubMed]
4. Vanhaesebroeck, B.; Guillermet-Guibert, J.; Graupera, M.; Bilanges, B. The emerging mechanisms of isoform specific PI3K signaling. *Nat. Rev. Mol. Cell Biol.* **2010**, *11*, 329–341. [CrossRef]
5. Engelman, J.A.; Luo, J.; Cantley, L.C. The evolution of phosphatidylinositol 3-kinases as regulators of growth and metabolism. *Nat. Rev. Genet.* **2006**, *7*, 606–619. [CrossRef] [PubMed]
6. Jimenez, C.; Hernandez, C.; Pimentel, B.; Carrera, A.C. The p85 regulatory subunit controls sequential activation of phosphoinositide 3-kinase by tyr kinases and ras. *J. Biol. Chem.* **2002**, *277*, 41556–41562. [CrossRef] [PubMed]
7. Brock, C.; Schaefer, M.; Reusch, H.P.; Czupalla, C.; Michalke, M.; Spicher, K.; Schultz, G.; Nurnberg, B. Roles of Gβγ in membrane recruitment and activation of p110γ/p101 phosphoinositide 3-kinase γ. *J. Cell Biol.* **2003**, *160*, 89–99. [CrossRef]
8. Okkenhaug, K.; Vanhaesebroeck, B. PI3K in lymphocyte development, differentiation and activation. *Nat. Rev. Immunol.* **2003**, *3*, 317–330. [CrossRef]

9. Liu, L.; Puri, K.D.; Penninger, J.M.; Kubes, P. Leukocyte PI3Kγ and PI3Kδ have temporally distinct roles for leukocyte recruitment in vivo. *Blood* **2007**, *110*, 1191–1198. [CrossRef]
10. Thomas, M.J.; Smith, A.; Head, D.H.; Milne, L.; Nicholls, A.; Pearce, W.; Vanhaesebroeck, B.; Wymann, M.P.; Hirsch, E.; Trifilieff, A.; et al. Airway inflammation: Chemokine-induced neutrophilia and the class I phosphoinositide 3-kinases. *Eur. J. Immunol.* **2005**, *35*, 1283–1291. [CrossRef]
11. Fruman, D.A.; Rommel, C. PI3K and cancer: Lessons, challenges and opportunities. *Nat. Rev. Drug Discov.* **2014**, *13*, 140–156. [CrossRef] [PubMed]
12. Thorpe, L.M.; Yuzugullu, H.; Zhao, J.J. PI3K in cancer: Divergent roles of isoforms, modes of activation and therapeutic targeting. *Nat. Rev. Cancer* **2015**, *15*, 7–24. [CrossRef] [PubMed]
13. Janku, F. Phosphoinositide 3-kinase (PI3K) pathway inhibitors in solid tumors: From laboratory to patients. *Cancer Treat. Rev.* **2017**, *59*, 93–101. [CrossRef] [PubMed]
14. Fruman, D.A.; Chiu, H.; Hopkins, B.D.; Bagrodia, S.; Cantley, L.C.; Abraham, R.T. The PI3K pathway in human disease. *Cell* **2017**, *170*, 605–635. [CrossRef]
15. Zhao, W.; Qiu, Y.; Kong, D. Class I phosphatidylinositol 3-kinase inhibitors for cancer therapy. *Acta Pharm. Sin. B* **2017**, *7*, 27–37. [CrossRef]
16. Garces, A.E.; Stocks, M.J. Class 1 PI3K clinical candidates and recent inhibitor design strategies: A medicinal chemistry perspective. *J. Med. Chem.* **2019**, *62*, 4815–4850. [CrossRef]
17. Knight, Z.A.; Gonzalez, B.; Feldman, M.E.; Zunder, E.R.; Goldenberg, D.D.; Williams, O.; Loewith, R.; Stokoe, D.; Balla, A.; Toth, B.; et al. A pharmacological map of the PI3-K family defines a role for P110α in insulin signaling. *Cell* **2006**, *125*, 733–747. [CrossRef]
18. Huang, X.; Liu, G.; Guo, J.; Su, Z. The PI3K/AKT Pathway in obesity and type 2 diabetes. *Int. J. Biol. Sci.* **2018**, *14*, 1483–1496. [CrossRef]
19. Jackson, S.P.; Schoenwaelder, S.M.; Goncalves, I.; Nesbitt, W.S.; Yap, C.L.; Wright, C.E.; Kenche, V.; Anderson, K.E.; Dopheide, S.M.; Yuan, Y.; et al. PI 3-Kinase P110β: A new target for antithrombotic therapy. *Nat. Med.* **2005**, *11*, 507–514. [CrossRef]
20. Jackson, S.P.; Schoenwaelder, S.M. Antithrombotic phosphoinositide 3-kinase β inhibitors in humans: A 'shear' delight! *J. Thromb. Haemostasis* **2012**, *10*, 2123–2126. [CrossRef]
21. Cushing, T.D.; Metz, D.P.; Whittington, D.A.; McGee, L.R. PI3Kδ and PI3Kγ as targets for autoimmune and inflammatory diseases. *J. Med. Chem.* **2012**, *55*, 8559–8581. [CrossRef] [PubMed]
22. Rowan, W.C.; Smith, J.L.; Affleck, K.; Amour, A. Targeting phosphoinositide 3-kinase δ for allergic asthma. *Biochem. Soc. Trans.* **2012**, *40*, 240–245. [CrossRef] [PubMed]
23. Yoo, E.J.; Ojiaku, C.A.; Sunder, K.; Panettieri, R.A. Phosphoinositide 3-kinase in asthma: Novel roles and therapeutic approaches. *Am. J. Respir. Cell Mol. Biol.* **2017**, *56*, 700–707. [CrossRef] [PubMed]
24. Perry, M.W.D.; Abdulai, R.; Mogemark, M.; Petersen, J.; Thomas, M.J.; Valastro, B.; Eriksson, A.W. Evolution of PI3Kγ and δ Inhibitors for inflammatory and autoimmune diseases. *J. Med. Chem.* **2019**, *62*, 4783–4814. [CrossRef]
25. Kracker, S.; Curtis, J.; Ibrahim, M.A.A.; Sediva, A.; Salisbury, J.; Campr, V.; Debré, M.; Edgar, J.D.M.; Imai, K.; Picard, C.; et al. Occurrence of B-cell lymphomas in patients with activated phosphoinositide 3-kinase δ syndrome. *J. Allergy Clin. Immunol.* **2014**, *134*, 233–236. [CrossRef]
26. Elkaim, E.; Neven, B.; Bruneau, J.; Mitsui-Sekinaka, K.; Stanislas, A.; Heurtier, L.; Lucas, C.L.; Matthews, H.; Deau, M.-C.; Sharapova, S.; et al. Clinical and immunologic phenotype associated with activated phosphoinositide 3-kinase δ syndrome 2: A cohort study. *J. Allergy Clin. Immunol.* **2016**, *138*, 210–218. [CrossRef]
27. Coulter, T.I.; Chandra, A.; Bacon, C.M.; Babar, J.; Curtis, J.; Screaton, N.; Goodlad, J.R.; Farmer, G.; Steele, C.L.; Leahy, T.R.; et al. Clinical spectrum and features of activated phosphoinositide 3-kinase δ syndrome: A large patient cohort study. *J. Allergy Clin. Immunol.* **2017**, *139*, 597–606. [CrossRef]
28. Conte, E.; Gili, E.; Fruciano, M.; Korfei, M.; Fagone, E.; Iemmolo, M.; Lo Furno, D.; Giuffrida, R.; Crimi, N.; Guenther, A.; et al. PI3K P110γ overexpression in idiopathic pulmonary fibrosis lung tissue and fibroblast cells: In vitro effects of its inhibition. *Lab. Investig.* **2013**, *93*, 566–576. [CrossRef]
29. Furman, R.R.; Sharman, J.P.; Coutre, S.E.; Cheson, B.D.; Pagel, J.M.; Hillmen, P.; Barrientos, J.C.; Zelenetz, A.D.; Kipps, T.J.; Flinn, I.; et al. Idelalisib and rituximab in relapsed chronic lymphocytic leukemia. *N. Engl. J. Med.* **2014**, *370*, 997–1007. [CrossRef]
30. Cheah, C.Y.; Fowler, N.H. Idelalisib in the management of lymphoma. *Blood* **2016**, *128*, 331–336. [CrossRef]

31. Vangapandu, H.V.; Jain, N.; Gandhi, V. Duvelisib: A phosphoinositide-3 kinase δ,γ inhibitor for chronic lymphocytic leukemia. *Expert Opin. Investig. Drugs* **2017**, *26*, 625–636. [CrossRef] [PubMed]
32. Greenwell, I.B.; Flowers, C.R.; Blumb, K.A.; Cohen, J.B. Clinical use of PI3K inhibitors in B-cell lymphoid malignancies: Today and tomorrow. *Expert Rev. Anticancer Ther.* **2017**, *17*, 271–279. [CrossRef] [PubMed]
33. Ma, C.-C.; Zhang, C.-M.; Tang, L.-Q.; Liu, Z.-P. Discovery of novel quinazolinone derivatives as high potent and selective PI3Kδ and PI3Kδ/γ inhibitors. *Eur. J. Med. Chem.* **2018**, *151*, 9–17. [CrossRef] [PubMed]
34. Khan, F.A.; Mushtaq, S.; Naz, S.; Farooq, U.; Zaidi, A.; Bukhari, S.M.; Rauf, A.; Mubarak, M.S. Sulfonamides as potential bioactive scaffolds. *Curr. Org. Chem.* **2018**, *22*, 818–830. [CrossRef]
35. Gulcin, I.; Taslimi, P. Sulfonamide inhibitors: A patent review 2013-present. *Expert Opin. Ther. Pat.* **2018**, *28*, 541–549. [CrossRef]
36. Zhao, C.; Rakesh, K.P.; Ravidar, L.; Fang, W.-Y.; Qin, H.-L. Pharmaceutical and medicinal significance of sulfur (S^{VI})-Containing motifs for drug discovery: A critical review. *Eur. J. Med. Chem.* **2019**, *162*, 679–734. [CrossRef]
37. Rassadin, V.A.; Tomashevskiy, A.A.; Sokolov, V.V.; Ringe, A.; Magull, J.; de Meijere, A. Facile access to bicyclic sultams with methyl-1-sulfonylcyclopropane-1-carboxylate moieties. *Eur. J. Org. Chem.* **2009**, 2635–2641. [CrossRef]
38. Murphy, R.C.; Ojo, K.K.; Larson, E.T.; Castellanos-Gonzalez, A.; Perera, B.G.; Keyloun, K.R.; Kim, J.E.; Bhandari, J.G.; Muller, N.R.; Verlinde, C.L.; et al. Discovery of potent and selective inhibitors of CDPK1 from *C. parvum* and *T. gondii*. *ACS Med. Chem. Lett.* **2010**, *1*, 331–335. [CrossRef]
39. Koresawa, M.; Okabe, T. High-throughput screening with quantitation of ATP consumption: A universal non-radioisotope, homogeneous assay for protein kinase. *Assay Drug Dev. Technol.* **2004**, *2*, 153–160. [CrossRef]
40. Raynaud, F.I.; Eccles, S.A.; Patel, S.; Alix, S.; Box, G.; Chuckowree, I.; Folkes, A.; Gowan, S.; De Haven Brandon, A.; Di Stefano, F.; et al. Biological properties of potent inhibitors of class I phosphatidylinositide 3-kinases: From PI-103 through PI-540, PI-620 to the oral agent GDC-0941. *Mol. Cancer Ther.* **2009**, *8*, 1725–1738. [CrossRef]
41. Freeman, J.H.; Wagner, E.C. 3,4-Dihydro-1,2,4-benzothiadiazine. *J. Org. Chem.* **1951**, *16*, 815–837. [CrossRef]
42. Berndt, A.; Miller, S.; Williams, O.; Le, D.D.; Houseman, B.T.; Pacold, J.I.; Gorrec, F.; Hon, W.C.; Ren, P.; Liu, Y.; et al. The p110δ structure: Mechanisms for selectivity and potency of new PI(3)K inhibitors. *Nat. Chem. Biol.* **2010**, *6*, 117–124. [CrossRef] [PubMed]

Sample Availability: Samples of the compounds **15a–j** and **16a–d** are available from the authors.

molecules

MDPI

Article

Design, Synthesis, and Biological Evaluation of Novel Thienopyrimidine Derivatives as PI3Kα Inhibitors

Lide Yu [1,2,†], Qinqin Wang [1,†], Caolin Wang [1], Binliang Zhang [1], Zunhua Yang [2], Yuanying Fang [2], Wufu Zhu [1,*] and Pengwu Zheng [1,*]

1 Jiangxi Provincial Key Laboratory of Drug Design and Evaluation, School of Pharmacy, Jiangxi Science & Technology Normal University, 605 Fenglin Road, Nanchang 330013, China; 20020680@jxutcm.edu.cn (L.Y.); m15180134379_2@163.com (Q.W.); wangcllw@163.com (C.W.); zbl1045762244@163.com (B.Z.)

2 College of Pharmacy, Jiangxi University of Traditional Chinese Medicine, Nanchang 330004, China; mtdzcool@163.com (Z.Y.); fangyuanying@163.com (Y.F.)

* Correspondence: zhuwf@jxstnu.edu.cn (W.Z.); zhengpw@126.com (P.Z.); Tel.: +86-791-8380-2393(W.Z.)

† These authors contributed equally to the paper.

Received: 23 August 2019; Accepted: 19 September 2019; Published: 20 September 2019

Abstract: Three series of novel thienopyrimidine derivatives **9a–l**, **15a–l**, and **18a–h** were designed and synthesized, and their IC_{50} values against four cancer cell lines HepG-2, A549, PC-3, and MCF-7 were evaluated. Most compounds show moderate cytotoxicity against the tested cancer cell lines. The most promising compound **9a** showed moderate activity with IC_{50} values of 12.32 ± 0.96, 11.30 ± 1.19, 14.69 ± 1.32, and 9.80 ± 0.93 μM, respectively. The inhibitory activities of compounds **9a** and **15a** against PI3Kα and mTOR kinase were further evaluated. Compound **9a** exhibited PI3Kα kinase inhibitory activity with IC_{50} of 9.47 ± 0.63 μM. In addition, docking studies of compounds **9a** and **15a** were also investigated.

Keywords: Thienopyrimidine; Pyrazole; PI3Kα inhibitor

1. Introduction

The PI3K-Akt-mTOR signaling pathway plays an important role in tumorigenesis and development [1,2]. The activation of related proteins in this pathway is closely related to the occurrence and development of tumors. In recent years, the development of small molecule drugs to effectively inhibit the overexpression of this pathway has become a research hotspot in cancer therapy [3]. Moreover, the study of the complex co-crystals structure of protein and small molecular Ligand also promoted the development of new drugs [4–6]. Many small molecule inhibitors targeting PI3K-Akt–mTOR signaling pathway have entered clinical studies, and some of them were even approved by FDA, such as PI3K inhibitor GDC-0941 [7]; AKT inhibitor GSK2110183 [8]; mTOR inhibitor AZD2014 (Figure 1) [9], Rapamycin, Deforolimus. PI3Kα is the most important isoform in cell proliferation in response to growth factor-tyrosine kinase pathway activation. There are currently more than ten PI3Kα inhibitors undergoing clinical trials. Many research groups are attempting to develop some more PI3Kα inhibitors.

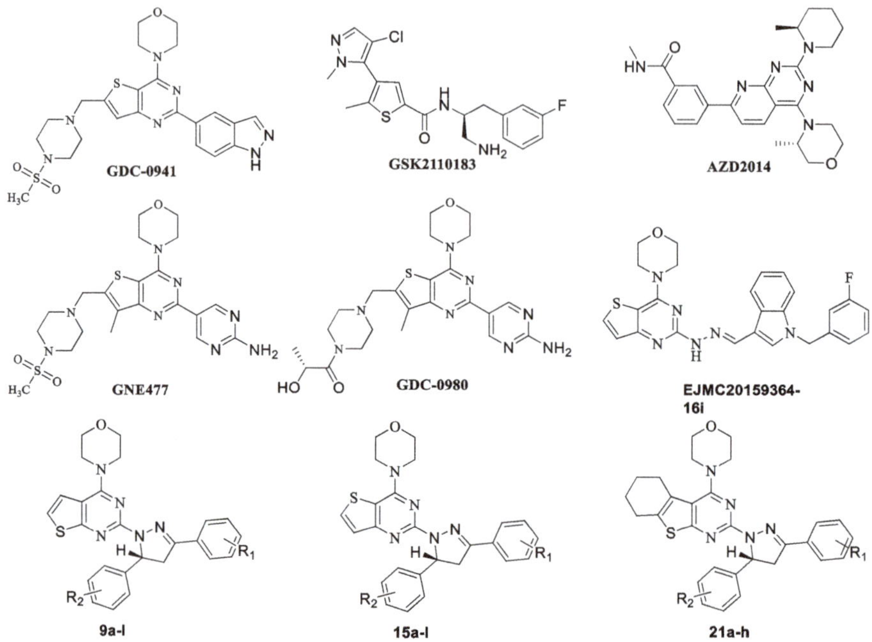

Figure 1. Structures of representative clinical PI3K/mTOR dual inhibitors and target compounds.

The thienopyrimidine core is widely used in small molecule inhibitors of the PI3K-Akt-mTOR signaling pathway. Among them, thienopyrimidine derivative GDC-0941 developed by Genentech, is the first PI3K inhibitor entering the clinical stage. Right after, several analogues of GDC-0941 were obtained. Two of them, GNE-477 and GDC-0980 (Figure 1), exhibited excellent activities and were regarded as potent PI3K/mTOR inhibitors [10,11]. Research showed that thienopyrimidines core were very important to the activity of these compounds, and it was considered to be an active pharmacophore.

In our previous research, several series of thienopyrimidine-containing compounds were designed and synthesized [12–14], one representative compound EJMC20159364-16i (Figure 1) exhibited the best in vitro cytotoxic activity and kinase inhibitory activity (PI3K, mTOR). SARs of this series of compounds were summarized. The results showed that the introduction of the flexible hydrazinyl linker at the pyrimidine 2 position helps to increase the cytotoxic activity of the target compounds. Continuous to this work, the hydrazinyl linker was kept unchanged in the new designed compounds, and we constructed a pyrazole ring on the hydrazinyl as a new flexible linker to connect with the aryl group, hoping to increase the compounds' inhibitory activity by improving the interaction of the compounds with the receptor (Figure 2). As a result, two series of thieno[2,3-*d*]pyrimidines and thieno[3,2-*d*]pyrimidines containing pyrazole unit (**9a–l**, **15a–l**) were designed and synthesized. Inspired by GDC-0084, in order to investigate the influence of the thienopyrimidine core to the activity, a flexible cyclohexane was introduced to the target compounds, resulting in a series of tricyclic thienopyrimidine compounds **21a–h**. It is expected to increase the cytotoxic activity and increase the interaction of the compounds with the enzyme to enhance the activity and selectivity. Finally, three series of thienopyrimidine derivatives containing pyrazole structure (**9a–l, 15a–l, 21a–h**) were designed, synthesized and evaluated for their cytotoxic activity.

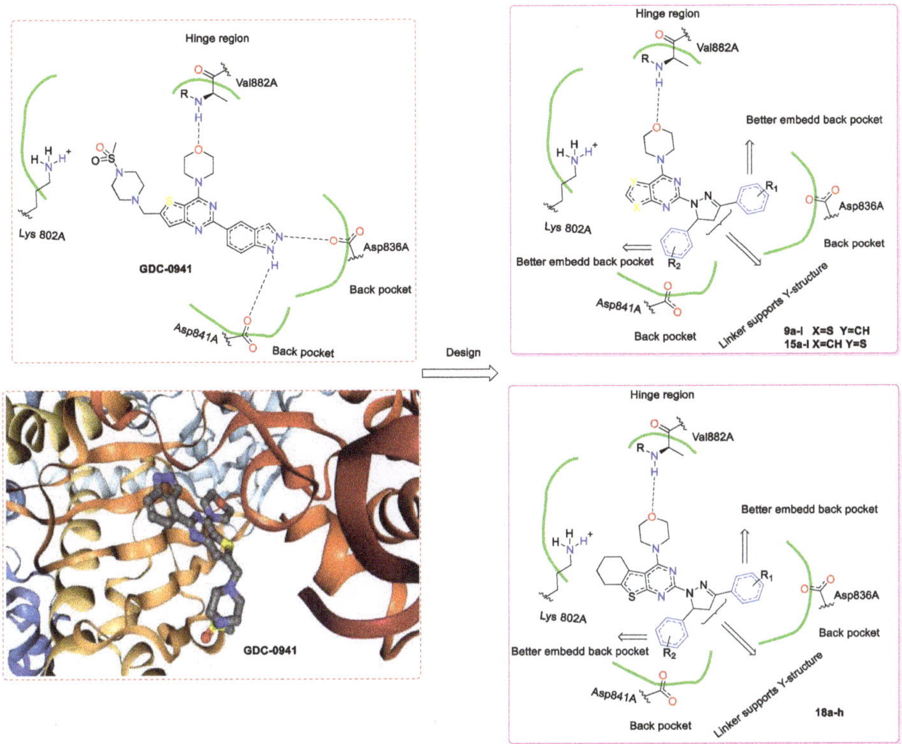

Figure 2. The design concept based on the co-crystal structure of GDC-0941 with protein.

2. Results and Discussion

2.1. Chemistry

The synthetic routes for thienopyrimidine derivatives **9a–l**, **15a–l**, and **21a–h** are outlined in Schemes 1 and 2. Condensation of the 4-substituted benzaldehydes (**1a–d**) with the 4-substituted acetophenones (**2a–e**) produced the corresponding chalcones **3a–l** (Scheme 1). Treatment of **5** with $POCl_3$ afforded 2,4-dichlorothieno[2,3-*d*]pyrimidine **6**, which was then treated with morpholine to give 4-(2-chlorothieno[2,3-*d*]pyrimidin-4-yl)morpholine **7**. Treatment of **7** with hydrazine gave the key intermediate **8**. Intermediate **8** condensed with the corresponding chalcones **3a–l** to afford the target compounds **9a–l**. The synthesis of compounds **15a–l** and **21a–h** was similar to that of compounds **9a–l** (Scheme 2). Generated by condensation reaction between **8** chalcone **3a–l**, there appears a chiral carbon atom at C-5 position of pyrazole of all of the compounds. The similar reaction was reported in previous research and the structures of target compounds can be easily identified. The structures of target compounds were confirmed by ^{1}H-NMR, ^{13}C-NMR, and TOF MS (ESI+), which were in agreement with the structures depicted.

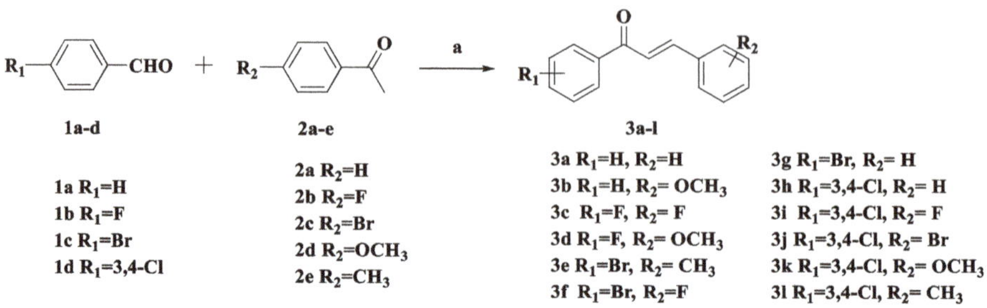

Scheme 1. Synthetic routes of chalcones **3a–l**. Reagents and conditions: **a** 10% NaOH, EtOH, r.t., 24 h.

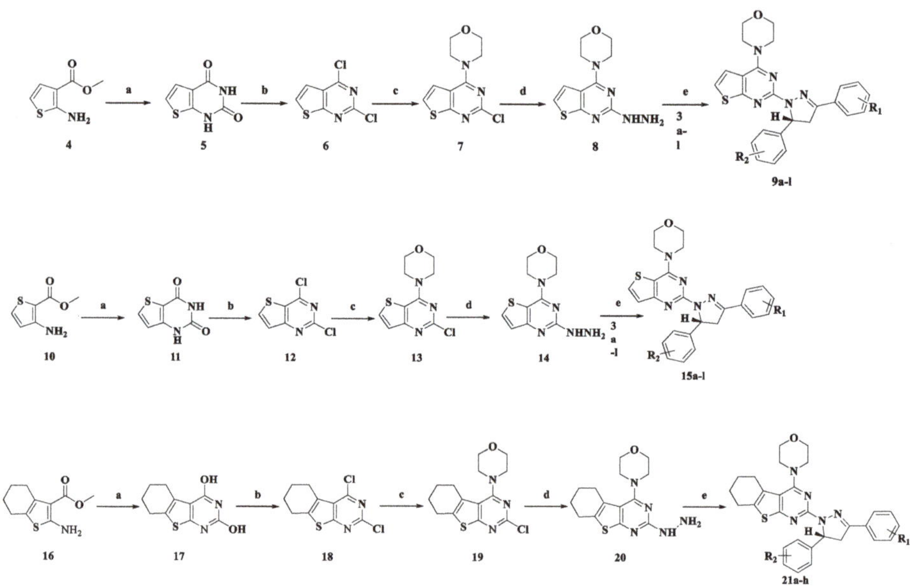

Scheme 2. Synthetic routes of target compounds **9a–l**, **15a–l**, and **21a–h**. Reagents and conditions: **a** 5 eq urea, 180 °C, 2h; **b** $POCl_3$, DMF (cat.), reflux, 8 h; **c** 2.1 eq morpholine, MeOH, 0 °C, 30 min, r.t., 2h; **d** 80% hydrazine monohydrate, reflux, 8h; **e** Glacial acetic acid, H_2SO_4 (78%), 100 °C.

2.2. Biological Discussion

All target compounds were evaluated for their cytotoxic activities against A549 (human lung cancer), PC-3 (human prostate cancer), MCF-7 (human breast cancer), HepG2 (human hepatoma) cell lines. In addition, the activity against PI3Kα/mTOR kinase of the most promising compounds **9a** and **15a** was further evaluated. The results expressed as IC_{50} were summarized in Tables 1–3.

Table 1. In vitro cytotoxic activities against different cancer cell lines of **9a–l** and **15a–l**.

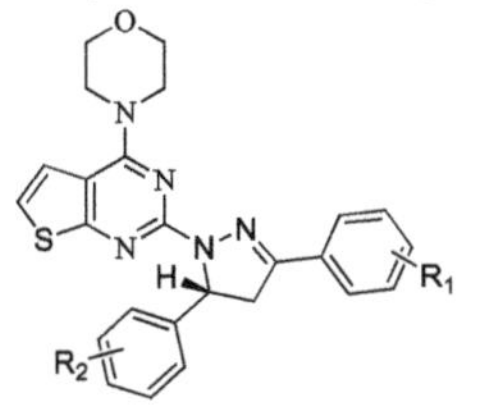

9a-l

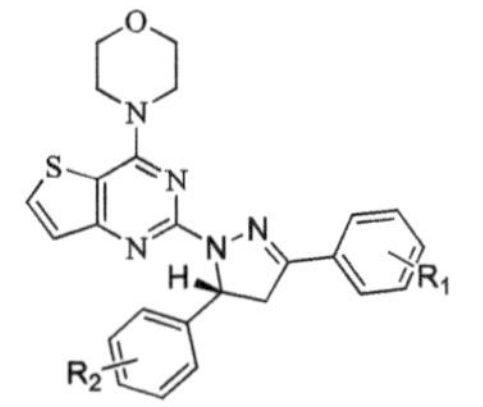

15a-l

Compd.	R_1	R_2	IC_{50} (μM) [a]				ClogP [b]	tPSA [b]
			PC-3	A549	MCF-7	HepG2		
9a	4-H	4-H	12.32 ± 0.96	11.30 ± 1.19	14.69 ± 1.32	9.80 ± 0.93	6.67	28.07
9b	4-H	4-OCH_3	15.36 ± 1.26	21.22 ± 2.75	14.12 ± 2.1	13.08 ± 1.20	6.59	37.3
9c	4-F	4-F	18.21 ± 1.55	24.23 ± 0.15	22.37 ± 0.17	17.36 ± 0.98	6.95	28.07
9d	4-F	4-OCH_3	22.15 ± 1.67	>50	20.62 ± 1.90	17.98 ± 2.12	6.73	37.3
9e	4-Br	4-CH_3	23.16 ± 1.96	>50	30.06 ± 2.86	21.63 ± 2.35	8.03	28.07
9f	4-Br	4-F	>50	15.37 ± 0.85	27.72 ± 2.71	13.49 ± 1.69	7.67	28.07
9g	4-Br	4-H	30.12 ± 3.01	22.78 ± 2.15	28.46 ± 3.9	28.85 ± 2.34	7.53	28.07
9h	3,4-di Cl	4-H	32.13 ± 2.96	38.53 ± 3.14	26.81 ± 2.13	23.70 ±2.08	7.97	28.07
9i	3,4-di Cl	4-F	27.65± 2.34	17.75 ± 1.64	29.53 ± 1.87	23.70 ± 2.11	8.12	28.07
9j	3,4-di Cl	4-Br	28.32 ± 2.16	>50	39.34 ± 2.51	>50	8.83	28.07
9k	3,4-di Cl	4-OCH_3	33.54 ± 3.26	40.65 ± 3.85	25.30 ± 2.20	20.88 ± 1.98	7.89	37.3
9l	3,4-di Cl	4-CH_3	28.36 ± 2.58	>50	>50	30.70 ± 0.15	8.47	28.07
15a	4-H	4-H	15.53 ± 1.21	16.90 ± 1.61	17.03 ± 1.68	13.14 ± 1.48	6.67	28.07
15b	4-H	4-OCH_3	25.45 ± 2.32	>50	>50	34.62 ± 2.82	6.58	37.3
15c	4-F	4-F	25.31 ± 2.39	39.03 ± 3.32	37.12 ± 2.99	18.90 ± 1.86	6.95	28.07
15d	4-F	4-OCH_3	22.13 ± 2.13	25.83 ± 1.99	35.15 ± 2.04	18.02 ± 1.30	6.73	37.3
15e	4-Br	4-CH_3	37.12 ± 3.16	45.78 ± 0.81	>50	24.41 ± 1.14	8.03	28.07
15f	4-Br	4-F	26.45 ± 2.57	42.09 ± 0.08	36.17 ± 1.13	19.90 ± 1.10	7.67	28.07
15g	4-Br	4-H	24.22 ± 2.26	21.73 ± 1.47	32.14 ± 0.89	21.36 ± 1.86	7.53	28.07
15h	3,4-di Cl	4-H	27.15 ± 2.53	33.23 ± 2.14	>50	21.15 ± 1.97	7.97	28.07
15i	3,4-di Cl	4-F	18.48 ± 1.73	>50	>50	15.56 ± 1.30	8.12	28.07
15j	3,4-di Cl	4-Br	32.97 ±3.22	41.78 ± 0.81	>50	28.97 ± 2.49	8.83	28.07
15k	3,4-di Cl	4-OCH_3	26.57 ± 2.38	31.05 ± 0.39	>50	19.86 ± 1.88	7.89	37.3
15l	3,4-di Cl	4-CH_3	23.68 ±1.94	31.79 ± 0.52	>50	21.59 ± 1.86	8.47	28.07
GDC-0941[c]	-	-	4.35 ± 0.33	6.99 ± 0.21	0.20 ± 0.08	0.07 ± 0.03	3.20	76.85

The value ">50" indicates that no inhibitory effect at 50 μM compound concentration. [a] The values are an average of two separate determinations; [b] Calculated by ChemBioDraw Ultra 15.0; [c] used as a positive control.

Table 2. In vitro cytotoxic activities against different cancer cell lines of **21a–h**.

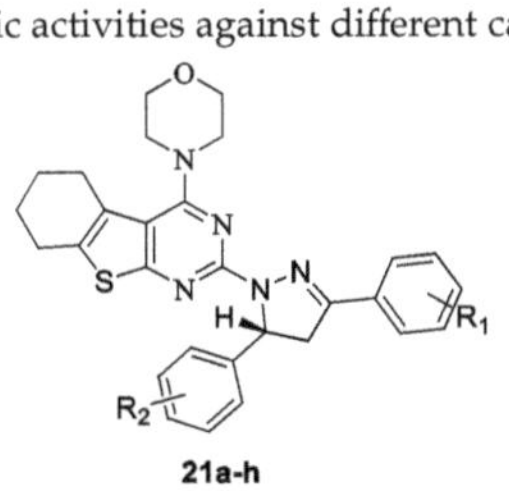

21a-h

Compd.	R1	R2	IC_{50} (μM) [a]				ClogP [b]	tPSA [b]
			PC-3	A549	MCF-7	HepG2		
21a	3,4-di Cl	4-OCH_3	31.75 ± 0.95	27.68 ± 0.10	>501	32.37 ± 1.84	8.23	28.07
21b	4-Br	4-CH_3	20.64 ± 0.63	11.59 ± 0.11	15.29 ± 0.83	12.43 ± 0.96	7.44	28.07
21c	4-H	4-H	>50	41.99 ± 1.49	>50	6>50	8.56	28.07
21d	4-F	4-OCH_3	25.28 ± 0.75	17.75± 1.1	29.53 ± 1.87	23.70 ± 0.11	8.79	28.07
21e	4-Br	4-F	>50	>50	>50	38.71 ± 1.72	7.86	28.07
21f	4-Br	4-H	>50	>50	>50	>50	8.84	28.07
21g	3,4-diCl	4-Br	>50	>50	>50	>50	8.63	28.07
21h	3,4-diCl	4-H	>50	23.53 ± 0.82	>50	>50	7.95	28.07
GDC-0941 [c]	-	-	4.35 ± 0.33	6.99 ± 0.21	0.20 ± 0.08	0.07 ± 0.03	3.20	76.85

The value ">50" indicates that no inhibitory effect at 50 μM compound concentration. [a] The values are an average of two separate determinations; [b] Calculated by ChemBioDraw Ultra 15.0; [c] used as a positive control.

Table 3. Enzymatic activities of compounds **9a** and **15a** against PI3Kα and mTOR (IC_{50}, μM).

Compd.	R1	R2	IC_{50} (μM) [a]	
			PI3Kα	mTOR
9a	4-H	4-H	9.47 ± 0.63	39.9 ± 7.6
15a	4-H	4-H	25.68 ± 2.33	>50
PI-103 [b]	-	-	0.019 ± 0.004	0.011 ± 0.002

[a] The values are an average of two separate determinations. [b] used as a positive control.

As illustrated in Tables 1 and 2, most of the target compounds exhibited moderate cytotoxic activities. The compounds whose skeleton are thieno[2,3-*d*]pyrimidine (**9a–1**) has slightly stronger inhibitory activity against the tested cancer cell lines than the compounds whose skeleton are thieno[3,2-*d*]pyrimidine (**15a–l** and **21a–h**). The most promising compound **9a** showed moderate to well inhibitory activity with IC_{50} values of 12.32 ± 0.96, 11.30 ± 1.19, 14.69 ± 1.32, and 9.80 ± 0.93 μM, respectively.

It is worth noting that when R_1 of the aryl group is an electron-withdrawing group (EWG) and R_2 is a H atom, the inhibitory activity of the compounds (**9g–h, 15g–h,** and **21a–h**) against cancer cells is decreased, especially for MCF-7 and A549 cells. The effect is greater than that of HepG2 and PC-3 cancer cell lines. Among them, the inhibitory activity of the compound **15h** against MCF-7 cells was $IC_{50} > 50$ μM, which means that the inhibitory activity was almost lost. When the C-3 and C-4 positions of the aryl group were both replaced by chlorine, the activity of the compounds (**9h–l, 15h–l**) is slightly lower than that of the compounds (**9b–g, 15b–g**) substituted by F or Br atoms.

When R_1 of the aryl group was hydrogen atom and R_2 was an electron-donating group, the inhibitory activities of the compounds **9b** and **15b** against the tested cancer cells decreased. The compound **15b** which contained the core skeleton thieno[3,2-*d*]pyrimidine was more obvious in this respect, and its IC_{50} values for A549 and MCF-7 were both higher than 50 μM. When R_1 of the aryl group was an electron withdrawing group, the inhibitory activity against cancer cells of the compounds **9c–l** and **15c–l** tended to decrease irrespective whether the substituent of R_2 was an electron withdrawing group or an electron donating group. Comparing the difference in activity between **9e–f** and **15e–f**, it is easily to find that the effect of the electron withdrawing group on the activity is slightly less than that of the electron-donating group. As shown in Table 3, compounds **21a–h** exhibited poor cytotoxic activity against the tested cell lines. This may attributed to the introduction of the tricyclic thieno-pyrimidine structure, resulting in an increase in steric hindrance which reduces the solubility of the compound at physiological pH and the relative molecular mass of the compound exceeds 500.

Finally, the inhibitory activity against PI3Kα kinase and mTOR kinase of selected compounds **9a** and **15a** were further examined. As shown in Table 3, enzymatic activity results of compounds **9a** and **15a** exhibited a moderate to excellent inhibitory activity against PI3Kα kinase. The inhibitory activity of the compounds against PI3Kα kinase is better than that of mTOR kinase.

*2.3. Molecular Docking Study of Compounds **9a** and **15a**.*

To further explore the binding modes of target compounds (**9a** and **15a**) with the active site of PI3Kα, molecular docking simulation studies were carried out by the AutoDock 4.2 software. Based on in vitro inhibition results, we selected compounds **9a** and **15a** as ligand examples, and the structures of PI3Kα (PDB code: 3TL5) were selected as the docking models. The best-scoring ligand–protein complex (Figure 3) was used for binding site analysis.

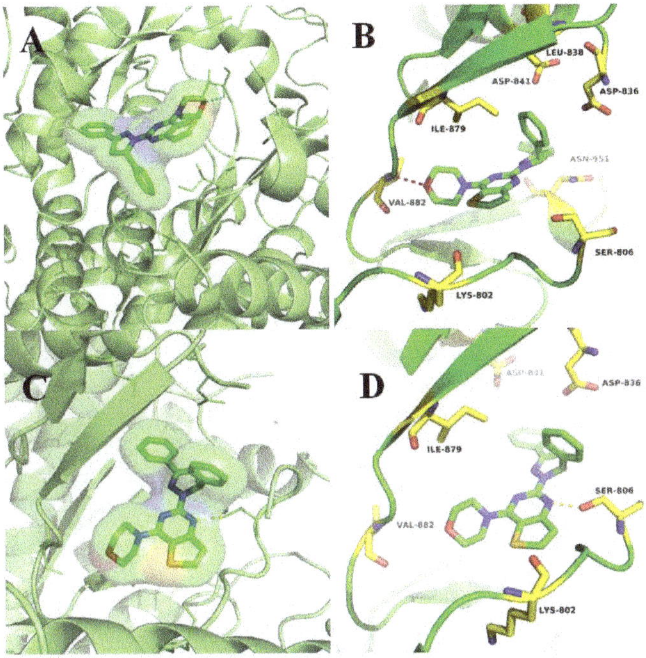

Figure 3. Docking modes of **9a** and **15a**. (**A**) Overview of the binding site of compound **9a** with PI3Kα (3TL5) kinase. (**B**) Binding model of compound **9a** with PI3Kα (3TL5) kinase. (**C**) Overview of the binding site of compound **15a** with PI3Kα (3TL5) kinase. (**D**) Binding model of compound **15a** with PI3Kα (3TL5) kinase.

The binding models of compounds **9a** and **15a** to the 3TL5 protein are approximately the same as our previously assumed binding model (Figure 3A,C). The detailed binding models of compounds **9a** and **15a** with the active site of PI3Kα kinase are shown in Figure 3. In the docking model of compound **9a** with PI3Kα (Figure 3B), we can easily see that the oxygen atom on the morphine ring formed a hydrogen bond with the hinge region residue VAL882. After careful observation of the binding model of compound **15a** with 3TL5 protein kinase (Figure 3D), it is not difficult to find that the N atom on the pyrimidine ring of thieno[3,2-*d*]pyrimidine formed a hydrogen bond interaction with residue SER806. Compared with the original ligand GDC-0980, the hydrogen bonding interaction between compounds **9a** and **15a** with protein is reduced, which may be one of the reasons why this series of compounds failed to achieve excellent cytotoxic activity.

3. Experimental Section

3.1. General Information

Unless otherwise required, all reagents used in the experiment were purchased as commercial analytical grade and used without further purification. Frequently used solvents (Ethanol, petroleum ether, ethyl acetate, dichloromethane, etc.) were absolutely anhydrous. All actions were monitored through GF_{254} thin-layer chromatography plate (Qingdao Haiyang Chemical Co., Ltd., Qingdao, China) and spots were visualized with iodine or light (in 254 nm or 365 nm). The structure of the target compound was confirmed by ^{1}H-NMR and ^{13}C-NMR spectra at room temperature on Bruker 400 MHz spectrometer (Bruker Bioscience, Billerica, MA, USA) with tetramethylsilane (TMS) as an internal standard. Mass spectrometry (MS) was performed on Waters High Resolution Quadrupole Time of Flight Tandem Mass Spectrometry (QTOF) (Waters Corporation, Milford, MA, USA). The purity of the compound was determined by Agilent 1260 liquid chromatograph (Agilent Technologies Inc., Palo Alto, CA, USA) fitted with an Inertex-C18 column. All target compounds had the purity of ≥95%.

3.2. Chemistry

3.2.1. General Procedure for the Preparation of Compounds **3a–l**

Compounds **3a–l** were synthesized according to the reported procedures by our research group [15].

3.2.2. General Procedure for the Preparation of Compounds **8**, **14** and **20**

Compound **5** was obtained by a cyclization reaction starting from commercially available methyl 2-aminothiophene-3-carboxylate (**4**) and urea. Subsequently, compound **5** is subjected to a chlorination reaction with $POCl_3$ to give compound **6**. Compound **6** was substituted by morphine and hydrazine hydrate respectively to obtain key intermediate **8**. Similarly, we used commercially available methyl 2-aminothiophene-3-carboxylate (**10**) or commercial available methyl 2-amino-4,5,6,7-tetrahydrobenzo[*b*]thiophene-3-carboxylate (**16**) as the starting material to obtain intermediates **14** or **20** through a similar reaction condition. Detailed synthesis of key intermediates **8**, **14**, and **20**, and their precursors **7**, **11**, **12**, and **13**. can be found in the article reported by our research group [13].

3.2.3. General Procedure for the Preparation of Target Compounds **9a–l**, **15a–l**, and **21a–h**.

A mixture of different substituted chalcone **3a–l** (1.5 mmol) and 4-(2-mercaptothieno[2,3-*d*] pyrimidin-4-yl) morpholine (**8**) or 4-(2-mercaptothieno[3,2-*d*]pyrimidin -4-yl)morpholine (**14**) or 4-(2-hydrazinyl-5,6,7,8-tetrahydrobenzo[4,5]thieno[2,3-*d*]pyrimidin-4-yl)morpholine (**20**) were dissolved (1.5 mmol, **8**/**14**/**20**) in 25 mL of glacial acetic acid. Subsequently, the reaction solution was stirred at 100–110 °C for 1.5 h under the action of 2–3 drops concentrated H_2SO_4 (78%) as a catalyst and monitored by thin-layer chromatography (TLC). The reaction mixture was concentrated under reduced pressure. After the completion of concentrated, the mixture was filtered and the precipitate was washed with ethanol. If the purify of the compound is not high enough, recrystallization by 95% EtOH or column chromatography (EtOAc:PE = 1:3) are needed. The obtained solids were then dried to give the target compounds **9a–l**, **15a–l**, and **18a–h** with the yield ranging from 30%–60%.

4-(2-(3-(3,4-dichlorophenyl)-5-(4-methoxyphenyl)-4,5-dihydro-1H-pyrazol-1-yl)thieno[2,3-d]pyrimidin-4-yl) morpholine (**9a**). Light yellow solid, mp 202–205 °C; ^{1}H NMR (400 MHz, DMSO-d_6) δ (ppm): 8.42 (d, *J* = 5.3 Hz, 1H), 7.95 (d, *J* = 8.7 Hz, 2H), 7.73 (s, 1H), 7.62 (m, *J* = 16.2, 7.0 Hz, 2H), 7.33 (d, *J* = 8.1 Hz, 1H), 7.12 (d, *J* = 8.4 Hz, 2H), 5.85–5.75 (m, 1H), 4.08 (m, *J* = 17.7, 11.6 Hz, 1H), 3.85 (s, 3H), 3.84–3.75 (m, 3H), 3.67 (s, 3H), 3.60–3.54 (m, 1H), 3.50–3.46 (m, 2H). HRMS (ESI): *m*/*z* calcd for $(C_{27}H_{25}N_3OS + H)^+$: 440.1797; found: 440.1834.

4-(2-(5-(4-bromophenyl)-3-(3,4-dichlorophenyl)-4,5-dihydro-1H-pyrazol-1-yl)thieno[2,3-d]pyrimidin-4-yl) morpholine (**9b**). Light yellow solid, m.p. 280–282 °C; ^{1}H NMR (400 MHz, DMSO-d_6) δ (ppm): 8.18 (d, *J* = 5.5 Hz, 1H), 7.90 (dd, *J* = 8.4, 5.5 Hz, 2H), 7.63 (dd, *J* = 8.4, 5.0 Hz, 2H), 7.37 (dd, *J* = 13.9, 7.0 Hz, 3H), 7.30–7.26 (m, 1H), 5.79 (dd, *J* = 12.1, 6.1 Hz, 1H), 3.95 (dd, *J* = 17.8, 12.2 Hz, 1H), 3.82–3.65 (m, 6H), 3.59 (d, *J* = 7.7 Hz, 3H). HRMS (ESI): *m*/*z* calcd for $(C_{28}H_{27}N_3O_2S + H)^+$: 470.1902; found: 470.1946.

4-(2-(3,5-bis(4-fluorophenyl)-4,5-dihydro-1H-pyrazol-1-yl)thieno[2,3-d]pyrimidin-4-yl)Morpholine (**9c**).Yellow solid, m.p. 225–227 °C; ^{1}H NMR (400 MHz, DMSO-d_6) δ (ppm): 8.47 (d, *J* = 5.6 Hz, 1H), 8.13 (s, 2H), 7.63 (s, 1H), 7.50–7.42 (m, 4H), 7.25 (t, *J* = 8.5 Hz, 2H), 5.88 (s, 1H), 4.13 (d, *J* = 12.1 Hz, 1H), 3.87 (s, 4H), 3.70 (s, 3H), 3.49 (s, 1H), 3.22 (s, 1H). HRMS (ESI): *m*/*z* calcd for $(C_{27}H_{23}F_2N_3OS + H)^+$: 476.1608; found: 476.1598.

4-(2-(3-(3,4-dichlorophenyl)-5-(4-fluorophenyl)-4,5-dihydro-1H-pyrazol-1-yl)thieno[2,3-d]pyrimidin-4-yl) morpholine (**9d**).Yellow solid, m.p. 286–289 °C; ^{1}H NMR (400 MHz, DMSO-d_6) δ (ppm): 7.73 (d,

J = 7.5 Hz, 2H), 7.54 (d, J = 7.9 Hz, 2H), 7.31 (d, J = 6.6 Hz, 3H), 7.25 (d, J = 7.8 Hz, 2H), 5.74 (d, J = 6.6 Hz, 1H), 3.95–3.84 (m, 1H), 3.76–3.63 (m, 6H), 3.59 (s, 2H), 3.49 (d, J = 5.9 Hz, 1H). HRMS (ESI): m/z calcd for $(C_{28}H_{26}FN_3O_2S + H)^+$: 488.1808; found: 488.1853.

4-(2-(3-(3,4-Dichlorophenyl)-5-phenyl-4,5-dihydro-1H-pyrazol-1-yl)thieno[2,3-d]pyrimidine-4-yl)morpholine (**9e**). Yellow solid, m.p. 228.3~229.1 °C; ^{1}H NMR (400 MHz, DMSO-d_6) δ (ppm): 8.07 (d, J = 5.4 Hz, 1H), 7.77 (d, J = 7.1 Hz, 2H), 7.55 (d, J = 8.4 Hz, 2H), 7.44 (d, J = 7.6 Hz, 3H), 7.25 (d, J = 5.5 Hz, 2H), 5.72 (dd, J = 12.1, 5.7 Hz, 1H), 3.87 (dd, J = 18.0, 12.3 Hz, 1H), 3.71 (s, 2H), 3.66–3.58 (m, 4H), 3.54 (s, 2H), 3.18 (dd, J = 18.1, 5.8 Hz, 1H). HRMS (ESI): m/z calcd for $(C_{28}H_{26}BrN_3OS + H)^+$: 534.1041; found: 534.0991.

4-(2-(5-(4-methoxyphenyl)-3-phenyl-4,5-dihydro-1H-pyrazol-1-yl)thieno[2,3-d]pyrimidine-4-yl)morpholine (**9f**). Orange solid, m.p. 237.6~239.1 °C; ^{1}H NMR (400 MHz, DMSO-d_6) δ (ppm): 8.17 (d, J = 4.9 Hz, 1H), 7.79 (d, J = 8.1 Hz, 2H), 7.35 (d, J = 4.7 Hz, 1H), 7.29 (d, J = 7.3 Hz, 2H), 7.24 (d, J = 7.7 Hz, 3H), 7.03 (d, J = 8.3 Hz, 2H), 5.69 (d, J = 6.4 Hz, 1H), 3.98–3.87 (m, 2H), 3.80 (s, 3H), 3.68 (s, 4H), 3.57 (s, 4H). HRMS (ESI): m/z calcd for $(C_{27}H_{23}BrFN_3OS + H)^+$: 538.0790; found: 538.0882.

4-(2-(3-(3,4-dichlorophenyl)-5-(p-tolyl)-4,5-dihydro-1H-pyrazol-1-yl)thieno[2,3-d]pyrimidin-4-yl)morpholine (**9g**). Yellow solid, m.p. 207.4~208.2 °C; ^{1}H NMR (400 MHz, DMSO-d_6) δ (ppm): 8.43 (d, J = 5.4 Hz, 1H), 7.90 (d, J = 7.6 Hz, 2H), 7.74 (s, 1H), 7.62 (dd, J = 15.4, 6.7 Hz, 2H), 7.41–7.29 (m, 3H), 5.80 (dd, J = 11.6, 6.2 Hz, 1H), 4.09 (dd, J = 18.2, 11.5 Hz, 1H), 3.82 (s, 4H), 3.67 (s, 3H), 3.48 (s, 2H), 2.40 (s, 3H). HRMS (ESI): m/z calcd for $(C_{27}H_{24}BrN_3OS + H)^+$: 520.0884; found: 520.0865.

4-(2-(3-(4-bromophenyl)-5-(p-tolyl)-4,5-dihydro-1H-pyrazol-1-yl)thieno[2,3-d]pyrimidine-4-yl)morpholine (**9h**). Light yellow solid, m.p. 222.8~223.9 °C; ^{1}H NMR (400 MHz, DMSO-d_6) δ (ppm): 8.11 (d, J = 5.0 Hz, 1H), 7.73 (d, J = 7.5 Hz, 2H), 7.54 (d, J = 7.9 Hz, 2H), 7.31 (d, J = 6.6 Hz, 3H), 7.25 (d, J = 7.8 Hz, 2H), 5.74 (d, J = 6.6 Hz, 1H), 3.95–3.84 (m, 1H), 3.76–3.63 (m, 6H), 3.59 (s, 2H), 3.13 (d, J = 13.7 Hz, 1H), 2.40 (s, 3H). ^{13}C NMR (101 MHz, DMSO-d_6) δ 163.89, 157.95, 156.29, 150.82, 145.81, 134.03, 132.46, 131.45, 131.41, 129.81, 129.71(2,C), 129.17, 128.43, 126.68(2,C), 126.29, 124.43, 106.60, 66.29(2,C), 61.90, 46.26(2,C).HRMS (ESI): m/z calcd for $(C_{27}H_{23}Cl_2N_3OS + H)^+$: 508.1017; found: 508.1059.

4-(2-(3,5-diphenyl-4,5-dihydro-1H-pyrazol-1-yl)thieno[2,3-d]pyrimidin-4-yl)morpholine (**9i**). Light yellow solid, m.p. 231.7~233.2 °C; ^{1}H NMR (400 MHz, DMSO-d_6) δ (ppm): 8.04 (d, J = 5.5 Hz, 1H), 7.77 (d, J = 7.6 Hz, 2H), 7.48–7.37 (m, 3H), 7.30–7.17 (m, 6H), 5.71 (dd, J = 12.0, 5.3 Hz, 1H), 3.87 (dd, J = 17.4, 12.2 Hz, 1H), 3.63 (dt, J = 19.1, 10.7 Hz, 6H), 3.49 (d, J = 13.7 Hz, 2H), 3.45–3.40 (m, 1H). HRMS (ESI): m/z calcd for $(C_{27}H_{22}Cl_2FN_3OS + H)^+$: 528.0898; found: 528.0891.

4-(2-(3-(4-fluorophenyl)-5-(4-methoxyphenyl)-4,5-dihydro-1H-pyrazol-1-yl)thieno[2,3-d]pyrimidin-4-yl) morpholine (**9j**). Light yellow solid, m.p. 215.8~216.8 °C; ^{1}H NMR (400 MHz, DMSO-d_6) δ (ppm): 7.91–7.86 (m, 2H), 7.50 (t, J = 5.0 Hz, 1H), 7.39–7.24 (m, 4H), 7.16 (t, J = 8.8 Hz, 1H), 7.06 (d, J = 8.6 Hz, 2H), 5.72 (dd, J = 11.0, 5.3 Hz, 1H), 4.07–3.96 (m, 1H), 3.82 (s, 3H), 3.74 (s, 4H), 3.65–3.56 (m, 3H), 3.48 (s, 2H). HRMS (ESI): m/z calcd for $(C_{27}H_{22}BrCl_2N_3OS + H)^+$: 588.0100; found: 588.0110.

4-(2-(3-(4-bromophenyl)-5-(4-fluorophenyl)-4,5-dihydro-1H-pyrazol-1-yl)thieno[2,3-d]Pyrimidin-4-yl) morpholine (**9k**). Yellow solid, m.p. 221.2~222.0 °C; ^{1}H -NMR (400 MHz, DMSO-d_6) δ (ppm): 8.14 (d, J = 5.6 Hz, 1H), 7.93–7.85 (m, 2H), 7.55 (d, J = 8.2 Hz, 2H), 7.39–7.30 (m, 3H), 7.27 (d, J = 8.3 Hz, 2H), 5.77 (dd, J = 11.9, 5.4 Hz, 1H), 3.93 (dd, J = 17.7, 12.3 Hz, 1H), 3.80–3.65 (m, 6H), 3.59 (d, J = 10.2 Hz, 2H), 3.19 (dd, J = 17.9, 5.8 Hz, 1H). HRMS (ESI): m/z calcd for $(C_{28}H_{25}Cl_2N_3O_2S + H)^+$: 538.1123; found: 538.1199.

4-(2-(3-(4-bromophenyl)-5-phenyl-4,5-dihydro-1H-pyrazol-1-yl)thieno[2,3-d]pyrimidine-4-Morpholine (**9l**). Light yellow solid, m.p. 221.2~222.0 °C; ^{1}H NMR (400 MHz, DMSO-d_6) δ (ppm): 8.05 (d, J = 5.5 Hz, 1H), 7.76 (d, J = 7.3 Hz, 2H), 7.50 7.39 (m, 5H), 7.21 (dd, J = 17.0, 6.8 Hz, 3H), 5.70 (d, J = 6.7 Hz, 1H), 3.86 (d, J = 5.2 Hz, 1H), 3.69 (t, J = 10.6 Hz, 2H), 3.64–3.57 (m, 4H), 3.53 (t, J = 9.8 Hz, 2H), 3.12 (d, J = 5.5 Hz, 1H). HRMS (ESI): m/z calcd for $(C_{28}H_{25}Cl_2N_3OS + H)^+$: 522.1174; found: 522.1203.

4-(2-(3-(3,4-dichlorophenyl)-5-(4-methoxyphenyl)-4,5-dihydro-1H-pyrazol-1-yl)thieno[3,2-d]pyrimidin-4-yl) morpholine (**15a**). Light yellow solid, m.p. 131.2~132.5 °C; ^{1}H NMR (400 MHz, DMSO-d_6) δ (ppm): 7.73 (d, J = 8.4 Hz, 2H), 7.57 (d, J = 8.1 Hz, 2H), 7.40 (d, J = 6.2 Hz, 1H), 7.19 (d, J = 6.0 Hz, 2H), 7.02 (d, J = 8.5 Hz, 2H), 5.69 (dd, J = 12.0, 5.5 Hz, 1H), 3.92–3.84 (m, 1H), 3.81 (s, 3H), 3.62 (dd, J = 22.9, 8.6 Hz, 6H), 3.51 (d, J = 8.6 Hz, 2H), 3.17 (dd, J = 17.7, 5.6 Hz, 1H). HRMS (ESI): m/z calcd for($C_{27}H_{25}N_3OS$ + H)$^+$: 440.1797; found: 440.1808.

4-(2-(5-(4-bromophenyl)-3-(3,4-dichlorophenyl)-4,5-dihydro-1H-pyrazol-1-yl)thieno[3,2-d]pyrimidin-4-yl) morpholine (**15b**). Light yellow solid, m.p. 265.3~266.3 °C; ^{1}H NMR (400 MHz, DMSO-d_6) δ (ppm): 7.69 (d, J = 7.8 Hz, 2H), 7.50 (d, J = 8.1 Hz, 2H), 7.40 (d, J = 6.2 Hz, 1H), 7.27 (d, J = 7.8 Hz, 2H), 7.20 (d, J = 7.8 Hz, 2H), 5.69 (dd, J = 12.2, 5.1 Hz, 1H), 3.93–3.82 (m, 1H), 3.62 (dd, J = 23.2, 8.0 Hz, 6H), 3.51 (d, J = 7.4 Hz, 2H), 3.12 (d, J = 18.1 Hz, 1H). HRMS (ESI): m/z calcd for ($C_{28}H_{27}N_3O_2S$ + H)$^+$: 470.1902; found: 470.1939.

4-(2-(3,5-bis(4-fluorophenyl)-4,5-dihydro-1H-pyrazol-1-yl)thieno[3,2-d]pyrimidin-4-yl)Morpholine (**15c**). Yellow solid, m.p. 254.7~255.4 °C; ^{1}H NMR (400 MHz, DMSO-d_6) δ (ppm): 7.88–7.82 (m, 2H), 7.39 (d, J = 6.1 Hz, 1H), 7.29 (dd, J = 16.3, 8.0 Hz, 4H), 7.19 (d, J = 6.1 Hz, 1H), 7.14 (d, J = 8.5 Hz, 2H), 5.73 (dd, J = 12.2, 5.2 Hz, 1H), 3.92–3.83 (m, 1H), 3.62 (dd, J = 20.8, 8.0 Hz, 6H), 3.51 (d, J = 8.0 Hz, 2H), 3.13 (dd, J = 18.0, 5.0 Hz, 1H). HRMS (ESI): m/z calcd for ($C_{27}H_{23}F_2N_3OS$ + H)$^+$: 476.1608; found: 476.1640.

4-(2-(3-(3,4-dichlorophenyl)-5-(4-fluorophenyl)-4,5-dihydro-1H-pyrazol-1-yl)thieno[3,2-d]pyrmidin-4-yl) morpholine (**15d**). Yellow solid, m.p. 237.7~238.8 °C; ^{1}H NMR (400 MHz, DMSO-d_6) δ (ppm): 7.60 (d, J = 7.9 Hz, 2H), 7.48 (d, J = 6.8 Hz, 2H), 7.31 (d, J = 5.8 Hz, 1H), 7.19 (d, J = 7.8 Hz, 2H), 7.11 (d, J = 6.4 Hz, 2H), 5.62 (d, J = 6.1 Hz, 1H), 3.82–3.73 (m, 1H), 3.55 (s, 2H), 3.51 (d, J = 7.4 Hz, 4H), 3.43 (d, J = 8.8 Hz, 2H), 3.08 (d, J = 12.8 Hz, 1H). ^{13}C NMR (101 MHz, DMSO-d_6) δ 162.70, 162.39, 161.13, 160.78, 157.90, 156.38, 140.04, 128.77, 128.03, 121.75, 115.91(2,C), 115.77(2,C), 114.63(3,C), 110.46, 66.28, 62.03, 55.83, 47.11, 42.77. HRMS (ESI): m/z calcd for ($C_{28}H_{26}FN_3O_2S$ + H)$^+$: 488.1808; found: 488.1842.

4-(2-(3-(3,4-Dichlorophenyl)-5-phenyl-4,5-dihydro-1H-pyrazol-1-yl)thieno[3,2-d]pyrimidine-4-yl)morpholine (**15e**). Yellow solid, m.p. 263–265 °C; ^{1}H NMR (400 MHz, DMSO-d_6) δ (ppm): 7.80 (d, J = 6.9 Hz, 2H), 7.61–7.55 (m, 2H), 7.49–7.44 (m, 3H), 7.43–7.39 (m, 1H), 7.21 (d, J = 6.2 Hz, 2H), 5.73 (dd, J = 12.2, 5.8 Hz, 1H), 3.89 (dd, J = 17.7, 12.2 Hz, 1H), 3.69–3.56 (m, 6H), 3.53–3.48 (m, 2H), 3.20 (dd, J = 17.8, 5.8 Hz, 1H). HRMS (ESI): m/z calcd for ($C_{28}H_{26}BrN_3OS$ + H)$^+$: 534.1041; found: 534.1008.

4-(2-(5-(4-methoxyphenyl)-3-phenyl-4,5-dihydro-1H-pyrazol-1-yl)thieno[3,2-d]pyrimidine-4-y)morpholine (**15f**). Yellow solid, m.p. 235–237 °C; ^{1}H NMR (400 MHz, DMSO-d_6) δ (ppm): 7.78 (d, J = 8.5 Hz, 2H), 7.42 (d, J = 6.1 Hz, 1H), 7.30 (d, J = 7.2 Hz, 2H), 7.25 (d, J = 6.2 Hz, 4H), 7.04 (d, J = 8.6 Hz, 2H), 5.73–5.65 (m, 1H), 3.91 (dd, J = 18.0, 12.1 Hz, 1H), 3.82 (s, 3H), 3.66–3.53 (m, 6H), 3.46 (s, 2H), 3.16 (d, J = 17.8 Hz, 1H). HRMS (ESI): m/z calcd for ($C_{27}H_{23}BrFN_3OS$ + H)$^+$: 538.0790; found: 538.0832.

4-(2-(3-(3,4-dichlorophenyl)-5-(p-tolyl)-4,5-dihydro-1H-pyrazol-1-yl)thieno[3,2-d]pyrimidin-4-yl)morpholine (**15g**). Yellow solid, m.p. 267–268 °C; ^{1}H NMR (400 MHz, DMSO-d_6) δ (ppm): 7.69 (d, J = 7.7 Hz, 2H), 7.57 (d, J = 8.2 Hz, 2H), 7.40 (d, J = 6.2 Hz, 1H), 7.28 (d, J = 8.0 Hz, 2H), 7.20 (d, J = 6.3 Hz, 2H), 5.70 (dd, J = 11.9, 5.6 Hz, 1H), 3.91–3.82 (m, 1H), 3.65–3.56 (m, 6H), 3.51 (d, J = 8.4 Hz, 2H), 3.21–3.13 (m, 1H), 2.35 (s, 3H). HRMS (ESI): m/z calcd for ($C_{27}H_{24}BrN_3OS$ + H)$^+$: 517.0823; found: 517.0798.

4-(2-(3-(4-bromophenyl)-5-(p-tolyl)-4,5-dihydro-1H-pyrazol-1-yl)thieno[3,2-d]pyrimidine-4-yl)morpholine (**15h**). Yellow solid, m.p. 255–257 °C; ^{1}H NMR (400 MHz, DMSO-d_6) δ (ppm): 7.68 (d, J = 8.1 Hz, 2H), 7.50 (d, J = 8.3 Hz, 2H), 7.40 (t, J = 6.6 Hz, 1H), 7.29 (d, J = 10.6 Hz, 2H), 7.22 – 7.17 (m, 3H), 5.69 (dd, J = 11.7, 4.7 Hz, 1H), 3.92–3.83 (m, 1H), 3.63–3.55 (m, 6H), 3.50 (d, J = 11.1 Hz, 2H), 3.09 (dd, J = 17.6, 5.7 Hz, 1H), 2.35 (s, 3H). ^{13}C NMR (101 MHz, DMSO-d_6) δ 171.77, 158.31, 154.66, 151.51, 145.64, 132.28, 131.46, 131.41, 129.95, 129.76, 129.17(2,C), 128.46, 126.76(2,C), 126.26, 121.64, 117.97, 110.41, 66.32(2,C), 61.88, 46.96(2,C), 42.01.HRMS (ESI): m/z calcd for ($C_{27}H_{23}Cl_2N_3OS$ + H)$^+$: 508.1017; found: 508.1044.

4-(2-(3,5-diphenyl-4,5-dihydro-1H-pyrazol-1-yl)thieno[3,2-d]pyrimidin-4-yl)morpholine (**15i**). Yellow solid, m.p. 266–267 °C; ^{1}H NMR (400 MHz, DMSO-d_6) δ (ppm): 8.04 (d, *J* = 5.5 Hz, 1H), 7.77 (d, *J* = 7.6 Hz, 2H), 7.56–7.35 (m, 3H), 7.32–7.15 (m, 6H), 5.71 (dd, *J* = 12.0, 5.3 Hz, 1H), 3.87 (dd, *J* = 17.4, 12.2 Hz, 1H), 3.70–3.54 (m, 6H), 3.50 (s, 2H), 3.09 (dd, *J* = 17.6, 5.3 Hz, 1H). HRMS (ESI): *m/z* calcd for $(C_{27}H_{22}Cl_2FN_3OS + H)^+$: 526.0923; found: 526.0889.

4-(2-(3-(4-fluorophenyl)-5-(4-methoxyphenyl)-4,5-dihydro-1H-pyrazol-1-yl)thieno[3,2-d]pyrimidin-4-yl) morpholine (**15j**). Yellow solid, m.p. 271–272 °C; ^{1}H NMR (400 MHz, DMSO-d_6) δ (ppm): 7.74 (d, *J* = 7.9 Hz, 2H), 7.35 (d, *J* = 6.0 Hz, 1H), 7.26–7.17 (m, 3H), 7.07 (d, *J* = 8.8 Hz, 2H), 6.95 (d, *J* = 8.6 Hz, 2H), 5.63 (dd, *J* = 11.8, 5.6 Hz, 1H), 3.85 (d, *J* = 17.8 Hz, 1H), 3.73 (s, 3H), 3.55 (dd, *J* = 25.4, 8.6 Hz, 7H), 3.09 (d, *J* = 16.8 Hz, 2H). HRMS (ESI): *m/z* calcd for $(C_{27}H_{22}BrCl_2N_3OS + H)^+$: 588.0100; found: 588.0132.

4-(2-(3-(4-bromophenyl)-5-(4-fluorophenyl)-4,5-dihydro-1H-pyrazol-1-yl)thieno[3,2-d]Pyrimidin-4-yl)morpholine (**15k**). Yellow solid, m.p. 251–252 °C; ^{1}H NMR (400 MHz, DMSO-d_6) δ (ppm): 7.75 (s, 2H), 7.41 (d, *J* = 7.6 Hz, 2H), 7.31 (d, *J* = 5.5 Hz, 1H), 7.21 (t, *J* = 8.0 Hz, 2H), 7.12 (d, *J* = 7.9 Hz, 3H), 5.62 (d, *J* = 6.8 Hz, 1H), 3.85–3.74 (m, 1H), 3.53 (d, *J* = 13.2 Hz, 6H), 3.44 (d, *J* = 8.9 Hz, 2H), 3.05 (d, *J* = 17.7 Hz, 1H). HRMS (ESI): *m/z* calcd for $(C_{28}H_{25}Cl_2N_3O_2S + H)^+$: 538.1123; found: 538.1161.

4-(2-(3-(4-bromophenyl)-5-phenyl-4,5-dihydro-1H-pyrazol-1-yl)thieno[3,2-d]pyrimidine-4-Morpholine (**15l**). Yellow solid, m.p. 244–245 °C; ^{1}H NMR (400 MHz, DMSO-d_6) δ (ppm): 7.79 (d, *J* = 7.3 Hz, 2H), 7.50 (d, *J* = 8.3 Hz, 2H), 7.44 (t, *J* = 8.0 Hz, 3H), 7.40 (d, *J* = 6.2 Hz, 1H), 7.24–7.18 (m, 3H), 5.71 (dd, *J* = 12.1, 5.7 Hz, 1H), 3.89 (dd, *J* = 17.5, 12.6 Hz, 1H), 3.62 (dd, *J* = 23.5, 8.5 Hz, 6H), 3.51 (d, *J* = 8.0 Hz, 2H), 3.13 (dd, *J* = 17.7, 5.6 Hz, 1H). HRMS (ESI): *m/z* calcd for $(C_{28}H_{25}Cl_2N_3OS + H)^+$: 522.1174; found: 522.1201.

4-(2-(3-(3,4-dichlorophenyl)-5-(4-methoxyphenyl)-4,5-dihydro-1H-pyrazol-1-yl)-5,6,7,8-tetrahydrobenzo [4,5]thieno[2,3-d]pyrimidin-4-yl)morpholine (**21a**). Dark blue solid, m.p. 252–253 °C; ESI-MS $[M + H]^+$ *m/z*: 594.5; ^{1}H NMR (400 MHz, DMSO-d_6) δ (ppm): 7.73 (d, *J* = 8.7 Hz, 2H), 7.56 (d, *J* = 7.0 Hz, 2H), 7.20 (d, *J* = 8.4 Hz, 1H), 7.02 (d, *J* = 7.0 Hz, 2H), 5.67 (d, *J* = 5.7 Hz, 1H), 3.88 (d, *J* = 17.1 Hz, 1H), 3.81 (s, 3H), 3.62 (d, *J* = 5.4 Hz, 2H), 3.58 (s, 2H), 3.18 (d, *J* = 12.1 Hz, 3H), 2.99 (s, 2H), 2.73 (s, 4H), 1.81 (s, 4H).

4-(2-(3-(4-bromophenyl)-5-(p-tolyl)-4,5-dihydro-1H-pyrazol-1-yl)-5,6,7,8-tetrahdrobenzo[4,5]thieno [2,3-d]pyrimidin-4-yl)morpholine (**21b**). Dark blue solid, m.p. 243–244 °C; ESI-MS $[M + H]^+$ *m/z*: 588.5; ^{1}H NMR (400 MHz, DMSO-d_6) δ (ppm): 7.69 (d, *J* = 7.9 Hz, 2H), 7.50 (d, *J* = 8.3 Hz, 2H), 7.27 (d, *J* = 7.7 Hz, 2H), 7.19 (d, *J* = 8.3 Hz, 2H), 5.70 (dd, *J* = 12.3, 5.4 Hz, 1H), 3.88 (dd, *J* = 17.7, 12.3 Hz, 1H), 3.64 (s, 2H), 3.57 (s, 2H), 3.15 (d, *J* = 16.2 Hz, 3H), 2.99 (s, 2H), 2.74 (s, 4H), 2.35 (s, 3H), 1.78 (d, *J* = 13.4 Hz, 4H).

4-(2-(3,5-diphenyl-4,5-dihydro-1H-pyrazol-1-yl)-5,6,7,8-tetrahydrobenzo[4,5]thiophene[2,3-d]pyramidin -4-yl)morpholine (**21c**). Dark blue solid, m.p. 212–213 °C; ESI-MS $[M + H]^+$ *m/z*: 495.6; ^{1}H NMR (400 MHz, DMSO-d_6) δ (ppm): 7.82–7.79 (m, 2H), 7.46 (d, *J* = 7.6 Hz, 3H), 7.29 (d, *J* = 7.3 Hz, 2H), 7.23 (dd, *J* = 9.2, 1.9 Hz, 3H), 5.73 (dd, *J* = 12.1, 5.5 Hz, 1H), 3.92 (dd, *J* = 17.7, 12.1 Hz, 1H), 3.65–3.60 (m, 2H), 3.55 (d, *J* = 6.5 Hz, 2H), 3.14 (dd, *J* = 17.7, 5.7 Hz, 3H), 3.02–2.94 (m, 2H), 2.74 (s, 4H), 1.80 (d, *J* = 28.8 Hz, 4H).

4-(2-(3-(4-fluorophenyl)-5-(4-methoxyphenyl)-4,5-dihydro-1H-pyrazol-1-yl)-5,6,7,8-tetrahydrobenzo [4,5]thieno[2,3-d]pyrimidin-4-yl)morpholine (**21d**). Dark blue solid, m.p. 189-193 °C; ESI-MS $[M + H]^+$ *m/z*: 543.6; ^{1}H NMR (400 MHz, DMSO-d_6) δ (ppm): 7.74 (d, *J* = 8.7 Hz, 2H), 7.28–7.23 (m, 2H), 7.12 (t, *J* = 8.8 Hz, 2H), 7.02 (d, *J* = 8.8 Hz, 2H), 5.71 (dd, *J* = 12.0, 5.4 Hz, 1H), 3.87 (d, *J* = 5.0 Hz, 1H), 3.81 (s, 3H), 3.68–3.61 (m, 2H), 3.57 (d, *J* = 6.4 Hz, 2H), 3.20–3.12 (m, 3H), 3.00 (s, 2H), 2.73 (s, 4H), 1.79 (d, *J* = 29.8 Hz, 4H).

4-(2-(3-(4-bromophenyl)-5-(4-fluorophenyl)-4,5-dihydro-1H-pyrazol-1-yl)-5,6,7,8-tetrahydrobenzo[4,5] thieno[2,3-d]pyrimidin-4-yl)morpholine (**21e**). Dark blue solid, m.p. 272–273 °C; ESI-MS $[M + H]^+$ *m/z*: 592.5; ^{1}H NMR (400 MHz, DMSO-d_6) δ (ppm): 7.85 (d, *J* = 6.4 Hz, 2H), 7.50 (d, *J* = 7.3 Hz, 2H), 7.30 (s,

2H), 7.20 (d, *J* = 8.0 Hz, 2H), 5.77–5.66 (m, 1H), 3.91 (t, *J* = 16.3 Hz, 1H), 3.63 (s, 2H), 3.58 (s, 2H), 3.18 (s, 3H), 3.01 (s, 2H), 2.74 (s, 4H), 1.79 (d, *J* = 18.0 Hz, 4H).

4-(2-(3-(4-bromophenyl)-5-phenyl-4,5-dihydro-1H-pyrazol-1-yl)-5,6,7,8-tetrahydrobenzo[4,5]thieno[2,3-d]pyrimidin-4-yl)morpholine (**21f**). Dark blue solid, m.p. 257–259 °C; ESI-MS $[M + H]^+$ *m/z*: 574.5; ^1H NMR (400 MHz, DMSO-d_6) δ (ppm): 7.80 (d, *J* = 7.8 Hz, 2H), 7.48 (dd, *J* = 17.6, 7.9 Hz, 5H), 7.20 (d, *J* = 8.4 Hz, 2H), 5.73 (dd, *J* = 11.9, 5.5 Hz, 1H), 3.91 (dd, *J* = 17.9, 12.1 Hz, 1H), 3.64 (d, *J* = 6.0 Hz, 2H), 3.57 (s, 2H), 3.15 (dd, *J* = 17.8, 5.5 Hz, 3H), 3.02 (s, 2H), 2.74 (s, 4H), 1.78 (d, *J* = 18.3 Hz, 4H).

4-(2-(5-(4-bromophenyl)-3-(3,4-dichlorophenyl)-4,5-dihydro-1H-pyrazol-1-yl)-5,6,7,8-tetrahydrobenzo[4,5]thieno[2,3-d]pyrimidin-4-yl)morpholine (**21g**). Dark blue solid, m.p. 231–234 °C; ESI-MS $[M + H]^+$ *m/z*: 643.4; ^1H NMR (400 MHz, DMSO-d_6) δ (ppm): 7.71 (d, *J* = 8.3 Hz, 2H), 7.63 (d, *J* = 8.3 Hz, 2H), 7.57 (d, *J* = 11.3 Hz, 2H), 7.22 (d, *J* = 8.8 Hz, 1H), 5.71 (dd, *J* = 11.9, 5.9 Hz, 1H), 3.89 (dd, *J* = 18.0, 12.5 Hz, 1H), 3.62 (s, 2H), 3.57 (s, 2H), 3.21 (dd, *J* = 17.9, 6.2 Hz, 3H), 2.99 (s, 2H), 2.73 (s, 4H), 1.78 (d, *J* = 37.6 Hz, 4H).

4-(2-(3-(3,4-dichlorophenyl)-5-phenyl-4,5-dihydro-1H-pyrazol-1-yl)-5,6,7,8-tetrahydrobenzo[4,5]thieno[2,3-d]pyrimidin-4-yl)morpholine (**21h**). Dark blue solid, m.p. 293–294 °C; ESI-MS $[M + H]^+$ *m/z*: 563.1; ^1H NMR (400 MHz, DMSO-d_6) δ (ppm): 7.80 (d, *J* = 6.5 Hz, 2H), 7.58 –7.55 (m, 2H), 7.46 (d, *J* = 7.6 Hz, 3H), 7.23–7.19(m, 1H), 5.73 (dd, *J* = 12.1, 5.9 Hz, 1H), 3.92 (dd, *J* = 17.8, 12.2 Hz, 1H), 3.63 (d, *J* = 6.2Hz, 2H), 3.58 (d, *J* = 6.4Hz, 2H), 3.21 (dd, *J* = 18.1, 6.3 Hz, 3H), 3.01 (s, 2H), 2.74 (s, 4H), 1.79 (d, *J* = 23.9 Hz, 4H).

3.3. *Cytotoxicity Assay In Vitro*

The *in vitro* cytotoxic activities of Compounds **9a–l**, **15a–l,** and **21a–h** were evaluated with A549, PC-3, HepG2, and MCF-7 cell lines by the standard MTT assay, with GDC-0941 as a positive control. The cancer cell lines were cultured in minimum essential medium (MEM) supplement with 10% fetal bovine serum (FBS). Approximately, 4×10^{3} cells, suspended in MEM medium, were plated onto each well of a 96-well plate and incubated in 5% CO_2 at 37 °C for 24 h. The test compounds at the indicated final concentrations were added to the culture medium, and cell cultures continued for 72 h. Fresh MTT was added to each well at a terminal concentration of 5 µg/mL and incubated with cells at 37 °C for 4 h. The formazan crystals were dissolved in 100 µL of DMSO in each well, and the absorbency at 492 nm (for absorbance of MTT formazan) and 630 nm (for the reference wavelength) was measured with an enzyme linked immunosorbent assay (ELISA) reader (MR-96A Mindray Elisa Microplate Reader, Guangzhou, China). All compounds were tested three times in each of the cell lines. The results expressed as inhibition rates or IC_{50} was the averages of two determinations and calculated using the Bacus Laboratories Inc. Slide Scanner (Bliss) software (the Bacus Laboratories Inc. Slide Scanner (BLISS) system, Lombard, IL, USA).

3.4. *mTOR Kinase Assay*

The potent compounds **9a** and **15a** were tested for their activities against mTOR enzyme using Kinase-Glo® Luminescent Kinase Assay (Promega, Madison, WI, USA), with NVPBEZ-235 and PI103 as positive controls. The kinase reaction was done in a 384-well black plate. Each well was loaded with 50 µL of test items (in 90% DMSO) and 5 µL reaction buffer containing 10 µg/mL PI substrate (L-α-phosphatidylinositol); Avanti Polar Lipids (Avanti Polar Lipids, Inc., Alabaster, AL, USA); prepared in 3% octyl-glucoside) and the mTOR protein 2.5 nM was then added to it. The reaction was started by the addition of 5 µL of 10 µM ATP prepared in the reaction buffer (50 mM HEPES pH 7.5, 1 mM EGTA, 3 mM $MnCl_2$, 10 mM $MgCl_2$, 2 mM DTT and 0.01% Tween-20) and was incubated for 60 min. It was terminated by the addition of 10 µL Kinase-Glo buffer. The plates were then read in Synergy 2 readers (BioTek, Winooski, VT, USA) for luminescence detection. The assay was repeated two times and the results expressed as IC_{50} (inhibitory concentration 50%) were the averages of two determinations.

3.5. PI3Kα Kinase Assay

The potent compounds **9a** and **15a** were tested for their activity against PI3Kα using a Kinase-Glo® Luminescent Kinase Assay (Promega, Madison, WI, USA), with GDC-0941 and PI103 as positive controls. The kinase reaction occurred in a 384-well black plate. Each well was loaded with 50 μL of test items (in 90% DMSO) and 5 μL of reaction buffer containing 10μg/mL PI substrate (L-α-phosphatidylinositol; Avanti Polar Lipids (Avanti Polar Lipids, Inc.); prepared in 3% octyl-glucoside), and the PI3Kα protein (10 nM) was then added to it. The reaction was started by the addition of 5 μL of 1 μM Adenosine triphosphate (ATP) prepared in the reaction buffer and incubated for 60 min for p110α. It was terminated by the addition of 10 μL of Kinase-Glo buffer. The plates were then read in a Synergy 2 reader (BioTek, Winooski, VT, USA) for luminescence detection. The assay was repeated two times and the results expressed as IC_{50} (inhibitory concentration 50%) were the averages of two determinations.

3.6. Docking Studies

Molecular docking simulation studies were carried out by the AutoDock 4.2 software (The Scripps Research Institute, San Diego, CA, USA). The docking tutorial we used and the detailed AutoDock basic operational methods can be found at: http://autodock.scripps.edu/faqs-help/tutorial. The protein preparation process of flexible docking mainly includes fixing the exact residues, adding hydrogen atoms, removing irrelevant water molecules, adding charges, etc. The potent compounds were selected as ligand examples, and the structures of PI3Kα (PDB code: 3TL5, http://www.pdb.org/) were selected as the docking models. Only the best-scoring ligand–protein complexes were used for the binding site analyses. All the docking results were processed and modified in Open-Source PyMOL 1.8.x software (https://pymol.org).

4. Conclusions

Three series of thienopyrimidine derivatives containing pyrazole structure were designed and synthesized. In addition, we evaluated their cytotoxic activities against four cancer cell lines *in vitro*. The pharmacological indicated that most of the compounds showed moderate cytotoxic activity against the tested cancer cell lines. What is more, the inhibitory activities of the compounds **9a** and **15a** against PI3Kα and mTOR kinase were further investigated. Compound **9a** exhibited moderate levels of inhibition activity against four cancer cell lines and PI3Kα kinase. Although compound **9a** did not reach the same level of inhibition as the positive control drug, it also gave us new direction for developing novel thienopyrimidines containing the pyrazole linker group as PI3Kα inhibitor.

Author Contributions: W.Z., Z.Y., and P.Z. provided and managed the project and supervise the progress of the project; L.Y., Q.W., B.Z., and Y.F. designed the chemical synthesis route and performed the experiments; L.Y., Q.W., and C.W. conducted experimental data analysis and software processing; L.Y., W.Z., and P.Z. started the project, and wrote and revised the paper.

Funding: We gratefully acknowledge the generous support provided by The National Natural Science Funds (No. 21967009); The Project Supported by Natural Science Foundation of Jiangxi, China (20171ACB21052 and 2018BBG70003); Natural Science Funds for Distinguished Young Scholar of Jiangxi Province, China (20171BCB23078); Key projects of the youth fund, Natural Science Funds of Jiangxi Province (20171ACB21052).

Conflicts of Interest: The authors declare no conflict of interest.

References

1. Dehnhardt, C.M.; Venkatesan, A.M.; Delos Santos, E.; Chen, Z.; Santos, O.; Ayral-Kaloustian, S.; Brooijmans, N.; Mallon, R.; Hollander, I.; Feldberg, L.; et al. Lead optimization of *N*-3-substituted 7-morpholinotriazolopyrimidines as dual phosphoinositide 3-kinase/mammalian target of rapamycin inhibitors: Discovery of PKI-402. *J. Med. Chem.* **2009**, *53*, 798–810. [CrossRef] [PubMed]
2. Guba, M.; von Breitenbuch, P.; Steinbauer, M.; Koehl, G.; Flegel, S.; Hornung, M.; Bruns, C.J.; Zuelke, C.; Farkas, S.; Anthuber, M.; et al. Rapamycin inhibits primary and metastatic tumor growth by antiangiogenesis: Involvement of vascular endothelial growth factor. *Nat. Med.* **2002**, *8*, 128. [CrossRef] [PubMed]

3. Marone, R.; Cmiljanovic, V.; Giese, B.; Wymann, M.P. Targeting phosphoinositide 3-kinase—Moving towards therapy. *Biochim. Biophys. Acta (BBA) Proteins Proteom.* **2008**, *1784*, 159–185. [CrossRef] [PubMed]
4. Lv, X.; Ma, X.; Hu, Y. Furthering the design and the discovery of small molecule ATP-competitive mTOR inhibitors as an effective cancer treatment. *Expert Opin. Drug Dis.* **2013**, *8*, 991–1012. [CrossRef] [PubMed]
5. Peng, W.; Tu, Z.C.; Long, Z.J.; Liu, Q.; Lu, G. Discovery of 2-(2-aminopyrimidin-5-yl)-4-morpholino -*N*-(pyridin-3-yl) quinazolin-7-amines as novel PI3K/mTOR inhibitors and anticancer agents. *Eur. J. Med. Chem.* **2016**, *108*, 644–654. [CrossRef] [PubMed]
6. Smith, M.C.; Mader, M.M.; Cook, J.A.; Iversen, P.; Ajamie, R.; Perkins, E.; Bloem, L.; Yip, Y.Y.; Barda, D.A.; Waid, P.P.; et al. Characterization of LY3023414, a novel PI3K/mTOR dual inhibitor eliciting transient target modulation to impede tumor growth. *Mol. Cancer ther.* **2016**, *15*, 2344–2356. [CrossRef] [PubMed]
7. Sarker, D.; Ang, J.E.; Baird, R.; Kristeleit, R.; Shah, K.; Moreno, V.; Clarke, P.A.; Raynaud, F.I.; Levy, G.; Ware, J.A.; et al. First-in-human phase I study of pictilisib (GDC-0941), a potent pan–class I phosphatidylinositol-3-kinase (PI3K) inhibitor, in patients with advanced solid tumors. *Clin. Cancer Res.* **2015**, *21*, 77–86. [CrossRef] [PubMed]
8. Spencer, A.; Yoon, S.S.; Harrison, S.J.; Morris, S.; Smith, D.; Freedman, S.J.; Brigandi, R.; Oliff, A.; Opalinska, J.B.; Chen, C. Novel AKT inhibitor GSK2110183 shows favorable safety, pharmacokinetics, and clinical activity in multiple myeloma. Preliminary results from a phase I first-time-in-human study. *Blood.* **2011**, *118*, 1856.
9. Huo, H.; Zhou, Z.; Wang, B.; Qin, J.; Liu, W.Y.; Gu, Y. Dramatic suppression of colorectal cancer cell growth by the dual mTORC1 and mTORC2 inhibitor AZD-2014. *Biochem. Bioph. Res. Commun.* **2014**, *443*, 406–412. [CrossRef] [PubMed]
10. Sutherlin, D.P.; Bao, L.; Berry, M.; Castanedo, G.; Chuckowree, I.; Dotson, J.; Folks, A.; Friedman, L.; Goldsmith, R.; Gunzner, J.; et al. Discovery of a potent, selective, and orally available class I phosphatidylinositol 3-kinase (PI3K)/mammalian target of rapamycin (mTOR) kinase inhibitor (GDC-0980) for the treatment of cancer. *J. Med. Chem.* **2011**, *54*, 7579–7587. [CrossRef] [PubMed]
11. Heffron, T.P.; Berry, M.; Castanedo, G.; Chang, C.; Chuckowree, I.; Dotson, J.; Folkes, A.; Gunzner, J.; Lesnick, J.D.; Lewis, C.; et al. Identification of GNE-477, a potent and efficacious dual PI3K/mTOR inhibitor. *Bioorg. Med. Chem. Lett.* **2010**, *20*, 2408–2411. [CrossRef] [PubMed]
12. Zhu, W.; Zhai, X.; Fu, Q.; Guo, F.; Bai, M.; Wang, J.; Wang, H.; Gong, P. Design, synthesis and anticancer activity of 4-morpholinothieno [3, 2-d] pyrimidine derivatives bearing arylmethylene hydrazine moiety. *Chem. Pharm. Bull.* **2012**, *60*, 1037–1045. [CrossRef] [PubMed]
13. Zhu, W.; Chen, C.; Sun, C.; Xu, S.; Wu, C.; Lei, F.; Xia, H.; Tu, Q.; Zheng, P. Design, synthesis and docking studies of novel thienopyrimidine derivatives bearing chromone moiety as mTOR/PI3Kα inhibitors. *Eur. J. Med. Chem.* **2015**, *93*, 64–73. [CrossRef] [PubMed]
14. Zhu, W.; Liu, Y.; Zhai, X.; Wang, X.; Zhu, Y.; Wu, D.; Zhou, H.; Gong, P.; Zhao, Y. Design, synthesis and 3D-QSAR analysis of novel 2-hydrazinyl-4-morpholinothieno [3, 2-d] pyrimidine derivatives as potential antitumor agents. *Eur. J. Med. Chem.* **2012**, *57*, 162–175. [CrossRef] [PubMed]
15. Wang, Q.; Li, X.; Sun, C.; Zhang, B.; Zheng, P.; Zhu, W.; Xu, S. Synthesis and Structure–Activity Relationships of 4-Morpholino-7, 8-Dihydro-5H-Thiopyrano [4, 3-d] pyrimidine Derivatives Bearing Pyrazoline Scaffold. *Molecules* **2017**, *22*, 1870. [CrossRef]

Sample Availability: Samples of the compounds **9a–l**, **15a–l**, and **21a–h** are available from the authors.

molecules

MDPI

Article

Potent Anti-Ovarian Cancer with Inhibitor Activities on Both Topoisomerase II and ^{V600E}BRAF of Synthesized Substituted Estrone Candidates

Mohamed El-Naggar [1], Abd El-Galil E. Amr [2,3,*], Ahmed A. Fayed [3,4], Elsayed A. Elsayed [5,6], Mohamed A. Al-Omar [2] and Mohamed M. Abdalla [7]

1 Chemistry Department, Faculty of Sciences, University of Sharjah, Sharjah 27272, UAE; m5elnaggar@yahoo.com
2 Drug Exploration & Development Chair (DEDC), Pharmaceutical Chemistry Department, College of Pharmacy, King Saud University, Riyadh 11451, Saudi Arabia; malomar1@ksu.edu.sa
3 Applied Organic Chemistry Department, National Research Center, Cairo 12622, Egypt; dr_ahmedfayed14@yahoo.com
4 Respiratory Therapy Department, College of Medical Rehabilitation Sciences, Taibah University, Madinah Munawara 22624, Saudi Arabia
5 Zoology Department, Bioproducts Research Chair, College of Science, King Saud University, Riyadh 11451, Saudi Arabia; eaelsayed@ksu.edu.sa
6 Chemistry of Natural and Microbial Products Department, National Research Centre, Cairo 12622, Egypt
7 Atos Pharma, Elkatyba Land, Belbis 44621, El Sharkya, Egypt; mmostafa201120@yahoo.com
* Correspondence: aamr@ksu.edu.sa; Tel.: +966-565-148-750

Received: 25 April 2019; Accepted: 28 May 2019; Published: 29 May 2019

Abstract: A series of 16-(α-alkoxyalkane)-17-hydrazino-estra-1(10),2,4-trien[17,16-c]-3-ol (**3a–l**) and estra-1(10),2,4-trien-[17,16-c]pyrazoline-3-ol derivatives (**4a–d**) were synthesized from corresponding arylidines **2a,b** which was prepared from estrone **1** as starting material. Condensation of 1 with aldehydes gave the corresponding arylidine derivatives **2a,b** which were treated with hydrazine derivatives in alcohols to give the corresponding derivatives **3a–l**, respectively. Additionally, treatment of **2a,b** with methyl- or phenylhydrazine in ethanolic potassium hydroxide afforded the corresponding N-substituted pyrazoline derivatives **4a–d**, respectively. All these derivatives showed potent anti-ovarian cancer both in vitro and in vivo. The mechanism of anti-ovarian cancer was suggested to process via topoisomerase II and ^{V600E}BRAF inhibition.

Keywords: estrone derivatives; hydrazine; N-substituted pyrazoline; anti-ovarian cancer; topoisomerase II inhibitor; kinase inhibitor

1. Introduction

Synthetic alterations of estrone lead to discovering of compounds with diverse biological activities, for example with antitumor effect [1], as anti-breast cancer agent [2] and with antioxidant activity [3]. Estrone derivatives with antitumor activities must be devoid completely of the estrogenic activities [4–6]. The inversion of the configuration at C-13 lead to estrone derivatives with antitumor activities devoid from hormonal actions due to conformational change for the overall molecule resulting from the cis junction of rings C and D [4,7]. Some recent publications report on the syntheses and in vitro biological evaluation of several 13α-estrone derivatives [8–11]. These derivatives exhibited biological activities with substantial anti-proliferative or enzyme inhibitory potentials. Most literature data are mainly focusing on 13α-estrone substitution in ring D, while modified derivatives with ring A substitutions are rarely reported [12].

Cancer is considered one of the most significant causes of death worldwide. Ovarian cancer is one of the major causes for death among adult females [13]. Cancer is characterized by abnormal cell proliferation bypassing normal cell growth and death mechanisms. Recently, DNA topoisomerase II inhibitors have been researched as a potential target, which interferes with cancer growth and development [14]. Topoisomerase II inhibition leads finally to cell cycle inhibition and apoptosis in abnormal cancer cells [15]. BRAF kinase inhibition is another possible control mechanism, which was also developed to interfere with cancer cell growth [16]. BRAF kinase constitutes a major signaling process integrated in the RAS-MEK proliferation process. The activation of MEK by BRAF signals finally induces cell proliferation and survival [17]. Inhibiting BRAF activity results in inhibition of the proliferation signals, and thus inhibiting cancer cell development and growth [18].

In view of these observations and in continuation of our previous work in heterocyclic chemistry [19–22], the current work aimed at evaluating the effect or remote long cage distortion caused by introducing some moieties in both 16 and 17 locations of ring D. We screened some of synthesized estrone candidates for their anti-ovarian cancer potential both in vitro and in vivo. Furthermore, the inhibitory effects of the synthesized compounds were investigated against topoisomerase II and ^{V600E}BRAF kinase inhibitors.

2. Results and Discussion

2.1. Results

2.1.1. Chenical Synthesis

A series of 17-hydrazino-estratrienol (**3a–l**) and pyrazolinestratrienol (**4a–d**) were synthesized from corresponding arylidines **2a,b** which was prepared from estrone **1** as starting material.

Treatment of aryledine derivatives **2a,b** with hydrazine hydrate, in refluxing methanol or ethanol afforded the corresponding 17-hydrazino-16-α-methoxymethane estrone derivatives **3a,b** and 17-hydrazino-16-α-ethoxyethane estrone derivatives **3c,d**, respectively.

Also, reaction of compounds **2a,b** with N-methyl hydrazine, in refluxing methanol or ethanol afford 17-N-methyl hydrazino-16-α-methoxymethane estrone derivatives **3e,f** and 17-*N*-methyl hydrazino-16-α-ethoxyethane estrone derivatives **3g,h** respectively.

Additionally, when compounds **2a,b** reacted with *N*-phenyl hydrazine, under the same conditions afford the corresponding 17-*N*-phenylhydrazino- 16-α-methoxymethane estrone derivatives **3i,j** and 17-*N*-phenylhydrazino- 16-α-ethoxyethane estrone derivatives **3k,l**, respectively. Finally, condensation of **2a,b** with CH_3NHNH_2 or $PhNHNH_2$ in refluxing dioxane afforded the corresponding N-substituted pyrazoline derivatives **4a–d**, respectively (Scheme 1).

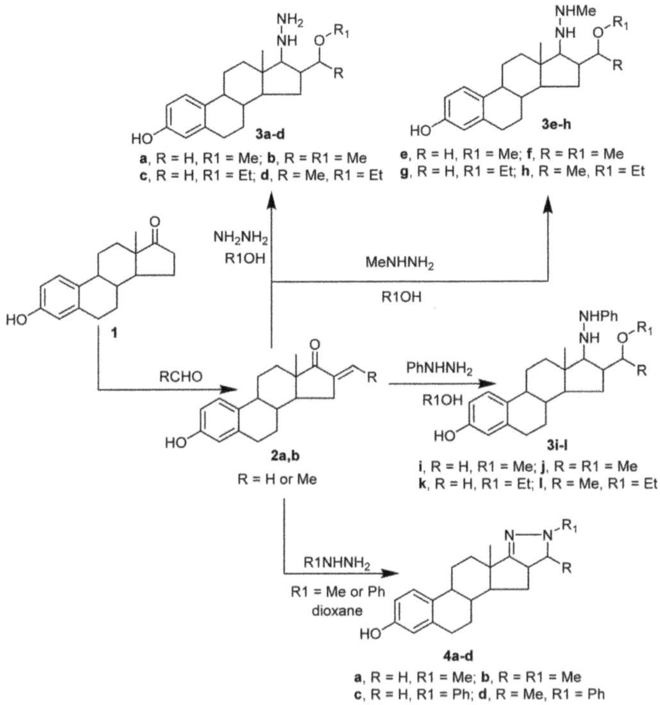

Scheme 1. Synthetic route for compounds **2–4**.

2.1.2. Biological Screening

In Vitro Cytotoxic Activities

The cytotoxicity of some synthesized derivatives against SKOV-3 cancer cell line in vitro was performed with the MTT assay. The obtained results showed that all synthesized compounds showed potent in vitro cytotoxic activities against SKOV-3 cells at the nanomolar level. Moreover, the effect of the synthesized compounds was dose-dependent. From the obtained IC_{50} values (Figure 1), prepared compounds can be arranged discerningly in the following order: **3a, 3b, 3c, 3d, 3e, 3f, 3g, 3h, 3i, 3j, 3k, 3l, 4a, 4b, 4c, 4d** (Figure 1). Compounds **3a–l** are characterized with the presence of hydrazine group rather than the pyrazoline group present in compounds **4a–d**. Furthermore, the alkyl group is found to be more active than the aromatic group. Generally Cpd. **3a** showed highest cytotoxic activity with IC_{50} value of 4.23 ± 0.12 nM, while Cpd. **4d** was the least active, where its IC_{50} value was about 9.5% of that obtained for Cpd. **3a**.

The effect of resveratrol (RES) and doxorubicin (DOX) on SKOV-3 showed IC_{50} of 55 and 250 nM, respectively.

The cytotoxicity of the newly synthesized compounds against fibroblast were as follow $\mathbf{IC_{50}}$ **3a** (1.2 μM), **3b** (2.45 μM), **3c** (5.67 μM), **3d** (7.44 μM), **3e** (8.11 μM), **3f** (9.20 μM), **3g** (11.18 μM), **3h**(16.22 μM), **3i** (15.13 μM), **3j** (16.20 μM), **3k** (17.78 μM), **3l** (20.21 μM), **4a** (23.34 μM), **4b** (24.55 μM), **4c** (25.55 μM), **4d** (30.34 μM).

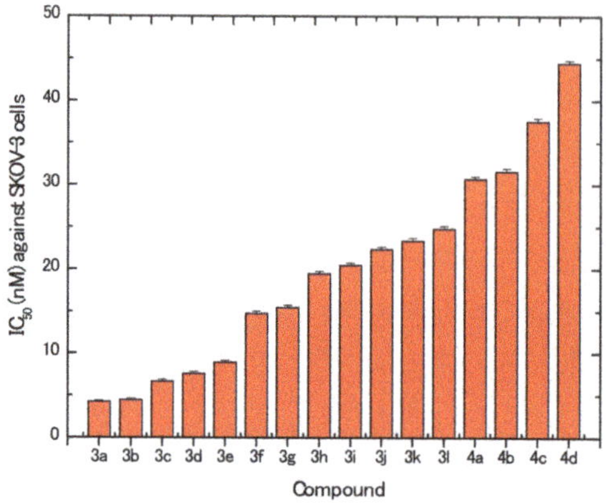

Figure 1. In vitro Cytotoxicity activities of the tested compounds against SKOV-3 cells.

In Vivo Anti-Ovarian Cancer

The in vivo anti-ovarian cancer activities of the tested compounds were evaluated using mouse xenograft model. Figure 2 represents the percentages of decrease in tumor growth upon treatment with different synthesized compounds. The obtained results showed that all compounds potentially reduced tumor growth over a period of 40 days of treatment, in comparison to control treatments, which showed normal tumor growth development. Moreover, it can be seen that the reduction in tumor size started directly from the 5th day of treatment, where the reduction percentage ranged from 45.7 ± 0.05% to 54.71 ± 0.01%. The reduction in tumor growth increased significantly reaching its maximal by the end of treatment period (40 days). The highest reduction in tumor growth was recorded for occurred Cpd. **3a**, which significantly decreased tumor growth by about 93.61 ± 0.7%. It can also be seen that Cpd. **3a**, was the most potent for in vivo treatment, where its effect was more obvious starting from day15 of treatment, where the reduction percentage in tumor size due to other compounds was more or less within the same range. We also can see that the in vivo results are coincided with those obtained for *in vitro* results, where the reduction in tumor size followed the same descending order: **3a**, **3b**, **3c**, **3d**, **3e**, **3f**, **3g**, **3h**, **3i**, **3j**, **3k**, **3l**, **4a**, **4b**, **4c**, and **4d**.

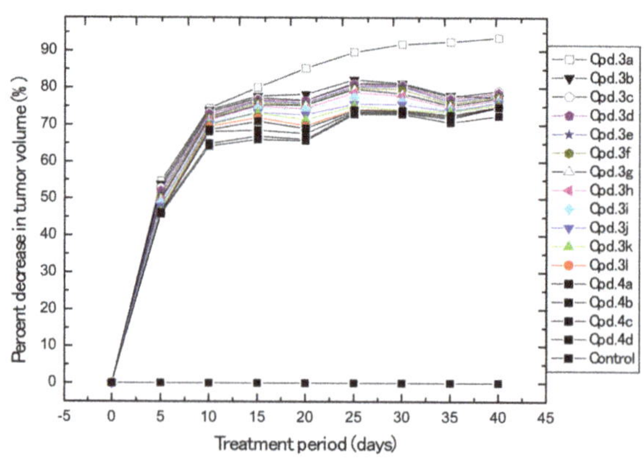

Figure 2. Percentages of decrease in tumor volume in nude mice in response to different synthesized derivatives.

2.1.3. Inhibition of Topoisomerase II Activities

In order to further investigate the possible mechanism of action of the newly synthesized derivatives, we investigated their inhibitory effects on topoisomerase II. Results obtained (Figure 3) showed that all synthesized compounds showed potential inhibitory effects against topoisomerase II. Furthermore, the inhibitory effect was also found to follow the same descending order obtained before during in vitro and in vivo investigation: **3a, 3b, 3c, 3d, 3e, 3f, 3g, 3h, 3i, 3j, 3k, 3l, 4a, 4b, 4c**, and **4d**. Cpd. **3a** showed the most inhibitory action for topoisomerase II with IC_{50} value of 3.45 ± 0.13 nM, which was about 7,9% of that obtained for the lest potent compound (IC_{50} for Cpd. **4d**: 43.56 ± 0.98 nM).

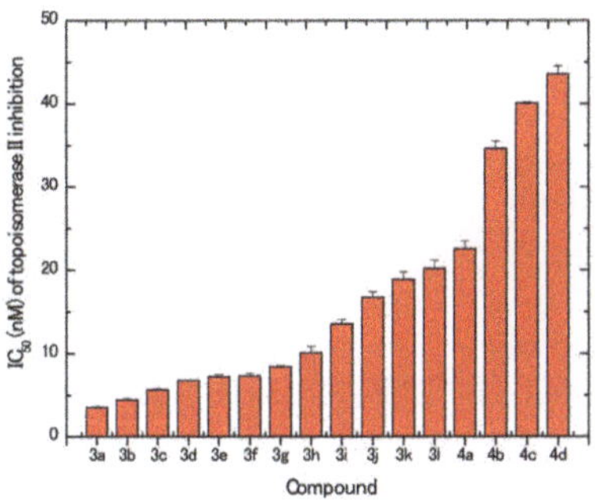

Figure 3. IC_{50} of Topoisomerase II Inhibitor activities of the tested compounds.

2.1.4. In Vitro Kinase Assay

The in vitro kinase assay of synthesized derivatives was investigated against both ^{WT}BRAF (BRAF kinase wild type) and ^{V600E}BRAF (mutant BRAF kinase). Results obtained in Figure 4 showed that all synthesized compounds were highly active inhibitors for ^{V600E}BRAF compared with moderate activities against ^{WT}BRAF. Again, the descending order of activities was as follow **3a, 3b, 3c, 3d, 3e, 3f, 3g, 3h, 3i, 3j, 3k, 3l, 4a, 4b, 4c**, and **4d**. Compound **3a** recorded the most active inhibition (IC_{50}: 0.041 ± 0.0016 and 4.23 ± 0.12 μM for mutant and wild type BRAF kinase, respectively. Furthermore, it can be seen that the inhibitory effect of Cpd. **3a** was much more superior to that obtained for different positive control drugs (0.48, 3.87 and 0.97 μM for Sorafenib, Dabrafenib and Vemurafenib, respectively.

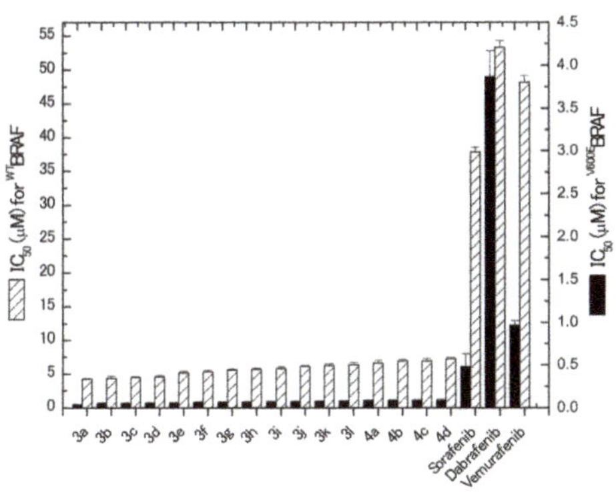

Figure 4. IC_{50} values of synthesized for both ^{WT}BRAF and ^{V600E}BRAF.

2.2. Discussion

Within the framework of the current work we synthesized new estrone derivatives from their corresponding arylidines. The newly synthesized derivatives showed potential cytotoxic activities against SKOV-3 cells. Moreover, in vivo investigations revealed that the synthesized compounds were able to potentially reduce tumor volume growth over a treatment period of 45 days.

The newly introduced 1-alkoxy benzyl moiety alone or combined with the 17- hydrazino- moities make remote destortion of the structure cage that completely elminate any hormonal activities of te estrone molceules and deviate the biological activities towards the aniticancer ones, so we investigated this property and tried to find the mechnisms of anticancer actions of these newly synthesized compounds.

In search for the possible mechanism of action of the anticancer activities of the tested compounds, we investigated the possibility of the compounds to inhibit both topoisomerase II and kinase enzymes. Results showed that the prepared compounds can potentially serve as inhibitors for these enzymes. The cytotoxic activities of the prepared estrone derivatives can be due to the inhibition of 17-hydroxysteroid dehydrogenases. We have previously reported on the anti-breast cancer activities of different estrone derivatives [23], and explained that their anticancer activities can be attributed to the inhibition of 17-hydroxysteroid dehydrogenase [24].

Concerning topoisomerase II and ^{V600E}BRAF kinase inhibition, our results suggest that the newly synthesized compounds exert their cytotoxic action against SKOV-3 cancer cells by interfering with the metabolic activity of these enzymes, thus preventing cancer cells from obtaining proliferation signaling molecules essential for their growth and survival [16,17]. Different activities of the prepared compounds may be attributed to the structure activity relationship of these compounds.

Hydrazine derivatives are generally potent than pyrazoline ones, due to their open chain structure as well as their higher electron density. Furthermore, it can be suggested that *N*-methyl derivatives are more active than *N*-phenyl ones. On the other hand, hydrazine derivatives can be divided into more active α-methoxyl derivatives and the less active α-ethoxyl, and then the least active *N*-phenyl derivatives. This can be explained due to the fact that phenyl group act as a withdrawing group. On the other hand, the weaker effect of α-ethoxyl derivatives than the α-methoxyl ones can be attributed to their bulky nature. This effect can be observed among different series of compound **3**. As the bulky nature of the substituted groups increase, accordingly more steric hindrance can be observed, leading to decreased cytotoxic activities.

3. Materials and Methods

3.1. Chemical Synthesis

"Melting points reported are inaccurate. IR spectra were registered on Shimadzu FT-IR 8300 E (Shimadzu Corporation, Kyoto, Japan) spectrophotometer using the (KBr) disk technique. The ^{1}H-NMR spectra were determined with bruker 600 MHz NMR spectrometer. The chemical shifts are expressed on the δ (ppm) scale using TMS as the standard reference. Mass spectra were recorded on Finnigan SSQ operating at 70 ev. Elemental analysis determined on a Perkin Elmer 240 (Microanalysis), Microanalysis Center, Cairo University, Cairo, Egypt".

3.1.1. Synthesis of 3-Hydroxy-16-[substituted]-estra-1(10),2,4-trien-17-ones (**2a**,**b**)

"A mixture of (**1**) (0.54 g, 20 mmol) and formaldehyde or acetaldehyde (20 mmol) in EtOH (50 mL) and aqueous KOH (10 mL, 30%) was stirred for 24 h at room temperature. The formed solid was collected by filtration, crystallized from ethanol to give compounds **2a** [25] and **2b**, respectively".

3-Hydroxy-16-[ethylene]-estra-1(10),2,4-trien-17-one (**2b**)

Yield 97%, mp 198–200 °C, $[\alpha]_D^{25}$ = + 71 (c 1, MeOH). IR (KBr, cm^{-1}): 3340 (OH), 2944 (CH, aliphatic), 1743 (C=O), 1642 (C=C). ^{1}H NMR: (600 MHz, $CDCl_3$): δ ppm 0.61 (1H, m, H-8β), 0.90 (3H, s, CH_3-18), 1.01 (1H, m, H-11β), 1.12 (1H, m, H-7α), 1.15 (1H, m, H-12α), 1.25 (1H, m, H-14α), 1.44 (1H, m, H-15β), 1.63 (1H, m, H-15α), 1.72 (1H, m, H-7β), 2.01 (1H, m, H-9α), 2.13 (1H, m, H-11α), 2.50 (1H, m, H-12β), 2.56 (1H, m, H-6α), 2.66 (1H, m, H-6β), 4.90 (1H, s, OH, disappeared with D_2O), 5.75 (1H, dd, H-2), 6.67 (1H, d, H-4), 2.08 (3H, d, CH_3, enone), 6.41 (1H, s, enone proton), 7.12 (1H, d, H-1). ^{13}C NMR: (150 MHz, $CDCl_3$): δ 13.52, 21.73, 25.51, 26.64, 27.48, 29.75, 36.35, 38.61, 43.81, 48.92, 50.43, 112.79, 115.53, 126.56, 128.48, 132.50, 137.02, 138.44, 153.82, 210.02 (20 C). MS (EI): *m/z* 296 (100%) [M$^+$]. Anal. Calcd for $C_{20}H_{24}O_2$ (296.40): Calcd C, 81.04; H, 8.16. Found C, 81.00; H, 8.10.

3.1.2. Synthesis of 16-(α-alkoxy-alkane)-17-hydrazino-estra-1(10),2,4-trien[17,16-c]-3-ol and their *N*-substituted derivatives (**3a–l**)

"A mixture of **2a,b** (14 mmol) and hydrazine derivatives, namely, hydrazine hydrate, methyl hydrazine or phenyl hydrazine (8 mmol) in absolute methanol or ethanol (30 mL) was refluxed for 5–10 h. The solvent was concentrated under reduced pressure, the formed precipitate was filtered off, washed with water, dried and crystallized from ethanol to give the corresponding derivatives **3a–l**, respectively".

16-(α-Methoxy-methane)-17-hydrazino-estra-1(10),2,4-trien-[17,16-c]-3-ol (**3a**)

Yield 80%, mp 199–201 °C, $[\alpha]_D^{25}$ = + 81 (c 1, MeOH). IR (KBr, cm^{-1}): 3444–3377 (NH, NH_2), 3345 (OH), 2951 (CH, aliphatic), 1638 (C=C). ^{1}H NMR: (600 MHz, $CDCl_3$): δ ppm 0.61 (1H, m, H-8β), 0.90 (3H, s, CH_3-18), 1.00 (1H, m, H-11β), 1.11 (1H, m, H-7α), 1.14 (1H, m, H-12α), 1.26 (1H, m, H-14 α), 1.39 (1H, m, H-15β), 1.58 (1H, m, H-15α), 1.68 (1H, m, H-7β), 2.01(1H, m, H-9α), 1.84 (1H, m, CH, 16-Hα), 2.11 (1H, m, H-11α), 2.49 (1H, m, H-12β), 2.61 (1H, m, H-6α), 2.66 (1H, m, H-6β), 2.83 (1H, d, H-17), 3.48 (3H, s, OCH_3), 4.65 (2H, m, NH_2, disappeared with D_2O), 4.80 (2H, d, CH_2-O), 4.87 (1H, s, OH, disappeared with D_2O), 5.70 (1H, dd, H-2), 6.61 (1H, d, H-4), 7.10 (1H, d, H-1), 7.70 (1H, br.s, NH, disappeared with D_2O). ^{13}C NMR: (150 MHz, $CDCl_3$): δ 13.58, 21.76, 25.57, 26.76, 28.00, 29.78, 36.38, 38.65, 43.89, 48.40, 50.45, 59.45, 69.11, 112.37, 115.56, 126.53, 132.81, 138.46, 153.84, 167.02 (20 C). MS (EI): *m/z* 330 (90%) [M$^+$]. Anal. Calcd for $C_{20}H_{30}N_2O_2$ (330.46): Calcd C, 72.69; H, 9.15; N, 8.48. Found C, 72.60; H, 9.10; N, 8.40.

16-(α-Methoxy-ethane)-17-hydrazino-estra-1(10),2,4-trien[17,16-c]-3-ol (**3b**)

Yield 57%, mp. 308–310 °C, $[\alpha]_D^{25}$ = + 112 (c 1, MeOH). IR (KBr, cm^{-1}): 3448-3377 (NH, NH_2), 3348 (OH), 2959 (CH, aliphatic), 1634 (C=C). ^{1}H NMR: (600 MHz, $CDCl_3$): δ ppm 0.59 (1H, m, H-8β), 0.91 (3H, s, CH_3-18), 1.01 (1H, m, H-11β), 1.12 (1H, m, H-7α), 1.14 (1H, m, H-12 α), 1.26 (1H, m, H-14 α), 1.39 (1H, m, H -15 β), 1.58 (1H, m, H-15α), 1.42 (3H, m, CH_3,C-16 ethane), 1.69 (1H, m, H-7β), 2.02(1H, m, H-9α), 1.83 (1H, m, CH, H-16α), 2.11 (1H, m, H-11α), 2.49 (1H, m, H-12β), 2.61 (1H, m, H-6α), 2.66 (1H, m, H-6β), 2.83 (1H, d, H-17), 3.48 (3H, s, OCH_3), 4.65 (2H, s, NH_2, disappeared with D_2O), 4.84 (1H, d, CH-O), 4.99 (1H, s, OH, disappeared with D_2O), 5.72 (1H, dd, H-2), 6.61 (1H, d, H-4), 7.11 (1H, d, H-1), 7.78 (1H, bs, NH, disappeared with D_2O). ^{13}C NMR: (150 MHz, $CDCl_3$): δ 13.58, 21.77, 22.22, 25.57, 26.47, 28.00, 29.78, 36.68, 38.47, 43.89, 48.69, 50.45, 59.45, 69.11, 112.37, 115.56, 126.55, 132.48, 138.46, 153.54, 167.76 (21 C). MS (EI): *m/z* 344 (11%) [M$^+$]. Anal. Calcd for $C_{21}H_{32}N_2O_2$ (344.49): Calcd C, 73.22; H, 9.36; N, 8.13. Found C, 73.18; H, 9.30; N, 8.10.

16-(α-Ethoxy-methane)-17-hydrazino-estra-1(10),2,4-trien-[17,16-c]-3-ol (**3c**)

Yield 56%, mp 219–221 °C, $[\alpha]_D^{25}$ = + 77 (c 1, MeOH). IR (KBr, cm^{-1}): 3445–3376 (NH, NH_2), 3346 (OH), 2951 (CH, aliphatic), 1638 (C=C). ^{1}H NMR: (600 MHz, $CDCl_3$): δ ppm 0.61 (1H, m, H-8β), 0.90 (3H, s, CH_3-18), 1.00 (1H, m, H-11β), 1.11 (1H, m, H-7α), 1.15 (1H, m, H-12α), 1.21 (3H, m, CH_3, ethoxyl), 1.25 (1H, m, H-14α), 1.36 (1H, m, H-15β), 1.57 (1H, m, H-15α), 1.68 (1H, m, H-7β), 2.01 (1H, m, H-9α), 1.84 (1H, m, CH, H-16α), 2.10 (1H, m, H-11α), 2.50 (1H, m, H-12β), 2.60 (1H, m, H-6α), 2.70 (1H, m, H-6β), 6.61 (1H, d, H-4), 2.80 (1H, d, H-17), 3.50 (2H, m, OCH_2), 4.70 (2H, m, NH_2, disappeared with D_2O), 4.80 (2H, d, CH-O), 4.87 (1H, s, OH, disappeared with D_2O), 5.70 (1H, dd, H-2), 7.10 (1H, d, H-1), 7.70 (1H, br.s, NH, disappeared with D_2O). ^{13}C NMR: (150 MHz, $CDCl_3$): δ 13.65, 18.74, 21.57, 25.17, 26.38, 28.04, 29.64, 36.54, 38.15, 44.11, 48.44, 50.54, 68.45, 69.11, 112.44, 115.67, 126.34, 131.11, 138.46, 153.84, 161.47 (21 C). MS (EI): *m/z* 344 (35%) [M^+]. Anal. Calcd for $C_{21}H_{32}N_2O_2$ (344.49): Calcd C, 73.22; H, 9.36; N, 8.13. Found C, 73.16; H, 9.30; N, 8.10.

16-(α-Ethoxy-ethane)-17-hydrazino-estra-1(10),2,4-trien-[17,16-c]-3-ol (**3d**)

Yield 90%, mp 223–225 °C, $[\alpha]_D^{25}$ = + 95 (c 1, MeOH). IR (KBr, cm^{-1}): 3440-3370 (NH, NH_2), 3350 (OH), 2951 (CH, aliphatic), 1631 (C=C). ^1H NMR: (600 MHz, $CDCl_3$): δ ppm 0.57 (1H, m, H-8β), 0.90 (3H, s, CH_3-18), 1.00 (1H, m, H-11β), 1.10 (1H, m, H-7α), 1.15 (1H, m, H-12α), 1.20 (3H, m, CH_3, ethoxyl), 1.24 (1H, m, H-14α), 1.36 (1H, m, H-15β), 1.45 (3H, m, CH_3,C-16 ethane), 1.59 (1H, m, H-15α), 1.71 (1H, m, H-7β), 1.96 (1H, m, H-9α), 1.82 (1H, m, CH, H-16α), 2.10 (1H, m, H-11α), 2.50 (1H, m, H-12β), 2.62 (1H, m, H-6α), 2.67 (1H, m, H-6β), 2.86 (1H, d, H-17), 3.48 (2H, m, OCH_2), 4.64 (2H, s, NH_2, disappeared with D_2O), 4.83 (1H, d, CH-O), 4.88 (1H, s, OH, disappeared with D_2O), 5.74 (1H, dd, H-2), 6.65 (1H, d, H-4), 7.12 (1H, d, H-1), 7.78 (1H, br.s, NH, disappeared with D_2O). ^{13}C NMR: (150 MHz, $CDCl_3$): δ 13.55, 18.79, 22.07, 22.28, 25.47, 26.52, 27.77, 28.09, 36.68, 37.97, 44.09, 48.11, 51.41, 68.43, 69.13, 112.56, 115.57, 126.37, 133.18, 137.87, 155.56, 162.74 (22 C). MS (EI): *m/z* 358 (45%) [M^+]. Anal. Calcd for $C_{22}H_{34}N_2O_2$ (358.51): Calcd C, 73.70; H, 9.56; N, 7.81. Found C, 73.64; H, 9.52; N, 7.75.

16-(α-Methoxy-methane)-17-[N-methyl-hydrazino]estra-1(10),2,4-trien[17,16-c]-3-ol (**3e**)

Yield 76%, mp 222–224 °C, $[\alpha]_D^{25}$ = + 66 (c 1, MeOH). IR (KBr, cm^{-1}): 3443–3371 (NH), 3344 (OH), 2953 (CH, aliphatic), 1634 (C=C). ^1H NMR: (600 MHz, $CDCl_3$): δ ppm 0.61 (1H, m, H-8β), 0.92 (3H, s, CH_3-18), 1.03 (1H, m, H-11β), 1.10 (1H, m, H-7α), 1.14 (1H, m, H-12α), 1.25 (1H, m, H-14α), 1.37 (1H, m, H-15β), 1.57 (1H, m, H-15α), 1.66 (1H, m, H-7β), 2.00 (1H, m, H-9α), 1.84 (1H, m, CH, H-16α), 2.13 (1H, m, H-11α), 2.32 (3H, s, NCH_3), 2.48 (1H, m, H-12β), 2.63 (1H, m, H-6α), 2.68 (1H, m, H-6β), 2.84 (1H, d, H-17), 3.49 (3H, s, OCH_3), 4.86 (2H, d, CH-O), 4.87 (1H, s, OH, disappeared with D_2O), 5.72 (1H, dd, H-2), 6.63 (1H, d, H-4), 7.11 (1H, d, H-1), 7.76 (1H, brs, NH, disappeared with D_2O), 7.99 (1H, bs, NH, disappeared with D_2O). ^{13}C NMR: (150 MHz, $CDCl_3$): δ 13.53, 21.44, 25.67, 26.36, 28.03, 29.23, 36.33, 38.43, 43.83, 47.47, 48.43, 50.34, 59.35, 69.31, 112.36, 115.67, 126.52, 132.32, 138.21, 153.45, 162.32 (21 C). MS (EI): *m/z* 344 (45%) [M^+]. Anal. Calcd for $C_{21}H_{32}N_2O_2$ (344.50): Calcd C, 73.22; H, 9.36; N, 8.13. Found C, 73.15; H, 9.31; N, 8.09.

16-(α-Methoxy-ethane)-17-[N-methyl-hydrazino]-estra-1(10),2,4-trien-[17,16-c]-3-ol (**3f**)

Yield 57%, mp 310–312 °C, $[\alpha]_D^{25}$ = + 112 (c 1, MeOH). IR (KBr, cm^{-1}): 3443–3374 (NH), 3344 (OH), 2955 (CH, aliphatic), 1628 (C=C). ^1H NMR: (600 MHz, $CDCl_3$): δ ppm 0.58 (1H, m, H-8β), 0.90 (3H, s, CH_3-18), 1.00 (1H, m, H-11β), 1.10 (1H, m, H-7α), 1.14 (1H, m, H-12α), 1.26 (1H, m, H-14 α), 1.39 (1H, m, H-15 β), 1.60 (1H, m, H-15α), 1.44 (3H, m, CH_3, C-16 ethane), 1.70 (1H, m, H-7β), 2.00 (1H, m, H-9α), 1.82 (1H, m, CH, H-16α), 2.11 (1H, m, H-11α), 2.36 (3H, s, NCH_3), 2.51 (1H, m, H-12β), 2.62 (1H, m, H-6α), 2.65 (1H, m, H-6β), 2.85 (1H, d, H-17), 3.44 (3H, s, OCH_3), 4.83 (1H, d, CH-O), 4.99 (1H, s, OH, disappeared with D_2O), 5.74 (1H, dd, H-2), 6.65 (1H, d, H-4), 7.13 (1H, d, H-1), 7.73 (1H, br.s, NH, disappeared with D_2O), 7.99 (1H, m, NH, disappeared with D_2O). ^{13}C NMR: (150 MHz, $CDCl_3$): δ 13.78, 21.54, 22.27, 25.97, 26.69, 28.03, 29.43, 36.45, 38.54, 43.68, 47.88, 48.57, 50.86, 59.46, 69.15, 112.54, 115.69, 126.46, 132.90, 138.75, 153.45, 163.60 (22 C). MS (EI): *m/z* 358 (100%) [M^+]. Anal. Calcd for $C_{22}H_{34}N_2O_2$ (358.50): Calcd C, 73.70; H, 9.56; N, 7.81. Found C, 73.60; H, 9.49; N, 7.75.

16-(α-Ethoxy-methane)-17-[N-methyl-hydrazino]-estra-1(10),2,4-trien-[17,16-c]-3-ol (**3g**)

Yield 90%, mp 286–288 °C, $[\alpha]_D^{25}$ = + 121 (c 1, MeOH). IR (KBr, cm^{-1}): 3441–3379 (NH), 3348 (OH), 2957 (CH, aliphatic), 1636 (C=C). ^1H NMR: (600 MHz, $CDCl_3$): δ ppm 0.61 (1H, m, H-8β), 0.91 (3H, s, CH_3-18), 1.01 (1H, m, H-11β), 1.13 (1H, m, H-7α), 1.15 (1H, m, H-12α), 1.22 (3H, m, CH_3, ethoxyl), 1.25 (1H, m, H-14α), 1.37 (1H, m, H-15β), 1.58 (1H, m, H-15α), 1.69 (1H, m, H-7β), 2.00 (1H, m, H-9 α), 1.81 (1H, m, CH, H-16α), 2.12 (1H, m, H-11α), 2.33 (3H, s, NCH_3), 2.54 (1H, m, H-12β), 2.65 (1H, m, H-6α), 2.76 (1H, m, H-6β), 2.87 (1H, d, H-17), 3.50 (2H, m, OCH_2), 4.85 (2H, d, CH_2-O), 4.98 (1H, s, OH, disappeared with D_2O), 5.74 (1H, dd, H-2), 6.65 (1H, d, H-4), 7.10 (1H, d, H-1), 7.76 (1H, br.s, NH, disappeared with D_2O), 7.95 (1H, m, NH, disappeared with D_2O). ^{13}C NMR: (150 MHz, $CDCl_3$): δ 13.35, 18.45, 21.43, 25.78, 26.80, 28.14, 29.88, 36.47, 38.90, 44.41, 47.37, 48.34, 50.54, 68.66, 69.67, 113.34, 115.55, 125.54, 131.53, 137.99, 154.44, 162.27 (22 C). MS (EI): *m/z* 358 (100%) [M^+]. Anal. Calcd for $C_{22}H_{34}N_2O_2$ (358.50): Calcd C, 73.70; H, 9.56; N, 7.81. Found C, 73.62; H, 9.50; N, 7.74.

16-(α-Ethoxy-ethane)-17-[N-methyl-hydrazino]-estra-1(10),2,4-trien-[17,16-c]-3-ol (**3h**)

Yield 78%, mp 280–282 °C, $[\alpha]_D^{25}$ = + 135 (c 1, MeOH). IR (KBr, cm^{-1}): 3441–3371 (NH), 3351 (OH), 2951 (CH, aliphatic), 1631 (C=C). ^1H NMR: (600 MHz, $CDCl_3$): δ ppm 0.60 (1H, m, H-8β), 0.93 (3H, s, CH_3-18), 1.04 (1H, m, H-11β), 1.11 (1H, m, H-7α), 1.16 (1H, m, H-12α), 1.19 (3H, m, CH_3,ethoxyl), 1.23 (1H, m, H-14α), 1.37 (1H, m, H-15β), 1.46 (3H, m, CH_3,C-16 ethane), 1.61 (1H, m, H-15α), 1.72 (1H, m, H-7β), 1.82 (1H, m, CH, H-16α), 1.93 (1H, m, H-9α), 2.10 (1H, m, H-11α), 2.50 (1H, m, H-12β), 2.34 (3H, s, NCH_3), 2.63 (1H, m, H-6α), 2.62 (1H, m, H-6β), 2.85 (1H, d, H-17), 3.43 (2H, m, OCH_2), 4.64 (1H, s, OH, disappeared with D_2O), 4.83 (1H, d, CH-O), 5.72 (1H, dd, H-2), 6.64 (1H, d, H-4), 7.10 (1H, d, H-1), 7.75 (1H, br.s, NH, disappeared with D_2O), 7.88 (1H, s, NH, disappeared with D_2O). ^{13}C NMR: (150 MHz, $CDCl_3$): δ 13.53, 18.67, 22.43, 22.90, 25.67, 26.78, 27.45, 28.29, 36.89, 37.65, 44.65, 47.35, 48.68, 51.90, 68.78, 69.13, 112.56, 115.56, 126.34, 133.55, 137.43, 155.34, 163.34 (23 C). MS (EI): *m/z* 372 (100%) [M^+]. Anal. Calcd for $C_{23}H_{36}N_2O_2$ (372.54): Calcd C, 74.15; H, 9.74; N, 7.52. Found C, 74.05; H, 9.68; N, 7.48.

16-(α-Methoxy-methane)-17-[N-phenyl-hydrazino]-estra-1(10),2,4-trien-[17,16-c]-3-ol (**3i**)

Yield 67%, mp 312–314 °C, $[\alpha]_D^{25}$ = + 95 (c 1, MeOH). IR (KBr, cm^{-1}): 3430–3367 (NH), 3345 (OH), 3068 (CH, aromatic), 2951 (CH, aliphatic), 1638 (C=C). ^1H NMR: (600 MHz, $CDCl_3$): δ ppm 0.61(1H, m, H-8β), 0.91 (3H, s, CH_3-18), 1.00 (1H, m, H-11β), 1.12 (1H, m, H-7α), 1.15 (1H, m, H-12α), 1.28 (1H, m, H-14α), 1.40 (1H, m, H-15β), 1.60 (1H, m, H-15α), 1.68 (1H, m, H-7β), 2.02 (1H, m, H-9α), 1.86 (1H, m, CH, H-16α), 2.12 (1H, m, H-11α), 2.49 (1H, m, H-12 β), 2.59 (1H, m, H-6α), 2.65 (1H, m, H-6β), 2.84 (1H, d, H-17), 3.47 (3H, s, OCH_3), 4.80 (2H, d, CH-O), 4.87 (1H, s, OH, disappeared with D_2O), 5.70 (1H, dd, H-2), 6.61 (1H, d, H-4), 7.10 (1H, d, H-1), 7.28-7.48 (5H, m, Ar-H), 7.76 (1H, br.s, NH, disappeared with D_2O), 7.99 (1H, s, NH, disappeared with D_2O). ^{13}C NMR: (150 MHz, $CDCl_3$): δ 13.45, 21.76, 25.76, 26.67, 28.45, 29.66, 36.43, 38.65, 43.45, 48.40, 50.87, 59.45, 69.67, 112.43, 112.76, 115.66, 119.11, 126.68, 129.45, 132.67, 138.53, 152.55, 153.79, 161.02 (26 C). MS (EI): *m/z* 406 (77%) [M^+]. Anal. Calcd for $C_{26}H_{34}N_2O_2$ (406.56): Calcd C, 76.81; H, 8.43; N, 6.89. Found C, 76.75; H, 8.40; N, 6.80.

16-(α-Methoxy-ethane)-17-[N-phenyl-hydrazino]-estra-1(10),2,4-trien-[17,16-c]-3-ol (**3j**)

Yield 66%, mp 229–231 °C, $[\alpha]_D^{25}$ = + 147 (c 1, MeOH). IR (KBr, cm^{-1}): 3433–3363 (NH), 3346 (OH), 3066 (CH, aromatic), 2955 (CH, aliphatic), 1635 (C=C). ^1H NMR: (600 MHz, $CDCl_3$): δ ppm 0.62 (1H, m, H-8β), 0.92 (3H, s, CH_3-18), 1.02 (1H, m, H-11β), 1.13 (1H, m, H-7α), 1.18 (1H, m, H-12α), 1.26 (1H, m, H-14α), 1.39 (1H, m, H-15β), 1.42 (3H, m, CH_3, C-16 ethane), 1.58 (1H, m, H-15α), 1.69 (1H, m, H-7β), 1.83 (1H, m, CH, H-16α), 2.03 (1H, m, H-9α), 2.10 (1H, m, H-11α), 2.52 (1H, m, H-12β), 2.62 (1H, m, H-6α), 2.65 (1H, m, H-6β), 2.85 (1H, d, H-17), 3.49 (3H, s, OCH_3), 4.86 (1H, d, CH-O), 4.89 (1H, s, OH, disappeared with D_2O), 5.71 (1H, dd, H-2), 6.61 (1H, d, H-4), 7.12 (1H, d, H-1), 7.27-7.49 (5H, m, Ar-H), 7.77 (1H, br.s, NH, disappeared with D_2O), 7.97 (2H, s, NH, disappeared with D_2O). ^{13}C NMR:

(150 MHz, $CDCl_3$): δ 13.52, 21.78, 22.92, 25.67, 26.45, 28.10, 29.90, 36.17, 38.47, 43.80, 48.69, 50.55, 59.25, 69.11, 112.12, 112.78, 115.54, 119.17, 126.46, 129.53, 132.79, 138.78, 152.42, 153.76, 163.11 (27 C). MS (EI): *m/z* 420 (81%) [M^+]. Anal. Calcd for $C_{27}H_{36}N_2O_2$ (420.58): Calcd C, 77.10; H, 8.63; N, 6.66. Found C, 77.00; H, 8.58; N, 6.60.

16-(α-Ethoxy-methane)-17-[N-phenyl-hydrazino]-estra-1(10),2,4-trien-[17,16-c]-3-ol (**3k**)

Yield 60%, mp 338–340 °C, $[\alpha]_D^{25}$ = + 155 (c 1, MeOH). IR (KBr, cm^{-1}): 3431–3362 (NH), 3343 (OH), 3064 (CH, aromatic), 2956 (CH, aliphatic), 1637 (C=C). ^1H NMR: (600 MHz, $CDCl_3$): δ ppm 0.63 (1H, m, H-8β), 0.90 (3H, s, CH_3-18), 1.01 (1H, m, H-11β), 1.11 (1H, m, H-7α), 1.16 (1H, m, H-12α), 1.21 (3H, m, CH_3, ethoxyl), 1.24 (1H, m, H-14α), 1.36 (1H, m, H-15β), 1.59 (1H, m, H-15α), 1.68 (1H, m, H-7β), 2.00 (1H, m, H-9α), 1.84 (1H, m, CH, H-16α), 2.11 (1H, m, H-11α), 2.50 (1H, m, H-12β), 2.61 (1H, m, H-6α), 2.70 (1H, m, H-6β), 6. disappeared (1H, d, H-4), 2.80 (1H, d, H-17), 3.53 (2H, m, OCH_2), 4.80 (2H, d, CH-O), 4.84 (1H, s, OH, exchangeable with D_2O), 5.70 (1H, dd, H-2), 7.15 (1H, d, H-1), 7.26-7.47 (5H, m, Ar-H), 7.76 (1H, br.s, NH, disappeared with D_2O), 7.98 (1H, m, NH, disappeared with D_2O). ^{13}C NMR: (150 MHz, $CDCl_3$): δ 13.64, 18.74, 21.57, 25.17, 26.30, 28.05, 29.64, 36.54, 38.15, 44.18, 48.46, 50.55, 68.43, 69.13, 112.49, 112.72, 115.60, 119.11, 126.34, 129.50, 131.11, 138.49, 152.40, 153.84, 162.47 (27 C). MS (EI): *m/z* 420 (88%) [M^+]. Anal. Calcd for $C_{27}H_{36}N_2O_2$ (420.58): Calcd C, 77.10; H, 8.63; N, 6.66. Found C, 77.02; H, 8.57; N, 6.61.

16-(α-Ethoxy-ethane)-17-[N-phenyl-hydrazino]-estra-1(10),2,4-trien-[17,16-c]-3-ol (**3l**)

Yield 96%, mp 288–300 °C, $[\alpha]_D^{25}$ = + 95 (c 1, MeOH). IR (KBr, cm^{-1}): 3431–3367 (NH), 3343 (OH), 3068 (CH, aromatic), 2951 (CH, aliphatic), 1631 (C=C). ^1H NMR: (600 MHz, $CDCl_3$): δ ppm 0.58 (1H, m, H-8β), 0.91 (3H, s, CH_3-18), 1.00 (1H, m, H-11β), 1.10 (1H, m, H-7α), 1.14 (1H, m, H-12α), 1.21 (3H, m, CH_3, ethoxyl), 1.24 (1H, m, H-14α), 1.36 (1H, m, H-15β), 1.44 (3H, m, CH_3, C-16 ethane), 1.60 (1H, m, H-15α), 1.71 (1H, m, H-7β), 1.97 (1H, m, H-9 α), 1.83 (1H, m, CH, H-16α), 2.11 (1H, m, H-11α), 2.51 (1H, m, H-12β), 2.62 (1H, m, H-6α), 2.67 (1H, m, H-6 β), 2.88 (1H, d, H-17), 3.49 (2H, m, OCH_2), 4.84 (1H, d, CH-O), 4.87 (1H, s, OH, disappeared with D_2O), 5.73 (1H, dd, H-2), 6.62 (1H, d, H-4), 7.13 (1H, d, H-1), 7.23-7.47 (5H, m, Ar-H), 7.77 (1H, br.s, NH, disappeared with D_2O), 7.87 (1H, m, NH, disappeared with D_2O). ^{13}C NMR: (150 MHz, $CDCl_3$): δ 13.56, 18.77, 22.27, 22.32, 25.76, 26.78, 27.34, 28.29, 36.54, 37.90, 44.21, 48.23, 51.32, 68.34, 69.56, 112.67, 112.77, 115.56, 119.10, 126.45, 129.50, 133.47, 137.23, 152.55, 155.51, 163.73 (28 C). MS (EI): *m/z* 434 (93%) [M^+]. Anal. Calcd for $C_{28}H_{38}N_2O_2$ (434.61): Calcd C, 77.38; H, 8.81; N, 6.45. Found C, 77.30; H, 8.75; N, 6.40.

3.1.3. Synthesis of pyrazoline-3-ol derivatives (**4a–d**)

A mixture of **2a,b** (4 mmol) and hydrazine derivatives, namely, methy hydrazine or phenyl hydrazine (16 mmol) in dioxane (25 mL) was refluxed for 5 h. The mixture was evaporated under vacuum, the residue formed was triturated with water, filtered off, washed with water, dried and crystallized from MeOH to give derivatives **4a–d**, respectively.

1′-Methyl-1′H-estra-1(10),2,4-trien-[17,16-c]pyrazoline-3-ol (**4a**)

Yield 96%, mp 117–119 °C, $[\alpha]_D^{25}$ = + 109 (c 1, MeOH). IR (KBr, cm^{-1}): 3351 (OH), 2946 (CH, aliphatic), 1627 (C=C), 1610 (C=N). ^1H NMR: (600 MHz, $CDCl_3$): δ ppm 0.61 (1H, m, H-8β), 0.94 (3H, s, CH_3-18), 1.08 (1H, m, H-11β), 1.13 (1H, m, H-7α), 1.18 (1H, m, H-12α), 1.27 (1H, m, H-14α), 1.41 (1H, m, H-15β), 1.66 (1H, m, H-15α), 1.74 (1H, m, H-7β), 1.84 (1H, m, CH, H-16α), 2.01 (1H, m, H-9α), 2.10 (3H, s, NCH_3), 2.22 (1H, m, H-11α), 2.42 (1H, m, H-12β), 2.52 (1H, m, H-6α), 2.66 (1H, m, H-6β), 2.84 (2H, d, pyrazoline-5′), 4.95 (1H, s, OH, disappeared with D_2O), 5.75 (1H, dd, H-2), 6.65 (1H, d, H-4), 7.15 (1H, d, H-1). ^{13}C NMR: (150 MHz, $CDCl_3$): δ 14.60, 22.56, 25.35, 26.46, 28.77, 29.56, 36.68, 38.68, 43.34, 45.36, 48.21, 50.24, 64.45, 112.46, 115.57, 126.44, 132.56, 138.45, 152.67, 156.46 (20 C). MS (EI): *m/z* 310 (100%)

[M+]. Anal. Calcd for $C_{20}H_{26}N_2O$ (310.43): Calcd C, 77.38; H, 8.44; N, 9.02. Found C, 77.29; H, 8.36; N, 8.98.

1′-Methyl -1′H-5′-methyl-estra-1(10),2,4-trien-[17,16-c]pyrazoline-3-ol (**4b**)

Yield 88%, mp 216–218 °C, $[\alpha]_D^{25}$ = + 111 (c 1, MeOH). IR (KBr, cm^{-1}): 3351 (OH), 2946 (CH, aliphatic), 1627 (C=C), 1617 (C=N). ^{1}H NMR: (600 MHz, $CDCl_3$): δ ppm 0.62 (1H, m, H-8β), 0.92 (3H, s, CH_3-18), 1.02 (1H, m, H-11β), 1.05 (3H, s, CH_3-5′-methyl), 1.10 (1H, m, H-7α), 1.14 (1H, m, H-12α), 1.25 (1H, m, H-14α), 1.40 (1H, m, H-15β), 1.66 (1H, m, H -15α), 1.77 (1H, m, H-7β), 1.88 (1H, m, CH, H-16α), 2.00 (1H, m, H-9α), 2.17 (3H, s, N-CH_3), 2.20 (1H, m, H-11α), 2.47 (1H, m, H-12β), 2.57 (1H, m, H-6α), 2.66 (1H, m, H-6β), 2.84 (1H, m, pyrazoline-5′), 4.88 (1H, s, OH, disappeared with D_2O), 5.79 (1H, dd, H-2), 6.68 (1H, d, H-4), 7.19 (1H, d, H-1). ^{13}C NMR: (150 MHz, $CDCl_3$): δ 13.35, 21.80, 24.27, 25.30, 26.07, 28.20, 29.77, 36.76, 38.70, 43.67, 45.67, 48.50, 50.70, 64.45, 112.37, 115.54, 126.46, 132.40, 138.77, 153.44, 155.42 (21 C). MS (EI): *m/z* 324 (100%) [M+]. Anal. Calcd for $C_{21}H_{28}N_2O$ (324.45): Calcd C, 77.74; H, 8.70; N, 8.63. Found C, 77.66; H, 8.64; N, 8.58.

1′-Phenyl-1′H-estra-1(10),2,4-trien-[17,16-c]pyrazoline-3-ol (**4c**)

Yield 70%, mp 255–257 °C, $[\alpha]_D^{25}$ = + 128 (c 1, MeOH). IR (KBr, cm^{-1}): 3347 (OH), 3071 and 3061 (CH, aromatic), 2931 (CH, aliphatic), 1633 (C=C), 1614 (C=N). ^{1}H NMR: (600 MHz, $CDCl_3$): δ ppm 0.60 (1H, m, H-8β), 0.90 (3H, s, CH_3-18), 1.00 (1H, m, H-11β), 1.10 (1H, m, H-7α), 1.20 (1H, m, H-12α), 1.28 (1H, m, H-14α), 1.49 (1H, m, H-15β), 1.68 (1H, m, H-15α), 1.77 (1H, m, H-7β), 1.86 (1H, m, CH, H-16α), 2.04 (1H, m, H-9α), 2.26 (1H, m, H-11α), 2.48 (1H, m, H -12β), 2.54 (1H, m, H-6α), 2.64 (1H, m, H-6β), 2.84 (2H, d, pyrazoline-5′), 5.00 (1H, s, OH, disappeared with D_2O), 5.71 (1H, dd, H-2), 6.70 (1H, d, H-4), 7.10 (1H, d, H-1), 7.28-7.40 (5H, m, Ar-H). ^{13}C NMR: (150 MHz, $CDCl_3$): δ 13.49, 21.24, 25.55, 26.46, 28.51, 29.67, 36.64, 38.45, 43.35, 50.73, 58.26, 64.45, 112.10, 112.48, 115.46, 119.31, 126.10, 129.20, 132.52, 138.79, 152.20, 153.13, 163.48 (25 C). MS (EI): *m/z* 372 (81%) [M+]. Anal. Calcd for $C_{25}H_{28}N_2O$ (372.50): Calcd C, 80.61; H, 7.58; N, 7.52. Found C, 80.52; H, 7.50; N, 7.48.

1′-Phenyl-1′H-5′-methyl-estra-1(10),2,4-trien-[17,16-c]pyrazoline-3-ol (**4d**)

Yield 75%, mp 214–216 °C, $[\alpha]_D^{25}$ = + 127 (c 1, MeOH). IR (KBr, cm^{-1}): 3345 (OH), 3068 (CH, aromatic), 2949 (CH, aliphatic), 1625 (C=C), 1614 (C=N). ^{1}H NMR: (600 MHz, $CDCl_3$): δ ppm 0.62 (1H, m, H-8β), 0.93 (3H, s, CH_3-18), 1.02 (1H, m, H-11β), 1.05 (3H, s, CH_3-5′-methyl), 1.12 (1H, m, H-7α), 1.17 (1H, m, H-12α), 1.27 (1H, m, H-14α), 1.41 (1H, m, H-15β), 1.71 (1H, m, H -15α), 1.77 (1H, m, H-7β), 1.87 (1H, m, CH, H-16α), 2.02 (1H, m, H-9α), 2.22 (1H, m, H-11α), 2.46 (1H, m, H -12β), 2.54 (1H, m, H-6α), 2.65 (1H, m, H-6β), 3.83 (1H, s, pyrazoline-5′), 4.91 (1H, s, OH, disappeared with D_2O), 5.81 (1H, dd, H-2), 6.73 (1H, d, H-4), 7.21 (1H, d, H-1), 7.28-7.48 (5H, m, Ar-H). ^{13}C NMR: (150 MHz, $CDCl_3$): δ 13.81, 21.89, 24.25, 25.80, 26.35, 28.34, 29.23, 36.56, 38.67, 43.34, 48.55, 50.67, 64.44, 112.70, 115.34, 119.10, 126.76, 129.50, 132.45, 138.56, 152.40, 154.36, 163.56, 164.55 (26 C). MS (EI): *m/z* 386 (23%) [M+]. Anal. Calcd for $C_{26}H_{30}N_2O$ (386.52): Calcd C, 80.79; H, 7.82; N, 7.25. Found C, 80.70; H, 7.76; N, 7.20.

3.2. *Biological Screening*

3.2.1. In Vitro Cytotoxic Activities

The cytotoxic activities of the synthesized derivatives against ovarian cancer cell lines (SKOV-3) were evaluated using standard MTT assay [26,27]. SKOV-3 cells cultivated on DMEM medium supplemented with 10% FBS, 100×, 1% antibiotic/antimycotic solution and 3.6 g/L $NaHCO_3$ were used. Cells were incubated under standard laboratory conditions [28,29]. Before testing compounds, cells were trypsinized, centrifuged and prepared as per our developed protocol [30,31]. MTT assay relies on the enzymatic conversion of the MTT substrate into purple formazan by living cells mitochondrial enzymes. Shortly, 96 well plates were seeded (10,000 cells/100 µL/well), then incubated for 24 h at standard conditions. Afterwards, cells were exposed to different concentrations from prepared compounds and incubated for another 24 h. Thereafter, MTT (10 μL, 5 mg/mL, PBS) were added to each well, and plates were incubated for 4 h. Supernatants were then replaced discarded with 200 μL of DMSO to dissolve the precipitated formazan crystals. Formazan absorbance, proportional to living cell number, was read at 550 nm using a microplate reader. Viability percentages were calculated and the corresponding IC_{50} values were obtained from the linear regression of the calibration curve. For comparison, doxorubicin (DOX) and resveratrol (RES) were used as positive controls. Furthermore, the effect of the newly synthesized derivatives was tested against normal fibroblast cell line to assess their toxicities.

3.2.2. In Vitro Anti-Ovarian Xenograft Model

Anti-ovarian cancer xenograft animal model was developed in nude mouse using SKOV-3 cells according to McCauley et al. [32]. Treatment protocol was approved by the University of South Dakota, Institutional Animal Care and Use Committee (study protocol 50-01-05-08B). Immunodeficient (athymic nude-Foxn1nu) female mice were inoculated (1×10^6 cells/site). Upon tumor development, (av. volume ~50 mm^3), 10-mice groups were implanted s.c. with constant release pellets containing tested compound (1 μM/gm) or placebo. Animal and tumor development were monitored measured every 5 days after pellet implantation, using standardized Caliper in two perpendicular diameters of the implant according to our previous work [2]. Due to large tumor volumes, (5-fold difference between largest and smallest tumor), relative tumor volumes were used for comparison. Relative tumor volume = $Vt_{\text{volume at time t}}/V0_{\text{initial volume}}$.

3.2.3. Topoisomerase II Inhibition

The inhibitory effects of the synthesized compounds against topoisomerase II were investigated using relaxation assay according to Goyeneche, et al. [33]. Topoisomerase II was purified from P388 cells, where enzyme unit corresponds to the activity required complete relaxation of 0.125 g of supercoiled pBR-322 DNA at 30 °C for 1 h. The assay was performed as per protocol and samples were subjected to electrophoresis (0.7% agarose gels, TBE buffer. Ethidium bromide-stained DNA was examined under UV light.

3.2.4. In Vitro Kinase Inhibition

Protein Expression and Purification

BRAF wild-type and V600E mutant kinase domains were expressed and purified according to Nakamura et al. [34]. Shortly, Sf 9 cells infected with BRAF kinase domain containing baculovirus were resuspended, sonicated, and then cleared using ultracentrifugation. Afterwards, the cleared lysate with mixed with equilibrated Talon resin, and the resin then washed with 10 column volumes of wash buffer and then eluted with buffer (25 mM Tris, pH 7.0, 250 mM NaCl, 160 mM imidazole, 10% glycerol). The eluant was then diluted, concentrated using Superdex 200 gel filtration column, purified as previously described and finally stored at −80 °C until use.

In Vitro ELISA-Based Kinase Assay

"This method was adopted from Nakamura et al. [34] and Qin et al. [35]. The previously prepared GST MEK-His protein was diluted in TTBS buffer (100 μL, 50 μg/mL), and then bound to 96-plate wells coated with glutathione (Pierce Biotechnology). Two DMSO-dilutions of each compound (1 μL) were added to 50 μL (50mM HEPES, pH7.0, 0.7 pmol of $BRAF^{V600E}$ kinase). Tubes were incubated at ambient temperature for 1 h, then added to GST-MEK-His-plate wells. Afterwards, 50 μL of phosphorylation buffer were added to start kinase reaction (37 °C/30 min/shaking). Reaction was stopped, then substrate was added, and the signal was recorded. The high throughput inhibitor screening was carried out according to standard assay conditions at different concentrations, to generate a sigmoidal dose response curve, a four-parameter logistic model using GraphPad Prism, for BRAF proteins, which was used to obtain corresponding IC_{50} values".

3.2.5. Statistical Analysis

"Measurements were carried out in thrice and data are represented as means ± SEM. Significance was calculated by Student's t-test using SPSS software (SPSS Inc., Paris, France). * $p < 0.05$, ** $p < 0.01$, *** $p < 0.001$. IC_{50} values were calculated using GraphPad Prism software, GraphPad Software, San Diego, CA, USA [36]".

4. Conclusions

During the current investigation, we synthesized a series of 17-hydrazino- and 17,16-c-pyrazoline estrone derivatives. Prepared compounds exhibited potential in vitro and in vivo anti-ovarian cancer activity against SKOV-3 cells. Compound **3a** was found to be the most potent with an IC_{50} value of 4.23 ± 0.12 nM. Additionally, in vivo xenograft ovarian cancer model showed that Cpd. **3a** was able to reduce tumor growth by 93.61 ± 0.7% after 40 days of treatment. Furthermore, the newly synthesized compounds were able to interfere with tumor proliferation through inhibiting the activity of topoisomerase II and ^{V600E}BRAF, where the obtained IC_{50} values for both enzymes were 3.45 ± 0.13 nM and 0.041 ± 0.0016 μM, respectively.

Author Contributions: M.E.-N., A.E.-G.E.A., A.A.F. performed most of the experiments; A.E.-G.E.A., M.A.A.-O., A.A.F. analyzed the data; E.A.E. and M.M.A. the contributed to the anticancer activity assays; All authors read and approved the final manuscript.

Funding: The authors are grateful to the Deanship of Scientific Research, king Saud University for funding through Vice Deanship of Scientific Research Chairs.

Acknowledgments: The authors are grateful to the Deanship of Scientific Research, king Saud University for funding through Vice Deanship of Scientific Research Chairs.

Conflicts of Interest: The authors declare no conflict of interest.

References

1. Gupta, A.; Kumar, B.S.; Negi, A.S. Current status on development of steroids as anticancer agents. *J. Steroid Biochem. Mol. Boil.* **2013**, *137*, 242–270. [CrossRef] [PubMed]
2. Amr, A.E.-G.E.; El-Naggar, M.; Al-Omar, M.A.; Elsayed, E.A.; Abdalla, M.M. In vitro and in vivo anti-breast cancer activities of some synthesized pyrazolinyl-estran-17-one candidates. *Molecules* **2018**, *23*, 1572. [CrossRef] [PubMed]
3. Afzal, M.; Al-Awadi, S.; Oommen, S. Antioxidant activity of biotransformed sex hormones facilitated by Bacillus stearothermophilus. In *Advanced Protocols in Oxidative Stress II, Methods in Molecular Biology*; Armstrong, D., Ed.; Springer: Basel, Switzerland, 2010.
4. Schönecker, B.; Lange, C.; Kötteritzsch, M.; Günther, W.; Weston, J.; Anders, E.; Görls, H. Conformational design for 13α-Steroids. *J. Org. Chem.* **2000**, *65*, 5487–5497. [CrossRef]
5. Jovanovic-Santa, S.; Petrović, J.; Andrić, S.; Kovačević, R.; Đurendić, E.; Sakač, M.; Lazar, D.; Stanković, S. Synthesis, structure, and screening of estrogenic and antiestrogenic activity of new 3,17-substituted-16,17-seco-estratriene derivatives. *Bioorg. Chem.* **2003**, *31*, 475–484. [CrossRef]
6. Minorics, R.; Bózsity, N.; Wölfling, J.; Mernyák, E.; Schneider, G.; Márki, A.; Falkay, G.; Ocsovszki, I.; Zupkó, I. Antiproliferative effect of normal and 13-epi-D-homoestrone and their 3-methyl ethers on human reproductive cancer cell lines. *J. Steroid Biochem. Mol. Biol.* **2013**, *132*, 168–175. [CrossRef] [PubMed]
7. Ayan, D.P.; Maltais, R.; Roy, J.; Poirier, D. Impact of estradiol structural modifications (18-methyl and/or 17-hydroxy inversion of configuration) on the in vitro and in vivo estrogenic activity. In Proceedings of the Endocrine Society's 93rd Annual Meeting & Expo, Boston, MA, USA, 4–7 June 2011; Volume 127.
8. Szabó, J.; Bacsa, I.; Wölfling, J.; Schneider, G.; Zupkó, I.; Varga, M.; Herman, B.E.; Kalmár, L.; Szécsi, M.; Mernyák, E. Synthesis and in vitro pharmacological evaluation of N-[(1-benzyl-1,2,3-triazol-4-yl)methyl]-

carboxamides on D-secoestrone scaffolds. *J. Enzyme Inhib. Med. Chem.* **2016**, *31*, 574–579. [CrossRef] [PubMed]

9. Szabó, J.; Jerkovics, N.; Schneider, G.; Wölfling, J.; Bózsity, N.; Minorics, R.; Zupkó, I.; Mernyák, E.; De Sousa, M.E. Synthesis and in vitro antiproliferative evaluation of c-13 epimers of triazolyl-d-secoestrone alcohols: the first potent 13α-d-secoestrone derivative. *Molecules* **2016**, *21*, 611. [CrossRef] [PubMed]
10. Szabó, J.; Pataki, Z.; Wölfling, J.; Schneider, G.; Bózsity, N.; Minorics, R.; Zupkó, I.; Mernyák, E. Synthesis and biological evaluation of 13α-estrone derivatives as potential antiproliferative agents. *Steroids* **2016**, *113*, 14–21. [CrossRef]
11. Mernyák, E.; Kovács, I.; Minorics, R.; Sere, P.; Czégány, D.; Sinka, I.; Wölfling, J.; Schneider, G.; Újfaludi, Z.; Boros, I.; et al. Synthesis of trans-16-triazolyl-13α-methyl-17-estradiol diastereomers and the effects of structural modifications on their in vitro antiproliferative activities. *J. Steroid Biochem. Mol. Boil.* **2015**, *150*, 123–134. [CrossRef]
12. Rao, P.N.; Cessac, J.W.; Tinley, T.L.; Mooberry, S.L. Synthesis and antimitotic activity of novel 2-methoxyestradiol analogs. *Steroids* **2002**, *67*, 1079–1089. [CrossRef]
13. Sundov, D.; Čarić, A.; Mrklić, I.; Gugic, D.; Čapkun, V.; Hofman, I.D.; Mise, B.P.; Tomic, S. P53, MAPK, topoisomerase II alpha and Ki67 immunohistochemical expression and KRAS/BRAF mutation in ovarian serous carcinomas. *Diagn. Pathol.* **2013**, *8*, 21. [CrossRef]
14. Kaur, P.V.; Kaur, S. DNA Topoisomerase II: promising target for anticancer drugs. In *Multi-Targeted Approach to Treatment of Cancer*; Gandhi, V., Ed.; Springer: Basel, Switzerland, 2015; pp. 323–338.
15. Nijenhuis, C.; Lucas, L.; Rosing, H.; Huitema, A.; Mergui-Roelvink, M.; Jamieson, G.C.; Fox, J.; Mould, D.; Schellens, J.; Beijnen, J. Metabolism and disposition of the anticancer quinolone derivative vosaroxin, a novel inhibitor of topoisomerase II. *Investig. New Drugs* **2017**, *35*, 478–490. [CrossRef]
16. Rahman, M.A.; Salajegheh, A.; Smith, R.A.; Lam, A.K.-Y.; Ariana, A. Inhibition of BRAF kinase suppresses cellular proliferation, but not enough for complete growth arrest in BRAF V600E mutated papillary and undifferentiated thyroid carcinomas. *Endocrine* **2016**, *54*, 129–138. [CrossRef]
17. Rahman, M.A.; Salajegheh, A.; Smith, R.A.; Lam, A.K.-Y.; Ariana, A. Multiple proliferation-survival signalling pathways are simultaneously active in BRAF V600E mutated thyroid carcinomas. *Exp. Mol. Pathol.* **2015**, *99*, 492–497. [CrossRef]
18. McCubrey, J.A.; Steelman, L.S.; Abrams, S.L.; Lee, J.T.; Chang, F.; Bertrand, F.E.; Navolanic, P.M.; Terrian, D.M.; Franklin, R.A.; D'Assoro, A.B.; et al. Roles of the RAF/MEK/ERK and PI3K/PTEN/AKT pathways in malignant transformation and drug resistance. *Adv. Enzym. Regul.* **2006**, *46*, 249–279. [CrossRef]
19. Ouf, N.H.; Amr, A.E. Synthesis and anti-inflammatory activity of some pyrimidines and thieno- pyrimidines using 1-(2-benzo[d][1,3]dioxol-5-yl)vinyl)-4-mercapto-6-methyl-pyrimidine-5-yl)-ethan-2- one as a starting material. *Monatsh. fur Chem.* **2008**, *139*, 579–585. [CrossRef]
20. Amr, A.E.; Abdulla, M.M. Synthesis and anti-inflammatory activities of new cynopyrane derivatives fused with steroidal nuclei. *Archiv. der Pharm.* **2008**, *339*, 88–95. [CrossRef]
21. Khalifa, N.M.; Al-Omar, M.A.; Amr, A.E.; Haiba, M.E. Antiviral activity of some new polycyclic nucleoside pyrene candidate against HIV-1 and HSV-1 virus. *Int. J. Biol. Macromol.* **2013**, *54*, 51. [CrossRef]
22. Abdel-Wahab, B.F.; Mohamed, S.F.; Amr, A.E.-G.E.; Abdalla, M.M. Synthesis and reactions of thiosemicarbazides, triazoles, and Schiff bases as antihypertensive α-blocking agents. *Monatsh. Chem.* **2008**, *139*, 1083–1090. [CrossRef]
23. Amr, A.E.-G.E.; Elsayed, E.A.; Al-Omar, M.A.; Eldin, H.O.B.; Nossier, E.S.; Abdallah, M.M.; Eldin, H.B. Design, synthesis, anticancer evaluation and molecular modeling of novel estrogen derivatives. *Molecules* **2019**, *24*, 416. [CrossRef]
24. Day, J.M.; Foster, P.A.; Tutill, H.J.; Schmidlin, F.; Sharland, C.M.; Hargrave, J.D.; Vicker, N.; Potter, B.V.L.; Reed, M.J.; Purohit, A. STX2171, a 17-hydroxysteroid dehydrogenase type 3 inhibitor, is efficacious in vivo in a novel hormone-dependent prostate cancer model. *Endocr. Relat. Cancer* **2013**, *20*, 53–64. [CrossRef]
25. Donald, P.; Ho-Jin, C.; Arezki, A.; Roch, P.B.; Sheng-Xiang, L. Estrone and estradiol C-16 derivatives as inhibitors of type 1 17β-hydroxysteroid dehydrogenase. *Mol. Cell. Endocrinol.* **2006**, *248*, 236–238.
26. Elsayed, E.A.; Sharaf-Eldin, M.; Wadaan, M. In vitro evaluation of cytotoxic activities of essential oil from moringa oleifera seeds on HeLa, HepG2, MCF-7, CACO-2 and L929 Cell Lines. *Asian Pac. J. Cancer Prev.* **2015**, *16*, 4671–4675. [CrossRef]

27. Elsayed, E.A.; Farooq, M.; Dailin, D.; El-Enshasy, H.A.; Othman, N.Z.; Malek, R.; Danial, E.; Wadaan, M. In vitro and in vivo biological screening of kefiran polysaccharide produced by Lactobacillus kefiranofaciens. *Biomed. Res.* **2017**, *28*, 594–600.
28. Al-Salahi, R.; Elsayed, E.A.; El Dib, R.A.; Wadaan, M.; Ezzeldin, E.; Marzouk, M. Synthesis, characterization and cytotoxicity evaluation of 5-hydrazono-[1,2,4]triazolo[1,5-a]quinazolines (Part I). *Lat. Am. J. Pharm.* **2016**, *35*, 58–65.
29. Al-Salahi, R.; Elsayed, E.A.; El Dib, R.A.; Wadaan, M.; Ezzeldin, E.; Marzouk, M. Cytotoxicity of new 5-hydrazono-[1,2,4]triazolo[1,5-a]quinazolines (Part II). *Lat. Am. J. Pharm.* **2016**, *35*, 66–73.
30. Elsayed, E.A.; Sharaf-Eldin, M.A.; El-Enshasy, H.A.; Wadaan, M. In vitro assessment of anticancer properties of Moringa peregrina essential seed oil on different cell lines. *Pak. J. Zool.* **2016**, *48*, 853–859.
31. Farooq, M.; Abu Taha, N.; Butorac, R.R.; Evans, D.A.; Elzatahry, A.A.; Elsayed, E.A.; Wadaan, M.A.M.; Al-Deyab, S.S.; Cowley, A.H.; Li, J. Biological screening of newly synthesized BIAN N-heterocyclic gold carbene complexes in zebrafish embryos. *Int. J. Mol. Sci.* **2015**, *16*, 24718–24731. [CrossRef]
32. McCauley, J.; Zivanovic, A.; Skropeta, D. Bioassays for anticancer activities. *Methods Mol. Biol.* **2013**, *1055*, 191–205.
33. Goyeneche, A.A.; Carón, R.W.; Telleria, C.M. Mifepristone inhibits ovarian cancer cancer cell growth in vitro and in vivo. *Clin. Cancer Res.* **2007**, *13*, 3370–3379. [CrossRef]
34. Nakamura, K.; Sugumi, H.; Yamaguchi, A.; Uenaka, T.; Kotake, Y.; Okada, T.; Kamata, J.; Niijima, J.; Nagasu, T.; Koyanagi, N.; et al. Antitumor activity of ER-37328, a novel carbazole topoisomerase II inhibitor. *Mol. Cancer Ther.* **2002**, *1*, 169–75.
35. Qin, J.; Xie, P.; Ventocilla, C.; Zhou, G.; Vultur, A.; Chen, Q.; Liu, Q.; Herlyn, M.; Winkler, J.; Marmorstein, R. Identification of a novel family of BRAF(V600E) inhibitors. *J. Med. Chem.* **2012**, *55*, 5220–5230. [CrossRef]
36. Stones, C.J.; Kim, J.E.; Joseph, W.R.; Leung, E.; Marshall, E.S.; Finlay, G.J.; Shelling, A.N.; Baguley, B.C. Comparison of responses of human melanoma cell lines to MEK and BRAF inhibitors. *Front. Genet.* **2013**, *4*, 66. [CrossRef]

Sample Availability: Samples of the compounds are available from the authors.

molecules

MDPI

Article

Synthesis, Biological Evaluation, and In Silico Studies of Novel Aminated Xanthones as Potential p53-Activating Agents

Agostinho Lemos [1], Ana Sara Gomes [2], Joana B. Loureiro [2], Pedro Brandão [1], Andreia Palmeira [1,3], Madalena M. M. Pinto [1,3], Lucília Saraiva [2,*] and Maria Emília Sousa [1,3,*]

1. Laboratory of Organic and Pharmaceutical Chemistry, Department of Chemical Sciences, Faculty of Pharmacy, University of Porto, Rua de Jorge Viterbo Ferreira, 228, 4050-313 Porto, Portugal; up201002662@ff.up.pt (A.L.); pedrocgbrandao@gmail.com (P.B.); andreiapalmeira@gmail.com (A.P.); madalena@ff.up.pt (M.M.M.P.)
2. UCIBIO/REQUIMTE, Laboratory of Microbiology, Department of Biological Sciences, Faculty of Pharmacy, University of Porto, Rua de Jorge Viterbo Ferreira, 228, 4050-313 Porto, Portugal; anasarag4@gmail.com (A.S.G.); up201407524@ff.up.pt (J.B.L.)
3. CIIMAR-Interdisciplinary Centre of Marine and Environmental Research, University of Porto, Novo Edificio do Terminal de Cruzeiros do Porto de Leixões, Avenida General Norton de Matos, S/N, 4450-208 Matosinhos, Portugal

* Correspondence: lucilia.saraiva@ff.up.pt (L.S.); esousa@ff.up.pt (M.E.S.); Tel.: +351-22-0428-584 (L.S.); +351-22-0428-689 (M.E.S.)

Academic Editor: Qiao-Hong Chen
Received: 7 May 2019; Accepted: 21 May 2019; Published: 22 May 2019

Abstract: Xanthone scaffold has been regarded as an attractive chemical tool in the search for bioactive molecules with antitumor activity, and in particular two xanthone derivatives, 12-hydroxy-2,2-dimethyl-3,4-dihydro-2*H*,6*H*-pyrano [3,2-*b*]xanthen-6-one (**4**) and 3,4-dimethoxy-9-oxo-9*H*-xanthene-1-carbaldehyde (**5**), were described as a murine double minute 2 (MDM2)-p53 inhibitor and a TAp73 activator, respectively. The xanthone **5** was used as a starting point for the construction of a library of 3,4-dioxygenated xanthones bearing chemical moieties of described MDM2-p53 inhibitors. Eleven aminated xanthones were successfully synthesized and initially screened for their ability to disrupt the MDM2-p53 interaction using a yeast cell-based assay. With this approach, xanthone **37** was identified as a putative p53-activating agent through inhibition of interaction with MDM2. Xanthone **37** inhibited the growth of human colon adenocarcinoma HCT116 cell lines in a p53-dependent manner. The growth inhibitory effect of xanthone **37** was associated with the induction of G1-phase cell cycle arrest and increased protein expression levels of p53 transcriptional targets. These results demonstrated the potential usefulness of coupling amine-containing structural motifs of known MDM2-p53 disruptors into a 3,4-dioxygenated xanthone scaffold in the design of novel and potent p53 activators with antitumor activity and favorable drug-like properties. Moreover, in silico docking studies were performed in order to predict the binding poses and residues involved in the potential MDM2-p53 interaction.

Keywords: antitumor activity; computational docking; MDM2-p53 interaction; xanthones; yeast-based assays

1. Introduction

The tumor suppressor p53 acts as a transcription factor, triggering the expression of multiple downstream target genes that play a pivotal role in the regulation of cell cycle arrest, apoptosis, senescence, and DNA repair [1–6]. Upon cellular stress stimuli, the activation of the p53 pathway may compromise the tumorigenesis, circumventing the proliferation of damaged cells with oncogenic potential. Inactivation of the p53 function represents one of the most common events in human cancers [7]. In approximately half of all human cancer cells, the p53 inactivation is caused by mutations within the p53 gene (*TP53*) or by post-translational modifications of its gene product [8]. In those tumors retaining the wild type (wt) p53 function, the tumor suppressor activity of p53 can be abolished by multiple mechanisms [9], mainly by direct interaction between p53 and its primary endogenous inhibitor, the murine double minute 2 (MDM2) protein [10,11]. The oncoprotein MDM2 physically interacts with the amino-terminal domain of p53 and negatively regulates its activity by blocking p53-mediated transactivation [12,13], by inducing the export of p53 from nucleus to the cytoplasm [14], and by promoting E3 ubiquitin ligase-mediated p53 degradation via the proteasomal pathway [15,16]. Targeting the MDM2-p53 interaction with small molecules has been regarded an attractive approach for the reactivation of the p53 pathway in wt p53-expressing tumors [17,18]. Since the seminal work of Vassilev et al. reporting the discovery of nutlin-3A (**1**, Figure 1) as the first inhibitor of MDM2-p53 interaction [19], an impressive number of MDM2-p53 disruptors from a huge diversity of chemical families have been identified in recent years, entering some of them into clinical trials [20,21].

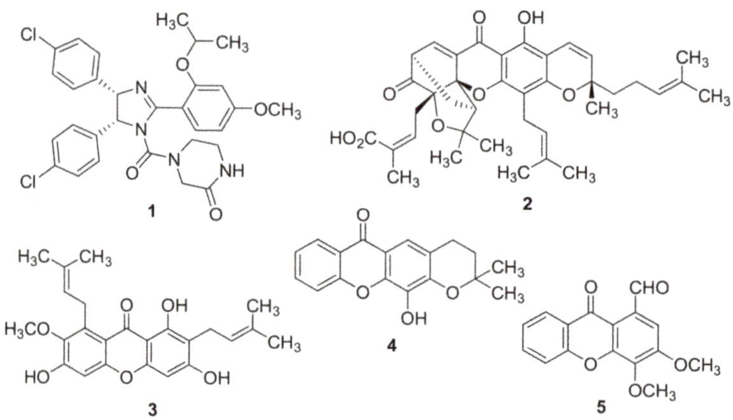

Figure 1. Chemical structures of nutlin-3A (**1**), gambogic acid (**2**), α-mangostin (**3**), 12-hydroxy-2,2-dimethyl-3,4-dihydro-2*H*,6*H*-pyrano[3,2-*b*]xanthen-6-one (**4**), and 3,4-dimethoxy-9-oxo-9*H*-xanthene-1-carbaldehyde (**5**).

Xanthones represent a privileged class of compounds with a multiplicity of biological activities, in particular with antitumor activity against several human tumor cell lines [22–36]. Intriguingly, our research group has demonstrated that the antitumor activity of some derivatives can be correlated to the disruption of the MDM2-p53 complex and the activation of a p53-dependent pathway [30,31]. In fact, implementing a yeast-based assay, the naturally occurring xanthones gambogic acid (**2**, Figure 1) and α-mangostin (**3**, Figure 1) were found to revert the inhibitory effect of MDM2 on p53-induced growth inhibition and on p53 transcriptional activity [30]. The synthetic xanthone 12-hydroxy-2,2-dimethyl-3,4-dihydro-2*H*,6*H*-pyrano [3,2-*b*]xanthen-6-one (**4**, Figure 1) was identified as a potential MDM2-p53 disruptor, using an in silico virtual screening strategy against MDM2 protein and a yeast-based assay [31]. Its molecular mechanism was corroborated in MDM2-overexpressing human tumor cell lines with wt p53. In fact, xanthone **4** selectively upregulated the p53 transcriptional activity, increasing the protein expression levels of p53-target genes in HCT116 human colon adenocarcinoma cells [31]. Nevertheless, xanthone **4** is highly hydrophobic and poorly water soluble, which could limit its in vivo use. Interestingly, Chen and co-workers explored the antitumor activity of xanthone **4** either in combination or hybridized with 5,6-dimethylxanthone-4-acetic acid (DMXAA) [37], a xanthone derivative with tumor-vascular disrupting activity. A very recent study reported the discovery of

3,4-dimethoxy-9-oxo-9*H*-xanthene-1-carbaldehyde (**5**, Figure 1) as a new TAp73 activator via disruption of its interaction with both MDM2 and mutant p53 [36].

Herein, based on the 3,4-oxygenated pattern of substitution of xanthones **4** and **5** (Figure 2A), and on chemical moieties derived from known MDM2-p53 disruptors, namely the molecules **1** [19], **6** [38], **7** [39], and **8** [40] (Figure 2B), we followed a molecular hybridization approach for the construction of novel 3,4-oxygenated xanthone derivatives (Figure 2D). In the present work, we opted to synthesize a library of aminated xanthones (Figure 2D) via a strategy of reductive amination of the xanthone **5** with a set of commercially available amine precursors (**9–19**) containing structural motifs of MDM2-p53 disruptors (Figure 2C). The introduction of amine moieties in the xanthone scaffold may contribute to a potential enhancement of drug-like properties, a critical parameter for the identification of promising drug candidates. The ability of the synthesized ligands to disrupt the MDM2-p53 interaction and to activate a p53-dependent pathway was further investigated using the previously established yeast-based assay and in human cancer cell lines. In silico docking studies were performed in order to predict the binding poses and residues involved in the potential MDM2-p53 interaction.

2. Results and Discussion

2.1. Chemistry

2.1.1. Synthesis of 3,4-dimethoxy-9-oxo-9*H*-xanthene-1-carbaldehyde (5)

In the present work, xanthone **5** was used as a starting precursor for the synthesis of a set of aminated xanthones with a 3,4-dioxygenated pattern of substitution. Recently, the multi-step synthesis of compound **5** has been reported [36] as consisting in: (i) a Friedel-Crafts acylation of 1,2,3-trimethoxybenzene (**20**) with the commercially available reagent 2-methoxybenzoyl chloride (**21**); (ii) an intramolecular nucleophilic aromatic substitution of (2-hydroxy-3,4-dimethoxyphenyl)(2-methoxyphenyl)methanone (**22**) and consecutive regioselective demethylation of the methoxy group at position C-4 under conventional heating; (iii) a Duff formylation at position C-1 of 4-hydroxy-3-methoxy-9*H*-xanthen-9-one (**23**); and (iv) a methylation of the hydroxyl group at position C-4 of 4-hydroxy-3-methoxy-9-oxo-9*H*-xanthene-1-carbaldehyde (**24**) (Scheme 1A). The difficulty in achieving a regioselective demethylation at position C-4 necessary for Duff formylation at position C-1 demanded the planning of an optimized synthetic route more appropriate for scaling-up. We hypothesized that the implementation of an analog precursor of **20** with a suitable substituent at position C-1 might provide a useful alternative for the synthesis of **5**, avoiding the troublesome demethylation and Duff formylation processes. Herein, the commercially available 1,2,3-trimethoxy-5-methylbenzene (**25**) was selected for the Friedel-Crafts acylation with the acyl chloride **21** and the Lewis acid aluminum chloride to furnish the intermediate (2-hydroxy-3,4-dimethoxy-6-methylphenyl)(2-methoxyphenyl)methanone (**26**). Subsequent intramolecular nucleophilic aromatic substitution followed by elimination of methanol under basic conditions and microwave (MW) irradiation provided the 3,4-dimethoxy-1-methyl-9*H*-xanthen-9-one (**27**) in good yield quantity. This two-step methodology for the construction of xanthone analogues of **27** has been previously described in the literature [32,41–43]. With the application of MW methodology in the basic cyclization of **26** instead of the conventional heating employed in the synthesis of **23**, the reaction time was reduced from 48 h to 6 h. Furthermore, xanthone **27** was obtained in higher reaction yield under MW irradiation (63% yield (**27**) vs. 38% yield (**23**)). Subsequently, the Vohl-Ziegler bromination of **27**, using dibenzoyl peroxide (DBP) and *N*-bromosuccinimide (NBS) as a radical initiator and a brominating agent, respectively, afforded the 1-(dibromomethyl)-3,4-dimethoxy-9*H*-xanthen-9-one (**28**) as the major product. A solvolytic displacement of bromine atoms of the xanthone **28** was effectively attained using 1-butyl-3-methylimidazolium tetrafluoroborate and water, under conventional heating, and furnished xanthone **5** in 64% yield quantity (Scheme 1B). Of note, the two-step procedure of Vohl-Ziegler bromination and subsequent solvolytic displacement required lower reaction times (4.5 h (2 steps from **27** to **5**) vs. 54 h (2 steps from **23** to **5**) and allowed the preparation of xanthone **5** in higher reaction yields (51% yield (2 steps from **27** to **5**) vs. 28% yield (2 steps from **23** to **5**)), compared to the Duff formylation/methylation pathway. Overall, the replacement of starting precursor **20** by the methylated derivative **25** at position C-1 of the aromatic ring was critical for the successful optimization of the preparation of xanthone **5**.

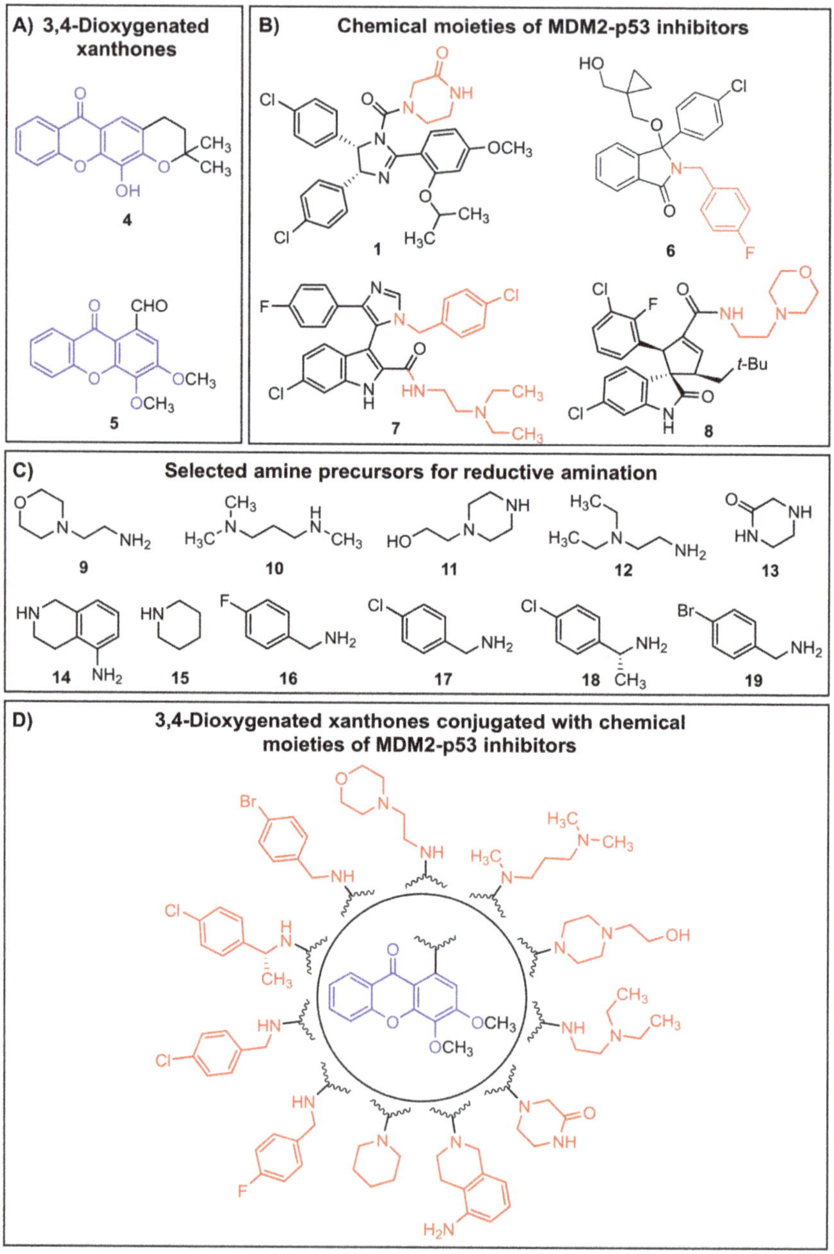

Figure 2. Strategy of molecular hybridization used for the construction of the library of aminated xanthones (**D**) by conjugation of the 3,4-dioxygenated substitution pattern of xanthones **4** and **5** (**A**) with the chemical moieties of known murine double minute 2 (MDM2)-p53 inhibitors (**C**), namely the molecules **1** (IC_{50} = 0.09 μM), **6** (IC_{50} = 2.6 μM), **7** (K_I = 0.656 μM), and **8** (K_I = 0.023 μM) (**B**).

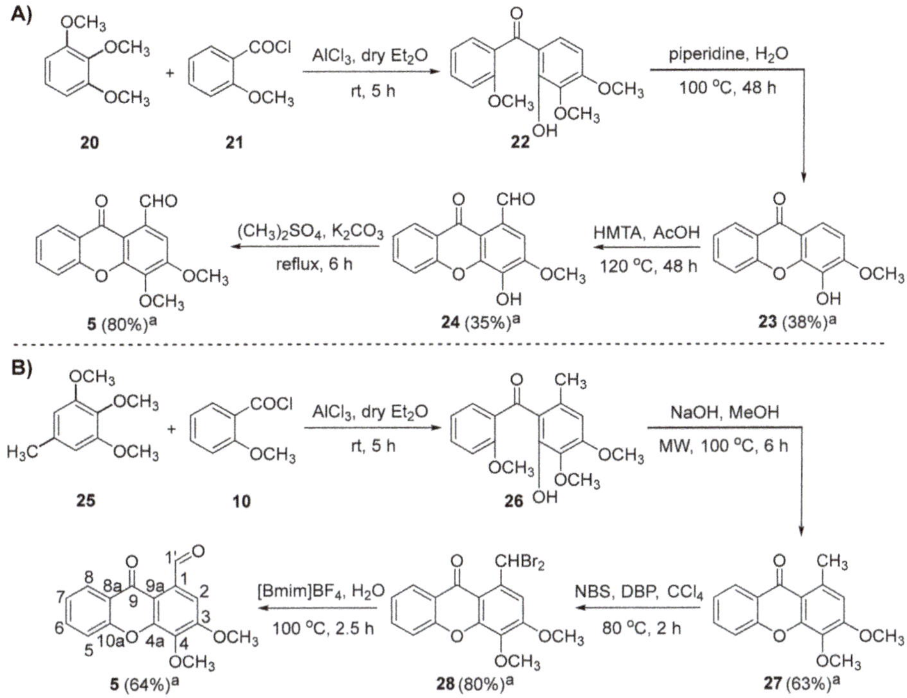

Scheme 1. (**A**) Synthetic route for the preparation of 3,4-dimethoxy-9-oxo-9*H*-xanthene-1-carbaldehyde (**5**) from 1,2,3-trimethoxybenzene (**20**). (**B**) Optimized synthetic route for the preparation of the xanthone **5** using the starting precursor 1,2,3-trimethoxy-5-methylbenzene (**25**). The compound numbering used concerns the nuclear magnetic resonance (NMR) assignments. Note: $[BmIm]BF_4$ = 1-butyl-3-methylimidazolium tetrafluoroborate; DBP = dibenzoyl peroxide; HMTA = hexamethylenetetramine; NBS = *N*-bromosuccinimide. [a] Isolated yields.

2.1.2. Synthesis of a Library of Aminated Xanthones (**30–40**)

A library of aminated xanthones **30–40** with a 3,4-dioxygenated pattern of substitution was obtained through a one-pot reductive amination of xanthone **5** with the appropriate amine precursors **9–19** (Scheme 2). In one-pot reductive aminations, the selection of the reducing agent is critical for their efficiency, since a suitable agent must reduce the Schiff base intermediate selectively over the carbonylated compounds. As an attempt to investigate the best reaction conditions, a solid-supported reactant containing borohydride ($MP\text{-}BH_4$) combined with methanol were initially employed, since it was successfully used in the reductive amination of a xanthone derivative (data not shown). When these conditions were applied to the reductive amination of **5**, the starting precursor was not completely consumed and the alcohol derivative 1-(hydroxymethyl)-3,4-dimethoxy-9*H*-xanthen-9-one (**29**) was the major product formed. The replacement of the above-mentioned conditions by the milder reducing agent sodium triacetoxyborohydride (STAB) and the solvent tetrahydrofuran allowed a total consumption of the xanthone **5**, favoring the one-pot amination/reduction pathway. Under the reaction conditions described in the Scheme 2, eleven aminated xanthones **30–40** were successfully synthesized in moderate to good yields (11 examples, 39–73% yields).

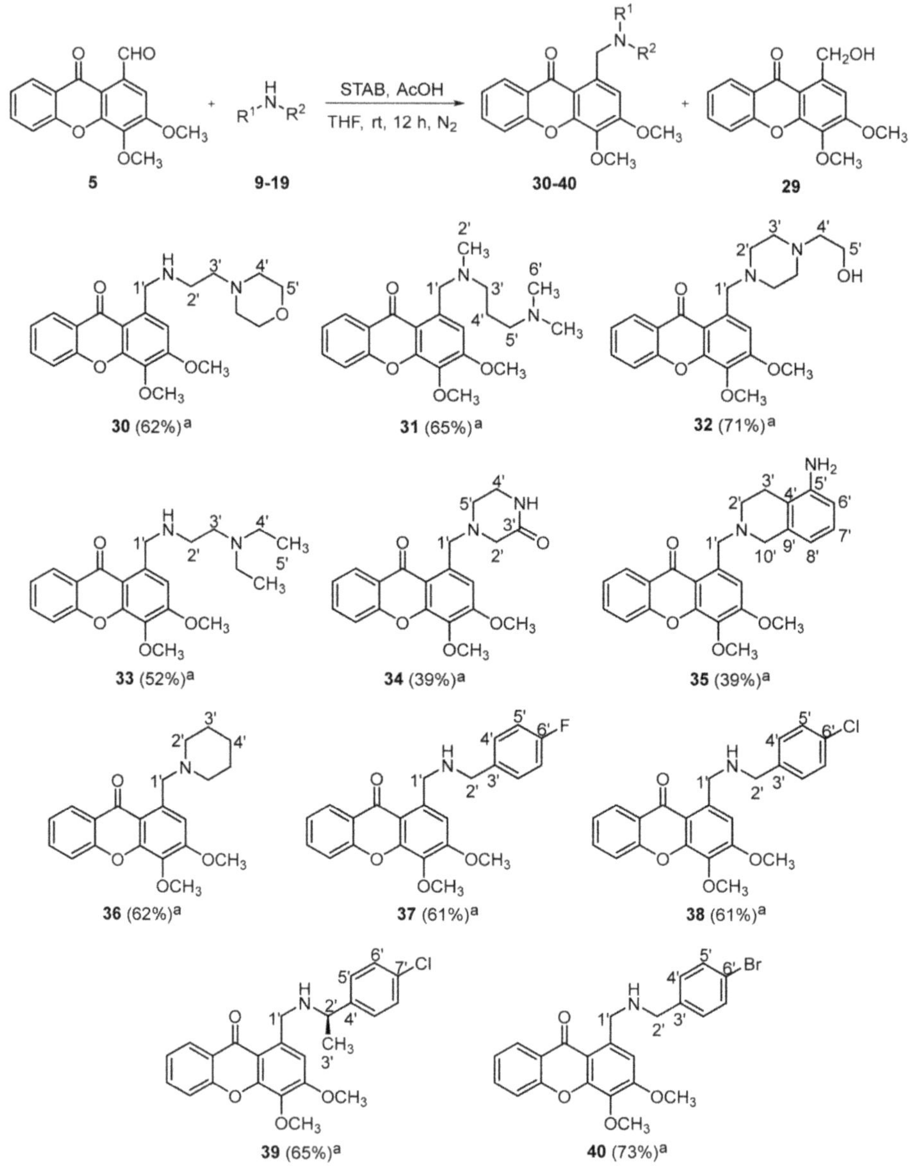

Scheme 2. Reductive amination of **5** with appropriate amine precursors **9–19** for the synthesis of aminated xanthones **30–40** with a 3,4-dioxygenated substitution pattern. The compound numbering used concerns the NMR assignments. [a] Isolated yields.

The structure elucidation of the xanthones **5** and **27–40** was established on the basis of high-resolution mass spectrometry (HRMS) (Figures S1–S15) and nuclear magnetic resonance (NMR) techniques (Figures S16–S45). The ^{13}C-NMR assignments were determined by bidimensional heteronuclear single quantum coherence (HSQC) and heteronuclear multiple bond correlation (HMBC) experiments (Supplementary Materials).

2.2. Biological Activity Evaluation

2.2.1. Effect of Synthesized Xanthone Derivatives **30–40** on the MDM2-p53 Interaction Using A Yeast-Based Screening Assay

Our group has previously developed a yeast-based screening assay to search for potential inhibitors of the MDM2-p53 interaction [30,31,44–46]. In this yeast cell system, the expression of human wt p53 induces a growth inhibition proportional to the degree of its activity (Figure 3, p53, dimethyl sulfoxide (DMSO)). On the other hand, this p53 inhibitory effect is reversed by yeast co-expression of human MDM2 (Figure 3, MDM2-p53, DMSO). This established yeast screening assay was used to study the potential inhibitory effect of 1-20 μM of xanthone derivatives **30–40** on the MDM2-p53 interaction. Figure 3 represents the maximal effect achieved with xanthone derivatives **30–40** at 10 μM. The results showed that only the xanthone **37** caused a significant reversion of the inhibitory effect of MDM2 on p53 (77.01 ± 7.35% of reversion, n = 3), with an almost complete reestablishment of the p53 growth inhibitory effect (63.55 ± 4.26% vs. 69.22 ± 2.23%; Figure 3, DMSO-treated p53-expressing yeast vs. xanthone **37**-treated MDM2-p53-expressing yeast). It should be noted that xanthone **37** did not interfere with the growth of control yeast (transformed with empty vectors) or yeast expressing human p53 alone (data not shown). As such, these results indicated that the xanthone **37** behaved as a potential p53-activating agent through inhibition of interaction with MDM2, and it was, therefore, selected for further investigation in human cancer cells.

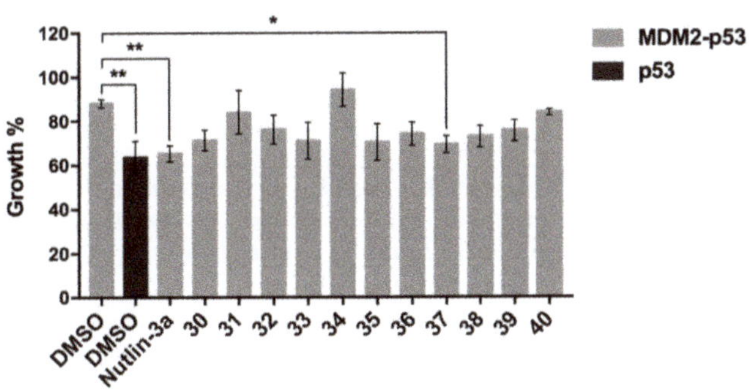

Figure 3. Effect of xanthones **30–40** on the MDM2-p53 interaction using a yeast-based assay. Effect of 10 μM xanthone derivatives **30–40** and nutlin-3A on the growth of yeast co-expressing p53 and MDM2 after 42 h treatment; results were plotted setting as 100% the growth of yeast transformed with the empty vector (control yeast); nutlin-3A (inhibitor of the MDM2-p53 interaction) was used as positive control. Data are mean ± standard error of the mean (SEM) of three independent experiments; mean values were statistically analyzed by one-way analysis of variance (ANOVA) with Tukey's multiple comparisons test, with significant differences from yeast co-expressing MDM2-p53 treated with DMSO. Note: * $p < 0.05$; ** $p < 0.01$.

2.2.2. Evaluation of the Antitumor Activity of Xanthone 37 in Human Cancer Cell Lines

Using the sulforhodamine B (SRB) assay, it was confirmed that xanthone **37** inhibited the growth of human HCT116 $p53^{+/+}$ colon cancer cells, with an IC_{50} (concentration that causes 50% growth inhibition) value of 8.67 ± 0.59 μM (n = 4), and of the MDM2-overexpressing human HepG2 liver carcinoma cells, with an IC_{50} value of 18.95 ± 0.39 μM (n = 4), after 48 h treatment.

To evaluate the dependency of the antitumor activity of xanthone **37** on the p53 pathway, we next determined the impact of xanthone **37** on the colony forming ability of HCT116 $p53^{+/+}$ cells and on the respective p53-knockout (HCT116 $p53^{-/-}$), using a colony formation assay (Figure 4A). The results showed a significant reduction of the growth inhibitory activity of xanthone **37**, at 3–5 μM in HCT116 $p53^{+/+}$ cells, demonstrating a p53-dependent antitumor effect of xanthone **37**. Accordingly, 10 and 20 μM of xanthone **37** caused a G1-phase cell cycle arrest in HCT116 $p53^{+/+}$ cells, but not in HCT116 p53$^{-/-}$ cells (Figure 4B) after 24 h treatment. It is of note that apoptosis analysis was also investigated by Annexin-V assay; nevertheless, apoptotic events were not detected at 10 and 20 µM of xanthone **37**, after 24 and 48 h treatment. In accordance with these results, we also observed that xanthone **37** upregulated the protein expression levels of MDM2, p53, and p21, in HCT116 p53$^{+/+}$ cells for 24 h treatment (Figure 4C).

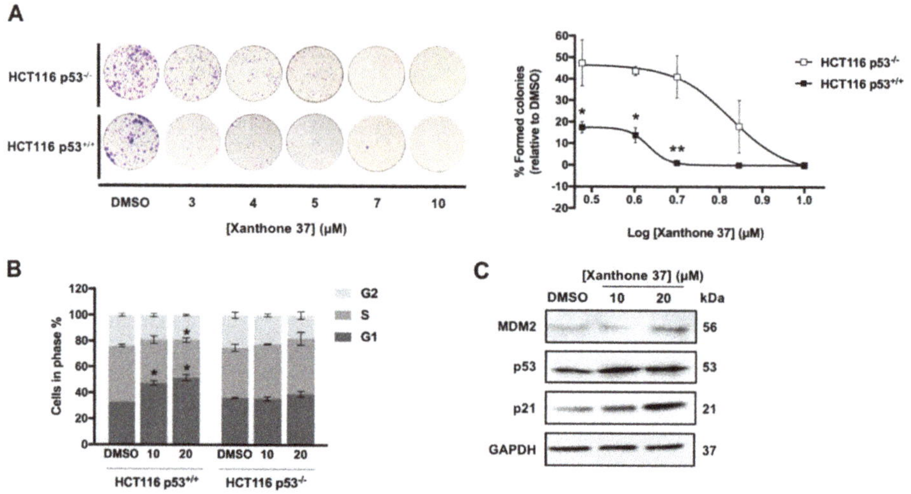

Figure 4. Xanthone **37** inhibits the colony forming capability of HCT116 cells through induction of cell cycle arrest and in a p53-dependent manner. (**A**) Evaluation of colony forming ability in HCT116 p53$^{+/+}$ and HCT116 p53$^{-/-}$ colon cancer cells after 11 days treatment with 3-10 µM of xanthone **37**; results were plotted setting as 100% the colonies formed after treatment with dimethyl sulfoxide (DMSO). (**B**) Effect of 10 and 20 µM of xanthone **37** on cell cycle progression of HCT116 p53$^{+/+}$ and HCT116 p53$^{-/-}$ cells, after 24 h treatment. (**C**) Effect of 10 and 20 µM of xanthone **37** on the expression levels of MDM2, p53, and p21 in HCT116 p53$^{+/+}$ cells analyzed by Western Blot after 24 h treatment. Immunoblots represent one of three independent experiments; Glyceraldehyde 3-phosphate dehydrogenase (GAPDH) was used as loading control. (**A**,**B**) Data are mean ± SEM of three independent experiments; values significantly different from HCT116 p53$^{-/-}$ cells using two-way ANOVA with Sidak's multiple comparisons test (**A**) or DMSO using Student's *t*-test (**B**) are indicated: * $p < 0.05$; ** $p < 0.01$.

Altogether, these results indicated that xanthone **37** had an in vitro p53-dependent antitumor activity mediated by induction of cell cycle arrest.

2.3. In Slico Studies

It is common knowledge that the amino-terminal (residues **18–26**) p53 α-helical peptide interacts with a deep hydrophobic cleft within the amino-terminal domain of MDM2 [47]. The MDM2 binding site consists of a large and a small pocket that interact with Phe19/Trp23 and Leu26 of p53, respectively (Figure 5A) [48]. The crystal structure of the MDM2 complexed with the transactivation domain of p53 (Protein Data Bank (PDB) id 1YCR [49]) allowed the visual inspection of the interactions between the Phe19, Trp23, and Leu26 residues of p53 and their respective pockets. Hydrogen-bonding interactions are established between the indole group of Trp23 and carbonyl backbone of Leu54, and between the NH backbone of Phe19 and the carbamoyl group of Gln72. Additional interactions are established between p53 and Leu57, Gly58, Ile61, Met62, Val75, Val93, and His96 residues of MDM2 (Figure 5B).

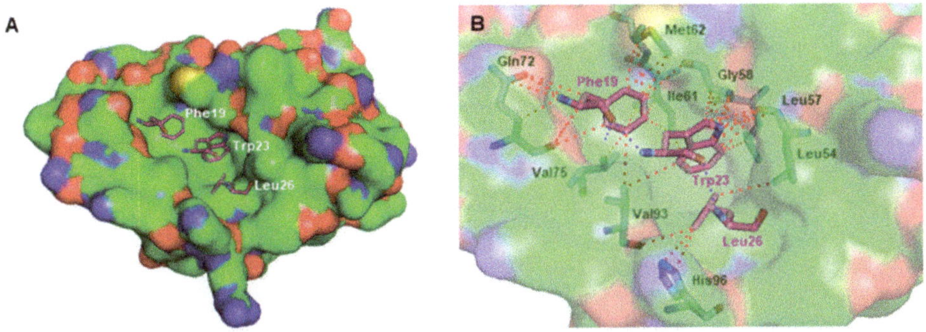

Figure 5. (**A**) Crystallographic p53 (for simplification, only Phe19, Trp23, and Leu26 residues are represented as purple sticks) bound to the three pockets of MDM2 (solid surface). (**B**) Binding mode of crystallographic p53 (for simplification, only residues Phe19, Trp23, and Leu26, are represented as purple sticks) in the hydrophobic cleft of MDM2 (transparent surface); MDM2 amino acid residues involved in interactions with p53 are represented as green sticks. Structural data were obtained from the X-ray crystal structure of MDM2-p53 complex (Protein Data Bank (PDB) id 1YCR). MDM2 is represented as surface, where carbon, oxygen, nitrogen, and sulfur are represented in green, red, blue, and yellow, respectively. Hydrogen-bonding interactions are depicted with a dashed blue line. Other types of interactions are represented as a dashed red line.

The 1.6 Å X-ray crystal structure of the small-molecule inhibitor of MDM2-p53 interaction **1** in complex with MDM2 (PDB id 4HG7 [50]) was selected for further molecular docking studies of the aminated xanthone derivatives **30–40** onto MDM2 protein, using the MDM2-p53 disruptors **1–4** as positive controls. In this work, AutoDock Vina [51] was the software chosen to predict docking conformations, as it has been described as being the best software in predicting crystallographic MDM2-p53 inhibitor poses (root-mean-square deviation (RMSD) < 1.0 Å) by redocking tests [52]. Docking scores for the most stable binding poses of xanthones **30–40** on MDM2 were determined using the AutoDock Vina software [51]. The predicted docking scores for known MDM2-p53 inhibitors (positive controls **1–4**) ranged from −7.7 to −8.0 kcal·mol^{-1} (Table 1). The most stable binding conformation of the synthesized xanthones **30–40** exhibited docking scores from −5.9 to −7.4 kcal· mol^{-1}, therefore being in the same range of binding affinity as the positive controls (Table 1).

Amongst the tested compounds, the xanthone **37** was identified as the most active compound in the yeast-based screening assay. In addition, the predicted free energy values for the most stable binding pose of xanthone **37** were more negative than the majority of the remaining ligands. Therefore, the xanthone **37** was further analyzed in terms of docking poses and residues potentially involved in the interaction with MDM2. Figure 6A shows the most stable conformation of xanthone **37** as suggested by the docking protocol. The xanthone **37** was predicted to interact within the p53-binding site, mimicking the key hydrophobic residues of p53 when bound to MDM2 (docking score of −7.3 kcal·mol^{-1}). Similarly to the binding mode of **1** within the p53-binding site (Figure 6B), no hydrogen-bonding interactions between the xanthone **37** and the MDM2 residues are predicted to be established. The *p*-fluorobenzylamino group of xanthone **37** occupies the Trp23 pocket and makes π-stacking interactions with Phe91 residue, amide-π interactions with the Leu57 and Gly58 residues, and CH-π interactions with the Leu54, Leu57, Gly58, Ile61, Val93, and Ile99 residues. Interestingly, the docking conformation of *p*-fluorobenzylamino group and the *p*-chlorophenyl ring of **1** are identical and superimposable (Figure 6A,B). The methoxy groups of the xanthone scaffold are oriented to the Leu26 pocket and make CH-CH interactions with the Leu54 residue. The adopted scaffold orientation of the xanthone **37** in the hydrophobic cleft where p53 is supposed to bind allows additional interactions to be formed, strengthening the binding of xanthone **37** to MDM2. For example, apart from the Gly58 residue of MDM2, the non-substituted aromatic ring of the xanthone scaffold is predicted to establish π-stacking interactions with the Phe55 residue, and amide-π and CH-π interactions with the Gln59 residue. The establishment of additional interactions within the MDM2 protein that are not observed in the MDM2-p53 binding have been described for a considerable number of high-affinity p53-activating agents [17]. The visual inspection of the xanthone **37** also suggests that an enhancement of its binding affinity towards MDM2 protein can be achieved by molecular modifications in the xanthone scaffold of **37** in order to optimize its interaction with the amino acid residues surrounding the Phe19 pocket.

Table 1. Docking scores (kcal·mol^{-1}) of xanthones **30–40** and positive controls **1–4** onto MDM2 target.

Xanthones 30–40	
Ligands	**Free Energy of the Ligand: MDM2 (kcal·mol^{-1})**
30	−6.6
31	−6.2
32	−6.6
33	−5.9
34	−6.9
35	−7.2
36	−6.6
37	−7.3
38	−7.1
39	−7.3
40	−7.4
Inhibitors of MDM2-p53 Interaction	
Ligands	**Free Energy of the Ligand: MDM2 (kcal·mol^{-1})**
1	−7.7
2	−8.0
3	−7.9
4	−8.0

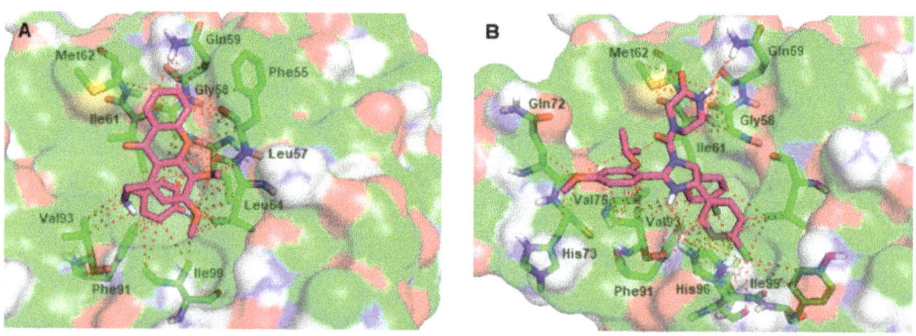

Figure 6. (**A**) Predicted binding pose of the xanthone **37** (purple sticks) in the binding site of MDM2. (**B**) MDM2 (transparent surface) in complex with the crystallographic nutlin-3A (**1**, purple sticks). MDM2 is represented as a transparent surface, where carbon, oxygen, nitrogen, and sulfur are represented in green, red, blue, and yellow, respectively. Small molecule-MDM2 interactions are depicted with a dashed red line. MDM2 residues involved in interactions with the ligands are represented as green sticks and labeled.

3. Materials and Methods

3.1. Chemistry

All reagents and solvents were purchased from Sigma Aldrich (Sigma-Aldrich Co. Ltd., Gillinghan, UK) and no further purification process was implemented. Solvents were evaporated using a rotary evaporator under reduced pressure, Buchi Waterchath B-480. Microwave (MW) reactions were performed using an Ethos MicroSYNTH 1600 Microwave Labstation from Milestone (Thermo Unicam, Portugal). The internal reaction temperature was controlled by a fiber optic probe sensor. All reactions were monitored by thin-layer chromatography (TLC) carried out on precoated plates with 0.2 mm of thickness using Merck silica gel 60 (GF_{254}) with appropriate mobile phases. Compounds **30–40** were easily detectable at 254 nm or 365 nm and after revelation with a solution of ninhydrin in ethanol 3 mg·mL^{-1} (activated by heat).

Flash column chromatography using silica gel 60 (0.040–0.063 mm, Merck, Darmstadt, Germany), flash cartridge chromatography (GraceResolv®, Grace Company, Deerfield, IL, USA), and Discovery® DSC-SCX SPE cationic exchange cartridge (Grace Company, Deerfield, IL, USA) were used in the purification of the synthesized compounds. Melting points (m.p.) were measured in a Köfler microscope (Wagner and Munz, Munich, Germany) and are uncorrected. ^{1}H- and ^{13}C-nuclear magnetic resonance (NMR) spectra were recorded at the University of Aveiro, Department of Chemistry in $CDCl_3$ or DMSO-d_6 (Deutero GmbH, Ely, UK) at room temperature on a Bruker Avance 300 spectrometer (300.13 MHz for ^{1}H and 75.47 MHz for ^{13}C, Bruker Biosciences Corporation, Billerica, MA, USA). Chemical shifts are expressed in δ (ppm) values relative to tetramethylsilane (TMS) as an internal reference. Coupling constants are reported in hertz (Hz). ^{13}C-NMR assignments were made by bidimensional heteronuclear single quantum coherence (HSQC) and heteronuclear multiple bond correlation (HMBC) NMR experiments (long-range C, H coupling constants were optimized to 7 Hz) or by comparison with the assignments of similar molecules. High-resolution mass spectroscopy (HRMS) spectra were measured on a Bruker FTMS APEX III mass spectrometer (Bruker Corporation, Billerica, MA, USA) and recorded as electrospray ionization (ESI) mode in Centro de Apoio Cientifico e Tecnolóxico á Investigación (CACTI, University of Vigo, Pontevedra, Spain). The following compounds were synthesized and purified by the described procedures.

3.1.1. Synthesis of 3,4-dimethoxy-1-methyl-9*H*-xanthen-9-one (**27**)

Xanthone **27** (9.34 g, 63% yield) was synthesized from 1,2,3-trimethoxy-5-methylbenzene (**25**) and characterized according to the previously described procedure [42].

3.1.2. Synthesis of 1-(dibromomethyl)-3,4-dimethoxy-9*H*-xanthen-9-one (**28**)

A mixture of **27** (2.52 g, 9.32 mmol), *N*-bromosuccinimide (3.32 g, 18.7 mmol), and dibenzoyl peroxide (0.68 g, 2.8 mmol) in carbon tetrachloride (25 mL) was refluxed (85 °C) for 2 h. The reaction was monitored using *n*-hexane/ethyl acetate in a proportion of 8:2. Once the reaction was completed, the resulting orange suspension was cooled at 0 °C and stirred for 30 min in an ice bath. The solid was filtered and washed with cold carbon tetrachloride. The filtrate was evaporated under reduced pressure and further purified by flash column chromatography (SiO_2, *n*-hexane/ethyl acetate in gradient) to obtain the **28** as a white powder.

For 1-(dibromomethyl)-3,4-dimethoxy-9*H*-xanthen-9-one (**28**): White powder (3.14 g, 80% yield); melting point (m.p.) 125–127 °C. ^{1}H-NMR ($CDCl_3$, 300.13 MHz): δ = 8.91 (1H, s, H-1), 8.30 (1H, dd, J = 8.0 and 1.6 Hz, H-8), 7.77 (1H, s, H-2), 7.73 (1H, ddd, J = 8.4, 7.0, and 1.6 Hz, H-6), 7.54 (1H, d, J = 8.4 Hz, H-5), 7.39 (1H, ddd, J = 7.5, H-7), 4.11 (3H, s, 4-OCH_3), 4.05 (3H, s, 3-OCH_3) ppm; ^{13}C-NMR ($CDCl_3$, 75.47 MHz): δ = 177.8 (C-9), 156.5 (C-3), 155.0 (C-10a), 150.4 (C-4a), 139.5 (C-4), 137.6 (C-1), 135.0 (C-6), 126.9 (C-8), 124.3 (C-7), 122.0 (C-8a), 117.6 (C-5), 111.9 (C-2), 110.8 (C-9a), 61.9 (3-OCH_3), 56.6 (4-OCH_3), 39.2 (C-1′) ppm. HRMS (ESI$^+$): *m/z* $[C_{16}H_{12}Br_2O_5 + H]^+$ calcd. for $[C_{16}H_{13}Br_2O_5]$: 426.91751; found: 426.91709.

3.1.3. Synthesis of 3,4-dimethoxy-9-oxo-9*H*-xanthene-1-carbaldehyde (**5**)

Xanthone **28** (3.14 g, 7.34 mmol) was added to a solution of 1-butyl-3-methylimidazolium tetrafluoroborate and water (6 mL, 5:1). The mixture was heated at 100 °C with stirring for 2.5 h. The reaction was monitored using *n*-hexane/ethyl acetate in a proportion of 7:3. After completion of the reaction, the resulting suspension was cooled at room temperature, diluted with water (10 mL), and extracted with ethyl acetate (5 × 100 mL). The combined organic layers were dried over anhydrous sodium sulfate, and after filtration of the solution, the solvent was evaporated under reduced pressure. The crude product was then purified by flash column chromatography (SiO_2, *n*-hexane/ethyl acetate in gradient). A light yellow powder corresponding to **5** was obtained.

For 3,4-dimethoxy-9-oxo-9*H*-xanthene-1-carbaldehyde (**5**): Light yellow powder (1.33 g, 64% yield); m.p. > 330 °C. ^{1}H-NMR ($CDCl_3$, 300.13 MHz): δ = 11.21 (1H, s, H-1′), 8.31 (1H, dd, *J* = 8.0 and 1.7 Hz, H-8), 7.77 (1H, ddd, *J* = 8.5, 7.0, and 1.7 Hz, H-6), 7.60 (1H, dd, *J* = 8.5 and 0.8 Hz, H-5), 7.56 (1H, s, H-2), 7.43 (1H, ddd, *J* = 8.0, 7.0, and 0.8 Hz, H-7), 4.11 (3H, s, 4-OCH_3), 4.07 (3H, s, 3-OCH_3) ppm; ^{13}C-NMR ($CDCl_3$, 75.47 MHz): δ = 192.8 (C-1′), 177.9 (C-9), 156.3 (C-3), 155.5 (C-10a), 150.9 (C-4a), 140.7 (C-4), 135.1 (C-6), 133.5 (C-1), 126.7 (C-8), 124.5 (C-7), 121.9 (C-8a), 117.8 (C-5), 116.1 (C-9a), 108.5 (C-2), 61.8 (4-OCH_3), 56.6 (3-OCH_3) ppm. HRMS (ESI$^+$): *m/z* $[C_{16}H_{12}O_5 + H]^+$ calcd. for $[C_{16}H_{13}O_5]$: 285.07575; found: 285.07598; $[C_{16}H_{12}O_5 + Na]^-$ calcd. for $[C_{16}H_{12}NaO_5]$: 307.05769; found 307.05750.

3.1.4. Synthesis of 1-(hydroxymethyl)-3,4-dimethoxy-9*H*-xanthen-9-one (**29**)

Xanthone **29** (52 mg, 52% yield) was synthesized from xanthone **5** and characterized according to the previously described procedure [36].

3.1.5. General Procedure for the Synthesis of Xanthones (**30–40**)

Xanthone **5** (40 mg, 0.141 mmol) was dissolved in tetrahydrofuran (3 mL) and the appropriate amine precursors **9–19** (0.197 mmol) were added to the solution under N_2 gas. After the addition of a 4.0 equimolar quantity of sodium triacetoxyborohydride (119 mg, 0.563 mmol), the resulting mixture was stirred at room temperature for 30 min. Subsequently, a 3.0 equimolar quantity of acetic acid (24 μL 0.423 mmol) was added to the solution, The reaction was carried out at room temperature for 12 h under N_2 gas. For monitoring the synthesis of xanthones **30–40** by TLC, two chromatographic systems were employed: (i) *n*-hexane/ethyl acetate (7:3) and methanol/triethylamine (10:0.1) for xanthones **30–36**; (ii) *n*-hexane/ethyl acetate (7:3) and chloroform/acetone/triethylamine (5:5:0.1) for xanthones **37–40**. Once completed of the reaction, three distinct work-up approaches were employed.

(a) For xanthones **30–32**: the solvent was evaporated under reduced pressure and the resulting crude product was basified with sodium hydroxide (10 mL, 5%, m/v) and extracted with chloroform (3 × 10 mL). The combined organic phases were then acidified and extracted with hydrochloric acid 5 M (3 × 30 mL). Afterwards, the aqueous phases were gathered and then basified with sodium hydroxide (100 mL, 20%, *m/v*). The crude product was extracted successively with chloroform (3 × 100 mL). The organic layers were gathered and dried over anhydrous sodium sulfate. After filtration, the solution was concentrated under reduced pressure, and the resulting crude product was purified by flash cartridge chromatography (SiO_2, chloroform/acetone/ammonium hydroxide, 90:10:1) to afford the xanthones 30, 31, and 32 as pure compounds.

For 3,4-dimethoxy-1-(((2-morpholinoethyl)amino)methyl)-9*H*-xanthen-9-one (**30**): Green powder (35 mg, 62% yield); m.p. 125–126 °C. ^{1}H-NMR ($CDCl_3$, 300.13 MHz): δ = 8.25 (1H, dd, *J* = 8.0 and 1.6 Hz, H-8), 7.72 (1H, ddd, *J* = 8.1, 7.0, and 1.6 Hz, H-6), 7.57 (1H, dd, *J* = 8.4 and 0.8 Hz, H-5), 7.38 (1H, ddd, *J* = 8.0, 7.1, and 0.9 Hz, H-7), 7.09 (1H, s, H-2), 4.34 (2H, s, H-1′); 4.04 (3H, s, 4-OCH_3), 4.01 (3H, s, 3-OCH_3), 3.66 (4H, t, *J* = 4.6 Hz, H-5′), 2.90 (2H, t, *J* = 6.1 Hz, H-2′), 2.60 (2H, t, *J* = 6.1 Hz, H-3′), 2.47 (4H, t, *J* = 4.3 Hz, H-4′) ppm; ^{13}C-NMR ($CDCl_3$, 75.47 MHz): δ = 178.0 (C-9), 156.5 (C-3), 155.3 (C-10a), 152.1 (C-4a), 137.0 (C-1), 136.0 (C-4), 134.6 (C-6), 126.5 (C-8), 124.1 (C-7), 122.1 (C-8a), 117.7 (C-5), 114.6 (C-9a), 111.6 (C-2), 67.0 (C-5′), 61.5 (4-OCH_3), 57.4 (C-2′), 56.4 (3-OCH_3), 53.7 (C-1′), 53.5 (C-4′), 45.3 (C-3′) ppm. HRMS (ESI$^+$): *m/z* $[C_{22}H_{26}N_2O_5 + H]^+$ calcd. for $[C_{22}H_{27}N_2O_5]$: 399.19145; found: 399.19060.

For 1-(((3-(dimethylamino)propyl)(methyl)amino)methyl)-3,4-dimethoxy-9*H*-xanthen-9-one (**31**): White powder (35 mg, 65% yield); m.p. 84–85 °C. ^{1}H-NMR ($CDCl_3$, 300.13 MHz): δ = 8.25 (1H, dd, *J* = 8.0 and 1.6 Hz, H-8), 7.69 (1H, ddd, *J* = 8.5, 7.0, and 1.6 Hz, H-6), 7.54 (1H, dd, *J*= 7.4 and 0.7, H-5), 7.53 (1H, s, H-2), 7.35 (1H, ddd, *J* = 8.0, 7.1, and 1.0 Hz, H-7), 4.36 (2H, s, H-1′); 4.05 (3H, s, 4-OCH_3),

4.02 (3H, s, 3-OCH$_3$), 2.65 (2H, t, J = 7.2 Hz, H-3′), 2.44 (2H, t, J = 7.5 Hz, H-5′), 2.39 (3H, s, H-2′), 2.28 (6H, s, H-6′), 1.82 (2H, m, J = 7.3 Hz, H-4′) ppm; ^{13}C-NMR (CDCl$_3$, 75.47 MHz): δ = 178.1 (C-9), 156.6 (C-3), 155.2 (C-10a), 151.9 (C-4a), 135.2 (C-1), 135.0 (C-4), 134.2 (C-6), 126.6 (C-8), 123.9 (C-7), 122.4 (C-8a), 117.6 (C-5), 114.5 (C-9a), 109.0 (C-2), 61.5 (4-OCH$_3$), 60.1 (C-1′), 57.8 (C-5′), 56.4 (3-OCH$_3$), 56.1 (C-3′), 45.3 (C-6′), 42.5 (C-2′), 25.3 (C-4′) ppm. HRMS (ESI$^+$): m/z [$C_{22}H_{28}N_2O_4$ + H]$^+$ calcd. for [$C_{22}H_{29}N_2O_4$]: 385.21218; found: 385.21139.

For 1-((4-(2-hydroxyethyl)piperazin-1-yl)methyl)-3,4-dimethoxy-9*H*-xanthen-9-one (**32**): Yellow powder (40 mg, 71% yield); m.p. 129–130 °C. ^{1}H-NMR (CDCl$_3$, 300.13 MHz): δ = 8.25 (1H, dd, J = 8.0 and 1.6 Hz, H-8), 7.68 (1H, ddd, J = 8.5, 7.0, and 1.6 Hz, H-6), 7.53 (1H, dd, J = 8.4 and 0.7 Hz, H-5), 7.48 (1H, s, H-2), 7.35 (1H, ddd, J = 8.0, 7.1, and 1.0 Hz, H-7), 4.32 (2H, s, H-1′), 4.03 (3H, s, 4-OCH$_3$), 4.01 (3H, s, 3-OCH$_3$), 3.63 (2H, t, J = 5.4 Hz), 2.58 (2H, t, J = 5.4 Hz) ppm; ^{13}C-NMR (CDCl$_3$, 75.47 MHz): δ = 178.1 (C-9), 156.5 (C-3), 155.2 (C-10a), 152.0 (C-4a), 138.8 (C-1), 134.8 (C-4), 134.2 (C-6), 126.6 (C-8), 123.9 (C-7), 122.5 (C-8a), 117.5 (C-5), 114.6 (C-9a), 108.2 (C-2), 61.5 (4-OCH$_3$), 60.2 (C-1′), 59.3 (C-5′), 57.7 (C-4′), 56.2 (3-OCH$_3$), 53.5 (C-3′), 53.2 (C-2′) ppm. HRMS (ESI$^+$): m/z [$C_{22}H_{26}N_2O_5$ + H]$^+$ calcd. for [$C_{22}H_{27}N_2O_5$]: 399.19145; found: 399.19059.

(b) For xanthones **33**–**36**: the solvent was evaporated under reduced pressure and the crude product was extracted with chloroform (3 × 10 mL). The organic phases were gathered, dried over anhydrous sodium sulfate, and after filtration, the resulting solution was concentrated under reduced pressure. Then, a solid phase extraction using a cation exchange cartridge Discovery® DSC-SCX was applied to further purify the crude product. Initially, an activation of the cartridge with methanol (100 mL) was carried out followed by loading the cartridge with the sample. Then, the elution was performed with the following solvents/solutions: (i) dichloromethane/methanol (5:5), (ii) methanol, and (iii) ammonium hydroxide/methanol (2%, *v/v*). The fractions obtained from the elution with ammonium hydroxide/methanol (2%, *v/v*) were gathered and the solvent was evaporated under reduced pressure. A flash cartridge chromatography with chloroform/acetone/ammonium hydroxide (90:10:1) was also performed to obtain the xanthones **33**, **34**, **35**, and **36** as pure compounds.

For 1-(((2-(diethylamino)ethyl)amino)methyl)-3,4-dimethoxy-9*H*-xanthen-9-one (**33**): Green powder (28 mg, 52% yield); m.p. 68–69 °C. ^{1}H-NMR (CDCl$_3$, 300.13 MHz): δ = 8.27 (1H, dd, J = 8.0 and 1.4 Hz, H-8), 7.71 (1H, ddd, J = 8.5, 7.0, and 1.6 Hz, H-6), 7.56 (1H, dd, J = 8.4 and 0.7 Hz, H-5), 7.37 (1H, ddd, J = 8.0, 7.1, and 1.0 Hz, H-7), 7.14 (1H, s, H-2), 4.39 (2H, s, H-1′); 4.05 (3H, s, 4-OCH$_3$), 4.01 (3H, s, 3-OCH$_3$), 2.87 (2H, t, J = 6.4 Hz, H-2′), 2.68 (2H, t, J = 6.4 Hz, H-3′), 2.55 (4H, m, J = 7.1 Hz, H-4′), 1.01 (6H, t, J = 7.1 Hz, H-5′) ppm; ^{13}C-NMR (CDCl$_3$, 75.47 MHz): δ = 178.1 (C-9), 156.5 (C-3), 155.3 (C-10a), 152.1 (C-4a), 137.4 (C-1), 135.8 (C-4), 134.5 (C-6), 126.6 (C-8), 124.0 (C-7), 122.2 (C-8a), 117.7 (C-5), 114.5 (C-9a), 111.1 (C-2), 61.5 (4-OCH$_3$), 56.4 (3-OCH$_3$), 53.4 (C-3′), 52.4 (C-1′), 46.9 (C-4′), 46.8 (C-2′), 11.6 (C-5′) ppm. HRMS (ESI$^+$): m/z [$C_{22}H_{28}N_2O_4$ + H]$^+$ calcd. for [$C_{22}H_{29}N_2O_4$]: 385.21218; found: 385.21150.

For 4-((3,4-dimethoxy-9-oxo-9*H*-xanthen-1-yl)methyl)piperazin-2-one (**34**): Orange powder (20 mg, 39% yield); m.p. 245–247 °C. ^{1}H-NMR (DMSO-d_6, 300.13 MHz): δ = 8.13 (1H, dd, J = 8.0 and 1.5 Hz, H-8), 7.82 (1H, ddd, J = 8.5, 7.0, and 1.6 Hz, H-6), 7.65 (1H, dd, J = 8.4 and 0.6, H-5), 7.45 (1H, ddd, J = 8.0, 7.1, and 1.0 Hz, H-7), 7.36 (1H, s, H-2), 4.24 (2H, s, H-1′); 3.98 (3H, s, 4-OCH$_3$), 3.90 (3H, s, 3-OCH$_3$), 3.20 (2H, t, J = 5.3 Hz, H-5′), 3.13 (2H, s, H-2′), 2.66 (2H, t, J = 5.3 Hz, H-4′) ppm; ^{13}C-NMR (DMSO-d_6, 75.47 MHz): δ = 176.7 (C-9), 168.0 (C-3′), 156.2 (C-3), 154.6 (C-10a), 151.8 (C-4a), 136.9 (C-1), 135.0 (C-4), 134.7 (C-6), 126.1 (C-8), 124.3 (C-7), 121.8 (C-8a), 117.7 (C-5), 113.7 (C-9a), 109.2 (C-2), 60.9 (4-OCH$_3$), 58.5 (C-1′), 57.2 (C-5′), 56.3 (3-OCH$_3$), 48.7 (C-2′), 30.7 (C-4′) ppm. HRMS (ESI$^+$): m/z [$C_{20}H_{20}N_2O_5$ + H]$^+$ calcd. for [$C_{20}H_{21}N_2O_5$]: 369.14450; found: 369.14369.

For 1-((5-amino-3,4-dihydroisoquinolin-2(1*H*)-yl)methyl)-3,4-dimethoxy-9*H*-xanthen-9-one (**35**): White powder (23 mg, 39% yield); m.p. 171–172 °C. ^{1}H-NMR (CDCl$_3$, 300.13 MHz): δ = 8.26 (1H, dd, J = 8.0 and 1.4 Hz, H-8), 7.69 (1H, ddd, J = 8.5, 7.0, and 1.6 Hz, H-6), 7.57 (1H, s, H-2), 7.54 (1H, dd, J = 8.4 and 0.7 Hz, H-5), 7.35 (1H, ddd, J = 8.0, 7.1, and 1.0 Hz, H-7), 6.99 (1H, t, J = 7.7 Hz, H-7′), 6.57 (1H, d, J = 7.8 Hz, H-6′), 6.53 (1H, d, J = 7.6 Hz, H-8′), 4.48 (2H, s, H-1′); 4.02 (3H, s, 4-OCH$_3$), 3.97

(3H, s, 3-OCH_3), 3.81 (2H, s, H-10′), 2.93 (2H, t, *J* = 5.9 Hz, H-2′), 2.66 (2H, t, *J* = 5.9 Hz, H-3′) ppm; ^{13}C-NMR ($CDCl_3$, 75.47 MHz): δ = 178.2 (C-9), 156.7 (C-3), 155.2 (C-10a), 151.9 (C-4a), 144.1 (C-5′), 139.3 (C-1), 136.3 (C-9′), 134.8 (C-4), 134.2 (C-6), 126.6 (C-8), 126.4 (C-7′), 123.8 (C-7), 122.5 (C-8a), 119.5 (C-4′), 117.6 (C-5), 117.1 (C-8′), 114.5 (C-9a), 112.7 (C-6′), 108.0 (C-2), 61.5 (4-OCH_3), 60.1 (C-1′), 56.7 (C-10′), 56.3 (3-OCH_3), 51.0 (C-2′), 24.9 (C-3′) ppm. HRMS (ESI$^+$): *m/z* [$C_{25}H_{24}N_2O_4$ + H]$^+$ calcd. for [$C_{25}H_{25}N_2O_4$]: 417.18088; found: 417.18018.

For 3,4-dimethoxy-1-(piperidin-1-ylmethyl)-9*H*-xanthen-9-one (**36**): Yellow powder (31 mg, 62% yield); m.p. 108-109 °C. ^{1}H-NMR ($CDCl_3$, 300.13 MHz): δ = 8.25 (1H, dd, *J* = 8.0 and 1.6 Hz, H-8), 7.66 (1H, ddd, *J* = 8.5, 8.0, and 1.6 Hz, H-6), 7.56 (1H, s, H-2), 7.52 (1H, dd, *J* = 8.3 and 0.7 Hz, H-5), 7.33 (1H, ddd, *J* = 7.9, 7.1, and 0.9 Hz, H-7), 4.26 (2H, s, H-1′); 4.03 (3H, s, 4-OCH_3), 4.01 (3H, s, 3-OCH_3), 2.57 (4H, t, *J* = 4.6 Hz, H-2′), 1.65 (4H, m, *J* = 5.5 Hz, H-3′), 1,50 (2H, m, *J* = 5.5 Hz, H-4′) ppm; ^{13}C-NMR ($CDCl_3$, 75.47 MHz) ppm: δ = 177.5 (C-9), 156.1 (C-3), 154.7 (C-10a), 151.3 (C-4a), 138.9 (C-4), 134.2 (C-1), 133.8 (C-6), 126.0 (C-8), 123.3 (C-7), 121.9 (C-8a), 117.1 (C-5), 113.9 (C-9a), 107.8 (C-2), 60.8 (4-OCH_3), 56.1 (3-OCH_3), 55.7 (C-2′), 54.3 (C-1′), 25.7 (C-3′), 23.8 (C-4′) ppm. HRMS (ESI$^+$): *m/z* [$C_{21}H_{23}NO_4$ + H]$^+$ calcd. for [$C_{21}H_{24}NO_4$]: 354.16998; found: 354.16939.

(c) For xanthones **37**–**40**: the solvent was evaporated under reduced pressure and the resulting crude product was basified with sodium hydroxide (10 mL, 5%, *m/v*) and extracted with chloroform (3 × 10 mL). The combined organic phases were then acidified and extracted with hydrochloric acid 5 M (3 × 30 mL). The resulting organic phase was dried over anhydrous sodium sulfate and, after filtration, the solution was concentrated under reduced pressure. Then, a solid phase extraction using a cation exchange cartridge Discovery® DSC-SCX was applied to further purify the crude product. Initially, an activation of the cartridge with methanol (100 mL) was carried out followed by loading the cartridge with the sample. Then, the elution was performed with the following solvents/solutions: (i) dichloromethane/methanol (5:5), (ii) methanol, and (iii) ammonium hydroxide/methanol (2%, *v/v*). The fractions obtained from the elution with ammonium hydroxide/methanol (2%, *v/v*) were gathered and the solvent was evaporated under reduced pressure to furnish the xanthones **37**, **38**, **39**, and **40** as pure compounds.

For 1-(((4-fluorobenzyl)amino)methyl)-3,4-dimethoxy-9*H*-xanthen-9-one (**37**): White powder, (34 mg, 61% yield); m.p. 163–165 °C. ^{1}H-NMR ($CDCl_3$, 300.13 MHz): δ = 8.28 (1H, dd, *J* = 8.0 and 1.6 Hz, H-8), 7.71 (1H, ddd, *J* = 8.5, 7.0, and 1.6 Hz, H-6), 7.55 (1H, dd, *J* = 8.5 and 0.8 Hz, H-5), 7.40 (1H, ddd, *J* = 8.0, 7.0, and 0.8 Hz, H-7), 7.36 (2H, m, H-5′), 7.01 (2H, m, H-4′), 6.96 (1H, s, H-2), 4.30 (2H, s, H-1′), 4.01 (3H, s, 4-OCH_3), 4.01 (3H, s, 3-OCH_3), 3.85 (2H, s, H-2′) ppm; ^{13}C-NMR ($CDCl_3$, 75.47 MHz): δ = 178.1 (C-9), 160.3 (C-6′), 156.3 (C-3), 155.3 (C-10a), 152.2 (C-4a), 138.6 (C-4), 135.9 (C-3′), 135.7 (C-1), 134.5 (C-6), 129.8 (C-5′), 126.7 (C-8), 124.0 (C-7), 122.2 (C-8a), 117.7 (C-5), 115.3 (C-4′), 114.7 (C-9a), 110.9 (C-2), 61.5 (4-OCH_3), 56.3 (3-OCH_3), 53.3 (C-1′), 52.5 (C-2′) ppm. HRMS (ESI$^+$): *m/z* [$C_{23}H_{20}FNO_4$ + H]$^+$ calcd. for [$C_{23}H_{21}FNO_4$]: 394.14491; found: 394.14410.

For 1-(((4-chlorobenzyl)amino)methyl)-3,4-dimethoxy-9*H*-xanthen-9-one (**38**): Light yellow powder (35 mg, 61% yield); m.p. 162–163 °C. ^{1}H-NMR ($CDCl_3$, 300.13 MHz): δ = 8.25 (1H, dd, *J* = 8.0 and 1.6 Hz, H-8), 7.79 (1H, ddd, *J* = 8.5, 7.0, and 1.6 Hz, H-6), 7.66 (2H, m, H-5′), 7.60 (1H, dd, *J* = 8.5 and 0.9 Hz, H-5), 7.43 (1H, ddd, *J* = 8.0, 7.0, and 0.9 Hz, H-7), 7.39 (1H, s, H-2), 7.38 (2H, m, H-4′), 4.53 (2H, s, H-2′); 4.33 (2H, s, H-1′), 4.07 (3H, s, 4-OCH_3), 4.01 (3H, s, 3-OCH_3) ppm; ^{13}C-NMR ($CDCl_3$, 75.47 MHz): δ = 179.6 (C-9), 157.0 (C-3), 155.5 (C-10a), 152.0 (C-4a), 137.7 (C-4), 135.8 (C-1), 135.6 (C-6), 131.7 (C-5′), 129.5 (C-4′), 129.4 (C-3′), 127.3 (C-6′), 126.6 (C-8), 124.6 (C-7), 121.3 (C-8a), 117.9 (C-5), 115.5 (C-2), 114.8 (C-9a), 61.6 (4-OCH_3), 57.1 (3-OCH_3), 51.3 (C-1′), 50.7 (C-2′) ppm. HRMS (ESI$^+$): *m/z* [$C_{23}H_{20}ClNO_4$ + H]$^+$ calcd. for [$C_{23}H_{21}ClNO_4$]: 410.11536; found: 410.11466.

For (*R*)-1-(((1-(4-chlorophenyl)ethyl)amino)methyl)-3,4-dimethoxy-9*H*-xanthen-9-one (**39**): White powder (39 mg, 65% yield); m.p. 163–164 °C. ^{1}H-NMR ($CDCl_3$, 300.13 MHz): δ = 8.26 (1H, dd, *J* = 8.0 and 1.6 Hz, H-8), 7.79 (1H, ddd, *J* = 8.5, 7.0, and 1.6 Hz, H-6), 7.70 (2H, m, H-6′), 7.59 (1H, dd, *J* = 8.5 and 0.8 Hz, H-5), 7.43 (1H, ddd, *J* = 8.0, 7.0, and 0.8 Hz, H-7), 7.42 (2H, m, H-5′), 7.25 (1H, s, H-2), 4.54 (2H, s, H-1′); 4.27 (1H, q, *J* = 6.8 Hz, H-1′), 4.04 (3H, s, 4-OCH_3), 4.01 (3H, s, 3-OCH_3),

1.83 (3H, d, J = 6.8 Hz, H-3′) ppm; ^{13}C-NMR ($CDCl_3$, 75.47 MHz): δ = 179.6 (C-9), 156.8 (C-3), 155.4 (C-10a), 151.9 (C-4a), 137.6 (C-4), 135.5 (C-6), 134.5 (C-1), 131.8 (C-7′), 129.8 (C-6′), 129.5 (C-5′), 127.3 (C-4′), 126.6 (C-8), 124.6 (C-7), 121.3 (C-8a), 117.9 (C-5), 115.6 (C-2), 114.9 (C-9a), 61.6 (4-OCH_3), 58.9 (C-2′), 57.0 (3-OCH_3), 50.2 (C-1′), 20.2 (C-3′) ppm. HRMS (ESI^+): *m/z* [$C_{24}H_{22}ClNO_4$ + H]$^+$ calcd. for [$C_{24}H_{23}ClNO_4$]: 424.13101; found: 424.13018.

For 1-(((4-bromobenzyl)amino)methyl)-3,4-dimethoxy-9*H*-xanthen-9-one (**40**): White powder (47 mg, 73% yield); m.p. 161–162 °C. ^{1}H-NMR ($CDCl_3$, 300.13 MHz): δ = 8.27 (1H, dd, J = 8.0 and 1.6 Hz, H-8), 7.73 (1H, ddd, J = 8.5, 7.0, and 1.6 Hz, H-6), 7.58 (1H, dd, J = 8.5 and 0.8 Hz, H-5), 7.48 (2H, m, H-5′), 7.39 (2H, m, H-4′), 7.38 (1H, ddd, J = 8.0, 7.0, and 0.8 Hz, H-7), 7.08 (1H, s, H-2), 4.31 (2H, s, H-1′); 4.01 (3H, s, 4-OCH_3), 4.01 (3H, s, 3-OCH_3), 3.88 (2H, s, H-2′) ppm; ^{13}C-NMR ($CDCl_3$, 75.47 MHz): δ = 178.6 (C-9), 156.5 (C-3), 155.3 (C-10a), 152.2 (C-4a), 136.4 (C-4), 136.2 (C-1), 134.9 (C-6), 131.8 (C-5′), 130.7 (C-4′), 128.4 (C-3′), 126.6 (C-8), 124.2 (C-7), 121.9 (C-8a), 121.8 (C-6′), 117.7 (C-5), 114.7 (C-9a), 112.5 (C-2), 61.6 (4-OCH_3), 56.7 (3-OCH_3), 52.7 (C-1′), 52.0 (C-2′) ppm. HRMS (ESI^+): *m/z* [$C_{23}H_{20}BrNO_4$ + H]$^+$ calcd. for [$C_{23}H_{21}BrNO_4$]: 454.06485; found: 454.06385.

3.2. Biological Evaluation

3.2.1. Yeast Strains and Growth Conditions

For the yeast assay, the previously obtained *Saccharomyces cerevisiae* cells co-expressing human p53 or human MDM2, as well as yeast control (transformed with empty vectors) [30,31], were used. To induce expression of human proteins, yeast cells were grown in selective induction medium with 2% (*w/w*) galactose and 2% (*w/w*) raffinose, in the presence of 1–20 μM of xanthones **30**–**40** or 0.1% DMSO, at 30 °C under continuous orbital shaking (200 rpm) for approximately 42 h, as described [30,31]. Yeast cell growth was analyzed by counting the number of colony-forming units (CFU) after 2 days incubation at 30 °C on Sabouraud Dextrose Agar plates from Liofilchem (Frilabo, Porto, Portugal). Results were estimated considering 100% growth as the number of CFU obtained with untreated yeast co-expressing p53 and MDM2.

3.2.2. Human Cancer Cell Lines and Culture Conditions

Human colon adenocarcinoma HCT116 cell lines expressing wt p53 (HCT116 p53$^{+/+}$) and its p53-null isogenic derivative (HCT116 p53$^{-/-}$) were provided by B. Vogelstein (The Johns Hopkins Kimmel Cancer Center, Baltimore, MD, USA). Human liver HepG2 carcinoma cell lines were purchased from ATCC (Rockville, MD, USA). Cancer cells were cultured in RPMI-1640 medium with ultraglutamine (Lonza, VWR, Carnaxide, Portugal), and supplemented with 10% fetal bovine serum (FBS; Merck Millipore, VWR). Cells were maintained at 37 °C in a humidified atmosphere of 5% CO_2.

3.2.3. Cell Proliferation Assay

Cell proliferation was determined using the SRB assay, as described [30,31]. Briefly, cells were seeded in 96-well plates at 5.0 × 10^3 cells/well for HCT116 p53$^{+/+}$ cells and 4.0 × 10^3 cells/well for HepG2 and 24 h later treated with serial dilutions (3.13–50 μM) of xanthone **37** or 0.25% DMSO for 48 h. IC_{50} values were determined from the concentration-response curves.

3.2.4. Colony Formation Assay

HCT116 p53$^{+/+}$ and HCT116 p53$^{-/-}$ cells were seeded in a 6-well plate at 1.0 × 10^3 cells/well and treated with 3, 4, 5, 7, and 10 μM of xanthone **37** or DMSO at the time of seeding. After 11 days incubation, colonies were fixed using 10% of methanol and 10% acetic acid for 10 min and stained with 0.5% crystal violet (Sigma-Aldrich) in 1:1 methanol/water for 15 min. Colonies with more than 20 cells were counted.

3.2.5. Cell Cycle Analysis

HCT116 $p53^{+/+}$ and HCT116 $p53^{-/-}$ cells were seeded in a 6-well plate at 1.5×10^5 cells/well for 24 h and treated with 10 and 20 μM of xanthone **37** or DMSO for 24 h. Cells were collected, fixed, and stained with propidium iodide (Fluka, Sigma-Aldrich). Cell cycle was analyzed by flow cytometry, as described [45].

3.2.6. Western Blot Analysis

HCT116 $p53^{+/+}$ were seeded in a 6-well plate at 1.5×10^5 cells/well for 24 h and treated with 10 and 20 μM of xanthone **37** or DMSO for 24 h. Total protein extracts of cancer cells were obtained and analyzed by Western blot, as described [45]. Membranes were probed with a mouse monoclonal anti-p53 (DO-1), anti-MDM2 (D-12), or with a rabbit polyclonal anti-p21 (C-19), followed by an anti-mouse or anti-rabbit horseradish-peroxidase (HRP)-conjugated secondary antibody. For loading control, membranes were stripped and re-probed with mouse monoclonal anti-GAPDH (6C5). All antibodies were purchased from Santa Cruz Biotechnology (Frilabo, Porto, Portugal). The signal was detected with enhanced chemiluminescence (ECL) Amersham Kit from GE Healthcare (VWR) and with Molecular Imager® ChemiDoc™ XRS+ System, using Image Lab™ software.

3.2.7. Statistical Analysis

Data's statistical analysis was performed using the Prism 7 program (GraphPad Software Inc., California, USA). Differences between means were tested for significance using one-way ANOVA with Tukey's multiple comparisons test, two-way ANOVA with Sidak's multiple comparisons test, and Student's *t*-test (* $p < 0.05$; ** $p < 0.01$).

3.3. *In Silico Studies onto MDM2*

The chemical structures of gambogic acid (**2**), α-mangostin (**3**), 12-hydroxy-2,2-dimethyl-3,4-dihydro-2*H*,6*H*-pyrano[3,2-*b*]xanthen-6-one (**4**), and the xanthones **30–40** were drawn using ChemSketch (Advanced Chemistry Development, Inc. (ACD/Labs), Canada); the structure of known MDM2-p53 inhibitor nutlin-3A (**1**) was obtained from PubChem [53]. The three-dimensional (3D) structures of the xanthones and **1** were minimized using the ArgusLab version 4.0.1 software for Windows by Hamiltonian (quantum mechanics) using the Parameterized Model number 3 (PM3) semi-empirical method [54]. The 3D structure of MDM2 was extracted from Protein Data Bank (PDB id 4HG7) [50]. Docking simulations involving MDM2 and the small molecules were undertaken in AutoDock Vina (Scripps Research Institute, USA) [51]. AutoDock Vina considered the macromolecular target conformation as a rigid unit, while the ligands were allowed to be flexible and adaptable to the target. Vina explored the lowest binding affinity conformations and returned nine different conformations for each ligand. AutoDock Vina was run using an exhaustiveness of 8 and a grid box with the dimensions of 19.7 Å, 26.1 Å, and 14.1 Å, engulfing the binding cavity occupied by the crystallographic nutlin-3A (PDB id 4HG7). Ligand conformations and interactions with the binding cavity were visualized using PyMOL version 1.3 [55]. In order to validate the docking approach for the macromolecular target structure used, nutlin-3A was docked onto the binding cavity of MDM2 using AutoDock Vina, and the obtained docking conformation was compared to crystallographic nutlin-3A (PDB id 4HG7) using RMSD (not shown). Docking scores of xanthones and positive controls were compared.

4. Conclusions

An alternative and efficient strategy for the preparation of carbaldehydic xanthones was successfully developed. The use of a precursor with a methyl substituent at position C-1 revealed to be crucial for the optimization of the synthesis of **5**. The newly described approach required lower reaction times and enabled the preparation of xanthone **5** in a higher global yield. In this work, a series of eleven aminated xanthones (**30–40**) possessing a 3,4-dioxygenated pattern of substitution was efficiently constructed in moderate to good yields. From this group of compounds, xanthone **37** was identified for the first time as a putative p53-activating agent, using a yeast-based screening assay. Xanthone **37** was revealed to inhibit the growth of human HCT116 $p53^{+/+}$ colon cancer cells, being that this effect is associated with cell cycle arrest through activation of the p53 pathway. Nevertheless, further studies are required to confirm the mechanism of action of **37**, which may lead to the identification of a novel xanthone derivative with promising antitumor activity.

These results demonstrated the potential usefulness of coupling amine-containing structural motifs of known MDM2-p53 disruptors into the 3,4-dioxygenated xanthone scaffold as a starting point for the design of novel and improved p53-activating agents with antitumor activity and drug-like properties.

Supplementary Materials: The following are available online. Figure S1–S15: HRMS spectra of the xanthone derivatives **5** and **27–40**. Figure S16–S45: 1H- and ^{13}C-NMR spectra of the xanthone derivatives **5** and **27–40**.

Author Contributions: A.L. performed the in silico studies and the synthesis of xanthones and wrote the manuscript. A.L., A.S.G., and J.B.L. performed biological experiments and analyzed the data. P.B. contributed to the experimental synthetic work. M.E.S. and L.S. conceived and designed the study, coordinated the experimental work, and wrote the manuscript. A.P. coordinated the in silico studies. M.M.M.P., M.E.S., and L.S. provided financial support for the study, analyzed the data, and wrote the manuscript.

Funding: The authors thank to national funds provided by FCT—Foundation for Science and Technology and European Regional Development Fund (ERDF) and COMPETE under the Strategic Funding UID/Multi/04423/2019, UID/QUI/50006/2019 (UCIBIO/REQUIMTE) the projects (3599-PPCDT) PTDC/DTP-FTO/1981/2014—POCI-01-0145-FEDER-016581, POCI-01-0145-FEDER-028736, and PTDC/MAR-BIO/4694/2014 (POCI-01-0145-FEDER-016790; 3599-PPCDT). FCT fellowships: PD/BD/114046/2015 (A.S. Gomes), SFRH/BD/128673/2017 (J. B. Loureiro), and the Programa Operacional Capital Humano (POCH), specifically the BiotechHealth Programme (PD/00016/2012).

Conflicts of Interest: The authors declare no conflict of interest. The funders had no role in the design of the study; in the collection, analyses, or interpretation of data; in the writing of the manuscript, or in the decision to publish the results.

References

1. Lane, D.P. Cancer. p53, guardian of the genome. *Nature* **1992**, *358*, 15–16. [CrossRef]
2. Shaw, P.H. The role of p53 in cell cycle regulation. *Pathol. Res. Pract.* **1996**, *192*, 669–675. [CrossRef]
3. Toledo, F.; Wahl, G.M. Regulating the p53 pathway: In vitro hypotheses, in vivo *veritas*. *Nat. Rev. Cancer* **2006**, *6*, 909–923. [CrossRef] [PubMed]
4. Vazquez, A.; Bond, E.E.; Levine, A.J.; Bond, G.L. The genetics of the p53 pathway, apoptosis and cancer therapy. *Nat. Rev. Drug Discov.* **2008**, *7*, 979–987. [CrossRef] [PubMed]
5. Rufini, A.; Tucci, P.; Celardo, I.; Melino, G. Senescence and aging: The critical roles of p53. *Oncogene* **2013**, *32*, 5129–5143. [CrossRef] [PubMed]
6. Williams, A.B.; Schumacher, B. p53 in the DNA-damage-repair process. *Cold Spring Harb. Perspect. Med.* **2016**, *6*, a026070. [CrossRef]
7. Vogelstein, B.; Lane, D.; Levine, A.J. Surfing the p53 network. *Nature (London, U.K.)* **2000**, *408*, 307–310. [CrossRef] [PubMed]
8. Hainaut, P.; Hollstein, M. p53 and human cancer: The first ten thousand mutations. *Adv. Cancer Res.* **1999**, *77*, 81–137.
9. Wang, X. p53 regulation: Teamwork between RING domains of MDM2 and MDMX. *Cell Cycle* **2011**, *10*, 4225–4229. [CrossRef] [PubMed]
10. Wu, X.; Bayle, J.H.; Olson, D.; Levine, A.J. The p53-MDM2 autoregulatory feedback loop. *Genes Dev.* **1993**, *7*, 1126–1132. [CrossRef] [PubMed]
11. Momand, J.; Wu, H.H.; Dasgupta, G. MDM2 - master regulator of the p53 tumor suppressor protein. *Gene* **2000**, *242*, 15–29. [CrossRef]
12. Momand, J.; Zambetti, G.P.; Olson, D.C.; George, D.; Levine, A.J. The MDM2 oncogene product forms a complex with the p53 protein and inhibits p53-mediated transactivation. *Cell* **1992**, *69*, 1237–1245. [CrossRef]
13. Oliner, J.D.; Pietenpol, J.A.; Thiagalingam, S.; Gyuris, J.; Kinzler, K.W.; Vogelstein, B. Oncoprotein MDM2 conceals the activation domain of tumor supressor p53. *Nature (London, U.K.)* **1993**, *362*, 857–860. [CrossRef]

14. Roth, J.; Dobbelstein, M.; Freedman, D.A.; Shenk, T.; Levine, A.J. Nucleo-cytoplasmic shuttling of the HDM2 oncoprotein regulated the levels of the p53 protein via a pathway used by the human immunodeficiency vírus ver protein. *EMBO J.* **1998**, *17*, 554–564. [CrossRef]
15. Haupt, Y.; Maya, R.; Kazaz, A.; Oren, M. MDM2 promotes the rapid degradation of p53. *Nature* **1997**, *387*, 296–299. [CrossRef] [PubMed]
16. Pant, V.; Lozano, G. Limiting the power of p53 through the ubiquitin proteasome pathway. *Genes Dev.* **2014**, *28*, 1739–1751. [CrossRef] [PubMed]
17. Zhao, Y.; Aguilar, A.; Bernard, D.; Wang, S. Small-molecule inhibitors of the MDM2-p53 protein-protein interaction (MDM2 inhibitors) in clinical trials for cancer treatment: Miniperspective. *J. Med. Chem.* **2014**, *58*, 1038–1052. [CrossRef] [PubMed]
18. Wang, S.; Zhao, Y.; Aguilar, A.; Bernard, D.; Yang, C.Y. Targeting the MDM2-p53 protein-protein interaction for new cancer therapy: Progress and challenges. *Cold Spring Harb. Perspect. Med.* **2017**, *7*, a026245. [CrossRef]
19. Vassilev, L.T.; Vu, B.T.; Graves, B.; Carvajal, D.; Podlaski, F.; Filipovic, Z.; Kong, N.; Kammlott, U.; Lukacs, C.; Klein, C.; Fotouhi, N.; Liu, E.A. In vivo activation of the p53 pathway by small-molecule antagonists of MDM2. *Science* **2004**, *303*, 844–848. [CrossRef]
20. Lemos, A.; Leão, M.; Soares, J.; Palmeira, A.; Pinto, M.; Saraiva, L.; Sousa, M.E. Medicinal chemistry strategies to disrupt p53-MDM2/MDMX interaction. *Med. Res. Rev.* **2016**, *36*, 789–844. [CrossRef]
21. Tisato, V.; Voltan, R.; Gonelli, A.; Secchiero, P.; Zauli, G. MDM2/X inhibitors under clinical evaluation: Perspectives for the management of hematological malignancies and pediatric cancer. *J. Hematol. Oncol.* **2017**, *10*, 133. [CrossRef] [PubMed]
22. Pinto, M.M.M.; Sousa, M.E.; Nascimento, M.S. Xanthone derivatives: New insights in biological activities. *Curr. Med. Chem.* **2005**, *12*, 2517–2538. [CrossRef] [PubMed]
23. Pouli, N.; Marakos, P. Fused xanthone derivatives as antiproliferative agents. *Anticancer Agents Med. Chem.* **2009**, *9*, 77–98. [CrossRef]
24. Pedro, M.; Cerqueira, F.; Sousa, M.E.; Nascimento, M.S.J.; Pinto, M. Xanthones as inhibitors of growth of human cancer cell lines and their effects on the proliferation of human lymphocytes in vitro. *Bioorg. Med. Chem.* **2002**, *10*, 3725–3730. [CrossRef]
25. Sousa, E.P.; Silva, A.M.S.; Pinto, M.M.M.; Pedro, M.M.; Cerqueira, F.A.M.; Nascimento, M.S.J. Isomeric kielcorins and dihydroxyxanthones: Synthesis, structure elucidation, and inhibitory activities of growth of human cancer cell lines and on the proliferation of human lymphocytes in vitro. *Helv. Chim. Acta* **2002**, *85*, 2862–2876. [CrossRef]
26. Castanheiro, R.A.; Pinto, M.M.; Silva, A.M.; Cravo, S.M.; Gales, L.; Damas, A.M.; Nazareth, N.; Nascimento, M.S.J.; Eaton, G. Dihydroxyxanthones prenylated derivatives: Synthesis, structure elucidation, and growth inhibitory activity on human tumor cell lines with improvement of selectivity for MCF-7. *Bioorg. Med. Chem.* **2007**, *15*, 6080–6088. [CrossRef]
27. Sousa, E.; Paiva, A.; Nazareth, N.; Gales, L.; Damas, A.M.; Nascimento, M.S.J.; Pinto, M. Bromoalkoxyxanthones as promising antitumor agents: Synthesis, crystal structure and effect on human tumor cell lines. *Eur. J. Med. Chem.* **2009**, *44*, 3830–3835. [CrossRef]
28. Palmeira, A.; Paiva, A.; Sousa, E.; Seca, H.; Almeida, G.M.; Lima, R.T.; Fernandes, M.X.; Pinto, M.; Vasconcelos, M.H. Insights into the in vitro antitumor mechanism of action of a new pyranoxanthone. *Chem. Biol. Drug Des.* **2010**, *76*, 43–58. [CrossRef]
29. Paiva, A.M.; Sousa, M.E.; Camoes, A.; Nascimento, M.S.J.; Pinto, M.M.M. Prenylated xanthones: Antiproliferative effects and enhancement of the growth inhibitory action of 4-hydroxytamoxifen in estrogen receptor-positive breast cancer cell line. *Med. Chem. Res.* **2012**, *21*, 552–558. [CrossRef]
30. Leão, M.; Gomes, S.; Pedraza-Chaverri, J.; Machado, N.; Sousa, E.; Pinto, M.; Inga, A.; Pereira, C.; Saraiva, L. α-Mangostin and gambogic acid as potential inhibitors of the p53-MDM2 interaction revealed by a yeast-based approach. *J. Nat. Prod.* **2013**, *76*, 774–778. [CrossRef]
31. Leão, M.; Pereira, C.; Bisio, A.; Ciribilli, Y.; Paiva, A.M.; Machado, N.; Palmeira, A.; Fernandes, M.X.; Sousa, E.; Pinto, M.; Inga, A.; Saraiva, L. Discovery of a new small-molecule inhibitor of p53-MDM2 interaction using a yeast-based approach. *Biochem. Pharmacol.* **2013**, *85*, 1234–1245. [CrossRef]

32. Fernandes, C.; Masawang, K.; Tiritan, M.E.; Sousa, E.; de Lima, V.; Afonso, C.; Bousbaa, H.; Sudprasert, W.; Pedro, M.; Pinto, M. New chiral derivatives of xanthones: Synthesis and investigation of enantioselectivity as inhibitors of growth of human tumor cell lines. *Bioorg. Med. Chem.* **2014**, *22*, 1049–1062. [CrossRef]
33. Barbosa, J.; Lima, R.T.; Sousa, D.; Gomes, A.S.; Palmeira, A.; Seca, H.; Choosang, K.; Pakkong, P.; Bousbaa, H.; Pinto, M.M.; et al. Screening a small library of xanthones for antitumor activity and identification of a hit compound which induces apoptosis. *Molecules* **2016**, *21*, 81. [CrossRef]
34. Cidade, H.; Rocha, V.; Palmeira, A.; Marques, C.; Tiritan, M.E.; Ferreira, H.; Lobo, J.S.; Almeida, I.F.; Sousa, M.E.; Pinto, M. In silico and in vitro antioxidant and cytotoxicity evaluation of oxygenated xanthone derivatives. *Arab. J. Chem.* **2017**. [CrossRef]
35. Alves, A.; Correia-da-Silva, M.; Nunes, C.; Campos, J.; Sousa, E.; Silva, P.M.A.; Bousbaa, H.; Rodrigues, F.; Ferreira, D.; Costa, P.C.; et al. Discovery of a new xanthone against glioma: Synthesis and development of (pro)liposome formulations. *Molecules* **2019**, *24*, 409. [CrossRef]
36. Gomes, S.; Raimundo, L.; Soares, J.; Loureiro, J.B.; Leão, M.; Ramos, H.; Monteiro, M.N.; Lemos, A.; Moreira, J.; Pinto, M.; et al. New inhibitor of the TAp73 interaction with MDM2 and mutant p53 with promising antitumor activity against neuroblastoma. *Cancer Lett.* **2019**, *446*, 90–102. [CrossRef]
37. Liu, J.; Zhou, F.; Zhang, L.; Wang, H.; Zhang, J.; Zhang, C.; Jiang, Z.; Li, Y.; Liu, Z.; Chen, H. DMXAA-pyranoxanthone hybrids enhance inhibition activities against human cancer cells with multi-target functions. *Eur. J. Med. Chem.* **2018**, *143*, 1768–1778. [CrossRef]
38. Hardcastle, I.R.; Liu, J.; Valeur, E.; Watson, A.; Ahmed, S.U.; Blackburn, T.J.; Bennaceur, K.; Clegg, W.; Drummond, C.; Endicott, J.A.; et al. Isoindolinone inhibitors of the murine double minute 2 (MDM2)-p53 protein-protein interaction: Structure-activity studies leading to improved potency. *J. Med. Chem.* **2011**, *54*, 1233–1243. [CrossRef]
39. Twarda-Ciapa, A.; Krzanik, S.; Kubica, K.; Guzik, K.; Labuzek, B.; Neochoritis, C.G.; Khoury, K.; Kowalska, K.; Czub, M.; Dubin, G.; et al. 1,4,5-Trisubstituted imidazole-based p53-MDM2/MDMX antagonists with aliphatic linkers for conjugation with biological carriers. *J. Med. Chem.* **2017**, *60*, 4234–4244. [CrossRef]
40. Gicquel, M.; Gomez, C.; Alvarez, M.C.G.; Pamlard, O.; Guérineau, V.; Jacquet, E.; Bignon, J.; Voituriez, A.; Marinetti, A. Inhibition of p53-murine double minute 2 (MDM2) interactions with 3,3′-spirocyclopentene oxindole derivatives. *J. Med. Chem.* **2018**, *61*, 9386–9392. [CrossRef]
41. Quillinan, A.J.; Schelnmann, F. Studies in the xanthone series. Part XII. A general synthesis of polyoxygenated xanthones from benzophenone precursors. *J. Chem. Soc. Perkin Trans.* **1973**, *1*, 1329–1337. [CrossRef]
42. Resende, D.I.S.P.; Pereira-Terra, P.; Inácio, Â.S.; da Costa, P.M.; Pinto, E.; Sousa, E.; Pinto, M.M.M. Lichen xanthones as models for new antifungal agents. *Molecules* **2018**, *23*, 2617. [CrossRef]
43. Martins, E.; Silva, V.; Lemos, A.; Palmeira, A.; Puthongking, P.; Sousa, E.; Rocha-Pereira, C.; Ghanem, C.I.; Carmo, H.; Remião, F.; et al. Newly synthesized oxygenated xanthones as potential P-glycoprotein activators: In vitro, ex vivo, and in silico studies. *Molecules* **2019**, *24*, 707. [CrossRef]
44. Soares, J.; Espadinha, M.; Raimundo, L.; Ramos, H.; Gomes, A.S.; Gomes, S.; Loureiro, J.B.; Inga, A.; Reis, F.; Gomes, C.; et al. DIMP53-1: A novel small-molecule dual inhibitor of p53-MDM2/X interactions with multifunctional p53-dependent anticancer properties. *Mol. Oncol.* **2017**, *11*, 612–627. [CrossRef]
45. Soares, J.; Pereira, N.A.; Monteiro, Â.; Leão, M.; Bessa, C.; dos Santos, D.J.; Raimundo, L.; Queiroz, G.; Bisio, A.; Inga, A.; et al. Oxazoloisoindolinones with in vitro antitumor activity selectively activate a p53-pathway through potential inhibition of the p53-MDM2 interaction. *Eur. J. Pharm. Sci.* **2015**, *66*, 138–147. [CrossRef]
46. Soares, J.; Raimundo, L.; Pereira, N.A.; dos Santos, D.J.; Pérez, M.; Queiroz, G.; Leão, M.; Santos, M.M.M.; Saraiva, L. A tryptophanol-derived oxazolopiperidone lactam is cytotoxic against tumors via inhibition of p53 interaction with murine double minute proteins. *Pharmacol. Res.* **2015**, *95–96*, 42–52. [CrossRef]
47. Chen, L.; Yin, H.; Farooqi, B.; Sebti, S.; Hamilton, A.D.; Chen, J. p53 α-helix mimetics antagonize p53/MDM2 interaction and activate p53. *Mol. Cancer Ther.* **2005**, *4*, 1019–1025. [CrossRef]
48. Kalid, O.; Ben-Tal, N. Study of MDM2 binding to p53-analogues: Affinity, helicity, and applicability to drug design. *J. Chem. Inf. Model.* **2009**, *49*, 865–876. [CrossRef]
49. Kussie, P.H.; Gorina, S.; Marechal, V.; Elenbaas, B.; Moreau, J.; Levine, A.J.; Pavletich, N.P. Structure of the MDM2 oncoprotein bound to the p53 tumor suppressor transactivation domain. *Science* **1996**, *274*, 948–953. [CrossRef]

50. Anil, B.; Riedinger, C.; Endicott, J.A.; Nobie, M.E. The structure of an MDM2-nutlin-3a complex solved by the use of a validated MDM2 surface-entropy reduction mutant. *Acta Crystallogr. D Biol. Crystallogr.* **2013**, *69*, 1358–1366. [CrossRef]
51. Trott, O.; Olson, A.J. AutoDock Vina: Improving the speed and the accuracy of docking with a new scoring function, efficient optimization and multithreading. *J. Comput. Chem.* **2010**, *31*, 455–461. [CrossRef] [PubMed]
52. Bharatham, N.; Bharatham, K.; Shelat, A.A.; Bashford, D. Ligand binding mode prediction by docking: MDM2/MDMX inhibitors as a case study. *J. Chem. Inf. Model.* **2014**, *54*, 648–659. [CrossRef] [PubMed]
53. Wang, Y.; Xiao, J.; Sujek, T.O.; Zhang, J.; Wang, J.; Bryant, S.H. PubChem: A public information system for analyzing bioactivities of small molecules. *Nucleic Acids Res.* **2009**, *37*, 623–633. [CrossRef] [PubMed]
54. Kini, R.M.; Evans, H.J. Molecular modeling of proteins: A strategy for energy minimization by molecular mechanics in the AMBER force field. *J. Biomol. Struct. Dyn.* **1991**, *9*, 475–488. [CrossRef] [PubMed]
55. Seeliger, D.; de Groot, B.L. Ligand docking and binding site analysis with PyMOL and AutoDock/Vina. *J. Comput. Aided Mol. Des.* **2010**, *24*, 417–422. [CrossRef] [PubMed]

Sample Availability: Samples of the compounds **5**, **16–40** are available from the authors.

molecules

MDPI

Article

Design and Synthesis of Indoleamine 2,3-Dioxygenase 1 Inhibitors and Evaluation of Their Use as Anti-Tumor Agents

Hui Wen †, Yuke Liu †, Shufang Wang, Ting Wang, Gang Zhang, Xiaoguang Chen, Yan Li, Huaqing Cui, Fangfang Lai * and Li Sheng *

State Key Laboratory of Bioactive Substances and Function of Natural Medicine, Institute of Materia Medica, Peking Union Medical College and Chinese Academy of Medical Sciences, Beijing 100050, China; wenhui@imm.ac.cn (H.W.); liuyuke@imm.ac.cn (Y.L.); wangshufang@imm.ac.cn (S.W.); wangtingdlf@imm.ac.cn (T.W.); gzhang@imm.ac.cn (G.Z.); chxg@imm.ac.cn (X.C.); yanli@imm.ac.cn (Y.L.); hcui@imm.ac.cn (H.C.)

* Correspondence: laifangfang@imm.ac.cn (F.L.); shengli@imm.ac.cn (L.S.); Tel.: +86-10-63165185 (F.L.); Fax: +86-10-63017757 (F.L.)

† These two authors contributed equally to this paper.

Academic Editor: Qiao-Hong Chen
Received: 14 May 2019; Accepted: 4 June 2019; Published: 5 June 2019

Abstract: Indoleamine 2,3-dioxygenase (IDO) 1 is the key enzyme for regulating tryptophan metabolism and is an important target for interrupting tumor immune escape. In this study, we designed four series of compounds as potential IDO1 inhibitors by attaching various fragments or ligands to indole or phenylimidazole scaffolds to improve binding to IDO1. The compounds were synthesized and their inhibitory activities against IDO1 and tryptophan 2,3-dioxygenase were evaluated. The cytotoxicities of the compounds against two tumor cell lines were also determined. Two compounds with a phenylimidazole scaffold (DX-03-12 and DX-03-13) showed potent IDO1 inhibition with IC_{50} values of 0.3–0.5 μM. These two IDO1 inhibitors showed low cell cytotoxicity, which indicated that they may exert their anti-tumor effect via immune modulation. Compound DX-03-12 was investigated further by determining the in vivo pharmacokinetic profile and anti-tumor efficacy. The pharmacokinetic study revealed that DX-03-12 had satisfactory properties in mice, with rapid absorption, moderate plasma clearance (~36% of hepatic blood flow), acceptable half-life (~4.6 h), and high oral bioavailability (~96%). Daily oral administration of 60 mg/kg of compound DX-03-12 decreased tumor growth by 72.2% after 19 days in a mouse melanoma cell B16-F10 xenograft model compared with the untreated control. Moreover, there was no obvious weight loss in DX-03-12-treated mice. In conclusion, compound DX-03-12 is a potent lead compound for developing IDO1 inhibitors and anti-tumor agents.

Keywords: indoleamine 2,3-dioxygenase; inhibitor; anti-tumor; immune modulation; tryptophan metabolism

1. Introduction

Tryptophan metabolism is an important pathway for cancer immunotherapy [1–3]. The accumulation of tryptophan can activate T cells, and a decrease in tryptophan concentration affects the regular function of T cells and interferes with the differentiation of naïve T cells. The accumulation of tryptophan metabolites, such as L-kynurenine and other downstream kynurenines (3-hydroxykynurenine and 3-hydroxyanthranilic acid), is toxic to T cells and induces T cell apoptosis. Thus, increasing tryptophan degradation inhibits the immune response [4–6].

Indoleamine 2,3-dioxygenase (IDO; E.C. 1.12.11.17) 1 is a monomeric 41 kDa enzyme that contains heme and converts L-tryptophan to *N*-formylkynurenine in non-hepatic tissues [7]. Tryptophan 2,3-dioxygenase (TDO; E.C. 1.13.11.11) also catalyzes the degradation of L-tryptophan to *N*-formylkynurenine [8]. However, these two enzymes are genetically distinct and have low sequence homology [8].

IDO1 is an important enzyme in tryptophan metabolism and contributes to creating peripheral immune tolerance by degrading L-tryptophan, which suppresses the function of T cells, and by producing *N*-formylkynurenine, which inhibits T cells [8]. In addition, IDO1 can also trigger other activators of anti-tumor immunity. Notably, IDO1 is overexpressed in a range of cancer tissues [4–6]. Thus, blocking the activity of IDO1 is a potential strategy for tumor immunotherapy.

The crystal structures of recombinant human IDO1 have been resolved [9,10], and biochemical studies have revealed that the heme iron in the active site of IDO1 binding and forms adducts with exogenous ligands including O_2^-, NO, CO, H_2S, and CN^- [9,11–14]. IDO1 tolerates various substrates, whereas TDO has strict substrate specificity. This difference can be used to develop selective IDO1 inhibitors [8].

During the development of anti-tumor drugs, potent IDO1 inhibitors were discovered, and intensive efforts have been made to develop potent IDO1/TDO inhibitors with various structural scaffolds. Some typical examples of IDO1/TDO inhibitors are shown in Figure 1 [1,15–21]. The indole and phenylimidazole scaffolds have produced several potent IDO1 inhibitors. For example, IDO1 inhibitors indoximod (pathway IC_{50} = 450 nM) and PF-0684003 (IDO1 IC_{50} = 410 nM) are indole derivatives [13], and GDC-0919 (IDO1 IC_{50} = 13 nM) and AMCL-17g (IDO1 IC_{50} = 77 nM) are phenylimidazole derivatives [20].

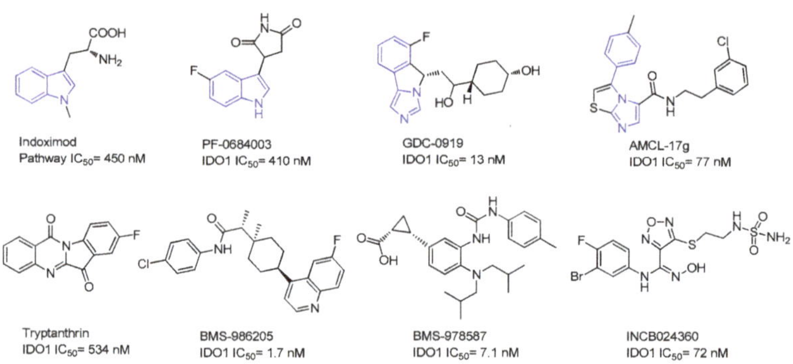

Figure 1. Reported IDO1 inhibitors. Indoximod and PF-0684003 have an indole scaffold and GDC-0919 and AMCL-17g have a phenylimidazole scaffold.

In this study, in the early stages of searching for new IDO1 inhibitors, we used indole and phenylimidazole as the core scaffolds. Four series of compounds were designed with different strategies. The compounds were synthesized and the IDO1/TDO inhibitory activities were determined. The in vivo pharmacokinetic profile and anti-tumor efficacy of a potent IDO1 inhibitor were evaluated to explore its potential as an anti-tumor agent.

2. Results and Discussion

2.1. Design Strategy for the Four Compound Series

Four series of compounds were designed (Figure 2) to explore the structure–activity relationship (SAR). The SAR information was used for further optimization. Indole is derived from tryptophan and phenylimidazole is an IDO1 inhibitor [18]. Thus, tryptophan and phenylimidazole fit into the active site of IDO1, and they were selected as the core scaffolds for designing the inhibitors. As we mentioned in the introduction, several exogenous ligands including hydroxylamine, O_2^-, NO, CO, H_2S, and CN^- were able to bind with the heme iron in the active site of IDO1 [9,11–14]. We attached various fragments and ligands to these scaffolds to strengthen the binding to the active site of IDO1.

In series 1, several ligands, such as hydroxylamine and SO, that interact strongly with heme iron were linked to the double bond of the indole scaffold. We hoped to observe a synergistic effect between the ligand and the indole ring in the IDO1 binding. Series 2 was based on compound PF-0684003 (Figure 1), which is an IDO1 inhibitor developed by Pfizer. The structure of PF-0684003 co-crystalized with IDO1 revealed that there was no interaction between PF-0684003 and the heme iron, which is usually observed between other IDO1 inhibitors and IDO1 [13]. Thus, several potential heme binding ligands, such as hydroxylamine and SO, were added to the structure of PF-0684003 to enhance the inhibitory activity.

Phenylimidazole is a weak IDO1 inhibitor. Crystal structures have revealed that the imidazole ring binds with the heme iron [18,19]. Thus, in series 3 and 4, we used phenylimidazole as the scaffold, and we attached fragments to either the imidazole ring (series 3) or the phenyl ring (series 4). These fragments were intended to improve the binding in the active site of IDO1 through various interactions, such as hydrogen bonds and π–π interactions.

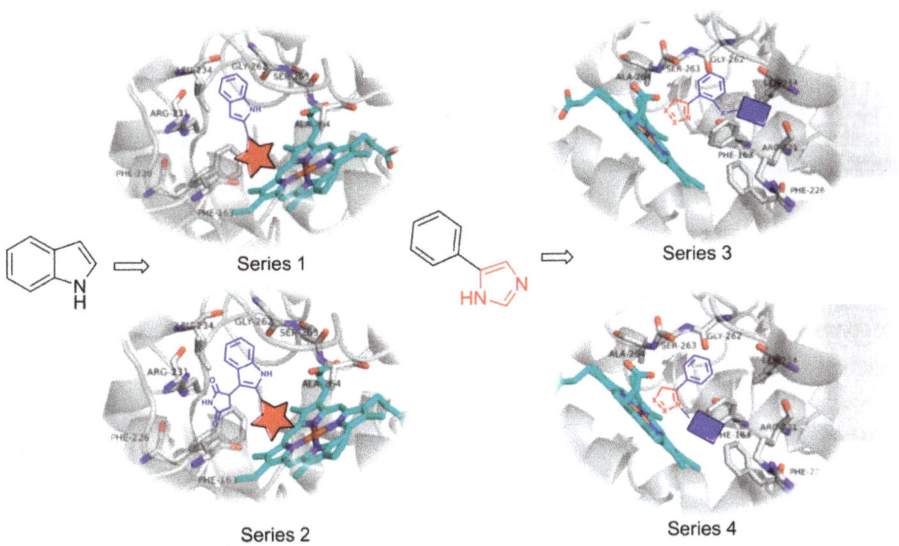

Figure 2. Design strategies of the four series of inhibitors. Because the parent compounds of series 1 and 2, indole and PF-0684003, respectively, do not interact with the heme iron, various heme binding ligands were attached to the indole scaffold. The imidazole ring interacts with the heme iron, and thus various fragments were attached to the phenyl ring in series 3 and the imidazole ring in series 4 to strengthen the binding to the active site of IDO1.

2.2. *Synthesis of Selected Compounds*

Although the compounds were classified into four series for examining the SAR, the structural diversity meant that they required a variety of synthetic routes. We describe representative synthetic schemes for four compounds. Syntheses for all the compounds are included in the Experimental section.

Scheme 1 shows the synthesis of DX-02-05. In the presence of a Lewis acid, ethyl 5-fluoro-1*H*-indole-2-carboxylate underwent a condensation reaction with 1*H*-pyrrole-2,5-dione to yield compound DX-02-03. Alcohol **1** was obtained by reducing DX-02-03, and then **1** was directly oxidized with MnO_2 to produce aldehyde **2**. Aldehyde **2** was condensed with hydroxylamine hydrochloride to obtain compound DX-02-04. Finally, the double bond in DX-02-04 was reduced with $NaBH_3CN$ to obtain compound DX-02-05.

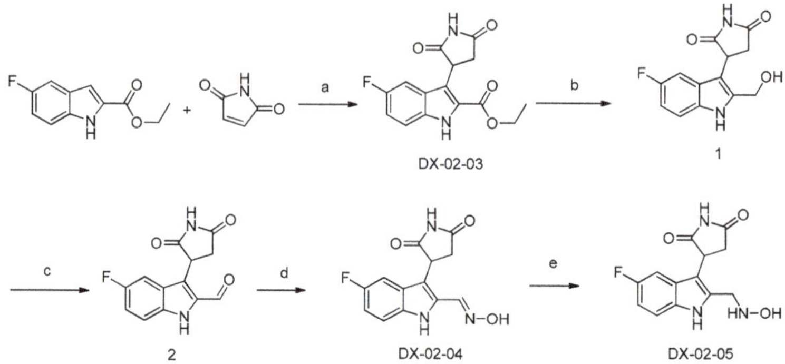

Scheme 1. Synthesis of DX-02-05. (a) BF_3-Et_2O, $ClCH_2CH_2Cl$, yield = 55%; (b) $LiAlH_4$, CH_3OH, yield = 86%; (c) MnO_2, dry dichloromethane, yield = 91%; (d) hydroxylamine hydrochloride, DIPEA, CH_3OH, yield = 66%; (e) $NaBH_3CN$, 12 N HCl, CH_3OH, yield = 43%.

Scheme 2 shows the synthesis of DX-02-07. Sulfur substitution of 5-fluoroindolin-2-one was performed with P_2S_5 to produce compound **3**. Under basic conditions, compound **4** was obtained through an SN_2 substitution reaction with CH_3I. A condensation reaction between **4** and 1*H*-pyrrole-2,5-dione was performed at 120 °C to obtain sulfide DX-02-06, which was oxidized to racemic sulfoxide DX-02-07.

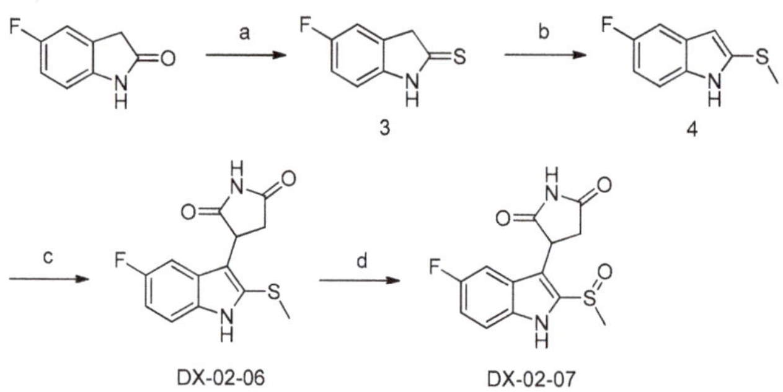

Scheme 2. Synthesis of DX-02-07. (a) P_2S_5, $NaHCO_3$, dry tetrahydrofuran, yield = 75%; (b) CH_3I, K_2CO_3, acetone, yield = 83%; (c) 1*H*-pyrrole-2,5-dione, CH_3CO_2H, yield = 61%; (d) m-CPBA, dry dichloromethane, yield = 35%.

Scheme 3 shows the synthesis of DX-03-12. First, the imidazole starting material was protected with trityl chloride to avoid various side reactions. Compound **6** was obtained by the Suzuki–Miyaura reaction with a boronic acid [22]. The methyl group was removed by BBr_3 to expose the hydroxyl group in compound **7**. Compound **8** was prepared in parallel by melting 3-chloropropylamine and isobenzofuran-1,3-dione together. Compounds **7** and **8** were subjected to an SN_2 nucleophilic reaction to obtain compound **9** under strong basic conditions. This step had a low yield, which was explained by the high steric hindrance of the large molecules and the weak nucleophilicity of compound **7**. The amine protecting group was removed with hydrazine hydrate to obtain compound **10**. Compound **10** was reacted with trifluoromethanesulfonylchloride under basic conditions to give compound **11**. Finally, DX-03-12 was obtained by removing the protecting group on the imidazole with acetic acid.

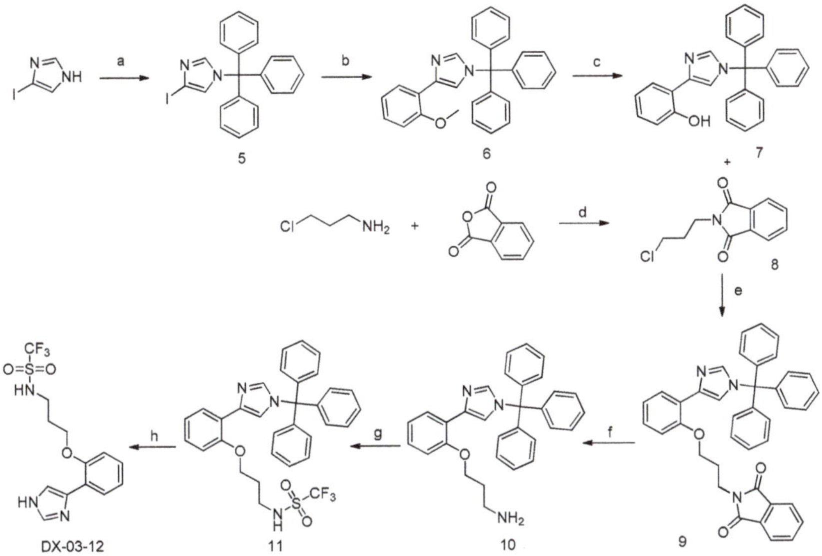

Scheme 3. Synthesis of DX-03-12. (a) Trityl Chloride, DIPEA, dry DMF, yield = 78%; (b) (2-methoxyphenyl)boronic acid, K_3PO_4, 14% $Pd(PPh_3)_4$, DMF, inert atmosphere, yield = 63%; (c) BBr_3, inert atmosphere, dry dichloromethane, yield = 65%; (d) solvent-free melt, yield = 55%; (e) KOH, dry DMF, yield = 71%; (f) hydrazine hydrate, CH_3OH; (g) trifluoromethanesulfonylchloride, DIPEA, dry dichloromethane, yield = 67%; (h) AcOH, CH_3OH, yield = 86%.

Scheme 4 shows the synthesis of DX-04-02. 2-Iodoimidazole was substituted with trifluoromethylbenzyl bromide to give compound **12**. Compound **12** underwent a Suzuki–Miyaura coupling reaction with (5-chloro-2-methoxyphenyl)boronic acid to obtain DX-04-01. Finally, the methyl group was removed with BBr_3 to obtain DX-04-02.

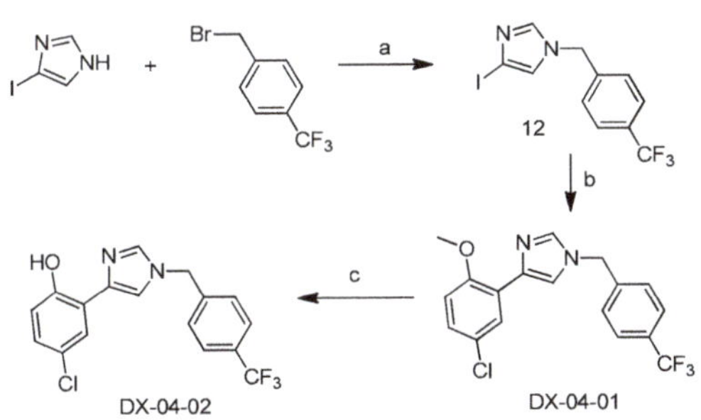

Scheme 4. Synthesis of DX-04-02. (a) DIPEA, dry DMF; (b) (5-chloro-2-methoxyphenyl)boronic acid, K_3PO_4, $Pd(PPh_3)_4$, DMF, inert atmosphere, yield = 72%; (c) BBr_3, inert atmosphere, yield = 53%.

2.3. *In Vitro Biological Evaluation*

We prepared the four series of compounds using the synthetic schemes in Section 2.2. Twelve commercially available compounds were purchased (see Section 3.1). In total, we screened 50 compounds in vitro for their IDO1 and TDO inhibitory activities and cell cytotoxicities against tumor cell lines H460 and MCF7 (Table 1). NLG919 was the reported potent IDO1/TDO inhibitor, and Taxol are known commercial anti-cancer drug. They were used as the reference compounds in this study.

Table 1. In vitro IDO1/TDO inhibitory activities and cell cytotoxicities of series 1.

Compound	Structure	IDO[a] IC_{50} or %	TDO [a] IC_{50} or %	H460 [a] IC_{50} or %	MCF7 [a] IC_{50} or %
DX-01-01	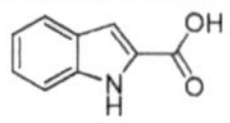	9.7%	8.9%	NA	NA
DX-01-02	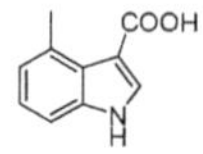	2.4%	10.0%	39.2%	43.1 μM
DX-01-03	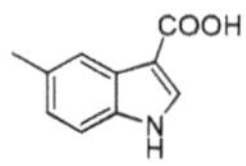	10.3%	10.1%	26.3%	37.6%
DX-01-04	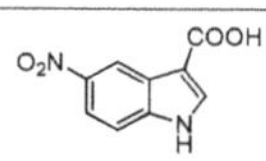	3.3%	6.0%	15.1%	24.3%
DX-01-05	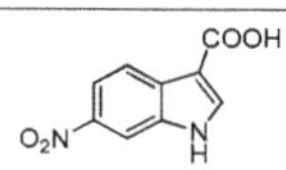	10.2%	10.5%	5.9%	29.7%
DX-01-06	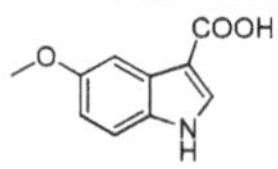	6.2%	8.4%	11.2%	25.7%
DX-01-07	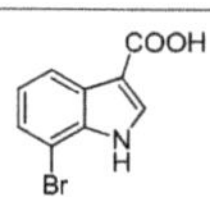	7.4%	16.9%	22.2%	34.6%
DX-01-08	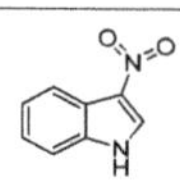	10.9%	3.2%	NA	NA
DX-01-09	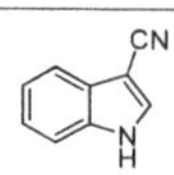	2.6%	7.8%	NA	NA
DX-01-10	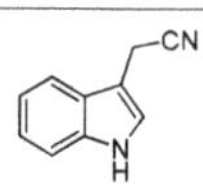	2.1%	8.9%	NA	NA
DX-01-11	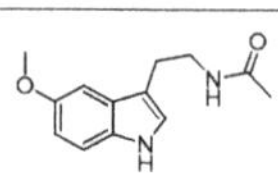	-	3.8%	NA	NA
DX-01-12	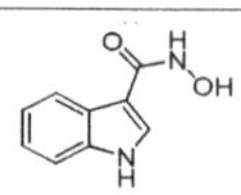	47.1%	33.9%	NA	NA
DX-01-13	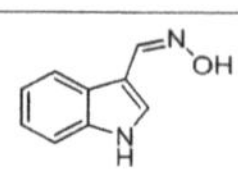	19.7%	8.1%	23.1%	10.1%
DX-01-14	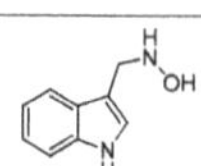	11.1 μM	38.2%	NA	NA

Table 1. *Cont.*

Compound	Structure	IDO[a] IC$_{50}$ or %	TDO [a] IC$_{50}$ or %	H460 [a] IC$_{50}$ or %	MCF7 [a] IC$_{50}$ or %
DX-01-15	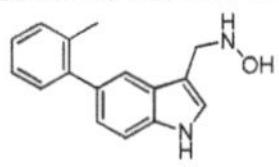	21.3 μM	35.4%	NA	NA
DX-01-16	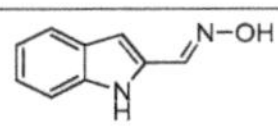	23.2 μM	19.7%	44.5%	20.9%
DX-01-17	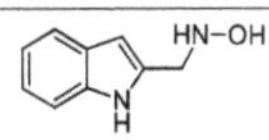	17.7 μM	42.2%	NA	NA
DX-01-18	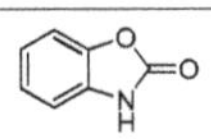	5.4%	-	NA	NA
DX-01-19	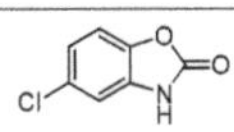	-	7.8%	NA	NA
DX-01-20	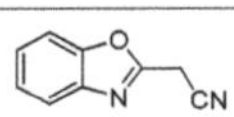	15.7%	3.8%	NA	NA
DX-01-21	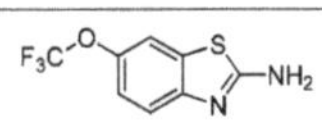	9.7%	9.2%	NA	NA
DX-01-22	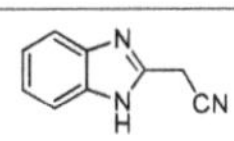	13.2%	4.5%	NA	NA
NLG919		0.064 μM	0.085 μM	NA	NA
Taxol		NA	NA	6 nM	15 nM

[a] When the calculated IC$_{50}$ of a compound is >50 μM, we show the inhibition rate (%) at 50 μM. -: no detectable inhibition. NA: not tested.

The IDO1 and TDO inhibitory activities of the 22 compounds in series 1 were measured (Table 1). The series 1 compounds contained heme binding fragments including CO, NO, CN, H_2S, imidazole, and hydroxylamine; however, the inhibition data showed that most compounds in series 1 exhibited marginal IDO1/TDO inhibition. However, four compounds (DX-01-14, DX-01-15, DX-01-16, and DX-01-17) containing hydroxylamine had moderate IDO1 inhibitory activities. The most active IDO1 inhibitor in series 1 was compound DX-01-14 with an IC$_{50}$ of 11.1 μM. In addition, cell cytotoxicity screening showed that most of the compounds were not toxic to mammalian cancer cell lines.

Generally speaking, these molecules have a rather low molecular weight, and the rather small moiety causes them hard to bind tightly inside the active center of IDO1. Thus, a poor SAR was observed for this series of compounds. Interestingly, for these four active compounds, they all contain the fragment of hydroxylamine. This may suggest that hydroxylamine is the ideal ligand to attach to the double bond of the indole scaffold, while still maintaining the binding with the heme iron.

Series 2 included seven compounds, which were all PF-0684003 derivatives (Table 2). However, the in vitro IDO1/TDO inhibitory activities of all these PF-0684003 derivatives were lower than that of the parent compound, and none were IDO1/TDO inhibitors. The cytotoxicity study demonstrated that these PF-0684003 derivatives were not toxic to cancer cell lines.

Table 2. In vitro IDO1/TDO inhibitory activities and cell cytotoxicities of series 2.

Compound	Structure	IDO [a] IC_{50} or %	TDO [a] IC_{50} or %	H460 [a] IC_{50} or %	MCF7 [a] IC_{50} or %
DX-02-01	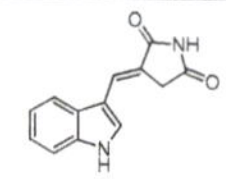	6.3%	-	NA	NA
DX-02-02	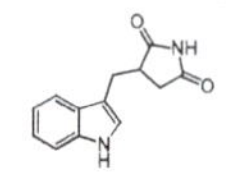	7.2%	2.3%	NA	NA
DX-02-03	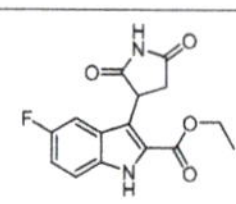	21.6%	15.4%	21.7%	22.1%
DX-02-04	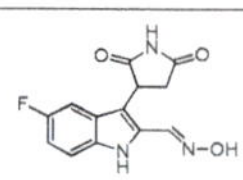	40.2%	14.5%	NA	NA
DX-02-05	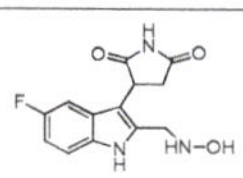	12.5%	16.3%	NA	NA
DX-02-06	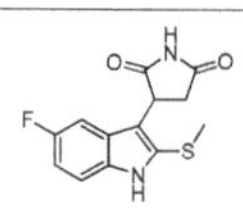	22.6%	19.6%	30.1%	19.9%
DX-02-07	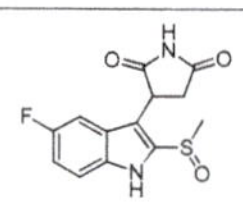	20.1%	13.9%	15.2%	11.0%
NLG919		0.064 µM	0.085 µM	NA	NA
Taxol		NA	NA	6 nM	15 nM

[a] When the calculated IC_{50} of a compound is >50 µM, we show the inhibition rate (%) at 50 µM. -: no detectable inhibition. NA: not tested.

The structure of PF-0684003 co-crystallized with IDO1 shows that PF-0684003 binds tightly in the active site of IDO1 but does not interact with the heme iron [18]. In the present study, the addition of the heme binding ligands [14] (SO and hydroxylamine in DX-02-07 and DX-02-05, respectively) to the double bond of the indole ring abrogated the IDO1 inhibition, similar to the optimization reported in a previous study.

Series 3 contains 13 phenylimidazole derivatives (Table 3). Compounds DX-03-01 to DX-03-10 showed marginal IDO1/TDO inhibition and weak cell cytotoxicities. However, compounds DX-03-11, DX-03-12, and DX-03-13 are potent IDO1 inhibitors with IC_{50} values of 0.3–2.4 µM. Interestingly, these three compounds show marginal TDO inhibition activity, and thus are IDO1/TDO selective inhibitors. In addition, these compounds are not toxic to mammalian cancer cell lines.

Compound DX-03-01 is a known compound [18], which binds to the active site in IDO1. The imidazole ring interacts with the heme iron, and the hydroxyl group binds to the nearby Ser167 in the active site [7]. However, the substitution of the hydroxyl group with hydroxylamine (DX-03-01 to DX-03-10) did not produce IDO1 inhibitors with higher activity. In DX-03-10 to DX-03-13, the hydroxyl group was used to attach an alkyl chain bearing terminal groups used in other reported IDO1 inhibitors [17,19]. The terminal fragments, such as sulfamide and urea, are important to maintain the binding [17,19].

Table 3. In vitro IDO1/TDO inhibitory activities and cell cytotoxicity of series 3.

Compound	Structure	IDO [a] IC_{50} or %	TDO [a] IC_{50} or %	H460 [a] IC_{50} or %	MCF7 [a] IC_{50} or %
DX-03-01	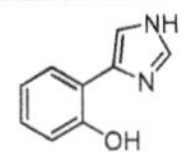	26.3%	10.3%	NA	NA
DX-03-02	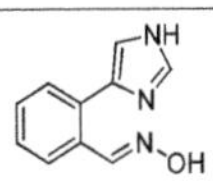	24.2%	13.9%	NA	NA
DX-03-03	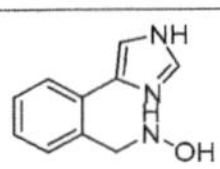	19.4%	11.1%	5.0%	22.2%
DX-03-04	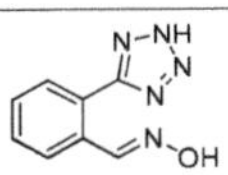	11.9%	20.3%	12.7%	34.7%
DX-03-05	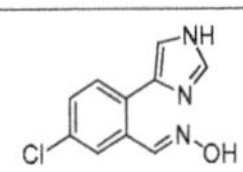	31.3%	12.1%	NA	NA
DX-03-06	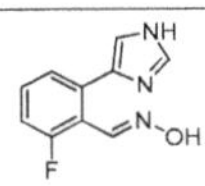	25.6%	12.9%	NA	NA
DX-03-07	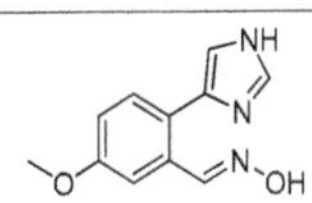	33.5%	15.1%	NA	NA
DX-03-08	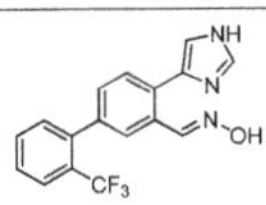	15.6%	11.1%	NA	NA
DX-03-09	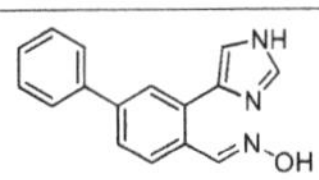	5.3%	6.4%	40.5%	37.7%
DX-03-10	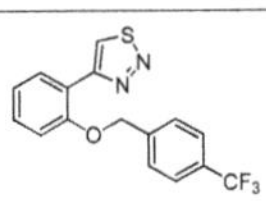	13.2%	21.5%	7.6%	24.7%
DX-03-11	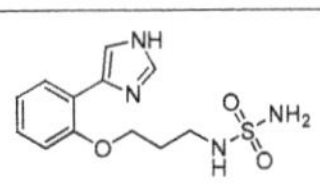	2.4 μM	38.2%	NA	NA
DX-03-12	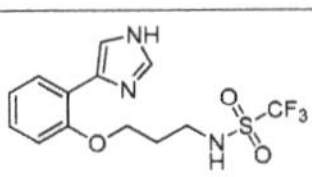	0.3 μM	36.4%	19.3%	6.6%
DX-03-13	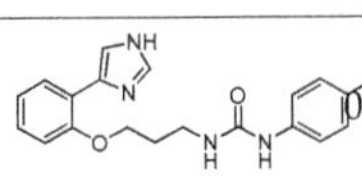	0.5 μM	38.9%	13.79	21.39
NLG919		0.064 μM	0.085 μM	NA	NA
Taxol		NA	NA	6 nM	15 nM

[a] When the calculated IC_{50} of a compound is >50 μM, we show the inhibition rate (%) at 50 μM. -: no detectable inhibition. NA: not tested.

Series 4 contains eight phenylimidazole derivatives (Table 4). Most compounds in this series showed marginal IDO1 inhibition, but compound DX-04-05 showed moderate IDO1 inhibition. However, compound DX-04-06, in which the hydroxyl group was methylated, showed decreased IDO1 inhibition. Most compounds in this series were toxic to the cancer cell lines H460 and MCF7 with an IC_{50} of around 10^{-5} M, which indicates the compounds also interrupt the function of other targets in the cells.

Table 4. In vitro IDO1/TDO inhibitory activities and cell cytotoxicities of series 4.

Compound	Structure	IDO [a] IC_{50} or %	TDO [a] IC_{50} or %	H460 [a] IC_{50} or %	MCF7 [a] IC_{50} or %
DX-04-01	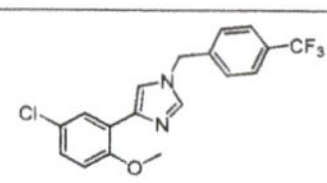	46.2%	26.5%	11.96 μM	8.53μM
DX-04-02	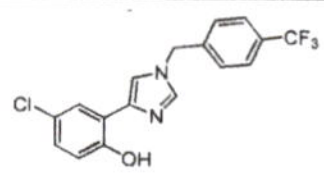	9.7%	18.0%	7.69 μM	35.72 μM
DX-04-03	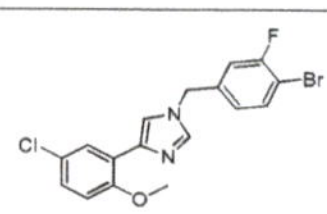	8.7%	17.3%	11.48 μM	15.44 μM
DX-04-04	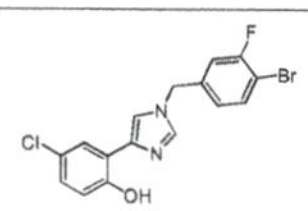	11.9%	23.8%	5.49 μM	20.95 μM
DX-04-05	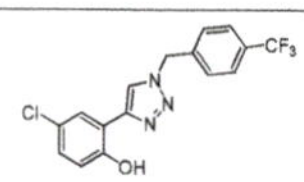	23 μM	22.4%	22.89 μM	42.55 μM
DX-04-06	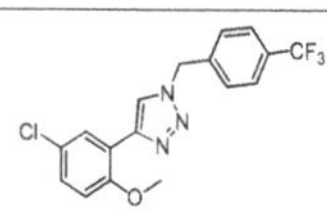	13.5%	23.6%	48.37 μM	49.34 μM
DX-04-07	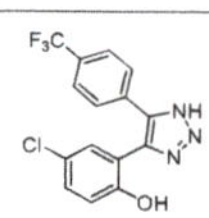	38.2%	21.4%	27.4 μM	12.28 μM
DX-04-08	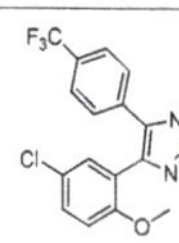	21.2%	11.2%	7.5%	24.9%
NLG919		0.064 μM	0.085 μM	NA	NA
Taxol		NA	NA	6 nM	15 nM

[a] When the calculated IC_{50} of a compound is >50 μM, we show the inhibition rate (%) at 50 μM. -: no detectable inhibition. NA: not tested.

In series 4, the design strategy was to attach fragments to the imidazole ring instead of the phenyl ring in series 3. However, this strategy does not maintain the IDO1 inhibitory activity. In addition, the free hydroxyl group in series 4 appears to be important for forming a hydrogen bond with an amino acid residue, such as Ser167 [7], in the active site; methylating this hydroxyl group decreased IDO1 inhibition (DX-04-05 versus DX-04-06).

In summary, based on the SAR study, compounds DX-03-12 and DX-03-13 showed potent IDO1 inhibition activity, and compound DX-03-13 has some structure similarity as previous published patent (WO2011/056652Al) [23]. Thus, the most potent IDO1 inhibitor DX-03-12 was used as the lead compound for further study.

2.4. Pharmacokinetic Study of DX-03-12

The in vivo pharmacokinetic properties of compound DX-03-12 were evaluated in male ICR mice. DX-03-12 was administered orally either as a bolus at a dose of 30 mg/kg or intravenously at a dose of 3 mg/kg. The plasma concentration-time profiles are shown in Figure 3. The pharmacokinetic parameters were determined by non-compartmental analysis (Table 5). After intravenous administration (3 mg/kg), compound DX-03-12 showed a moderate clearance of 33.3 mL/min/kg, which was approximately 36% of mouse hepatic blood flow (90 mL/min/kg). The volume of distribution in the steady state was 10 L/kg, suggesting that there was an extensive distribution of compound DX-03-12 in tissues. Compound DX-03-12 was rapidly absorbed after oral administration of 30 mg/kg. The plasma concentration was quantifiable at the first sampling time point (5 min) and remained detectable at 24 h. The maximum plasma concentration of compound DX-03-12 of 2963 ng/mL was observed 1 h post-dose. Compound DX-03-12 was eliminated relatively slowly with a half-life of 4.6 h. The oral bioavailability of compound DX-03-12 was calculated to be 96%.

The pharmacokinetic study revealed that compound DX-03-12 showed rapid absorption and almost complete oral bioavailability in mice. After oral administration of 30 mg/kg in mice, it exhibited a long half-life (4.6 h) due to moderate plasma clearance. The pharmacokinetic properties of compound DX-03-12 in mice indicate that it has the potential to be a once-a-day drug.

Table 5. Pharmacokinetic parameters of DX-03-12 after a single oral or intravenous dose in male ICR mice.

Parameters	Units	PO 30 mg/kg	iv 3 mg/kg
$t_{1/2\beta}$	h	4.61	3.49
T_{max}	h	1	0.033
C_{max}	ng/mL	2963	2138
$AUC_{(0-t)}$	h*ng/mL	12,902	1346
$AUC_{(0-\infty)}$	h*ng/mL	13,094	1500
V_{ss}	L/kg	-	10.1
Cl	mL/min/kg	-	33.3
F%		96	-

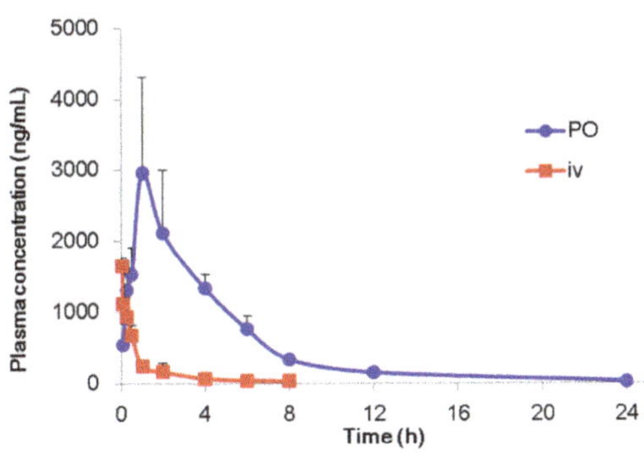

Figure 3. Mean plasma concentration-time profile in male ICR mice after administration of a single oral (30 mg/kg) or intravenous (3 mg/kg) dose of compound DX-03-12. PO stands for per os, which means oral administration of drug; iv stands for intravenous administration of drug.

2.5. *In Vivo Anti-Tumor Efficacy Study of Compound DX-03-12*

To determine whether the compound was effective against tumors in vivo, the anti-tumor effect of DX-03-12 was evaluated in a B16F10 subcutaneous xenograft model in syngeneic mice (Figure 4). Oral and intraperitoneal (i.p.) administration (30 or 60 mg/kg/day) of DX-03-12 significantly decreased the growth of melanoma B16F10 xenograft tumors in a dose-dependent manner. DX-03-12 oral treatment resulted in a 72.2% decrease in tumor weight and i.p. treatment resulted in a 72.3% decrease at a dose of 60 mg/kg compared with the control tumor after 19 days treatment. DX-03-12 had no obvious effect on the body weight of the mice and the peripheral white blood cells, which indicated that DX-03-12 had low toxicity in mice. In this study, the classic first line anti-cancer drug cyclophosphamide (CTX) was used as the reference drug.

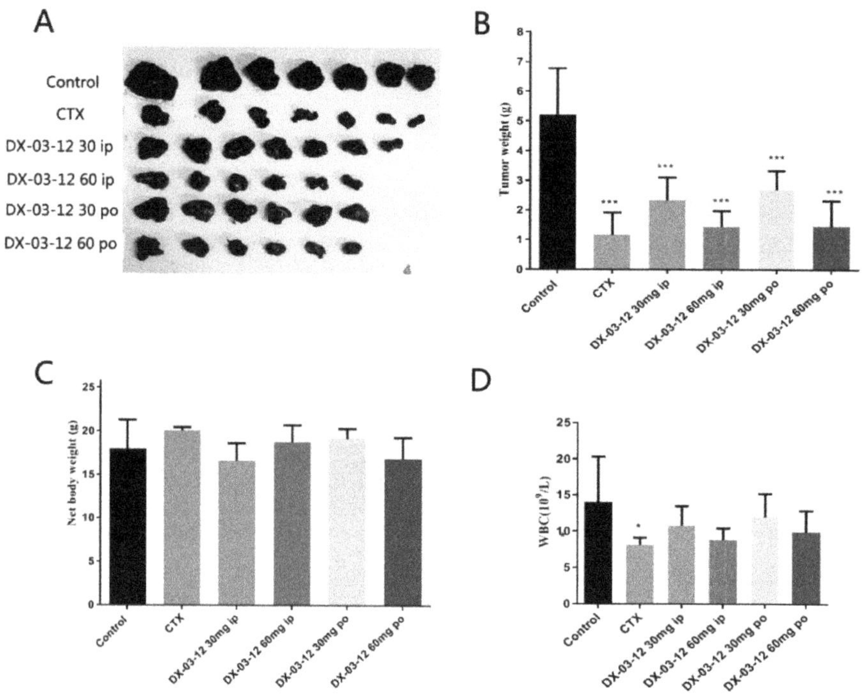

Figure 4. In vivo anti-tumor activity of DX-03-12 in B16F10 xenograft mice. (**A**,**B**) Tumors from each group after 19 days of treatment. Mice bearing B16F10 xenografts were dosed orally or i.p. with vehicle (0.5% methylcellulose), CTX (Cyclophosphamide, orally, 60 mg/kg twice a week), DX-03-12 (i.p., 30 mg/kg/day), DX-03-12 (i.p., 60 mg/kg/day), DX-03-12 (orally, 30 mg/kg/day), or DX-03-12 (orally, 60 mg/kg/day). Results are expressed as the mean ± SD (n = 5–7 for each group). * $p < 0.05$ and *** $p < 0.001$ versus vehicle. (**C**) The body weight from each group after the treatment. There is no obvious body weight difference among all of the groups. (**D**) The white blood cells detected in the blood of all groups of animals. There is also no obvious WBC difference among all of the groups.

3. Experiment Section

3.1. *Chemistry*

Reagents and solvents were obtained from commercial suppliers and used as received. ^{1}H-NMR spectra were obtained on an NMR spectrometer (Mercury, Varian, San Diego, CA, USA; 400 MHz). Electrospray ionization (ESI) mass spectra and high-resolution mass spectroscopy (HRMS) were performed with a liquid chromatograph/mass selective detector time-of-flight mass spectrometer

(LC/MSD TOF, Agilent Technologies, Santa Clara, CA, USA). silica gel column chromatography was performed with silica gel 60G (Qingdao Haiyang Chemical, Qingdao, China). Purity was determined using HPLC, LC/MS and NMR spectroscopy. All of the synthesized compounds have the purity over than 95%.

Several commercial available compounds were purchased from Beijing innochem Co. Ltd. (Beijing, China). They are DX-01-01, DX-01-08, DX-01-09, DX-01-10, DX-01-11, DX-01-12, DX-01-18, DX-01-19, DX-01-20, DX-01-21, DX-01-22, DX-03-01.

3.1.1. Preparation of (*R/S*) 3-(5-fluoro-2-((hydroxyamino)methyl)-1*H*-indol-3-yl)pyrrolidine-2,5-dione (DX-02-05)

Preparation of (*R/S*) Ethyl 3-(2,5-dioxopyrrolidin-3-yl)-5-fluoro-1*H*-indole-2-carboxylate (DX-02-03)

Ethyl 5-fluoro-1*H*-indole-2-carboxylate (2 g, 9.7 mmol) and 1*H*-pyrrole-2,5-dione (1.40 g, 14.4 mmol) were added to dry 1,2-dichloroethane (50 mL), and 46.5% BF_3-Et_2O (3.54 g, 11.6 mmol) was added to reaction mixture at 20 °C. After the reaction mixture was stirred at 90 °C, until the starting material disappeared in thin layer chromatography (TLC), the reaction mixture was distilled in vacuo, and dichloromethane (50 mL) was added to the mixture. The organic extract was washed twice with saturated aqueous $NaHCO_3$ and NaCl (20 mL) respectively, and the organic extract was dried over Na_2SO_4. After solvent was removed under vacuum, the product was purified as a white solid by silica gel column chromatography, 1.62 g, yield 55%. ^{1}H-NMR (400 MHz, DMSO-d_6): δ = 12.00 (s, 1H, NH-indolyl), 11.31 (s, 1H, NH), 7.49–7.45 (m, 2H, H-indolyl), 7.18 (td, *J* = 9.2, 2.6 Hz, 1H, H-indolyl), 4.82 (dd, *J* = 9.6, 6.6 Hz, 1H, CH), 4.33–4.27 (m, 2H, CH_2), 3.08 (dd, *J* = 17.7, 9.6 Hz, 1H, $\underline{CH'}$H"), 2.70 (dd, *J* = 17.7, 6.6 Hz, 1H, CH'$\underline{H''}$), 1.30 (t, *J* = 7.1 Hz, 3H, CH_3). ^{13}C-NMR (101 MHz, CD_3OD): δ =182.17, 180.15, 162.66, 160.66, 134.24, 129.01, 126.54, 119.11, 115.66, 114.82, 104.78, 62.19, 39.68, 39.37, 14.63. HRMS (ESI): *m/z* $[M + H]^+$ calculated for $C_{15}H_{14}O_4N_2F$: 305.09321; found: 305.09290.

Preparation of (*R/S*) 3-(5-fluoro-2-(hydroxymethyl)-1*H*-indol-3-yl) pyrrolidine-2,5-dione (**1**)

Ethyl 3-(2,5-dioxopyrrolidin-3-yl)-5-fluoro-1*H*-indole-2-carboxylate (DX-02-03, 1.3 g, 4.3 mmol) were added to dry CH_3OH (20 mL), $LiAlH_4$ (0.13 g, 4.3 mmol) was added to reaction mixture gradually at 20 °C. The reaction mixture was stirred at 20 °C until the starting material disappeared in TLC. The reaction mixture was distilled in vacuo, and ethyl acetate (50 mL) was added to the mixture. The organic extract was washed twice with saturated aqueous NaCl (20 mL), and the organic extract was dried over Na_2SO_4. After solvent was removed under vacuum, the product was purified as a white solid by silica gel column chromatography, 0.97 g, yield 86%. ^{1}H-NMR (400 MHz, CD_3OD): δ = 7.30 (dd, *J* = 8.8, 4.4 Hz, 1H, H-phenyl), 6.93 (dd, *J* = 9.9, 2.4 Hz, 1H, H-phenyl), 6.89–6.83 (m, 1H, H-phenyl), 4.72 (d, *J* = 1.3 Hz, 2H, CH_2), 4.46 (dd, *J* = 9.7, 5.6 Hz, 1H, CH), 3.20 (dd, *J* = 18.4, 9.7 Hz, 1H, $\underline{CH'}$H"), 2.81 (dd, *J* = 18.4, 5.6 Hz, 1H, CH'$\underline{H''}$). ^{13}C-NMR (101 MHz, CD_3OD): δ = 182.67, 180.16, 160.22, 157.85, 139.57, 133.85, 127.82, 113.46, 110.70, 103.45, 56.67, 39.93, 39.00. HRMS (ESI): *m/z* $[M + H]^+$ calculated for $C_{13}H_{12}N_2O_3F$: 263.08265; found: 263.08160.

Preparation of (*R/S*) 3-(2,5-dioxopyrrolidin-3-yl)-5-fluoro-1*H*-indole-2-carbaldehyde (**2**)

3-(5-Fluoro-2-(hydroxymethyl)-1*H*-indol-3-yl)pyrrolidine-2,5-dione (**1**, 0.8 g, 3.1 mmol) was added to dry dichloridemethane (20 mL), MnO_2 (0.36 g, 4.1 mmol) was added to reaction mixture gradually at 20 °C. The reaction mixture was stirred at 20 °C until the starting material disappeared in TLC. The reaction mixture was filtered, the solvent was removed under vacuum, and the product was purified as a white solid by silica gel column chromatography, 0.73g, yield 91%. ^{1}H-NMR (400 MHz, CD_3OD): δ = 10.00 (s, 1H, CHO), 7.50 (dd, *J* = 9.1, 4.3 Hz, 1H, H-phenyl), 7.27 (dd, *J* = 9.5, 2.3 Hz, 1H, H-phenyl), 7.19 (td, *J* = 9.1, 2.4 Hz, 1H, H-phenyl), 4.91 (dd, *J* = 9.7, 6.0 Hz, 1H, CH), 3.29–3.21 (m, 1H, $\underline{CH'}$H"), 2.84 (dd, *J* = 18.1, 6.0 Hz, 1H, CH'$\underline{H''}$). ^{13}C-NMR (101 MHz, CD_3OD): δ = 183.66,

181.23, 179.66, 160.59, 158.30, 135.75, 135.36, 127.61, 117.26, 115.66, 105.59, 39.77, 39.35. HRMS (ESI): *m/z* $[M + H]^+$ calculated for $C_{13}H_{10}N_2O_3F$: 261.06700; found: 261.06638.

Preparation of (*R/S*) (*E*)-3-(2,5-dioxopyrrolidin-3-yl)-5-fluoro-1*H*-indole-2-carbaldehyde oxime (DX-02-04)

3-(2,5-Dioxopyrrolidin-3-yl)-5-fluoro-1*H*-indole-2-carbaldehyde (0.5 g, 1.92 mmol) was added to dry CH_3OH (30 mL), then *N,N*-Diisopropylethylamine (0.5 g, 3.84 mmol) and hydroxylamine hydro -chloride (0.13 g, 1.92 mmol) were added respectively at 20 °C. The reaction mixture was stirred at 60 °C until the starting material disappeared in TLC. After solvent was removed under vacuum, the product was purified as a white solid by silica gel column chromatography, 0.35 g, yield 66%. ^{1}H-NMR (400 MHz, CD_3OD): δ = 8.22 (s, 1H, =CH), 7.32 (dd, *J* = 8.8, 4.4 Hz, 1H, H-indolyl), 7.06–6.86 (m, 2H, H-indolyl), 4.63 (dd, *J* = 9.7, 5.9 Hz, 1H, CH), 3.19 (dd, *J* = 18.3, 9.7 Hz, 1H, C$\underline{H'}$H"), 2.81 (dd, *J* = 18.7, 6.2 Hz, 1H, CH'$\underline{H''}$). ^{13}C-NMR (101 MHz, CD_3OD): δ =181.92, 179.89, 160.31, 157.98, 141.03, 136.51, 134.81, 132.30, 113.78, 112.58, 103.95, 39.83, 38.66. HRMS (ESI): *m/z* $[M + H]^+$ calculated for $C_{13}H_{11}N_3O_3F$: 276.07790; found: 276.07718.

Preparation of (*R/S*) 3-(5-fluoro-2-((hydroxyamino)methyl)-1*H*-indol-3-yl) pyrrolidine-2,5-dione (DX-02-05)

3-(2,5-Dioxopyrrolidin-3-yl)-5-fluoro-1*H*-indole-2-carbaldehyde oxime (DX-02-04, 0.3 g, 1.1 mmol) was added to CH_3OH (20 mL), then $NaBH_3CN$ (0.07 g, 1.1 mmol) was added at 20 °C. 12N HCl was added to reaction mixture continuously to keep acidic. The reaction mixture was stirred at 20 °C until the starting material disappeared in TLC. After solvent was removed under vacuum, the product was purified as a white solid by silica gel column chromatography, 0.13 g, yield 43%. ^{1}H-NMR (400 MHz, CD_3OD): δ = 7.30 (dd, *J* = 8.8, 4.5 Hz, 1H, H-indolyl), 6.93–6.88 (m, 1H, H-indolyl), 6.88–6.82 (m, 1H, H-indolyl), 4.50 (dd, *J* = 9.7, 5.5 Hz, 1H, CH), 4.12 (d, *J* = 3.6 Hz, 2H, $\underline{CH_2}$NH), 3.21 (dd, *J* = 18.5, 9.7 Hz, 1H, C$\underline{H'}$H"), 2.85 (dd, *J* = 18.5, 5.5 Hz, 1H, CH'$\underline{H''}$). ^{13}C-NMR (101 MHz, CD_3OD): δ = 160.27, 157.92, 135.20, 130.85, 130.02, 113.00, 110.85, 110.54, 104.55, 104.31, 50.48, 38.34, 30.37. HRMS (ESI): *m/z* $[M + H]^+$ calculated for $C_{13}H_{13}N_3O_3F$: 278.09355; found: 278.09291.

3.1.2. Preparation of (*R/S*) 3-(5-fluoro-2-(methylsulfinyl)-1*H*-indol-3-yl)pyrrolidine-2,5-dione (DX-02-07)

Preparation of 5-fluoroindoline-2-thione (**3**)

5-fluoroindolin-2-one (2 g, 13 mmol) and P_2S_5 (2.92 g, 13 mmol) were added to dry tetrahydrofuran (30 mL). After the reaction mixture was stirred at room temperature for 1 h. Until the starting material disappeared in thin layer chromatography (TLC), the $NaHCO_3$ (3.43 g, 39 mmol) was added gradually. After stirring at room temperature for 1 h, the reaction mixture was distilled in vacuo, dichloromethane (50 mL) was added to the mixture. The organic extract was washed twice with saturated aqueous NaCl (20 mL), and the organic extract was dried over Na_2SO_4. After solvent was removed under vacuum, the product was obtained as yellow crystals by re-crystallization using ethanol, 1.62 g, yield 75%. ^{1}H-NMR (400 MHz, $CDCl_3$): δ = 10.14 (s, 1H, NH), 7.05–6.95 (m, 1H, H-phenyl), 6.94–6.89 (m, 1H, H-phenyl), 4.08 (s, 1H, CH_2). ^{13}C-NMR (101 MHz, $CDCl_3$)): δ = 203.39, 159.10, 140.24, 132.15, 114.87, 112.47, 110.47, 49.15. HRMS (ESI): *m/z* $[M + H]^+$ calculated for C_8H_7NFS: 168.02777; found: 168.02773.

Preparation of 5-fluoro-2-(methylthio)-1*H*-indole (**4**)

5-fluoroindoline-2-thione (**3**, 1 g, 6 mmol), CH_3I (0.99 g, 7 mmol) and K_2CO_3 (0.97 g, 7 mmol) were added to acetone (30 mL), and the reaction mixture was stirred at room temperature until the starting material disappeared in TLC. The reaction mixture was distilled in vacuo, ethyl acetate (50 mL) was added to the mixture. The organic extract was washed twice with saturated aqueous NaCl (20 mL), and the organic extract was dried over Na_2SO_4. After solvent was removed under vacuum, the product was purified as a white solid by silica gel column chromatography, 0.90 g, yield 83%. ^{1}H-NMR (400 MHz, $CDCl_3$): δ = 8.04 (s, 1H, NH), 7.23–7.13 (m, 2H, H-indolyl), 6.91 (s, 1H, H-indolyl), 6.49 (s, 1H, H-indolyl), 2.52 (s, 3H, CH_3). ^{13}C-NMR (101 MHz, $CDCl_3$): δ = 159.18, 156.85, 133.57, 129.02, 110.94, 110.47, 105.31, 104.73, 18.86. HRMS (ESI): *m/z* $[M + H]^+$ calculated for C_9H_9NFS: 182.04342; found: 182.04425.

Preparation of (*R/S*) 3-(5-fluoro-2-(methylthio)-1*H*-indol-3-yl)pyrrolidine-2,5-dione (DX-02-06)

5-Fluoro-2-(methylthio)-1*H*-indole (**4**, 0.5 g, 2.7 mmol) and 1*H*-pyrrole-2,5-dione (0.54 g, 5.4 mmol) were added to dry CH_3CO_2H (30 mL), and the reaction mixture was stirred at 120 °C until the starting material disappeared in TLC. The reaction mixture was distilled in vacuo, ethyl acetate (100 mL) was added to the mixture. The organic extract was washed twice with saturated aqueous NaCl (30 mL), and the organic extract was dried over Na_2SO_4. After solvent was removed under vacuum, the product was purified as a white solid by silica gel column chromatography, 0.47 g, yield 61%. ^{1}H-NMR (400MHz, CD_3OD): δ = 7.28 (dd, *J* = 8.9, 4.5 Hz, 1H, H-phenyl), 7.00 (dd, *J* = 9.7, 2.4 Hz, 1H, H-phenyl), 6.91 (td, *J* = 9.2, 2.5 Hz, 1H, H-phenyl), 4.56 (dd, *J* = 9.8, 5.6 Hz, 1H, CH), 3.22 (dd, *J* = 18.3, 9.8 Hz, 1H, C$\underline{H'}$H"), 2.77 (dd, *J* = 18.3, 5.6 Hz, 1H, CH'$\underline{H"}$), 2.41 (s, 3H, CH_3). ^{13}C-NMR (101 MHz, CD_3OD): δ = 182.38, 180.11, 160.26, 135.05, 132.13, 127.67, 116.34, 113.18, 111.70, 103.25, 40.35, 39.10, 19.59. HRMS (ESI): *m/z* $[M + H]^+$ calculated for $C_{13}H_{12}O_2N_2FS$: 279.05980; found: 279.05930.

Preparation of (*R/S*) 3-(5-fluoro-2-(methylsulfinyl)-1*H*-indol-3-yl)pyrrolidine-2,5-dione (DX-02-07)

3-(5-Fluoro-2-(methylthio)-1*H*-indol-3-yl)pyrrolidine-2,5-dione (DX-02-06, 0.2 g, 0.7 mmol) was added to dry dichloridemethane (20 mL), and 3-Chloroperoxybenzoic acid (0.15 g, 0.9 mmol) was added gradually at 0 °C. The reaction mixture was stirred at 0 °C until the starting material disappeared in TLC, and $Na_2S_2O_3$ (0.11 g, 0.7 mmol) was added to the mixture. After reaction mixture was stirred for 20 min, the reaction mixture was washed twice with saturated aqueous NaCl (20 mL), and the organic extract was dried over Na_2SO_4. After solvent was removed under vacuum, the product was purified as a white solid by silica gel column chromatography, 0.074 g, yield 35%. ^{1}H-NMR (400MHz, DMSO-d_6): δ = 12.28 (s, 1H, NH), 11.51 (s, 1H, NH), 7.51–7.48 (m, 1H, H-phenyl), 7.19–7.13 (m, 2H, H-phenyl), 4.61 (ddd, *J* = 26.8, 9.7, 5.8 Hz, 1H, CH), 3.18 (ddd, *J* = 18.0, 9.7, 2.3 Hz, 1H, C$\underline{H'}$H"), 2.98 (d, *J* = 16.7 Hz, 3H, CH_3), 2.76 (ddd, *J* = 41.8, 18.1, 5.8 Hz, 1H, CH'$\underline{H"}$). ^{13}C-NMR (101 MHz, DMSO-d_6): δ = 179.74, 177.94, 158.72, 138.29, 134.14, 125.83, 114.50, 113.93, 113.53, 104.46, 41.67, 38.62, 38.11. HRMS (ESI): *m/z* $[M + H]^+$ calculated for $C_{13}H_{12}O_3N_2FS$: 295.05472; found: 295.05508.

3.1.3. Preparation of *N*-(3-(2-(1*H*-imidazol-5-yl)phenoxy)propyl)-1,1,1-trifluoromethane sulfonamide (DX-03-12)

Preparation of 4-iodo-1-trityl-1*H*-imidazole (**5**)

4-Iodo-1*H*-imidazole (5 g, 25.8 mmol) and *N,N*-diisopropylethylamine (6.65 g, 51.5 mmol) were added to dry dimethylformamide (30 mL), and (chloromethanetriyl)tribenzene (7.89 g, 28.4 mmol) was added to reaction mixture gradually at 20 °C. After the reaction mixture was stirred at 20 °C until the starting material disappeared in thin layer chromatography (TLC), the reaction mixture was distilled in vacuo, ethyl acetate (200 mL) was added to the mixture. The organic extract was washed twice with saturated aqueous NaCl (40 mL), and the organic extract was dried over Na_2SO_4. After solvent was removed under vacuum, the product was purified as a white solid by silica gel column chromatography, 8.77 g, yield 78%. ^{1}H-NMR (400 MHz, $CDCl_3$): δ = 7.38–7.33 (m, 10H, H-phenyl, H-imidazolyl), 7.13–7.09 (m, 6H, H-phenyl), 6.92 (d, *J* = 1.4 Hz, 1H, H-imidazolyl). ^{13}C-NMR (101 MHz, $CDCl_3$): δ = 141.83, 140.56, 129.72 (6C), 128.29 (3C), 128.18 (6C), 127.91, 126.89 (3C), 75.84. HRMS (ESI): *m/z* $[M + H]^+$ calculated for $C_{22}H_{18}N_2I$: 437.05092; found: 437.04934.

Preparation of 4-(2-methoxyphenyl)-1-trityl-1*H*-imidazole (**6**)

4-Iodo-1-trityl-1*H*-imidazole (**5**, 2 g, 4.58 mmol), (5-chloro-2-methoxyphenyl)boronic acid (0.852 g, 4.58 mmol), K_3PO_4 (2.9 g, 13.7 mmol), $Pd(PPh_3)_4$ (0.74 g, 0.64 mmol) were added to dry dimethylformamide (30 mL). The reaction mixture was stirred at 100 °C under inert atmosphere, until the starting material disappeared in TLC. The reaction mixture was distilled in vacuo, and ethyl acetate (100 mL) was added to the mixture. The organic extract was washed twice with saturated aqueous NaCl (20 mL), and the organic extract was dried over Na_2SO_4. After solvent was removed under vacuum, the product was purified as a white solid by silica gel column chromatography, 1.2 g, yield 63%. ^{1}H-NMR (400 MHz, $CDCl_3$): δ = 7.51–7.32 (m, 12H, H-phenyl, H-imidazolyl), 7.15–7.04 (m, 8H, H-phenyl, H-imidazolyl), 6.94 (d, *J* = 8.1 Hz, 1H, H-phenyl), 3.99 (s, 3H, CH_3). HRMS (ESI): *m/z* $[M + H]^+$ calculated for $C_{29}H_{25}N_2O$: 417.19614; found: 417.19647.

Preparation of 2-(1-trityl-1*H*-imidazol-4-yl)phenol (**7**)

4-(2-Methoxyphenyl)-1-trityl-1*H*-imidazole (**6**, 1.0 g, 2.4 mmol) was added to dry dichloridemethane (20 mL), BBr_3 (0.71 g, 2.9 mmol) was added to reaction mixture gradually at −70 °C. The reaction mixture was stirred under inert atmosphere until the starting material disappeared in TLC. The reaction mixture was diluted with dichloridemethane (50 mL), and was washed twice with saturated aqueous NaCl (20 mL), then the organic extract was dried over Na_2SO_4. After solvent was removed under vacuum, the product was purified as a white solid by silica gel column chromatography, 0.63 g, yield 65%. ^{1}H-NMR (400 MHz, DMSO-d_6): δ = 11.19 (s, 1H, OH), 7.49–7.36 (m, 2H, H-phenyl), 7.33–7.10 (m, 16H, H-phenyl, H-imidazolyl), 6.84–6.70 (m, 2H, H-phenyl), 6.45 (s, 1H, H-phenyl). ^{13}C-NMR (101 MHz, DMSO-d_6): δ = 147.24, 141.47, 137.70, 136.55, 128.71 (6C), 127.80 (6C), 127.56, 127.24 (3C), 126.99 (3C), 126.10, 118.39, 117.87, 115.68, 74.61. HRMS (ESI): *m/z* $[M + H]^+$ calculated for $C_{28}H_{23}N_2O$: 403.18049; found: 403.18134.

Preparation of 2-(3-chloropropyl)isoindoline-1,3-dione (**8**)

3-Chloropropan-1-amine (3.77 g, 40.5 mmol) and isobenzofuran-1,3-dione (2 g, 13.5 mmol) were mixed without solvent, and the reaction mixture was stirred at 140 °C (molten condition), until the starting material disappeared in TLC. The reaction mixture was distilled in vacuo, ethyl acetate (100 mL) was added to the mixture. The organic extract was washed twice with saturated aqueous NaCl (20 mL), and the organic extract was dried over Na_2SO_4. After solvent was removed under vacuum, the product was purified as a white solid by silica gel column chromatography, 1.66 g, yield 55%. ^{1}H-NMR (400 MHz, DMSO-d_6): δ = 7.85–7.78 (m, 4H, H-phenyl), 3.73–3.62 (m, 4H, CH_2, CH_2), 2.08–2.01(m, 2H, CH_2). ^{13}C-NMR (101 MHz, DMSO-d_6): δ = 167.38 (2C), 133.75 (2C), 131.19 (2C), 122.43 (2C), 42.31, 34.60, 30.39. HRMS (ESI): *m/z* $[M + H]^+$ calculated for $C_{11}H_{11}ClNO_2$: 224.04728; found: 224.04683.

Preparation of 2-(3-(2-(1-trityl-1*H*-imidazol-5-yl)phenoxy)propyl)isoindoline-1,3-dione (**9**)

2-(1-Trityl-1*H*-imidazol-4-yl)phenol (**7**, 0.5 g, 1.2 mmol) and KOH (0.14 g, 2.5 mmol) were added to dry dimethylformamide (20 mL), after the reaction mixture was stirred at 20 °C for 15 min, 2-(3-chloropropyl)isoindoline-1,3-dione (**8**, 0.294 g, 1.32 mmol) was added to reaction mixture at 20 °C. After the reaction mixture was stirred at 60 °C until the starting material disappeared in thin layer chromatography (TLC), the reaction mixture was distilled in vacuo, ethyl acetate (100 mL) was added to the mixture. The organic extract was washed twice with saturated aqueous NaCl (20 mL), and the organic extract was dried over Na_2SO_4. After solvent was removed under vacuum, the product was purified as a white solid by silica gel column chromatography, 0.5 g, yield 71%. ^{1}H-NMR (400 MHz, DMSO-d_6): δ = 8.08 (dd, *J* = 7.7, 1.6 Hz, 1H, H-phenyl), 7.88–7.81 (m, 4H, H-phenyl, H-imidazolyl), 7.44–7.35 (m, 10H, H-phenyl), 7.17–7.13 (m, 7H, H-phenyl, H-imidazolyl), 7.12–7.08 (m, 1H, H-phenyl), 6.97 (t, *J* = 7.5 Hz, 1H, H-phenyl), 6.92 (d, *J* = 8.2 Hz, 1H, H-phenyl), 3.93 (t, *J* = 6.4 Hz, 2H, CH_2), 3.43 (t, *J* = 6.5 Hz, 2H, CH_2), 1.82–1.69 (m, 2H, CH_2). ^{13}C-NMR (101 MHz, DMSO-d_6): δ = 167.25, 154.09,

141.77, 137.17, 134.72, 133.82, 131.11, 128.71 (6C), 128.65 (3C), 127.69, 127.66 (6C), 127.46, 127.36 (3C), 126.71, 125.92, 122.47, 121.86, 121.01, 120.60, 119.93, 111.33, 74.14, 64.42, 33.61, 27.54. HRMS (ESI): *m/z* $[M + H]^+$ calculated for $C_{39}H_{32}N_3O_3$: 590.24382; found: 590.24541.

Preparation of 3-(2-(1-trityl-1*H*-imidazol-4-yl)phenoxy)propan-1-amine (**10**)

2-(3-(2-(1-Trityl-1*H*-imidazol-4-yl)phenoxy)propyl)isoindoline-1,3-dione (**9**, 0.4 g, 0.68 mmol) and 35% hydrazine hydrate (0.12 g, 1.35 mmol) were added to CH_3OH, and the reaction mixture was stirred at 50 °C under inert atmosphere. After the starting material disappeared in thin layer chromatography (TLC), the reaction mixture was distilled in vacuo, ethyl acetate (100 mL) was added to the mixture. The organic extract was washed twice with saturated aqueous $NaHCO_3$ and NaCl (20 mL) respectively, and the organic extract was dried over Na_2SO_4. After solvent was removed under vacuum, the unpurified product was added to the next step directly.

Preparation of 1,1,1-trifluoro-*N*-(3-(2-(1-trityl-1*H*-imidazol-4-yl)phenoxy)propyl) Methane Sulfonamide (**11**)

3-(2-(1-Trityl-1*H*-imidazol-4-yl)phenoxy)propan-1-amine (crude **10**, 0.3 g, 0.65 mmol) and *N,N*-diisopropylethylamine (0.168 g, 1.3 mmol) were added to dry dichloridemethane (20 mL), and trifluoromethanesulfonylchloride (0.12 g, 0.71 mmol) was added to reaction mixture gradually at 20 °C. After the starting material disappeared in thin layer chromatography (TLC), the reaction mixture was distilled in vacuo, the reaction mixture was diluted with dichloridemethane (50 mL), and the organic extract was washed twice with saturated aqueous NaCl (20 mL), and the organic extract was dried over Na_2SO_4. After solvent was removed under vacuum, the product **11** was purified as a white solid by silica gel column chromatography, 0.257 g, yield 67%. ^{1}H-NMR (400 MHz, $CDCl_3$): δ = 7.80 (s, 1H, NH), 7.43–7.32 (m, 10H, H-phenyl, H-imidazolyl), 7.23–7.16 (m, 8H, H-phenyl, H-imidazol), 7.07 (d, *J* = 1.5 Hz, 1H, H-phenyl), 6.97–6.86 (m, 2H, H-phenyl), 4.16 (t, *J* = 5.2 Hz, 2H, CH_2), 3.57–3.46 (m, 2H, CH_2), 2.19–2.06 (m, 2H, CH_2). ^{13}C-NMR (101 MHz, $CDCl_3$): δ= 154.95, 142.08, 139.92, 138.22, 129.77 (6C), 128.56 (3C), 128.36, 128.15 (3C), 128.09 (6C), 121.68, 120.87, 119.04, 118.47, 111.86, 75.75, 67.83, 43.24, 29.80. HRMS (ESI): *m/z* $[M + H]^+$ calculated for $C_{32}H_{29}N_3O_3F_3S$: 592.18762; found: 592.18616.

Preparation of *N*-(3-(2-(1*H*-imidazol-5-yl)phenoxy)propyl)-1,1,1-trifluoromethane Sulfonamide (DX-03-12)

1,1,1-Trifluoro-*N*-(3-(2-(1-trityl-1*H*-imidazol-4-yl)phenoxy)propyl)methanesulfonamide (**11**, 0.2 g, 0.34 mmol) and AcOH (0.5 mL) were added to CH_3OH (10 mL), and the reaction mixture was stirred at 20 °C. After the starting material disappeared in thin layer chromatography (TLC), the reaction mixture was distilled in vacuo, the product was purified as a white solid by silica gel column chromatography, 0.101 g, yield 86%. ^{1}H-NMR (400 MHz, DMSO-d_6): δ =7.99 (d, *J* = 7.4 Hz, 1H, H-phenyl), 7.72 (s, 1H, H-imidazolyl), 7.49 (s, 1H, H-imidazolyl), 7.18 (t, *J* = 7.8 Hz, 1H, H-phenyl), 7.03 (d, *J* = 8.1 Hz, 1H, H-phenyl), 6.98 (t, *J* = 7.5 Hz, 1H, H-phenyl), 4.15 (t, *J* = 6.0 Hz, 2H, CH_2), 3.40 (t, *J* = 6.8 Hz, 2H, CH_2), 2.06–2.09 (m, 2H, CH_2). ^{13}C-NMR (101 MHz, DMSO-d_6): δ = 154.86, 135.47, 134.49, 127.46, 127.25, 124.99, 122.69, 120.97, 118.57, 112.34, 65.09, 41.39, 30.14. HRMS (ESI): *m/z* $[M + H]^+$ calculated for $C_{13}H_{15}O_3N_3F_3S$: 350.07807; found: 350.07782.

3.1.4. Preparation of 4-chloro-2-(1-(4-(trifluoromethyl)benzyl)-1*H*-imidazol-4-yl) Phenol (DX-04-02)

Preparation of 4-iodo-1-(4-(trifluoromethyl)benzyl)-1*H*-imidazole (**12**)

4-Iodo-1*H*-imidazole (1 g, 5.2 mmol) and *N,N*-diisopropylethylamine (1.34 g, 10.4 mmol) were added to dry dimethylformamide (20 mL), and 1-(bromomethyl)-4-(trifluoromethyl)benzene (1.48 g, 6.2 mmol) was added to reaction mixture at 20 °C. After the reaction mixture was stirred at 20 °C until the starting material disappeared in thin layer chromatography (TLC), the reaction mixture was distilled in vacuo, dichloromethane (50 mL) was added to the mixture. The organic extract was washed twice with saturated aqueous $NaHCO_3$ and NaCl (20 mL) respectively, and the organic extract was dried over Na_2SO_4. After solvent was removed under vacuum, the unpurified product was added to the next step directly.

Preparation of 4-(5-chloro-2-methoxyphenyl)-1-(4-(trifluoromethyl)benzyl)-1*H*-imidazole (DX-04-01)

4-Iodo-1-(4-(trifluoromethyl)benzyl)-1*H*-imidazole (crude **12**, 0.5 g, 1.4 mmol), (5-chloro-2-methoxyphenyl)boronic acid (0.27 g, 1.4 mmol), K_3PO_4 (0.9 g, 4.3 mmol), $Pd(PPh_3)_4$ (0.23 g, 0.2 mmol) were added to dry dimethylformamide (10 mL). The reaction mixture was stirred at 100 °C under inert atmosphere, until the starting material disappeared in TLC. The reaction mixture was distilled in vacuo, ethyl acetate (50 mL) was added to the mixture. The organic extract was washed twice with saturated aqueous NaCl (20 mL), and the organic extract was dried over Na_2SO_4. After solvent was removed under vacuum, DX-04-01 was purified as a white solid by silica gel column chromatography, 0.37 g, yield 72%. ^{1}H-NMR (400 MHz, CD_3OD): δ = 7.94 (d, *J* = 2.5 Hz, 1H, H-phenyl), 7.81 (s, 1H, H-imidazolyl), 7.65–7.63 (m, 3H, H-imidazolyl, H-phenyl), 7.40 (d, *J* = 8.0 Hz, 2H, H-phenyl), 7.15 (dd, *J* = 8.7, 2.5 Hz, 1H, H-phenyl), 6.96 (d, *J* = 8.8 Hz, 1H, H-phenyl), 5.34 (s, 2H, CH_2), 3.86 (s, 3H, CH_3). ^{13}C-NMR (101 MHz, CD_3OD): δ = 156.09, 142.76, 138.77, 137.13, 131.46, 129.05 (2C), 128.22, 127.44, 126.92 (2C), 124.85, 124.18, 121.78, 113.52, 112.48, 56.17, 51.22. HRMS (ESI): *m/z* $[M + H]^+$ calculated for$C_{18}H_{15}ON_2ClF_3$: 367.08195; found: 367.08374.

Preparation of 4-chloro-2-(1-(4-(trifluoromethyl)benzyl)-1*H*-imidazol-4-yl)phenol (DX-04-02)

4-(5-Chloro-2-methoxyphenyl)-1-(4-(trifluoromethyl)benzyl)-1*H*-imidazole (DX-04-01, 0.3 g, 0.82 mmol) was added to dry dichloridemethane (20 mL), BBr_3 (0.24 g, 0.98 mmol) was added to reaction mixture gradually at −70 °C. The reaction mixture was stirred under inert atmosphere until the starting material disappeared in TLC. The reaction mixture was diluted with dichloridemethane (50 mL), and was washed twice with saturated aqueous NaCl (20 mL), then the organic extract was dried over Na_2SO_4. After solvent was removed under vacuum, DX-04-02 was purified as a white solid by silica gel column chromatography, 0.15 g, yield 53%. ^{1}H-NMR (400 MHz, CD_3OD): δ = 7.85 (s, 1H, H-imidazolyl), 7.70–7.65 (m, 3H, H-imidazolyl, H-phenyl), 7.63 (d, *J* = 2.6 Hz, 1H, H-phenyl), 7.45 (d, *J* = 8.1 Hz, 2H, H-phenyl), 7.02 (dd, *J* = 8.7, 2.6 Hz, 1H, H-phenyl), 6.80 (d, *J* = 8.7 Hz, 1H, H-phenyl), 5.37 (s, 2H, CH_2). ^{13}C-NMR (101 MHz, CD_3OD): δ = 155.21, 142.66, 140.49, 137.67, 129.87, 129.60, 129.12 (2C), 128.42, 126.89 (2C), 126.06, 125.01, 121.01, 118.79, 118.28, 51.17. HRMS (ESI): *m/z* $[M + H]^+$ calculated for$C_{17}H_{13}ON_2ClF_3$: 353.06630; found: 353.06635.

3.1.5. Preparation of 4-methyl-1*H*-indole-3-carboxylic Acid (DX-01-02)

Methyl 4-methyl-1*H*-indole-3-carboxylate (200 mg, 1.06 mmol) used hydrolysis reaction (2 N NaOH water solution) to afford DX-01-02 (white solid, 151 mg, yield 82%). ^{1}H-NMR (400 MHz, CD_3OD): δ = 8.18 (dd, *J* = 3.9, 1.9 Hz, 1H, H-indolyl), 7.30 (d, *J* = 8.0 Hz, 1H, H-indolyl), 7.17 (t, *J* = 7.7 Hz, 1H, H-indolyl), 7.01 (dd, *J* = 7.3, 0.7 Hz, 1H, H-indolyl), 2.77 (s, 3H, CH_3). ^{13}C-NMR (101 MHz, CD_3OD): δ = 139.17, 133.89, 126.39, 125.96, 125.68, 120.61, 117.71, 112.19, 111.02, 23.30. HRMS (ESI): *m/z* $[M + H]^+$ calculated for $C_{10}H_{10}NO_2$: 176.07061; found: 176.07129.

3.1.6. Preparation of 5-methyl-1*H*-indole-3-carboxylic Acid (DX-01-03)

Methyl 5-methyl-1*H*-indole-3-carboxylate (200 mg, 1.06 mmol) used hydrolysis reaction (2 N NaOH water solution) to afford DX-01-03 (white solid, 150 mg, yield 81%). ^{1}H-NMR (400 MHz, CD_3OD): δ = 8.15 (d, *J* = 1.8 Hz, 1H, H-indolyl), 8.07 (s, 1H, H-indolyl), 7.39 (d, *J* = 8.3 Hz, 1H, H-indolyl), 7.15 (dd, *J* = 8.3, 1.1 Hz, 1H, H-indolyl), 2.46 (s, 3H, CH_3). ^{13}C-NMR (101 MHz, CD_3OD): δ = 137.41, 134.35, 127.80, 127.00, 122.51, 120.09, 117.20, 113.08, 110.78, 21.77. HRMS (ESI): *m/z* $[M + H]^+$ calculated for $C_{10}H_{10}NO_2$: 176.07061; found: 176.07094.

3.1.7. Preparation of 5-nitro-1*H*-indole-3-carboxylic Acid (DX-01-04)

Methyl 5-nitro-1*H*-indole-3-carboxylate (200 mg, 0.91 mmol) used hydrolysis reaction (2 N NaOH water solution) to afford DX-01-04 (white solid, 172 mg, yield 92%). ^{1}H-NMR (400 MHz, CD_3OD): δ = 8.99 (d, *J* = 2.2 Hz, 1H, H-indolyl), 8.14 (s, 1H, H-indolyl), 8.12 (dd, *J* = 9.0, 2.3 Hz, 1H, H-indolyl), 7.58 (d, *J* = 9.0 Hz, 1H, H-indolyl). ^{13}C-NMR (101 MHz, CD_3OD): δ = 167.81, 144.32, 141.16, 136.51, 127.01, 118.93, 118.80, 113.45, 111.10, 49.00. HRMS (ESI): *m/z* $[M + H]^+$ calculated for $C_9H_7N_2O_4$: 207.04003; found: 207.03940.

3.1.8. Preparation of 6-nitro-1*H*-indole-3-carboxylic Acid (DX-01-05)

Methyl 6-nitro-1*H*-indole-3-carboxylate (200 mg, 0.91 mmol) used hydrolysis reaction (2 N NaOH water solution) to afford DX-01-05 (white solid, 168 mg, yield 90%). ^{1}H-NMR (400 MHz, CD_3OD): δ = 8.38 (d, *J* = 1.5 Hz, 1H, H-indolyl), 8.22 (s, 1H, H-indolyl), 8.18 (d, *J* = 8.9 Hz, 1H, H-indolyl), 8.05 (dd, *J* = 8.8, 1.7 Hz, 1H, H-indolyl). ^{13}C-NMR (101 MHz, CD_3OD): δ = 167.87, 144.97, 138.31, 136.78, 132.29, 122.19, 117.33, 109.89, 109.69. HRMS (ESI): *m/z* $[M + H]^+$ calculated for $C_9H_7N_2O_4$: 207.04003; found: 207.03949.

3.1.9. Preparation of 5-methoxy-1*H*-indole-3-carboxylic Acid (DX-01-06)

Methyl 5-methoxy-1*H*-indole-3-carboxylate (200 mg, 0.97 mmol) used hydrolysis reaction (2 N NaOH water solution) to afford DX-01-06 (white solid, 140 mg, yield 75%). ^{1}H-NMR (400 MHz, CD_3OD): δ = 7.88 (s, 1H, H-indolyl), 7.57 (d, *J* = 2.4 Hz, 1H, H-indolyl), 7.31 (d, *J* = 8.8 Hz, 1H, H-indolyl), 6.83 (dd, *J* = 8.8, 2.5 Hz, 1H, H-indolyl), 3.83 (s, 3H, CH_3). ^{13}C-NMR (101 MHz, CD_3OD): δ = 156.99, 133.58, 128.36, 115.37, 114.23, 113.88, 113.61, 104.51, 103.64, 56.06. HRMS (ESI): *m/z* $[M + H]^+$ calculated for $C_{10}H_{10}NO_3$: 192.06552; found: 192.06645.

3.1.10. Preparation of 7-bromo-1*H*-indole-3-carboxylic Acid (DX-01-07)

Methyl 7-bromo-1*H*-indole-3-carboxylate (200 mg, 0.79 mmol) used hydrolysis reaction (2 N NaOH water solution) to afford DX-01-07 (white solid, 160 mg, yield 85%). ^{1}H-NMR (400 MHz, CD_3OD): δ = 8.06 (dd, *J* = 8.0, 0.9 Hz, 1H, H-indolyl), 7.98 (s, 1H, H-indolyl), 7.36 (dd, *J* = 7.6, 0.7 Hz, 1H, H-indolyl), 7.08 (t, *J* = 7.8 Hz, 1H, H-indolyl). ^{13}C-NMR (101 MHz, CD_3OD): δ = 168.56, 138.29, 134.03, 129.07, 126.24, 123.59, 121.46, 117.02, 106.02. HRMS (ESI): *m/z* $[M + H]^+$ calculated for $C_9H_7NO_2Br$: 239.96547; found: 239.96452.

3.1.11. Preparation of (*E*) 1*H*-indole-3-carbaldehyde Oxime (DX-01-13)

1*H*-indole-3-carbaldehyde (200 mg, 1.38 mmol) following the similar procedure described for the preparation of DX-02-04 afforded DX-01-13 (white solid, 158 mg, yield 72%). ^{1}H-NMR (400 MHz, DMSO-d_6): δ = 11.56 (s, 1H, OH), 11.17 (s, 1H, NH), 8.26 (s, 1H, =CH), 8.22 (d, *J* = 1.3 Hz, 1H, H-indolyl), 7.97 (d, *J* = 7.9 Hz, 1H, H-indolyl), 7.44 (d, *J* = 8.1 Hz, 1H, H-indolyl), 7.16 (t, *J* = 7.5 Hz, 2H, H-indolyl). ^{13}C-NMR (101 MHz, CD_3OD): δ = 146.89, 138.66, 132.19, 127.98, 123.30, 121.40, 118.79, 112.59, 107.56. HRMS (ESI): *m/z* $[M + H]^+$ calculated for $C_9H_9ON_2$: 161.07094; found: 161.07076.

3.1.12. Preparation of *N*-((1*H*-indol-3-yl)methyl)hydroxylamine (DX-01-14)

DX-01-13 (100 mg, 0.62 mmol) following the similar procedure described for the preparation of DX-02-05 afforded DX-01-14 (white solid, 70 mg, yield 69%). ^{1}H-NMR (400 MHz, DMSO-d_6): δ = 10.87 (s, 1H, NH-indolyl), 7.58 (d, *J* = 7.8 Hz, 1H, H-indolyl), 7.34 (d, *J* = 8.1 Hz, 1H, H-indolyl), 7.29 (br, 1H, NH), 7.24 (s, 1H, H-indolyl), 7.06 (t, *J* = 8.0 Hz, 1H, H-indolyl), 6.99–6.95 (m, 1H, H-indolyl), 5.66 (br, 1H, OH), 4.04 (s, 2H, CH_2). ^{13}C-NMR (101 MHz, CD_3OD): δ = 138.02, 128.61, 125.94, 122.58, 120.11, 119.41, 112.28, 110.24, 55.80. HRMS (ESI): *m/z* $[M + H]^+$ calculated for $C_9H_{11}ON_2$: 163.08659; found: 163.08611.

3.1.13. Preparation of *N*-((5-(o-tolyl)-1*H*-indol-3-yl)methyl)hydroxylamine (DX-01-15)

5-Bromo-1*H*-indole-3-carbaldehyde (300 mg, 1.34 mmol) and o-tolylboronic acid (183 mg, 1.34 mmol) following the similar procedure described for the preparation of DX-03-12 and DX-02-05 afforded DX-01-15 (white solid, 145 mg, yield 43% from 5-bromo-1*H*-indole-3-carbaldehyde). ^{1}H-NMR (400 MHz, CD_3OD): δ = 7.57–7.39 (m, 3H, H-phenyl, H-indolyl), 7.26–7.04 (m, 5H, H-phenyl, H-indolyl), 5.13 (s, 2H, CH_2), 2.24 (s, 3H, CH_3). ^{13}C-NMR (101 MHz, CD_3OD): δ = 144.63, 137.29, 136.60, 135.38, 131.19, 131.12, 128.56, 127.79, 126.62, 125.69, 124.87, 119.47, 112.33, 107.61, 62.12, 29.31. HRMS (ESI): *m/z* $[M + H]^+$ calculated for $C_{16}H_{17}N_2O$: 253.13354; found: 253.13471.

3.1.14. Preparation of (*E*)-1*H*-indole-2-carbaldehyde Oxime (DX-01-16)

1*H*-indole-2-carbaldehyde (200 mg, 1.38 mmol) following the similar procedure described for the preparation of DX-02-04 afforded DX-01-16 (white solid, 117 mg, yield 53%). ^{1}H-NMR (400 MHz, DMSO-d_6): δ = 11.29 (s, 1H, OH), 11.17 (s, 1H, NH), 8.14 (s, 1H, =CH), 7.52 (d, *J* = 8.0 Hz, 1H, H-indolyl), 7.37 (d, *J* = 8.2 Hz, 1H, H-indolyl), 7.12 (t, *J* = 7.6 Hz, 1H, H-indolyl), 6.98 (t, *J* = 7.5 Hz, 1H, H-indolyl), 6.56 (s, 1H, H-indolyl). ^{13}C-NMR (101 MHz, CD_3OD): δ = 142.67, 138.93, 132.77, 129.48, 124.71, 122.20, 120.89, 112.84, 108.61. HRMS (ESI): *m/z* $[M + H]^+$ calculated for $C_9H_9ON_2$: 161.07094; found: 161.07077.

3.1.15. Preparation of *N*-((1*H*-indol-2-yl)methyl)hydroxylamine (DX-01-17)

DX-01-16 (60 mg, 0.37 mmol) following the similar procedure described for the preparation of DX-02-05 afforded DX-01-17 (white solid, 39 mg, yield 65%). ^{1}H-NMR (400 MHz, DMSO-d_6): δ = 10.88 (s, 1H, NH-indolyl), 7.46–7.39 (m, 2H, H-indolyl, NH), 7.32 (d, *J* = 8.3 Hz, 1H, H-indolyl), 7.03–6.97 (m, 1H, H-indolyl), 6.93 (t, *J* = 8.1 Hz, 1H), 6.28 (s, 1H, H-indolyl), 6.17 (br, 1H, OH), 4.00 (s, 2H, CH_2). ^{13}C-NMR (101 MHz, CD_3OD): δ = 137.98, 136.56, 122.09, 120.86, 120.84, 120.01, 111.84, 101.86, 51.98. HRMS (ESI): *m/z* $[M + H]^+$ calculated for $C_9H_{11}ON_2$: 163.08659; found: 163.08636.

3.1.16. Preparation of (*E*)-3-((1*H*-indol-3-yl)methylene)pyrrolidine-2,5-dione (DX-02-01)

1*H*-indole-3-carbaldehyde (500 mg, 3.45 mmol) and 1*H*-pyrrole-2,5-dione (401 mg, 4.14 mmol) following the similar procedure described for the preparation of DX-02-04 afforded DX-02-01 (white solid, 398 mg, yield 51% from 1*H*-indole-3-carbaldehyde). ^{1}H-NMR (400 MHz, DMSO-d_6): δ = 11.94 (s, 1H, NH-indolyl), 11.18 (s, 1H, NH), 7.81 (dd, *J* = 12.1, 5.1 Hz, 2H, H-indolyl, =CH), 7.70 (t, *J* = 2.1 Hz, 1H, H-indolyl), 7.54–7.41 (m, 1H, H-indolyl), 7.21–7.16 (m, 2H, H-indolyl), 3.52 (d, *J* = 2.2 Hz, 2H). HRMS (ESI): *m/z* $[M + H]^+$ calculated for $C_{13}H_{11}O_2N_2$: 227.08150; found: 227.08134.

3.1.17. Preparation of (*R/S*) 3-((1*H*-indol-3-yl)methyl)pyrrolidine-2,5-dione (DX-02-02)

DX-02-01 (200 mg, 3.45 mmol) following the similar procedure described for the preparation of DX-02-04 afforded DX-02-02 (white solid, 65 mg, yield 32%). ^{1}H-NMR (400 MHz, DMSO-d_6): δ = 11.06 (s, 1H, NH-indolyl), 10.91 (s, 1H, NH), 7.51 (d, *J* = 7.8 Hz, 1H, H-indolyl), 7.33 (d, *J* = 8.0 Hz, 1H, H-indolyl), 7.16 (s, 1H, H-indolyl), 7.06 (t, *J* = 7.5 Hz, 1H, H-indolyl), 6.97 (t, *J* = 7.5 Hz, 1H, H-indolyl), 3.20–3.12 (m, 1H, CH'H"), 2.95 (dd, *J* = 14.0, 8.5 Hz, 1H, CH'H"), 2.70–2.61 (m, 2H, H-pyrrolidine-2,5-dione), 2.34 (dd, *J* = 18.0, 3.5 Hz, 1H, H-pyrrolidine-2,5-dione). HRMS (ESI): *m/z* $[M + H]^+$ calculated for $C_{13}H_{13}N_2O_2$: 229.09715; found: 229.09663

3.1.18. Preparation of (*E*) 2-(1*H*-imidazol-4-yl)benzaldehyde Oxime (DX-03-02)

Compound **5** (400 mg, 0.92 mmol) and (2-formylphenyl)boronic acid (138 mg, 0.92 mmol) following the similar procedure described for the preparation of DX-03-12 and DX-02-04 afforded DX-03-02 (white solid, 98 mg, yield 57% from (2-formylphenyl)boronic acid). ^{1}H-NMR (400 MHz, CD_3OD): δ = 8.32 (s, 1H, =CH), 7.85–7.84 (m, 1H, H-phenyl), 7.79 (s, 1H, H-imidazolyl), 7.52 (d, *J* = 7.7 Hz, 1H, H-phenyl), 7.42–7.38 (m, 1H, H-phenyl), 7.34–7.30 (m, 1H, H-phenyl), 7.12 (s, 1H, H-imidazolyl).

^{13}C-NMR (100 MHz, DMSO-d_6): δ = 148.70, 136.36, 133.83, 130.10, 129.50, 129.27, 128.72, 128.34, 127.09, 126.20. HRMS (ESI): *m/z* $[M + H]^+$ calculated for $C_{10}H_{10}ON_3$: 188.08184; found: 188.08191.

3.1.19. Preparation of *N*-(2-(1*H*-imidazol-4-yl)benzyl)hydroxylamine (DX-03-03)

Compound DX-03-02 (50 mg, 0.27 mmol) following the similar procedure described for the preparation of DX-02-04 afforded DX-03-03 (white solid, 32 mg, yield 63%). ^{1}H-NMR (400 MHz, CD_3OD): δ = 7.75 (s, 1H, H-imidazolyl), 7.53 (d, *J* = 1.7 Hz, 1H, H-phenyl), 7.47–7.44 (m, 1H, H-phenyl), 7.35–7.27 (m, 3H, H-imidazolyl, H-phenyl), 4.04 (s, 2H). HRMS (ESI): *m/z* $[M + H]^+$ calculated for $C_{10}H_{12}ON_3$: 190.09749; found: 190.09737.

3.1.20. Preparation of (*E*) 2-(2*H*-tetrazol-5-yl)benzaldehyde Oxime (DX-03-04)

2-(2H-tetrazol-5-yl)benzaldehyde (200 mg, 1.15 mmol) following the similar procedure described for the preparation of DX-03-12 and DX-02-04 afforded DX-03-04 (white solid, 78 mg, yield 36% from 2-(2*H*-tetrazol-5-yl)benzaldehyde). ^{1}H-NMR (400 MHz, DMSO-d_6): δ = 11.23 (s, 1H, OH), 11.07 (s, 1H, H-tetrazolyl), 8.29 (s, 1H, =CH), 7.73–7.56 (m, 4H, H-phenyl). ^{13}C-NMR (101 MHz, DMSO-d_6): δ = 156.17, 137.81, 132.14, 130.64, 129.27, 127.64, 116.84, 110.69. HRMS (ESI): *m/z* $[M + H]^+$ calculated for $C_8H_8N_5O$: 190.07234; found: 190.07158.

3.1.21. Preparation of (*E*) 5-chloro-2-(1*H*-imidazol-4-yl)benzaldehyde Oxime (DX-03-05)

Compound **5** (300 mg, 0.69 mmol) and (4-chloro-2-formylphenyl)boronic acid (127 mg, 0.69 mmol) following the similar procedure described for the preparation of DX-03-12 and DX-02-04 afforded DX-03-05 (white solid, 70 mg, yield 46% from (4-chloro-2-formylphenyl)boronic acid). ^{1}H-NMR (400 MHz, DMSO-d_6): δ = 12.38 (s, 1H, OH), 11.32 (s, 1H, NH-imidazolyl), 8.77 (s, 1H, =CH), 7.80 (s, 1H, H-imidazolyl), 7.74 (s, 1H, H-imidazolyl), 7.63 (d, *J* = 2.4 Hz, 1H, H-phenyl), 7.44–7.42 (m, 2H, H-phenyl). ^{13}C-NMR (101 MHz, DMSO-d_6): δ = 147.77, 138.56, 136.60, 133.12, 131.72, 131.48, 131.05, 129.25, 125.42, 116.28. HRMS (ESI): *m/z* $[M + H]^+$ calculated for $C_{10}H_9ClN_3O$: 222.04287; found: 222.04330.

3.1.22. Preparation of (*E*) 2-fluoro-6-(1*H*-imidazol-4-yl)benzaldehyde Oxime (DX-03-06)

Compound **5** (300 mg, 0.69 mmol) and (3-fluoro-2-formylphenyl)boronic acid (116 mg, 0.69 mmol) following the similar procedure described for the preparation of DX-03-12 and DX-02-04 afforded DX-03-06 (white solid, 75 mg, yield 53% from (3-fluoro-2-formylphenyl)boronic acid). ^{1}H-NMR (400 MHz, DMSO-d_6): δ = 12.37 (s, 1H, OH), 11.24 (s, 1H, NH-imidazolyl), 8.37 (s, 1H, =CH), 7.76 (s, 1H, H-imidazolyl), 7.52 (s, 1H, H-imidazolyl), 7.36–7.13 (m, 3H, H-phenyl). ^{13}C-NMR (101 MHz, DMSO-d_6): δ = 161.48, 159.00, 144.68, 136.29, 130.27, 124.36, 122.95, 117.89, 116.35, 113.98. HRMS (ESI): *m/z* $[M + H]^+$ calculated for $C_{10}H_9FN_3O$: 206.07242; found: 206.07250.

3.1.23. Preparation of (*E*) 2-(1*H*-imidazol-4-yl)-5-methoxybenzaldehyde Oxime (DX-03-07)

Compound **5** (300 mg, 0.69 mmol) and (2-formyl-4-methoxyphenyl)boronic acid (124 mg, 0.69 mmol) following the similar procedure described for the preparation of DX-03-12 and DX-02-04 afforded DX-03-07 (white solid, 113 mg, yield 76% from (2-formyl-4-methoxyphenyl)boronic acid). ^{1}H-NMR (400 MHz, CD_3OD): δ = 8.73 (s, 1H, H-imidazolyl), 7.78 (s, 1H, H-imidazolyl), 7.52–7.38 (m, 3H, H-phenyl), 7.15 (s, 1H, H-phenyl), 7.10–6.96 (m, 4H, H-phenyl), 3.85 (s, 3H, CH_3). ^{13}C-NMR (101 MHz, CD_3OD): δ = 141.55, 137.87, 133.07, 132.61, 121.44, 118.60, 117.79, 116.37, 113.90, 110.95, 55.90. HRMS (ESI): *m/z* $[M + H]^+$ calculated for $C_{11}H_{12}N_3O_2$: 218.09240; found: 218.09206.

3.1.24. Preparation of (*E*) 4-(1*H*-imidazol-4-yl)-2′-(trifluoromethyl)-[1,1′-biphenyl]-3-carbaldehyde Oxime (DX-03-08)

Compound **5** (300 mg, 0.69 mmol) and (3-formyl-2′-(trifluoromethyl)-[1,1′-biphenyl]-4-yl) boronic acid (202 mg, 0.69 mmol) following the similar procedure described for the preparation of DX-03-12 and DX-02-04 afforded DX-03-08 (white solid, 82mg, yield 36% from (3-formyl-2′-(trifluoromethyl)-[1,1′-biphenyl]-4-yl)boronic acid). ^{1}H-NMR (400 MHz, DMSO-d_6): δ = 12.38 (s, 1H, OH), 11.14 (s, 1H, NH-imidazolyl), 8.85(s, 1H, H-imidazolyl), 7.86–7.79 (m, 2H, H-imidazolyl, H-phenyl), 7.73–7.63 (m, 4H, H-phenyl), 7.46 (br, 2H, H-phenyl), 7.33 (s, 1H, H-phenyl). ^{13}C-NMR (101 MHz, DMSO-d_6): δ = 148.54, 140.58, 137.83, 136.56, 132.89, 132.57, 130.11, 129.84, 129.53, 128.94, 128.64, 126.58, 126.32, 126.23, 126.04, 123.22, 116.04. HRMS (ESI): *m/z* [M + H]$^+$ calculated for $C_{17}H_{13}F_3N_3O$: 332.10052; found: 332.10123.

3.1.25. Preparation of (*E*) 3-(1*H*-imidazol-4-yl)-[1,1′-biphenyl]-4-carbaldehyde Oxime (DX-03-09)

Compound **5** (300 mg, 0.69 mmol) and (4-formyl-[1,1′-biphenyl]-3-yl)boronic acid (156 mg, 0.69 mmol) following the similar procedure described for the preparation of DX-03-12 and DX-02-04 afforded DX-03-09 (white solid, 81 mg, yield 45% from (4-formyl-[1,1′-biphenyl]-3-yl)boronic acid). ^{1}H-NMR (400 MHz, DMSO-d_6): δ = 11.01 (s, 1H, OH), 10.34 (s, 1H, NH-imidazolyl), 8.55 (s, 1H, =CH), 8.39 (s, 1H, H-imidazolyl), 8.12 (s, 1H, H-imidazolyl), 7.58 (br, 1H, H-phenyl), 7.48–7.22 (m, 2H, H-phenyl), 7.11–7.02 (m, 2H, H-phenyl), 6.87–6,81 (m, 2H, H-phenyl), 6.50 (s, 1H, H-phenyl). HRMS (ESI): *m/z* [M + H]$^+$ calculated for $C_{16}H_{14}N_3O$: 264.11314; found: 264.11346.

3.1.26. Preparation of 4-(2-((4-(trifluoromethyl)benzyl)oxy)phenyl)-1,2,3-thiadiazole (DX-03-10)

2-(1,2,3-Thiadiazol-4-yl)phenol (100 mg, 0.56 mmol) and 1-(bromomethyl)-4-(trifluoromethyl)benzene (134 mg, 0.56 mmol) following the similar procedure described for the preparation of **12** afforded DX-03-10 (white solid, 128 mg, yield 68%). ^{1}H-NMR (400 MHz, DMSO-d_6): δ = 9.39 (s, 1H, H-thiadiazolyl), 8.26 (d, *J* = 7.5 Hz, 1H, H-phenyl), 7.76 (d, *J* = 8.2 Hz, 2H, H-phenyl), 7.70 (d, *J* = 8.5 Hz, 2H, H-phenyl), 7.48–7.43 (m, 1H, H-phenyl), 7.31 (d, *J* = 7.7 Hz, 1H, H-phenyl), 7.17 (t, *J* = 7.5 Hz, 1H, H-phenyl), 5.44 (s, 2H, CH_2). HRMS (ESI): *m/z* [M + H]$^+$ calculated for $C_{16}H_{12}F_3N_2OS$: 337.06169; found: 337.06116.

3.1.27. Preparation of *N*-(3-(2-(1*H*-imidazol-5-yl)phenoxy)propyl)-aminesulfonamide (DX-03-11)

Compound **9** (200 mg, 0.34 mmol) following the similar procedure described for the preparation of DX-03-12 afforded DX-03-11 (white solid, 45 mg, yield 45% from compound **9**). ^{1}H-NMR (400 MHz, CD_3OD): δ = 8.67 (s, 1H, NH-imidazolyl), 8.08 (s, 1H, H-imidazolyl), 7.83 (s, 1H, H-imidazolyl), 7.69 (d, *J* = 7.7 Hz, 1H, H-phenyl), 7.40 (t, *J* = 7.1 Hz, 1H, H-phenyl), 7.16 (d, *J* = 8.2 Hz, 1H, H-phenyl), 7.08 (t, *J* = 7.4 Hz, 1H, H-phenyl), 4.20 (t, *J* = 6.0 Hz, 2H, CH_2), 3.44 (t, *J* = 6.9 Hz, 2H, CH_2), 2.11–2.03 (m, 2H, CH_2). HRMS (ESI): *m/z* [M + H]$^+$ calculated for $C_{12}H_{17}O_3N_4S$: 297.10159; found: 297.10115.

3.1.28. Preparation of 1-(3-(2-(1*H*-imidazol-5-yl)phenoxy)propyl)-3-(4-(trifluoromethyl) phenyl)urea (DX-03-13)

Compound **9** (200 mg, 0.34 mmol) following the similar procedure described for the preparation of DX-03-12 afforded DX-03-13 (white solid, 77 mg, yield 56% from compound **9**). ^{1}H-NMR (400 MHz, DMSO-d_6): δ = 12.24 (s, 1H, NH-imidazolyl), 8.90 (s, 1H, H-imidazolyl), 8.01 (d, *J* = 7.4 Hz, 1H, H-phenyl), 7.75 (s, 1H, H-imidazolyl), 7.61–7.54 (m, 5H, H-phenyl), 7.21–7.15 (m, 1H, H-phenyl), 7.06 (d, *J* = 7.8 Hz, 1H, H-phenyl), 7.02–6.94 (m, 1H, H-phenyl), 6.48 (t, *J* = 5.7 Hz, 1H, H-phenyl), 4.14 (t, *J* = 6.1 Hz, 2H, CH_2), 3.38–3.32 (m, 2H, CH_2), 2.08–1.97 (m, 2H, CH_2). ^{13}C-NMR (101 MHz, DMSO-d_6): δ = 155.42, 155.08, 144.71, 135.42, 129.17, 127.38, 127.13, 126.38 (2C), 123.78, 122.81, 121.53, 121.21, 120.86, 117.71 (2C), 112.33, 65.82, 36.89, 29.98. HRMS (ESI): *m/z* [M + H]$^+$ calculated for $C_{20}H_{20}O_2N_4F_3$: 405.15329; found: 405.15302.

3.1.29. Preparation of 1-(3-bromo-4-fluorobenzyl)-4-(5-chloro-2-methoxyphenyl)-1*H*-imidazole (DX-04-03)

2-Bromo-4-(bromomethyl)-1-fluorobenzene (500 mg, 1.88 mmol) following the similar procedure described for the preparation of DX-04-02 afforded DX-04-03 (white solid, 480 mg, yield 65% from 2-bromo-4-(bromomethyl)-1-fluorobenzene). ^{1}H-NMR (400 MHz, CD_3OD): δ = 7.95 (d, *J* = 2.7 Hz, 1H, H-phenyl), 7.78 (d, *J* = 1.3 Hz, 1H, H-imidazolyl), 7.64 (d, *J* = 1.3 Hz, 1H, H-imidazolyl), 7.57 (dd, *J* = 6.5, 2.2 Hz, 1H, H-phenyl), 7.30–7.24 (m, 1H, H-phenyl), 7.20 (d, *J* = 8.5 Hz, 1H, H-phenyl), 7.16 (dd, *J* = 8.8, 2.7 Hz, 1H, H-phenyl), 6.98 (d, *J* = 8.8 Hz, 1H, H-phenyl), 5.22 (s, 2H, CH_2), 3.88 (s, 3H, CH_3). ^{13}C-NMR (101 MHz, CD_3OD): δ = 161.35, 158.96, 156.10, 138.33, 137.40, 133.91, 129.70, 128.04, 127.36, 126.81, 125.19, 121.53, 117.84, 113.47, 110.01, 56.13, 50.30. HRMS (ESI): *m/z* $[M + H]^+$ calculated for $C_{17}H_{14}ON_2BrClF$: 394.99566; found: 394.99728.

3.1.30. Preparation of 2-(1-(3-bromo-4-fluorobenzyl)-1*H*-imidazol-4-yl)-4-chlorophenol (DX-04-04)

DX-04-03 (200 mg, 0.51 mmol) following the similar procedure described for the preparation of DX-04-02 afforded DX-04-04 (white solid, 116 mg, yield 60%). ^{1}H-NMR (400 MHz, DMSO-d_6): δ = 9.12 (s, 1H, H-imidazolyl), 8.40 (s, 1H, H-imidazolyl), 8.01 (s, 1H, H-imidazolyl), 7.89 (dd, *J* = 6.5, 1.7 Hz, 1H, H-phenyl), 7.56–7.49 (m, 1H, H-phenyl), 7.45 (t, *J* = 8.6 Hz, 1H, H-phenyl), 7.34 (dd, *J* = 8.8, 2.5 Hz, 1H, H-phenyl), 7.00 (d, *J* = 8.8 Hz, 1H, H-phenyl), 5.42 (s, 2H, CH_2). ^{13}C-NMR (101 MHz, CD_3OD): δ = 161.85, 159.35, 154.93, 136.62, 134.79, 130.61, 130.34, 126.90, 125.53, 119.70, 118.77, 118.32, 118.09, 117.92, 110.27, 51.71. HRMS (ESI): *m/z* $[M + H]^+$ calculated for $C_{16}H_{12}ON_2BrClF$: 380.98001; found: 380.98065.

3.1.31. Preparation of 4-chloro-2-(1-(4-(trifluoromethyl)benzyl)-1*H*-1,2,3-triazol-4-yl)phenol (DX-04-05)

DX-04-06 (300 mg, 0.81 mmol) following the similar procedure described for the preparation of DX-04-02 afforded DX-04-05 (white solid, 176 mg, yield 61%). ^{1}H-NMR (400 MHz, DMSO-d_6): δ = 10.49 (s, 1H, OH), 7.85 (s, 1H, H-triazolyl), 7.64 (d, *J* = 8.1 Hz, 2H, H-phenyl), 7.34 (dd, *J* = 8.8, 2.7 Hz, 1H, H-phenyl), 7.20 (d, *J* = 8.1 Hz, 2H, H-phenyl), 7.16 (d, *J* = 2.7 Hz, 1H, H-phenyl), 6.98 (d, *J* = 8.8 Hz, 1H, H-phenyl), 5.62 (s, 2H, CH_2). ^{13}C-NMR (101 MHz, CD_3OD): δ = 155.39, 140.99, 136.49, 134.75, 132.46, 131.76, 131.11, 129.36 (2C), 126.49 (2C), 125.38, 124.09, 118.30, 116.15, 53.27. HRMS (ESI): *m/z* $[M + H]^+$ calculated for $C_{16}H_{12}ON_3ClF_3$: 354.06155; found: 354.06015.

3.1.32. Preparation of 4-(5-chloro-2-methoxyphenyl)-1-(4-(trifluoromethyl)benzyl)-1*H*-1,2,3-triazole (DX-04-06)

4-chloro-2-ethynyl-1-methoxybenzene (500 mg, 3.01 mmol) and 1-(bromomethyl)-4-(trifluoromethyl)benzene (717 mg, 3.01 mmol) following the similar procedure described for the preparation of DX-04-02 afforded DX-04-06 (white solid, 675 mg, yield 61% from 4-chloro-2-ethynyl-1-methoxybenzene). ^{1}H-NMR (400 MHz, CD_3OD): δ = 7.71 (s, 1H, H-triazolyl), 7.50 (d, *J* = 8.1 Hz, 2H, H-phenyl), 7.40 (dd, *J* = 8.9, 2.7 Hz, 1H, H-phenyl), 7.14 (d, *J* = 8.1 Hz, 2H, H-phenyl), 7.09 (d, *J* = 2.6 Hz, 1H, H-phenyl), 7.03 (d, *J* = 8.9 Hz, 1H, H-phenyl), 5.55 (s, 2H, CH_2), 3.64 (s, 3H, CH_3). ^{13}C-NMR (101 MHz, CD_3OD): δ = 154.74, 143.61, 131.20, 130.91, 129.93 (2C), 129.81, 129.39, 127.59, 127.02 (2C), 125.98, 125.64, 118.63, 117.43, 55.31, 55.04. HRMS (ESI): *m/z* $[M + H]^+$ calculated for $C_{17}H_{14}ON_3ClF_3$: 368.07720; found: 368.07599.

3.1.33. Preparation of 4-chloro-2-(5-(4-(trifluoromethyl)phenyl)-1*H*-1,2,3-triazol-4-yl)phenol (DX-04-07)

DX-04-08 (200 mg, 0.57 mmol) following the similar procedure described for the preparation of DX-04-02 afforded DX-04-07 (white solid, 144 mg, yield 75%). ^{1}H-NMR (400 MHz, DMSO-d_6): δ = 15.28 (s, 1H, H-triazolyl), 9.91 (s, 1H, NH-triazolyl), 7.75–7.68 (m, 4H, H-phenyl), 7.37 (br, 2H, H-phenyl), 6.94 (s, 1H, H-phenyl). ^{13}C-NMR (101 MHz, CD_3OD): δ = 155.58, 142.95, 137.77, 136.14, 131.62, 131.27,

130.86, 128.63 (2C), 126.43 (2C), 125.31, 124.28, 119.14, 118.53. HRMS (ESI): *m/z* $[M + H]^+$ calculated for $C_{15}H_{10}ON_3ClF_3$: 340.04590; found: 340.04453.

3.1.34. Preparation of 4-(5-chloro-2-methoxyphenyl)-5-(4-(trifluoromethyl)phenyl)-1*H*-1,2,3-triazole (DX-04-08)

4-chloro-2-ethynyl-1-methoxybenzene (300 mg, 1.81 mmol) and 1-iodo-4-(trifluoromethyl)benzene (491 mg, 1.81 mmol) following the similar procedure described for the preparation of DX-04-02 afforded DX-04-08 (white solid, 338 mg, yield 53% from 4-chloro-2-ethynyl-1-methoxybenzene). ^{1}H-NMR (400 MHz, DMSO-d_6): δ = 15.41 (s, 1H, NH-triazolyl), 7.74 (d, *J* = 8.1 Hz, 2H, H-phenyl), 7.68–7.59 (m, 2H, H-phenyl), 7.54 (d, *J* = 8.9 Hz, 1H, H-phenyl), 7.48 (d, *J* = 2.7 Hz, 1H, H-phenyl), 7.15 (s, 1H, H-phenyl), 3.42 (s, 3H, CH_3). ^{13}C-NMR (101 MHz, CD_3OD): δ = 157.20, 136.42, 131.71, 131.59, 131.14, 129.65, 128.37 (2C), 126.96, 126.75, 126.40 (2C), 124.27, 121.57, 114.17, 55.99. HRMS (ESI): *m/z* $[M + H]^+$ calculated for $C_{16}H_{12}ON_3ClF_3$: 354.06155; found: 354.06079.

3.2. Pharmacological Method

3.2.1. Enzyme-Based IDO1s or TDOs Activity Assay

The compounds on IDO1 or TDO activity were determined as follows [16,24,25]: A standard reaction mixture (100 μL) containing 100 mM potassium phosphate buffer (pH 6.5), 40 mM ascorbic acid (neutralized with NaOH), 200 μg/mL catalase, 20 μM methylene blue and 0.05 μM rhIDO1 or rhTDO was added to the solution containing the substrate L-tryptophan and the test sample at a determined concentration. The reaction was carried out at 37 °C for 45 min and stopped by adding 20 μL of 30% (*w/v*) trichloroacetic acid. After heating at 65 °C for 15 min, 100 μL of 2% (*w/v*) p-dimethylaminobenzaldehyde in acetic acid was added to each well. The yellow pigment derived from kynurenine was measured at 492 nm using a SYNERGY-H1 microplate reader (Biotek Instruments, Inc., Winooski, VT, USA). IC_{50} was analyzed using the GraphPad Prism 8.0 software (GraphPad Software, San Diego, CA, USA).

3.2.2. Cell Culture

B16-F10 mouse melanoma cells, NCI-H460 human lung cancer cell line and MCF7 were obtained from American Type Culture Collection (ATCC). All the cell lines were cultured with Dulbecco' modified Eagle's medium (DMEM) (Invitrogen Corporation, Waltham, MA, USA) supplemented with 10% fetal bovine serum (FBS) (Hyclone, Waltham, MA, USA) and 1% penicillin streptomycin (Invitrogen) at 37 °C in 5% CO_2.

3.2.3. Cell Viability Assay

The in vitro inhibitory effects of the compounds were measured by MTT assay [26]. Briefly, different kinds of cells were plated in 96-well plates at a density of 2000/well. After attachment for overnight at 37 °C, the cells were treated with the compounds at various concentrations. After 72 h culture, the MTT reagent was added to each well, and plates were incubated for another 4 h at 37 °C. Then, the blue-purple crystal formamidine was dissolved in DMSO after discarding the supernatant. Samples were measured using microplate reader at a wavelength of 570 nm (Biotek Instruments, Inc., Winooski, VT, USA). IC_{50} values were calculated with GraphPad Prism 8.0 software.

3.2.4. Mice

C57BL/6 mice were obtained from Beijing Vital River Laboratory Animal Technology Co., Ltd. (Beijing Vital River Laboratory Animal Technology Co., Ltd, Beijing, China). Studies involving mice were approved by the Experimental Animal Management and Welfare Committee at the Institute of Materia Medica, Peking Union Medical College.

3.2.5. Pharmacokinetic Studies

The animal Care and Welfare Committee of Institute of Materia Medica, Chinese Academy of Medical Sciences approved all animal care, housing, and laboratory procedures. Male ICR mice were used in the single dose pharmacokinetic studies. Compound DX-03-12 was prepared as 3 mg/mL suspension with 0.5% CMC (containing 0.3% Tween 80) for oral use and was formulated as 3 mg/mL solution with 5% DMSO in saline for intravenous injection. Twenty mice were divided into two groups, 10 in each group. After fasting 12 h with free access to water, mice were treated with a 3 mg/kg i.v. or 30 mg/kg oral dose of compound DX-03-12. Blood samples (50 μL) were collected at 5, 15, 30 min, 1, 2, 4, 6, 8, 12 and 24 h after oral administration and 2, 5, 15, 30 min, 1, 2, 4, 6, 8, 12 and 24 h after intravenous injection. After centrifugation, the plasma samples (15 μL) were precipitated by five volumes of acetonitrile. The supernatant were analyzed by liquid chromatography/tandem mass spectrometry (Agilent Technologies, Santa Clara, CA, USA) with a Zobax C18 column (50 mm × 2.1 mm, 3.5 μm). Compound detection was performed with the mass spectrometer in MRM (multiple reaction monitoring, Agilent Technologies, Santa Clara, CA, USA) negative ionization mode. The selected reaction monitoring transitions were *m/z* 348.5→160 for compound DX-03-12. The pharmacokinetic parameters were calculated with WinNonlin software V6.3 using non-compartmental analysis (Pharsight Corporation, Mountain View, CA, USA).

3.2.6. In Vivo Studies

The mouse melanoma cells B16F10 were cultured and harvested in saline. At day 0 of the experiment, 1×10^6 cells were injected subcutaneously into mice, and treatment was initiated at day 1 following the mice enrolled randomly in control and experimental groups [27]. For control group, 0.5% CMCNa was orally administered every day. Compound DX-03-12 was dissolved in 0.5% CMC for oral treatment or dissolved in saline for intraperitoneal treatment. When the mice were sacrificed, the tumors were stripped and weighted. The tumor growth inhibition (TGI) was calculated as TGI = (1 − tumor weight $_{\text{treatment}}$/tumor weight $_{\text{vehicle}}$) × 100%. The statistical analysis was performed with GraphPad Prism 8.0 software and the significance level was evaluated with a one-way ANOVA model.

4. Conclusions

We designed four series of IDO1 inhibitors using indole and phenylimidazole as the scaffolds. The design strategies were based on the mechanism of IDO1, focusing on the interaction between the inhibitor and the heme iron. The four series of compounds were synthesized and their IDO1 and TDO inhibition was evaluated. Most compounds showed marginal IDO1 inhibition, but eight compounds showed moderate IDO1 inhibition. In particular, DX-03-12 and DX-03-13 showed IDO1 inhibition with IC_{50}s of 0.3 and 0.5 μM and low cell cytotoxicities against two cancer cell lines. A pharmacokinetic study showed that DX-03-12 had satisfactory properties, with rapid absorption, moderate plasma clearance, acceptable half-life, and high oral bioavailability. The in vivo anti-tumor efficacy in a B16F10 subcutaneous xenograft mouse model showed that DX-03-12 orally administered at a dose of 60 mg/kg inhibited tumor growth by 72.2% compared with the control tumors. In summary, IDO1 inhibitor DX-03-12 exhibits promising drug like properties, good pharmacokinetic properties, low cellular toxicity, and impressive in vivo anti-tumor efficacy.

Author Contributions: L.S., F.L., and H.C. conceived and designed the experiments; H.W., Y.L. (Yuke Liu), S.W., T.W., and G.Z. performed the experiments, analyzed the data; Y.L. (Yan Li), and X.C. checked the data; L.S., F.L., and H.C. wrote the paper. Please contact L.S. for pharmacokinetic study, F.L. for pharmacology study and H.C. for medicinal chemistry.

Funding: The research leading to these results has received funding from The CAMS Innovation Fund for Medical Sciences (2017-I2M-1-010), The Drug Innovation Major Project (2018ZX09711001), National Natural Science Foundation of China (81603190).

Acknowledgments: We would like to express our appreciation to Jie Li of Beijing Chao-Yang Hospital for the clinical issue discussion.

Conflicts of Interest: The authors declare no conflict of interest.

References

1. Weng, T.; Qiu, X.; Wang, J.; Li, Z.; Bian, J. Recent discovery of indoleamine-2,3-dioxygenase 1 inhibitors targeting cancer immunotherapy. *Eur. J. Med. Chem.* **2018**, *143*, 656–669. [CrossRef] [PubMed]
2. Muller, A.J.; DuHadaway, J.B.; Donover, P.S.; Sutanto-Ward, E.; Prendergast, G.C. Inhibition of indoleamine 2,3-dioxygenase, an immunoregulatory target of the cancer suppression gene Bin1, potentiates cancer chemotherapy. *Nat. Med.* **2005**, *11*, 312–319. [CrossRef] [PubMed]
3. Platten, M.; Nollen, E.A.A.; Rohrig, U.F.; Fallarino, F.; Opitz, C.A. Tryptophan metabolism as a common therapeutic target in cancer, neurodegeneration and beyond. *Nat. Rev. Drug Discov* **2019**, *18*, 379–401. [CrossRef] [PubMed]
4. Cervenka, I.; Agudelo, L.; Ruas, J. Kynurenines: Tryptophan's metabolites in exercise, inflammation, and mental health. *Science* **2017**, *357*. [CrossRef] [PubMed]
5. Abdulla, A.-B.B. Kynurenine Pathway of Tryptophan Metabolism: Regulatory and Functional Aspects. *Int. J. Tryptophan. Res.* **2017**, *10*. [CrossRef]
6. Zhai, L.; Spranger, S.; Binder, D.C.; Gritsina, G.; Lauing, K.L.; Giles, F.J.; Wainwright, D.A. Molecular Pathways: Targeting IDO1 and Other Tryptophan Dioxygenases for Cancer Immunotherapy. *Clin. Cancer Res.* **2015**, *21*, 5427–5433. [CrossRef] [PubMed]
7. Chauhan, N.; Basran, J.; Efimov, I.; Svistunenko, D.A.; Seward, H.E.; Moody, P.C.; Raven, E.L. The role of serine 167 in human indoleamine 2,3-dioxygenase: A comparison with tryptophan 2,3-dioxygenase. *Biochemistry* **2008**, *47*, 4761–4769. [CrossRef] [PubMed]
8. Batabyal, D.; Yeh, S.R. Human tryptophan dioxygenase: A comparison to indoleamine 2,3-dioxygenase. *J. Am. Chem. Soc.* **2007**, *129*, 15690–15701. [CrossRef]
9. Sugimoto, H.; Oda, S.; Otsuki, T.; Hino, T.; Yoshida, T.; Shiro, Y. Crystal structure of human indoleamine 2,3-dioxygenase: Catalytic mechanism of O2 incorporation by a heme-containing dioxygenase. *Proc. Natl. Acad. Sci. USA* **2006**, *103*, 2611–2616. [CrossRef]
10. Rohrig, U.F.; Zoete, V.; Michielin, O. The Binding Mode of *N*-Hydroxyamidines to Indoleamine 2,3-Dioxygenase 1 (IDO1). *Biochemistry* **2017**, *56*, 4323–4325. [CrossRef]
11. Samelson-Jones, B.J.; Yeh, S.R. Interactions between nitric oxide and indoleamine 2,3-dioxygenase. *Biochemistry* **2006**, *45*, 8527–8538. [CrossRef] [PubMed]
12. Yanagisawa, S.; Sugimoto, H.; Shiro, Y.; Ogura, T. A specific interaction of L-tryptophan with CO of CO-bound indoleamine 2,3-dioxygenase identified by resonance Raman spectroscopy. *Biochemistry* **2010**, *49*, 10081–10088. [CrossRef] [PubMed]
13. Crosignani, S.; Bingham, P.; Bottemanne, P.; Cannelle, H.; Cauwenberghs, S.; Cordonnier, M.; Dalvie, D.; Deroose, F.; Feng, J.L.; Gomes, B.; et al. Discovery of a Novel and Selective Indoleamine 2,3-Dioxygenase (IDO-1) Inhibitor 3-(5-Fluoro-1*H*-indol-3-yl)pyrrolidine-2,5-dione (EOS200271/PF-06840003) and Its Characterization as a Potential Clinical Candidate. *J. Med. Chem.* **2017**, *60*, 9617–9629. [CrossRef] [PubMed]
14. Yang, D.; Li, T.; Li, Y.; Zhang, S.; Li, W.; Liang, H.; Xing, Z.; Du, L.; He, J.; Kuang, C.; et al. H_2S suppresses indoleamine 2, 3-dioxygenase 1 and exhibits immunotherapeutic efficacy in murine hepatocellular carcinoma. *J. Exp. Clin. Cancer Res.* **2019**, *38*, 88. [CrossRef] [PubMed]
15. Pham, K.N.; Yeh, S.R. Mapping the Binding Trajectory of a Suicide Inhibitor in Human Indoleamine 2,3-Dioxygenase 1. *J. Am. Chem. Soc.* **2018**, *140*, 14538–14541. [CrossRef] [PubMed]
16. Yang, S.; Li, X.; Hu, F.; Li, Y.; Yang, Y.; Yan, J.; Kuang, C.; Yang, Q. Discovery of tryptanthrin derivatives as potent inhibitors of indoleamine 2,3-dioxygenase with therapeutic activity in Lewis lung cancer (LLC) tumor-bearing mice. *J. Med. Chem.* **2013**, *56*, 8321–8331. [CrossRef] [PubMed]
17. Yue, E.W.; Douty, B.; Wayland, B.; Bower, M.; Liu, X.; Leffet, L.; Wang, Q.; Bowman, K.J.; Hansbury, M.J.; Liu, C.; et al. Discovery of potent competitive inhibitors of indoleamine 2,3-dioxygenase with in vivo pharmacodynamic activity and efficacy in a mouse melanoma model. *J. Med. Chem.* **2009**, *52*, 7364–7367. [CrossRef] [PubMed]

18. Kumar, S.; Jaller, D.; Patel, B.; LaLonde, J.M.; DuHadaway, J.B.; Malachowski, W.P.; Prendergast, G.C.; Muller, A.J. Structure based development of phenylimidazole-derived inhibitors of indoleamine 2,3-dioxygenase. *J. Med. Chem.* **2008**, *51*, 4968–4977. [CrossRef]
19. Rohrig, U.F.; Majjigapu, S.R.; Grosdidier, A.; Bron, S.; Stroobant, V.; Pilotte, L.; Colau, D.; Vogel, P.; Van den Eynde, B.J.; Zoete, V.; et al. Rational design of 4-aryl-1,2,3-triazoles for indoleamine 2,3-dioxygenase 1 inhibition. *J. Med. Chem.* **2012**, *55*, 5270–5290. [CrossRef]
20. Tojo, S.; Kohno, T.; Tanaka, T.; Kamioka, S.; Ota, Y.; Ishii, T.; Kamimoto, K.; Asano, S.; Isobe, Y. Crystal Structures and Structure-Activity Relationships of Imidazothiazole Derivatives as IDO1 Inhibitors. *ACS Med. Chem. Lett.* **2014**, *5*, 1119–1123. [CrossRef]
21. Zhu, M.M.T.; Dancsok, A.R.; Nielsen, T.O. Indoleamine Dioxygenase Inhibitors: Clinical Rationale and Current Development. *Curr. Oncol. Rep.* **2019**, *21*, 2. [CrossRef]
22. Yan, N.; He, Y.; Wen, H.; Lai, F.; Yin, D.; Cui, H. A Suzuki-Miyaura method for labelling proliferating cells containing incorporated BrdU. *Analyst* **2018**, *143*, 1224–1233. [CrossRef] [PubMed]
23. Mautino, M.; Kumar, S.; Jaipuri, F.; Kesharwani, T.; Zhang, X. Imidazole Derivatives as IDO inhibitors. WO2011056652A1, 12 May 2011.
24. Austin, C.J.; Mizdrak, J.; Matin, A.; Sirijovski, N.; Kosim-Satyaputra, P.; Willows, R.D.; Roberts, T.H.; Truscott, R.J.; Polekhina, G.; Parker, M.W.; et al. Optimised expression and purification of recombinant human indoleamine 2,3-dioxygenase. *Protein Expr. Purif.* **2004**, *37*, 392–398. [CrossRef] [PubMed]
25. Littlejohn, T.K.; Takikawa, O.; Skylas, D.; Jamie, J.F.; Walker, M.J.; Truscott, R.J. Expression and purification of recombinant human indoleamine 2, 3-dioxygenase. *Protein Expr. Purif.* **2000**, *19*, 22–29. [CrossRef]
26. Lai, F.; Shen, Z.; Wen, H.; Chen, J.; Zhang, X.; Lin, P.; Yin, D.; Cui, H.; Chen, X. A Morphological identification cell cytotoxicity assay using cytoplasm-localized fluorescent probe (CLFP) to distinguish living and dead cells. *Biochem. Biophys. Res. Commun.* **2017**, *482*, 257–263. [CrossRef] [PubMed]
27. He, Y.; Wen, J.; Cui, Q.; Lai, F.; Yin, D.; Cui, H. Quantitative Evaluation of in Vivo Target Efficacy of Anti-tumor Agents via an Immunofluorescence and EdU Labeling Strategy. *Front. Pharmacol.* **2018**, *9*, 812. [CrossRef] [PubMed]

Sample Availability: Samples of the compounds are available from the authors.

molecules

MDPI

Article

Synthesis and Cytotoxicity of 7,9-*O*-Linked Macrocyclic C-Seco Taxoids

Yu Zhao [1], Tian-En Wang [1], Alberto Mills [2], Federico Gago [2] and Wei-Shuo Fang [1,*]

1 State Key Laboratory of Bioactive Substances and Functions of Natural Medicines, Institute of Materia Medica, Chinese Academy of Medical Sciences and Peking Union Medical College, 2A Nan Wei Road, Beijing 100050, China; zhaoyu8410@126.com (Y.Z.); wangtianen@imm.ac.cn (T.-E.W.)

2 Department of Biomedical Sciences and "Unidad Asociada IQM-CSIC", School of Medicine and Health Sciences, University of Alcalá, E-28805 Alcalá de Henares, Madrid, Spain; albertomillsfernandez@gmail.com (A.M.); federico.gago@uah.es (F.G.)

* Correspondence: wfang@imm.ac.cn; Tel.: +86-10-6316-5229

Academic Editor: Qiao-Hong Chen
Received: 23 May 2019; Accepted: 6 June 2019; Published: 8 June 2019

Abstract: A series of novel 7,9-*O*-linked macrocyclic taxoids together with modification at the C2 position were synthesized, and their cytotoxicities against drug-sensitive and P-glycoprotein and βIII-tubulin overexpressed drug-resistant cancer cell lines were evaluated. It is demonstrated that C-seco taxoids conformationally constrained via carbonate containing-linked macrocyclization display increased cytotoxicity on drug-resistant tumors overexpressing both βIII and P-gp, among which compound **22b**, bearing a 2-m-methoxybenzoyl group together with a five-atom linker, was identified as the most potent. Molecular modeling suggested the improved cytotoxicity of **22b** results from enhanced favorable interactions with the T7 loop region of βIII.

Keywords: taxoids; βIII-tubulin; P-glycoprotein; drug resistance

1. Introduction

Antitubulin agent paclitaxel (**1a**, Figure 1) and its semi-synthetic derivative docetaxel (**1b**, Figure 1) are successfully used in the clinic for the treatment of ovarian, breast, and non-small cell lung and prostate cancers and Kaposi's sarcoma.

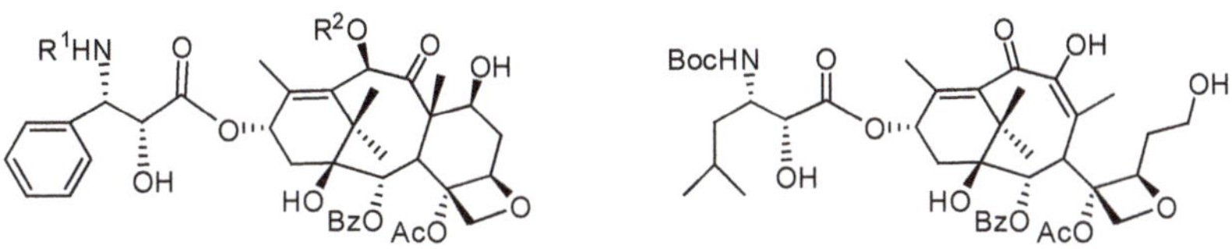

1a R^1 = Bz, R^2 = Ac
1b R^1 = Boc, R^2 = H

2

Figure 1. Structures of paclitaxel (**1a**), docetaxel (**1b**), and IDN5390 (**2**).

However, their clinical uses are severely restricted by drug resistance. Various resistance mechanisms toward taxane-based anticancer drugs have been revealed, among which only overexpression of P-glycoprotein (P-gp) and βIII-tubulin have been confirmed clinically [1–4].

A great deal of effort has been made to overcome multi-drug resistance (MDR) mediated by overexpression of P-gp. Nevertheless, many taxane-based drug candidates targeting P-gp overexpression did not achieve the expected efficacy in clinical trials [5,6].

A correlation between βIII-tubulin overexpression and poor prognosis has been reported in several human tumors, including various advanced malignancies upon treatment of taxanes, such as breast, non-small cell lung, and ovarian cancers [7–10]. It was reported that a C-seco taxane IDN5390 (**2**, Figure 1) is more active than paclitaxel in several paclitaxel-resistant human ovarian adenocarcinoma cell lines (e.g., A2780TC1, A2780TC3, and OVCAR-3), expressing high βIII-tubulin and P-gp levels. However, IDN5390 was nearly 10-fold less active than paclitaxel in paclitaxel-sensitive cells [11].

To find a modified taxane effective against both paclitaxel-sensitive and -resistant tumors, the 7,9-*O*-linked C-seco taxoid **3** (Figure 2) was synthesized in our lab and shown to exhibit significant activity enhancement against drug-sensitive Hela and βIII-tubulin overexpressing HeLa-βIII tumor cells compared to the C-seco paclitaxel derivative **4** (an analog of IDN5390, Figure 2) [12]. Those macrocyclic taxoids provided a successful example for the compromise between structural pre-organization and sufficient flexibility in the C ring of C-seco taxoids to improve the cytotoxicity against tumor cells that overexpress βIII tubulin [12].

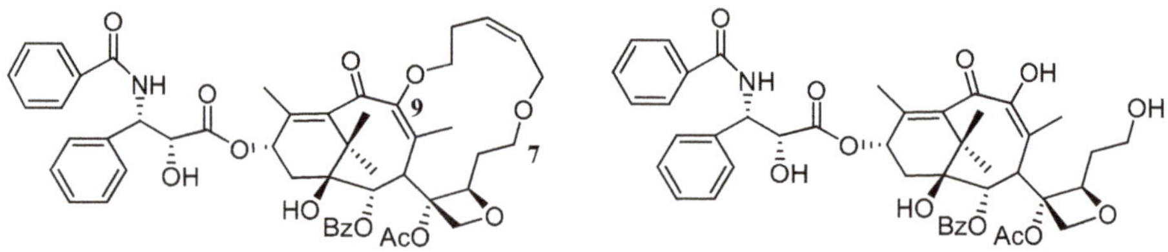

3 **4**

Figure 2. Structures of the 7,9-*O*-linked C-seco taxoid **3** and C-seco paclitaxel derivative **4**.

It has long been observed that modification of taxane at the C2 position could play a critical role in its interaction with tubulin. Consistent with this observation, the 7,9-*O*-linked C-seco taxoid with C2 modification **5** (Figure 3) was much more cytotoxic than the C-seco taxoid **6** (Figure 3) in drug-resistant A2780AD and KB-V1 cells (P-gp overexpression) and Hela-βIII (βIII overexpression) [12]. It was demonstrated that the *meta*-substitution (i.e., -OMe, -F, -Cl) of the C2-benzoate moiety of C-seco taxoids derivatives **7a–c** (Figure 3) could increase the interaction of C-seco-taxoids with βIII-tubulin to overcome paclitaxel-resistance [13].

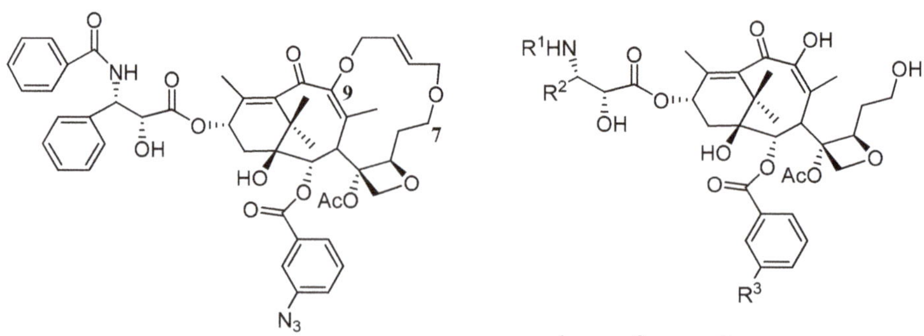

5

6 $R^1 = Ph$, $R^2 = Ph$, $R^3 = N_3$
7a $R^1 = Boc$, $R^2 = (CH_3)_2CHCH_2$, $R^3 = OCH_3$
7b $R^1 = Boc$, $R^2 = (CH_3)_2CHCH_2$, $R^3 = F$
7c $R^1 = Boc$, $R^2 = (CH_3)_2CHCH_2$, $R^3 = Cl$

Figure 3. Structures of the 7,9-*O*-linked C-seco taxoid **5** and C-seco taxoids **6, 7a–c**.

In order to explore the effect of macrocyclization in a different way from that employed in our previous study (i.e., via the carbonate formation to restrict the conformation), the synthesis and biological activity assessment of a series of 7,9-*O*-linked macrocyclic taxoids together with modification at the C2 position were performed and are reported here.

2. Results and Discussion

2.1. Chemistry

Our synthesis began with the preparation of 2′-*tert*-butyldimethylsilyl-paclitaxel **12a**, which was then converted to 10-deacetylpaclitaxel **13a** upon treatment with hydrazine hydrate in methanol. Synthesis of the analogues **12b–e** of 2′-*tert*-butyldimethylsilyl-paclitaxel with modifications at the C2 positions was then realized by selective C2 debenzoylation and then elaboration with various *m*-substituted benzoyl group. C2-modified 10-deacetylpaclitaxel **13b–e** were afforded in the same manner as compound **13a**. Then the compounds **13a–e** were oxidized by copper (II) diacetate to furnish **14a–e** as a mixture of two epimers. Reductive trapping of the ring C-seco tautomers **15a–e** were obtained by treatment with L-selectride. Subsequent deprotection with pyridine hydrofluoride (HF-pyridine) afforded **16a–e**. The 9-OH in **15a–e** was hydroxylalkylated by 2-bromoethanol or 3-bromo-1-propanol in the presence of potassium carbonate and potassium iodide in *N*,*N*-dimethylformamide (DMF). Cyclization of compounds **17a–e** could be accomplished by treatment with a slight excess of triphosgene, affording the cyclic carbonate analogues **19a–e**. Desilylation of **19a–e** with HF-pyridine afforded macrocyclic analogues **21a–e**. Accordingly, macrocyclic taxoids **22a–e** bearing a linkage with one more carbon atom were synthesized from **18a–e** in a similar manner (Scheme 1).

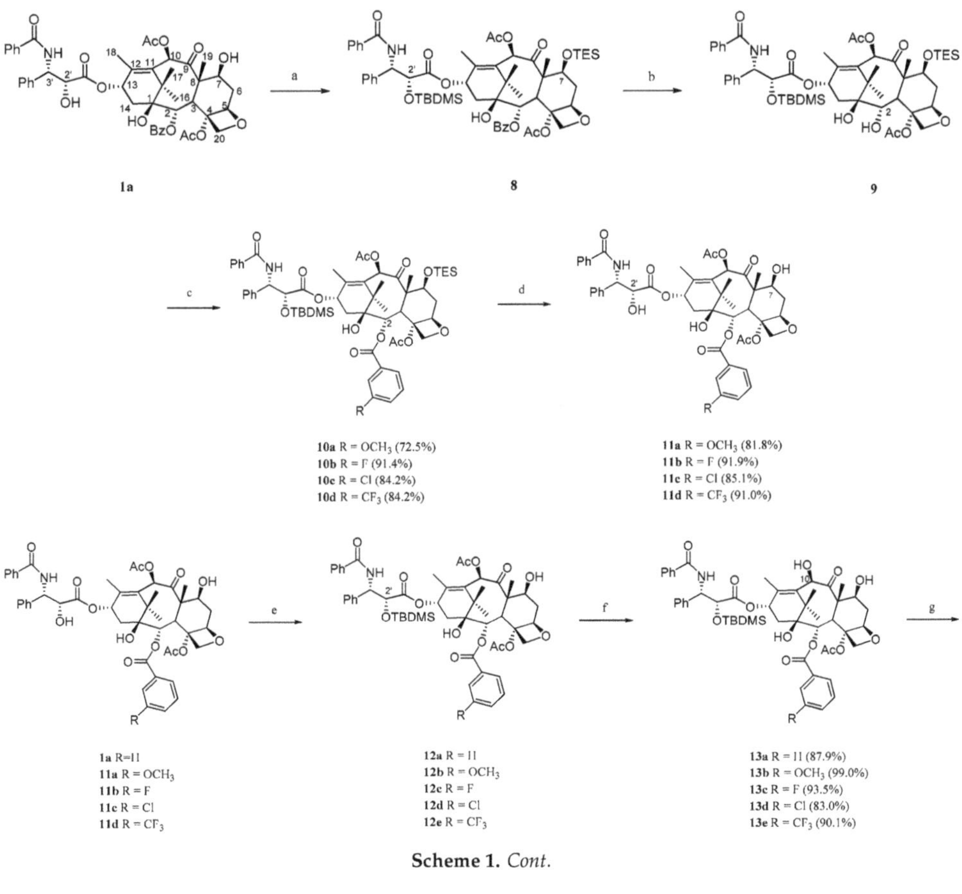

Scheme 1. *Cont.*

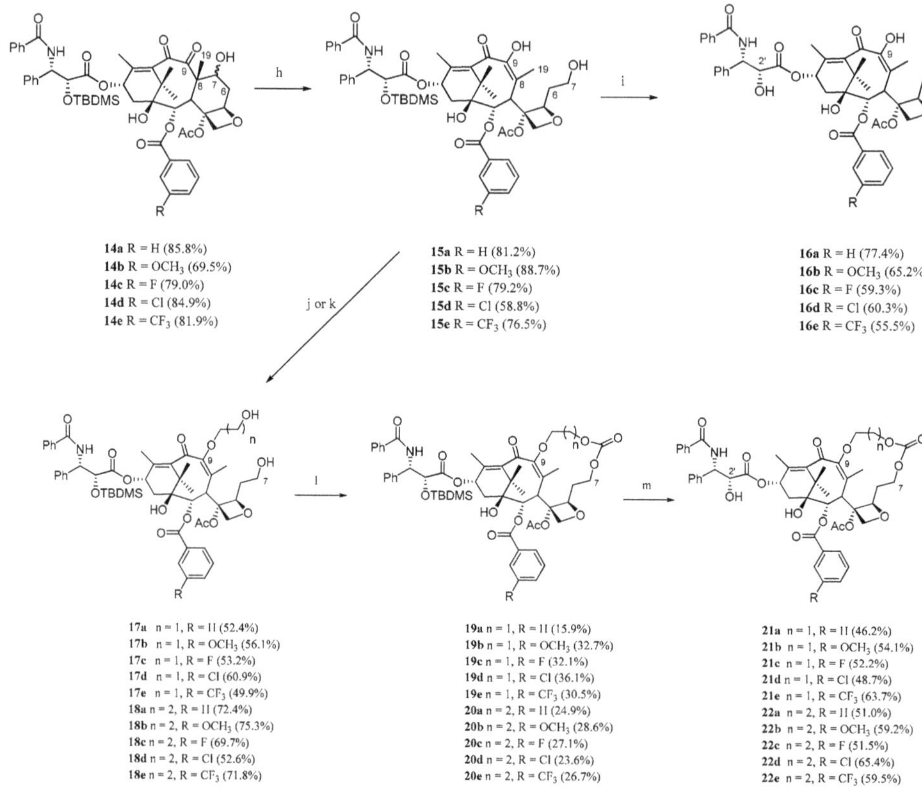

Scheme 1. (a) tert-ButyldiMethylsilyl chloride (TBDMSCl), imidazole, DMF, 2 h, 60 °C, and; triethylchlorosilane (TESCl), imidazole, DMF, overnight, r.t., 90.1%; (b) Triton-B, tetrahydrofuran (THF), 15 min, −40 °C, 47.7%; (c) (**10a**) m-anisic acid, N, N′-diisopropylcarbodiimide (DIC), 4-dimethylaminopyridine (DMAP), toluene, overnight, 60 °C, 72.5%; (**10b**) m-fluorobenzoic acid, DIC, DMAP, toluene, overnight, 60 °C, 91.4%; (**10c**) m-chlorobenzoic acid, DIC, DMAP, toluene, overnight, 60 °C, 84.2%; (**10d**) m-trifluoromethyl acid, DIC, DMAP, toluene, overnight, 60 °C, 84.2%; (d) HF -pyridine, THF, overnight, r.t.; (**11a**) 81.8%; (**11b**) 91.9%; (**11c**) 85.1%; (**11d**) 91.0%; (e) TBDMSCl, imidazole, DMF, 4 h, r.t.; (f) $NH_2NH_2{\cdot}H_2O$, C_2H_5OH, 2 h, r.t. (e and f two steps), (**13a**) 87.9%, (**13b**) 99.0%; (**13c**) 93.5%; (**13d**) 83.0%; (**13e**) 90.1%; (g) $Cu(OAc)_2{\cdot}H_2O$, CH_3OH, overnight, r.t., (**14a**) 85.8%; (**14b**) 69.5%; (**14c**) 79.0%; (**14d**) 84.9%; (**14e**) 81.9%; (h) L-selectride, THF, 15 min, −20 °C, (**15a**) 81.2%; (**15b**) 88.7%; (**15c**) 79.2%; (**15d**) 58.8%; (**15e**) 76.5%; (i) HF/Py, THF, overnight, r.t., (**16a**) 77.4%; (**16b**) 65.2%; (**16c**) 59.3%; (**16d**) 60.3%; (**16e**) 55.5%; (j) 2-bromoethanol, K_2CO_3, KI, DMF, 5–9 h, r.t., (**17a**) 52.4%; (**17b**) 56.1%; (**17c**) 53.2%; (**17d**) 60.9%; (**17e**) 49.9%; (k) 3-bromo-1-propanol, K_2CO_3, KI, DMF, 4–9 h, r.t., (**18a**) 72.4%; (**18b**) 75.3%; (**18c**) 69.7%; (**18d**) 52.6%; (**18e**) 71.8%; (l) triphosgene, pyridine, DCM, 3–5 h, 0 °C to r.t., (**19a**) 15.9%; (**19b**) 32.7%; (**19c**) 32.1%; (**19d**) 36.1%; (**19e**) 30.5%; (**20a**) 24.9%; (**20b**) 28.6%; (**20c**) 27.1%; (**20d**) 23.6%; (**20e**) 26.7%; (m) HF/Py, THF, 30 h, r.t., (**21a**) 46.2%; (**21b**) 54.1%; (**21c**) 52.2%; (**21d**) 48.7%; (**21e**) 63.7%; (**22a**) 51.0%; (**22b**) 59.2%; (**22c**) 51.5%; (**22d**) 65.4%; (**22e**) 59.5%.

2.2. *Bioactivity Evaluation of Taxoids* **21a–e** *and* **22a–e**

Taxoids **21a–e**, **22a–e**, and **16a–e** were evaluated for their in vitro cytotoxicities against cervical carcinoma HeLa cells and their corresponding drug-resistant cell lines (HeLa-βIII).

As shown in Table 1, all the 7,9-*O*-linked macrocyclic analogues (**21a–e, 22a–e**) possessed a remarkably higher potency against HeLa and HeLa-βIII cells than their corresponding C-seco taxoids analogues **16a–e**. The R/S values (IC_{50} in drug resistant cells/IC_{50} in drug sensitive cells) of all macrocyclic analogues were lower than those of their corresponding C-seco taxoids analogues **16a–e**. These findings demonstrate that conformational restraint via carbonate-containing linked macrocyclization can improve the cytotoxicity against human carcinoma cell lines overexpressing βIII tubulin.

Furthermore, all of the 7,9-*O*-linked macrocyclic analogues bearing the four-atom linker (**21a–e**) turned out to be generally more potent against sensitive HeLa cells and HeLa-βIII cells than the corresponding macrocyclic analogues bearing the five-atom linker (**22a–e**). Since the cytotoxicity of **21a–d** was approximately equal to that of paclitaxel, these results suggest that a four-atom tether is optimal in these macrocyclic C-seco taxoids.

For the effect of C2 modifications in these macrocyclic C-seco taxoids, we found similar results as previously reported [12,13]. Pepe et al. studied the cytotoxicity of a series of C-seco taxoids, whereby the introduction of a substituent (-OMe, -F, -Cl) to the *meta*-position of the C2 benzoyl moiety increased potency against the βIII-tubulin-overexpressing, paclitaxel-resistant cell line A2780TC3 [13]. Taxoid **6** bearing a 2-(*m*-azido) benzyloxy group and synthesized in our lab exhibited higher binding affinity for microtubulin (MT) than its corresponding taxoids bearing a 2-benzyloxy group [12]. The 7,9-*O*-linked C-seco taxoid bearing a 2-(*m*-azido) benzyloxy group **5** was significantly more active than **6** on drug-resistant A2780AD, HeLa-βIII, and KB-V1 cells [12].

We investigated this effect in the 7,9-*O*-linked C-seco taxoids **21b–e** and **22b–e** reported here. Thus, introduction of a *meta* substituent (-OMe, -F, -Cl) on derivatives bearing the four-atom linker showed similar cytotoxicity against HeLa sensitive cell lines and Hela-βIII cells lines as their corresponding C-seco taxoid **21a** bearing a 2-benzyloxy group. In contrast, the *meta*-substituted (-OMe, -F, -Cl) derivatives bearing five-atom linker possessed higher potency against HeLa-βIII cells lines than its corresponding C-seco taxoid **22a** (by a factor of 3.1–8.9). Nonetheless, the 2-*m*-CF_3 analogues **21e** and **22e** were considerably less cytotoxic against both drug sensitive and resistant cells by one to two orders of magnitude.

The growth inhibition effects of the 7,9-*O*-linked macrocyclic analogues were also measured on human breast cancer MCF-7 cells and their corresponding P-gp-overexpressing drug-resistant MCF-7/R cells. As shown in Table 1, the 7,9-*O*-linked macrocyclic analogues possessed remarkable potency against MCF-7/R cells compared to their C-seco counterparts, except for the 2-*m*-CF_3 derivatives. Strikingly, macrocyclic taxoids bearing the five-atom linker were almost inactive. The cytotoxicity against MCF-7/R cells of the 7,9-*O*-linked macrocyclic derivatives (-OMe, -F, -Cl) bearing the five-atom linker were slightly higher than that of the compouds bearing the four-atom linker. Compounds **22b–d** (-OMe, -F, -Cl) bearing the five-atom linker and **21a**, **21d** (-H, -Cl) bearing the four-atom linker displayed lower R/S values than that of paclitaxel. All in all, **22b** turned out to be the best compound in the whole series.

Table 1. Cytotoxicity of taxoids **16a–e**, **21a–e**, and **22a–e**.

Compound	Cytotoxicity (IC_{50}, nM)		Ratio	Cytotoxicity (IC_{50}, nM)		Ratio
	HeLa	HeLa-βIII	R/S	MCF-7	MCF-7/R	R/S
21a	5.97 ± 1.13	29.92 ± 2.85	5.01 ± 0.48	11.82 ± 1.10	6291.33 ± 1252.19	532.26 ± 105.94
21b	5.90 ± 1.47	17.61 ± 2.13	3.17 ± 0.25	9.93 ± 2.70	6440.00 ± 1040.85	648.76 ± 104.85
21c	7.82 ± 3.10	22.14 ± 6.36	2.83 ± 0.81	7.70 ± 1.68	6411.67 ± 645.71	832.68 ± 83.86
21d	7.75 ± 2.24	19.02 ± 9.60	2.46 ± 1.24	9.36 ± 1.76	4126.33 ± 91.92	440.85 ± 9.82
21e	186.03 ± 48.30	503.40 ± 132.41	2.61 ± 0.98	159.80 ± 33.91	>10,000	
22a	28.28 ± 0.47	162.33 ± 58.80	5.74 ± 2.08	19.16 ± 2.39	>10,000	
22b	7.97 ± 1.79	18.11 ± 2.91	1.52 ± 1.34	5.15 ± 0.96	2769.00 ± 399.24	538.02 ± 77.57
22c	12.07 ± 0.93	52.40 ± 16.98	4.34 ± 1.41	9.33 ± 1.44	4756.33 ± 443.24	509.79 ± 47.51
22d	11.53 ± 1.98	50.11 ± 16.92	4.35 ± 1.47	14.48 ± 3.37	3704.67 ± 539.43	255.79 ± 37.24
22e	89.71 ± 29.80	267.20 ± 65.38	2.77 ± 0.89	86.00 ± 9.28	>10,000	
16a	149.57 ± 31.70	1423.67 ± 291.75	8.55 ± 1.75	103.53 ± 22.21	>10,000	
16b	13.63 ± 2.09	142.90 ± 5.66	10.48 ± 0.42	7.53 ± 0.19	>10,000	
16c	22.78 ± 2.20	467.13 ± 171.75	20.50 ± 7.54	16.90 ± 4.04	>10,000	
16d	17.73 ± 1.70	181.17 ± 18.92	10.22 ± 1.07	15.08 ± 1.65	>10,000	
16e	110.14 ± 17.40	525.87 ± 88.76	4.77 ± 0.81	110.90 ± 13.25	>10,000	
Paclitaxel	4.59 ± 0.55	12.31 ± 1.27	2.68 ± 0.28	6.21 ± 1.85	3450.00 ± 509.99	555.56 ± 82.12

2.3. *Binding Mode of* **22b** *and Rationale for the Increased Affinity for the βIII Isotype*

Inspection of the paclitaxel-β-tubulin complex in high-resolution cryo-electron microscopy (cryo-EM) structures of mammalian microtubules reveals a very tight fit between the bulky drug and the taxane-binding site, in which the M-loop is structured as an α-helix [14]. The oxetane ring oxygen of paclitaxel (**1a**) accepts a hydrogen bond from the backbone NH of Thr276, whereas the C-3′ benzamide carbonyl oxygen acts as a hydrogen bond acceptor for N^{ε} of His229. These two hydrogen bonds are likely to be present in the **22b**:β-tubulin complex as well (Figure 4), and definitely contribute to the binding affinity, but these two residues are common to both βIIB and βIII isotypes. In the search for sequence differences that can account for the resistance to taxanes, a lot of emphasis has been placed on the Ser→Ala replacement at position 277, but we believe that the most important replacement in relation to drug resistance possibly involves Cys241→Ser. The reason is that, as a consequence of this substitution, disulfide bond formation with Cys356 is precluded in the βIII isotype and the T7 loop region, which closes over the bound taxane, is likely to be more flexible. By directing the macrocyclic region of **22b** towards this loop, favorable interactions within the taxane-binding site are enhanced and the affinity towards the βIII isotype is improved. We hypothesize that the improved cytotoxicity of **22b** relative to **1a**, and the other taxanes described here, results from enhanced favorable interactions with the T7 loop region of βIII, an isotype in which Cys356 cannot engage in a disulfide bond with the amino acid present at position 241 (Ser).

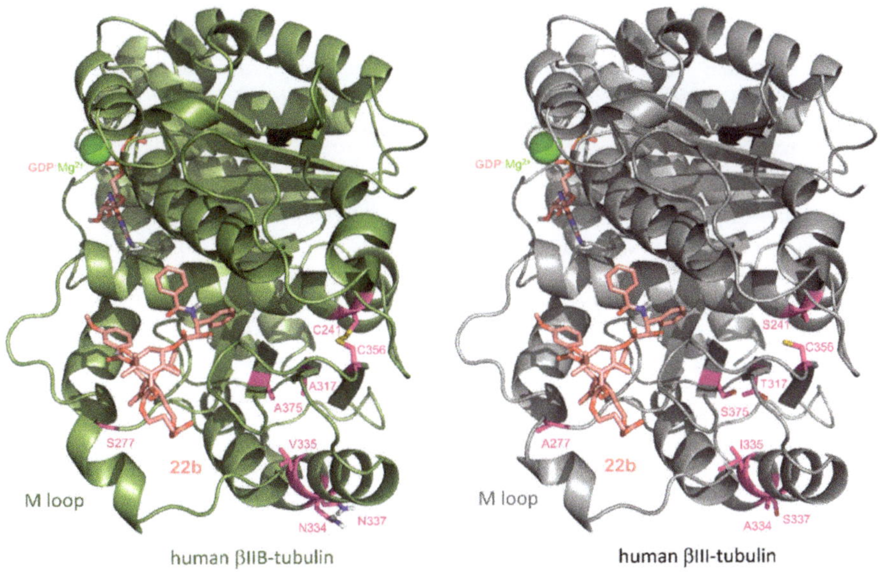

Figure 4. 22b docked into homology models of human tubulins IIb and III bound to guanosine diphosphate (GDP)-Mg^{2+}. Colored in magenta and labeled are those residues close to the taxane-binding site that differ between these two isotypes.

As shown in this modelling study, the binding of these taxoids to microtubules are similar to that of paclitaxel. Although cyclization does increase the cytotoxicity either in drug-sensitive and -resistant cells in most cases, the 7,9-*O*-linked macrocyclic taxoids only showed comparable cytotoxicity to that of paclitaxel. The enhanced activity is not only arisen from the known C-2 modifications [15,16], but also from the cyclization of the cleaved C-ring of taxane.

3. Experimental

3.1. Chemical Synthesis

3.1.1. General Methods

All chemicals and reagents were purchased from Beijing Innochem Science and Technology Co. Ltd. (Beijing, China), Sinopharm Chemical Reagent Co. Ltd. (Beijing, China), and thin-layer chromatography (TCI). The 200–300 mesh silica gel used for flash column chromatography was purchased from Rushanshi Shuangbang Xincailiao Co. Ltd. (Rushan, Shandong, China). Visualization on TLC (analytical thin layer chromatography) was achieved by the use of UV light (254 nm) and treatment with phosphomolybdic acid or $KMnO_4$ followed by heating. All solvents were purified and dried according to the standard procedures. The purification was performed on flash column chromatography. The high performance liquid chromatography (HPLC)- electrospray ionization (ESI)-mass spectrometry (MS) analysis was carried out in an Agilent 1260 Infinity HPLC system (Agilent Technologies, Waldbronn, Germany) equipped with a reversed phase 4.68 × 50 mm (1.8 um) XDB-C18 Column and consisted of a binary solvent delivery system, an auto sampler, a column temperature controller, and an UV detector. The mass spectra were acquired by a 6120 Quadrupole LC-MS mass spectrometer (Agilent Technologies, Waldbronn, Germany) connected to the HPLC system via an ESI interface. Proton and carbon magnetic resonance spectra (^{1}H-NMR and ^{13}C-NMR) were recorded on a Bruker BioSpin AG 300 or 400 MHz spectrometer or Varian 300, 400, or 600 MHz spectrometer.^{1}H-NMR data were reported as follows: Chemical shifts, multiplicity (s = singlet, d = doublet, t = triplet, q = quartet, m=multiplet), coupling constant(s) in Hz, integration. All tested compounds **16a–e**, **21a–e**, and **22a–e** were ≥95% pure by HPLC (column XDB C18 4.6 × 50 mm 1.8 μm, mobile phase: acetonitrile-water (10:90–100:0 gradient in 4.5 min), flow rate 1.0 mL/min, detected at 220 nm).

3.1.2. General Experimental Procedure for Compounds **14a–e**

2′-O-(tert-Butyldimethylsilyl)-10-dehydro-10-deacetylpaclitaxel (**14a**). To a solution of **13a** (261.3 mg, 0.282 mmol) in methanol (8 mL) was added $Cu(OAc)_2{\cdot}H_2O$ (282 mg, 1.41 mmol). The suspension was stirred at room temperature overnight (open air) and then diluted with ethyl acetate. The organic phase was washed sequentially with saturated aqueous NaCl (50 mL), 2 N NH_3 to remove copper salts and saturated aqueous NH_4Cl. After drying (Na_2SO_4) and evaporation under reduced pressure, the crude product was purified by silica gel chromatography (ethyl acetate: petroleum ether = 1:2) to give a 4:1 mixture of epimers **14a** (14-β-OH and 14-α-OH, 223.8 mg, 85.8% total yield). ^{1}H-NMR ($CDCl_3$, 600 MHz) δ: 8.19 (d, *J* = 7.8 Hz, 1H, Ar-H), 7.73 (d, *J* = 7.8 Hz, 2H, Ar-H), 7.48 (m, 11H, Ar-H), 7.06 (d, *J* = 9.0 Hz, 1H, NH), 6.28 (t, *J* = 8.7 Hz, 1H, H-13), 5.87 (d, *J* = 7.2 Hz, 1H, H-2), 5.79 (dd, *J* = 1.5, 8.7 Hz, 1H, H-3′), 4.93 (m, 1H, H-5), 4.67 (d, *J* = 1.8 Hz, 1H, H-2′), 4.50 (d, *J* = 11.4 Hz, 1H, H-7), 4.44 (d, *J* = 8.4 Hz, 1H, H- 20a), 4.38 (d, *J* = 9.0 Hz, 1H, H-20b), 4.04 (d, *J* = 7.2 Hz, 1H, H-3), 3.88 (m, 1H, OH-7), 2.67 (s, 3H, CH_3), 2.48 (dd, *J* = 9.6, 15.6 Hz, 1H, H-6a), 2.29 (m, 2H, H-14b, H-14a), 2.19 (m, 1H, H-6b), 1.86 (s, 3H, CH_3), 1.75 (s, 3H, CH_3), 1.21 (s, 3H, CH_3), 1.13 (s, 3H, CH_3), 0.79 (s, 9H, $SiC(CH_3)_3$), −0.04 (s, 3H, $Si(CH_3)$), −0.30 (s, 3H, $Si(CH_3)$). (For the chemical characterization refer to http://dx.doi.org/10.1016/j.ejmech.2017.06.001)

2′-O-(tert-Butyldimethylsilyl)-2-debenzoyl-2-(3-methoxybenzoyl)-7-epi-10-dehydro-10-deacetylpaclitaxel (**14b**). 69.5% yield as a 4:1 mixture of two epimers; ^{1}H-NMR ($CDCl_3$, 400 MHz) δ: 7.80 (d, *J* = 7.7 Hz, 1H, Ar-H), 7.74 (d, *J* = 7.2 Hz, 2H, Ar-H), 7.41 (m, 10H, Ar-H), 7.21 (dd, *J* = 2.0, 8.0 Hz, Ar-H), 7.09 (d, *J* = 9.1 Hz, 1H, NH), 6.27 (t, *J* = 8.9 Hz, 1H, H-13), 5.89 (d, *J* = 7.2 Hz, 1H, H-2), 5.79 (dd, *J* = 2.2, 9.4 Hz, 1H, H-3′), 4.94 (m, 1H, H-5), 4.67 (d, *J* = 2.0 Hz, 1H, H-2′), 4.50 (d, *J* = 11.2 Hz, 1H, H-7), 4.47 (d, *J* = 8.8 Hz, 1H, H- 20a), 4.38 (d, *J* = 8.6 Hz, 1H, H-20b), 4.05 (d, *J* = 7.1 Hz, 1H, H-3), 3.90 (s, 3H, OCH_3), 3.88 (m, 1H, OH-7), 2.67 (s, 3H, CH_3), 2.49 (dd, *J* = 9.8, 15.4 Hz, 1H, H-6a), 2.29 (m, 2H, H-14b, H-14a), 1.86 (s, 3H, CH_3), 2.25 (m, 1H, H-6b), 1.75 (s, 3H, CH_3), 1.21(s, 3H, CH_3), 1.13 (s, 3H, CH_3), 0.81 (s, 9H, $SiC(CH_3)_3$), −0.02 (s, 3H, $Si(CH_3)$), −0.26 (s, 3H, $Si(CH_3)$); ^{13}C-NMR ($CDCl_3$, 100 MHz) δ: 207.8, 188.7,

172.2, 170.9, 167.0, 166.9, 159.8, 143.3, 141.1, 138.2, 134.1, 131.9, 130.3, 130.0, 128.8 (2C), 128.1, 127.0, 126.4, 122.7, 120.5, 114.4, 82.7, 81.8, 79.2, 77.4, 75.3, 75.1, 70.7, 57.2, 55.5 (2C), 40.3, 39.4, 36.3, 35.4, 26.9, 26.1, 25.5, 22.9, 18.2, 15.0, 14.4, −5.2, −5.8; LC-MS (ESI, *m/z*): [M + 1], found 954.4, [M + 23], found 976.4, $C_{52}H_{63}NO_{14}Si$: 953.40 (see supplementary materials).

2′-O-(tert-Butyldimethylsilyl)-2-debenzoyl-2-(3-fluorobenzoyl)-7-epi-10-dehydro-10-deacetylpaclitaxel (**14c**). 79.0% yield as a 4:1 mixture of two epimers; ^{1}H-NMR ($CDCl_3$, 400 MHz) δ: 8.02 (d, *J* = 8.0 Hz, 1H, Ar-H), 7.89–7.86 (m, 1H, Ar-H), 7.73 (d, *J* = 7.2 Hz, 2H, Ar-H), 7.59–7.33 (m, 10H, Ar-H), 7.07 (d, *J* = 9.2 Hz, 1H, BzNH), 6.27 (t, *J* = 8.8 Hz, 1H, H-13), 5.86 (d, *J* = 7.2 Hz, 1H, H-2), 5.80 (dd, *J* = 2.0, 9.2 Hz, 1H, H-3′), 4.95 (dd, *J* = 4.0, 8.0 Hz, 1H, H-5), 4.68 (d, *J* = 2.4 Hz, 1H, H-2′), 4.48 (d, *J* = 11.2 Hz, 1H, H-7), 4.44 (d, *J* = 8.8 Hz, 1H, H- 20a), 4.36 (d, *J* = 8.8 Hz, 1H, H-20b), 4.05 (d, *J* = 7.2 Hz, 1H, H-3), 3.92–3.88 (m, 1H, OH-7), 2.68 (s, 3H, $COCH_3$), 2.48 (dd, *J* = 9.6, 15.2 Hz, 1H, H-6a), 2.31–2.29 (m, 2H, H-14b, H-14a), 2.22 (dd, *J* = 8.4, 15.6 Hz, 1H, H-6b), 1.99 (br, 1H, OH), 1.86 (s, 3H, CH_3), 1.76 (s, 3H, CH_3), 1.22 (s, 3H, CH_3), 1.13 (s, 3H, CH_3), 0.81 (s, 9H, $SiC(CH_3)$)), −0.02 (s, 3H, $Si(CH_3)$)), −0.26 (s, 3H, $Si(CH_3)_2$); ^{13}C-NMR ($CDCl_3$, 100 MHz) δ: 207.8, 188.6, 172.3, 171.2, 170.9, 167.0, 165.9 (d, $^4J_{C\text{-}F}$ = 2.9 Hz), 162.7 (d, $^1J_{C\text{-}F}$ = 246.5 Hz), 143.5, 140.9, 138.2, 134.1, 131.9, 131.3 (d, $^3J_{C\text{-}F}$ = 7.3 Hz), 130.7 (d, $^3J_{C\text{-}F}$ = 7.6 Hz), 128.83 (2C), 128.77 (2C), 128.1, 127.0 (2C), 126.4 (2C), 126.1 (d, $^4J_{C\text{-}F}$ = 3.1 Hz), 120.0 (d, $^2J_{C\text{-}F}$ = 21.1 Hz), 117.1 (d, $^2J_{C\text{-}F}$ = 23.1 Hz), 82.8, 81.7, 79.4, 75.5, 75.3, 70.6, 57.2, 55.6, 40.3, 39.5, 36.3, 35.4, 26.1, 25.5 (3C), 22.9 (2C), 18.2, 15.0, 14.5, 14.2, −5.2, −5.8; LC-MS (ESI, *m/z*): [M + 1], found 942.4, [M + 23], found 964.3, $C_{51}H_{60}FNO_{13}Si$: 941.38.

2′-O-(tert-Butyldimethylsilyl)-2-debenzoyl-2-(3-chlorobenzoyl)-7-epi-10-dehydro-10-deacetylpaclitaxel (**14d**). 84.9% yield as a 4:1 mixture of two epimers; ^{1}H-NMR ($CDCl_3$, 400 MHz) δ: 8.18 (s, 1H, Ar-H), 8.11 (d, *J* = 7.6 Hz, 1H, Ar-H), 7.73 (d, *J* = 7.6 Hz, 2H, Ar-H), 7.62 (d, *J* = 7.6 Hz, 1H, Ar-H), 7.55–7.50 (m, 2H, Ar-H), 7.44–7.35 (m, 7H, Ar-H), 7.08 (d, *J* = 8.8 Hz, 1H, BzNH), 6.25 (t, *J* = 8.8 Hz, 1H, H-13), 5.84 (d, *J* = 7.2 Hz, 1H, H-2), 5.79 (dd, *J* = 8.8 Hz, 1H, H-3′), 4.96 (m, 1H, H-5), 4.67 (d, *J* = 2.0 Hz, 1H, H-2′), 4.47 (d, *J* = 11.2 Hz, 1H, H-7), 4.44 (d, *J* = 8.4 Hz, 1H, H- 20a), 4.35 (d, *J* = 8.4 Hz, 1H, H-20b), 4.05 (d, *J* = 7.2 Hz, 1H, H-3), 3.89 (m, 1H, OH-7), 2.68 (s, 3H, CH_3), 2.48 (dd, *J* = 10.0, 15.4 Hz, 1H, H-6a), 2.29 (m, 2H, H-14b, H-14a), 2.23 (m, 1H, H-6b), 1.86 (s, 3H, CH_3), 1.76 (s, 3H, CH_3), 1.22 (s, 3H, CH_3), 1.13 (s, 3H, CH_3), 0.82 (s, 9H, $SiC(CH_3)_3$), −0.02 (s, 3H, $Si(CH_3)$)), −0.26 (s, 3H, $Si(CH_3)$)); ^{13}C-NMR ($CDCl_3$, 100 MHz) δ: 207.8, 188.6, 172.2, 170.9, 165.7, 143.5, 140.9, 138.2, 134.9, 134.1, 133.9, 131.9, 130.9, 130.4, 130.3, 128.83 (2C), 128.77 (2C), 128.5, 128.1, 127.0 (2C), 126.5 (2C), 82.7, 81.7, 79.4, 75.4, 75.3, 70.7, 60.4, 57.2, 55.6, 40.2, 39.4, 36.3, 35.3, 29.7, 26.1, 25.5 (2C), 22.9, 22.8, 18.2, 14.9, 14.5, −5.2, −5.8; LC-MS (ESI, *m/z*): [M + 1], found 958.4, [M + 23], found 980.4, $C_{51}H_{60}ClNO_{13}Si$: 957.35.

2′-O-(tert-Butyldimethylsilyl)-2-debenzoyl-2-(3-trifluoromethyl)-7-epi-10-dehydro-10-deacetylpaclitaxel (**14e**). 81.9% yield as a 4:1 mixture of two epimers; ^{1}H-NMR ($CDCl_3$, 400 MHz) δ: 8.50 (s, 1H, Ar-H), 8.43 (d, *J* = 7.6 Hz, 1H, Ar-H), 7.91 (d, *J* = 8.0 Hz, 1H, Ar-H), 7.72 (d, *J* = 7.8 Hz, 3H, Ar-H), 7.51 (m, 1H, Ar-H), 7.41 (m, 7H, Ar-H), 7.06 (d, *J* = 9.2 Hz, 1H, BzNH), 6.24 (t, *J* = 8.6 Hz, 1H, H-13), 5.88 (d, *J* = 7.6 Hz, 1H, H-2), 5.78 (dd, *J* = 1.6, 9.2 Hz, 1H, H-3′), 4.97 (m, 1H, H-5), 4.67 (d, *J* = 2.0 Hz, 1H, H-2′), 4.45 (d, *J* = 11.2 Hz, 1H, H-7), 4.42 (d, *J* = 8.5 Hz, 1H, H-20a), 4.37 (d, *J* = 8.6 Hz, 1H, H-20b), 4.09 (d, *J* = 7.6 Hz, 1H, H-3), 3.90 (m, 1H, OH-7), 2.66 (s, 3H, CH_3), 2.51 (dd, *J* = 9.6, 15.5 Hz, 1H, H-6a), 2.30 (m, 2H, H-14b, H-14a), 2.26 (m, 1H, H-6b), 1.87 (s, 3H, CH_3), 1.77 (s, 3H, CH_3), 1.23 (s, 3H, CH_3), 1.15 (s, 3H, CH_3), 0.83 (s, 9H, $SiC(CH_3)_3$), −0.02 (s, 3H, $Si(CH_3)$)), −0.24 (s, 3H, $Si(CH_3)$)); ^{13}C-NMR ($CDCl_3$, 100 MHz) δ: 207.7, 188.6, 172.1, 171.0, 167.1, 165.6, 143.6, 140.9, 138.3, 134.2, 133.6, 131.9, 131.4 (q, $^2J_{C\text{-}F}$ = 33.2 Hz), 130.3 (q, ^3J = 3.4 Hz), 130.3, 130.1, 129.9, 128.9, 128.8, 128.1, 127.1 (q, $^3J_{C\text{-}F}$ = 4.0 Hz), 127.0, 126.5, 123.7 (q, $^1J_{C\text{-}F}$ = 273.6 Hz), 82.8, 81.7, 79.5, 75.6, 75.3, 70.7, 57.2, 55.6, 40.3, 39.5, 36.3, 35.4, 26.1, 25.6, 22.9, 22.7, 18.2, 14.9, 14.5, −5.2, −5.8; LC-MS (ESI, *m/z*): [M + 1], found 992.0, $C_{52}H_{60}F_3NO_{13}Si$: 991.38.

3.1.3. General Experimental Procedure for Compounds **15a–e**

2′-tert-Butyldimethylsilyl-10-dehydro-7-8-seco-10-deacetylpaclitaxel (**15a**). L-selectride (1M solution in THF, 0.8 mL) was added, dropwise, to a solution of **14a** (171.5 mg, 0.186 mmol) in THF (4.1 mL) at −20 °C. After 15 min, the reaction was quenched by addition of cold ethyl acetate (50.0 mL) and 2 N H_2SO_4 (4.0 mL). The reaction mixture was extracted with ethyl acetate and the combined organic phases were washed with a saturated aqueous $NaHCO_3$ and saturated aqueous NH_4Cl. The resulting solution was dried over anhydrous $MgSO_4$ and the solvent evaporated under reduced pressure to give a crude product. The crude product was purified by silica gel chromatography (ethyl acetate: petroleum ether = 1:1) which gave product **15a** (139.5 mg, 81.2% yield) as a white solid

2′-tert-Butyldimethylsilyl-2-debenzoyl-2-(3-methoxybenzoyl)-10-dehydro-7,8-seco-10-deacetylpaclitaxel (**15b**). White solid; yield 88.7%; ^{1}H-NMR ($CDCl_3$, 400 MHz) δ: 7.73–7.70 (m, 3H, Ar-H), 7.55 (s, 1H, Ar-H), 7.42 (m, 10H, Ar-H), 7.14 (dd, *J* = 2.3, 8.2 Hz, 1H, BzNH), 6.47 (s, 1H, OH-9), 6.29 (t, *J* = 8.0 Hz, 1H, H-13), 5.91 (d, *J* = 8.8 Hz, 1H, H-3′), 5.60 (d, *J* = 9.2 Hz, 1H, H-2), 5.24 (brs, 2H, H-5, H-20a), 4.72 (d, *J* = 1.6 Hz, 1H, H-2′), 4.29 (d, *J* = 6.8 Hz, 1H, H-3), 4.20 (brs, 1H, H-7a), 3.96 (brs, 1H, OH), 3.85 (s, 4H, OCH_3, H-7b), 2.82 (brs, 1H, H-6a), 2.71 (brs, 1H, OH), 2.26 (dd, *J* = 9.6, 15.6 Hz, 2H, H-14a, H-14b), 2.09–2.02 (m, 4H, CH_3, H-6b), 1.87 (brs, 6H, 2 × CH_3), 1.28 (s, 3H, CH_3), 1.10 (s, 3H, CH_3), 0.79 (s, 9H, $SiC(CH_3)_3$), −0.11 (s, 3H, $Si(CH_3)$), −0.28 (s, 3H, $Si(CH_3)$); ^{13}C-NMR ($CDCl_3$, 100 MHz) δ: 191.2, 171.2, 171.1, 168.9, 167.4, 167.2, 159.8, 148.9, 142.1, 138.2, 133.9, 131.9, 130.5, 130.3, 128.7 (4C), 128.0, 127.1 (2C), 126.7 (2C), 124.6, 122.2, 119.5, 115.0, 86.3, 76.1, 75.1, 70.6, 59.2, 55.8, 55.5, 43.1, 36.6, 25.5 (3C), 23.4, 22.2, 21.5, 18.3, 14.8, 14.4, −5.6, −6.0; LC-MS (ESI, *m/z*): [M + 1], found 956.4, [M + 23], found 978.4, $C_{52}H_{65}NO_{14}Si$: 955.42.

2′-tert-Butyldimethylsilyl-2-debenzoyl-2-(3-fluorobenzoyl)-10-dehydro-7,8-seco-10-deacetylpaclitaxel (**15c**). White solid; yield 79.2%; ^{1}H-NMR ($CDCl_3$, 400 MHz) δ: 7.94 (d, *J* = 7.8 Hz, 1H, Ar-H), 7.76 (d, *J* = 8.7 Hz, 1H, Ar-H), 7.68 (d, *J* = 7.4 Hz, 2H, Ar-H), 7.53–7.44 (m, 3H, Ar-H), 7.40–7.30 (m, 8H, NH, Ar-H), 6.48 (s, 1H, OH-9), 6.30 (t, *J* = 8.0 Hz, 1H, H-13), 5.92 (d, *J* = 9.0 Hz, 1H, H-3′), 5.60 (d, *J* = 9.5 Hz, 1H, H-2), 5.25 (brs, 2H, H-5, H-20a), 4.71 (d, *J* = 2.1 Hz, 1H, H-2′), 4.30 (d, *J* = 7.8 Hz, 1H, H-3), 4.19 (brs, 1H, H-20b), 3.96 (brs, 1H, H-7a), 3.80 (brs, 1H, H-7b), 2.78 (brs, 1H, H-6a), 2.69 (brs, 1H, H-14a), 2.26 (dd, *J* = 9.5, 15.6 Hz, 1H, H-14b), 2.10–2.00 (ovelap, 1H, H-6b), 1.90 (s, 3H, CH_3), 1.86 (overlap and brs, 6H, 2 × CH_3), 1.27 (s, 3H, CH_3), 1.10 (s, 3H, CH_3), 0.78 (s, 9H, $SiC(CH_3)_3$), −0.09 (s, 3H, $Si(CH_3)$), −0.29 (s, 3H, $Si(CH_3)$); ^{13}C-NMR ($CDCl_3$, 100 MHz) δ: 191.1, 171.2, 171.0, 168.8, 167.4, 166.4, 131.0 (d, $^1J_{C\text{-}F}$ = 248.1 Hz), 128.8 (2C), 128.1, 127.1, 126.7, 125.8 (d, $^4J_{C\text{-}F}$ = 2.6 Hz), 124.6, 121.1 (d, $^2J_{C\text{-}F}$ = 21.3 Hz), 116.7 (d, $^2J_{C\text{-}F}$ = 22.6 Hz), 86.5, 80.7, 76.1, 75.5, 70.5, 59.0, 55.8, 44.5, 43.2, 36.7, 25.6, 22.3, 21.6, 18.3, 14.9, 14.5, −5.4, −5.9; LC-MS (ESI, *m/z*): [M + 1], found 944.4, [M + 23], found 966.4, $C_{51}H_{62}FNO_{13}Si$: 943.40.

2′-tert-Butyldimethylsilyl-2-debenzoyl-2-(3-chlorobenzoyl)-10-dehydro-7,8-seco-10-deacetylpaclitaxel (**15d**). White solid; yield 58.8%; ^{1}H-NMR ($CDCl_3$, 400 MHz) δ: 8.05 (d, *J* = 7.6 Hz, 2H, Ar-H), 8.01 (s, 1H, Ar-H), 7.68 (d, *J* = 7.6 Hz, 2H, Ar-H), 7.57 (d, *J* = 8.0 Hz, 1H, Ar-H), 7.41–7.31 (m, 9H, NH, Ar-H), 6.49 (s, 1H, OH-9), 6.29 (t, *J* = 8.4 Hz, 1H, H-13), 5.92 (d, *J* = 9.3 Hz, 1H, H-3′), 5.59 (d, *J* = 9.5 Hz, 1H, H-2), 5.23 (brs, 2H, H-5, H-20a), 4.71 (d, *J* = 1.6 Hz, 1H, H-2′), 4.30 (d, *J* = 6.9 Hz, 1H, H-3), 4.18 (brs, 1H, H- 20b), 3.98 (brs, 1H, H-7a), 3.83 (brs, 1H, H-7b), 2.78 (brs, 1H, H-6a), 2.67 (brs, 1H, H-14a), 2.25 (dd, *J* = 9.6, 15.6 Hz, 1H, H-14b), 2.05 (m, 1H, H-6b), 1.89 (s, 3H, CH_3), 1.85 (brs, 6H, 2 × CH_3), 1.26 (s, 3H, CH_3), 1.10 (s, 3H, CH_3), 0.78 (s, 9H, $SiC(CH_3)_3$), −0.11 (s, 3H, $Si(CH_3)$), −0.28 (s, 3H, $Si(CH_3)$); ^{13}C-NMR ($CDCl_3$, 100 MHz) δ: 191.1, 171.0, 168.7, 167.4, 166.3, 148.9, 142.0, 138.0, 137.1, 135.0, 133.9, 131.9, 131.0, 130.6, 129.6, 128.7 (2C), 128.1, 128.0, 127.0 (2C), 126.7 (2C), 124.5, 86.4, 87.0, 80.5, 76.0, 75.4, 70.5, 55.7, 43.1, 36.6, 29.7, 26.9, 25.5 (3C), 22.2, 21.5, 18.3, 14.8, 14.5, −5.5, −6.0; LC-MS (ESI, *m/z*): [M + 1], found 960.0, [M + 23], found 981.9, $C_{51}H_{62}ClNO_{13}Si$: 959.37.

2′-tert-Butyldimethylsilyl-2-debenzoyl-2-(3-trifluoromethylbenzoyl)-10-dehydro-7,8-seco-10-deacetylpaclitaxel (**15e**). White solid; yield 76.5%; ^{1}H-NMR ($CDCl_3$, 400 MHz) δ: 8.38 (d, *J* = 7.9 Hz, 2H, Ar-H), 7.84 (d, *J* = 7.9 Hz, 2H, Ar-H), 7.48 (m, 11H, NH, Ar-H), 6.51 (s, 1H, OH-9), 6.29 (t, *J* = 8.4 Hz, 1H, H-13), 5.89 (d,

J = 9.3 Hz, 1H, H-3′), 5.62 (d, J = 9.4 Hz, 1H, H-2), 5.25 (brs, 2H, H-5, H-20a), 4.72 (brs, 1H, H-2′), 4.32 (d, J = 6.8 Hz, 1H, H-3), 4.24 (brs, 1H, H- 20b), 3.94 (brs, 1H, H-7a), 3.76 (brs, 1H, H-7b), 2.78 (brs, 1H, H-6a), 2.66 (brs, 1H, H-14a), 2.28 (dd, J = 9.5, 15.6 Hz, 1H, H-14b), 2.05 (m, 1H, H-6b), 1.92 (s, 3H, CH_3), 1.85 (brs, 6H, 2 × CH_3), 1.27 (s, 3H, CH_3), 1.11 (s, 3H, CH_3), 0.78 (s, 9H, $SiC(CH_3)_3$), −0.08 (s, 3H, $Si(CH_3)$), −0.29 (s, 3H, $Si(CH_3)$); ^{13}C-NMR ($CDCl_3$, 100 MHz) δ: 191.0, 170.9, 167.5, 166.2, 148.9, 142.1, 137.9, 133.9, 133.1, 131.9, 131.4 (q, $^2J_{C\text{-}F}$ = 33.3 Hz), 130.2, 128.7, 128.0, 126.9, 126.7 (q, $^3J_{C\text{-}F}$ = 4.1 Hz), 126.5, 123.5 (q, $^1J_{C\text{-}F}$ = 273.7 Hz), 87.2, 86.3, 80.6, 75.8, 75.6, 74.5, 70.4, 67.6, 59.0, 55.7, 44.4, 43.2, 38.3, 36.6, 29.7, 29.1, 25.5, 22.1, 21.5, 18.2, 14.8, 14.4, −5.5, −6.0; LC-MS (ESI, *m/z*): [M + 1], found 994.3, [M + 23], found 1016.3, $C_{52}H_{62}F_3NO_{13}Si$: 993.39.

3.1.4. General Experimental Procedure for Compounds **16a–e**

10-Dehydro-7,8-seco-10-deacetylpaclitaxel (**16a**). To a solution of of **15a** (19.8 mg, 0.0214 mmol) in THF (1.4 mL) was added, dropwise, 0.3 mL of HF-pyridine (*v/v* = 1:2) at 0 °C, and the reaction mixture was stirred at room temperature for 30 h. The reaction was quenched with saturated aqueous $NaHCO_3$, diluted with ethyl acetate, washed with saturated NH_4Cl. The organic layer dried over anhydrous Na_2SO_4 and then concentrated under reduced pressure. Purification of the crude product by silica gel chromatography (ethyl acetate: petroleum ether = 2:1) gave product **16a** as a white solid (13.4 mg, 77.4% yield). ^{1}H-NMR ($CDCl_3$, 400 MHz) δ: 8.04 (d, J = 7.6 Hz, 2H, Ar-H), 7.69 (d, J = 7.2 Hz, 2H, Ar-H), 7.57 (t, J = 7.4 Hz, 1H, Ar-H), 7.48–7.44 (m, 5H, Ar-H), 7.38–7.27 (m, 6H, NH, Ar-H), 6.47 (s, 1H, OH-9), 6.16 (t, J = 7.5 Hz, 1H, H-13), 5.86 (dd, J = 2.8, 9.4 Hz, 1H, H-3′), 5.60 (d, J = 9.5 Hz, 1H, H-2), 5.20 (brs, 1H, H-5), 5.16 (d, J = 11.4 Hz, 1H, H-20a), 4.78 (d, J = 3.0 Hz, 1H, H-2′), 4.27 (d, J = 8.1 Hz, 1H, H-3), 4.20 (brs, 1H, H-20b), 3.89 (brs, 1H, H-7a), 3.68 (dt, J = 6.2, 10.1 Hz, 1H, H-7b), 2.77 (brs, 1H, H-6a), 2.61 (brs, 1H, H-14a), 2.38 (dd, J = 9.7, 15.9 Hz, 1H, H-14b), 2.29 (brs, 1H, OH), 2.10–2.07 (m, 1H, H-6b), 1.83 (brs, 6H, 2 × CH_3), 1.75 (s, 3H, CH_3), 1.20 (s, 3H, CH_3), 1.07 (s, 3H, CH_3); ^{13}C-NMR ($CDCl_3$, 100 MHz) δ: 191.0, 172.4, 169.0, 167.3, 167.2, 148.8, 142.2, 138.0, 136.7, 133.8, 133.6, 132.0, 129.7, 129.3, 129.0, 128.8, 128.7, 128.1, 127.1, 127.0, 124.6, 86.9, 86.2, 80.5, 74.8, 73.7, 70.7, 59.6, 54.8, 43.0, 36.6, 29.7, 24.9, 22.1, 21.2, 18.4, 14.6, 14.5; LC-MS (ESI, *m/z*): [M + 1], found 812.0, [M + 23], found 834.0, $C_{45}H_{49}NO_{13}$: 811.32.

2-Debenzoyl-2-(3-methoxybenzoyl)-10-dehydro-7,8-seco-10-deacetylpaclitaxel (**16b**). White solid; yield 65.2%; ^{1}H-NMR ($CDCl_3$, 400 MHz) δ: 7.72 (d, J = 7.6 Hz, 2H, Ar-H), 7.60 (d, J = 7.1 Hz, 1H, Ar-H), 7.47–7.43 (m, 5H, Ar-H), 7.36–7.31 (m, 5H, Ar-H), 7.29–7.25 (m, 1H, Ar-H), 7.10 (d, J = 8.1 Hz, 1H, NH), 6.49 (brs, 1H, OH-9), 6.09 (t, J = 7.4 Hz, 1H, H-13), 5.81 (d, J = 9.2 Hz, 1H, H-3′), 5.58 (d, J = 9.5 Hz, 1H, H-2), 5.20 (brs, 1H, H-5), 5.14 (d, J = 11.3 Hz, 1H, H-20a), 4.73 (brs, 1H, H-2′), 4.24 (d, J = 7.2 Hz, 1H, H-3), 4.19 (brs, 1H, H-20b), 3.87 (brs, 1H, H-7a), 3.79 (s, 3H, OCH_3), 3.65 (brs, 1H, H-7b), 2.74 (brs, 1H, H-6a), 2.56 (brs, 1H, H-14a), 2.40 (dd, J = 9.9, 15.9 Hz, 1H, H-14b), 2.35 (brs, 1H, OH-1), 2.09 (m, 1H, H-6b), 1.83 (brs, 6H, 2 × CH_3), 1.69 (s, 3H, CH_3), 1.17 (s, 3H, CH_3), 1.06 (s, 3H, CH_3); ^{13}C-NMR ($CDCl_3$, 100 MHz) δ: 191.1, 172.4, 169.0, 167.1, 159.8, 148.8, 142.1, 138.1, 136.7, 133.6, 131.9, 130.7, 130.1, 129.0, 128.7, 128.6, 128.2, 128.1, 127.1, 124.5, 121.8, 119.5, 114.8, 86.9, 86.1, 80.4, 74.8, 73.7, 70.5, 59.7, 55.5, 55.0, 44.5, 42.9, 36.6, 29.8, 29.7, 24.9, 22.2, 21.1, 14.6, 14.5; LC-MS (ESI, *m/z*): [M + 1], found 842.4, [M + 23], found 864.3, $C_{46}H_{51}NO_{14}$: 841.33.

2-Debenzoyl-2-(3-fluorobenzoyl)-10-dehydro-7, 8-seco-10-deacetylpaclitaxel (**16c**). White solid; yield 59.3%, ^{1}H-NMR ($CDCl_3$, 300 MHz) δ: 7.90 (d, J = 7.7 Hz, 1H, Ar-H), 7.75–7.68 (m, 3H, Ar-H), 7.48–7.44 (m, 4H, Ar-H), 7.41–7.31 (m, 6H, Ar-H), 7.24 (d, J = 8.0 Hz, 1H, NH), 6.46 (brs, 1H, OH-9), 6.20 (t, J = 7.9Hz, 1H, H-13), 5.88 (d, J = 7.6 Hz, 1H, H-3′), 5.59 (d, J =9.5 Hz, 1H, H-2), 5.19 (overlap, J = 11.5 Hz, 2H, H-20a, H-5), 4.81 (brs, 1H, H-2′), 4.46 (brs, 1H, OH), 4.29 (d, J = 7.9Hz, 1H, H-3), 4.22 (brs, 1H, H-20b), 3.92 (brs, 1H, H-7a), 3.70 (brs, 1H, H-7b), 3.39 (brs, 1H, OH), 2.77 (brs, 1H, H-6a), 2.60 (brs, 1H, H-14a), 2.37 (dd, J = 9.7, 15.8 Hz, 1H, H-14b), 2.09 (m, 1H, H-6b), 1.85 (brs, 6H, 2 × CH_3), 1.78 (s, 3H, CH_3), 1.64 (brs, 1H, OH-1), 1.22 (s, 3H, CH_3), 1.09 (s, 3H, CH_3); ^{13}C-NMR ($CDCl_3$, 75 MHz) δ: 190.9, 172.4, 167.2, 166.2, 162.7 (d, $^1J_{C\text{-}F}$ = 248.7 Hz), 148.9, 142.1, 137.9, 133.6, 132.0, 131.4 (d, $^2J_{C\text{-}F}$ = 7.4 Hz), 130.8 (d, $^3J_{C\text{-}F}$ = 7.9 Hz), 128.9, 128.7, 128.2, 127.0, 126.9, 125.5, 124.4, 121.0 (d, $^2J_{C\text{-}F}$ = 21.2 Hz), 116.5 (d,

$^{2}J_{C\text{-}F}$ = 23.5 Hz), 86.8, 86.2, 80.5, 75.2, 74.7, 73.6, 70.7, 59.5, 54.6, 42.9, 36.5, 29.7, 29.3, 24.9, 22.1, 21.2, 14.7, 14.5; LC-MS (ESI, *m/z*): [M + 1], found 830.3, [M + 23], found 852.3, $C_{45}H_{48}FNO_{13}$: 829.31.

2-Debenzoyl-2-(3-chlorobenzoyl)-10-dehydro-7, 8-seco-10-deacetylpaclitaxel (**16d**). White solid; yield 60.3%; ^{1}H-NMR ($CDCl_3$, 400 MHz) δ: 7.98 (d, *J* = 7.5 Hz, 2H, Ar-H), 7.72 (d, *J* = 7.0 Hz, 2H, Ar-H), 7.56 (d, *J* = 8.4 Hz, 1H, Ar-H), 7.47–7.42 (m, 4H, Ar-H), 7.40–7.29 (m, 6H, NH, Ar-H), 6.49 (brs, 1H, OH-9), 6.15 (t, *J* = 7.8 Hz, 1H, H-13), 5.86 (d, *J* = 8.1 Hz, 1H, H-3′), 5.58 (d, *J* = 9.5 Hz, 1H, H-2), 5.21 (brs, 1H, H-5), 5.14 (d, *J* =11.0 Hz, 1H, H-20a), 4.79 (d, *J* = 2.8 Hz, 1H, H-2′), 4.27 (d, *J* =7.8 Hz, 1H, H-3), 4.20 (brs, 1H, H-20b), 3.89 (brs, 1H, H-7a), 3.71–3.67 (m, 1H, H-7b), 2.75 (brs, 1H, H-6a), 2.59 (brs, 1H, H-14a), 2.38 (dd, *J* = 9.7, 15.8 Hz, 1H, H-14b), 2.25 (brs, 1H, OH), 2.09 (m, 1H, H-6b), 2.00 (m, 1H, OH), 1.84 (brs, 6H, 2 × CH_3), 1.74 (s, 3H, CH_3), 1.20 (s, 3H, CH_3), 1.07 (s, 3H, CH_3); ^{13}C-NMR ($CDCl_3$, 100 MHz) δ: 191.0, 172.5, 167.2, 166.0, 148.9, 142.1, 138.1, 135.0, 133.8, 133.7, 132.0, 131.1, 130.4, 129.5, 128.8, 128.7, 128.1, 127.9, 127.0, 124.3, 86.9, 86.2, 80.4, 75.3, 74.7, 73.6, 70.6, 59.6, 54.8, 50.8, 42.9, 36.6, 29.7, 29.5, 29.3, 24.9, 22.2, 21.2, 14.6, 14.5; LC-MS (ESI, *m/z*): [M + 1], found 845.9, [M + 23], found 867.8, $C_{45}H_{48}ClNO_{13}$: 845.28.

2-Debenzoyl-2-(3-trifluoromethylbenzoyl)-10-dehydro-7,8-seco-10-deacetylpaclitaxel (**16e**). White solid; yield 55.5%; ^{1}H-NMR ($CDCl_3$, 400 MHz) δ: 8.33 (d, *J* = 7.7 Hz, 1H, Ar-H), 8.25 (brs, 1H, NH), 7.85 (d, *J* = 7.4 Hz, 1H, Ar-H), 7.68–7.62 (m, 3H, Ar-H), 7.48–7.45 (m, 3H, Ar-H), 7.40–7.29 (m, 6H, Ar-H), 6.47 (brs, 1H, OH-9), 6.18 (t, *J* = 7.9 Hz, 1H, H-13), 5.87 (d, *J* = 7.6 Hz, 1H, H-3′), 5.62 (d, *J* = 9.4 Hz, 1H, H-2), 5.18 (overlap, *J* = 11.5 Hz, 2H, H-20a, H-5), 4.80 (d, *J* = 2.8 Hz, 1H, H-2′), 4.62 (brs, 1H, OH), 4.28 (d, *J* = 7.6 Hz, 1H, H-3), 4.24 (brs, 1H, H-20b), 3.90 (brs, 1H, H-7a), 3.68 (brs, 1H, H-7b), 3.38 (brs, 1H, OH), 2.77 (brs, 1H, H-6a), 2.58 (brs, 1H, H-14a), 2.37 (dd, *J* = 9.7, 15.7 Hz, 1H, H-14b), 2.05 (brs, 1H, OH), 2.03–1.98 (m, 1H, H-6b), 1.84 (brs, 6H, 2 × CH_3), 1.78 (s, 3H, CH_3), 1.22 (s, 3H, CH_3), 1.09 (s, 3H, CH_3); ^{13}C-NMR ($CDCl_3$, 100 MHz) δ: 190.9, 172.4, 167.2, 166.0, 148.9, 142.1, 138.0, 133.7, 133.0, 132.0, 131.7, 130.3, 130.0, 129.7, 128.9, 128.7, 128.2, 127.0 (2C), 126.4, 124.8, 124.2, 122.1, 86.9, 86.2, 80.5, 75.4, 74.7, 73.5, 70.7, 59.6, 54.7, 43.0, 36.6, 31.9, 29.7, 25.5, 22.1, 21.2, 14.6, 14.4; LC-MS (ESI, *m/z*): [M + 1], found 880.0, [M + 23], found 901.9, $C_{46}H_{48}F_3NO_{13}$: 879.31.

3.1.5. General Experimental Procedure for Compounds **17a–e**

2′-O-(tert-Butyldimethylsilyl)-9-O-(2-hydroxyethyl)-10-dehydro-7, 8-seco-10-deacetylpaclitaxel (**17a**). To a mixture of **15a** (50 mg, 0.0540 mmol), potassium carbonate (104 mg, 0.754 mmol), and potassium iodide (18 mg, 0.108 mmol) in DMF (0.9 mL) was added 2-bromoethanol (54 μL 0.762 mmol), dropwise, at 0 °C. The reaction mixture was stirred for 9 h at room temperature and then was diluted with ethyl acetate. The organic phase was washed with saturated aqueous NH_4Cl. The organic layer was dried over anhydrous Na_2SO_4 and then concentrated under reduced pressure. Purification of the crude product by silica gel chromatography (ethyl acetate: petroleum ether = 1:1) gave product **17a** as a white solid (19 mg, 52.4% yield). ^{1}H-NMR ($CDCl_3$, 300 MHz) δ: 8.09 (d, *J* = 7.2 Hz, 2H, Ar-H), 7.62 (d, *J* = 7.2 Hz, 2H, Ar-H), 7.57 (d, *J* = 7.5 Hz, 1H, Ar-H), 7.49 (t, *J* = 7.5 Hz, 2H, Ar-H), 7.36 (m, 8H, Ar-H), 6.30 (t, *J* = 8.4 Hz, 1H, H-13), 5.88 (d, *J* = 9.0 Hz, 1H, H-3′), 5.57 (d, *J* = 9.6 Hz, 1H, H-2), 5.28 (overlap, 2H, H-5, H-20a), 4.69 (d, *J* = 1.8 Hz, 1H, H-2′), 4.26 (d, *J* = 7.8 Hz, 1H, H-3), 4.20 (m, 2H, H-20b, OCH$_2$<u>CH$_2$</u>OCO), 3.94 (m, 1H, OCH$_2$<u>CH$_2$</u>OCO), 3.87 (m, *J* = 1.8, 6.3, 8.7, 12.0 Hz, 1H, H-7a), 3.74 (overlap, 2H, H-7b, <u>OCH$_2$</u>CH$_2$OCO), 3.62 (m, 1H, <u>OCH$_2$</u>CH$_2$OCO), 2.71 (m, 2H, H-6a, H-14a), 2.25 (dd, *J* = 9.3, 15.9 Hz, 2H, H-6b, H-14b), 1.97 (s, 3H, CH_3), 1.92 (s, 3H, CH_3), 1.82 (s, 3H, CH_3), 1.27 (s, 3H, CH_3), 1.16 (s, 3H, CH_3), 0.76 (s, 9H, $SiC(CH_3)_3$), −0.08 (s, 3H, $Si(CH_3)$), −0.33 (s, 3H, $Si(CH_3)$); ^{13}C-NMR ($CDCl_3$, 100 MHz) δ: 192.3, 170.7, 168.7, 167.3, 153.8, 144.0, 139.4, 138.0, 133.7 (2C), 131.8, 129.9 (2C), 128.9 (2C), 128.6 (4C), 127.9, 126.9 (2C), 126.4 (2C), 87.1, 87.7, 85.7, 79.9, 75.6, 75.4, 74.6, 73.8, 70.5, 61.8, 58.7, 55.6, 42.9, 36.6, 25.4 (3C), 22.9, 22.0, 18.1, 15.3, 14.6, −5.5, −6.1; LC-MS (ESI, *m/z*): [M + 1], found 970.5, [M + 23], found 992.4, $C_{53}H_{67}NO_{14}Si$: 969.43.

2′-O-(tert-Butyldimethylsilyl)-2-debenzoyl-2-(3-methoxybenzoyl)-9-O-(2-hydroxyethyl)-10-dehydro-7,8-seco-10-deacetylpaclitaxel (**17b**). White solid; yield 56.1%; ^{1}H-NMR ($CDCl_3$, 400 MHz) δ: 7.72–7.66 (m, 3H, Ar-H), 7.54 (s, 1H, Ar-H), 7.47–7.43 (m, 2H, Ar-H), 7.42–7.29 (m, 8H, Ar-H), 7.12 (dd, J = 2.0, 8.4 Hz, 1H, BzNH), 6.29 (t, J = 8.5 Hz, 1H, H-13), 5.88 (d, J = 9.3 Hz, 1H, H-3′), 5.59 (d, J = 9.6 Hz, 1H, H-2), 5.26 (overlap, 2H, H-5, H-20a), 4.72 (s, 1H, H-2′), 4.26 (d, J = 6.4 Hz, 1H, H-3), 4.19–4.15 (m, 1H, H-20b), 3.94–3.64 (m, 9H, OCH_3, OCH_2CH_2OH, H-7a, H-7b), 2.61 (br, 2H, H-6b, H-14b), 2.25 (dd, J = 9.6, 15.6 Hz, 2H, H-6a, H-14a), 2.03 (s, 3H, OAc), 1.93 (s, 6H, 2 × CH_3), 1.26 (s, 3H, CH_3), 1.16 (s, 3H, CH_3), 0.77 (s, 9H, $SiC(CH_3)_3$), −0.10 (s, 3H, $Si(CH_3)$), −0.30 (s, 3H, $Si(CH_3)$); ^{13}C-NMR ($CDCl_3$, 100 MHz) δ: 192.4, 171.2, 170.9, 168.8, 167.3, 167.0, 162.6, 159.7, 144.1, 138.1, 133.8, 131.8, 130.4, 130.2, 128.6 (2C), 127.9, 127.0 (2C), 126.6 (2C), 122.2, 119.5, 114.9, 85.7, 79.8, 75.8, 74.8, 61.8, 58.9, 55.7, 55.5, 42.9, 36.6, 36.5, 31.9, 31.4, 29.7, 25.5 (3C), 22.9, 22.1, 18.2, 15.2, 14.6, −5.5, −6.1; LC-MS (ESI, *m/z*): [M + 1], found 1000.5, [M + 23], found 1022.5, $C_{54}H_{69}NO_{16}Si$: 999.44.

2′-O-(tert-Butyldimethylsilyl)-2-debenzoyl-2-(3-fluorobenzoyl)-9-O-(2-hydroxyethyl)-10-dehydro-7,8-seco-10-deacetylpaclitaxel (**17c**). White solid; yield 53.2%; ^{1}H-NMR ($CDCl_3$, 400 MHz) δ: 7.93 (d, J = 7.8 Hz, 1H, Ar-H), 7.76 (d, J = 8.8 Hz, 1H, Ar-H), 7.63 (d, J = 7.6 Hz, 2H, Ar-H), 7.52–7.28 (m, 11H, NH, Ar-H), 6.29 (t, J = 8.1 Hz, 1H, H-13), 5.89 (d, J = 9.2 Hz, 1H, H-3′), 5.58 (d, J = 9.6 Hz, 1H, H-2), 5.35–5.15 (overlap, 2H, H-5, H-20a), 4.70 (d, J = 1.9 Hz, 1H, H-2′), 4.26 (d, J = 7.6 Hz, 1H, H-3), 4.20–4.16 (m, 2H, H-20b, OCH_2CH_2OCO), 3.95 (brs, 1H, OCH_2CH_2OCO), 3.89–3.84 (ddd, J = 2.3, 6.8, 8.7, 12.4 Hz, 1H, H-7a), 3.80–3.70 (overlap, 2H, H-7b, OCH_2CH_2OCO), 3.60–3.58 (m, 1H, OCH_2CH_2OCO), 2.71–2.63 (m, 2H, H-6a, H-14a), 2.25 (dd, J = 9.6, 15.8 Hz, 2H, H-6b, H-14b), 2.03 (s, 3H, CH_3), 1.91(s, 3H, CH_3), 1.87 (brs, 3H, CH_3), 1.83 (brs, 2H, 2 × OH), 1.26 (s, 3H, CH_3), 1.15 (s, 3H, CH_3), 0.73 (s, 9H, $SiC(CH_3)_3$), −0.08 (s, 3H, $Si(CH_3)$), −0.32 (s, 3H, $Si(CH_3)$); ^{13}C-NMR ($CDCl_3$, 100 MHz) δ: 192.3, 171.2, 170.8, 168.6, 167.4, 166.2, 162.7 (d, $^1J_{C\text{-}F}$ = 248.3 Hz), 144.0, 137.9, 133.9, 131.9, 131.2 (d, $^3J_{C\text{-}F}$ = 7.4 Hz), 131.0 (d, $^3J_{C\text{-}F}$ = 7.7 Hz), 128.7 (2C), 128.0, 127.0, 126.5, 125.8 (d, $^4J_{C\text{-}F}$ = 2.6 Hz), 121.0 (d, $^2J_{C\text{-}F}$ = 21.2 Hz), 116.3 (d, $^2J_{C\text{-}F}$ = 22.9 Hz), 85.8, 80.0, 75.7, 75.2, 70.5, 61.9, 58.7, 55.6, 45.7, 42.9, 36.7, 25.5, 22.9, 22.1, 18.2, 15.3, 14.6, 13.7, −5.4, −6.0; LC-MS (ESI, *m/z*): [M + 1], found 988.0, $C_{53}H_{66}FNO_{14}Si$: 987.42.

2′-O-(tert-Butyldimethylsilyl)-2-debenzoyl-2-(3-chlorobenzoyl)-9-O-(2-hydroxyethyl)-10-dehydro-7,8-seco-10-deacetylpaclitaxel (**17d**). White solid; yield 60.9%; ^{1}H-NMR ($CDCl_3$, 400 MHz) δ: 8.06 (d, J = 8.8 Hz, 2H, Ar-H), 7.63 (d, J = 7.5 Hz, 2H, Ar-H), 7.57 (d, J = 8.2 Hz, 1H, Ar-H), 7.50–7.43 (m, 3H, Ar-H), 7.43–7.33 (m, 8H, Ar-H, BzNH), 6.31 (t, J = 8.0 Hz, 1H, H-13), 5.90 (d, J = 9.2 Hz, 1H, H-3′), 5.59 (d, J = 9.6 Hz, 1H, H-2), 5.32–5.28 (overlap, 2H, H-5, H-20b), 4.71 (d, J = 1.9 Hz, 1H, H-2′), 4.28 (d, J = 7.6 Hz, 1H, H-3), 4.24–4.20 (m, 2H, H-20a, OCH_2CH_2OH), 3.98–3.95 (m, 1H, OCH_2CH_2OH), 3.93–3.89 (m, 1H, H-7b), 3.78–3.72 (overlap, 2H, H-7a, OCH_2CH_2OH), 3.65 (br, 1H, OCH_2CH_2OH), 2.72–2.68 (m, 2H, H-6b, H-14b), 2.26 (dd, J = 7.2, 13.4 Hz, 2H, H-6a, H-14a), 1.98 (s, 3H, CH_3), 1.93 (brs, 1H, OH), 1.85 (brs, 2H, OH), 1.29 (brs, 6H, CH_3), 1.18 (s, 3H, CH_3), 0.78 (s, 9H, $SiC(CH_3)_3$), −0.08 (s, 3H, $Si(CH_3)$), −0.30 (s, 3H, $Si(CH_3)$); ^{13}C-NMR ($CDCl_3$, 100 MHz) δ: 192.3, 170.8, 167.4, 166.3, 144.0, 137.9, 135.0, 133.9 (2C), 132.0, 130.8, 130.7, 129.7, 128.8 (2C), 128.7 (2C), 128.2, 128.1, 127.0 (2C), 126.6 (2C), 85.9, 75.8, 75.3, 70.5, 62.0, 55.6, 43.0, 36.7, 32.0, 29.7, 29.4, 27.3, 25.5 (3C), 23.0, 22.7, 22.2, 18.3, 15.3, 14.7, 14.2, −5.4, −6.0; LC-MS (ESI, *m/z*): [M + 1], found 1004.4, [M + 23], found 1026.4, $C_{53}H_{66}ClNO_{14}Si$: 1003.39.

2′-O-(tert-Butyldimethylsilyl)-2-debenzoyl-2-(3-trifluoromethylbenzoyl)-9-O-(2-hydroxyethyl)-10-dehydro-7,8-seco-10-deacetylpaclitaxel (**17e**). White solid; yield 49.9%; ^{1}H-NMR ($CDCl_3$, 400 MHz) δ: 7.83 (d, J = 7.7 Hz, 2H, Ar-H), 7.68 (t, J = 7.8 Hz, 1H, Ar-H), 7.58 (d, J = 7.3 Hz, 1H, Ar-H), 7.45 (t, J = 7.4 Hz, 2H, Ar-H), 7.35 (m, 8H, Ar-H), 6.29 (t, J = 8.2 Hz, 1H, H-13), 5.87 (d, J = 8.7 Hz, 1H, H-3′), 5.60 (d, J = 9.65 Hz, 1H, H-2), 5.26 (overlap, 2H, H-5, H-20a), 4.70 (d, J = 1.3 Hz, 1H, H-2′), 4.28 (d, J = 6.8 Hz, 1H, H-3), 4.19 (m, 2H, H-20b, OCH_2CH_2OCO), 3.98 (m, 1H, OCH_2CH_2OCO), 3.87 (m, J = 1.8, 6.3, 8.7, 12.0 Hz, 1H, H-7a), 3.75 (overlap, 2H, H-7b, OCH_2CH_2OCO), 3.66 (m, 1H, OCH_2CH_2OCO), 2.65 (m, 2H, H-6a, H-14a), 2.24 (dd, J = 6.7, 16.3 Hz, 2H, H-6b, H-14b), 1.97 (s, 3H, CH_3), 1.92 (s, 3H, CH_3), 1.82 (s, 3H, CH_3), 1.26 (s, 3H, CH_3), 1.17 (s, 3H, CH_3), 0.77 (s, 9H, $SiC(CH_3)_3$), −0.08 (s, 3H, $Si(CH_3)$), −0.32 (s, 3H, $Si(CH_3)$); ^{13}C-NMR ($CDCl_3$, 100 MHz) δ: 192.3, 170.8, 167.6, 166.1, 144.1, 137.8, 133.9, 133.2,

132.0, 131.4 (q, $^2J_{C\text{-}F}$ = 33.2 Hz), 130.3, 130.2 (q, $^3J_{C\text{-}F}$ = 3.5 Hz), 130.0, 128.8, 128.7, 128.1, 126.9, 126.8 (q, $^3J_{C\text{-}F}$ = 3.6 Hz), 126.5, 123.6 (q, $^1J_{C\text{-}F}$ = 273.8 Hz), 85.8, 75.6, 75.4, 70.5, 62.0, 58.4, 55.6, 43.0, 36.7, 31.9, 29.8, 29.7, 29.6 (2C), 29.3 (2C), 27.2, 25.5, 23.0, 22.7, 22.1, 18.4, 18.2, 15.3, 14.6, 14.1, −5.4, −6.0; LC-MS (ESI, *m/z*): [M + 1], found 1038.4, [M + 23], found 1060.4, $C_{54}H_{66}F_3NO_{14}Si$: 1037.42.

3.1.6. General Experimental Procedure for Compounds **19a–e**

2′-O-(tert-Butyldimethylsilyl)-macrocyclic taxoid (**19a**). To a solution of **17a** (19 mg, 0.0196 mmol) in dichloromethane (4.2 mL) was added, dropwise, pyridine (22 μL, 0.266 mmol) and triphosgene (8.7 mg, 0.0293 mmol) at 0 °C, then the reaction mixture was stirred at room temperature for 5 h. The reaction was diluted with ethyl acetate, washed with saturated NaCl. The organic layer was dried over anhydrous Na_2SO_4 and then concentrated under reduced pressure. Purification of the crude product by silica gel chromatography (ethyl acetate: petroleum ether = 1:3) gave product **19a** as a white solid (3.1 mg, 15.9% yield). ^{1}H-NMR ($CDCl_3$, 400 MHz) δ: 8.17 (d, *J* = 7.2 Hz, 2H, Ar-H), 7.75 (d, *J* = 7.2 Hz, 2H, Ar-H), 7.63 (t, *J* = 7.2 Hz, 1H, Ar-H), 7.54 (t, *J* = 7.6 Hz, 2H, Ar-H), 7.50 (d, *J* = 7.6 Hz, 1H, Ar-H), 7.43 (d, *J* = 7.6 Hz, 2H, Ar-H), 7.39 (t, *J* = 7.2 Hz, 2H, Ar-H), 7.34–7.29 (m, 3H, Ar-H), 7.08 (d, *J* = 9.2 Hz, 1H, NH), 6.27 (t, *J* = 8.8 Hz, 1H, H-13), 5.76 (d, *J* = 8.4 Hz, 1H, H-3′), 5.60 (d, *J* = 7.6 Hz, 1H, H-2), 4.84 (overlap, 2H, H-5, $O\underline{CH_2}CH_2OCO$), 4.79 (d, *J* = 7.6 Hz, 1H, H-3), 4.67 (d, *J* = 2.0 Hz, 1H, H-2′), 4.57 (dd, *J* = 6.8, 12.0 Hz, 1H, $\overline{OCH_2CH_2}OCO$), 4.49 (dd, *J* = 6.8, 12.0 Hz, 1H, $OCH_2\underline{CH_2}OCO$), 4.46 (d, *J* = 8.4 Hz, 1H, H-20a), 4.35 (d, *J* = 8.4 Hz, 1H, H-20b), 4.32 (dd, *J* = 5.2, 13.6 Hz, 1H, $\overline{OCH_2}CH_2OCO$), 4.13 (ddd, *J* = 6.4, 10.8, 17.2 Hz, 1H, H-7a), 4.02 (ddd, *J* = 8.8, 11.6, 17.2 Hz, 1H, H-7b), 2.55 (s, 3H, 4-OAc), 2.35 (m, 3H, H-6a, H-6b, H-14a), 2.18 (dd, *J* = 8.8, 15.2 Hz, 1H, H-14b), 1.84 (s, 3H, CH_3), 1.25 (s, 3H, CH_3), 1.24 (s, 3H, CH_3), 1.19 (s, 3H, CH_3), 0.79 (s, 9H, $SiC(CH_3)_3$), −0.03 (s, 3H, $Si(CH_3)$), −0.30 (s, 3H, $Si(CH_3)$); ^{13}C-NMR ($CDCl_3$, 150 MHz) δ: 192.1, 171.0, 169.4, 166.9, 166.8, 152.4, 151.5, 144.5, 139.7, 138.3, 134.6, 134.1, 133.8, 131.8, 130.2 (2C), 129.0, 128.8 (2C), 128.7, 127.9, 127.0 (2C), 126.3 (2C), 89.6, 84.7, 78.6, 76.1, 75.3, 75.2, 71.4, 70.6, 68.9, 65.9, 55.6, 42.9, 42.4, 36.5, 31.0, 26.2, 25.5 (3C), 22.9, 21.6, 18.1, 14.4, 13.6, −5.3, −5.9; LC-MS (ESI, *m/z*): [M + 1], found 996.4, [M + 23], found 1018.4, $C_{54}H_{65}NO_{15}Si$: 995.41.

2′-O-(tert-Butyldimethylsilyl)-2-debenzoyl-2-(3-methoxybenzoyl)-macrocyclic taxoid (**19b**). White solid; yield 32.7%; ^{1}H-NMR ($CDCl_3$, 400 MHz) δ: 7.80 (d, *J* = 1.2, 7.6 Hz, 1H, Ar-H), 7.77 (d, *J* = 6.8 Hz, 2H, Ar-H), 7.67 (dd, *J* = 1.5, 2.5 Hz, 1H, Ar-H), 7.55–7.51 (m, 1H, Ar-H), 7.49–7.39 (m, 3H, Ar-H), 7.40–7.31 (m, 5H, Ar-H), 7.20–7.17 (m, 1H, Ar-H), 7.08 (d, *J* = 9.2 Hz, 1H, BzNH), 6.28 (t, 1H, H-13), 5.76 (dd, *J* = 1.6, 8.9 Hz, H-3′), 5.62 (d, *J* = 7.5 Hz, 1H, H-2), 4.87 (d, *J* = 7.6 Hz, 1H, H-20b), 4.85 (d, *J* = 4.8 Hz, 1H, H-5), 4.81 (d, *J* = 7.5 Hz, 1H, H-20a), 4.68 (d, *J* = 2.0 Hz, 1H, H-2′), 4.60–4.32 (m, 5H, H-7a, H-7b, H-16a, H-16b, H-3), 4.18–4.03 (m, H-15a, H-15b), 3.91 (s, 3H, OCH_3), 2.55 (d, *J* = 1.3 Hz, 6H, 2 × CH_3), 2.41–2.35 (m, 3H, H-14b, H-6a, H-6b), 2.24–2.20 (m, 1H, H-14a), 1.84 (d, *J* = 1.2 Hz, 3H, $COCH_3$), 1.26 (s, 3H, CH_3), 1.21 (s, 3H, CH_3), 0.81 (s, 9H, $SiC(CH_3)_3$), −0.008 (s, 3H, $Si(CH_3)$), −0.28 (s, 3H, $Si(CH_3)$); ^{13}C-NMR ($CDCl_3$, 100 MHz) δ: 192.2, 171.1, 169.4, 166.9, 166.8, 159.8, 152.5, 151.6, 144.6, 139.7, 138.4, 134.7, 134.2, 131.9, 130.4, 130.0, 128.82 (2C), 128.78 (2C), 128.0, 127.0 (2C), 126.4 (2C), 122.6, 120.3, 114.7, 89.6, 84.8, 78.5, 75.4, 75.3, 71.5, 70.7, 69.0, 65.9, 55.6, 43.0, 42.5, 36.5, 31.1, 29.7, 26.3, 25.6 (3C), 22.9, 21.6, 18.2, 14.4, 13.7, −5.2,−5.8; LC-MS (ESI, *m/z*): [M + 1], found 1026.4, [M + 23], found 1048.4, $C_{55}H_{67}NO_{16}Si$: 1025.42.

2′-O-(tert-Butyldimethylsilyl)-2-debenzoyl-2-(3-fluorobenzoyl)-macrocyclic taxoid (**19c**). White solid; yield 32.1%; ^{1}H-NMR ($CDCl_3$, 400 MHz) δ: 8.01(d, *J* = 7.8 Hz, 1H, Ar-H), 7.84–7.87 (m, 1H, Ar-H), 7.75–7.73 (m, 2 H, Ar-H), 7. 56–7.49 (m, 2H, Ar-H), 7.44–7.31 (m, 8H, Ar-H), 7.09 (d, *J* = 9.0 Hz, 1H, NH), 6.28 (t, *J* = 8.8 Hz,1H, H-13), 5.78 (dd, *J* = 1.4, 9.1 Hz, 1H, H-3′), 5.61 (d, *J* = 7.6 Hz, 1H, H-2), 4.87–4.82 (overlap, 2H, $O\underline{CH_2}CH_2OCO$, H-5), 4.83 (d, *J* = 7.5 Hz, 1H, H-3), 4.69 (d, *J* = 2.0 Hz, 1H, H-2′), 4.58 (dd, *J* = 6.4, 11.9 Hz, 1H, $OCH_2\underline{CH_2}OCO$), 4.51 (dd, *J* = 6.4, 13.7 Hz, 1H, $OCH_2\underline{CH_2}OCO$), 4.46 (d, *J* = 8.2 Hz, 1H, H-20a), 4.36–4.30 (overlap, 2H, $O\underline{CH_2}CH_2OCO$, H-20b), 4.16–4.09 (m, 1H, H-7a), 4.06–3.99 (m, 17.2 Hz, 1H, H-7b), 2.57 (s, 3H, $COCH_3$), 2.56 (s, 3H, 4-OAc), 2.39–2.31 (m, 3H, H-6a, H-6b, H-14a), 2.18 (dd, *J* = 8.4, 15.4 Hz, 1H, H-14b), 1.90 (brs, 1H, OH), 1.84 (s, 3H, CH_3), 1.23 (s, 3H, CH_3), 1.19 (s, 3H, CH_3), 0.80 (s, 9H, $SiC(CH_3)_3$), −0.29 (s, 3H, $Si(CH_3)$), −0.03 (s, 3H, $Si(CH_3)$); ^{13}C-NMR ($CDCl_3$, 100 MHz) δ: 192.1, 171.1, 169.4, 167.0, 165.7, 162.7 (d, $^{1}J_{C\text{-}F}$ = 247.8 Hz), 152.5, 151.6, 144.5, 139.8, 138.4, 134.5, 134.2, 131.9, 131.3 (d, $^{3}J_{C\text{-}F}$ = 7.6Hz), 130.6 (d, $^{3}J_{C\text{-}F}$ = 7.6 Hz), 128.8 (2C), 128.0, 127.0, 126.5, 126.0 (d, $^{4}J_{C\text{-}F}$ = 3.0 Hz), 121.0 (d, $^{2}J_{C\text{-}F}$ = 21.4 Hz), 117.1 (d, $^{2}J_{C\text{-}F}$ = 23.3 Hz), 89.6, 84.7, 78.6, 76.1, 75.7, 75.3, 71.5, 70.7, 68.9, 65.9, 55.6, 43.0, 42.5, 36.4, 31.0, 26.3, 25.6, 22.8, 21.6, 18.2, 14.4, 13.6, −5.2, −5.8; LC-MS (ESI, *m/z*): [M + 1], found 1014.4, [M + 23], found 1036.4, $C_{54}H_{64}FNO_{15}Si$: 1013.40.

2′-O-(tert-Butyldimethylsilyl)-2-debenzoyl-2-(3-chlorobenzoyl)-macrocyclic taxoid (**19d**). White solid; yield 36.1%; ^{1}H-NMR ($CDCl_3$, 400 MHz) δ: 8.19 (t, *J* = 1.6 Hz, 1H, Ar-H), 8.10–8.07 (m, 1H, Ar-H), 7.77–7.75 (m, 2H, Ar-H), 7.64–7.61 (m, 1H, Ar-H), 7.55–7.49 (m, 2H, Ar-H), 7.46–7.33 (m, 7H, Ar-H), 7.08 (d, *J* = 9.2 Hz, 1H, BzNH), 6.25 (m, 1H, H-13), 5.76 (dd, *J* = 1.6, 9.0 Hz, 1H, H-3′), 5.59 (d, *J* = 7.6 Hz, 1H, H-2), 4.89–4.81 (m, 3H, $\underline{OCH_2}CH_2OCO$, H-5, H-3), 4.68 (d, *J* = 2.0 Hz, 1H, H-2′), 4.57 (dd, *J* = 6.6, 11.9 Hz, 1H, $OCH_2CH_2\underline{OCO}$), 4.50 (dd, *J* = 6.5, 11.8 Hz, 1H, $OCH_2\underline{CH_2}OCO$), 4.44 (d, *J* = 8.0 Hz, 1H, H-20a), 4.38–4.32 (m, 2H, $\underline{OCH_2}CH_2OCO$, H-20b), 4.15–4.10 (m, 1H, H-7a), 4.07–4.01 (m, *J* = 17.2 Hz, 1H, H-7b), 2.56 (s, 3H, CH_3), 2.55 (s, 3H, CH_3), 2.41–2.30 (m, 3H, H-6a, H-6b, H-14a), 2.25–2.18 (m, 1H, H-14b), 1.84 (d, *J* = 1.2 Hz, 3H, CH_3), 1.25 (s, 3H, CH_3), 1.20 (s, 3H, CH_3), 0.82 (s, 9H, $SiC(CH_3)_3$), −0.01 (s, 3H, $Si(CH_3)$), −0.26 (s, 3H, $Si(CH_3)$); ^{13}C-NMR ($CDCl_3$, 100 MHz) δ: 192.1, 171.1, 169.4, 165.6, 152.5, 151.7, 144.5, 139.8, 138.4, 134.9, 134.5, 133.6, 131.8, 131.0, 130.3, 128.81 (2C), 128.79 (2C), 128.4, 128.0, 127.0 (2C), 126.5 (2C), 89.6, 84.7, 78.7, 77.3, 75.6, 75.3, 70.8, 69.0, 55.7, 43.0, 42.5, 36.4, 29.7, 26.3, 25.6 (3C), 22.8, 21.6, 18.2, 14.4, 13.6, −5.2, −5.8; LC-MS (ESI, *m/z*): [M + 1], found 1030.4, [M + 23], found 1052.4, $C_{54}H_{64}ClNO_{15}Si$: 1029.37.

2′-O-(tert-Butyldimethylsilyl)-2-debenzoyl-2-(3-trifluoromethylbenzoyl)-macrocyclic taxoid (**19e**). White solid; yield 30.5%; ^{1}H-NMR ($CDCl_3$, 400 MHz) δ: 8.51 (s, 1H, Ar-H), 8.41 (d, *J* = 7.8 Hz, 1H, Ar-H), 7.92 (d, *J* = 7.8 Hz, 1H, Ar-H), 7.76–7.72 (m, 3H, Ar-H), 7.55–7.51 (m, 1H, Ar-H), 7.47–7.40 (m, 4H, Ar-H), 7.37–7.33 (m, 3H, Ar-H), 7.09 (d, *J* = 9.1 Hz, 1H, NH), 6.24 (t, *J* = 8.8 Hz, 1H, H-13), 5.76 (dd, *J* = 1.0, 9.0 Hz, 1H, H-3′), 5.63 (d, *J* = 7.6 Hz, 1H, H-2), 4.91–4.84 (m, 3H, H-3, H-5, $\underline{OCH_2}CH_2OCO$), 4.67 (d, *J* = 1.8 Hz, 1H, H-2′), 4.58 (dd, *J* = 6.8, 11.8 Hz, 1H, $OCH_2\underline{CH_2}OCO$), 4.52 (dd, *J* = 6.8, 13.7 Hz, 1H, $\underline{OCH_2}CH_2OCO$), 4.44 (d, *J* = 8.1 Hz, 1H, H-20a), 4.38–4.33 (m, 2H, $OCH_2\underline{CH_2}OCO$, H-20b), 4.11–4.18 (m, 1H, H-7a), 4.09–4.02 (m, *J* = 17.2 Hz, 1H, H-7b), 2.55 (s, 3H, 4-OAc), 2.42–2.36 (m, 3H, H-6a, H-6b, H-14a), 2.29–2.20 (m,1H, H-14b), 1.94 (s, 1H, OH), 1.86 (d, *J* = 1.04 Hz, 3H, CH_3), 1.29 (s, 3H, CH_3), 1.26 (s, 3H, CH_3), 1.22 (s, 3H, CH_3), 0.84 (s, 9H, $SiC(CH_3)_3$), −0.004 (s, 3H, $Si(CH_3)$), −0.24 (s, 3H, $Si(CH_3)$); ^{13}C-NMR ($CDCl_3$, 100 MHz) δ: 192.0, 171.1, 169.3, 167.0, 165.4, 152.5, 151.6, 144.5, 139.8, 138.4, 134.4, 134.3, 133.6, 131.8, 131.4 (q, $^{2}J_{C\text{-}F}$ = 33.2 Hz), 130.3 (q, $^{3}J_{C\text{-}F}$ = 3.4 Hz), 130.2, 129.7, 128.8, 128.0, 127.0, 126.9 (q, $^{3}J_{C\text{-}F}$ = 4.3 Hz), 126.5, 123.7 (q, $^{1}J_{C\text{-}F}$ = 273.8 Hz), 89.6, 84.7, 78.7, 76.0, 75.8, 75.2, 71.5, 70.8, 69.0, 65.9, 55.7, 43.0, 42.4, 36.4, 31.0, 29.0, 26.3, 25.6, 22.7, 21.6, 18.2, 14.4, 13.6, −5.2,−5.8; LC-MS (ESI, *m/z*): [M + 1], found 1064.4, [M + 23], found 1086.4, $C_{55}H_{64}F_3NO_{15}Si$: 1063.40.

3.1.7. General Procedure for the Syntheses of Compounds **21a–e**

Macrocyclic taxoid (**21a**)

To a solution of of **19a** (32.3 mg, 0.0464 mmol) in THF (8 mL) was added, dropwise, 1.53 mL of HF-pyridine (*v/v* = 1:2) at 0 °C, and the reaction mixture was stirred at room temperature for 30 h. The reaction was quenched with saturated aqueous $NaHCO_3$, diluted with ethyl acetate, and washed with saturated NH_4Cl. The organic layer was dried over anhydrous Na_2SO_4 and then concentrated under reduced pressure. Purification of the crude product by silica gel chromatography (ethyl acetate: petroleum ether = 2:1) gave product **21a** as a white solid (13.2 mg, 46.2% yield). ^{1}H-NMR ($CDCl_3$, 400 MHz) δ: 8.14 (d, *J* = 7.0 Hz, 2H, Ar-H), 7.73 (d, *J* = 8.6 Hz, 2H, Ar-H), 7.62 (t, *J* = 7.5 Hz, 1H, Ar-H), 7.52–7.45 (m, 5H, Ar-H), 7.40–7.30 (m, 5H, Ar-H), 7.22 (d, *J* = 9.1 Hz, 1H, NH), 6.20 (t, *J* = 8.5 Hz, 1H, H-13), 5.78 (dd, *J* = 2.5, 9.1 Hz, 1H, H-3′), 5.58 (d, *J* = 7.5 Hz, 1H, H-2), 4.80–4.74 (overlap, 4H, H-5, H-2′, H-3, $\underline{OCH_2}CH_2OCO$), 4.52 (dd, *J* = 6.4, 12.0 Hz, 1H, $OCH_2\underline{CH_2}OCO$), 4.45–4.44 (overlap, 2H, H-20a, $OCH_2\underline{CH_2}OCO$), 4.31-4.25 (overlap, 2H, H-20b, $\underline{OCH_2}CH_2\underline{OCO}$), 4.07–3.91 (overlap, 2H, H-7b, H-7a),

2.56 (br, 1H, OH-2′), 2.51 (s, 3H, CH_3), 2.35 (s, 3H, CH_3), 2.33–2.25 (overlap, 4H, H-14a, H-14b, H-6a, H-6b), 1.68 (s, 3H, CH_3), 1.18 (s, 3H, CH_3), 1.16 (s, 3H, CH_3); ^{13}C-NMR ($CDCl_3$, 150 MHz) δ: 191.8, 172.4, 169.7, 166.9, 166.8, 152.4, 151.5, 144.8, 138.6, 137.9, 135.0, 133.9, 133.6, 132.0, 130.1 (2C), 129.0 (2C), 128.8 (4C), 128.3, 127.0 (2C), 89.4, 84.7, 78.4, 76.1, 75.1, 73.1, 71.8, 71.5, 68.9, 65.8, 54.8, 42.8, 42.4, 36.4, 30.9, 29.7, 26.3, 22.5, 21.2, 14.0, 13.7; LC-MS (ESI, *m/z*): [M + 1], found 882.8, [M + 23], found 904.4, $C_{48}H_{51}NO_{15}$: 881.33.

2-Debenzoyl-2-(3-methoxybenzoyl)-macrocyclic taxoid (**21b**). White solid; yield 54.1%; ^{1}H-NMR ($CDCl_3$, 400 MHz) δ: 7.76–7.74 (m, 3H, Ar-H), 7.66–7.65 (m, 1H, Ar-H), 7.53–7.46 (m, 8H, Ar-H), 7.36–7.32 (m, 1H, Ar-H), 7.03 (d, *J* = 8.9 Hz, 1H, NH), 6.17 (t, *J* = 8.2 Hz, 1H, H-13), 5.79 (dd, *J* = 2.3, 9.0 Hz, 1H, H-3′), 5.59 (d, *J* = 7.5 Hz, 1H, H-2), 4.84–4.77 (overlap, 4H, H-5, H-2′, H-3, OCH_2CH_2OCO), 4.55 (dd, *J* = 6.5, 11.9 Hz, 1H, OCH_2CH_2OCO), 4.45 (dd, *J* = 6.6, 13.2 Hz, 1H, OCH_2CH_2OCO), 4.43 (d, *J* = 7.5 Hz, 1H, H-20a), 4.36 (d, *J* = 8.29 Hz, 1H, H-20b), 4.32 (dd, *J* = 5.2, 13.8 Hz, 1H, OCH_2CH_2OCO), 4.12–3.96 (m, 2H, H-7b, H-7a), 3.88 (s, 3H, OAc), 3.62 (brs, 1H, OH-2′), 2.53 (s, 3H, CH_3), 2.36 (s, 3H, CH_3), 2.40–2.27 (overlap, 4H, H-14a, H-14b, H-6a, H-6b), 1.93 (brs, 1H, OH-1), 1.68 (d, 3H, CH_3), 1.23 (s, 3H, CH_3), 1.18 (s, 3H, CH_3); ^{13}C-NMR ($CDCl_3$, 100 MHz) δ: 191.9, 172.4, 169.7, 167.0, 166.7, 159.8, 152.4, 151.5, 144.8, 138.6, 138.0, 135.1, 133.7, 132.0, 130.3 (2C), 130.0, 129.8, 129.7, 129.0 (2C), 128.7 (4C), 128.3, 127.0 (2C), 122.5, 120.0, 115.0, 89.4, 84.7, 78.4, 76.2, 75.3, 73.2, 71.7, 71.5, 68.9, 65.8, 55.5, 54.9, 42.8, 42.4, 36.4, 31.9, 30.9, 29.7, 26.3, 22.5, 21.2, 14.0, 13.7; LC-MS (ESI, *m/z*): [M + 1], found 912.3, [M + 23], found 934.3, $C_{49}H_{53}NO_{16}$: 911.34.

2-Debenzoyl-2-(3-fluorobenzoyl)-macrocyclic taxoid (**21c**). White solid; yield 52.2%; ^{1}H-NMR ($CDCl_3$, 400 MHz) δ: 7.97–7.92 (m, 1H, Ar-H), 7.86–7.83 (ddd, *J* = 1.5, 2.5, 9.2 Hz, 1H, Ar-H), 7.75–7.72 (m, 2H, Ar-H), 7.54–7.47 (m, 4H, Ar-H), 7.43–7.39 (m, 4 H, Ar-H), 7.37–7.32 (m, 2H, Ar-H), 7.02 (d, *J* = 9.1 Hz, 1H, NH), 6.17 (dd, *J* = 7.5, 8.8 Hz, 1H, H-13), 5.79 (dd, *J* = 2.4, 9.0 Hz, 1H, H-3′), 5.57 (d, *J* = 7.6 Hz, 1H, H-2), 4.84–4.78 (overlap, 4H, H-5, H-2′, H-3, OCH_2CH_2OCO), 4.55 (dd, *J* = 6.4, 11.9 Hz, 1H, OCH_2CH_2OCO), 4.47–4.40 (m, 2H, H-20b, H-20a), 4.34–4.29 (m, 2H, OCH_2CH_2OCO), 4.12–3.96 (m, 2H, H-7b, H-7a), 3.62 (d, *J* = 4.9 Hz, 1H, OH-2′), 2.53 (s, 3H, CH_3), 2.36 (s, 3H, CH_3), 2.35–2.25 (m, 4H, H-14a, H-14b, H-6a, H-6b), 1.93 (brs, 1H, OH-1), 1.68 (d, *J* = 1.2 Hz, 3H, CH_3), 1.23 (s, 3H, CH_3), 1.18 (s, 3H, CH_3); ^{13}C-NMR ($CDCl_3$, 100 MHz) δ: 191.8, 172.4, 169.6, 167.1, 165.6 (d, $J_{C\text{-}F}$ = 3.2 Hz, CO), 162.4 (d, $^1J_{C\text{-}F}$ = 247.8 Hz), 152.4, 151.6, 144.7, 138.7, 138.0, 134.8, 133.7, 132.0, 131.3 (d, $^3J_{C\text{-}F}$ = 7.6 Hz), 130.5 (d, $^3J_{C\text{-}F}$ = 7.8 Hz), 129.9 (d, $^4J_{C\text{-}F}$ = 3.9 Hz), 129.7, 129.0, 128.7, 128.4, 127.0, 126.0, 121.0 (d, $^2J_{C\text{-}F}$ = 21.3 Hz), 117.0 (d, $^2J_{C\text{-}F}$ = 23.3 Hz), 89.5, 84.7, 78.5, 76.0, 75.5, 73.2, 71.7, 71.5, 68.9, 65.7, 55.0, 42.8, 42.4, 36.3, 30.9, 26.3, 25.5, 22.7, 22.4, 21.2, 14.1, 14.0, 13.6; LC-MS (ESI, *m/z*): [M + 1], found 900.0, [M + 23], found 922.0, $C_{48}H_{50}FNO_{15}$: 899.32.

2-Debenzoyl-2-(3-chlorobenzoyl)-macrocyclic taxoid (**21d**). White solid; yield 48.7%; ^{1}H-NMR ($CDCl_3$, 400 MHz) δ: 8.16 (t, 1H, Ar-H), 8.06–8.03 (m, 1H, Ar-H), 7.75–7.72 (m, 2H, Ar-H), 7.61 (ddd, *J* = 1.1, 2.1, 8.0 Hz, 1H, Ar-H), 7.53–7.45 (m, 4H, Ar-H), 7.43–7.39 (m, 4 H, Ar-H), 7.36–7.32 (m, 1H, Ar-H), 7.01 (d, *J* = 9.1 Hz, 1H, NH), 6.17 (td, *J* =1.3, 8.7 Hz, 1H, H-13), 5.78 (dd, *J* = 2.3, 9.0 Hz, 1H, H-3′), 5.56 (d, *J* = 7.6 Hz, 1H, H-2), 4.84–4.78 (overlap,4H, H-5, H-2′, H-3, OCH_2CH_2OCO), 4.55 (dd, *J* = 6.4, 11.9 Hz, 1H, OCH_2CH_2OCO), 4.47–4.38 (m, 2 H, H-20b, H20a), 4.34–4.29 (m, 2H, OCH_2CH_2OCO), 4.11–3.96 (m, 2H, H-7b, H-7a), 3.62 (brs, 1H, OH-2′), 2.52 (s, 3H, CH_3), 2.37 (s, 3H, CH_3), 2.42–2.27 (overlap, 4H, H-14a, H-14b, H-6a, H-6b), 2.0 (brs, 1H, OH-1), 1.68 (d, *J* = 1.2 Hz, 3H, CH_3), 1.23 (s, 3H, CH_3), 1.18 (s, 3H, CH_3); ^{13}C-NMR ($CDCl_3$, 100 MHz) δ: 191.8, 172.4, 169.6, 167.1, 165.5, 152.4, 151.6, 144.7, 138.7, 138.0, 134.8 (2C), 133.8, 133.7, 132.0, 130.9, 130.2 (2C), 129.0, 128.7, 128.4 (2C), 127.1, 127.0, 89.4, 84.7, 78.4, 76.0, 75.5, 73.1, 71.7, 71.5, 68.9, 65.7, 55.0, 42.8, 42.4, 36.3, 30.9, 26.2, 22.4, 21.2, 14.0, 13.6; LC-MS (ESI, *m/z*): [M + 1], found 916.3, [M + 23], found 938.3, $C_{48}H_{50}ClNO_{15}$: 915.29.

2-Debenzoyl-2-(3-trifluoromethylbenzoyl)-macrocyclic taxoid (**21e**). White solid; yield 63.7%; ^{1}H-NMR ($CDCl_3$, 400 MHz) δ: 8.47 (s, 1H, Ar-H), 8.36 (d, *J* = 7.9 Hz, 1H, Ar-H), 7.90 (d, *J* = 7.8 Hz, 1H, Ar-H), 7.73–7.67 (m, 3H, Ar-H), 7.46–7.52 (m, 3 H, Ar-H), 7.43–7.32 (m, 5H, Ar-H), 6.94 (d, *J* = 9.0 Hz, 1H,

NH), 6.16 (dd, *J* = 7.5, 8.8 Hz, 1H, H-13), 5.77 (dd, *J* = 2.0, 8.9 Hz, 1H, H-3′), 5.60 (d, *J* = 7.5 Hz, 1H, H-2), 4.85–4.78 (overlap, 4H, H-5, H-2′, H-3, OCH_2CH_2OCO), 4.55 (dd, *J* = 6.6, 12.0 Hz, 1H, OCH_2CH_2OCO), 4.45 (dd, *J* = 6.7, 13.6 Hz, 1H, OCH_2CH_2OCO), 4.39 (d, *J* = 8.0 Hz, 1 H, H-20b), 4.33 (dd, 1H, OCH_2CH_2OCO), 4.31 (d, *J* = 7.7 Hz, 1H, H-20a),4.12-3.97 (m, 2H, H-7b, H-7a), 3.53 (d, *J* = 6.9 Hz, 1H, OH-2′), 2.53 (s, 3H, CH_3), 2.34 (s, 3H, CH_3), 2.46–2.28 (m, 4H, H-14a, H-14b, H-6a, H-6b), 1.93 (brs, 1H, OH-1), 1.70 (d, *J* = 1.2 Hz, 3H, CH_3), 1.24 (s, 3H, CH_3),1.15 (s, 3H, CH_3); ^{13}C-NMR ($CDCl_3$, 100 MHz) δ: 192.0, 171.1, 169.3, 167.0, 165.4, 152.5, 151.6, 144.5, 139.8, 138.4, 134.4, 134.3, 133.6, 131.8, 131.4 (q, $^2J_{C\text{-}F}$ = 33.2 Hz), 130.3 (q, $^3J_{C\text{-}F}$ = 3.4 Hz), 130.2, 129.7, 128.8, 128.0, 127.0, 126.9 (q, $^3J_{C\text{-}F}$ = 4.3 Hz), 126.5, 123.7 (q, $^1J_{C\text{-}F}$ = 273.8 Hz), 89.6, 84.7, 78.7, 76.0, 75.8, 75.2, 71.5, 70.8, 69.0, 65.9, 55.7, 43.0, 42.4, 36.4, 31.0, 29.0, 26.3, 25.6, 22.7, 21.6, 18.2, 14.4, 13.6, −5.2, −5.8; LC-MS (ESI, *m/z*): [M + 1], found 950.3, [M + 23], found 972.3, $C_{49}H_{50}F_3NO_{15}$: 949.31.

3.1.8. General Experimental Procedure for Compounds **18a–e**

2′-O-(tert-Butyldimethylsilyl)-9-O-(3-hydroxyethyl)-10-dehydro-7, 8-seco-10-deacetylpaclitaxel (**18a**). To a mixture of **15a** (65 mg, 0.0703 mmol), potassium carbonate (67.8 mg, 0.491 mmol) and potassium iodide (11.7 mg, 0.0705 mmol) in DMF (0.65 mL) was added 3-bromo-1-propanol (44 μL 0.487 mmol), dropwise, at 0 °C. The reaction mixture was stirred for 4 h at room temperature and then was diluted with ethyl acetate. The organic phase was washed with saturated aqueous NH_4Cl. The organic layer was dried over anhydrous Na_2SO_4 and then concentrated under reduced pressure. Purification of the crude product by silica gel chromatography (ethyl acetate: petroleum ether = 1:1) gave product **18a** as a white solid (50 mg, 72.4% yield). ^{1}H-NMR ($CDCl_3$, 400 MHz) δ: 8.10 (d, *J* = 7.6 Hz, 2H, Ar-H), 7.62 (d, *J* = 7.6 Hz, 2H, Ar-H), 7.58 (t, *J* = 7.2 Hz, 1H, Ar-H), 7.47 (dd, *J* = 7.6, 14.8 Hz, 2H, Ar-H), 7.43–7.40 (m, 1H, Ar-H), 7.38–7.36 (m, 4H, Ar-H), 7.30–7.29 (m, 3H, Ar-H), 6.30 (t, *J* = 8.4 Hz, 1H, H-13), 5.88 (d, *J* = 9.6 Hz, 1H, H-3′), 5.57 (d, *J* = 9.6 Hz, 1H, H-2), 5.30–5.27 (overlap, 2H, H-5, H-20a), 4.69 (d, *J* = 2.0 Hz, 1H, H-2′), 4.26 (d, *J* = 7.6 Hz, 1H, H-3), 4.20 (brs, 1H, H-20b), 4.00-3.95 (m, 2H, $OCH_2CH_2\underline{CH_2}OCO$), 3.91–3.83 (m, 3H, $O\underline{CH_2}CH_2CH_2OCO$, H-7a), 3.76 (brs, 1H, H-7b), 2.75–2.64 (m, 2H, H-6a, H-14a), 2.27–2.21 (m, 2H, H-6b, H-14b), 1.92–1.90 (m, 5H, CH_3, $OCH_2\underline{CH_2}CH_2OCO$), 1.96 (s, 3H, CH_3), 1.81 (brs, 3H, CH_3), 1.27 (s, 3H, CH_3), 1.18 (s, 3H, CH_3), 0.76 (s, 9H, $Si\underline{C(CH_3)_3}$), −0.08 (s, 3H, $Si(CH_3)$), −0.33 (s, 3H, $Si(CH_3)$); ^{13}C-NMR ($CDCl_3$, 100 MHz) δ: 191.6, 170.7, 168.7, 167.3 (2C), 153.1, 152.8, 144.1, 137.9, 133.8, 133.7, 131.9, 129.9 (2C), 128.9 (2C), 128.7 (4C), 128.6, 127.9 (2C), 126.5 (2C), 82.1, 79.9, 75.7, 74.7, 70.5, 68.8, 60.4, 59.3, 58.8, 55.6, 42.8, 36.6, 32.2, 25.4 (3C), 23.2, 22.1, 18.2, 14.9, 14.2, −5.5, −6.1; LC-MS (ESI, *m/z*): [M + 23], found 1006.0, $C_{54}H_{69}NO_{14}Si$: 983.45.

2′-O-(tert-Butyldimethylsilyl)-2-debenzoyl-2-(3-methoxybenzoyl)-9-O-(3-hydroxyethyl)-10-dehydro-7,8-seco-10-deacetylpaclitaxel (**18b**). White solid; yield 75.3%; ^{1}H-NMR ($CDCl_3$, 400 MHz) δ: 7.71–7.65 (m, 3H, Ar-H), 7.53 (m, 1H, Ar-H), 7.46–7.41 (m, 2H, Ar-H), 7.11 (dd, *J* = 2.4, 8.0 Hz, 1H, BzNH), 6.28 (t, *J* = 8.6 Hz, 1H, H-13), 5.87 (d, *J* = 9.2 Hz, 1H, H-3′), 5.58 (d, *J* = 9.5 Hz, 1H, H-2), 5.29–5.26 (overlap, 2H, H-5, H-20a), 4.72 (d, *J* = 2.1 Hz, 1H, H-2′), 4.26 (d, *J* = 6.6 Hz, 1H, H-3), 4.21 (brs, 1H, H-20b), 4.00-3.95 (m, 2H, $OCH_2CH_2\underline{CH_2}O$), 3.98–3.86 (m, 3H, $O\underline{CH_2}CH_2CH_2O$, H-7b), 3.83 (overlap, 4H, OCH_3, H-7a), 2.77–2.66 (m, 2H, H-6b, H-14b), 2.27–2.21 (m, 2H, H-6a, H-14a), 1.96 (s, 3H, CH_3), 1.92 (brs, 2H, $OCH_2\underline{CH_2}CH_2O$), 1.83 (m, 2H, OH), 1.84 (brs, 3H, CH_3), 1.26 (s, 3H, CH_3), 1.19 (s, 3H, CH_3), 0.78 (s, 9H, $Si\underline{C(CH_3)_3}$), −0.09 (s, 3H, $Si(CH_3)$), −0.29 (s, 3H, $Si(CH_3)$); ^{13}C-NMR ($CDCl_3$, 100 MHz) δ: 191.6, 171.2, 170.9, 168.9, 167.3, 167.2, 159.8, 144.4, 138.1, 133.8, 131.9, 130.4, 130.3, 128.7 (2C), 128.7 (2C), 128.0, 127.0 (2C), 126.7 (2C), 122.3, 119.6, 114.9, 85.8, 79.9, 75.8, 74.9, 70.7, 68.8, 59.3, 59.0, 55.7, 55.5, 42.8, 36.6, 32.3, 25.5 (3C), 25.2, 23.2, 22.2, 18.2, 14.9, 14.5, −5.5, −6.0; LC-MS (ESI, *m/z*): [M + 1], found 1014.4, [M + 23], found 1036.4, $C_{55}H_{71}NO_{16}Si$: 1013.46.

2′-O-(tert-Butyldimethylsilyl)-2-debenzoyl-2-(3-fluorobenzoyl)-9-O-(3-hydroxyethyl)-10-dehydro-7, 8-seco-10-deacetylpaclitaxel (**18c**). White solid; yield 69.7%; ^{1}H-NMR ($CDCl_3$, 400 MHz) δ: 7.93 (d, *J* = 7.6 Hz, 1H, Ar-H), 7.75 (d, *J* = 8.9 Hz, 1H, Ar-H), 7.63 (d, *J* = 7.5 Hz, 1H, Ar-H), 7.52–7.28 (m, 11H, NH, Ar-H), 6.29 (t, *J* = 8.1 Hz, 1H, H-13), 5.89 (d, *J* = 9.2 Hz, 1H, H-3′), 5.57 (d, *J* = 9.6 Hz, 1H, H-2), 5.28–5.26

(overlap, 2H, H-5, H-20a), 4.70 (d, J = 2.0 Hz, 1H, H-2′), 4.27 (d, J = 8.1 Hz, 1H, H-3), 4.19 (brs, 1H, H-20b), 3.99–3.94 (m, 2H, $OCH_2CH_2CH_2OH$), 3.88–3.81 (m, 3H, $OCH_2CH_2CH_2OH$, H-7a), 3.76 (brs, 1H, H-7b), 2.72–2.63 (m, 2H, H-6a, H-14a), 2.24 (dd, 1H, J = 9.5, 15.8 Hz, H-14b), 2.06– 1.98 (overlap, 1 H, H-6b), 1.95 (s, 3H, CH_3), 1.93–1.87 (m, 4H, CH_3, $OCH_2CH_2CH_2OH$), 1.83 (brs, 3H, CH_3), 1.26 (brs, 3H, CH_3), 1.17 (s, 3H, CH_3), 0.77 (s, 9H, $SiC(CH_3)_3$), −0.09 (s, 3H, $Si(CH_3)$), −0.32 (s, 3H, $Si(CH_3)$); ^{13}C-NMR ($CDCl_3$, 100 MHz) δ: 191.5, 171.2, 170.8, 168.6, 167.4, 166.3, 162.7 (d, $^1J_{C\text{-}F}$ = 248.2 Hz), 144.3, 137.9, 133.9, 131.9, 131.2 (d, $^2J_{C\text{-}F}$ = 7.3 Hz), 131.0 (d, $^3J_{C\text{-}F}$ = 7.7 Hz), 128.8, 128.7, 128.0, 127.0, 126.5, 125.8 (d, $^4J_{C\text{-}F}$ = 2.6 Hz), 121.0 (d, $^2J_{C\text{-}F}$ = 21.2 Hz), 116.6 (d, $^2J_{C\text{-}F}$ = 22.8 Hz), 85.9, 80.0, 75.8, 75.2, 70.5, 68.9, 59.3, 55.6, 42.8, 36.7, 32.3, 25.5, 23.2, 22.1, 18.2, 15.0, 14.5, −5.4, −6.0; LC-MS (ESI, *m/z*): [M + 1], found 1002.0, [M + 23], found 1025.0, $C_{54}H_{68}FNO_{14}Si$: 1001.44.

2′-O-(tert-Butyldimethylsilyl)-2-debenzoyl-2-(3-chlorobenzoyl)-9-O-(3-hydroxyethyl)-10-dehydro-7,8-seco-10-deacetylpaclitaxel (**18d**). White solid; yield 52.6%; ^{1}H-NMR ($CDCl_3$, 400 MHz) δ: 8.03 (d, J = 7.6 Hz, 1H, Ar-H), 8.00–7.96 (m, J = 7.6 Hz, 1H, Ar-H), 7.65 (d, J = 7.6 Hz, 2H, Ar-H), 7.54 (t, J = 7.2 Hz, 1H, Ar-H), 7.48–7.44 (m, 2H, Ar-H), 7.43–7.40 (m, 1H, Ar-H), 7.38–7.36 (m, 4H, Ar-H), 7.39–7.28 (m, 7H, Ar-H), 6.30 (t, J = 8.4 Hz, 1H, H-13), 5.88 (d, J = 9.6 Hz, 1H, H-3′), 5.57 (d, J = 9.6 Hz, 1H, H-2), 5.30–5.27 (overlap, 2H, H-5, H-20a), 4.71 (s, 1H, H-2′), 4.26 (d, J = 7.6 Hz, 1H, H-3), 4.18 (brs, 1H, H-20b), 3.99–3.93 (m, 2H, $OCH_2CH_2CH_2O$), 3.79–3.40 (m, 3H, $OCH_2CH_2CH_2O$, H-7a), 3.73–3.64 (brs, 1H, H-7b), 2.94 (s, 3H, CH_3), 2.84 (s, 3H, CH_3), 2.66 (br, 2H, H-6a, H-14a), 2.29–2.22 (m, 2H, H-6b, H-14b), 1.93 (s, 3H, CH_3), 1.93–1.86 (m, 5H, CH_3, $OCH_2CH_2CH_2O$), 1.82 (brs, 3H, CH_3), 1.24 (s, 3H, CH_3), 1.16 (s, 3H, CH_3), 0.76 (s, 9H, $SiC(CH_3)_3$), −0.11 (s, 3H, $Si(CH_3)$), −0.31 (s, 3H, $Si(CH_3)$); ^{13}C-NMR ($CDCl_3$, 100 MHz) δ: 191.5, 171.1, 170.8, 167.4, 165.9, 162.5, 144.3, 137.9, 134.8, 133.9, 133.7, 131.8, 131.0, 130.6, 129.5, 128.7 (2C), 128.6 (2C), 128.1, 127.9, 126.9 (2C), 126.5 (2C), 85.8, 75.7, 75.2, 70.5, 68.8, 67.9, 60.4, 59.2, 55.6, 42.7, 36.6, 36.4, 32.3, 31.4, 25.4 (3C), 23.2, 22.1, 21.0, 18.2, 14.5, 14.2, −5.5, −6.1; LC-MS (ESI, *m/z*): [M + 1], found 1018.4, [M + 23], found 1040.4, $C_{54}H_{68}ClNO_{14}Si$: 1017.41.

2′-O-(tert-Butyldimethylsilyl)-2-debenzoyl-2-(3-trifluoromethylbenzoyl)-9-O-(3-hydroxyethyl)-10-dehydro-7,8-seco-10-deacetylpaclitaxel (**18e**). White solid; yield 71.8%; ^{1}H-NMR ($CDCl_3$, 400 MHz): δ 8.38 (d, J = 7.8 Hz, 2H, Ar-H), 7.83 (d, J = 7.7 Hz, 2H, Ar-H), 7.68 (t, J = 7.8 Hz, 1H, Ar-H), 7.44 (dd, J = 15.4, 8.0 Hz, 2H, Ar-H), 7.47–7.41 (m, 1H, Ar-H), 7.40–7.36 (m, 4H, Ar-H), 7.30–7.29 (m, 3H, Ar-H), 6.29 (t, J = 8.5 Hz, 1H, H-13), 5.86 (d, J = 8.6 Hz, 1H, H-3′), 5.59 (d, J = 9.5 Hz, 1H, H-2), 5.26 (overlap, 2H, H-5, H-20a), 4.70 (d, J = 2.0 Hz, 1H, H-2′), 4.29 (d, J = 7.3 Hz, 1H, H-3), 4.21 (brs, 1H, H-20b), 4.00–3.96 (m, 2H, $OCH_2CH_2CH_2OH$), 3.90–3.87 (m, 3H, $OCH_2CH_2CH_2OH$, H-7a), 3.75 (brs, 1H, H-7b), 2.70–2.60 (m, 2H, H-6a, H-14a), 2.28–2.22 (m, 2H, H-6b, H-14b), 1.97 (s, 3H, CH_3), 1.94–1.92 (m, 5H, CH_3, $OCH_2CH_2CH_2OH$), 1.81 (brs, 3H, CH_3), 1.27 (s, 3H, CH_3), 1.19 (s, 3H, CH_3), 0.76 (s, 9H, $SiC(CH_3)_3$), −0.08 (s, 3H, $Si(CH_3)$), −0.32 (s, 3H, $Si(CH_3)$); ^{13}C-NMR ($CDCl_3$, 100 MHz) δ: 191.5, 170.8, 167.5, 144.3, 137.9, 133.9, 133.2, 132.0, 131.4 (q, $^2J_{C\text{-}F}$ = 33.3 Hz), 130.2 (q, $^3J_{C\text{-}F}$ = 4.0 Hz), 130.0, 128.8, 128.1, 126.9, 126.8 (q, $^3J_{C\text{-}F}$ = 3.9 Hz), 126.5, 123.6 (q, $^1J_{C\text{-}F}$ = 274.2 Hz), 85.9, 75.6, 75.4, 70.5, 59.4, 55.6, 42.9, 36.7, 32.3, 25.5, 18.2, 14.6, −5.4, −6.0; LC-MS (ESI, *m/z*): [M + 1], found 1052.4, [M + 23], found 1074.4, $C_{55}H_{68}NO_{14}F_3Si$: 1051.44.

3.1.9. General Experimental Procedure for Compounds **20a–e**

2′-O-(tert-Butyldimethylsilyl)-macrocyclic taxoid (**20a**). To a solution of **18a** (26.2 mg, 0.0266 mmol) in dichloromethane (5.7 mL) was added, dropwise, pyridine (11 μL, 0.133 mmol) and triphosgene (8.7 mg, 0.0293 mmol) at 0 °C, then the reaction mixture was stirred at room temperature for 3.5 h. The reaction was diluted with ethyl acetate, then washed with saturated NaCl. The organic layer was dried over anhydrous Na_2SO_4 and then concentrated under reduced pressure. Purification of the crude product by silica gel chromatography (ethyl acetate: petroleum ether = 1:3) gave product **20a** as a white solid (6.7 mg, 24.9% yield). ^{1}H-NMR ($CDCl_3$, 400 MHz) δ: 8.17 (d, J = 8.0 Hz, 2H, Ar-H), 7.75 (d, J = 7.6 Hz, 2H, Ar-H), 7.63 (t, J = 7.2 Hz, 1H, Ar-H), 7.56–7.49 (m, 3H, Ar-H), 7.44–7.29 (m, 7H, Ar-H), 7.09 (d, J = 9.2 Hz, 1H, NH), 6.27 (t, J = 8.8 Hz, 1H, H-13), 5.76 (d, J = 8.8 Hz, 1H, H-3′), 5.60 (d, J = 8.0 Hz, 1H,

H-2), 4.80 (d, *J* = 7.6 Hz, 2H, H-5, H-3), 4.67 (brs, 1H, H-2′), 4.63 (m, 1H, $O\underline{CH_2}CH_2CH_2OCO$), 4.53 (dd, *J* = 6.4, 11.6 Hz, 1H, $OCH_2CH_2\underline{CH_2}OCO$), 4.47 (d, *J* = 8.4 Hz, 1H, H-20a), 4.42 (dd, *J* = 4.0, 7.2 Hz, 1H, $OCH_2CH_2\underline{CH_2}OCO$), 4.34 (d, *J* = 8.4 Hz, 1H, H-20b), 4.11 (overlap, 2H, H-7a, $O\underline{CH_2}CH_2CH_2OCO$), 3.98 (dt, *J* = 6.0, 11.6 Hz, 1H, H-7b), 2.66 (m, 1H, H-6a), 2.56 (s, 3H, CH_3), 2.52 (s, 3H, CH_3), 2.42–2.11 (m, 5H, H-6b, H-14a, H-14b, $OCH_2\underline{CH_2}CH_2O$), 1.82 (s, 3H, CH_3), 1.24 (s, 3H, CH_3), 1.17 (s, 3H, CH_3), 0.79 (s, 9H, $SiC(CH_3)_3$), −0.04 (s, 3H, $Si(CH_3)$), −0.31 (s, 3H, $Si(CH_3)$); ^{13}C-NMR ($CDCl_3$, 150 MHz) δ: 191.6, 170.7, 169.7, 169.3, 166.7, 166.6, 153.6, 152.4, 144.1, 138.8, 138.1, 135.5, 133.6, 131.6, 130.2 (2C), 130.0, 128.7, 128.6, 128.5, 127.7, 126.8 (2C), 126.1 (2C), 90.3, 84.4, 78.4, 76.1, 75.2, 75.0, 70.4, 68.9, 65.8, 64.2, 55.4, 42.6 (2C), 36.4, 30.8, 28.8, 25.9, 25.3 (3C), 22.5, 21.5, 17.9, 14.5, 14.1, −5.5, −6.1; LC-MS (ESI, *m/z*): [M + 23], found 1032.0, $C_{55}H_{67}NO_{15}Si$: 1009.43.

2′-O-(tert-Butyldimethylsilyl)-2-debenzoyl-2-(3-methoxybenzoyl)-macrocyclic taxoid (**20b**). White solid; yield 28.6%; ^1H-NMR ($CDCl_3$, 400MHz) δ: 7.79 (d, *J* = 7.6 Hz, 1H, Ar-H), 7.76 (d, *J* = 7.2 Hz, 2H, Ar-H), 7.67–7.66 (m, 1H, Ar-H), 7.55–7.50 (m, 1H, Ar-H), 7.48–7.42 (m, 3H, Ar-H), 7.40–7.29 (m, 5H, Ar-H), 7.19–7.16 (m, 1H, Ar-H), 7.09 (d, *J* = 8.8 Hz, 1H, BzNH), 6.27 (t, *J* = 8.8 Hz, 1H, H-13), 5.76 (dd, *J* = 1.5, 9.0 Hz, 1H, H-3′), 5.62 (d, *J* = 7.64 Hz, 1H, H-2), 4.85–4.82 (m, 2H, H-5, H-3), 4.69–4.63 (m, 2H, H-2′, $O\underline{CH_2}CH_2CH_2OCO$), 4.56–4.51 (m, 1H, $OCH_2CH_2\underline{CH_2}OCO$), 4.48–4.38 (m, 3H, H-20a, H-20b, $OCH_2\underline{CH_2}\underline{CH_2}OCO$), 4.16–4.07 (m, 2H, H-7a, $O\underline{CH_2}CH_2\underline{CH_2}OCO$), 4.01–3.96 (m, 1H, H-7b), 3.90 (s, 3H, OCH_3), 2.72–2.62 (m, 1H, H-6a), 2.57 (s, 3H, CH_3), 2.53 (s, 3H, CH_3), 2.43–2.36 (m, 1H, H-6b), 2.35–2.28 (m, 1H, H-14a), 2.16–2.14 (m, 2H, H-14b, $OCH_2\underline{CH_2}CH_2O$), 1.82 (d, *J* = 1.1 Hz, 3H, CH_3), 1.25 (s, 3H, CH_3), 1.18 (s, 3H, CH_3), 0.88 (s, 9H, $SiC(CH_3)_3$), −0.014 (s, 3H, $Si(CH_3)$), −0.29 (s, 3H, $Si(CH_3)$); ^{13}C-NMR ($CDCl_3$, 100 MHz) δ: 190.8, 171.3, 171.2, 169.2, 166.9, 166.8, 159.8, 144.8, 138.3, 134.2, 131.8, 130.6, 130.1, 128.8 (2C), 128.7 (2C), 128.0, 127.0 (2C), 126.6 (2C), 122.3, 120.0, 114.5, 85.1, 77.4, 77.3, 76.8, 75.3, 74.9, 70.8, 67.8, 60.4, 55.8, 55.5, 42.8, 41.6, 40.4, 36.6, 33.0, 29.7, 25.5 (3C), 23.2, 22.4, 21.0, 18.2, 14.5, 14.2, −5.3,−5.8; LC-MS (ESI, *m/z*): [M + 1], found 1040.5, [M + 23], found 1062.5, $C_{56}H_{69}NO_{16}Si$: 1039.44.

2′-O-(tert-Butyldimethylsilyl)-2-debenzoyl-2-(3-fluorobenzoyl)-macrocyclic taxoid (**20c**). White solid; yield 27.1%; ^1H-NMR ($CDCl_3$, 400 MHz) δ: 8.00 (d, *J* = 7.7 Hz, 1H, Ar-H), 7.87 (d, *J* = 8.8 Hz, 1H, Ar-H), 7.77 (d, *J* = 7.32 Hz, 1H, Ar-H), 7.57–7.51 (m, 2H, Ar-H), 7.46–7.33 (m, 8H, Ar-H), 7.10 (d, *J* = 9.0 Hz, 1H, NH), 6.26 (t, *J* = 8.5 Hz, 1H, H-13), 5.78 (d, *J* = 8.5 Hz, 1H, H-3′), 5.60 (d, *J* = 7.7 Hz, 1H, H-2), 4.85–4.82 (overlap, 2H, H-5, H-3), 4.72–4.63 (overlap, 2H, $O\underline{CH_2}CH_2CH_2OCO$, H-2′), 4.55 (dt, *J* = 5.5, 10.3 Hz, 1H, $OCH_2CH_2\underline{CH_2}OCO$), 4.47–4.42 (overlap, 2H, $OCH_2CH_2\underline{CH_2}OCO$, H-20a), 4.37 (d, *J* = 8.2 Hz, 1H, H-20b), 4.14–4.10 (overlap, 2H, H-7a, $O\underline{CH_2}CH_2CH_2OCO$), 3.99 (dt, *J* = 6.4, 11.3 Hz, 1H, H-7b), 2.73–2.64 (m, 1H, H-6a), 2.57 (s, 3H, CH_3), 2.54 (s, 3H, CH_3), 2.42–2.18 (m, 5H, H-6b, H-14a, H-14b, $OCH_2\underline{CH_2}CH_2O$), 2.10 (brs, 1H, OH), 1.83 (s, 3H, CH_3), 1.25 (s, 3H, CH_3), 1.18 (s, 3H, CH_3), 0.82 (s, 9H, $SiC(CH_3)_3$), −0.008 (s, 3H, $Si(CH_3)$), −0.27 (s, 3H, $Si(CH_3)$); ^{13}C-NMR ($CDCl_3$, 100 MHz) δ: 191.8, 171.0, 169.5, 166.9, 165.7 (d, $^5J_{C\text{-}F}$ = 3.0 Hz, ArCO), 162.6 (d, $^1J_{C\text{-}F}$ = 247.8 Hz), 153.8, 152.6, 144.3, 139.1, 138.4, 135.5, 134.2, 131.8, 131.3 (d, $^3J_{C\text{-}F}$ = 7.5 Hz), 130.6 (d, $^3J_{C\text{-}F}$ = 7.7 Hz), 128.8, 128.7, 127.9, 127.0, 126.4, 126.0 (d, $^4J_{C\text{-}F}$ = 2.6 Hz), 120.9 (d, $^2J_{C\text{-}F}$ = 21.1 Hz), 117.0 (d, $^2J_{C\text{-}F}$ = 23.2 Hz), 90.6, 84.6, 78.6, 77.4, 77.1, 76.7, 76.2, 75.8, 75.3, 70.6, 69.2, 66.0, 64.4, 55.6, 42.8 (2C), 36.5, 31.0, 29.0, 26.1, 25.5 (3C), 22.7, 21.7, 18.2, 14.7, 14.4, −5.2, −5.8; LC-MS (ESI, *m/z*): [M + 1], found 1028.4, [M + 23], found 1050.4, $C_{55}H_{66}FNO_{15}Si$: 1027.42.

2′-O-(tert-Butyldimethylsilyl)-2-debenzoyl-2-(3-chlorobenzoyl)-macrocyclic taxoid (**20d**). White solid; yield 23.6%; ^1H-NMR ($CDCl_3$, 400 MHz) δ: 8.20 (t, *J* = 1.6 Hz, 1H, Ar-H), 8.12–8.09 (m, 1H, Ar-H), 7.77 (d, *J* = 7.2 Hz, 1H, Ar-H), 7.65–7.62 (m, 1H, Ar-H), 7.56–7.51 (m, 2H, Ar-H), 7.47–7.33 (m, 7H, Ar-H), 7.09 (d, *J* = 9.0 Hz, 1H, BzNH), 6.26 (t, *J* = 8.8 Hz, 1H, H-13), 5.77 (dd, *J* = 1.5, 8.98 Hz, 1H, H-3′), 5.60 (d, *J* = 7.8 Hz, 1H, H-2), 4.85–4.82 (dd, *J* = 3.5, 11.0 Hz, 2H, H-5, H-17b), 4.72–4.64 (m, 2H, $O\underline{CH_2}CH_2CH_2OCO$, H-2′), 4.59–4.53 (m, 1H, $OCH_2CH_2\underline{CH_2}OCO$), 4.49–4.43 (m, 2H, $OCH_2CH_2\underline{CH_2}OCO$, H-20a), 4.38 (d, *J* = 8.4 Hz, 1H, H-20b), 4.15–4.10 (m, 2H, $OCH_2CH_2\underline{CH_2}OCO$, H-20a), 4.02–3.96 (m, 1H, H-7b), 2.74–2.65 (m, 1H, H-6a), 2.57 (s, 3H, CH_3), 2.55 (s, 3H, CH_3), 2.42–2.20 (m, 5H, H-6b, H-14a, H-14b, $OCH_2\underline{CH_2}CH_2O$), 1.84 (d, *J* = 1.0 Hz, 3H, CH_3), 1.26 (s, 3H, CH_3), 1.19 (s, 3H, CH_3), 0.83 (s, 9H,

$SiC(CH_3)_3$), −0.005 (s, 3H, $Si(CH_3)$), −0.26 (s, 3H, $Si(CH_3)$); ^{13}C-NMR ($CDCl_3$, 100 MHz) δ: 190.7, 171.2, 169.1, 167.0, 165.7, 144.8, 138.3, 135.5, 135.0, 134.3, 133.9, 131.8, 131.1, 130.5, 129.9, 128.8 (2C), 128.7 (2C), 128.2, 128.0, 127.0 (2C), 126.7 (2C), 90.6, 84.6, 78.7, 76.2, 75.8, 75.3, 70.7, 67.8, 55.7, 42.8, 41.6, 36.5, 34.7, 31.6, 29.7, 25.6 (3C), 22.7, 22.4, 18.2, 14.5, 14.1, −5.3, −5.8; LC-MS (ESI, *m/z*): [M + 1], found 1044.0, [M + 23], found 1065.9, $C_{55}H_{66}ClNO_{15}Si$: 1043.39.

2′-O-(tert-Butyldimethylsilyl)-2-debenzoyl-2-(3-trifluoromethylbenzoyl)-macrocyclic taxoid (**20e**). White solid; yield 26.7%; ^{1}H-NMR ($CDCl_3$, 400MHz) δ: 8.50 (s, 1H, Ar-H), 8.41 (d, *J* = 7.8 Hz, 1H, Ar-H), 7.92 (d, *J* = 7.9 Hz, 1H, Ar-H), 7.55–7.51 (m, 1H, Ar-H), 7.48–7.33 (m, 8H, Ar-H), 7.09 (d, *J* = 9.0 Hz, 1H, NH), 6.26–6.21 (m, 1H, H-13), 5.76 (dd, *J* =1.4, 9.1 Hz, 1H, H-3′), 5.64 (d, *J* = 7.8 Hz, 1H, H-2), 4.89–4.83 (m, 2H, H-5, H-3), 4.69–4.63 (m, 2H, $O\underline{CH_2}CH_2CH_2OCO$, H-2′), 4.60–4.55 (m, 1H, $OCH_2CH_2\underline{CH_2}OCO$), 4.49–4.43 (m, 2H, $OCH_2CH_2\underline{CH_2}\overline{OCO}$, H-20a), 4.37 (d, *J* = 8.0 Hz,1H, H-20b), 4.13 (t, *J* = 7.7 Hz, 2H, H-7a, $O\underline{CH_2}CH_2CH_2OCO$), 2.75–2.67 (m, 1H, H-6a), 4.02–3.96 (m, 1H, H-7b), 2.58 (s, 3H, CH_3), 2.53 (s, 3H, CH_3), 2.45–2.18 (m, 5H, H-6b, H-14a, H-14b, $OCH_2\underline{CH_2}CH_2O$), 1.84 (d, *J* =1.0 Hz, 1H, CH_3), 1.26 (s, 3H, CH_3), 1.25 (s, 3H, CH_3), 1.20 (s, 3H, CH_3), 0.83 (s, 9H, $SiC(CH_3)_3$), −0.006 (s, 3H, $Si(CH_3)$), −0.25 (s, 3H, $Si(CH_3)$); ^{13}C-NMR ($CDCl_3$, 100 MHz) δ: 191.7, 171.1, 167.0, 165.5, 153.9, 152.7, 135.4, 134.3, 133.6, 131.8, 131.4 (q, ^2J = 33.3 Hz), 130.9, 130.3 (q, ^3J = 3.9 Hz), 130.2, 129.7, 128.8, 128.0, 127.0, 126.9 (q, ^3J = 3.8 Hz), 126.5, 123.7 (q, ^1J = 273.8 Hz), 90.6, 84.7, 78.7, 76.2, 75.8, 75.3, 70.8, 69.2, 66.0, 64.5, 55.7, 42.9, 42.8, 36.5, 31.0, 29.0, 26.1, 22.6, 21.6, 18.2, 14.6, 14.4, −5.2, −5.8; LC-MS (ESI, *m/z*): [M + 1], found 1078.4, [M + 23], found 1100.4, $C_{56}H_{66}F_3NO_{15}Si$: 1077.42.

3.1.10. General Procedure for the Syntheses of Compounds **22a–e**

Macrocyclic taxoid (**22a**)

To a solution of of **20a** (29.6 mg, 0.0293 mmol) in THF (8 mL) was added, dropwise, 0.47 mL of HF-pyridine (*v/v* = 1:2) at 0 °C, and the reaction mixture was stirred at room temperature for 30 h. The reaction was quenched with saturated aqueous $NaHCO_3$, diluted with ethyl acetate, and washed with saturated NH_4Cl. The organic layer was dried over anhydrous Na_2SO_4 and then concentrated under reduced pressure. Purification of the crude product by silica gel chromatography (ethyl acetate: petroleum ether = 2:1) gave product **22a** as a white solid (13.4 mg, 51.0% yield). ^{1}H-NMR ($CDCl_3$, 400 MHz) δ: 7.16 (d, *J* = 7.1 Hz, 2H, Ar-H), 7.75 (d, *J* = 7.0 Hz, 2H, Ar-H), 7.64 (t, *J* = 7.5 Hz, 1H, Ar-H), 7.54–7.50 (m, 3H, Ar-H), 7.49–7.47 (m, 2H, Ar-H), 7.43–7.39 (m, 4H, Ar-H), 7.36–7.32 (m,1H, Ar-H), 7.04 (d, *J* = 9.1 Hz, 1H, NH), 6.18 (dd, *J* = 8.7 Hz, 1H, H-13), 5.81 (dd, *J* = 2.4, 9.1 Hz, 1H, H-3′), 5.59 (d, *J* = 7.7 Hz, 1H, H-2), 4.81–4.79 (overlap, 3H, H-5, H-3, H-2′), 4.61 (dt, *J* = 5.4, 11.0 Hz, 1H, $O\underline{CH_2}CH_2CH_2OCO$), 4.52 (dt, *J* = 6.9, 12.0 Hz, 1H, $OCH_2CH_2\underline{CH_2}OCO$), 4.44 (overlap, 2H, H-20a, $OCH_2CH_2\underline{CH_2}OCO$), 4.41–4.33 (m, 1H, H-20b), 4.34–4.28 (overlap, *J* = 6.7 Hz, H-7a), 4.08 (overlap, 2H, H-7a, $O\underline{CH_2}CH_2CH_2OCO$), 3.95 (m, 1H, H-7b), 3.58 (brs, 1H, OH-2′), 2.66–2.61 (m, 1H, H-6a), 2.55 (s, 3H, CH_3), 2.37–2.33 (brs, 3H, CH_3), 2.30–2.12 (overlap, 3H, H-6b, H-14a, H-14b), 1.67 (brs, 2H, $OCH_2\underline{CH_2}CH_2OCO$), 1.23 (s, 3H, CH_3), 1.16 (s, 3H, CH_3); ^{13}C-NMR ($CDCl_3$, 100 MHz) δ: 191.6, 172.4, 169.8, 167.0, 166.9, 153.8, 152.6, 144.6, 138.0 (2C), 136.1, 133.9, 133.7, 130.2 (2C), 129.1, 129.0 (2C), 128.9, 128.8 (2C), 128.7 (2C), 128.3, 127.0 (2C), 90.5, 84.7, 78.5, 76.3, 75.3, 73.2, 71.7, 69.2, 65.6, 64.4, 54.8, 42.9, 42.7, 36.5, 31.0, 29.0, 26.2, 22.4, 21.3, 14.7, 14.0; LC-MS (ESI, *m/z*): [M + 1], found 896.3, [M + 23], found 918.3, $C_{49}H_{53}NO_{15}$: 895.34.

2-Debenzoyl-2-(3-methoxybenzoyl)-macrocyclic taxoid (**22b**). White solid; yield 59.2%; ^{1}H-NMR ($CDCl_3$, 400 MHz) δ: 7.75 (d, *J* = 7.4 Hz, 3H, Ar-H), 7.65 (dd, *J* =1.42, 2.3 Hz, 1H, Ar-H), 7.52–7.38 (m, 9H, Ar-H), 7.17 (dd, *J* = 2.1, 8.2 Hz, 1H, Ar-H), 7.06 (d, *J* = 9.0 Hz, 1H, NH), 6.15 (t, *J* = 8.2 Hz, 1H, H-13), 5.78 (dd, *J* = 2.1, 8.9 Hz, 1H, H-3′), 5.59 (d, *J* = 7.6 Hz, 1H, H-2), 4.80–4.76 (overlap, 3H, H-5, H-3, H-2′), 4.60 (dt, *J* = 5.6, 11.2 Hz, 1H, $O\underline{CH_2}CH_2CH_2OCO$), 4.51 (dt, *J* = 5.7, 11.2 Hz, 1H, $OCH_2CH_2\underline{CH_2}OCO$), 4.44–4.37 (overlap, *J* = 5.6 Hz, 2H, $OCH_2CH_2\underline{CH_2}OCO$, H-20a), 4.36 (d, *J* = 8.3 Hz, 1H, H-20b), 4.07 (overlap, 2H, H-7a, $O\underline{CH_2}CH_2CH_2OCO$), 3.97–3.91 (m, 1H, H-7b), 3.87 (s, 3H, OCH_3), 3.66 (d, *J* = 4.1 Hz, 1H, OH-2′),

2.67–2.56 (m, 1H, H-6a), 2.55 (s, 3H, CH_3), 2.34 (s, 3H, CH_3), 2.40–2.30 (m, 2H, $OCH_2\underline{CH_2}CH_2OCO$), 2.28–2.12 (m, 3H, H-6b, H-14a, H-14b), 2.02 (brs, 1H, OH-1), 1.65 (s, 3H, CH_3), 1.22 (s, 3H, CH_3), 1.15 (s, 3H, CH_3); ^{13}C-NMR ($CDCl_3$, 100 MHz) δ: 191.6, 172.3, 169.8, 167.0, 166.8, 159.8, 153.7, 152.6, 144.6, 138.1, 137.9, 136.1, 133.7, 132.0, 130.3, 129.8, 129.0, 128.7, 128.3, 127.1, 127.0, 122.4, 112.0, 115.0, 90.4, 84.7, 78.4, 76.3, 75.3, 73.3, 71.7, 69.2, 66.0, 64.4, 55.5, 54.9, 42.8, 42.7, 36.5, 31.0, 29.0, 26.1, 22.4, 21.2, 14.7, 14.0; LC-MS (ESI, *m/z*): [M + 1], found 926.3, [M + 23], found 948.3, $C_{50}H_{55}NO_{16}$: 925.35.

2-Debenzoyl-2-(3-fluorobenzoyl)-macrocyclic taxoid (**22c**). White solid; yield 51.5%; ^{1}H-NMR ($CDCl_3$, 400 MHz) δ: 7.96 (d, *J* = 7.69 Hz, 1 H, Ar-H), 7.84 (d, *J* = 9.1 Hz, 1H, Ar-H), 7.74 (d, *J* = 7.7 Hz, 2H, Ar-H), 7.53–7.46 (m, 4 H, Ar-H), 7.40 (t, *J* = 7.5 Hz, 4H, Ar-H), 7.36–7.32 (m, 2H, Ar-H), 7.05 (d, *J* = 9.0 Hz, 1H, NH), 6.15 (t, *J* = 8.6 Hz, 1H, H-13), 5.78 (dd, *J* = 2.0, 9.0 Hz, 1H, H-3′), 5.57 (d, *J* = 7.7 Hz, 1H, H-2), 4.81–4.79 (overlap, 3H, H-5, H-3, H-2′), 4.60 (dt, *J* = 5.3, 10.7 Hz, 1H, $\underline{OCH_2}CH_2CH_2OCO$), 4.52 (dt, *J* = 5.4, 10.8 Hz, 1H, $OCH_2CH_2\underline{CH_2}OCO$), 4.44–4.40 (ovelap, 2H, H-7a, $\overline{OCH_2}CH_2\underline{CH_2}OCO$), 4.40 (d, *J* = 8.0 Hz, 1H, H-20a), 4.32 (d, *J* = 8.1 Hz, 1H, H-20b), 4.07 (t, *J* = 7.5 Hz, 2H, $O\underline{CH_2}\overline{CH_2}CH_2OCO$), 3.93 (dt, *J* = 5.9, 11.9 Hz, 1H, H-7b), 3.69 (brs, 1H, OH-2′), 2.68–2.58 (m, 1H, H-6a), 2.54 (s, 3H, CH_3), 2.34 (s, 3H, CH_3), 2.33–2.26 (m, 2H, $OCH_2CH_2CH_2OCO$), 2.24–2.16 (m, 3H, H-6b, H-14a, H-14b), 1.97 (brs, 1H, OH-1), 1.65 (br, 3H, CH_3), 1.22 (s, 3H, CH_3), 1.15 (s, 3H, CH_3); ^{13}C-NMR ($CDCl_3$, 100 MHz) δ: 191.5, 172.4, 169.7, 167.0, 165.7 (d, $J_{C\text{-}F}$ = 2.8 Hz, CO), 162.6 (d, $^1J_{C\text{-}F}$ =247.9 Hz), 153.8, 152.6, 144.5, 138.1 (2C), 135.9, 133.8, 131.9, 131.3 (d, $^3J_{C\text{-}F}$ = 7.5 Hz), 130.5 (d, $^3J_{C\text{-}F}$ = 7.6 Hz), 129.0, 128.7, 128.3, 127.0 (2C), 126.0 (d, $^4J_{C\text{-}F}$ = 2.9 Hz), 121.0 (d, $^2J_{C\text{-}F}$ = 21.3 Hz), 116.9 (d, $^2J_{C\text{-}F}$ = 23.3 Hz), 90.5, 84.6, 78.5, 76.2, 75.6, 73.3, 71.6, 69.2, 66.0, 64.4, 55.0, 42.8, 42.7, 36.4, 30.9, 29.3, 29.0, 26.1, 22.3, 21.3, 14.6, 14.0; LC-MS (ESI, *m/z*): [M + 1], found 914.3, [M + 23], found 936.3, $C_{49}H_{52}FNO_{15}$: 913.33.

2-Debenzoyl-2-(3-chlorobenzoyl)-macrocyclic taxoid (**22d**). White solid; yield 65.4%; ^{1}H-NMR ($CDCl_3$, 400 MHz) δ: 8.16 (t, *J* = 1.8 Hz, 1H, Ar), 8.06–8.04 (m, 1 H, Ar-H), 7.75–7.73 (m, 2H, Ar-H), 7.61 (ddd, *J* =1.0, 2.0, 8.0 Hz, 1H, Ar-H), 7.43–7.39 (m, 4H, Ar-H), 7.52–7.45 (m, 4 H, Ar-H), 7.37–7.32 (m, 1H, Ar-H), 7.01 (d, *J* = 9.0 Hz, 1H, NH), 6.15 (dd, *J* = 7.4, 8.7 Hz, 1H, H-13), 5.78 (dd, *J* = 2.3, 9.0 Hz, 1H, H-3′), 5.57 (d, *J* = 7.7 Hz, 1H, H-2), 4.81–4.79 (overlap, 3H, H-5, H-3, H-2′), 4.60 (dt, *J* = 5.3, 10.7 Hz, 1H, $\underline{OCH_2}CH_2CH_2OCO$), 4.53 (dt, *J* = 5.5, 11.3 Hz, 1H, $OCH_2CH_2\underline{CH_2}OCO$), 4.45–4.44 (m, 1H, $OCH_2CH_2\underline{CH_2}OCO$), 4.39 (d, *J* = 8.2 Hz, 1H, H-20a), 4.33 (d, *J* = 8.2 Hz, 1H, H-20b), 4.08 (overlap, *J* = 7.62 Hz, 2H, H-7a, $\underline{OCH_2}CH_2CH_2OCO$), 3.96–3.90 (m, 1H, H-7b), 3.60 (brs, 1H, OH-2′), 2.68–2.58 (m, 1H, H-6a), 2.54 (s, 3H, CH_3), 2.35 (s, 3H, CH_3), 2.44–2.30 (m, 2H, $OCH_2\underline{CH_2}CH_2OCO$), 2.28–2.16 (m, 3H, H-6b, H-14a, H-14b), 1.97 (brs, 1H, OH-1), 1.65 (d, *J* =1.7 Hz, 3H, CH_3), 1.23 (s, 3H, CH_3), 1.16 (s, 3H, CH_3); ^{13}C-NMR ($CDCl_3$, 100 MHz) δ: 191.5, 172.4, 169.7, 167.0, 165.5, 153.8, 152.6, 144.5, 138.0, 135.9, 134.8, 133.8, 133.7, 132.0, 130.9, 130.2 (2C), 129.0, 128.7, 128.4, 127.1, 127.0, 90.4, 84.6, 78.5, 76.1, 75.5, 73.2, 71.7, 69.2, 65.9, 64.4, 55.0, 42.8, 42.7, 36.4, 30.9, 29.0, 26.1, 22.3, 21.2, 14.6, 14.0; LC-MS (ESI, *m/z*): [M + 1], found 930.3, [M + 23], found 952.3, $C_{49}H_{52}ClNO_{15}$: 929.30.

2-Debenzoyl-2-(3-trifluoromethylbenzoyl)-macrocyclic taxoid (**22e**). White solid; yield 59.5%; ^{1}H-NMR ($CDCl_3$, 400 MHz) δ: 8.46 (s, 1 H, Ar), 8.36 (d, *J* = 7.8 Hz, 1H, Ar-H), 7.90 (d, *J* =7.7 Hz, 1H, Ar-H), 7.73–7.67 (m, 3 H, Ar-H), 7.51–7.47 (m, 3H, Ar-H), 7.42–7.32 (m, 5H, Ar-H), 6.98 (d, *J* = 9.0 Hz, 1H, NH), 6.15 (t, *J* = 8.1 Hz, 1H, H-13), 5.77 (dd, *J* = 2.0, 9.0 Hz, 1H, H-3′), 5.61 (d, *J* = 7.7 Hz, 1H, H-2), 4.84–4.78 (overlap, 3H, H-5, H-3, H-2′), 4.62–4.51 (m, 2H, $\underline{OCH_2}CH_2\underline{CH_2}OCO$), 4.45–4.41 (m, 2H, H-7a, $OCH_2CH_2\underline{CH_2}OCO$), 4.39 (d, *J* = 8.0 Hz, 1H, H-20a), 4.31 (d, *J* = 8.2 Hz, 1H, H-20b), 4.07 (t, *J* = 7.6 Hz, 1H, $\underline{OCH_2}\overline{CH_2}CH_2OCO$), 3.93 (dt, *J* = 6.9, 11.6 Hz, 1H, H-7b), 3.62 (brs, 1H, OH-2′), 2.66–2.58 (m, 1H, H-6a), 2.54 (s, 3H, CH_3), 2.44–2.35 (m, 2H, $OCH_2\underline{CH_2}CH_2OCO$), 2.32 (s, 3H, CH_3), 2.28–2.16 (m, 3H, H-6b, H-14a, H-14b), 1.97 (brs, 1H, OH-1), 1.67 (br, 3H, CH_3), 1.23 (s, 3H, CH_3), 1.17 (s, 3H, CH_3); ^{13}C-NMR ($CDCl_3$, 75 MHz) δ: 191.6, 172.4, 169.7, 167.0, 165.4, 153.7, 152.6, 144.5, 138.1 (2C), 135.8, 133.7, 133.6, 131.9, 131.3 (d, $^2J_{C\text{-}F}$ = 33.2 Hz), 130.3 (d, $^3J_{C\text{-}F}$ = 3.7 Hz), 130.1, 129.6, 129.0, 128.7, 128.4, 127.1, 127.0, 126.9 (d, $^3J_{C\text{-}F}$ = 3.2 Hz), 125.5, 90.5, 84.6, 78.5, 76.1, 75.6, 73.1, 71.7, 69.2, 66.0, 64.4, 55.0, 42.8, 42.7, 36.3, 30.9, 29.3, 28.9, 26.1, 22.2, 21.2, 14.6, 14.0; LC-MS (ESI, *m/z*): [M + 1], found 964.4, [M + 23], found 986.3, $C_{50}H_{52}F_3NO_{15}$: 963.33.

3.2. Cell Assays

Cell viability after taxoids treatment was evaluated using CCK-8 assay. Briefly, 3000 cells per well were seeded in 96-well plates and incubated under normal conditions for 24 h. Cells were treated with different concentrations of the test agent for 72 h, then the medium was removed, 100 μL of CCK-8 working solution was added to each well for 1 h at 37 °C. The absorbance was measured at 450 nm with a microplate reader (Tecan Trading, AG, Switzerland). Vehicle-only treated cells served as the indicator of 100% cell viability. The 50% inhibitory concentration (IC_{50}) was defined as the concentration that reduced the absorbance of the vehicle-only treated wells by 50% in the 3-(4,5-dimethylthiazol-2-yl)-2,5-diphenyltetrazolium bromide (MTT) assay.

3.3. Model Building and Molecular Dynamics Simulations

The X-ray crystal structure of paclitaxel provided a template for the construction of **18b** and **22b** using the molecular editing tools implemented in PyMOL [17]. Geometry optimization of **18b** and **22b** was achieved by means of the updated AM1 hamiltonian implemented in the *sqm* program, which also produced atomic charge distributions for both ligands that can reproduce the molecular electrostatic potential. The ff14SB AMBER force field was used to assign bonded and non-bonded parameters to protein and ligand atoms [18,19]. **18b** was immersed in a cubic box containing TIP3P water molecules and simulated under periodic boundary conditions for 50 ns at 300 K. Subsequent gradual cooling, from 300 to 273 K over 1 ns, of snapshots taken regularly every 2.5 ns, followed by energy minimization until the root-mean-square of the Cartesian elements of the gradient was less than 0.1 kcal·mol^{-1}·Å^{-1}, provided representative structures of this molecule; those displaying the shortest distance between the free hydroxyl groups were chosen to build **22b** by means of a C=O linkage. The simulated macromolecular ensemble representing a short piece of a microtubule with bound **22b** was constructed as previously reported for D-seco taxol derivatives [20].

4. Conclusions

In summary, this study demonstrated that C-seco taxoids conformationally constrained via carbonate-containing linked macrocyclization display increased cytotoxicity on drug-resistant tumors overexpressing both βIII and P-gp, compared to the non-cyclized C-seco taxoid counterparts Among them, compound **22b**, bearing a 2-*m*-methoxybenzoyl group together with a five-atom linker, was identified as the most potent compound in the series.

Supplementary Materials: The supplementary materials are available online, cell lines and culture [21], establishment of model multidrug-resistant breast cancer cell line MCF-7/ADR. Copies of ESI-MS, HPLC, ^{1}H-NMR and ^{13}C-NMR spectra for representative compounds.

Author Contributions: Y.Z. performed most of the experiments; T.-N.W. carried out the bioassays; A.M. and F.G. carried out the molecular modeling studies; writing—original draft preparation, Y.Z., T.-N.W. and A.M.; writing—review and editing, W.-S.F. and F.G.; W.-S.F. planned, designed, and organized the whole research of this study. All authors read and approved the final version of the manuscript.

Funding: CAMS Innovation Fund for Medical Sciences (CIFMS Grant No. 2016-I2M-1-01) and the Drug Innovation Major Project (Grant Nos. 2018ZX09711001-001-001 and 2018ZX09711001-001-003) by MOST of China (W.-S.F.) and Spanish MEC/MICINN for grant SAF2015-64629-C2-2 (F.G.) are acknowledged.

Conflicts of Interest: The authors declare no conflicts of interest regarding the publication of this paper.

References

1. Fojo, T.; Coley, H.M. The role of efflux pumps in drug-resistant metastatic breast cancer: New insights and treatment strategies. *Clin. Breast Cancer* **2007**, *7*, 749–756. [CrossRef] [PubMed]
2. Kavallaris, M. Microtubules and resistance to tubulin-binding agents. *Nat. Rev. Cancer* **2010**, *10*, 194–204. [CrossRef] [PubMed]
3. Kamath, K.; Wilson, L.; Cabral, F.; Jordan, M.A. βIII-tubulin induces paclitaxel resistance in association with reduced effects on microtubule dynamic instability. *J. Biol. Chem.* **2005**, *280*, 12902–12907. [CrossRef] [PubMed]

4. Orr, G.A.; Verdier-Pinard, P.; McDaid, H.; Horwitz, S.B. Mechanisms of Taxol resistance related to microtubules. *Oncogene* **2003**, *22*, 7280–7295. [CrossRef] [PubMed]
5. Ferlini, C.; Gallo, D.; Scambia, G. New taxanes in development. *Expert Opin. Investig. Drugs* **2008**, *17*, 335–347. [CrossRef] [PubMed]
6. Ojima, I.; Lichtenthal, B.; Lee, S.; Wang, C.; Wang, X. Taxane anticancer agents: A patent perspective. *Expert Opin. Ther. Pat.* **2016**, *26*, 1–20. [CrossRef] [PubMed]
7. Paradiso, A.; Mangia, A.; Chiratti, A.; Tommasi, S.; Zito, A.; Latorre, A.; Schittulli, F.; Lorusso, V. Biomarkers predictive for clinical efficacy of taxol-based chemotherapy in advanced breast cancer. *Ann. Oncol.* **2005**, *16*, 14–19. [CrossRef] [PubMed]
8. Seve, P.; Mackey, J.; Isaac, S.; Tredan, O.; Souquet, P.-J.; Perol, M.; Lai, R.; Voloch, A.; Dumontet, C. Class III β-tubulin expression in tumor cells predicts response and outcome in patients with non-small cell lung cancer receiving paclitaxel. *Mol. Cancer Ther.* **2005**, *4*, 2001–2007. [CrossRef] [PubMed]
9. Mozzett, S.; Ferlini, C.; Conocolino, P.; Filippetti, F.; Raspaglio, G.; Prislei, S.; Gallo, D.; Martinelli, E.; Ranelletti, F.O.; Ferrandina, G.; et al. Class III β-tubulin overexpression is a prominent mechanism of paclitaxel resistance in ovarian cancer patients. *Clin. Cancer Res.* **2005**, *11*, 298–305.
10. Ferrandina, G.; Zannoni, G.F.; Martinelli, E.; Paglia, A.; Gallotta, V.; Mozzetti, S.; Scambia, G.; Ferlini, C. Class III β-tubulin overexpression is a marker of poor clinical outcome in advanced ovarian cancer patients. *Clin. Cancer Res.* **2006**, *12*, 2774–2779. [CrossRef]
11. Ferlini, C.; Raspaglio, G.; Mozzetti, S.; Cicchillitti, L.; Filippetti, F.; Gallo, D.; Fattorusso, C.; Campiani, G.; Scambia, G. The Seco-Taxane IDN5390 Is able to target class III β-Tubulin and to overcome paclitaxel resistance. *Cancer Res.* **2005**, *65*, 2397–2405. [CrossRef]
12. Tang, Y.; Rodriguez-Salarichs, J.; Zhao, Y.; Cai, P.; Estevez-Gallego, J.; Balaguer-Perez, F.; Horcajo, M.R.; Lucena-Agell, D.; Barasoain, I.; Diaz, J.F.; et al. Modification of C-seco taxoids through ring tethering and substituent replacement leading to effective agents against tumor drug resistance mediated by βIII-Tubulin and P-glycoprotein (P-gp) overexpressions. *Eur. J. Med. Chem.* **2017**, *137*, 488–503. [CrossRef] [PubMed]
13. Pepe, A.; Sun, L.; Zanardi, I.; Wu, X.Y.; Ferlini, C.; Fontana, G.; Bombardelli, E.; Ojima, I. Novel C-seco-taxoids possessing high potency against paclitaxel-resistant cancer cell lines overexpressing class III β-tubulin. *Bioorg. Med. Chem. Lett.* **2009**, *19*, 3300–3304. [CrossRef] [PubMed]
14. Alushin, G.M.; Lander, G.C.; Kellogg, E.H.; Zhang, R.; Baker, D.; Nogales, E. High resolution microtubule structures reveal the structural transitions in alpha-beta tubulin upon GTP hydrolysis. *Cell* **2014**, *157*, 1117–1129. [CrossRef] [PubMed]
15. Chaudhary, A.G.; Gharpure, M.M.; Rimoldi, J.M.; Chordia, M.D.; Gunatilaka, A.A.L.; Kingston, D.G.I. Unexpectedly facile hydrolysis of the 2-benzoate group of taxol and syntheses of analogs with increased activities. *J. Am. Chem. Soc.* **1994**, *116*, 4097–4098. [CrossRef]
16. Kingston, D.G.I.; Chaudhary, A.G.; Chordia, M.D. Synthesis and biological evaluation of 2-acyl analogues of paclitaxel (taxol). *J. Med. Chem.* **1998**, *41*, 3715–3726. [CrossRef] [PubMed]
17. Vella-Zarb, L.; Baisch, U.; Dinnebier, R.E. Small molecule, big difference: The role of water in the crystallization of paclitaxel. *J. Pharm. Sci.* **2013**, *102*, 674–683. [CrossRef]
18. Walker, R.C.; Crowley, M.F.; Case, D.A. The implementation of a fast and accurate QM/MM potential method in Amber. *J. Comput. Chem.* **2008**, *29*, 1019–1031. [CrossRef]
19. Kaus, J.W.; Pierce, L.T.; Walker, R.C.; McCammon, J.A. Improving the efficiency of free energy calculations in the Amber molecular dynamics package. *J. Chem. Theory Comput.* **2013**, *9*, 4131–4139. [CrossRef]
20. Wang, S.R.; Yang, C.G.; Sánchez-Murcia, P.A.; Snyder, J.P.; Yan, N.; Sáez-Calvo, G.; Díaz, J.F.; Gago, F.; Fang, W.S. Restoration of Microtubule Interaction and Cytotoxicity in D-seco Taxanes upon Incorporation of 20-Hydroxymethyl-4-allyloxy Groups. *Org. Lett.* **2015**, *17*, 6098–6101. [CrossRef]
21. Cai, P.; Lu, P.; Sharom, F.J.; Fang, W.S. A semisynthetic taxane Yg-3-46a effectively evades P-glycoprotein and beta-III tubulin mediated tumor drug resistance in vitro. *Cancer Lett.* **2013**, *341*, 214–223. [CrossRef] [PubMed]

Sample Availability: Not available.

molecules

MDPI

Article

New Zampanolide Mimics: Design, Synthesis, and Antiproliferative Evaluation

Guanglin Chen [1], Ziran Jiang [1], Qiang Zhang [2], Guangdi Wang [2] and Qiao-Hong Chen [1,*]

[1] Department of Chemistry, California State University, Fresno, CA 93740, USA; chen.bmc@gmail.com (G.C.); ziranjiang@mail.fresnostate.edu (Z.J.)

[2] Department of Chemistry and RCMI Cancer Research Center, Xavier University of Louisiana, New Orleans, LA 70125, USA; qzhang1@xula.edu (Q.Z.); gwang@xula.edu (G.W.)

* Correspondence: qchen@csufresno.edu; Tel.: +1-559-278-2394

Received: 26 December 2019; Accepted: 14 January 2020; Published: 15 January 2020

Abstract: Zampanolide is a promising microtubule-stabilizing agent (MSA) with a unique chemical structure. It is superior to the current clinically used MSAs due to the covalent nature of its binding to β-tubulin and high cytotoxic potency toward multidrug-resistant cancer cells. However, its further development as a viable drug candidate is hindered by its limited availability. More importantly, conversion of its chemically fragile side chain into a stabilized bioisostere is envisioned to enable zampanolide to possess more drug-like properties. As part of our ongoing project aiming to develop its mimics with a stable side chain using straightforward synthetic approaches, 2-fluorobenzyl alcohol was designed as a bioisosteric surrogate for the side chain based on its binding conformation as confirmed by the X-ray structure of tubulin complexed with zampanolide. Two new zampanolide mimics with the newly designed side chain have been successfully synthesized through a 25-step chemical transformation for each. Yamaguchi esterification and intramolecular Horner–Wadsworth–Emmons condensation were used as key reactions to construct the lactone core. The chiral centers at C17 and C18 were introduced by the Sharpless asymmetric dihydroxylation. Our WST-1 cell proliferation assay data in both docetaxel-resistant and docetaxel-naive prostate cancer cell lines revealed that compound **6** is the optimal mimic and the newly designed side chain can serve as a bioisostere for the chemically fragile *N*-acetyl hemiaminal side chain in zampanolide.

Keywords: natural product; anticancer agent; synthesis; zampanolide

1. Introduction

Prostate cancer is still one of the big health concerns, as evidenced by its high incidence and mortality rate in American men. In 2019, 174,650 new prostate cancer cases that account for nearly 20% of all cancer cases and 31,620 prostate cancer deaths are projected to occur in the United States [1]. Prostate cancer is driven by the androgen receptor (AR)-regulated gene expression that is initiated by the binding of androgen to the AR [2]. Androgen deprivation therapy (ADT) has thus been the main treatment for prostate cancer over 70 years. However, the median duration of ADT response is merely 18–24 months due to inevitable progression to castration-resistant prostate cancer (CRPC) [3]. Consequently, approximately 30,000 prostate cancer deaths in the United State each year are caused by CRPC as well as resistance to the current treatments. The critical driving force for the continued progression of lethal CRPC is the reactivation of AR transcriptional activity [4,5]. The current first-line and second-line chemotherapeutics for CRPC are two microtubule-stabilizing cytotoxic agents (MSA), docetaxel and cabazitaxel [6–8]. Promotion of mitotic arrest is the initially well-established mechanism underlying the action of MSAs as anticancer agents [9]. The MSAs were recently revealed to impair AR transcriptional activity by suppressing nuclear importation of AR as downstream of microtubule stabilization [10]. This alternative mechanism is independent of MSA-induced mitotic arrest and can explain in part the efficacy of MSA in AR-driven CRPC.

The marine macrolide (−)-zampanolide (**1**, Figure 1) [11] has been demonstrated as a unique and promising MSA, which distinguishes it from the current clinically used MSAs due to (1) the covalent nature of its binding to the taxane pocket in β-tubulin as confirmed by a high-resolution X-ray structure of zampanolide in complex with α,β-tubulin, and (2) the very high cytotoxic potency as evidenced by low nanomolar IC_{50} values in suppressing multidrug-resistant cancer cell proliferation [12].

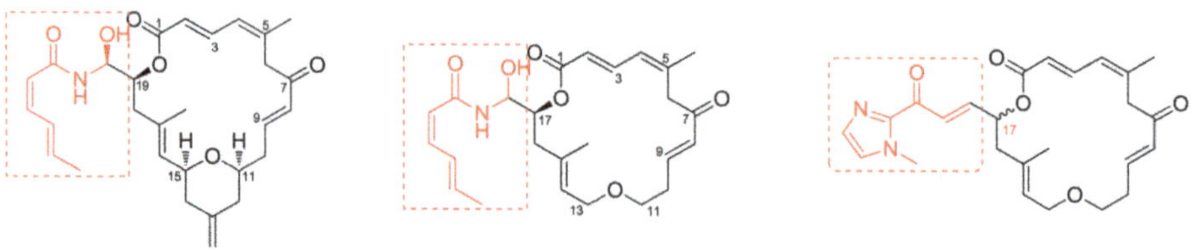

(-)-zampanolide (**1**) desTHP-(-)-zampanolide (**2**) desTHPzampanolide mimic **3**, 17S desTHPzampanolide mimic **4**, 17R

Figure 1. Zampanolide, desTHP-(−)-zampanolide, desTHPzampanolide mimics **3** and **4**.

Although (−)-zampanolide has shown great potential in becoming a more effective chemotherapeutic for CRPC, no in vivo assessment of its antitumor efficacy, pharmacokinetics, and toxicity in animal models has so far been reported yet mainly because of its limited supply. Unfortunately, the supply issue of (−)-zampanolide cannot be addressed either by isolation from marine sponge sources or by current reported total syntheses. The best yield for isolation of (−)-zampanolide from marine sponge sources is merely 0.001% [12,13], and the highest yield for its syntheses is only 0.9% [14–18]. More importantly, the chemically fragile *N*-acyl hemiaminal side chain of zampanolide can compromise its pharmacokinetic profiles as well as the feasibility as a viable drug candidate. The easy cleavage of the *N*-acyl hemiaminal side chain has been confirmed by a thermolysis reaction carried out by Professor Smith and his coworkers [16], and the instability of zampanolide in $CDCl_3$ has been reported by Higa and coworkers when they first identified its structure [13]. The *N*-acyl hemiaminal side chain of zampanolide is, however, very vital to retain its excellent cytotoxic potency, and the derivative without the side chain has 10- to 1000-fold less potency in certain cell models [12,19,20]. Our previous study has confirmed that a suitably designed side chain (e.g., the side chain in desTHPzampanoide mimics **3** and **4**) can function as a bioisostere for the chemically unstable *N*-acyl hemiaminal side chain in desTHPzampanolide (**2**) [21]. However, the bioisosteric side chains that we reported previously do not contain a hydroxyl substituent, corresponding to the C20 alcohol of zampanolide that is hydrogen-bonded to the carbonyl oxygen of Thr276 in β-tubulin. As part of our ongoing project to develop simplified and stabilized zampanolide mimics, this paper presents the design, total synthesis, and antiproliferative evaluation of zampanolide mimics in which the *N*-acyl hemiaminal side chain is substituted by more stable 2-fluorobenzyl alcohol appendages.

2. Results and Discussion

2.1. Design of New Zampanolide Mimics

The first group of side chains in the zampanolide mimics (e.g., **3**–**4**) previously published by us [21] do not contain a hydroxyl group in order to render a more simplified synthesis. However, the binding conformation confirmed by the high-resolution crystal structure of zampanolide tubulin complex [22] indicates the hydroxyl group at the C20 position in zampanolide is hydrogen-bonded to the carbonyl oxygen of Thr276 in β-tubulin. With this point in mind, a new side chain (S-2) was designed as a bioisosteric substitution for the N-acyl hemiaminal side chain, an unstable moiety in zampanolide but important for its potent cytotoxic properties. The stabilized side chain (S-2) was designed to replace the chemically fragile N-acylhemiaminal moiety (blue circle in Figure 2) with a benzyl alcohol. The 20OH group is retained in the target side chain so that it can be hydrogen-bonded to the main-chain carbonyl oxygen of Thr^{276} in β-tubulin. The 1′O atom of zampanolide's side chain is replaced with fluorine atom in the designed side chain so that it can be hydrogen-bonded to the NH group of Thr^{276} in β-tubulin. The E,Z-hexadienoyl amide in zampanolide side chain is replaced with a planar conjugate phenyl ring to preserve the hydrophobic contacts between the proposed side chain and residues of β-tubulin. The Almann's desTHP-dactylolide and its enantiomer [23] were further adopted as the core structure of the new zampanolide mimics (**5** and **6**) in the current study because of the acceptable in vitro potency of desTHP-(−)-zampanolide (**2**) and the practical synthesis of the core. Consequently, we set **5** and **6** as our new target mimics of zampanolide in this study.

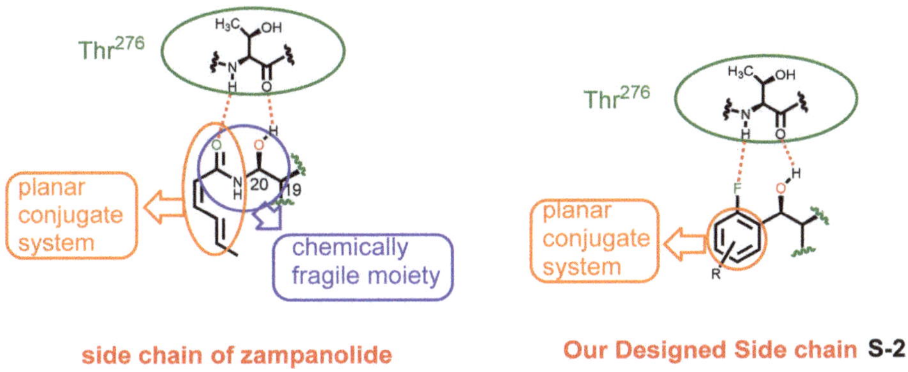

Figure 2. Design of a new stabilized side chain for zampanolide mimics.

2.2. Synthesis

Our retrosynthetic analysis of the zampanolide mimics **5** and **6**, using Yamaguchi esterification and intramolecular Horner–Wadsworth–Emmons condensation as key reactions, is illustrated in Scheme 1. The Yamaguchi esterification was employed to connect Fragment C1–C8 (carboxylic acid **9**) with Fragment C9–C18 (alcohol **7** or **8**) via the ester bond between C1 and C17. The intramolecular Horner–Wadsworth–Emmons condensation was used to close the macrolactone ring at C8–C9. These two key reactions were successfully applied to our syntheses of desTHPdactylolide and the mimics of desTHPzampanolides [21,23]. The known Fragment C1–C8 (**9**) was readily synthesized via 10 steps from commercially available 2-butyn-1-ol according to the reported procedure [24].

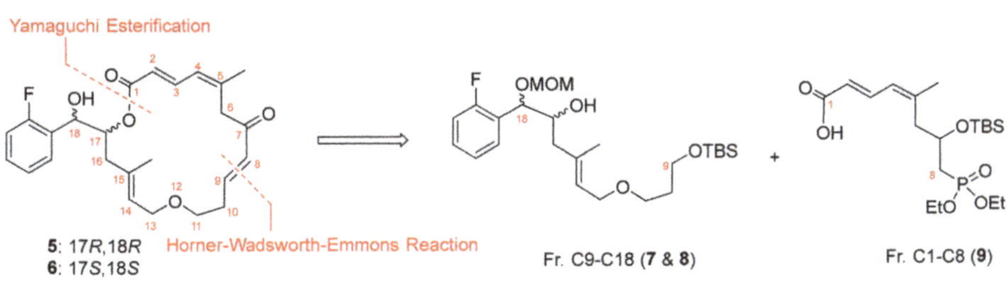

Scheme 1. Retrosynthetic analysis of zampanolide mimics **5** and **6**.

The preparation of Fragment C9–C18 (**7** and **8**) with the desired side chain is shown in Scheme 2. The chiral centers at C17 and C18 in the Fragment C9–C18 (**7** and **8**) were introduced by the Sharpless asymmetric dihydroxylation using the commercially available AD-mix formulations (AD-mix-α and AD-mix-β, respectively) with the ligand and the osmium salt as the critical trace component (0.6%

by wt) and ferricyanide and carbonate as the bulk ingredient (99.4% by wt.) [25]. Compound (*E*)-ethyl 3-(2-fluorophenyl)acrylate was synthesized by the Wittig reaction of the commercially available 2-fluorobenzaldehyde (**10**) with ethyl 2-(triphenyl- phosphoranylidene)acetate (**11**) according to the procedure described in the literature [26]. (*E*)-3-(2-Fluorophenyl)prop-2-en-1-ol (**13**) was synthesized by reducing (*E*)-ethyl 3-(2-fluorophenyl)acrylate (**12**) with diisobutylaluminium hydride (DIBAL) based on the procedure reported in the literature [27]. The Sharpless asymmetric dihydroxylation of the allylic alcohol (**13**) with AD-mix-α or AD-mix-β was performed following the standard experimental procedure reported in the literature and sulfonamide was used to accelerate the hydrolysis of osmate ester [25]. Epoxy alcohols (**18** with *R,R* configuration, **19** with *S,S* configuration) have been synthesized by sequential selective mesylation of primary alcohol (**14** or **15**) and intermolecular Williamson ether synthesis [28]. The hydroxy group in epoxy alcohols (**18** with *R,R* configuration, **19** with *S,S* configuration) was then protected as the corresponding methoxymethyl (MOM) ethers (**20** with *R,R* configuration, **21** with *S,S* configuration). Iodo ether **22** was prepared using the optimized protocol previously developed in our laboratory [23]. Its lithiation with *tert*-butyllithium followed by nucleophilic reaction with epoxy MOM ether (**20** with *R,R* configuration, **21** with *S,S* configuration) in toluene at −90 °C mediated by boron trifluoride etherate furnished Fragment C9–C18 (**7** with *R,R* configuration, **8** with *S,S* configuration) in 22–23% overall yield from **22**.

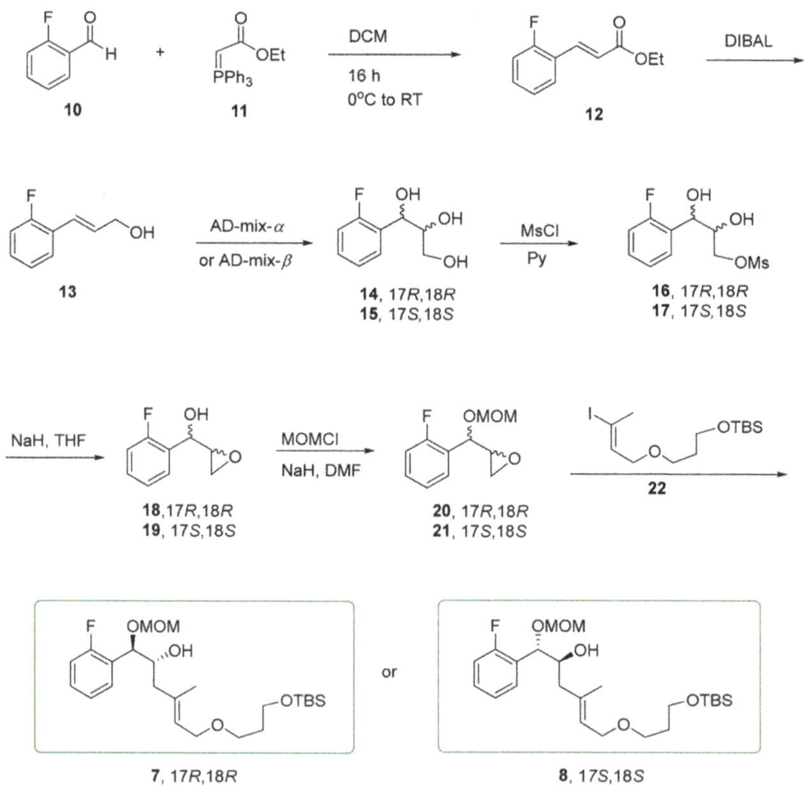

Scheme 2. Synthesis of Fragment C9–C18 (**7** and **8**).

As illustrated in Scheme 3, the union of Fragment C1–C8 (alcohol **9**) and Fragment C9–C18 (carboxylic acid, **7** with *R,R* configuration, **8** with *S,S* configuration) has been accomplished by the Yamaguchi esterification to yield bis-TBS ethers (**23** with *R,R* configuration, **24** with *S,S* configuration). Removal of the protecting TBS groups at C7 and C9 with HF-pyridine complex followed by double oxidation of the corresponding diol (**25** with *R*,*R* configuration and **26** with *S*,*S* configuration) with Dess–Martin periodinane afforded the keto aldehydes (**27** with *R*,*R* configuration, **28** with *S*,*S* configuration). Without further chromatographic purification, the crude keto aldehydes were directly subjected to the synthesis of zampanolide mimics (**29** with *R*,*R* configuration, **30** with *S*,*S* configuration) through the intramolecular HWE condensation catalyzed by $Ba(OH)_2$. Since extractive work-up resulted in significant hydrolysis of the ester [21], the reaction was quenched by filtration of the reaction mixture through a pad of silica gel and the crude product was subjected to preparative TLC purification. The MOM group in **29** was initially planned to be removed using methanolic HCl, but the methanol participated in a Michael addition to the enone, which resulted in the byproduct **31** (Scheme 4). The removal of the MOM with HCl was, therefore, carried out using THF rather than methanol as solvent, leading to the desired zampanolide mimics (**5** with *R*,*R* configuration at C17 and C18, **6** with *S*,*S* configuration at C17 and C18).

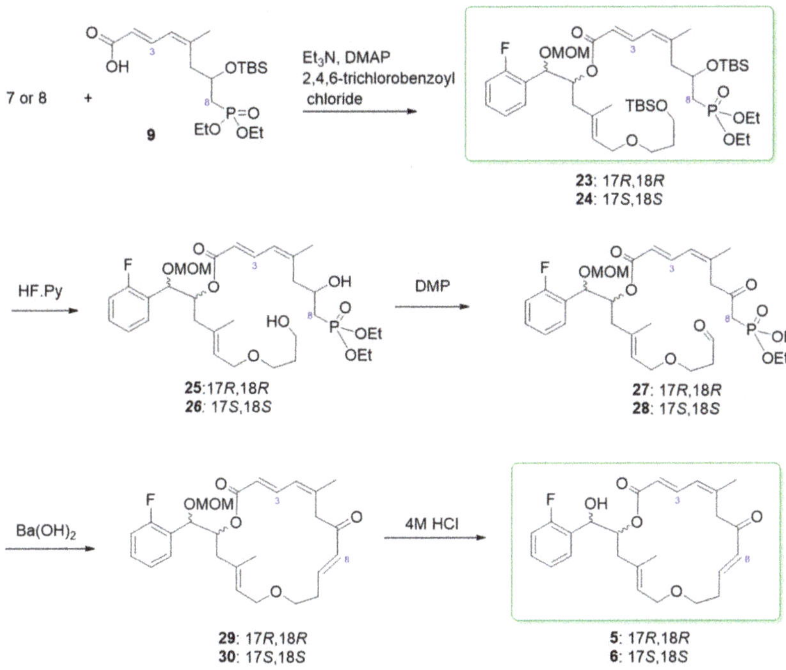

Scheme 3. Synthesis of zampanolide mimics 5 and 6.

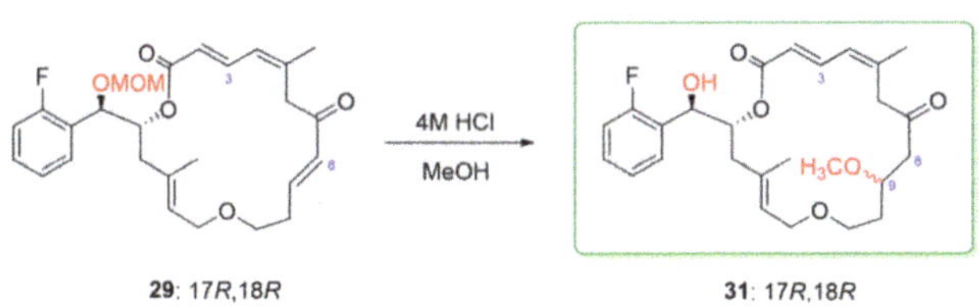

Scheme 4. Deprotection of MOM ether 29 with methanolic HCl.

2.3. Antiproliferative Activity toward Prostate Cancer Cell Lines

The in vitro antiproliferative activity of two pairs of enantiomeric macrolides, **5** and **6**, **29** and **30**, has been assessed against a panel of prostate cancer cell lines, including three docetaxel-sensitive prostate cancer cell models (PC-3 DU145, and LNCaP) and two docetaxel-resistant prostate cancer cell lines (PC-3/DTX and DU145/DTX). WST-1 cell proliferation assay was used for the in vitro evaluation according to the procedure described in the Experimental Section. Docetaxel was used as a positive control while DMSO as a negative control. The half-maximal inhibitory concentrations (IC_{50} values) were measured by WST-1 cell proliferation assay after 3 days of exposure, calculated from the dose–response curves, and presented as the mean ± standard deviation of the mean in Table 1. The IC_{50} values for these four new zampanolide mimics are in the range of 1.00–9.36 μM. Mimic **6** has a set of smallest IC_{50} values (1.00–3.91 μM) among the four test macrolides. As summarized in Figure 3, the IC_{50} values of new mimic **6** are very close to those for mimic **3** (0.86–2.97 μM) and mimic **32** (1.92–3.16 μM). The mimic **3** has been evidenced to have similar potency as desTHPzampanolide **2** with the *N*-acetyl hemiaminal side chain of zampanolide against prostate cancer cells [21]. The side chain in mimic **6** was thus identified as a new bioisostere for the chemically unstable *N*-acetyl hemiaminal side chain of zampanolide. The relative resistance for Mimic **6** of PC-3/DTX over PC-3 and DU145/DTX over DU145 is 0.59 and 0.44, respectively.

Table 1. Antiproliferative potency of zampanolide mimics against docetaxel-sensitive and docetaxel-resistant prostate cancer cells.

Compounds	IC_{50}: (μM) [a]		R/S [a]	IC_{50}: (μM) [a]		R/S [a]	IC_{50}: (μM)
	PC-3	PC-3/DTX		DU145	DU145/DTX		LNCaP
Docetaxel	0.0019 ± 0.0006	2.34 ± 0.25	1232	0.0012 ± 0.0003	8.58 ± 0.39	7150	0.0002 ± 0.00005
3 [b]	0.88 ± 0.19	2.97 ± 0.09	1.3	0.86 ± 0.25	2.78 ± 0.16	3.2	0.76 ± 0.29
4 [b]	0.35 ± 0.05	0.30 ± 0.05	0.9	0.29 ± 0.03	0.46 ± 0.10	1.6	0.35 ± 0.02
29	9.36 ± 0.15	3.97 ± 0.24	0.42	3.98 ± 0.57	4.42 ± 0.55	1.1	5.29 ± 0.49
5	8.72 ± 2.21	3.63 ± 0.11	0.42	3.87 ± 0.23	5.03 ± 1.11	1.3	6.51 ± 0.60
30	5.80 ± 0.21	3.71 ± 0.72	0.64	2.28 ± 0.51	4.30 ± 0.79	1.9	3.15 ± 0.19
6	3.91 ± 0.73	2.31 ± 0.32	0.59	2.27 ± 0.39	1.00 ± 0.91	0.44	1.92 ± 0.29

[a] The relative resistance of the two cell lines obtained by dividing the IC_{50} value of the resistance cell line by that of the parental cell line. [b] These data were reported in our previous paper [21].

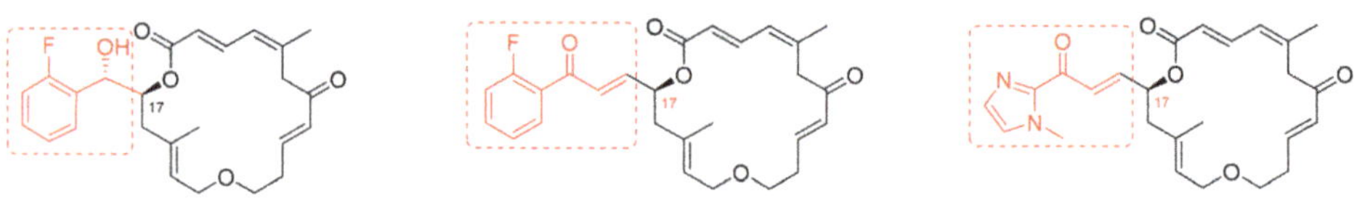

6
IC_{50} Values in the five cell lines:
1.00 - 3.91 μM

32
IC_{50} Values in the five cell lines:
1.92 - 3.16 μM

3
IC_{50} Values in the five cell lines:
0.86 - 2.97 μM

Figure 3. Comparison of antiproliferative potency among different zampanolide mimics.

3. Materials and Methods

3.1. General Procedures

Optical rotations were measured on a RUDOLPH Research Analytical Autopol III Automatic Polarimeter (RUDOLPH Research Analytical, Hackettstown, NJ, USA). IR spectra were recorded on a Nicolet Nexus 470 FTIR spectrophotometer (Thermo Fisher Scientific, Waltham, MA, USA). High-Resolution MS were obtained on an Orbitrap mass spectrometer (Thermo Fisher Scientific, Waltham, MA, USA) with electrospray ionization (ESI). NMR spectra (see Supplementary Materials) were obtained on a Bruker Fourier 300 spectrometer (Billerica, MA, USA) in $CDCl_3$. The chemical shifts are given in ppm referenced to the respective solvent peak, and coupling constants are reported in Hz. Anhydrous THF and dichloromethane were purified by PureSolv MD 7 Solvent Purification System from Innovative Technologies (MB-SPS-800) (Herndon, VA, USA). All other reagents and solvents were purchased from commercial sources (Fisher Scientific, Portland, OR, USA) and were used without further purification. Silica gel column chromatography was performed using silica gel (32–63 μM). Preparative thin-layer chromatography (PTLC) separations were carried out on thin-layer chromatography plates loaded with silica gel 60 GF254 (EMD Millipore Corporation, Berlington, MA, USA). Starting materials **22** and **9** were synthesized using the procedure previously described by us [23]. (*E*)-ethyl 3-(2-fluorophenyl)acrylate (**12**) was prepared from commercially available 2-fluorobenzaldehyde (**10**, CAS 446-52-6) according to the reported procedure [26]. (*E*)-3-(2-Fluorophenyl)prop-2-en-1-ol (**13**) was synthesized by reducing (*E*)-ethyl 3-(2-fluorophenyl)acrylate (**12**) with DIBAL based on the procedure reported in the literature [27]. Its structure was confirmed by ^{1}H NMR and high resolution mass spectrometry (HRMS) data (calculated for $C_9H_{10}FO$ (M + H): 153.0716; Found: 153.0710).

3.2. *Synthesis of (1R,2R)-1-(2-Fluorophenyl)propane-1,2,3-triol [(17R,18R) triol* **14***]*

AD-mix-α (5.9 g) was dissolved in a mixture of *tert*-butyl alcohol (21 mL) and water (21 mL). The solution was stirred vigorously at room temperature until two clear phases were observed. At this point, the lower aqueous phase emerged as bright yellow. Methanesulfonamide (399 mg, 4.2 mmol, 1 equiv) was added and the reaction mixture was cooled down to 0 °C. A solution of 13 (640 mg, 4.2 mmol, 1 equiv) in 1 mL of *tert*-butyl alcohol was then added. The resulting mixture was stirred vigorously at 0 °C overnight and the reaction progress was monitored with TLC. The reaction was quenched by adding solid sodium sulfate (6.3 g) at 0 °C. The mixture was warmed to room temperature and stirred for 30–60 min. The *tert*-butyl alcohol was removed under vacuum, and saturated sodium bicarbonate (30 mL) and water (300 mL) were added to the residue. The mixture was stirred for additional 30 min and then extracted with ethyl acetate (150 mL × 3). The combined extracts were rinsed with brine, dried over anhydrous sodium sulfate, and concentrated. The crude product was purified through column chromatography eluting with ethyl acetate. The product after purification, with quantitative yield, still contained a trace amount of methanesulfonamide, which is good enough to be used for the next-step reaction. ^{1}H NMR (300 MHz, $CDCl_3$) δ. 7.38 (t, *J* = 7.2 Hz, 1H, aromatic H), 7.21 (dd, *J* = 13.5, 5.7 Hz, 1H, aromatic H), 7.06 (t, *J* = 7.5 Hz, 1H, aromatic H), 6.95 (t, *J* = 8.4 Hz, 1H, aromatic H), 4.88 (d, *J* = 6.3 Hz, 1H, H-18), 4.23 (br.s, 3H, 3 × OH), 3.77 (q, *J* = 5.1 Hz, 1H, H-17), 3.45 (d, *J* = 4.8 Hz, 2H, H_2-16). ^{13}C NMR (75 MHz, $CDCl_3$) δ 159.9 (d, J_{CF} = 243.8 Hz), 129.6, 128.5, 127.9 (d, J_{CF} = 12.8 Hz), 124.6, 115.4 (d, J_{CF} = 21.8 Hz), 75.3, 68.8, 63.5. IR (film) ν_{max}: 3384, 2988, 1617, 1490, 1455, 1320, 1222, 1054 cm^{-1}. HRMS (ESI): *m/z* calculated for $C_9H_{12}FO_3$ [M + H]$^+$: 187.0770. Found: 187.0766.

3.3. *Synthesis of (2R,3R)-3-(2-Fluorophenyl)-2,3-dihydroxypropyl methanesulfonate [(17R,18R) mesylate* **16***]*

To a solution of triol **14** (1.37 g, 7.39 mmol) in pyridine (15 mL, 0.5 M), methane sulfonyl chloride (0.57 mL, 7.39 mmol) was added dropwise at 0 °C under argon. The reaction mixture was stirred at room temperature for 20 h and the reaction progress was monitored by TLC (Hexane/EtOAc, 1:1, *v*/*v*). The reaction was quenched by diluting with ethyl acetate (800 mL), and the resulting solution was rinsed with brine (50 mL × 3) and dried over anhydrous sodium sulfate. After removing the organic solvent, the residue was subjected to column chromatography, using 40% ethyl acetate in hexane as eluent, to give the desired product. Colorless oil; 81% yield. ^{1}H NMR (300 MHz, $CDCl_3$) δ 7.47 (dt, *J* = 7.5, 1.8 Hz, 1H, aromatic H), 7.34–7.27 (m, 1H, aromatic H), 7.17 (dt, *J* = 7.5, 0.9 Hz, 1H, aromatic H), 7.04 (ddd, *J* = 10.5, 8.1, 0.9 Hz, 1H, aromatic H), 5.00 (d, *J* = 5.7 Hz, 1H, H-18), 4.27–4.16 (m, 2H, H_2-16), 4.06–4.01 (m, 1H, H-17), 3.18 (br.s, 2H, 2 × OH), 3.03 (s, 3H, SO_2CH_3). ^{13}C NMR (75 MHz, $CDCl_3$) δ 159.9 (d, J_{CF} = 244.3 Hz), 130.1 (d, J_{CF} = 8.3 Hz), 128.4 (d, J_{CF} = 3.8 Hz), 127.0 (d, J_{CF} = 12.8 Hz), 124.8 (d, J_{CF} = 3.8 Hz), 115.7 (d, J_{CF} = 21.8 Hz), 72.9, 70.4, 67.9 (d, J_{CF} = 2.3 Hz), 37.6. IR (film) ν_{max}: 3502, 3029, 2940, 1617, 1587, 1490, 1456, 1346, 1171 cm^{-1}. HRMS (ESI): *m/z* calculated for $C_{10}H_{14}FO_5S$ [M + H]$^+$: 265.0546. Found: 265.0547.

3.4. *Synthesis of (R)-(2-Fluorophenyl)((R)-oxiran-2-yl)methanol [(17R,18R) epoxide* **18***]*

To a suspension of sodium hydride (275 mg, 60%, 6.87 mmol, 1.5 equiv) in anhydrous THF (36 mL), a solution of **16** (1.21 g, 4.58 mmol, 1 equiv) in anhydrous THF was added at about −30 °C under argon. The reaction mixture was stirred at 0 °C overnight and the reaction progress was monitored with TLC (hexane:EtOAc, 3:1). The mixture was filtered through a silica gel pad eluting with ethyl acetate. After concentration to remove the solvent, the residue was subjected to PTLC purification eluting with toluene:EtOAc (3:1, *v*/*v*) to furnish the desired epoxide. Colorless oil; 57% yield. ^{1}H NMR (300 MHz, $CDCl_3$) δ 7.57 (dd, J = 7.8, 1.8 Hz, 1H, aromatic H), 7.35–7.28 (m, 1H, aromatic H), 7.20 (dt, J = 7.5, 1.2 Hz, 1H, aromatic H), 7.06 (ddd, J = 10.5, 8.1, 1.2 Hz, 1H, aromatic H), 4.84 (t, J = 6.6 Hz, 1H, H-18), 3.26–3.22 (m, 1H, H-17), 2.92–2.85 (overlapped, 2H, H_2-16), 2.47 (d, J = 5.7 Hz, 1H, OH). ^{13}C NMR (75 MHz, $CDCl_3$) δ 159.9 (d, J_{CF} = 244.5 Hz), 129.6 (d, J_{CF} = 8.3 Hz), 127.9 (d, J_{CF} = 4.5 Hz), 127.3 (d, J_{CF} = 13.5 Hz), 124.5 (d, J_{CF} = 3.8 Hz), 115.4 (d, J_{CF} = 21.8 Hz), 68.7 (d, J_{CF} = 2.3 Hz), 55.6, 45.5 (d, J = 2.3 Hz). IR (film) ν_{max}: 3420, 3067, 3002, 2928, 1617, 1586 1488, 1456, 1224 cm^{-1}. HRMS (ESI): *m*/*z* calculated for $C_9H_{10}FO_2$ $[M + H]^+$: 169.0665. Found: 169.0657.

3.5. *Synthesis of (R)-2-((R)-(2-Fluorophenyl)(methoxymethoxy)methyl)oxirane [(17R,18R)MOM ether* **20***]*

To a solution of alcohol **18** (716 mg, 4.3 mmol) in DMF (4.2 mL), sodium hydride (204 mg, 60%, 5.1 mmol) was added at 4 °C, and the mixture was stirred at 4 °C for 30 min. Methoxymethyl chloride (0.39 mL, 5.1 mmol) followed by tetrabutylammonium iodide (157 mg, 0.43 mmol) was added to the reaction mixture. The reaction was proceeded with stirring at room temperature for 20 h. The reaction mixture was diluted with ethyl acetate (300 mL) and diethyl ether (300 mL) and then rinsed with brine (50 mL × 3). The organic layer was dried over anhydrous sodium sulfate and concentrated to give a crude mass, which was purified by column chromatography eluting with hexane/ethyl acetate (3:1, *v*/*v*) to furnish the MOM ether **20** as a pale-yellow oil in 67% yield. ^{1}H NMR (300 MHz, $CDCl_3$) δ 7.51 (dt, J = 7.2, 1.8 Hz, 1H, aromatic H), 7.33–7.25 (m, 1H, aromatic H), 7.17 (dt, J = 7.5, 1.2 Hz, 1H, aromatic H), 7.04 (ddd, J = 9.9, 8.1, 1.2 Hz, 1H, aromatic H), 4.75 (d, J = 6.9 Hz, 1H, OCH_2OCH_3), 4.67 (d, J = 6.9 Hz, 1H, OCH_2OCH_3), 4.62 (d, J = 6.6 Hz, 1H, H-18), 3.36 (s, 3H, OCH_3), 3.26–3.22 (m, 1H, H-17), 2.73–2.72 (overlapped, 2H, H_2-16). ^{13}C NMR (75 MHz, $CDCl_3$) δ 160.3 (d, J = 244.5 Hz), 129.8 (d, J = 8.3 Hz), 128.6 (d, J = 4.5 Hz), 125.2 (d, J = 14.3 Hz), 124.4 (d, J = 3.0 Hz), 115.5 (d, J = 21.8 Hz), 94.6, 73.0, 55.6, 54.4, 44.2 (d, J = 2.3 Hz). IR (film) ν_{max}: 2891, 1615, 1587, 1488, 1455, 1022 cm^{-1}. HRMS (ESI): *m*/*z* calculated for $C_{11}H_{14}FO_3$ $[M + H]^+$: 213.0927. Found: 213.0921.

3.6. *Synthesis of (5R,6R,E)-5-(2-Fluorophenyl)-8,16,16,17,17-pentamethyl-2,4,11,15-tetraoxa-16-silaoctadec-8-en-6-ol [(17R,18R) Fragment C9–C18 (***7***)]*

To a solution of vinyliodide **22** (164 mg, 0.44 mmol; co-evaporated twice with pentane) in toluene (3 mL) at −78 °C, *tert*-butyllithium (0.46 mL, 1.9 M, 0.89 mmol) was added, and the mixture was stirred at −78 °C for 45 min prior to being cooled down to −90 °C. Epoxide **20** (188 mg, 0.89 mmol; co-evaporated twice with pentane) in toluene (1.5 mL) was added dropwise to make sure that interior temperature lower than −78 °C. The reaction solution was re-cooled to −90 °C before BF_3•OEt_2 (0.11 mL, 0.89 mmoL) was added dropwise. The resulting solution was then stirred at −78 °C overnight prior to being quenched with ethyl acetate (15 mL) and saturated aqueous sodium bicarbonate (35 mL) was added. The organic layer was separated and the aqueous layer was extracted with ethyl acetate (60 mL × 3). The combined organic layers were dried over anhydrous sodium sulfate and concentrated *in Vacuum* to remove ethyl acetate. The crude mass was subjected to PTLC purification over silica gel using hexane/ethyl acetate (4:1, *v*/*v*) as eluent to yield secondary alcohol **7** as a pale-yellow oil in 23% yield. ^{1}H NMR (300 MHz, $CDCl_3$) δ. 7.41 (dt, J = 7.2, 1.5 Hz, 1H, aromatic H), 7.32–7.24 (m, 1H, aromatic H), 7.15 (dt, J = 7.5, 0.9 Hz, 1H, aromatic H), 7.53 (ddd, J = 9.9, 8.1, 0.9 Hz, 1H, aromatic H), 5.41 (t, J = 6.6 Hz, 1H, H-14), 4.81 (d, J = 6.3 Hz, 1H, H-17), 4.62 (d, J = 6.9 Hz, 1H, OCH_2OCH_3), 4.58 (d, J = 6.6 Hz, 1H, OCH_2OCH_3), 3.94 (d, J = 6.6 Hz, 2H, H_2-13), 3.67 (t, J = 6.3 Hz, 2H, H_2-11), 3.46 (t, J = 6.3 Hz, 2H, H_2-9), 3.36 (s, 3H), OCH_3), 1.75 (quin, J = 6.3 Hz, 2H, H_2-10), 1.64 (s, 3H, 15-CH_3), 0.87 (s, 9H, TBS), 0.03 (s, 6H, TBS). ^{13}C NMR (75 MHz, $CDCl_3$) δ 160.9 (d, J_{CF} = 244.8 Hz), 136.4, 129.8, 129.1, 128.7, 126.1 (d, J_{CF} = 13.5 Hz), 124.5 (d, J_{CF} = 3.8 Hz), 115.6 (d, J_{CF} = 21.8 Hz), 95.3, 75.6, 72.5 (d, J_{CF} = 12.1 Hz), 67.3, 67.0, 60.2, 56.2, 43.0, 33.2, 26.1, 26.07, 18.5, 16.6, 16.5. IR (film) ν_{max}: 3420, 2929,

1715, 1647, 1615, 1488, 1029 cm^{-1}. HRMS (ESI): *m/z* calculated for $C_{24}H_{42}FO_5Si$ $[M + H]^+$: 457.2786. Found: 457.2780.

3.7. Synthesis of (2E,4Z)-(5R,6R,E)-5-(2-Fluorophenyl)-8,16,16,17,17-pentamethyl-2,4,11,15-tetraoxa-16-silaoctadec-8-en-6-yl 7-((tert-butyldimethylsilyl)oxy)-8-(diethoxyphosphoryl)-5- methylocta-2,4-dienoate [(17R,18R) ester **23***]*

To a solution of Fragment C1–C8 (**9**, 37 mg, 0.09 mmol; co-evaporated with pentane twice) in toluene (0.5 mL) at room temperature, trimethylamine (28 µL, 0.20 mmol) and 2,4,6-trichlorobenzoyl chloride (18 µL, 0.12 mmol) was sequentially added, and the reaction mixture was stirred at room temperature for 1.5 h. A solution of alcohol **7** (35 mg, 0.08 mmol) and DMAP (9.3 mg, 0.08 mmol) in toluene (0.5 mL) was then added to the reaction mixture. The reaction was allowed to proceed with stirring at room temperature for 19 h prior to being quenched with water (5 mL) and saturated aqueous sodium bicarbonate (5 mL). The mixture was extracted with ethyl acetate (5 mL × 3), the combined organic extracts were dried over anhydrous sodium sulfate and concentrated *in vacuum*. PTLC purification of the crude product over silica gel eluting with hexane/ethyl acetate (60:40, *v/v*) yielded the ester **23** as a mixture of diastereoisomers in a 1:1 ratio as a colorless oil in 77% yield. ^1H NMR (300 MHz, $CDCl_3$) δ 7.50 (dd, *J* = 15.0, 11.7 Hz, H-3), 7.42 (t, *J* = 7.5 Hz, 1H, aromatic H), 7.25–7.20 (m, 1H, aromatic H), 7.10 (t, *J* = 7.5 Hz, 1H, aromatic H), 7.00 (t, *J* = 8.4 Hz, 1H, aromatic H), 6.03 (d, *J* = 11.4 Hz, H-4), 5.75 (d, *J* = 15.3 Hz, 1H, H-2), 5.43–5.37 (m, 1H, H-17), 5.33 (t, *J* = 6.6 Hz, 1H, H-14), 5.08 (d, *J* = 5.4 Hz, 1H, H-18), 4.58 (d, *J* = 6.6 Hz, 1H, -OCH_2OCH_3), 4.51 (d, *J* = 6.6 Hz, 1H, OCH_2OCH_3), 4.18–4.04 (overlapped, 5H, 2 x OCH_2CH_3, H-7), 3.93–3.79 (m, 2H, H_2-13), 3.64 (t, *J* = 6.3 Hz, 2H, H_2-11), 3.40 (t, *J* = 6.3 Hz, 2H, H_2-9), 3.32 (s, 3H, -OCH_2OCH_3), 2.58–2.48 (m, 2H, H_2-16), 2.33–2.24 (m, 2H, H_2-8), 2.00–1.92 (m, 2H, H_2-6), 1.87 (s, 3H, 5-CH_3), 1.72 (quin, *J* = 6.3 Hz, 2H, H_2-10), 1.64 (1.63) (s, 3H, 15-CH_3), 1.31 (t, *J* = 7.2 Hz, 6H, 2 × OCH_2CH_3), 0.86 (s, 9H, TBS), 0.81 (0.80) (s, 9H, TBS), 0.04 (0.03) (s, 3H, TBS), 0.01 (s, 6H, TBS), −0.04(−0.05) (s, 3H, TBS). ^{13}C NMR (75 MHz, $CDCl_3$) δ 166.8 (166.7), 160.8 (d, *J* = 244.5 Hz), 146.4 (d, *J* = 9.8 Hz), 141.6, 135.2 (d, *J* = 3.8 Hz), 129.7, 129.0, 126.8, 125.7 (d, *J* = 13.5 Hz), 125.1, 124.3, 119.3, 115.6 (115.3), 95.0, 72.9, 72.3, 67.3, 66.8, 61.7(61.6), 60.5, 60.1, 56.1, 41.8 (41.2), 36.1, 34.3, 33.1, 27.0, 26.11, 26.05, 25.90, 25.87, 25.2, 25.0, 18.5, 18.0, 16.6 (16.5), −4.6, −5.2. IR (film) ν_{max}: 2929, 2856, 1716, 1489, 1251, 1020 cm^{-1}. HRMS (ESI): *m/z* calculated for $C_{43}H_{77}FO_{10}PSi_2$ $[M + H]^+$: 859.4777. Found: 859.4756.

3.8. Synthesis of (2E,4Z)-(1R,2R,E)-1-(2-Fluorophenyl)-6-(3-hydroxypropoxy)-1-(methoxymethoxy) -4-methylhex-4-en-2-yl 8-(diethoxyphosphoryl)-7-hydroxy-5-methylocta-2,4-dienoate [(17R,18R) diol **25***]*

To a solution of di-TBS ether **23** (90 mg, 0.105 mmol) in THF (4.2 mL) at 0 °C in a plastic bottle, hydrogen fluoride-pyridine complex (70%, 1.0 mL) was added dropwise. The solution was stirred at 0 °C for 5 min and then at room temperature for 16 h. Saturated sodium bicarbonate (30 mL) was added to quench the reaction and the suspension was extracted with ethyl acetate (30 mL × 3). The combined organic extracts were dried over anhydrous sodium sulfate and the dried extract was concentrated under vacuum. The crude product was purified by PTLC, eluting with dichloromethane/methanol (93:7. *v/v*), and the pure diol was washed out from the PTLC silica gel with acetone as a pale-yellow oil in 92% yield. ^1H NMR (300 MHz, $CDCl_3$) δ 7.50 (7.49) (dd, *J* = 15.3, 11.7 Hz, 1H, H-3), 7.43 (t, *J* = 9.0 Hz, 1H, aromatic H), 7.30–7.23 (m, 1H, aromatic H), 7.13 (7.12) (t, *J* = 7.5 Hz, 1H, aromatic H), 7.031 (7.028) (dd, *J* = 10.2, 9.0 Hz, 1H, aromatic H), 6.11 (d, *J* = 11.4 Hz, 1H, H-4), 5.80 (d, *J* = 15.3 Hz, 1H, H-2), 5.47–5.40 (m, 1H, H-17), 5.32 (t, *J* = 5.7 Hz, 1H, H-14), 5.09 (d, *J* = 5.7 Hz, 1H, H-18), 4.58 (d, *J* = 6.9 Hz, 1H, -OCH_2OCH_3), 4.51 (d, *J* = 6.9 Hz, 1H, OCH_2OCH_3), 4.18–4.06 (overlapped, 5H, 2 × OCH_2CH_3, H-7), 3.90 (t, *J* = 5.7 Hz, 2H, H_2-13), 3.69 (3.68) (t, *J* = 5.7 Hz, 2H, H_2-11), 3.48 (3.47) (t, *J* = 5.7 Hz, 2H, H_2-9), 3.33 (3.32) (s, 3H, -OCH_2OCH_3), 3.03 (s, 2H, 2 × OH), 2.66–2.53 (m, 1H, H-16), 2.46–2.19 (m, 3H, H_2-8 & H-16), 1.92 (S, 3H, 5-CH_3), 1.96–1.88 (m, 2H, H_2-6), 1.75 (quin, *J* = 5.7 Hz, 2H, H_2-10), 1.65 (s, 3H, 15-CH_3), 1.33 (t, *J* = 7.2 Hz, 6H, 2 × OCH_2CH_3). ^{13}C NMR (75 MHz, $CDCl_3$) δ 167.0 (166.8), 160.9 (d, *J* = 247.5 Hz), 146.0, 140.8 (d, *J* = 17.3 Hz), 135.7 (d, *J* = 9.0 Hz), 129.8, 129.0,

126.8, 125.6 (d, *J* = 12.8 Hz), 124.8 (d, *J* = 11.3 Hz), 124.4, 119.7 (d, *J* = 11.3 Hz), 115.7 (115.4), 94.9, 73.0, 72.4, 68.8, 67.4, 65.3, 62.2, 61.8, 56.1, 41.1, 34.6 (34.5), 32.7, 32.3, 25.3, 25.0, 16.6 (16.5). IR (film) ν_{max}: 3366, 2929, 1711, 1633, 1488, 1222, 1019 cm^{-1}. HRMS (ESI): *m/z* calculated for $C_{31}H_{49}FO_{10}P$ [M + H]$^+$: 631.3048. Found: 631.3041.

*3.9. Synthesis of (R,3E,9E,11Z,15E)-6-((R)-(2-Fluorophenyl)(methoxymethoxy)methyl)-4,12-dimethyl-1,7-dioxacyclooctadeca-3,9,11,15-tetraene-8,14-dione [(17R,18R) macrolactone **29**]*

To a solution of diol **25** (65 mg, 0.10 mmol) in dichloromethane (6.2 mL) at room temperature, Dess–Martin periodinane (DMP, 131 mg, 0.30 mmol) was added. The reaction mixture was stirred for 30 min before a second portion of DMP (131 mg, 0.30 mmol) was added. The reaction was allowed to proceed with stirring at room temperature for an additional 1 h. The reaction mixture was poured into a stirred mixture of saturated sodium bicarbonate (30 mL) and saturated sodium thiosulfate (30 mL), and the resulting suspension was stirred for 30 min before being extracted with dichloromethane (30 mL × 3). The combined organic extracts were dried over anhydrous sodium sulfate and the dried extract was concentrated under vacuum. The crude product was used for the next reaction without further purification. To a solution of the crude ketoaldehyde (0.10 mmol) obtained above in THF (103 mL) at 0 °C was added water (2.2 mL) followed by activated barium hydroxide (15 mg, 0.08 mmol). The reaction mixture was stirred at 0 °C for 30 min and at room temperature for 2.5 h, then was filtered through a pad of sodium sulfate and a pad of silica gel that was rinsed with ethyl acetate. After evaporation of the solvent, the crude product was subjected to PTLC purification, using hexane/ethyl acetate (73:37) as eluent, to yield the pure macrolactone **29**. Colorless oil, 46% yield for two steps. [α]: −15.6 (*c* = 0.23, MeOH). ^{1}H NMR (300 MHz, $CDCl_3$) δ 7.60 (dd, *J* = 15.0, 11.4 Hz, 1H, H-3), 7.46 (dt, *J* = 7.5, 1.8 Hz, 1H, aromatic H), 7.33–7.25 (m, 1H, aromatic H), 7.16 (dt, *J* = 7.5, 1.2 Hz, 1H, aromatic H), 7.05 (ddd, *J* = 9.9, 8.4, 1.2 Hz, 1H, aromatic H), 6.82 (dt, *J* = 16.2, 6.6 Hz, 1H, H-9), 6.12 (d, *J* = 11.4 Hz, 1H, H-4), 6.01 (d, *J* = 16.2 Hz, 1H, H-8), 5.91 (d, *J* = 15.0 Hz, 1H, H-2), 5.51 (ddd, *J* = 11.4, 6.3, 1.2 Hz, 1H, H-17), 5.27 (dd, *J* = 7.8, 4.8 Hz, 1H, H-14), 5.12 (d, *J* = 6.3 Hz, 1H, H-18), 4.60 (d, *J* = 6.9 Hz, 1H, *O-CH*$_2$OCH$_3$), 4.53 (d, *J* = 6.9 Hz, 1H, O*CH*$_2$OCH$_3$), 3.99 (dd, *J* = 12.0, 8.1 Hz, 1H, H-16), 3.88–3.81 (m, 2H, H_2-13), 3.47–3.28 (m, 2H, H_2-11), 3.34 (s, 3H, OCH$_2$O*CH*$_3$), 3.14 (d, *J* = 12.6 Hz, 1H, H-16), 2.43–2.36 (m, 2H, H_2-10), 2.33 (d, *J* = 12.0 Hz, 1H, H-6), 2.05 (d, *J* = 12.1 Hz, 1H, H-6), 1.83 (s, 3H, 5-CH_3), 1.63 (S, 3H, 15-CH_3). ^{13}C NMR (75 MHz, $CDCl_3$) δ 197.2, 166.6, 160.9 (d, *J* = 244.5 Hz), 146.8, 142.5, 139.7, 138.9, 134.3, 130.3, 128.9 125.9 (d, *J* = 7.5 Hz), 125.6 (d, *J* = 13.5 Hz), 125.2 (d, *J* = 5.6 Hz), 124.5, 120.9 (d, *J* = 5.3 Hz), 115.6 (d, *J* = 21.8 Hz), 94.9, 72.9, 72.6, 67.9, 67.8, 56.0, 46.0, 41.4, 33.1, 24.09, 16.7. IR (film) ν_{max}: 2931, 1713, 1633, 1489, 1358, 1226, 1030 cm^{-1}. HRMS (ESI): *m/z* calculated for $C_{27}H_{34}FO_6$ [M + H]$^+$: 473.2339. Found: 473.2333.

*3.10. Synthesis of (R,3E,9E,11Z,15E)-6-((R)-(2-Fluorophenyl)(hydroxy)methyl)-4,12-dimethyl-1,7-dioxacyclooctadeca-3,9,11,15-tetraene-8,14-dione [(17R,18R) macrolactone **5**]*

To a solution of **29** (30 mg, 0.064 mmol) in a mixture of tetrahydrofuran/water (0.92 mL, 1:1, *v/v*), concentrated hydrochloric acid (130 μL) was added. The two more portions of concentrated hydrochloric acid (130 μL × 2) were added sequentially after each one-hour stirring at room temperature. The reaction mixture was stirred at room temperature overnight before the reaction was quenched by adding saturated ammonium chloride (60 mL). The subsequent mixture was extracted with ethyl acetate (40 mL × 3). The combined extracts were dried over anhydrous sodium sulfate and the solvents were evaporated *in vacuum*. The crude product was purified over preparative thin layer chromatography eluting with toluene/ethyl acetate (3:1, *v/v*) to furnish the desired product (11 mg). Colorless syrup, 41% yield. ^{1}H NMR (300 MHz, $CDCl_3$) δ 7.62 (dd, *J* = 15.0, 11.7 Hz, 1H, H-3), 7.49 (dt, *J* = 7.5, 1.8 Hz, 1H, aromatic H), 7.31–7.27 (m, 1H, aromatic H), 7.17 (dt, *J* = 7.5, 1.2 Hz, 1H), 7.05 (ddd, *J* = 10.2, 8.1, 0.9 Hz, 1H), 6.83 (dt, *J* = 15.9, 6.9 Hz, 1H, H-9), 6.12 (d, *J* = 11.4 Hz, 1H, H-4), 6.02 (d, *J* = 16.2 Hz, 1H, H-8), 5.91 (d, *J* = 15.0 Hz, 1H, H-2), 5.48–5.38 (m, 1H, H-17), 5.27 (t, *J* = 6.0 Hz, 1H, H-14), 5.10 (d, *J* = 6.3 Hz, 1H, H-18), 3.99 (dd, *J* = 12.0, 8.1 Hz, 1H, H-16), 3.86 (br.s, 1H, H-13), 3.82 (br.s, 1H, H-13),

3.51–3.36 (m, 2H, H_2-11), 3.18 (d, *J* = 12.9 Hz, 1H, H-16), 2.44–2.34 (m, 3H, H_2-10, H-6), 2.06 (d, *J* = 14.4 Hz, 1H, H-6), 1.83 (s, 3H, 5-CH_3), 1.62 (s, 3H, 15-CH_3). ^{13}C NMR (75 MHz, $CDCl_3$) δ 197.2, 167.0, 160.1 (d, J_{CF} = 244.5 Hz), 146.9, 143.0, 140.1 (d, J_{CF} = 12.8 Hz), 134.2, 130.2, 129.9, 128.8, 127.6 (d, J_{CF} = 12.8 Hz), 126.0, 125.2, 124.6, 120.7, 115.6 (d, J_{CF} = 21.8 Hz), 79.4, 74.4, 70.3, 68.0, 45.9, 41.4, 33.0, 24.1, 16.7. [α]: −15.2 (*c* = 0.16, MeOH). IR (film) ν_{max}: 3428, 2924, 2854, 1706, 1633, 1558, 1488, 1360, 1221, 1036 cm^{-1}. HRMS (ESI): *m/z* calculated for $C_{25}H_{30}FO_5$ [M + H]$^+$: 429.2077. Found: 429.2074.

3.11. *Synthesis of (1S,2S)-1-(2-Fluorophenyl)propane-1,2,3-triol [(17S,18S) triol* **15***]*

Triol **15** was prepared in 68% yield from 13 catalyzed by AD-mix-β using a similar procedure used to synthesize its antipode **14**. ^{1}H NMR (300 MHz, $CDCl_3$) δ 7.39 (t, *J* = 7.5 Hz, 1H, aromatic H), 7.22 (dd, *J* = 13.8, 7.2 Hz, 1H, aromatic H), 7.07 (t, *J* = 7.5 Hz, 1H, aromatic H), 6.96 (t, *J* = 9.3 Hz, 1H, aromatic H), 4.90 (d, *J* = 6.3 Hz, 1H, H-18), 4.21 (br.s, 3H, 3 × OH), 3.78 (dd, *J* = 10.2, 4.8 Hz, 1H, H-17), 3.48 (d, *J* = 4.8 Hz, 2H, H_2-16). ^{13}C NMR (75 MHz, $CDCl_3$) δ 160.0 (d, J_{CF} = 244.5 Hz), 129.6, 128.5 (d, J_{CF} = 16.5 Hz), 127.8 (d, J_{CF} = 12.8 Hz), 124.6, 115.5 (d, J_{CF} = 21.8 Hz), 75.4, 68.8, 63.4. IR (film) ν_{max}: 3375, 2930, 1781, 1489, 1456, 1319 cm^{-1}. HRMS (ESI): *m/z* calculated for $C_9H_{12}FO_3$ [M + H]$^+$: 187.0770. Found: 187.0765.

3.12. *Synthesis of (2S,3S)-3-(2-Fluorophenyl)-2,3-dihydroxypropyl methanesulfonate [(17S,18S) mesylate* **17***]*

Mesylate **17** was prepared from triol **15** as a colorless oil in 72% yield, employing a procedure similar to that used for the mesylation of triol **14**. ^{1}H NMR (300 MHz, $CDCl_3$) δ 7.48 (dt, *J* = 7.5, 1.8 Hz, 1H, Aromatic H), 7.32–7.29 (m, 1H, aromatic H), 7.18 (dt, *J* = 8.4, 0.9 Hz, 1H, aromatic H), 7.05 (ddd, *J* = 9.3, 8.1, 0.9 Hz, 1H, aromatic H), 5.01 (d, *J* = 5.7 Hz, 1H, H-18), 4.28–4.15 (m, 2H, H_2-16), 4.08–4.03 (m, 1H, H-17), 3.04 (s, 3H, SO_2CH_3). ^{13}C NMR (75 MHz, $CDCl_3$) δ 159.9 (d, J_{CF} = 244.5 Hz, 1H), 130.1, 128.4, 127.0 (d, J_{CF} = 12.8 Hz, 1H), 124.8, 115.7 (d, J_{CF} = 21.8 Hz, 1H), 72.9, 70.3, 67.9, 37.6. IR (film) ν_{max}: 3482, 3029, 2939, 1616, 1587, 1489, 1456, 1332, 1168 cm^{-1}. HRMS (ESI): *m/z* calculated for $C_{10}H_{14}FO_5S$ [M + H]$^+$: 265.0546. Found: 265.0542.

3.13. *Synthesis of (S)-(2-Fluorophenyl)((S)-oxiran-2-yl)methanol [(17S,18S) epoxide* **19***]*

Epoxide **19** (52%, pale yellow oil) was obtained from mesylate **17** according to the internal Williamson ether synthesis procedure employed for the conversion of mesylate **16** to epoxide **18**. ^{1}H NMR (300 MHz, $CDCl_3$) δ 7.57 (dt, *J* = 7.5, 1.8 Hz, 1H, aromatic H), 7.35–7.25 (m, 1H, aromatic H), 7.20 (dt, *J* = 7.5, 1.2 Hz, 1H, aromatic H), 7.06 (ddd, *J* = 10.5, 8.1, 1.2 Hz, 1H, aromatic H), 4.83 (d, *J* = 5.1 Hz, 1H, H-18), 3.26–3.21 (m, 1H, H-17), 2.92–2.84 (m, 2H, H_2-16). ^{13}C NMR (75 MHz, $CDCl_3$) δ 160.0 (d, J_{CF} = 244.5 Hz), 129.8, 127.6 (d, J_{CF} = 9.0 Hz), 127.4 (d, J_{CF} = 13.5 Hz), 124.7, 115.6 (d, J_{CF} = 21.0 Hz), 68.6, 55.4, 45.6. IR (film) ν_{max}: 3482, 3029, 2939, 1617, 1587, 1489, 1456, 1331, 1168 cm^{-1}. HRMS (ESI): *m/z* calculated for $C_9H_{10}FO_2$ [M + H]$^+$: 169.0665. Found: 169.0659.

3.14. *Synthesis of (S)-2-((S)-(2-Fluorophenyl)(methoxymethoxy)methyl)oxirane [(17S,18S) MOM ether* **21***]*

MOM ether **21** was prepared from epoxide **19** as a pale-yellow oil in 73% yield employing a procedure similar to that used for conversion of **18**. ^{1}H NMR (300 MHz, $CDCl_3$) δ 7.44 (dt, *J* = 7.5, 1.8 Hz, 1H, aromatic H), 7.32–7.27 (m, 1H, aromatic H), 7.17 (dt, *J* = 7.5, 0.9 Hz, 1H, aromatic H), 7.05 (ddd, *J* = 10.2, 8.4, 1.2 Hz, 1H, aromatic H), 4.76 (d, *J* = 6.6 Hz, 1H, -OCH_2OCH_3), 4.68 (d, *J* = 6.9 Hz, 1H, H-18), 4.63 (d, *J* = 6.6 Hz, 1H, -OCH_2OCH_3), 3.37 (s, 3H, -OCH_2OCH_3), 3.27 – 3.23 (m, 1H, H-17), 2.75–2.73 (m, 2H, H_2-16). ^{13}C NMR (75 MHz, $CDCl_3$) δ 160 (d, J_{CF} = 245.3 Hz), 129.9 (d, J_{CF} = 8.3 Hz), 128.7 (d, J_{CF} = 3.8 Hz), 125.3 (d, J_{CF} = 14.3 Hz), 124.5 (d, J_{CF} = 3.8 Hz), 115.7 (d, J_{CF} = 21.8 Hz), 94.8, 73.1, 55.8, 54.6, 44.4. IR (film) ν_{max}: 2891, 2825, 1616, 1587, 1488, 1455, 1149, 1022 cm^{-1}. HRMS (ESI): *m/z* calculated for $C_{11}H_{14}FO_3$ [M + H]$^+$: 213.0927. Found: 213.0920.

*3.15. Synthesis of (5S,6S,E)-5-(2-Fluorophenyl)-8,16,16,17,17-pentamethyl-2,4,11,15-tetraoxa-16-silaoctadec-8-en-6-ol [(17S, 18S) Fragment C9–C18 (**8**)]*

(17*S*,18*S*) Fragment C9–C18 (**8**) was synthesized as a colorless oil in 22% yield from MOM ether **21** in a similar way to the synthesis of its antipode (17*R*,18*R*) Fragment C9–C18 (7). ^{1}H NMR (300 MHz, $CDCl_3$) δ 7.41 (dt, *J* = 7.5, 1.8 Hz, 1H, aromatic H), 7.32–7.24 (m, 1H, aromatic H), 7.15 (dt, *J* = 7.5, 1.2 Hz, 1H, aromatic H), 7.03 (ddd, *J* = 10.2, 8.4, 1.2 Hz, 1H, aromatic H), 5.41 (t, *J* = 6.6 Hz, 1H, H-14), 4.81 (d, *J* = 6.6 Hz, 1H, H-18), 4.63 (d, *J* = 6.6 Hz, 1H, OCH_2OCH_3), 4.58 (d, *J* = 6.6 Hz, 1H, OCH_2OCH_3), 3.95 (d, *J* = 6.6 Hz, 2H, H_2-13), 3.82 (dt, *J* = 10.2, 5.7 Hz, 1H, H-17), 3.67 (t, *J* = 6.0 Hz, 2H, H_2-11), 3.46 (t, *J* = 6.6 Hz, 2H, H_2-9), 3.36 (s, 3H, OCH_3), 2.23 (dd, *J* = 12.6, 9.6 Hz, 1H, H-16), 2.05 (dd, *J* = 12.6, 2.7 Hz, 1H, H-16), 1.76 (quin, *J* = 6.3 Hz, 2H, H_2-10), 1.64 (s, 3H, 15-CH_3), 0.87 (s, 9H, TBS), 0.03 (s, 6H, TBS). ^{13}C NMR (75 MHz, $CDCl_3$) δ 160.9 (d, J_{CF} = 244.7 Hz), 136.4, 129.2, 128.9, 128.6, 126.1 (d, J_{CF} = 12.8 Hz), 124.5, 115.5, 95.3, 75.6, 72.7, 67.3, 67.0, 60.2, 56.2, 43.0, 33.2, 26.0, 18.5, 16.6, 16.5. IR (film) ν_{max}: 3461, 2928, 2855, 1616, 1586, 1252, 1090, 1031 cm^{-1}. HRMS (ESI): *m/z* calculated for $C_{24}H_{42}FO_5Si$ [M + H]$^+$: 457.2786. Found: 457.2782.

*3.16. Synthesis of (2E,4Z)-(5S,6S,E)-5-(2-Fluorophenyl)-8,16,16,17,17-pentamethyl-2,4,11,15-tetraoxa-16-silaoctadec-8-en-6-yl 7-((tert-butyldimethylsilyl)oxy)-8-(diethoxyphosphoryl)-5-methylocta-2,4-dienoate [(17S,18S) ester **24**]*

(17*S*,18*S*) Ester **24** was obtained as a pale-yellow oil in 91% yield from (17*S*,18*S*) Fragment C9–C18 (**8**) and Fragment C1–C8 (**9**), according to the esterification procedure employed for the preparation of ester **23**. ^{1}H NMR (300 MHz, $CDCl_3$) δ 7.50 (dd, *J* = 14.4, 12.0 Hz, 1H, H-3), 7.42 (t, *J* = 7.2 Hz, 1H, aromatic H), 7.34–7.21 (m, 1H, aromatic H), 7.10 (t, *J* = 7.5 Hz, 1H, aromatic H), 7.01 (t, *J* = 9.3 Hz, 1H, aromatic H), 6.03 (d, *J* = 11.7 Hz, 1H, H-4), 5.76 (d, *J* = 15.0 Hz, 1H, H-2), 5.45–5.37 (m, 1H, H-17), 5.33 (t, *J* = 6.0 Hz, 1H, H-14), 5.08 (d, *J* = 5.1 Hz, 1H, H-18), 4.58 (d, *J* = 6.9 Hz, 1H, OCH_2OCH_3), 4.51 (d, *J* = 6.6 Hz, 1H, OCH_2OCH_3), 4.23–4.04 (m, 5H, 2 × OCH_2CH_3, H-7), 3.93–3.80 (m, 2H, H_2-13), 3.65 (t, *J* = 6.6 Hz, 2H, H_2-11), 3.41 (t, *J* = 6.3 Hz, H_2-9), 3.32 (s, 3H, OCH_2OCH_3), 2.58–2.54 (m, 2H, H_2-16), 2.33–2.28 (m, 2H, H_2-8), 2.03–1.93 (m, 2H, H_2-6), 1.87 (s, 3H, 5-CH_3), 1.77–1.70 (m, 2H. H_2-10), 1.64 (s, 3H, 15-CH_3), 1.31 (t, *J* = 6.9 Hz, 6H, 2 × OCH_2CH_3), 0.90 (0.88) (s, 3H, TBS), 0.86 (s, 6H, TBS), 0.81 (0.80) (s, 9H, TBS), 0.08 (0.04) (s, 6H, TBS), 0.02 (-0.04) (s, 6H, TBS). ^{13}C NMR (75 MHz, $CDCl_3$) δ 166.7, 160.8 (d, J_{CF} = 245.3 Hz), 146.5 (146.4), 146.3 (146.2), 135.7 (135.2), 129.8, 129.0, 126.8, 125.8 (125.6),125.1 (124.7), 124.3 119.2, 115.5 (d, J_{CF} = 27.5 Hz), 95.0, 72.9, 72.3, 68.9, 66.8, 61.8, 61.7, 60.1, 56.1, 41.7 (41.2), 36.0 (34.2), 33.1, 32.3, 29.8, 27.0, 26.0, 25.9, 25.8, 24.9, 18.5, 18.1, 18.0, 16.6, 16.5. IR (film) ν_{max}: 2928, 2856, 1714, 1636, 1250, 1020 cm^{-1}. HRMS (ESI): *m/z* calculated for $C_{43}H_{77}FO_{10}PSi_2$ [M + H]$^+$: 859.4777. Found: 859.4774.

*3.17. Synthesis of (2E,4Z)-(1S,2S,E)-1-(2-Fluorophenyl)-6-(3-hydroxypropoxy)-1-(methoxymethoxy)-4-methylhex-4-en-2-yl 8-(diethoxyphosphoryl)-7-hydroxy-5-methylocta-2,4-dienoate [(17S,18S) diol **26**]*

(17*S*,18*S*) Diol **26** was obtained as a colorless syrup in 65% yield according to the TBS deprotection procedure used for the conversion of (17*R*,18*R*) ester **23** to (17*R*,18*R*) diol **25**. ^{1}H NMR (300 MHz, CD_3COCD_3) δ 7.63–7.55 (m, 1H, H-3), 7.52 (t, *J* = 7.8 Hz, 1H, aromatic H), 7.41–7.33 (m, 1H, aromatic H), 7.23 (t, *J* = 7.2 Hz, 1H, aromatic H), 7.14 (t, *J* = 9.0 Hz, 1H, aromatic H), 6.16 (d, *J* = 11.4 Hz, 1H, H-4), 5.80 (d, *J* = 15.0 Hz, 1H, H-2), 5.46 (quin, *J* = 5.1 Hz, 1H, H-17), 5.31 (t, *J* = 6.6 Hz, 1H, H-14), 5.10 (d, *J* = 5.7 Hz, 1H, H-18), 4.61 (d, *J* = 6.6 Hz, 1H, -OCH_2OCH_3), 4.51 (d, *J* = 6.6 Hz, 1H, -OCH_2OCH_3), 4.22–4.04 (overlapped, 5H, 2 × –OCH_2CH_3, H-7), 3.88 (d, *J* = 6.0 Hz, 2H, H_2-13), 3.57 (t, *J* = 4.8 Hz, 2H, H_2-11), 3.40 (t, *J* = 6.3 Hz, 2H, H_2-9), 3.30 (s, 3H, -OCH_2OCH_3), 2.92 (br.s, 2H, 2 × OH), 2.60–2.57(overlapped, 2H, H_2-16), 2.29 (d, *J* = 9.3 Hz, 2H, H_2-8), 2.07–2.04 (m, 2H, H_2-6), 1.95 (s, 3H, 5-CH_3), 1.68 (quin, *J* = 6.0 Hz, H_2-10), 1.65 (s, 3H, 15-CH_3), 1.29 (t, *J* = 7.2 Hz, 6H, 2 × –OCH_2CH_3). ^{13}C NMR (75 MHz, $CDCl_3$) δ 166.0, 160.7 (d, J_{CF} = 243.8 Hz), 147.0 (d, J_{CF} = 9.8 Hz), 140.8, 134.2, 129.8, 129.3, 125.8 (d, J_{CF} = 9.8 Hz), 125.6, 125.4 (d, J_{CF} = 4.5 Hz), 124.3, 119.1, 115.3 (115.0), 94.7, 72.3, 66.8, 66.7, 65.5, 61.4(61.3), 61.2 (61.1), 59.1, 55.1, 41.2, 40.7, 34.6, 33.02(32.98), 32.0, 24.4, 15.91(15.86), 15.7(15.6). IR (film) ν_{max}: 3381,

2927, 1709, 1633, 1488, 1019 cm^{-1}. HRMS (ESI): *m/z* calculated for $C_{31}H_{49}FO_{10}P$ [M + H]$^+$: 631.3048. Found: 631.3045.

3.18. Synthesis of (2E,4Z)-(1S,2S,E)-1-(2-Fluorophenyl)-1-(methoxymethoxy)-4-methyl-6-(3-oxopropoxy) hex-4-en-2-yl 8-(diethoxyphosphoryl)-5-methyl-7-oxoocta-2,4-dienoate [ketoaldehyde (17S,18S) **28***]*

The crude product was obtained from (17*S*,18S) diol **26** employing the oxidation procedure used for the synthesis of its antipode **27**. After being confirmed by its ^{1}H NMR data, the crude product was directly used for the next step reaction without further purification. ^{1}H NMR (300 MHz, $CDCl_3$) δ 9.72 (t, *J* = 1.8 Hz, 1H, CHO), 7.41 (dt, *J* = 7.5, 1.8 Hz, 1H, aromatic H), 7.31 (dd, *J* = 15.0, 11.7 Hz, 1H, H-3), 7.29–7.22 (m, 1H), 7.11 (dt, *J* = 7.5, 0.9 Hz, 1H), 7.51 (ddd, *J* = 10.2, 8.1, 0.9 Hz, 1H), 6.17 (d, *J* = 11.1 Hz, 1H, H-4), 5.83 (d, *J* = 15.0 Hz, 1H, H-2), 5.45–5.38 (m, 1H), 5.31 (t, *J* = 5.7 Hz, 1H, H-14), 5.07 (d, *J* = 5.4 Hz, 1H), 4.57 (d, *J* = 6.9 Hz, 1H, OCH_2OCH_3), 4.50 (d, *J* = 6.9 Hz, 1 H, OCH_2OCH_3), 4.20–4.11 (m, 5H, 2 × OCH_2CH_3, H-7), 3.90 (t, *J* = 7.2 Hz, 2H, H_2-13), 3.65 (t, *J* = 6.0 Hz, 2H, H_2-11), 3.31 (s, 3H, OCH_3), 3.10 (d, *J* = 22.8 Hz, 2H, H_2-8), 2.39–2.19 (m, 2H, H_2-10), 1.87 (s, 3H, 5-CH_3), 1.63 (s, 3H, 15-CH_3).

3.19. Synthesis of (S,3E,9E,11Z,15E)-6-((S)-(2-Fluorophenyl)(methoxymethoxy)methyl)-4,12-dimethyl-1,7-dioxacyclooctadeca-3,9,11,15-tetraene-8,14-dione [(17S,18S) macrolide **30***]*

(17*S*,18*S*) Macrolide **30** was synthesized according to the HWE ring closing procedure employed for the conversion of **27** to **29**. Colorless syrup, 68% yield for two steps. [α]: +8.1 (*c* = 0.22, MeOH). ^{1}H NMR (300 MHz, $CDCl_3$) δ 7.59 (dd, *J* = 15.0, 11.4 Hz, 1H, H-3), 7.46 (dt, *J* = 7.5, 1.8 Hz, 1H, aromatic H), 7.36–7.25 (m, 1H, aromatic H), 7.15 (dt, *J* = 7.5, 1.2 Hz, 1H, aromatic H), 7.04 (ddd, *J* = 9.9, 8.1, 1.2 Hz, 1H, aromatic H), 6.81 (dt, *J* = 15.9, 6.9 Hz, 1H, H-9), 6.11 (d, *J* = 11.4 Hz, 1H, H-4), 6.00 (d, *J* = 16.2 Hz, 1H, H-8), 5.90 (d, *J* = 15.0 Hz, 1H, H-2), 5.50 (dd, *J* = 11.4, 6.3 Hz, 1H, H-17), 5.26 (dd, *J* = 7.5, 4.5 Hz, 1H, H-14), 5.11 (d, *J* = 6.3 Hz, 1H, H-18), 4.59 (d, *J* = 6.9 Hz, 1H,–OCH_2OCH_3), 4.52 (d, *J* = 6.6 Hz, 1H, –OCH_2OCH_3), 3.98 (dd, *J* = 12.0, 8.1 Hz, 1H, H-16), 3.88 – 3.81 (overlapped, 2H, H_2-13), 3.46 – 3.31 (overlapped, 2H, H_2-11), 3.33 (s, 3H, OCH_3), 3.14 (d, *J* = 12.6 Hz, 1H, H-16), 2.42–2.35 (m, 2H, H_2-10), 2.33 (d, *J* = 11.7 Hz, 1H, H-6), 2.04 (d, *J* = 11.7 Hz, 1H, H-6), 1.82 (s, 3H, 5-CH_3), 1.63 (s, 3H, 15-CH_3). ^{13}C NMR (75 MHz, $CDCl_3$) δ 197.1, 166.6, 160.9 (d, J_{CF} = 244.5 Hz), 146.8, 142.5, 139.8, 134.3, 130.2, 129.9, 129.0, 125.9 (d, J_{CF} = 7.5 Hz), 125.5 (d, *J* = 13.5 Hz), 125.2 (d, J_{CF} = 4.5 Hz), 124.5, 120.9 (d, J_{CF} = 3.8 Hz), 115.6 (d, J_{CF} = 21.0 Hz), 94.9, 72.9, 72.6, 67.9, 67.8, 56.0, 45.9, 41.4, 33.1, 24.1, 16.7. IR (film) ν_{max}: 2925, 2854, 1714, 1669, 1634, 1489, 1359, 1280 cm^{-1}. HRMS (ESI): *m/z* calculated for $C_{27}H_{34}FO_6$ [M + H]$^+$: 473.2339. Found: 473.2332.

3.20. Synthesis of (S,3E,9E,11Z,15E)-6-((S)-(2-Fluorophenyl)(hydroxy)methyl)-4,12-dimethyl-1,7-dioxacyclooctadeca-3,9,11,15-tetraene-8,14-dione [(17S,18S) zampanolide mimic **6***]*

(17*S*,18*S*) Zampanolide mimic **6** was obtained according to the MOM deprotection procedure used for the conversion of (17*R*,18*R*) macrolide **29** to (17S,18S) zampanolide mimic **5**. Colorless syrup, 45% yield. [α]: +15.6 (*c* = 0.15, MeOH). ^{1}H NMR (300 MHz, CD_3COCD_3) δ 7.61 (dd, *J* = 15.0, 11.1 Hz, 1H, H-3), 7.34 (dd, *J* = 14.4, 7.2 Hz, 1H, aromatic H), 7.21 (t, *J* = 7.5 Hz, 1H, aromatic H), 7.10 (dd, *J* = 10.5, 8.1 Hz, 1H, aromatic H), 6.83 (dt, *J* = 16.2, 6.3 Hz, 1H, H-9), 6.20 (d, *J* = 11.1 Hz, 1H, H-4), 6.06 (d, *J* = 15.9 Hz, H-8), 5.88 (d, *J* = 12.6 Hz, 1H, H-2), 5.44 (dd, *J* = 11.1, 5.4 Hz, 1H, H-17), 5.27 (t, *J* = 5.4 Hz, 1H, H-14), 5.17 (t, *J* = 5.4 Hz, 1H, H-18), 4.81 (d, *J* = 5.4 Hz, 1H, OH), 4.07–3.97 (m, 1H, H-16), 3.90 (d, *J* = 12.9 Hz, 1H, H-13), 3.83 (dd, *J* = 12.3, 4.5 Hz, 1H, H-13), 3.48– 3.32 (m, 2H, H_2-11), 3.17 (d, *J* = 12.6 Hz, 1H, H-16), 2.42–2.33 (overlapped, 3H, H_2-10, H-6), 2.19 (d, *J* = 13.8 Hz, 1H, H-6), 1.81 (s, 3H, 5-CH_3), 1.64 (s, 3H, 15-CH_3). ^{13}C NMR (75 MHz, CD_3COCD_3) δ 196.5, 166.5, 160.5 (d, J_{CF} = 242.3 Hz), 146.6, 142.7, 139.8, 134.7, 130.6, 129.7, 129.5, 126.3, 126.2, 125.7, 124.8, 121.7, 115.6, 73.8, 69.0, 68.9, 68.2, 45.8, 41.6, 33.2, 23.8, 16.3. IR (film) ν_{max}: 3447, 2916, 2855, 1710, 1669, 1633, 1489, 1456, 1359, 1281, 1148 cm^{-1}. HRMS (ESI): *m/z* calculated for $C_{25}H_{30}FO_5$ [M + H]$^+$: 429.2077. Found: 429.2073.

3.21. Cell Culture

All cell lines were initially purchased from American Type Culture Collection (ATCC). The PC-3, PC-3/DTX, and LNCaP prostate cancer cell lines were routinely cultured in RPMI-1640 medium supplemented with 10% FBS and 1% penicillin/streptomycin. Cultures were maintained in a high humidity environment supplemented with 5% carbon dioxide at a temperature of 37 °C. The DU145 and DU145/DTX prostate cancer cells were routinely cultured in Eagle's Minimum Essential Medium (EMEM) supplemented with 10% FBS and 1% penicillin/streptomycin.

The procedure illustrated in the literature [29,30] was adapted to establish docetaxel-resistant prostate cancer cell lines. Specifically, docetaxel-resistant DU145 and PC-3 cell lines (DU145/DTX and PC-3/DTX) were developed over a period of one year by stepwise increased concentrations of docetaxel. Cells were repeatedly conserved in an appropriate concentration of docetaxel, starting with IC_{50} value of the respective parent cell lines. Docetaxel-containing media will be replaced every 2–3 days. The concentration of docetaxel was increased when cells exhibited resistance to treatments.

3.22. WST-1 Cell Proliferation Assay

PC-3, PC-3/DTX, DU145, DU145/DTX, or LNCaP cells were placed in 96-well plates at a density of 3200 cells each well in 200 μL of culture medium. The cells were then treated with synthesized mimics, or positive reference separately at different doses for 3 days, while equal treatment volumes of DMSO were used as vehicle control. After the cells were cultured in a CO_2 incubator at 37 °C for three days, the premixed WST-1 cell proliferation reagent (10 μL, Clontech) was added to each well. The cells were incubated for additional 3 h at 37 °C before mixing gently for one minute on an orbital shaker to ensure homogeneous distribution of color. A microplate-reader (Synergy HT, BioTek) was used to measure the absorbance of each well at a wavelength of 430 nm. The half-maximal inhibitory concentration (IC_{50} value) is the concentration of each compound that inhibits cell proliferation by 50% under the experimental conditions. Each of IC_{50} value is represented as the average from triplicate determinations that were reproducible and statistically significant. The IC_{50} values were calculated based on dose–response curves from at least five dosages for each compound.

3.23. Statistical Analysis

All data are represented as the mean ± standard deviation (S.D.) for the number of experiments indicated. Other differences between treated and control groups were analyzed using the Student's t-test. A p-value < 0.05 was considered statistically significant.

4. Conclusions

In summary, two new zampanolide mimics have been designed and each of them has been achieved through a 25-step chemical transformation starting from commercially available 2-butyn-1-ol. Yamaguchi esterification and intramolecular Horner–Wadsworth–Emmons condensation were employed as crucial reactions to build up the C-17 and C-1 ester moiety and to close the lactone ring. The chiral centers at C17 and C18 in the Fragment C9–C18 (**7** and **8**) were introduced by the Sharpless asymmetric dihydroxylation using the commercially available AD-mix formulations. Our WST-1 cell proliferation assay data in both docetaxel-resistant and docetaxel-sensitive prostate cancer cell lines revealed that compound **6** is the optimal mimic and the newly designed side chain can act as a bioisostere for the chemically fragile *N*-acetyl hemiminal side chain in zampanolide.

Supplementary Materials: The following are available online at http://www.mdpi.com/1420-3049/25/2/362/s1, NMR spectra (^{1}H and ^{13}C) of the zampanolide mimics **5** and **6**, as well as the macrolides **30** and **31**, and intermediates **7–8**, **14–21**, and **23–26**.

Author Contributions: Conceptualization and design, Q.C.; experimentation and data analysis, G.C., Z.J., Q.Z., G.W., and Q.-H.C.; funding acquisition, Q.-H.C. and G.W.; all authors finally reviewed and approved the manuscript. All authors have read and agreed to the published version of the manuscript.

Funding: This research was funded by the National Institutes of Health (National Institute of General Medical Sciences) under Award Number SC2GM121185 (Q. Chen). HRMS were supported by the National Institutes of Health RCMI program at Xavier University of Louisiana through Grant 2G12MD007595 (G. Wang).

Acknowledgments: We thank the Department of Chemistry and College of Science and Mathematics at CSU-Fresno for all administrative support.

Conflicts of Interest: The authors declare no conflict of interest. The funders had no role in the design of the study; in the collection, analyses, or interpretation of data; in the writing of the manuscript; or in the decision to publish the results.

References

1. Siegel, R.L.; Miller, K.D.; Jamal, A. Cancer Statistics, 2019. *CA Cancer J. Clin.* **2019**, *69*, 7–34. [CrossRef] [PubMed]
2. Tan, M.H.; Li, J.; Xu, H.E.; Melcher, K.; Yong, E.-L. Androgen receptor: Structure, role in prostate cancer, and drug discovery. *Acta Pharmacol. Sin.* **2015**, *36*, 3–23. [CrossRef] [PubMed]
3. Elshan, N.G.R.D.; Rettig, M.B.; Jung, M.E. Molecules targeting the androgen receptor (AR) signaling axis beyond the AR-ligand binding domain. *Med. Res. Rev.* **2019**, *39*, 910–960. [CrossRef] [PubMed]
4. Ojo, D.; Lin, X.; Wong, N.; Gu, Y.; Tang, D. Prostate cancer stem-like cells contribute to the development of castration-resistant prostate cancer. *Cancers* **2015**, *7*, 2290–2308. [CrossRef] [PubMed]
5. Schweizer, M.T.; Yu, E.Y. Persistent androgen receptor addiction in castration-resistant prostate cancer. *J. Hematol. Oncol.* **2015**, *8*, 128. [CrossRef] [PubMed]
6. De Bono, J.S.; Oudard, S.; Ozguroglu, M.; Hansen, S.; Machiels, J.-P.; Kocak, I.; Gravis, G.; Bodrogi, I.; Mackenzie, M.; Shen, L.; et al. Prednisone plus cabazitaxel or mitoxantrone for metastatic castration-resistant prostate cancer progressing after docetaxel treatment: A randomized open-label trial. *Lancet* **2010**, *376*, 1147–1154. [CrossRef]
7. Tannock, I.F.; de Wit, R.; Berry, W.R.; Horti, J.; Pluzanska, A.; Chi, K.N.; Oudard, S.; Theodore, C.; James, N.D.; Turesson, I.; et al. Docetaxel plus prednisone or mitoxantrone plus prednisone for advanced prostate cancer. *Engl. J. Med.* **2004**, *351*, 1502–1512. [CrossRef]
8. Petrylak, D.P.; Tangen, C.M.; Hussain, M.H.A.; Lara, P.N.; Jones, J.A.; Taplin, M.E.; Burch, P.A.; Berry, D.; Moinpour, C.; Kohli, M.; et al. Docetaxel and estramustine compared with mitoxantrone and prednisone for advanced refractory prostate cancer. *N. Engl. J. Med.* **2004**, *351*, 1513–1520. [CrossRef]
9. Jordan, M.A.; Wilson, L. Microtubules as a target for anticancer drugs. *Nat. Rev. Cancer* **2004**, *4*, 253–265. [CrossRef]
10. Thadani-Mulero, M.; Nanus, D.M.; Giannakakou, P. Androgen receptor on the move: Boarding the microtubule expressway to the nucleus. *Cancer Res.* **2012**, *72*, 4611–4615. [CrossRef]
11. Chen, Q.-H.; Kingston, D.G.I. Zampanolide and dactylolide: Cytotoxic tubulin-assembly agents and promising anticancer leads. *Nat. Prod. Rep.* **2014**, *31*, 1202–1226. [CrossRef] [PubMed]
12. Field, J.J.; Singh, A.J.; Kanakkanthara, A.; Halafihi, T.I.; Northcote, P.T.; Miller, J.H. Microtubule stabilizing activity of zampanolide, a potent macrolide isolated from the Tongan marine sponge Cacospongia mycofijensis. *J. Med. Chem.* **2009**, *52*, 7328–7332. [CrossRef] [PubMed]
13. Tanaka, J.; Higa, T. Zampanolide, a new cytotoxic macrolide from a marine sponge. *Tetrahedron Lett.* **1996**, *37*, 5535–5538. [CrossRef]
14. Hoye, T.R.; Hu, M. Macrolactonization via Ti(IV)-mediated epoxy-acid coupling: A total synthesis of (−)-dactylolide [and zampanolide]. *J. Am. Chem. Soc.* **2003**, *125*, 9576–9577. [CrossRef]
15. Ghosh, A.K.; Cheng, X. Enantioselective total synthesis of (−)-zampanolide, a potent microtubule-stabilizing agent. *Org. Lett.* **2011**, *13*, 4108–4111. [CrossRef]
16. Smith, A.B.; Safonov, I.G.; Corbett, R.M. Total synthesis of (+)-zampanolide and (+)-dactylolide. *J. Am. Chem. Soc.* **2002**, *124*, 11102–11113. [CrossRef]
17. Uenishi, J.; Iwamoto, T.; Tanaka, J. Total synthesis of (−)-zampanolide and questionable existence of (−)-dactylolide as the elusive biosynthetic precursor of (−)-zampanolide in an Okinwan sponge. *Org. Lett.* **2009**, *11*, 3262–3265. [CrossRef]
18. Zurwerra, D.; Glaus, F.; Betschart, L.; Schuster, J.; Gertsch, J.; Ganci, W.; Altmann, K.-H. Total synthesis of (−)-zampanolide and structure-activity relationship studies on (−)-dactylolide derivatives. *Chem. Eur. J.* **2012**, *18*, 16868–16883. [CrossRef]

19. Field, J.J.; Pera, B.; Calvo, E.; Canales, A.; Zurwerra, D.; Trigili, C.; Rodriguez-Salarichs, J.; Matesanz, R.; Kanakkanthara, A.; Wakefield, S.J.; et al. Zampanolide, a potent new microtubule-stabilizing agent, covalently reacts with the taxane luminal site in tubulin α, β-heterodimers and microtubules. *Chem. Biol.* **2012**, *19*, 686–698. [CrossRef]
20. Ding, F.; Jennings, M.P. Total synthesis of (−)-dactylolide and formal synthesis of (−)-zampanolide via target oriented β-C-glycoside formation. *J. Org. Chem.* **2008**, *73*, 5965–5976. [CrossRef]
21. Chen, G.; Patanapongpibu, M.; Jiang, Z.; Zhang, Q.; Zheng, S.; Wang, G.; White, J.D.; Chen, Q.-H. Synthesis and antiproliferative evaluation of new zampanolide mimics. *Org. Biomole. Chem.* **2019**, *10*, 3830–3844. [CrossRef] [PubMed]
22. Prota, A.E.; Bargsten, K.; Zurwerra, D.; Field, J.J.; Diaz, J.F.; Altmann, K.-H.; Steinmetz, M.O. Molecular mechanism of action of microtubule-stabilizing anticancer agents. *Science* **2013**, *339*, 587–590. [CrossRef] [PubMed]
23. Chen, G.; Wang, R.; Vue, B.; Patanapongpibul, M.; Zhang, Q.; Zheng, S.; Wang, G.; White, J.D.; Chen, Q.-H. Optimized synthesis and antiproliferative activity of desTHPdactylolides. *Bioorg. Med. Chem.* **2018**, *26*, 3514–3520. [CrossRef] [PubMed]
24. Zurwerra, D.; Gertsch, J.; Altmann, K.-H. Synthesis of (−)-dactylolide and 13-desmethylene-(−)-dactylolide and their effects on tubulin. *Org. Lett.* **2010**, *12*, 2302–2305. [CrossRef] [PubMed]
25. Sharpless, K.B.; Amberg, W.; Bennani, Y.L.; Crispino, G.A.; Hartung, J.; Jeong, K.-S.; Kwong, H.-L.; Morikawa, K.; Wang, Z.M.; Xu, D.; et al. The osmium-catalyzed asymmetric dihydroxylation: A new ligand class and a process improvement. *J. Org. Chem.* **1992**, *57*, 2768–2771. [CrossRef]
26. Lad, N.P.; Kulkarni, S.; Sharma, R.; Mascarenhas, M.; Kulkarni, M.R.; Pandit, S.S. Piperlongumine derived cyclic sulfonamides (sultams): Synthesis and in vitro exploration for therapeutic potential against HeLa cancer cell lines. *Eur. J. Med. Chem.* **2017**, *126*, 870–878. [CrossRef] [PubMed]
27. Huang, J.; Wang, W.; He, H.-Y.; Jian, L.; Fu, H.-Y.; Zheng, X.-L.; Li, R.-X. An approach to the synthesis of 1-propenylnaphthols and 3-arylnaphtho[2,1-*b*]furans. *J. Org. Chem.* **2017**, *82*, 2523–2534. [CrossRef]
28. Banwell, M.G.; Chand, S.; Savage, G.P. An enantioselective total synthesis of the stilbenolignan (−)-aiphanol and the determination of its absolute stereochemistry. *Tetrahedron Asymmetry* **2005**, *16*, 1645–1654. [CrossRef]
29. O'Neill, A.J.; Prencipe, M.; Dowline, C.; Fan, Y.; Mulrane, L.; Gallagher, W.M.; O'Connor, D.; Devery, A.; Corcoran, C.; Rani, S.; et al. Characterisation and manipulation of docetaxel resistant prostate cancer cell lines. *Mol. Cancer* **2011**, *10*, 126. [CrossRef]
30. Shiota, M.; Kashiwagi, E.; Yokomizo, A.; Takeuchi, A.; Dejima, T.; Song, Y.; Tatsugami, K.; Inokuchi, J.; Uchiumi, T.; Naito, S. Interaction between docetaxel resistance and castration resistance in prostate cancer: Implications of twistI, YB-I, and androgen receptor. *Prostate* **2013**, *73*, 1336–1344. [CrossRef]

Sample Availability: Samples of the compounds **5, 6, 29 and 30** are available from the authors.

molecules

MDPI

Article

Synthesis and Antiproliferative Screening Of Novel Analogs of Regioselectively Demethylated Colchicine and Thiocolchicine

Dominika Czerwonka [1], Szymon Sobczak [2], Ewa Maj [3], Joanna Wietrzyk [3], Andrzej Katrusiak [2] and Adam Huczyński [1,*]

1 Department of Medical Chemistry, Faculty of Chemistry, Adam Mickiewicz University, Uniwersytetu Poznańskiego 8, 61-614 Poznan, Poland; dominika.czerwonka@amu.edu.pl
2 Department of Materials Chemistry, Faculty of Chemistry Adam Mickiewicz University, Uniwersytetu Poznańskiego 8, 61-614 Poznań, Poland; szymon.sobczak@amu.edu.pl (S.S.); katran@amu.edu.pl (A.K.)
3 Hirszfeld Institute of Immunology and Experimental Therapy, Polish Academy of Sciences, Rudolfa Weigla 12, 53-114 Wrocław, Poland; ewa.maj@hirszfeld.pl (E.M.); joanna.wietrzyk@hirszfeld.pl (J.W.)
* Correspondence: adhucz@amu.edu.pl; Tel.: +48-618291673

Academic Editor: Qiao-Hong Chen
Received: 29 January 2020; Accepted: 3 March 2020; Published: 5 March 2020

Abstract: Colchicine, a pseudoalkaloid isolated from *Colchicum autumnale*, has been identified as a potent anticancer agent because of its strong antimitotic activity. It was shown that colchicine modifications by regioselective demethylation affected its biological properties. For demethylated colchicine analogs, 10-demethylcolchicine (colchiceine, **1**) and 1-demethylthiocolchicine (**3**), a series of 12 colchicine derivatives including 5 novel esters (**2b–c** and **4b–d**) and 4 carbonates (**2e–f** and **4e–f**) were synthesized. The antiproliferative activity assay, together with in silico evaluation of physicochemical properties, confirmed attractive biological profiles for all obtained compounds. The substitutions of H-donor and H-acceptor sites at C1 in thiocolchicine position provide an efficient control of the hydration affinity and solubility, as demonstrated for anhydrate **3**, hemihydrate **4e** and monohydrate **4a**.

Keywords: colchicine analogs; thiocolchicine; colchiceine; antimitotic agents; antiproliferative activity; hydrates

1. Introduction

Colchicine (Figure 1) is a pseudoalkaloid produced by *Colchicum autumnale* [1]. Its beneficial applications have been known for centuries, as colchicine was used by ancient Greeks and Egyptians to treat swelling and inflammation [2]. Presently, colchicine is considered as the first-line therapy for gout, pericarditis and familial Mediterranean fever [1,3–5]. The most interesting property of colchicine is its high affinity for binding to the tubulin in cancer cells, leading to the inhibition of microtubule polymerization and mitosis arrest [6–8]. These unique properties have attracted great interest to colchicine as an anticancer-drug candidate, however its use is limited by its toxicity towards normal cells [9–11]. For this reason, new derivatives obtained through chemical modifications guided by structure–activity relations are intensively investigated. This research is aimed at reducing the colchicine toxicity and preserving the antimitotic and anticancer properties [12–24]. As it turns out, tubulin interacts with trimethoxyphenyl ring A and tropolone ring C, making the methoxy groups at C1, C2 and C10, as well as the C9-keto group, crucial for colchicine's antimitotic activity [25–27].

Unfortunately, colchicine is also prone to isomerization, resulting in isocolchicine (Figure 1) with 500 times lower affinity for binding to tubulin than colchicine itself [28].

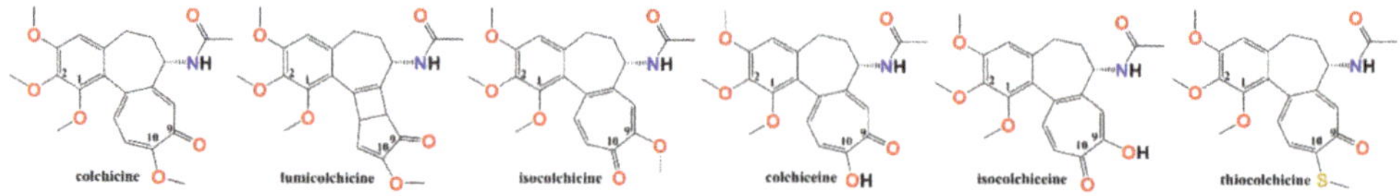

Figure 1. Structures of colchicine, lumicolchicine, isocolchicine, colchiceine, isocolchiceine and thiocolchicine.

Colchiceine (Figure 1) is a C10 demethylated colchicine analog characterized by much lower toxicity [29,30]. It is, next to lumicolchicine (Figure 1), the main product of colchicine degradation and can naturally occur in plant extracts together with colchicine [31]. Elguero et al. [32] have established that colchiceine (as well as its C10-acylated analog) can occur in two tautomeric forms, from which the isoform is slightly more dominant. This equilibrium between colchiceine and isocolchiceine (Figure 1) exists also in the solid state, which has been confirmed by X-ray diffraction studies [33]. The tendency of colchiceine towards tautomerization, in combination with the loss of the C10-methoxy group, may be responsible for its poor antimitotic activity. In contrast, colchiceine shows better bacteriostatic and antifungal activity than colchicine, because its free hydroxyl group may increase its binding affinity towards the cell walls of pathogens [29,33].Interestingly, the replacement of the C10-methoxy group with thiomethyl in a colchicine analog thiocolchicine (Figure 1) decreases its isomerization. Thiocolchicine is more stable, exhibits lower toxicity and has a higher binding affinity to tubulin [34–36]. As could be expected, demethylation of thiocolchicine at C1/C2/C3 positions leads to a lower binding ability to tubulin and lower toxicity [37–39]. As the removal of the methoxy groups from colchicine's structure reduces its toxicity but also lowers its binding affinity to tubulin, we decided to replace these groups with a bigger substituent, such as an ester or carbonate moiety, to investigate an effect of this modification on biological activity [40].

For this reason, we carried out a series of regioselective demethylation reactions of colchicine and thiocolchicine, in order to to obtain colchiceine (**1**) and 1-demethylthiocolchicine (**3**). On the basis of **1** and **3**, we synthesized a series of 12 mono- and double-modified colchicine analogs. Within these analogs, we present 5 novel esters (**2b–c** and **4b–d**) and 4 novel carbonates (**2e–f** and **4e–f**). The pathways used for these syntheses are depicted in Scheme 1.

We also evaluated the antiproliferative activity of these derivatives using three human cancer cell lines, human lung adenocarcinoma (A549), human breast adenocarcinoma (MCF-7) and human colon adenocarcinoma cell line (LoVo), and one normal murine embryonic fibroblast cell line (BALB/3T3). Moreover, on the basis of the in silico calculations, we were able to predict the physicochemical properties of the obtained compounds and check their compliance with Lipiński's rule of 5, permitting evaluation of its drug-likeness.

2. Results and Discussion

2.1. Chemistry

A series of colchicine esters and carbonates substituted at C1 and C10 positions in colchicine were synthesized by performing regioselective demethylation reactions of C1 and C10 methoxy groups, respectively. At first, we performed regioselective demethylation of the colchicine C10 methoxy group by treating colchicine with a mixture of glacial acetic acid and 0.1N hydrochloric acid (i). Reaction resulted in precipitation of yellow solid [41], which was further recrystallized in acetone, leading to growth of good quality, large single crystals. Performed X-ray diffraction analysis proved them to be a colchiceine (**1**, Scheme 1) hemihydrate of the same structure as that reported by Mackay et al. [33], in which the unit-cell accommodates two tautomeric forms: colchiceine and isocolchiceine.

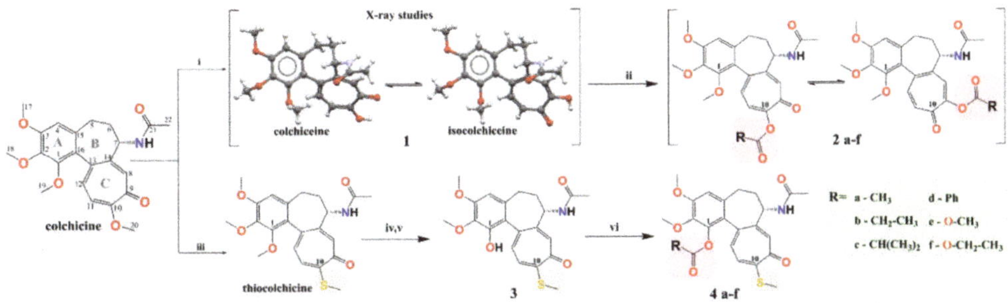

Scheme 1. Synthesis of novel colchicine analogs. The obtained crystal structure of **1** was identical to the one proposed by Mackey et al. [33]. Reagents and conditions: (i) glacial acetic acid, hydrochloric acid, 100 °C, 6h; (iii) MeOH/H_2O, CH_3SNa, RT, 24h; (iv) DCM, acetyl chloride, $SnCl_4$, 0 °C → RT, 48h; (v) MeOH/H_2O, LiOH, RT, 1h; (ii,vi) DCM, Et_3N, respective acyl chloride/chloroformate, 0 °C → RT, 24h.

Colchicine was also treated with sodium methanethiolate (**iii**) to obtain thiocolchicine [42]. By using a slightly modified method proposed by Bladé-Font [43] (**iv,v**), thiocolchicine was regioselectively demethylated at the C1 methoxy group, leading to 1-demethylthiocolchicine (3) with 40% yield. This regioselective demethylation was confirmed by X-ray analysis (Figure 2). Finally, compounds **1** and **3** were treated with respective acyl chlorides or chloroformates (**ii, vi**) to give single modified derivatives **2a–f** and double modified derivatives **4a–f** with 38%–58% yields (Scheme 1).

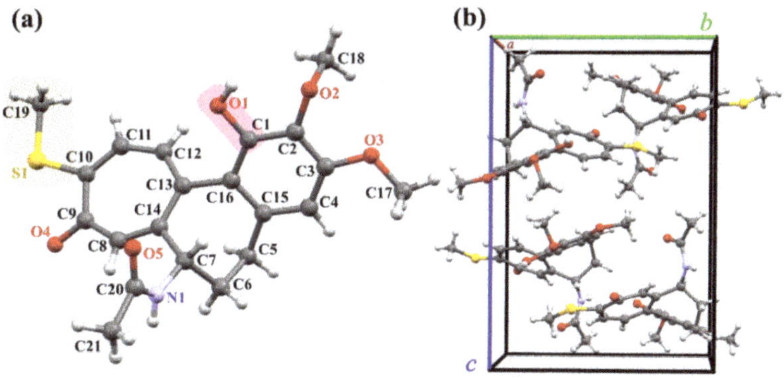

Figure 2. (**a**) Molecule of 1-demethylthiocolchicine (**3**) and (**b**) its crystal structure projected along the crystal direction [100].

The purity and structure of synthesized colchicine derivatives **1**, **2a–f**, **3** and **4a–f** were determined on the basis of ESI-MS, NMR and X-ray analysis. The specific data can be found in Section 3 and in Supplementary Materials. The disappearance of the signal at about 56.5 ppm in the ^{13}C NMR spectrum of colchicine, assigned to the C10 methoxy group, is the evidence of the formation of colchiceine (**1**). Moreover, in the spectra of derivatives **2a–2f**, an additional signal from the carbonyl group can be observed in the range 164.1–174.3 ppm for esters **2a–2d**, and 151.9–152.5 ppm for carbonates **2e–f**. A shift of the signal corresponding to the C10 methoxy group from 56.5 to 15.1 ppm is evidence for the introduction of the thiomethyl group at position C10, and the absence of one of the signals around 61 ppm assigned to the C1 methoxy group is evidence of 1-demethylthiocolchicine (**3**) formation. An additional signal corresponding to the carbonyl carbon atom can be observed in the range 168.3–174.7 ppm for esters **4a–4d** and in the range 152.8–152.9 ppm for carbonates **4e–f**.

2.2. *In Silico Calculations of the Physicochemical Properties*

We used the Molinspiration online database (http://www.molinspiration.com, free of charge) to predict the physicochemical properties of all synthesized compounds and collected them in Table 1 [44].

Table 1. Physicochemical properties of the synthesized compounds based on the Molinspiration database [44].

Compound	MW	clog*P*	tPSA	n(O,N)	N(OH,NH)	Rotb	MV
1	385.42	0.83	94.10	7	2	4	346.63
2a	427.45	0.60	100.18	8	1	6	383.14
2b	441.48	1.27	100.18	8	1	7	399.94
2c	455.51	1.51	100.18	8	1	7	416.53
2d	489.52	2.92	100.18	8	1	7	437.99
2e	443.45	0.95	109.41	9	1	7	392.12
2f	457.48	1.33	109.41	9	1	8	408.93
3	401.48	1.89	84.86	6	2	4	355.77
4a	443.52	1.66	90.94	7	1	6	392.28
4b	457.55	2.33	90.94	7	1	7	409.08
4c	471.57	2.57	90.94	7	1	7	425.67
4d	505.59	3.98	90.94	7	1	7	447.13
4e	459.52	2.02	100.18	8	1	7	401.27
4f	473.55	2.39	100.18	8	1	8	418.07
colchicine	399.44	1.10	83.11	7	1	5	364.15

MW: Molecular weight; clog*P*: calculated log octanol/water partition coefficient; tPSA: total polar surface area; n(O,N): number of hydrogen acceptors; n(OH,NH): number of hydrogen donors; Rotb: rotatable bonds; MV: molecular volume.

According to Lipinski's rule of 5, most "drug-like" molecules should have log$P \leq 5$, molecular weight ≤ 500, number of hydrogen bond acceptors ≤ 10 and number of hydrogen bond donors ≤ 5. Additionally, it was demonstrated that a total polar surface area (tPSA) < 140 and number of rotatable bonds < 10, in combination with log$P < 5$, are crucial for both good bioavailability and permeability through biological membranes [45].

The demethylation of the C1 and C10 position of colchicine, both in **1** and **3**, increases the number of H-donor sites while the substitution of colchicine's C10 methoxy group with thiomethyl results in a decreased number of H-acceptor sites in **3**. Additionally, the demethylation of the C1 and C10 position of colchicine reduces the number of rotatable bonds. Substitution of a hydroxyl group, both in **1** and **3**, with an ester or carbonate substituent, increases the number of H-acceptor sites and reduces the number of H-donor sites to that of colchicine. According to the performed calculations, all synthesized compounds **2a–e** and **4a–e** have a rather lipophilic character, with the clog*P* values between 0.60 and 3.98. Conducted syntheses allowed us to obtain compounds with less lipophilic character than that of colchicine for compounds **1**, **2a** and **2e**, with clog*P* values 0.83, 060 and 0.95, respectively. Interestingly, esters and carbonates in the C10 position (**2a–e**) are in general less lipophilic than corresponding esters and carbonates in the C1 position (**4a–e**). Except for **4d**, whose molecular weight is above 500, the calculations for all colchicine analogs are in agreement with Lipinski's descriptors. Importantly, in order to be active, a drug should not have more than one violation [46]. This, in combination with the number of rotatable bonds between 4 and 8, as well as tPSA between 84.86 and 100.18, confirm good physicochemical profiles of all obtained compounds.

2.3. *X-ray Analysis*

The structures of compounds **3**, **4a** and **4e** were additionally confirmed by X-ray diffraction. Selected crystallographic data are collected in Table 2, and more detailed information can be found in Supplementary Information. The single crystals of **3**, **4a**, **4e** were obtained by slow evaporation from an ethyl acetate mixture. The 1-Demethylthiocolchicine (**3**) crystallizes in the orthorhombic space group $P2_12_12_1$ (Figure 2) while the crystals of **4a** and **4e** are monoclinic, space group $P2_1$. The substitution at the C1 atom with acetyl ester (**4a**) and methyl carbonate (**4e**), and the following change in the ratio between H-bond acceptors and donors, increases the tendency of these colchicine derivatives to co-crystallize with water; hence, monohydrate **4a**·H_2O and hemihydrate **4e**·½H_2O were obtained.

Molecules **4a** and **4e** significantly differ in conformation (Figure 3).The arrangement of the C2 methoxy group, which can be described by the C1-C2-O2-C18 torsion angle, changed from −122.36° to 108.75° in **4a** and **4e**, respectively. Together with increasing mass of the C1 moiety, the twist between the planar phenyl and tropolone rings around the C13-C16 bond increases, altering the C1-C16-C13-C12 angle from 45.43° in **3**, through 58.54° in **4a**, to 60.11° in **4e**.

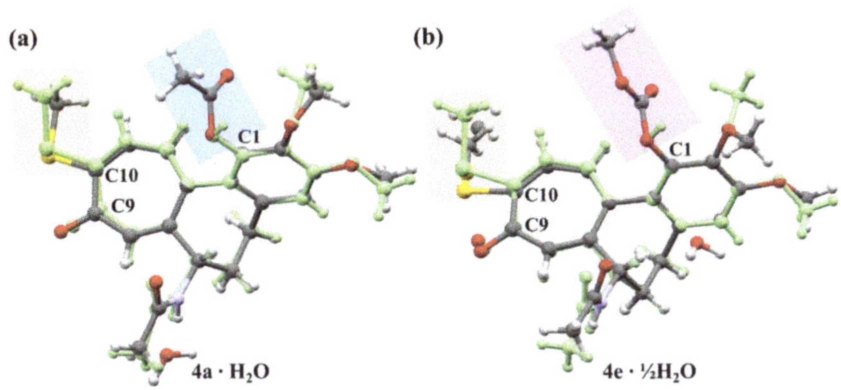

Figure 3. Comparison of the molecular conformation from the X-ray analysis studies between (**a**) molecule **4a** and (**b**) **4e**, superimposed with respect to the benzene ring on the 1-demethylthiocolchicine (molecule **3**), highlighted with a light-green color.

Table 2. Selected crystallographic data for compounds **3**, **4a·H_2O** and **4e·½H_2O**.

Label		3	4a·H_2O	4e·1/2H_2O
Formula		$C_{21}H_{22}NO_5S$	$C_{23}H_{25}NO_6S \cdot H_2O$	$C_{23}H_{25}NO_7S \cdot 1/2H_2O$
CCDC number		1966196	1966194	1966195
Crystal system		orthorhombic	monoclinic	monoclinic
Space group		$P2_12_12_1$	$P2_1$	$P2_1$
Unit cell dimensions	*a* (Å)	9.1005(17)	10.600(2)	10.8835(10)
	b (Å)	11.866(2)	6.9635(11)	9.2158(6)
	c (Å)	17.881(4)	16.712(3)	12.0632(12)
	β (°)	90	107.07(2)	104.613(9)
Volume (Å^3)		1930.8(7)	1179.2(4)	1170.80(18)
Z/Z′		4/1	2/1	2/1
D_x (g/cm^3)		1.378	1.300	1.329

The presence of water significantly alters the pattern of H-bonds between **3** and **4a·H_2O** and **4e·½H_2O**. Although in all structures amide nitrogen participates in the formation of intermolecular contacts, only in **3** are the NH···S, of 2.793(2) Å, and NH···O4, of 2.370(3) Å,bonds formed. In a monohydrate crystal **4a·H_2O**, water interrupts the NH···O4 interaction observed in the crystal structure of **3**, accepting NH amide proton, of 2.086(1) Å and further donating its H-atoms to the HO-H···O4′, of 2.007(3) Å, and HO-H···O5′, of 1.994(3) Å bond. Much weaker H-bonds are present in the crystal structure of **4e·½H_2O**. Despite the presence of a water molecule in the crystal structure of **4e·½H_2O**, the strong NH···O5′ bond, of 2.033(2) Å is present again. The disordered by location at half-occupied sites water molecule is involved in formation of a weak HO-H···O5′′ interaction of 2.538(1) Åand the H-bond at the disordered terminal carbonyl at C9. Due to the HO-H···O4′ of 2.241(1) Å bond, the occupational disorder of H_2O is passed onto the orientation of **4e** molecules as illustrated in Figure 3.

Depending on the presence or absence of this water molecule, its adjacent molecule **4e** is slightly shifted in the crystal structure. This disorder is most apparent for the terminal carbonyl at C9 (dislocated by 0.358 Å) and thiomethyl at C10 (dislocated by 0.625 Å).

2.4. Antiproliferative Activity

The antiproliferative activity of all synthesized colchicine analogs **1**, **2a–f**, **3**, **4a–f** was *tested in vitro* against three human cancer cell lines: human lung adenocarcinoma (A549), human breast adenocarcinoma (MCF-7) and human colon adenocarcinoma cell line (LoVo). For a more accurate evaluation of cytotoxic activity, the effect on normal murine embryonic fibroblast cell line (BALB/3T3) was also tested according to the previously published procedure [12]. Detailed information concerning antiproliferation assay can be found in Supplementary Materials. The mean values of IC_{50} ± SD of the tested compounds are collected in Table 3.

Table 3. Antiproliferative activity (IC_{50}) of 10-demethylcolchicine (colchiceine, **1**), 1-demethylthiocolchicine (**3**) and their derivatives(**2a–f**, **4a–f**) compared to the antiproliferative activity of colchicine and standard anticancer drugs doxorubicin and cisplatin and the calculated values of selectivity index (SI).

Compound	A549	SI	MCF-7	SI	LoVo	SI	BALB/3T3
	IC_{50} (μM)		IC_{50} (μM)		IC_{50} (μM)		IC_{50} (μM)
1	12.99 ± 1.79	0.79	11.23 ± 2.52	0.91	6.00 ± 1.88	1.71	10.25 ± 0.96
2a	12.47 ± 2.77	0.68	10.03 ± 2.18	0.85	6.18 ± 1.48	1.37	8.50 ± 0.50
2b	9.97 ± 0.70	0.75	7.56 ± 2.84	0.99	2.39 ± 1.20	3.13	7.47 ± 0.50
2c	20.39 ± 11.30	0.41	11.95 ± 1.54	0.70	6.47 ± 0.35	1.30	8.42 ± 1.14
2d	8.75 ± 0.33	1.02	8.21 ± 3.35	1.09	4.87 ± 2.17	1.83	8.92 ± 3.93
2e	0.98 ± 0.16	0.84	0.98 ± 0.33	0.84	0.48 ± 0.32	1.70	0.82 ± 0.11
2f	9.67 ± 0.84	0.86	9.07 ± 1.90	0.92	6.41 ± 1.57	1.30	8.36 ± 0.17
3	0.82 ± 0.02	0.74	0.12 ± 0.05	4.92	0.11 ± 0.03	5.38	0.61 ± 0.14
4a	0.48 ± 0.15	1.36	0.10 ± 0.02	6.85	0.11 ± 0.02	5.92	0.65 ± 0.12
4b	0.97 ± 0.04	0.77	0.96 ± 0.13	0.78	0.50 ± 0.19	1.53	0.75 ± 0.10
4c	0.89 ± 0.07	0.80	0.86 ± 0.10	0.83	0.56 ± 0.06	1.27	0.71 ± 0.03
4d	0.60 ± 0.31	0.75	0.78 ± 0.22	0.58	0.10 ± 0.08	4.71	0.45 ± 0.23
4e	0.90 ± 0.09	0.87	1.02 ± 0.10	0.77	0.43 ± 0.19	1.84	0.78 ± 0.06
4f	0.96 ± 0.13	1.08	0.95 ± 0.20	1.09	0.79 ± 0.16	1.31	1.03 ± 0.20
colchicine	0.07 ± 0.01	0.63	0.01 ± 0.01	4.30	0.01 ± 0.01	5.38	0.04 ± 0.01
cisplatin	3.60 ± 0.25	0.81	3.05 ± 0.67	0.95	3.80 ± 0.28	0.77	2.91 ± 1.83
doxorubicin	0.16 ± 0.03	0.25	0.15 ± 0.05	0.26	0.08 ± 0.03	0.49	0.04 ± 0.03

The IC_{50} value is defined as the concentration of a compound at which 50% growth inhibition is observed. Human lung adenocarcinoma (A549), human breast adenocarcinoma (MCF-7), human colon adenocarcinoma cell line (LoVo) and normal murine embryonic fibroblast cell line (BALB/3T3). The SI (Selectivity Index) was calculated for each compound, using the formula SI = IC_{50} for normal cell line BALB/3T3/IC_{50} for the respective cancerous cell line. A beneficial SI > 1.0 indicates a drug with efficacy against tumor cells greater than the toxicity against normal cells.

All colchicine analogs showed stronger antiproliferative activity against all tested cancer cell lines than the conventional chemotherapeutic, cisplatin. In general, the IC_{50} values are better for colchicines doubly modified at C1 and C10 positions (**3**, **4a–f**) than for the analogs singly modified at position C10 only (**1**, **2a–f**). Compound **4a**, with a thiomethyl group at position C10 and an acetyl ester substituent at C1, showed the highest activity against all tested cell lines (IC_{50} = 0.48 ± 0.15, 0.10 ± 0.02, 0.11 ± 0.02 μM for A549, MCF-7, LoVo cancer cell lines, respectively).

All tested colchicine analogs exhibit higher SI values than doxorubicin, which indicates the therapeutic potential of the synthesized compounds. Compound **3**, 1-demethylthiocolchicine, as well as its acylated analog **4a**, showed high SI values against MCF-7 (SI = 4.92, SI = 6.88) as well as LoVo cell lines (SI = 5.36, SI = 5.95). From among analogs modified exclusively at position C10, compound **2b** with propionyl ester substituent revealed a higher SI value towards LoVo cell line (SI = 3.13).

3. Materials and Methods

3.1. General

Information concerning reagents and solvents, as well as equipment used for measurements, can be found in the Supplementary Materials.

3.1.1. Synthesis and Characterization of 10-Demethylcolchicine (colchiceine, 1), Thiocolchicine and 1-Demethylthiocolchicine (3)

Information concerning the synthesis of 10-demethylcolchicine (colchiceine, **1**), thiocolchicine and 1-demethylthiocolchicine (**3**) can be found in Supplementary Materials.

3.1.2. General Route for Synthesis of Compounds 2a–f and 4a–f

To a solution of **1** or **3** (100 mg, 0.25 mmol) in dichloromethane (DCM, 10 mL) cooled to 0 °C, Et_3N (1 mL, 7 mmol) and respective acyl chloride or chloroformate were added (excess). The mixture was first stirred at 0 °C for 30 min and then for the next 24h at RT. Reaction time was determined by TLC. After that time the solution was filtered to remove triethylamine hydrochloride, the DCM was evaporated under reduced pressure and the residue was purified by CombiFlash® (chloroform/acetone, increasing concentration gradient) to give respective compounds as amorphous yellow solids.

3.1.3. Characterization of Acetyl Ester of Colchiceine 2a

Amorphous yellow solid, yield 49%, m.p 120–122 °C; ^{1}H NMR ($CDCl_3$, 400 MHz) δ 7.50 (1H, s), 7.31 (1H, d, *J* = 11.3 Hz), 7.22 (1H, d, *J* = 11.3 Hz), 6.53 (1H, s), 4.60 (1H, dt, *J* = 12.7, 6.5 Hz), 3.91 (3H, s), 3.88 (3H, s), 3.66 (3H, s, 2.50 (1H, dd, J = 13.6, 6.3 Hz), 2.35 (3H, s), 2.26–2.17 (1H, m), 1.96 (3H, s), 1.87 (1H, td, *J* = 12.1, 6.9 Hz). ^{13}C NMR ($CDCl_3$, 101 MHz) δ 169.9, 168.2, 153.9, 151.0, 148.6, 141.8, 141.5, 137.0, 134.5, 131.2, 130.3, 125.2, 107.4, 61.6, 61.3, 56.0, 52.1, 36.8, 29.7, 22.7, 20.7. ESI-MS (m/z): $[M + H]^+$ 428, $[M + Na]^+$ 450, $[M + K]^+$ 466, $[2M + Na]^+$ 877.

3.1.4. Characterization of Propionyl Ester of Colchiceine 2b

Amorphous yellow solid, yield 52%, m.p 133-135 °C; ^{1}H NMR ($CDCl_3$, 400 MHz) δ 7.50 (1H, s), 7.30 (1H, d, *J* = 11.3 Hz), 7.22 (1H, d, *J* = 11.2 Hz), 6.52 (1H, s), 4.66–4.57 (1H, m), 3.91 (3H, s), 3.88 (3H, s), 3.66 (3H, s), 2.66 (2H, q, *J* = 7.4 Hz), 2.50 (1H, dd, *J* = 13.5, 6.3 Hz), 2.35 (1H, ddd, *J* = 12.7, 10.3, 6.0 Hz), 2.24–2.16 (1H, m), 1.97 (3H, s), 1.87 (2H, td, *J* = 12.0, 6.7 Hz), 1.26 (3H, t, *J* = 7.6 Hz). ^{13}C NMR ($CDCl_3$, 101 MHz) δ 171.8, 169.9, 153.9, 151.1, 148.9, 141.7, 141.6, 136.7, 134.5, 130.9, 130.5, 125.2, 107.4, 61.7, 61.4, 56.1, 52.1, 36.9, 29.8, 27.4, 22.8, 9.0. ESI-MS (m/z): $[M + Na]^+$ 464, $[2M + Na]^+$ 905.

3.1.5. Characterization of Isobutyryl Ester of Colchiceine 2c

Yellowish brown oil, yield 55%; ^{1}H NMR ($CDCl_3$, 400 MHz) δ 7.56 (1H, s), 7.28 (1H, d, *J* = 11.0 Hz), 7.23 (1H, d, *J* = 10.6 Hz), 6.52 (1H, s), 4.64 (1H, dt, *J* = 12.2, 6.8 Hz), 3.91 (3H, s), 3.88 (3H, s), 3.65 (3H, s), 2.90–2.82 (1H, m), 2.54–2.47 (1H, m), 2.36 (1H, td, *J* = 13.2, 6.9 Hz), 2.24–2.12 (2H, m), 1.96 (3H, s), 1.92–1.85 (1H, m), 1.35 (3H, d, *J* = 1.4 Hz), 1.33 (3H, d, *J* = 1.3 Hz). ^{13}C NMR ($CDCl_3$, 101 MHz) δ 174.3, 170.0, 153.9, 151.1, 150.3, 142.1, 141.5, 136.0, 134.5, 131.6, 130.1, 125.2, 107.4, 61.7, 61.3, 56.0, 52.1, 36.6, 34.0, 29.8, 26.4, 22.7, 19.0. ESI-MS (m/z): $[M + Na]^+$ 478, $[2M + Na]^+$ 933.

3.1.6. Characterization of Benzyl Ester of Colchiceine 2d

Amorphous yellow solid, yield 41%, m.p 123–125 °C; ^{1}H NMR ($CDCl_3$, 400 MHz) δ 8.18 (2H, d, *J* = 7.4 Hz), 7.65–7.60 (2H, m), 7.49 (1H, ddd, *J* = 4.8, 3.1, 1.1 Hz), 7.34 (2H, s), 6.53 (1H, s), 4.66–4.58 (1H, m), 3.93 (3H, d, *J* = 0.9 Hz,), 3.90 (3H, d, *J* = 0.7 Hz), 3.68 (3H, d, *J* = 1.1 Hz), 2.49 (1H, dd, *J* = 13.4, 4.9 Hz), 2.42–2.32 (1H, m), 2.17–2.06 (1H, m), 1.86 (3H, d, *J* = 4.0 Hz), 1.84–1.78 (1H, m). ^{13}C NMR

($CDCl_3$, 101 MHz) δ 169.9, 164.1, 153.9, 151.1, 142.0, 141.6, 134.5, 133.8, 130.4, 128.9, 128.5, 125.3, 107.4, 61.7, 61.4, 56.1, 52.0, 36.9, 29.8, 22.7. ESI-MS (m/z): $[M + H]^+$ 490, $[M + Na]^+$ 512, $[M + K]^+$ 528.

3.1.7. Characterization of Methyl Carbonate of Colchiceine 2e

Amorphous yellowish brown solid, yield 58%, m.p 115–118 °C; ^{1}H NMR ($CDCl_3$, 400 MHz) δ 7.57 (1H, s), 7.32 (1H, d, *J* = 20.5 Hz), 6.54 (1H, s), 4.62 (1H, dt, *J* = 11.8, 6.0 Hz), 3.92 (3H, s)*, 3.92 (3H, s)*, 3.89 (3H, s), 3.68 (3H, s), 2.52 (1H, dd, *J* = 13.4, 6.1 Hz), 2.37 (1H, td, *J* = 13.0, 6.7 Hz), 2.29–2.18 (1H, m), 1.99 (3H, s), 1.91 (1H, dd, *J* = 19.0, 12.2 Hz). ^{13}C NMR ($CDCl_3$, 101 MHz) δ 169.9, 154.1, 152.5, 151.1, 141.6, 134.5, 125.1, 107.4, 61.7, 61.3, 56.1, 55.8, 52.2, 37.2, 29.8, 22.8. ESI-MS (m/z): $[M + H]^+$ 444, $[M + Na]^+$ 466, $[M + K]^+$ 482, $[2M + Na]^+$ 909.

3.1.8. Characterization of Ethyl Carbonate of Colchiceine 2f

Yellowish brown oil, yield 55%; ^{1}H NMR ($CDCl_3$, 400 MHz) δ 7.46 (1H, s), 7.40–7.32 (1H, m, *J* = 6.2 Hz), 7.30–7.21 (1H, m), 6.55 (1H, s), 4.62 (1H, dt, *J* = 12.6, 6.4 Hz), 4.36 (2H, q, *J* = 7.1 Hz), 3.93 (3H, s, *J* = 2.9 Hz), 3.90 (3H, s), 3.68 (3H, s), 2.54 (1H, dd, *J* = 13.6, 6.4 Hz), 2.41 (1H, td, *J* = 13.1, 7.1 Hz), 2.32–2.21 (1H, m), 2.01 (3H, s), 1.94–1.84 (1H, m), 1.41 (3H, t, *J* = 7.1 Hz). ^{13}C NMR ($CDCl_3$, 101 MHz) δ 169.9, 154.0, 151.9, 151.1, 141.6, 134.5, 125.1, 107.4, 65.4, 61.7, 61.3, 56.1, 52.1, 37.2, 29.8, 22.8, 14.1. ESI-MS (*m/z*): $[M + H]^+$ 458, $[M + Na]^+$ 480, $[M + K]^+$ 496, $[2M + Na]^+$ 937.

3.1.9. Characterization of Acetyl Ester of 1-demethylthiocolchicine 4a

Amorphous yellow solid, yield 45%, m.p 168-172 °C; ^{1}H NMR (DMSO-d_6, 400 MHz) δ 8.51 (1H, d, *J* = 7.7 Hz), 7.23 (1H, d, *J* = 10.8 Hz), 7.02 (1H, s), 6.97 (1H, s), 6.92 (1H, d, *J* = 10.3 Hz), 3.89 (3H, s), 3.74 (3H, s), 2.65 (1H, dd, *J* = 13.5, 6.0 Hz), 2.41 (3H, s), 2.32–2.24 (1H, m), 2.22 (3H, s), 2.12–2.01 (1H, m), 1.85 (3H, s, *J* = 6.3 Hz), 1.84–1.77 (1H, m, *J* = 12.1, 6.8 Hz). ^{13}C NMR (DMSO-d_6, 101 MHz) δ 181.2, 168.9, 168.2, 157.7, 152.8, 150.4, 140.8, 139.3, 136.4, 134.4, 132.7, 128.2, 126.4, 124.6, 109.9, 60.1, 56.0, 50.7, 36.2, 29.1, 22.5, 20.3, 14. ESI-MS (m/z): $[M + Na]^+$ 466, $[2M + Na]^+$ 909.

3.1.10. Characterization of Propionyl Ester of 1-demethylthiocolchicine 4b

Amorphous yellow solid, yield 47%, m.p 136-140 °C; ^{1}H NMR (DMSO-d_6, 400 MHz) δ 8.52 (1H, d, *J* = 7.7 Hz), 7.23 (1H, d, *J* = 10.7 Hz), 7.03 (1H, s), 6.98 (1H, s), 6.92 (1H, d, *J* = 10.2 Hz), 4.34 (1H, dt, *J* = 11.8, 7.1 Hz), 3.90 (3H, s), 3.76–3.71 (3H, m), 2.66 (1H, dd, *J* = 13.2, 6.4 Hz), 2.41 (3H, s), 2.33–2.19 (2H, m), 2.08 (2H, ddd, *J* = 11.4, 9.8, 5.4 Hz), 1.84–1.78 (1H, m), 1.11 (3H, t, *J* = 7.5 Hz). ^{13}C NMR (DMSO-d_6, 101 MHz) δ 181.2, 172.3, 168.3, 157.7, 152.8, 150.5, 140.9, 139.2, 136.4, 134.4, 132.9, 128.3, 126.4, 124.7, 109.9, 60.1, 56.0, 50.7, 36.2, 29.1, 26.7, 22.6, 14.5, 9.2. ESI-MS (m/z): $[M + H]^+$ 458, $[M + Na]^+$ 480, $[M + K]^+$ 496, $[2M + Na]^+$ 937.

3.1.11. Characterization of Isobutyryl Ester of 1-demethylthiocolchicine 4c

Amorphous yellow solid, yield 49%, m.p 165-167 °C; ^{1}H NMR (DMSO-d_6, 101 MHz) δ 8.50 (1H, d, *J* = 7.8 Hz), 7.22 (1H, d, *J* = 10.6 Hz), 7.03 (1H, s), 6.98 (1H, s), 6.91 (1H, d, *J* = 8.8 Hz), 4.35 (1H, dt, *J* = 11.7, 7.3 Hz), 3.90 (3H, s), 3.72 (3H, s), 2.74 (1H, dt, *J* = 13.9, 6.9 Hz), 2.66 (1H, dd, *J* = 13.6, 6.1 Hz), 2.39 (3H, s), 2.34–2.25 (1H, m), 2.09 (1H, td, *J* = 12.7, 5.9 Hz), 1.86 (3H, s), 1.81 (1H, dd, *J* = 12.0, 6.9 Hz, 1.16 (3H, d, *J* = 3.5 Hz), 1.14 (3H, d, *J* = 3.5 Hz). ^{13}C NMR (DMSO-d_6, 101 MHz) δ 181.2, 174.7, 168.3, 157.7, 152.7, 150.4, 140.8, 139.2, 136.4, 134.4, 132.9, 128.3, 126.3, 124.8, 109.9, 60.1, 56.1, 50.7, 36.2, 33.3, 29.1, 22.6, 18.8, 14.6. ESI-MS (m/z): $[M + Na]^+$ 494, $[2M + Na]^+$ 965.

3.1.12. Characterization of Benzyl Ester of 1-demethylthiocolchicine 4d

Amorphous yellow solid, yield 38%, m.p 166-170 °C; ^{1}H NMR (DMSO-d_6, 101 MHz) δ 8.52 (1H, s), 8.07 (2H, d, *J* = 7.3 Hz), 7.77–7.71 (1H, m), 7.63–7.56 (2H, m), 7.22–7.12 (1H, m), 7.06 (1H, s), 7.02 (1H, s), 4.49–4.40 (1H, m), 3.94 (3H, s), 3.74 (3H, s), 2.72 (1H, dd, *J* = 13.0, 5.9 Hz), 2.36 (1H, dd, *J* = 7.4,

5.5 Hz,), 2.31 (3H, s), 2.13 (2H, ddd, J = 19.4, 12.8, 6.9 Hz,), 1.87 (3H, s).^{13}C NMR (DMSO-d_6, 101 MHz) δ 181.1, 168.3, 157.7, 152.9, 150.6, 141.0, 139.4, 136.3, 134.6, 134.2, 129.8, 129.1, 128.4, 128.3, 126.2, 124.9, 110.2, 60.3, 56.1, 50.8, 36.3, 29.2, 22.6, 14.5. ESI-MS (m/z): [M + Na]$^+$ 528, [2M + Na]$^+$ 1033.

3.1.13. Characterization of Methyl Carbonate of 1-demethylthiocolchicine 4e

Amorphous yellow solid, yield 53%, m.p 158-162 °C; ^{1}H NMR (DMSO-d_6, 101 MHz) δ 8.55 (1H d, J = 7.6 Hz), 7.26 (1H, d, J = 10.6 Hz), 7.05–6.99 (3H, m), 4.34 (1H, dt, J = 11.8, 7.0 Hz), 3.91 (3H, s), 3.82 (3H, s), 3.79 (3H, s), 2.69 (1H, dd, J = 13.5, 6.2 Hz), 2.43 (3H, s), 2.29 (1H, ddd, J = 18.6, 12.3, 5.4 Hz), 2.09 (1H, ddd, J = 18.7, 12.5, 6.2 Hz), 1.88 (3H, s), 1.86–1.80 (1H, m). ^{13}C NMR (DMSO-d_6, 101 MHz) δ 181.2, 168.4, 157.9, 152.9, 152.8, 150.5, 140.8, 139.3, 136.0, 134.5, 133.2, 128.2, 126.4, 124.3, 110.2, 60.4, 56.14, 56.07, 50.8, 36.1, 29.1, 22.6, 14.4. ESI-MS (m/z): [M + H]$^+$ 460, [M + Na]$^+$ 482, [M + K]$^+$ 498, [2M + Na]$^+$ 941.

3.1.14. Characterization of Ethyl Carbonate of 1-demethylthiocolchicine 4f

Amorphous yellow solid, yield 48%, m.p 165-167 °C; ^{1}H NMR (DMSO-d_6, 400 MHz) δ 8.52 (1H, d, J = 7.6 Hz), 7.23 (1H, d, J = 10.7 Hz), 7.01 (3H, t, J = 10.3 Hz), 4.33 (1H, dt, J = 12.6, 7.5 Hz), 4.27–4.20 (2H, m), 3.90 (3H, s), 3.78 (3H, s), 2.67 (1H, dd, J = 13.2, 6.6 Hz), 2.41 (3H, s), 2.34–2.23 (1H, m), 2.08 (3H, s), 1.87 (3H, s), 1.85–1.78 (1H, m), 1.22 (3H, t, J = 7.1 Hz). ^{13}C NMR (DMSO-d_6, 101 MHz) δ 181.2, 168.4, 157.9, 152.8, 152.4, 150.5, 140.8, 139.3, 136.2, 134.5, 133.1, 128.2, 126.3, 124.4, 110.2, 65.1, 60.3, 56.1, 50.8, 36.1, 29.1, 22.6, 14.4, 14.0. ESI-MS (m/z): [M + Na]$^+$ 496, [M + K]$^+$ 512, [2M + Na]$^+$ 969.

3.2. *Antiproliferative Activity*

Detailed information concerning antiproliferative activity assay is given in Supplementary Materials.

3.3. *X-ray Measurements*

X-ray measurements and detailed crystallographic data are given in Supplementary Materials.

4. Conclusions

On the basis of regioselectively demethylated colchicine analogs, colchiceine (**1**) and 1-demethylthiocolchicine (**3**), we have designed and synthesized a series of **12** colchicine derivatives bearing ester and carbonate substituents, including **9** entirely novel derivatives (**2b**,**c**,**e**,**f** and **4b**,**c**,**d**,**e**,**f**). Derivatives **4a**·H_2O and **4e**·½H_2O, with acetyl ester and methyl carbonate moieties, display reduced hydrophilic properties and crystallize as hydrates, which affects their biological activity and increases their solubility. The control over water co-crystallization from monohydrate to hemihydrate has been achieved through the number of H-donor and acceptor sites. These features can be invaluable for the regulation of the bioaccessibility and pharmaceutical processing of this group of compounds [47]. The synthesized derivatives exhibit a considerable in vitro antiproliferative activity against three human cancer cell lines. Compound 4a, carrying the thiomethyl group at position C10 and acetyl ester substituent at C1, showed the highest activity and selectivity index values. The biological evaluation has been supported by prediction of physicochemical properties, which are consistent with Lipinski's rule of five for all synthesized analogs.

Supplementary Materials: The following are available online: General procedures, experimental details, as well as an elaborate description of the X-ray diffraction sudies and in vitro methods used.

Author Contributions: Conceptualization, D.C. and A.H.; methodology, D.C., A.H., S.S. and E.M. validation, A.H., A.K. and J.W.; investigation, D.C, S.S. and E.M. resources, A.H., A.K. and J.W. data curation, D.C., S.S and E.M writing—original draft preparation, D.C. and S.S writing—review and editing, A.H., A.K. and J.W. visualization, D.C.; supervision, A.H.; project administration, A.H.; funding acquisition, A.H. All authors have read and agreed to the published version of the manuscript.

Funding: Financial support with a grant from the Polish National Science Centre (NCN)—No. 2016/21/B/ST5/00111 is gratefully acknowledged.

Acknowledgments: D.C. and S.S. acknowledge a scholarship (No. POWR. 03.02.00-00-I026/16 and POWR. 03.02.00-00-I023/17, respectively) co-financed by the European Union through the European Social Fund under the Operational Program Knowledge Education Development.

Conflicts of Interest: The authors declare that they have no conflict of interest.

References

1. Slobodnick, A.; Shah, B.; Pillinger, M.H.; Krasnokutsky, S. Colchicine: Old and New. *Am. J. Med.* **2015**, *128*, 461–470. [CrossRef] [PubMed]
2. Graham, W.; Roberts, J.B. Intravenous colchicine in the management of gouty arthritis. *Ann. Rheum. Dis.* **1953**, *12*, 16–19. [CrossRef] [PubMed]
3. Khanna, D.; Fitzgerald, J.D.; Khanna, P.P.; Bae, S.; Singh, M.K.; Neogi, T.; Pillinger, M.H.; Merill, J.; Lee, S.; Prakash, S.; et al. American college of rheumatology guidelines for management of gout. Part 1: Systematic nonpharmacologic and pharmacologic therapeutic approaches to hyperuricemia. *Arthritis Care Res.* **2012**, *64*, 1431–1446. [CrossRef]
4. Grattagliano, I.; Bonfrate, L.; Ruggiero, V.; Scaccianoce, G.; Palasciano, G.; Portincasa, P. Novel therapeutics for the treatment of familial mediterranean fever: From colchicine to biologics. *Clin. Pharmacol. Ther.* **2014**, *95*, 89–97. [CrossRef]
5. Imazio, M.; Gaita, F.; LeWinter, M. Evaluation and treatment of pericarditis: A systematic review. *J. Am. Med. Assoc.* **2015**, *314*, 1498–1506. [CrossRef]
6. Vindya, N.G.; Sharma, M.; Yadav, M.; Ethiraj, K.R. Tubulins—The Target for Anticancer Therapy. *Curr. Top. Med. Chem.* **2015**, *15*, 73–82. [CrossRef]
7. Seligmann, J.; Twelves, C. Tubulin: An example of targeted chemotherapy. *Future Med. Chem.* **2013**, *5*, 339–352. [CrossRef]
8. Katsetos, C.D.; Draber, P. Tubulins as Therapeutic Targets in Cancer: From Bench to Bedside. *Curr. Pharm. Des.* **2012**, *18*, 2778–2792. [CrossRef]
9. Cocco, G.; Chu, D.C.C.; Pandolfi, S. Colchicine in clinical medicine. A guide for internists. *Eur. J. Intern. Med.* **2010**, *21*, 503–508. [CrossRef]
10. Yang, L.P.H. Oral Colchicine (Colcrys): In the treatment and prophylaxis of gout. *Drugs* **2010**, *70*, 1603–1613. [CrossRef]
11. Avendaño, C.; Menéndez, J.C. *Medicinal Chemistry of Anticancer Drugs*; Elsevier: Amsterdam, The Netherlands, 2008. [CrossRef]
12. Majcher, U.; Klejborowska, G.; Kaik, M.; Maj, E.; Wietrzyk, J.; Moshari, M.; Preto, J.; Tuszynski, J.; Huczyński, A. Synthesis and Biological Evaluation of Novel Triple-Modified Colchicine Derivatives as Potent Tubulin-Targeting Anticancer Agents. *Cells* **2018**, *7*, 216. [CrossRef] [PubMed]
13. Klejborowska, G.; Urbaniak, A.; Preto, J.; Maj, E.; Moshari, M.; Wietrzyk, J.; Tuszynski, J.; Chambers, T.C.; Huczyński, A. Synthesis, biological evaluation and molecular docking studies of new amides of 4-bromothiocolchicine as anticancer agents. *Bioorg. Med. Chem.* **2019**, *23*, 115–144. [CrossRef] [PubMed]
14. Nakagawa-Goto, K.; Chen, C.X.; Hamel, E.; Wu, C.C.; Bastow, K.F.; Brossi, A.; Lee, K.H. Antitumor agents. Part 236: Synthesis of water-soluble colchicine derivatives. *Bioorg. Med. Chem. Lett.* **2015**, *15*, 235–238. [CrossRef]
15. Shchegravina, E.S.; Maleev, A.A.; Ignatov, S.K.; Gracheva, I.A.; Stein, A.; Schmalz, H.G.; Gavryushin, A.E.; Zubareva, A.A.; Svirshchevskaya, E.V.; Fedorov, A.Y. Synthesis and biological evaluation of novel non-racemic indole-containing allocolchicinoids. *Eur. J. Med. Chem.* **2017**, *141*, 51–60. [CrossRef]
16. Yasobu, N.; Kitajima, M.; Kogure, N.; Shishido, Y.; Matsuzaki, T.; Nagaoka, M.; Takayama, H. Design, synthesis, and antitumor activity of 4-halocolchicines and their pro-drugs activated by cathepsin B. *ACS Med. Chem. Lett.* **2011**, *2*, 348–352. [CrossRef]
17. Huczyński, A.; Majcher, U.; Maj, E.; Wietrzyk, J.; Janczak, J.; Moshari, M.; Tuszynski, J.A.; Bartl, F. Synthesis, antiproliferative activity and molecular docking of Colchicine derivatives. *Bioorg. Chem.* **2016**, *64*, 103–112. [CrossRef]
18. Zhang, X.; Kong, Y.; Zhang, J.; Su, M.; Zhou, Y.; Zang, Y.; Li, J.; Chen, Y.; Fang, Y.; Zhang, X.; et al. Design, synthesis and biological evaluation of colchicine derivatives as novel tubulin and histone deacetylase dual inhibitors. *Eur. J. Med. Chem.* **2015**, *95*, 127–135. [CrossRef]

19. Nicolaou, K.C.; Valiulin, R.A.; Pokorski, J.K.; Chang, V.; Chen, J.S. Bio-inspired synthesis and biological evaluation of a colchicine-related compound library. *Bioorg. Med. Chem. Lett.* **2012**, *22*, 3776–3780. [CrossRef]
20. Chang, D.J.; Yoon, E.Y.; Lee, G.B.; Kim, S.O.; Kim, W.J.; Kim, Y.M.; Jung, J.W.; An, H.; Suh, Y.G. Design, synthesis and identification of novel colchicine-derived immunosuppressant. *Bioorg. Med. Chem. Lett.* **2009**, *19*, 4416–4420. [CrossRef]
21. Marzo-Mas, A.; Barbier, P.; Breuzard, G.; Allegro, D.; Falomir, E.; Murga, J.; Carda, M.; Peyrot, V.; Marco, J.A. Interactions of long-chain homologues of colchicine with tubulin. *Eur. J. Med. Chem.* **2017**, *126*, 526–535. [CrossRef] [PubMed]
22. Johnson, L.; Goping, I.S.; Rieger, A.; Mane, J.Y.; Huzil, T.; Banerjee, A.; Luduena, R.; Hassani, B.; Winter, P.; Tuszynski, J.A. Novel Colchicine Derivatives and their Anti-cancer Activity. *Curr. Top. Med. Chem.* **2017**, *17*. [CrossRef] [PubMed]
23. Kumar, A.; Sharma, P.R.; Mondhe, D.M. Potential anticancer role of colchicine-based derivatives: An overview. *Anticancer Drugs* **2016**, *28*, 250–262. [CrossRef]
24. Kozaka, T.; Nakagawa-Goto, K.; Shi, Q.; Lai, C.Y.; Hamel, E.; Bastow, K.F.; Brossi, A.; Lee, K.H. Antitumor agents 273. Design and synthesis of N-alkyl-thiocolchicinoids as potential antitumor agents. *Bioorg. Med. Chem. Lett.* **2010**, *20*, 4091–4094. [CrossRef]
25. Andreu, J.M.; Timasheff, S.N. Tubulin bound to colchicine forms polymers different from microtubules. *Proc. Natl. Acad. Sci. USA* **1982**, *79*, 6753–6756. [CrossRef]
26. Cortese, F.; Bhattacharyya, B.; Wolff, J. Podophyllotoxin as a probe for the colchicine binding site of tubulin. *J. Biol. Chem.* **1977**, *252*, 1134–1140.
27. Chen, J.; Liu, T.; Dong, X.; Hu, Y. Recent Development and SAR Analysis of Colchicine Binding Site Inhibitors. *Mini Rev. Med. Chem.* **2009**, *9*, 1174–1190. [CrossRef]
28. Hastie, S.B.; Williams, R.C.; Puett, D.; Macdonald, T.L. The binding of isocolchicine to tubulin. Mechanisms of ligand association with tubulin. *J. Biol. Chem.* **1989**, *264*, 6682–6688.
29. Gohar, M.A.; Makkawi, M. The Antibacterial Action of Colchicine and Colchiceine. *J. Pharm. Pharmacol.* **1951**, *3*, 415–419. [CrossRef]
30. Boyland, E.; Mawson, E.H. The conversion of colchicine into colchiceine. *Biochem. J.* **1938**, *32*, 1204–1206. [CrossRef]
31. Klein, A.E.; Davis, P.J. Determination of Colchicine and Colchiceine in Microbial Cultures by High-Performance Liquid Chromatography. *Anal. Chem.* **1980**, *52*, 2432–2435. [CrossRef]
32. Elguero, J.; Muller, R.N.; Blade-Font, A.; Faure, R.; Vincent, E.J. Carbon-13 Magnetic Resonance Spectroscopy. A Study Of Colchicine And Related Compounds. *Bull. Soc. Chim. Belges* **1980**, *89*, 193–204. [CrossRef]
33. Mackay, M.F.; Morrison, J.D.; Gulbis, J.M. Crystal Structure of Triclinic Colchiceine Hemihydrate. *Aust. J. Phys.* **1985**, *38*, 413. [CrossRef]
34. Kurek, J.; Barczynski, P. Colchiceine complexes with lithium, sodium and potassium salts-spectroscopic studies. *Croat. Chem. Acta* **2016**, *89*, 297–308. [CrossRef]
35. Shi, Q.; Verdier-Pinard, P.; Brossi, A.; Hamel, E.; Lee, K.H. Antitumor Agents-CLXXV. Anti-tubulin action of (+)-thiocolchicine prepared by partial synthesis. *Bioorg. Med. Chem.* **1997**, *5*, 2277–2282. [CrossRef]
36. Prajapati, P.B.; Bodiwala, K.B.; Marolia, B.P.; Bhingradiya, N.; Shah, S. Oxidative Degradation Kinetic Study of Thiocolchicoside using Stability Indicating High Performance Thin Layer Chromatographic Method. *Pharm. Methods* **2014**, *5*, 69–78. [CrossRef]
37. Banerjee, A.; Kasmala, L.T.; Hamel, E.; Sun, L.; Lee, K.H. Interaction of novel thiocolchicine analogs with the tubulin isoforms from bovine brain. *Biochem. Biophys. Res. Commun.* **1999**, *254*, 334–337. [CrossRef]
38. Kerekes, P.; Sharma, P.N.; Brossi, A.; Chignell, C.F.; Quinn, F.R. Synthesis and Biological Effects of Novel Thiocolchicines. 3. Evaluation of N-Acyldeacetylthiocolchicines, N-(Alkoxycarbonyl)deacetylthiocolchicines, and O-Ethyldemethylthiocolchicines. New Synthesis of Thiodemecolcine and Antileukemic Effects of 2-Demeth. *J. Med. Chem.* **1985**, *28*, 1204–1208. [CrossRef]
39. Alkadi, H.; Khubeiz, M.J. Colchicine: A Review About Chemical Structure and Clinical Using. *Infect. Disord. Drug Targets* **2017**, 17. [CrossRef]
40. Shi, Q.; Chen, K.; Morris-Natschke, S.L.; Lee, K.H. Recent progress in the development of tubulin inhibitors as antimitotic antitumor agents. *Curr. Pharm. Des.* **1998**, *4*, 219–248.

41. Dumont, R.; Brossi, A.; Chignell, C.F.; Quinn, F.R.; Suffness, M. A Novel Synthesis of Colchicide and Analogues from Thiocolchicine and Congeners: Reevaluation of Colchicide as a Potential Antitumor Agent. *J. Med. Chem.* **1987**, *30*, 732–735. [CrossRef] [PubMed]
42. Voitovich, Y.V.; Shegravina, E.S.; Sitnikov, N.S.; Faerman, V.I.; Fokin, V.V.; Schmalz, H.G.; Combes, S.; Allegro, D.; Barbier, P.; Beletskaya, I.P.; et al. Synthesis and biological evaluation of furanoallocolchicinoids. *J. Med. Chem.* **2015**, *58*, 692–704. [CrossRef] [PubMed]
43. Blade-Font, A. New chemistry of colchicine and related compounds IV. Selective demethylation of colchicine with Lewis acids and tge structure of Zeisel's dimethylcolchicinic acid. *Afinidad* **1979**, *36*, 329.
44. Molinspiration Property Calculation Service. Available online: http://www.molinspiration.com (accessed on 15 January 2020).
45. Lipinski, C. Lead-and drug-like compounds: The rule-of-five revolution. *Drug Discov. Today Technol.* **2004**, *4*, 337–341. [CrossRef]
46. Lipinski, C.; Lombardo, F.; Dominy, B.W.; Feeney, P.J. Experimental and Computational Approaches to Estimate Solubility and Permeability in Drug Discovery and Development Settings. *Adv. Drug Deliv. Rev.* **1997**, *23*, 3–25. [CrossRef]
47. Khankari, R.K.; Grant, D.J.W. Pharmaceutical hydrates. *Thermochim. Acta* **1995**, *248*, 61–79. [CrossRef]

Sample Availability: Samples of the compounds **1**, **2a–f**, **3** and **4a–f** are available from the authors.

molecules

MDPI

Article

Synthesis, Antiproliferative Activity and Molecular Docking Studies of Novel Doubly Modified Colchicine Amides and Sulfonamides as Anticancer Agents

Julia Krzywik [1,2], Witold Mozga [2], Maral Aminpour [3], Jan Janczak [4], Ewa Maj [5], Joanna Wietrzyk [5], Jack A. Tuszyński [3,6] and Adam Huczyński [1,*]

1. Department of Medical Chemistry, Faculty of Chemistry, Adam Mickiewicz University, Uniwersytetu Poznańskiego 8, 61–614 Poznań, Poland; julia.krzywik@amu.edu.pl
2. TriMen Chemicals, Piłsudskiego 141, 92–318 Łódź, Poland; mozga@trimen.pl
3. Department of Oncology, University of Alberta, Edmonton, AB T6G 1Z2, Canada; aminpour@ualberta.ca (M.A.); jack.tuszynski@gmail.com (J.A.T.)
4. Institute of Low Temperature and Structure Research, Polish Academy of Sciences, PO Box 1410, 50–950 Wrocław, Poland; j.janczak@intibs.pl
5. Hirszfeld Institute of Immunology and Experimental Therapy, Polish Academy of Sciences, Rudolfa Weigla 12, 53–114 Wrocław, Poland; ewa.maj@hirszfeld.pl (E.M.); joanna.wietrzyk@hirszfeld.pl (J.W.)
6. DIMEAS, Politecnico di Torino, Corso Duca degli Abruzzi, 24, 10129 Torino, Italy

* Correspondence: adhucz@amu.edu.pl; Tel.: +48618291673

Academic Editor: Qiao-Hong Chen
Received: 16 March 2020; Accepted: 11 April 2020; Published: 14 April 2020

Abstract: Colchicine is a well-known compound with strong antiproliferative activity that has had limited use in chemotherapy because of its toxicity. In order to create more potent anticancer agents, a series of novel colchicine derivatives have been obtained by simultaneous modification at C7 (amides and sulfonamides) and at C10 (methylamino group) positions and characterized by spectroscopic methods. All the synthesized compounds have been tested in vitro to evaluate their cytotoxicity toward A549, MCF-7, LoVo, LoVo/DX and BALB/3T3 cell lines. Additionally, the activity of the studied compounds was investigated using computational methods involving molecular docking of the colchicine derivatives to β-tubulin. The majority of the obtained derivatives exhibited higher cytotoxicity than colchicine, doxorubicin or cisplatin against tested cancer cell lines. Furthermore, molecular modeling studies of the obtained compounds revealed their possible binding modes into the colchicine binding site of tubulin.

Keywords: anticancer agents; colchicine amide; colchicine sulfonamide; tubulin inhibitors; docking studies; crystal structure

1. Introduction

Microtubules, which are composed of α- and β-tubulin heterodimers, are involved in a large number of processes, such as intracellular transport, cell shape development, cell division and cell motility. During cell division microtubules form the mitotic spindle that in normal cells correctly separates the chromosomes into two daughter cells. In cancer cells the rate of mitosis is typically increased but chromosome segregation is imperfect leading to aneuploidy. Microtubules formed during mitosis are considered as an ideal target for anticancer drugs since no cell can divide without the force generated by microtubules. Therefore, many inhibitors of microtubule dynamics have been investigated for their potential use as cancer chemotherapy drugs [1–7]. One of these compounds is colchicine **1** (see Scheme 1), a well–known tropolone alkaloid isolated from *Colchicum autumnale*, which has been shown to exhibit very high cytotoxic effects. It binds to tubulin at the colchicine binding site and induces conformational change in the tubulin dimer making it incompetent for microtubule assembly. As a result, the cell cycle is blocked and apoptosis is induced [8–14]. Unfortunately, colchicine is too toxic to be useful as an antitumor agent [8,15–21]. Nevertheless, it has found use in therapy, e.g., for the treatment of familial Mediterranean fever, Behcet's disease or acute gout [22–27].

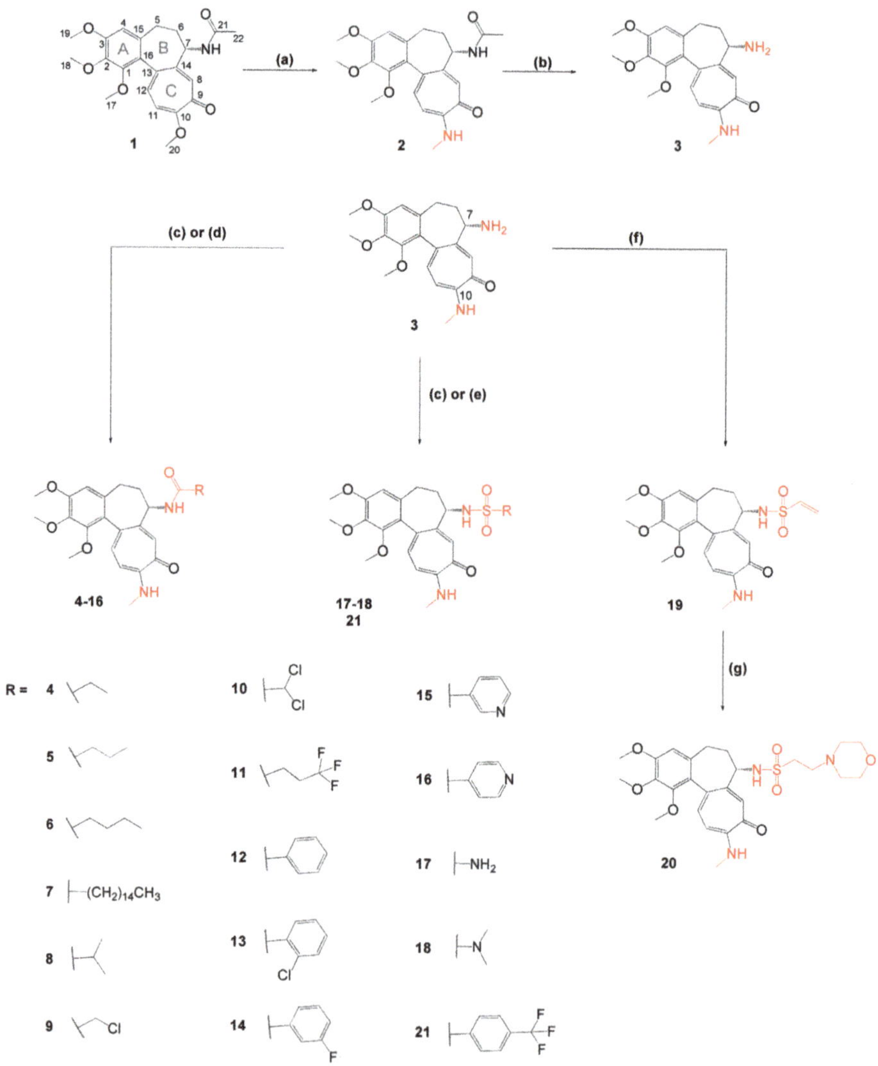

Scheme 1. Synthesis of doubly modified colchicine derivatives (**2–21**), changes at C7 and C10 positions are highlighted in red. Reagents and conditions: (**a**) $NHCH_3$/EtOH, reflux; (**b**) 2M HCl, reflux; (**c**) RC(O)Cl or RSO_2Cl, Et_3N, DCM, 0 °C to RT for **4**, **8**, **13**, **15–16**, **18** and **21**; (**d**) RCOOH, EDCI, DCM, RT for **5–7**, **9–12** and **14**; (**e**) (1) *N*-(*tert*-butoxycarbonyl)-*N*-[4-(dimethylazaniumylidene)-1,4-dihydropyridin-1-ylsulfonyl]azanide, DCM, RT, (2) 4M HCl/EtOAc, RT for **17**; (**f**) $ClCH_2CH_2SO_2Cl$, Et_3N, DCM, 0 °C to RT; (**g**) morpholine, DCM, RT.

Therefore, over the past few decades much interest has been focused on structural modifications of **1** in the hope of improving its therapeutic index [28–31]. Numerous double-modified colchicine derivatives have been synthesized with the group at position C7 substituted by various amide and sulfonamide moieties as well as with replacement of the methoxy group at position C10 by a group containing either a nitrogen or a sulfur atom and their biological activities have been determined [28,29,32–36]. These results have shown that new derivatives may have lower toxicity with respect to normal cells while maintaining high antitumor activity. In addition, from the chemical point of view, such a change at position C10 allows obtaining compounds more resistant to acid hydrolysis [29,30,33]. We have decided to check various amide and sulfonamide moieties because they have long been valued for their rich biological and chemical profiles and have emerged as a promising class of compounds in drug discovery [37–41].

Herein, we report the synthesis, crystallographic and spectroscopic analysis of a series of structurally different derivatives of colchicine obtained by its modification at position C7 (various amide, sulfonamide or sulfamide moieties) and at position C10 (methylamino group). We also describe the results of in vitro antiproliferative activity evaluation of colchicine (**1**) and the obtained colchicine derivatives (**2–21**) against four human cancer cell lines and one normal murine embryonic fibroblast cell line. To acquire more knowledge about the molecular mechanism of action of the investigated compounds (**1–21**), we also present results of *in silico* molecular docking study of the colchicine binding site (CBS) of β-tubulin.

2. Results and Discussion

2.1. Chemistry

To investigate the effect of methylamino group at position C10 and, at the same time, various amide, sulfonamide and sulfamide moieties at position C7 of colchicine **1** on its antiproliferative activity, eighteen new derivatives (**4–21**) were synthesized. To facilitate the structure-activity relationship analysis (SAR) we designed compounds with different side chains at position C7: alkyl chains of various length, straight and branched (**4–8**), unsaturated alkyl chain (**19**), alkyl chains of various lengths containing halogen atoms (**9–11**), an aromatic group without or with substituents (**12–16**, **21**), and compounds containing an amino group **17–18** and **20**.

The general route for the synthesis of colchicine derivatives **2–21** is depicted in Scheme 1. Colchicine (**1**) was treated with methylamine solution in ethanol to give 10-methylamino-10-demethoxycolchicine (**2**) with 80% yield, according to the method described earlier [42]. The replacement of water solution of methylamine by ethanol solution eliminated the work up after the reaction and permitted obtaining comparable final yields. Next, hydrolysis of **2** with 2M HCl yielded *N*-deacetyl-10-methylamino-10-demethoxycolchicine (**3**). Compounds **4–16**, **18–19** and **21** were readily available from **3** by treatment with respective acid/ sulfonamide/ sulfamide chloride in the presence of triethylamine or with the corresponding carboxylic acid and carbodiimide as a condensing agent. Compound **17** was prepared using a *N*-(*tert*-butoxycarbonyl)-*N*-[4-(dimethylazaniumylidene)-1,4-dihydropyridin-1-ylsulfonyl]azanide and further modified by removal of the *tert*-butoxycarbonyl group from amine with HCl [43]. Vinylsulfonamide **19** was synthesized from 2-chloroethanesulfonyl chloride and **3** through sulfonylation and in situ β-elimination of HCl. Compound **19** was used as the Michael acceptor with an electron-deficient double bond for the reaction with morpholine to produce compound **20** [44,45]. All synthesized compounds were isolated in pure form after column chromatography.

The purity and structures of the obtained compounds **2–21** were determined using the LC-MS, ^{1}H and ^{13}C NMR methods and are shown in the Supplementary Materials and discussed below. The characteristic signals of -OCH_3 group at position C10 of **1** in the ^{1}H NMR and ^{13}C NMR spectra were observed as a singlet at 4.0 ppm and at 56.5 ppm, respectively. These signals vanish after the reaction of colchicine with methylamine proving the substitution of the -OCH_3 group in the tropolone ring of **1**. After the introduction of -NHCH_3 at position C10 the signals of this group in the obtained derivatives (**2–21**) were visible approx. at 3.1 ppm as a doublet and approx. at 7.4 ppm as a quartet in ^{1}H NMR and approx. at 29.5 ppm in ^{13}C NMR. The chemical shifts of the amide moiety can be found in the range 7.9–9.7 ppm in ^{1}H NMR and in the range 164.2–175.2 ppm in ^{13}C NMR, depending on the substituent used. The ESI mass spectrometry confirmed the structure of the obtained compounds by the presence of an *m*/*z* signals assigned to the corresponding pseudomolecular ions of these compounds.

2.2. X-ray Crystal Analysis

Structural characterization of the colchicine derivatives is very important in order to understand their anticancer properties stemming from their interaction with tubulin as well as to enable structure–activity relationship analysis (SAR) and related investigation. Therefore, structural analyses of all crystals that were suitable for X-ray analysis of single crystals were performed. Crystals of **6, 11, 12, 14, 18** and **19** suitable for the X-ray single crystal analysis were obtained by recrystallization of the respective colchicine derivatives from acetonitrile, whereas crystals **15** and **16** from ethyl acetate solutions. All crystals were measured at room (295 K) and low (100 K) temperature. Details of the data collection parameters, crystallographic data and the final agreement parameters are listed in Supplementary Table S1. In the temperature range from 295 K to 100 K, no structural phase transitions were observed in the crystals studied, although for colchicine derivative **11** at low temperature some disorder of the -CF_3 group in the -CH_2-CH_2-CF_3 group at atom C21 could be observed. Colchicine derivatives **6, 11, 12, 14, 15,** and **16** crystallize in the $P3_221$ space group of the trigonal system while derivative **18** crystallizes in the $P2_12_12_1$ space group of the orthorhombic system and derivative **19** crystallizes in the $P2_1$ space group of the monoclinic system. These space groups are chiral since the compounds contain an asymmetric carbon (C7) atom. The absolute configuration at the C7 atom is *S* in all structures. The molecular structures of all colchicine derivatives (**6, 11, 12, 14, 15, 16, 18** and **19**) are illustrated in Supplementary Figure S60. The planar phenyl A and tropolone C rings in all colchicine derivatives (**6, 11, 12, 14, 15, 16, 18** and **19**) are twisted around the C13–C16 bond with the torsion angle describing the twisting conformation C1–C16–C13–C12 between ~53° and ~56° at 100 K and they do not differ significantly from the values at room temperature (Table 1). Ring B in all colchicine derivatives exhibits a similar puckering pattern and the extent of its non-planarity is such that it adopts a conformation, which is close to the twist-boat with a flattening caused by the fusion of rings A and C (see Supplementary Figure S60). So the conformation of the fused A, B and C rings of colchicine skeleton in the investigated derivatives is quite similar to that in colchicine itself [46].

Table 1. Selected torsion angles (°) of colchicine derivatives **6, 11, 12, 14, 15, 16, 18** and **19** obtained by X-ray analysis and DFT computation for a comparison.

		6	11	12	14	15	16	18	19
	100 K	53.1(4)	55.5(6)	53.7(3)	54.0(5)	53.6(4)	54.1(3)	56.1(4)	55.3(3)
C1–C16–C13–C12	295 K	55.2(4)	55.5(6)	55.0(3)	54.4(4)	54.7(4)	55.0(3)	56.1(4)	55.9(4)
	DFT value	53.1	52.3	53.4	53.5	52.9	53.3	54.5	56.0
	100 K	−79.0(4)	−86.4(6)	−89.3(3)	−90.6(5)	−87.3(4)	−86.8(4)	−108.6(3)	66.2(3)
C17–O1–C1–C2	295 K	−86.5(4)	−86.4(6)	−86.4(4)	−87.4(5)	−87.8(4)	−86.4(4)	−106.8(3)	65.6(4)
	DFT value	−73.0	−70.7	−80.3	−80.0	−72.9	−79.4	−74.8	59.2
	100 K	108.0(3)	105.2(6)	96.1(2)	95.5(4)	99.7(4)	94.5(3)	−77.5(4)	−102.7(3)
C18–O2–C2–C3	295 K	106.9(4)	105.2(6)	98.7(3)	98.0(4)	101.4(4)	98.7(3)	−74.0(4)	−100.6(4)
	DFT value	70.1	68.8	82.1	82.3	71.1	81.1	−59.6	−77.2
	100 K	−14.1(5)	−10.5(9)	8.6(4)	14.4(6)	−6.0(6)	7.4(6)	1.2(5)	7.7(4)
C19–O3–C3–C4	295 K	−8.1(7)	−10.5(10)	6.9(6)	11.4(7)	−2.3(6)	6.9(6)	0.2(5)	6.8(5)
	DFT value	−4.0	−3.7	−2.0	−1.9	−3.8	−1.9	0.7	3.1
	100 K	7.7(5)	8.8(8)	4.6(3)	4.4(6)	5.0(5)	6.6(4)	−0.2(5)	4.7(4)
C20–N1–C10–C11	295 K	6.8(6)	8.7(9)	7.5(4)	5.0(6)	5.2(5)	7.5(4)	−1.7(5)	4.0(7)
	DFT value	−0.9	−0.9	−1.4	−1.0	−1.2	−1.3	0.2	−1.6

The methoxy group -OCH_3 linked to the phenyl ring at C3 is almost coplanar with the ring in all structures of colchicine derivatives, whereas the other two methoxy groups linked at C1 and

C2 atoms of the phenyl ring have different orientations in some colchicine derivatives (Table 1). The *N*-methylamino group (-$NHCH_3$) linked to tropolone C ring at C10 atom is almost coplanar with the ring. The differences between the conformations of the investigated colchicine derivatives are illustrated in Figure 1 and Table 1. For clarity, the colchicine derivatives have been divided into two groups, according to the substituent in ring B at position C7; one group comprises the derivatives with a chain substituent (Figure 1a) and the other group comprises the derivatives with a substituent containing an aromatic ring (Figure 1b). Analysis of these results reveals a significant difference in the torsion angle C17-O1-C1-C2 in compounds 18 (~−109°) and 19 (~66°) or the difference between the calculated (~−103°) and measured (~−77°) torsion angle C18-O2 -C2-C3 in compound 19. These differences result from different approach to the description of the molecule conformations, the X-ray analysis values refer to the conformation of molecules in crystals, in which the intermolecular interactions play a significant role and leads crystallization and specific crystal packing, while the DFT values refer to a single isolated molecule in the gas state with the intermolecular interactions not taken into account.

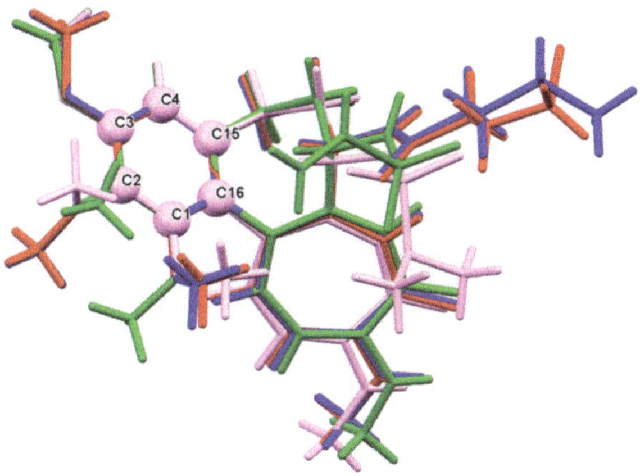

(a)

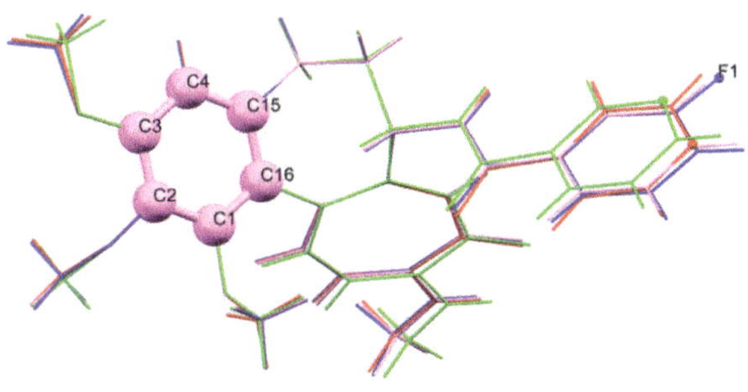

(b)

Figure 1. Comparison of the X-ray structure of (**a**) derivatives with a chain substituent at position C7: **6** (blue), **11** (red), **18** (pink) and **19** (green) and (**b**) derivatives with a substituent containing an aromatic ring at position C7: **12** (pink), **14** (blue), **15** (green) and **16** (red) showing the conformation of the colchicine skeleton. The molecules are overlapped one over another so that the ring C1-C2-C3-C4-C15-C16 is at the same position.

2.3. Molecular Electrostatic Potential Map Analysis

The role of the trimethoxyphenyl ring A of colchicine as well as that of the tropolone ring C in tubulin binding have been studied in great details. The tropolonoic ring C of the colchicine skeleton is found to be crucial for the interaction with tubulin [47,48]. The molecular electrostatic potential map (MESP) correlated with the electronic density in a molecule and is a powerful tool for analyzing interactions [49–51]. It was, therefore, calculated for all structurally characterized colchicine derivatives. Additionally, the gas-phase structures of all molecules were determined using the DFT optimization with the Gaussian09 program package [52]. All calculations were carried out by the DFT method using the Becke3-Lee–Yang–Parr correlation functional (B3LYP) [53–56] with the 6–31 + G basis set, starting from the X-ray geometry of molecules. The gas-phase optimized conformations of all colchicine derivatives are, in general, in good agreement with those obtained from the X-ray single crystal investigation, however the optimized torsion angle C18–O2–C2–C3 describing the orientation of the methoxy group is significantly smaller than that provided by the X-ray analysis (Table 1 and for more details see Supplementary Table S2).

The region of tubulin that interacts with colchicine is near the αβ-tubulin/dimer interface [57]. In order to better understand the interaction of the colchicine derivatives with tubulin, the molecular electrostatic potential was calculated for all structurally characterized colchicine derivatives as well as, for comparison, for colchicine itself. The three-dimensional MESP maps for colchicine derivatives and for colchicine itself were calculated on the basis of the DFT (B3LYP) optimized geometries of molecules and mapped onto the total electron density isosurface (0.008 $eÅ^{-3}$) for both molecules using the GaussView 5.0 program (Figure 2). The color coding of MESP is in the range of −0.05 (red) to 0.05 $eÅ^{-1}$ (blue). For all colchicine derivatives, the regions of negative MESP are usually associated with the lone pair of electronegative atoms (O and N), whereas the regions of positive MESP are associated with the electropositive atoms (Figure 2).

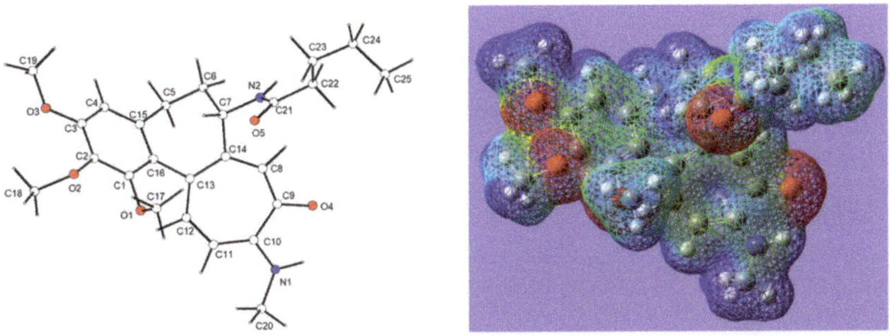

a (**6**)

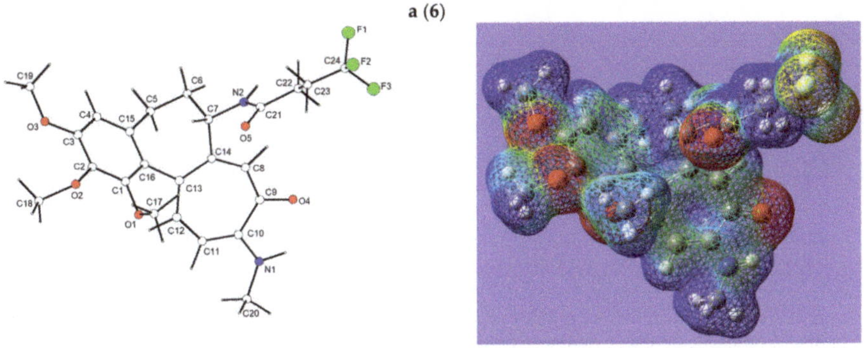

b (**11**)

Figure 2. *Cont.*

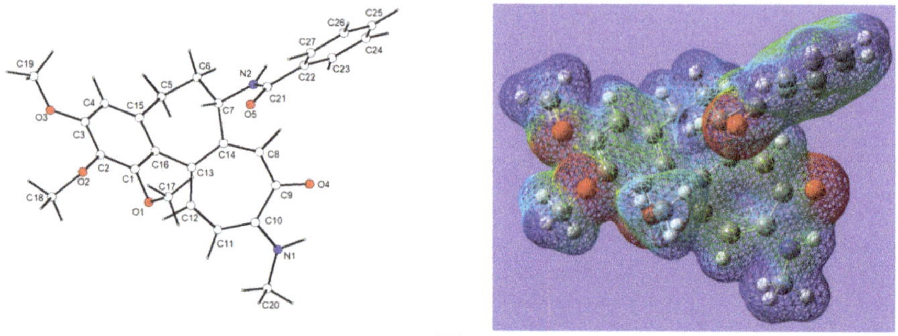

c (12)

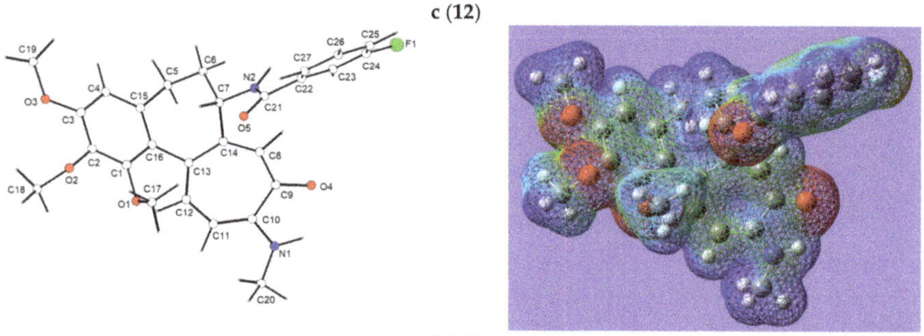

d (14)

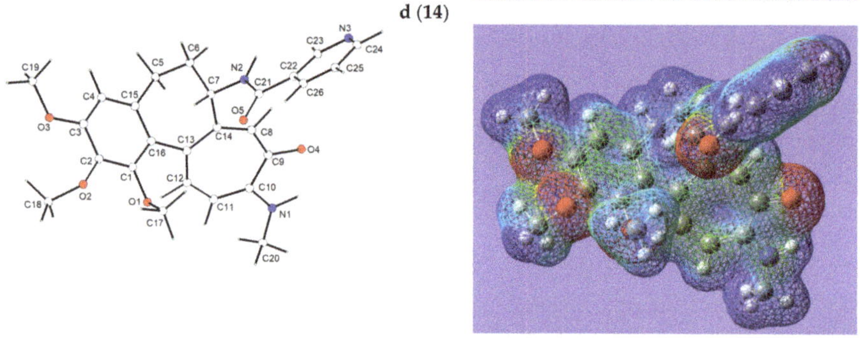

e (15)

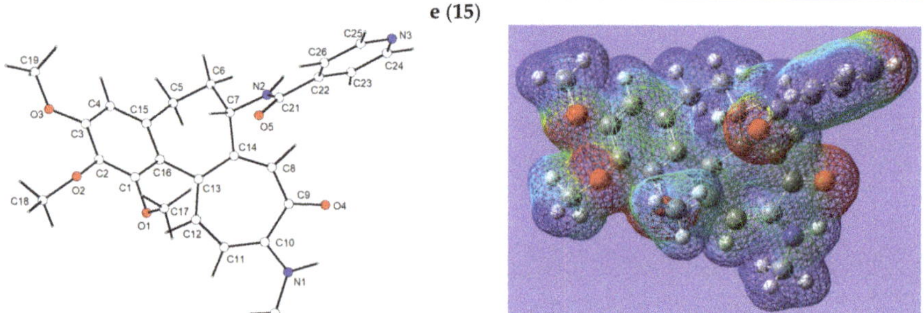

f (16)

Figure 2. *Cont.*

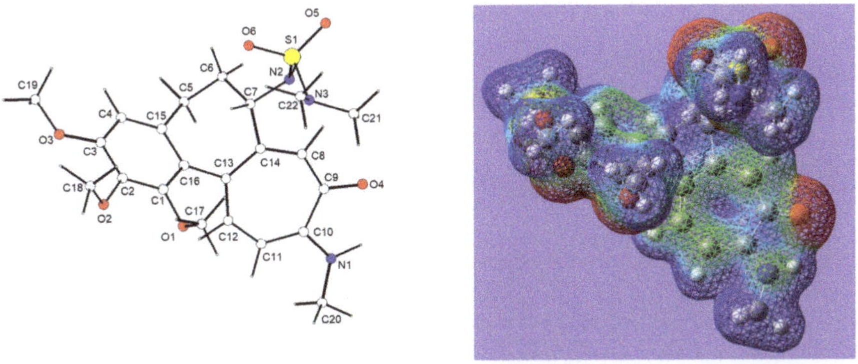

g (18)

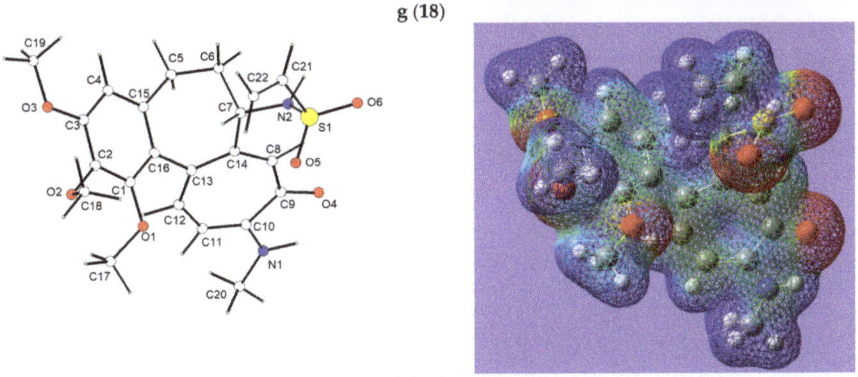

h (19)

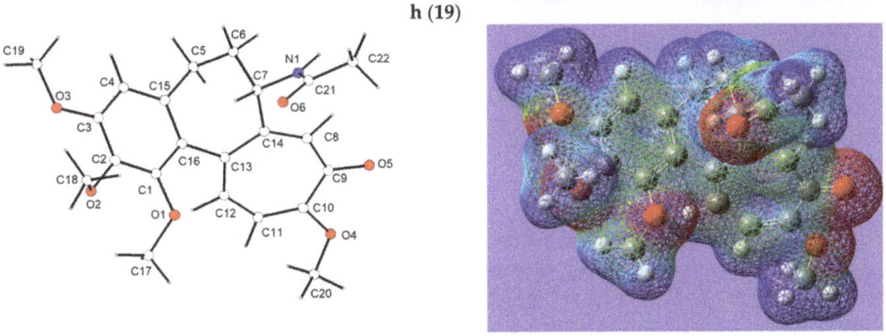

i (colchicine **1**)

Figure 2. Optimized conformation (left) and three-dimensional molecular electrostatic potential map (right) for colchicine derivatives (**a–h**) and colchicine itself (**i**), for comparison. Color code: $-0.05\ e\text{Å}^{-1}$ (red) to $+0.05\ e\text{Å}^{-1}$ (blue).

The nucleophilic regions in colchicine derivatives are observed near oxygen atoms of all methoxy and carbonyl groups. In addition, significantly less negative value of MESP than that near the oxygen atoms spreads across the aromatic phenyl rings. The planar conformation of tropolone ring C, showing the alternating single and double C-C bonds, is manifested as partial delocalization of the π electrons resulting in a slightly negative value of MESP on both sides of the planar fragment of colchicine derivatives. The molecular electrostatic potential for colchicine itself was also calculated for comparison (Figure 2i). In all colchicine derivatives the methoxy (-OCH_3) substituent in the tropolone C ring is replaced by *N*-methylamino substituent (-$NHCH_3$), therefore, MESP maps show a less negative area near this group (Figure 2a–h) compared to the MESP map of colchicine itself (Figure 2i).

Additionally, the replacement in colchicine molecule of the -NHC(O)CH_3 group in ring B at C7 atom with various substituents modified the size of the molecule and the maps of electrostatic potential. This is particularly visible for derivatives **11**, **14** and **18**, **19** in which the -NHC(O)CH_3 group is replaced by -NHC(O)$C_2H_4CF_3$, -NHC(O)C_6H_4F in **11** and **14**, respectively, and in **18** and **19** by the substituents containing sulfonyl group (-SO_2R).

The DFT results, especially the three-dimensional molecular electrostatic potential map (MESP) providing information on the distribution of the electron density of molecules are useful for predictions of interactions between the tested compounds and homology modeled tubulin βI. The formation of guest-host complexes (colchicine derivatives as guest and tubulin as host) depends on the guest's fit into the host cavity and their interactions that result from the mutual matching of electrostatic interactions.

2.4. *In Vitro Determination of Drug-Induced Inhibition of Human Cancer Cell Line Growth*

The synthesized colchicine derivatives **2–21** and starting material **1** were evaluated for their in vitro antiproliferative effect on four human cancer cell lines, including one cell line displaying various levels of drug resistance and additionally one normal murine embryonic fibroblast cells.

The majority of new derivatives of **1** showed antiproliferative activity in the nanomolar range and were characterized by lower IC_{50} values than unmodified colchicine **1**, as well as doxorubicin and cisplatin, commonly used as antitumor agents in cancer chemotherapy (Table 2). From the set of tested compounds, the ones most active against A549 tumor cell line were **2**, **4–6**, **8–14** and **18–19** ($IC_{50} \leq 15$ nM), against MCF-7 tumor cell line-were **2**, **9–17** and **19** ($IC_{50} \leq 13$ nM), against LoVo tumor cell line-were **2**, **4–6**, **8–16**, **18–19** ($IC_{50} \leq 11$ nM) of which the lowest IC_{50} values were shown by compounds **9–10** and **13** (IC_{50} = 0.7–1.8 nM). Moreover, compound **13** was observed to be most active towards the LoVo/DX line (IC_{50} = 9.6 nM), approx. 170 times more potent than unmodified colchicine **1** (IC_{50} = 1646.6 nM). Compound **7** from amides and compound **20** from sulfonamides showed the weakest activity (the highest IC_{50} values) against all cancer cell lines tested. The decrease in cytotoxicity of compound **7** could be related to an increase in hydrophobicity (high calculated octanol/water partition coefficient clog*P* = 8.7, see Table 3). It is well known that high clog*P* value and therefore low hydrophilicity are responsible for poor absorption and permeation to the colchicine binding pocket in β-tubulin. The high IC_{50} value for compound **20** may be due to the presence of a morpholine ring which is a large volume substituent and can adopt different conformations. Although these compounds were the least potent out of the whole series of tested derivatives (**1–21**), their IC_{50} values were in the micromolar range (see Table 2).

Table 2. Antiproliferative activity (IC_{50}) of colchicine (**1**) and its derivatives (**2–21**) compared with antiproliferative activity of standard anticancer drugs doxorubicin and cisplatin and the calculated values of the resistance index (RI) of tested compounds.

Compound	A549	MCF-7	LoVo	LoVo/DX		BALB/3T3
	IC_{50} [nM]	IC_{50} [nM]	IC_{50} [nM]	IC_{50} [nM]	RI	IC_{50} [nM]
1	115.3 ± 23.6	22.6 ± 1.3	17.5 ± 2.5	1646.6 ± 314.0	93.9	115.3 ± 36.8
2	10.8 ± 1.3	8.6 ± 1.3	4.3 ± 1.3	271.3 ± 99.9	63.0	10.8 ± 1.3
3	16.9 ± 2.8	19.7 ± 1.7	14.0 ± 1.7	129.2 ± 11.8	9.2	19.7 ± 7.0
4	14.6 ± 2.4	14.6 ± 1.5	9.7 ± 1.5	271.8 ± 104.4	28.0	19.4 ± 4.1
5	14.1 ± 2.4	14.1 ± 1.4	9.6 ± 0.5	194.8 ± 51.9	20.2	16.4 ± 3.5
6	13.6 ± 1.4	15.9 ± 6.6	6.8 ± 3.9	102.3 ± 20.7	15.0	13.6 ± 2.3
7	613.8 ± 194.4	464.8 ± 186.7	62.4 ± 16.9	2435.7 ± 923.4	39.0	545.9 ± 104.4
8	11.7 ± 1.4	18.8 ± 9.9	7.0 ± 1.4	171.2 ± 41.3	24.3	28.1 ± 10.8
9	11.6 ± 2.8	9.2 ± 1.4	1.8 ± 0.4	62.4 ± 6.7	35.2	11.6 ± 2.3
10	8.6 ± 1.3	8.6 ± 1.2	1.5 ± 0.5	38.5 ± 21.6	25.8	10.7 ± 1.3
11	14.6 ± 2.1	12.7 ± 0.4	10.4 ± 1.3	289.6 ± 165.2	27.8	81.3 ± 20.4
12	13.0 ± 1.3	13.0 ± 1.3	8.5 ± 0.4	99.9 ± 10.0	11.8	13.0 ± 3.3
13	6.3 ± 3.2	9.2 ± 0.8	0.7 ± 0.1	9.6 ± 3.3	14.0	6.2 ± 1.6
14	10.7 ± 0.6	12.6 ± 1.3	8.6 ± 0.8	102.5 ± 24.9	12.0	12.6 ± 2.1
15	36.8 ± 12.1	13.0 ± 2.2	10.8 ± 1.3	832.1 ± 292.7	76.8	43.3 ± 29.7
16	17.3 ± 3.7	12.8 ± 0.9	10.8 ± 1.3	946.9 ± 260.5	87.4	52.0 ± 29.3

Table 2. *Cont.*

17	56.6 ± 14.7	10.3 ± 3.9	21.1 ± 17.5	6466.0 ± 264.2	306.0	100.1 ± 24.1
18	10.6 ± 0.6	15.5 ± 1.7	9.3 ± 1.1	540.2 ± 107.2	57.8	14.2 ± 13.2
19	11.4 ± 1.7	13.0 ± 4.3	8.4 ± 0.7	306.7 ± 144.9	36.7	8.3 ± 3.8
20	800.3 ± 130.0	150.0 ± 25.3	268.4 ± 94.0	44385.7 ± 23852.0	165.4	991.1 ± 280.5
21	85.5 ± 5.4	134.3 ± 41.5	73.5 ± 15.7	6122.0 ± 825.1	83.3	87.6 ± 13.5
Doxorubicin	141.7 ± 46.0	204.2 ± 47.8	99.4 ± 41.0	8732.0 ± 2540.7	87.9	149.0 ±126.8
Cisplatin	5741.0 ± 968.0	7139.8 ± 1218.7	7076.3 ± 1596.2	8336.5 ± 1119.2	1.2	5665.1 ± 31.8

The IC_{50} value is defined as the concentration of a compound at which 50% growth inhibition is observed. The IC_{50} values shown are mean ± SD. Human lung adenocarcinoma (A549), human breast adenocarcinoma (MCF-7), human colon adenocarcinoma cell line (LoVo) and doxorubicin-resistant subline (LoVo/DX), normal murine embryonic fibroblast cell line (BALB/3T3). The RI (Resistance Index) indicates how many times more chemoresistant is a resistant subline relative to its parental cell line. The RI was calculated for each compound using the formula: RI = (IC_{50} for LoVo/DX cell line)/(IC_{50} for LoVo cell line). When RI is 0–2, the cells are sensitive to the compound tested, RI in the range 2–10 means that the cells shows moderate sensitivity to the drug tested, RI above 10 indicates strong drug resistance.

Table 3. Computational predictions of interactions between tested compounds (**1–21**) and homology modeled tubulin βI. 3D representation and 2D layout of colchicine derivatives–tubulin protein complex, binding energy (BE), calculated octanol/water partition coefficient (clog*P*) and active residues are tabulated.

Compound	3D Representation of the Interactions	2D Representation of the Interactions	Binding Energy [kcal/mol]	clog*P*	Active Residues
1	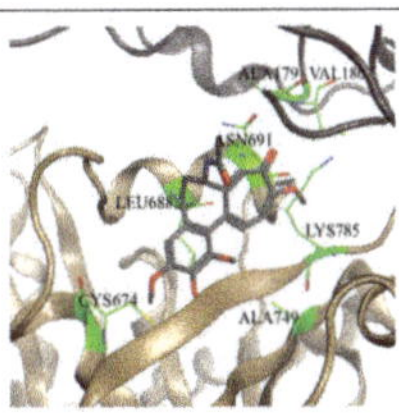	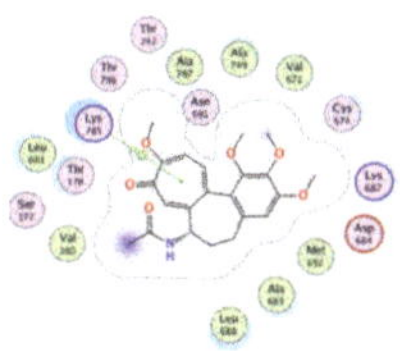	−41.0	1.1	Ala179 Val180 **Cys674** **Leu688** Asn691 Ala749 **Lys785**
2	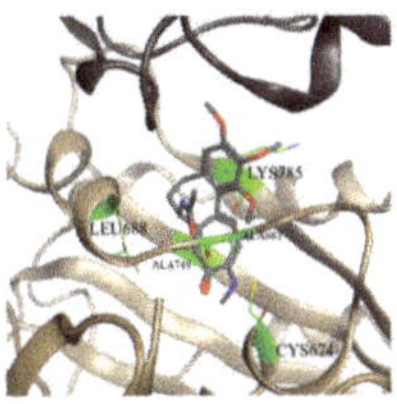	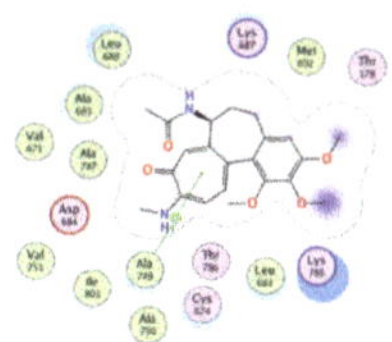	−39.3	1.6	Cys674 Ala683 **Leu688** **Lys785**
3	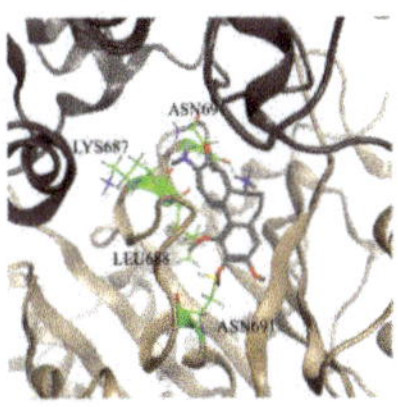	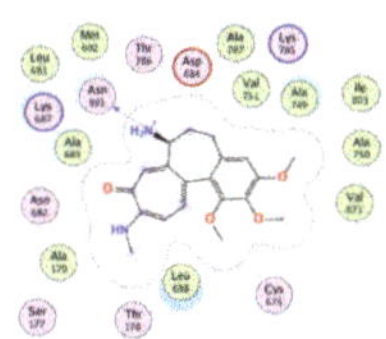	−4.0	0.9	Cys674 Lys687 **Leu688** **Asn691**
4	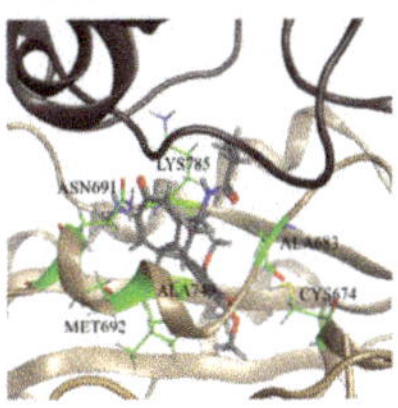	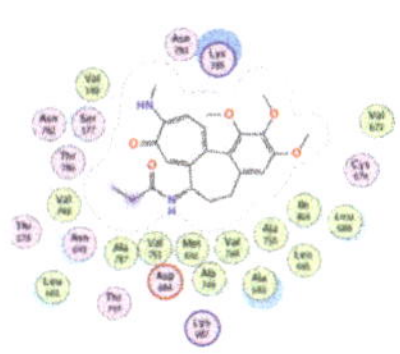	−43.4	1.9	Cys674 Ala683 **Leu688** Asn691 Met692 Ala749 **Lys785**

Table 3. *Cont.*

Compound	3D Representation of the Interactions	2D Representation of the Interactions	Binding Energy [kcal/mol]	clog*P*	Active Residues
5	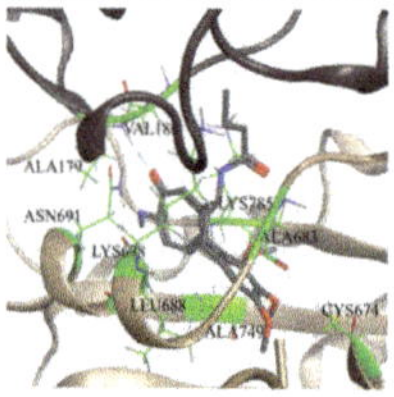	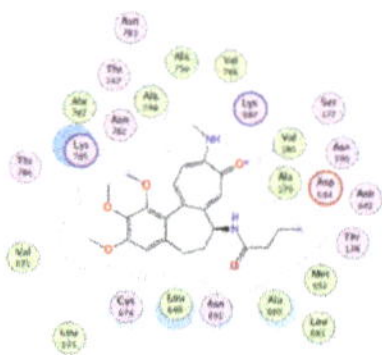	−43.0	2.5	Ala179 Val180 **Cys674** **Leu688** Asn691 Ala749 **Lys785**
6	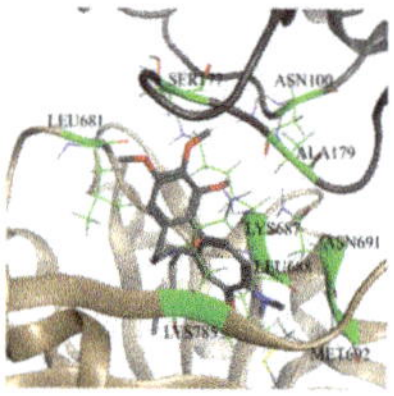	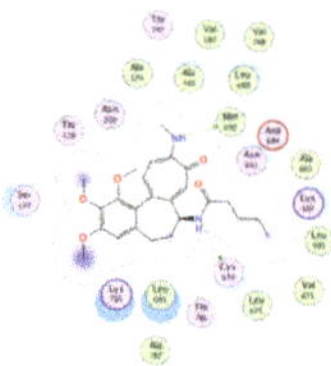	−37.2	3.0	Asn100 Ser177 Ala179 Leu681 **Lys687** Leu688 Asn691 **Lys785**
7	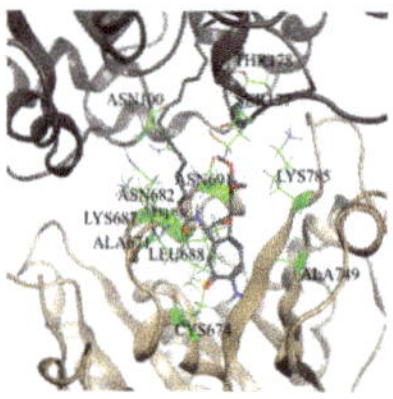	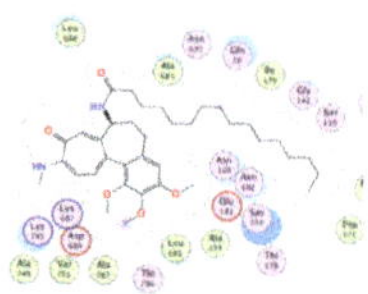	−53.7	8.7	Gln10 Asn100 Ser177 Thr178 Cys674 Leu681 Asn682 Ala683 **Lys687** **Leu688** Asn691 Ala749 **Lys785**
8	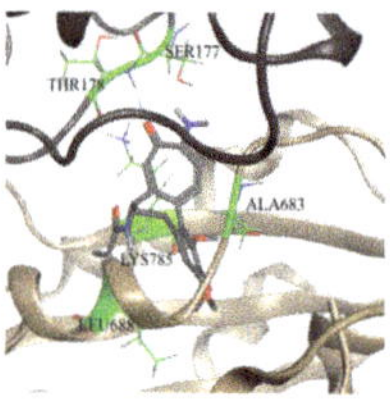	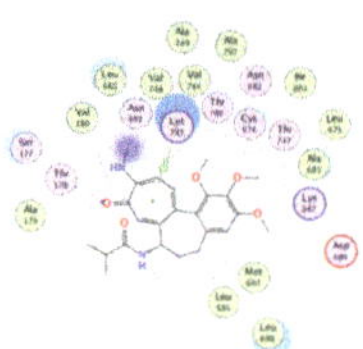	−32.3	2.7	Ser177 Leu681 Ala683 **Leu688** **Lys785**
9	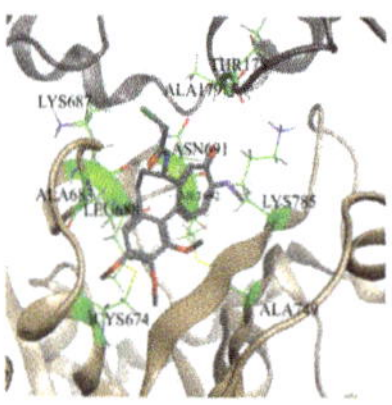	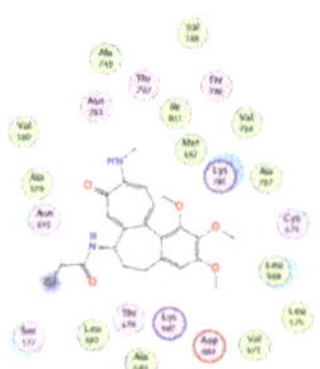	−44.0	2.2	Ala179 Cys674 Ala683 Lys687 **Leu688** Asn691 Met693 Ala749 **Lys785**
10	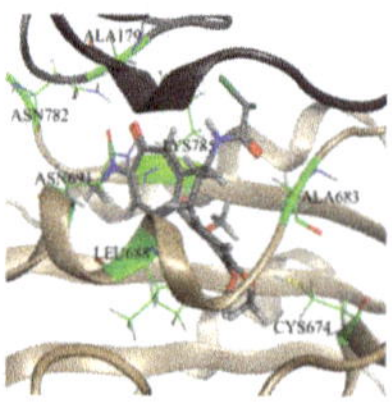	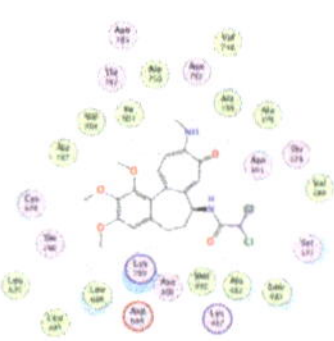	−41.8	2.7	Ala179 Cys674 Ala683 **Leu688** Asn691 Asn782 **Lys785**

Table 3. *Cont.*

Compound	3D Representation of the Interactions	2D Representation of the Interactions	Binding Energy [kcal/mol]	clog*P*	Active Residues
11	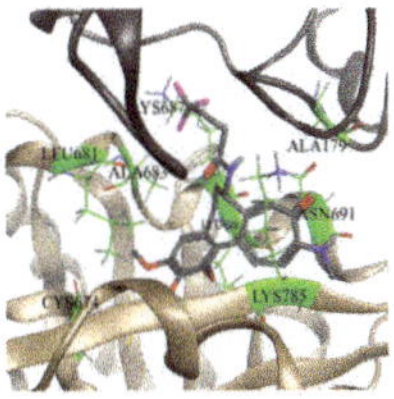	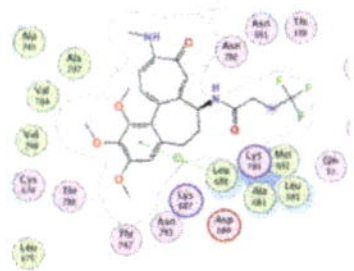	−34.7	3.0	Ala179 Cys674 Leu681 Ala683 Lys687 **Leu688** Asn691 **Lys785**
12	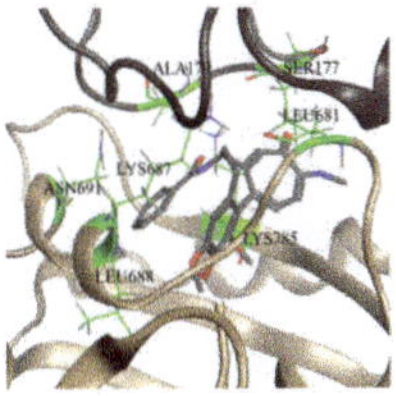	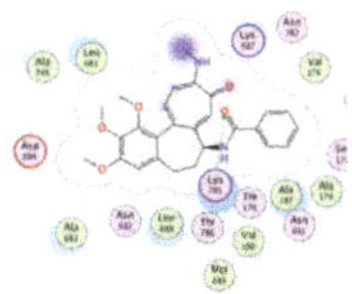	−35.2	3.3	Ser177 Ala179 Leu681 Lys687 **Leu688** Asn691 **Lys785**
13	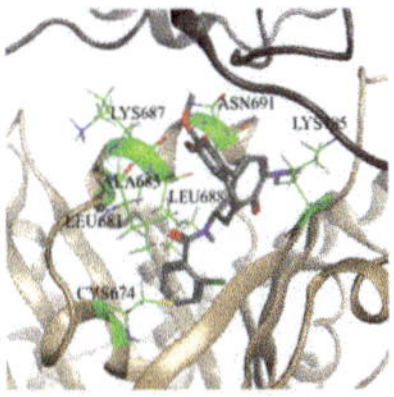	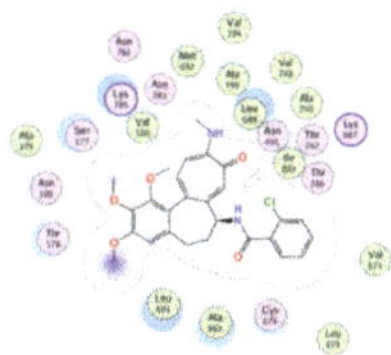	−40.1	3.9	Cys674 Leu681 Ala683 **Lys687** **Leu688** Asn691 **Lys785**
14	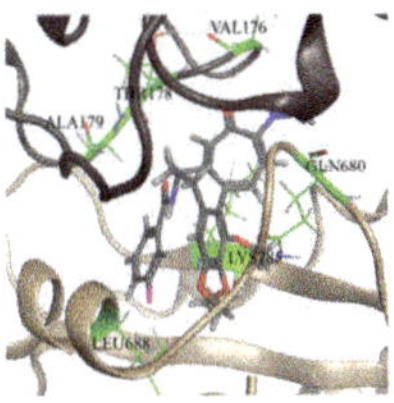	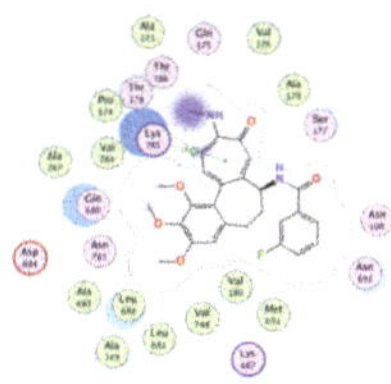	−34.3	3.4	Val176 Ser177 Thr178 Ala179 **Gln680** Leu688 **Lys785**
15	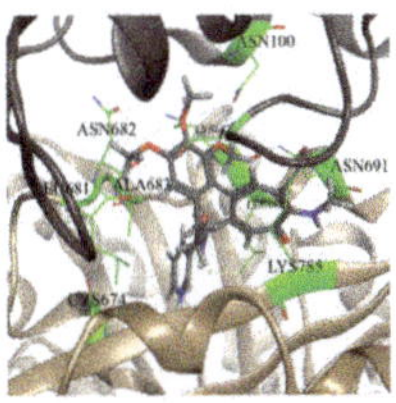	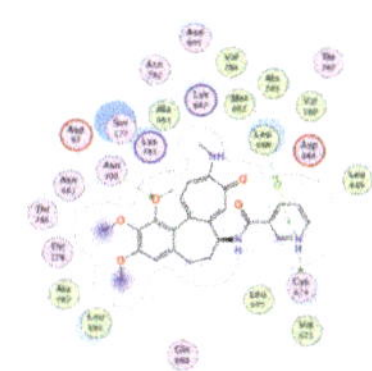	−43.9	2.0	**Asn100** **Ser177** Cys674 **Leu681** Asn682 Ala683 **Lys687** **Leu688** Asn691 **Lys785**
16	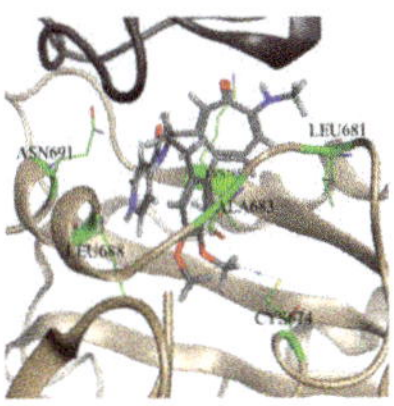	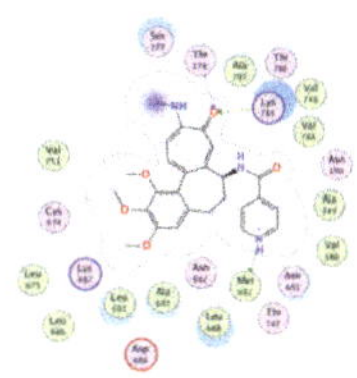	−38.3	2.0	Ser177 Thr178 Cys674 Leu681 Ala683 **Leu688** Asn691 **Lys785**

Table 3. *Cont.*

Compound	3D Representation of the Interactions	2D Representation of the Interactions	Binding Energy [kcal/mol]	clog*P*	Active Residues
17	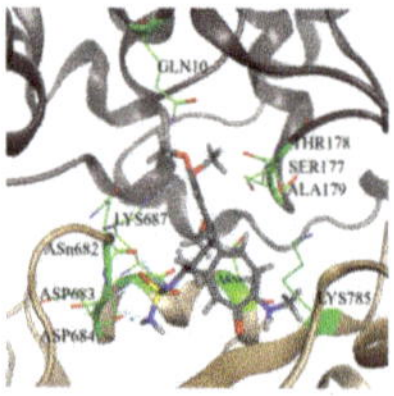	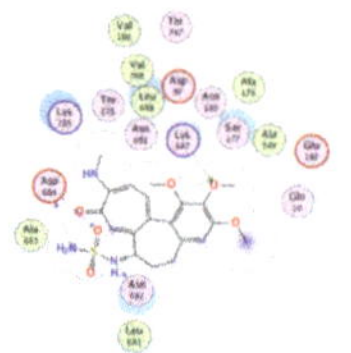	−34.8	1.9	**Gln10** **Ser177** Thr178 Ala179 Asn682 Ala683 **Asp684** **Lys687** Asn691 Lys785
18	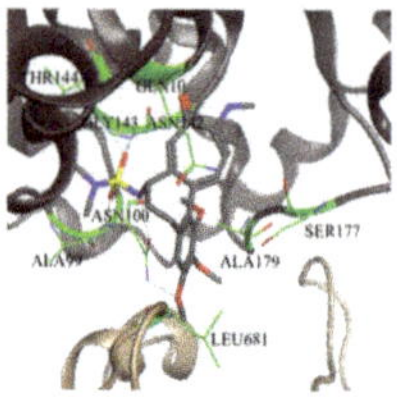	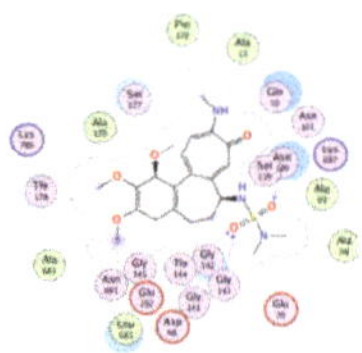	−54.6	2.5	**Gln10** Ala99 Asn100 **Gly142** **Gly143** **Thr144** **Ser177** Thr178 Ala179 Leu681
19	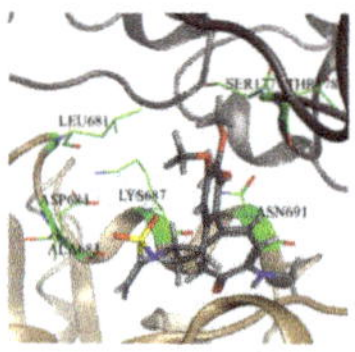	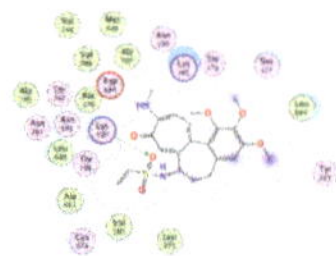	−23.4	2..8	**Ser177** Thr178 **Leu681** Ala683 Asp684 **Lys687** Asn691 **Lys785**
20	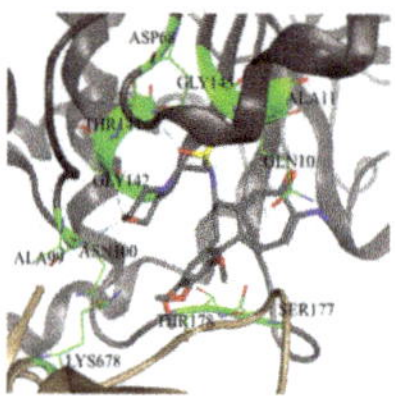	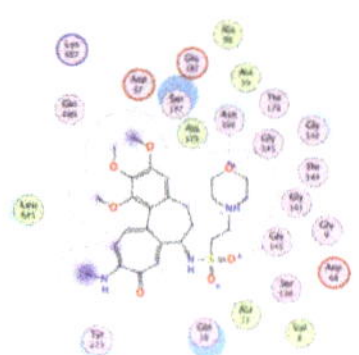	−59.6	2.4	Gly9 Gln10 Ala11 **Asp68** Ala99 **Asn100** Gly142 Gly143 Thr144 **Gly145** Ser177 Thr178 **Lys687**
21	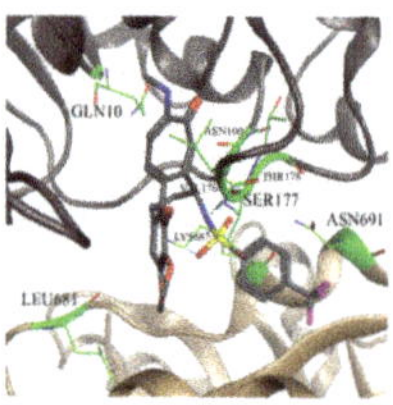	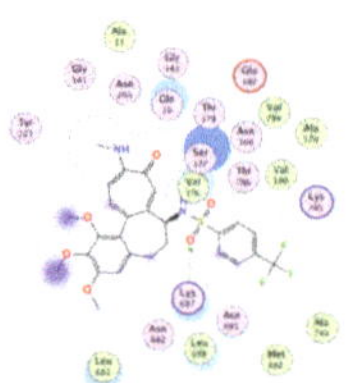	−29.8	4.9	Ala179 Val180 **Cys674** **Leu688** Asn691 Ala749 **Lys785**

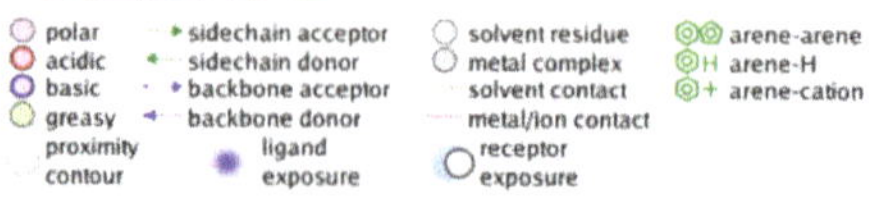

Although the synthesized compounds are effective toward cancer cells, their potential is limited against cells with developed drug resistance. The data presented in Table 2 show that unmodified colchicine **1** and all of the colchicine derivatives **2–21** less effectively inhibited the proliferation of the doxorubicin-resistant subline LoVo/DX than the sensitive LoVo cell line. The calculated values of RI clearly confirmed that none of the tested amides and sulfonamides was able to overcome the drug resistance of LoVo/DX cell line (RI ranges from 11.8 to 306.0). It can be explained by the upregulated expression of efflux transporters in these cells, playing an important role in drug transport in many organs and determining the drug resistance of cancer cells. Because this type of resistance is one of the mechanisms of cancer resistance [58], compounds **1–2** and **4–21** are probably good substrates for such pumps. Increased efflux of compounds makes it impossible to reach their adequate concentrations in the cell and consequently to exert efficient cytotoxic effect. The only compound which showed RI < 10 was derivative **3**, having at position C7 a free amino group. Keeping in mind its good activity (IC_{50} < 20 nM for three cancer cells, see Table 2) it can be still considered as a good starting point for the chase after antitumor agents active against drug resistant lines.

The selectivity index (SI) was calculated to evaluate the toxicity of the compounds studied against normal cells and to predict their therapeutic potential (see Figure 3). High SI values result from large differences between the cytotoxicity against cancer and normal cells and this means that cancer cells will be killed at a higher rate than normal ones. From the set of tested compounds with methylamino group at position C10 and alkyl chains at position C7 (**2, 4–8, 19**) the best selectivity index for A549, MCF-7 and LoVo cells (SI = 1.5–4.0) showed **8** with short and branched substituent (isobutyric acid derivative). The 4,4,4-trifluorobutyric acid derivative **11** (from compounds with alkyl chains of various lengths containing halogen atoms **9–11**) showed outstanding selectivity for three out of four cancer cells (SI = 5.6–7.8). It should be emphasized that compound **11** was the only compound with SI values greater than that of unmodified colchicine **1** for all tumor cell lines. Despite the fact that compounds **9, 10,** and **13** stood out from the synthesized compounds in terms of IC_{50} values, their selectivity indices were high only for LoVo lines (SI = 6.5–9.1), they were very cytotoxic also to non-cancerous BALB/3T3 cells (IC_{50} = 6.2–11.6 nM). Among aryl amides and sulfonamides **12–16** and **21**, distinctive SI values were derived for colchicine derivatives containingnicotinic and isonicotinic amide residue (SI ranges 3.0 to 4.8). These results are noteworthy and suggest that extended and more detailed research of similar derivatives is necessary to determine the importance of ring aromaticity, its size or heteroatom type. Especially high SI values for MCF-7 were obtained for sulfamide **17** (SI = 9.8) and sulfonamide containing a morpholine ring **20** (SI = 6.6). These results deserve special attention and require further studies to determine whether the conversion of an amide bond to a sulfonamide bond with an appropriate substituent would allow obtaining compounds highly selective towards MCF7 cells, compared to colchicine **1**. As many as thirteen of the obtained derivatives exhibited SI ≥ 2 for LoVo cell line (see Figure 3). The results indicated that properly designed doubly modified (at C7 and C10 positions) colchicine derivatives can have greater selectivity towards cancer cells than the parental compound.

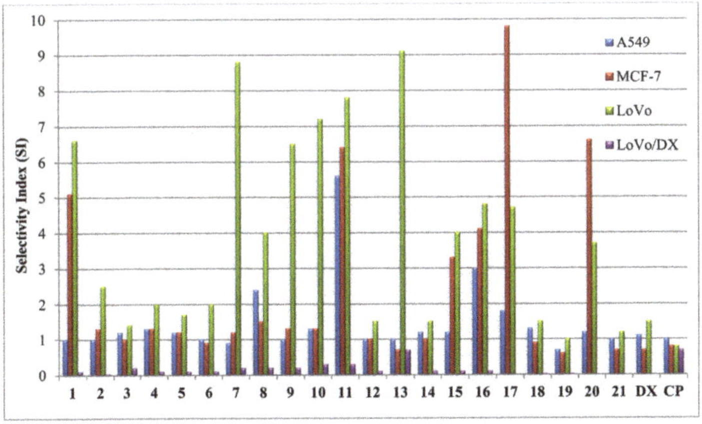

Figure 3. Comparison of selectivity index (SI) values of the tested compounds. The SI was calculated for each compound using the formula: SI = (IC_{50} for normal cell line BALB/3T3)/(IC_{50} for respective cancerous cell line). A favorable SI > 1.0 indicates a drug with efficacy against tumor cells greater than the toxicity against normal cells.

2.5. In Silico Determination of the Molecular Mode of Action

In the present study, computational investigation including molecular docking, molecular dynamics (MD) simulations, molecular mechanics generalized Born/surface area (MM/GBSA) binding free energy calculations and decomposition of pair-wise free energy on a per-residue basis were conducted to deeply explore the molecular basis for the binding of twenty novel double modified colchicine amides and sulfonamides to β-tubulin. The latter is one of the subunits of microtubules in the cytoskeleton structure of every eukaryotic cell, which is the target of many anticancer drugs. The twenty structures of colchicine derivatives described above were docked into the βI-tubulin (the most abundant isotype in most cancer tumors) colchicine binding site.

On the basis of our computational predictions, according to increasing binding energy, the compounds are ordered as follows: **20** (−59.6), **18** (−54.6), **7** (−53.7), **9** (−44.0), **15** (−43.9), **4** (−43.4), **5** (−43.1), **10** (−41.8), **1** (−41.1), **13** (−40.1), **2** (−39.3), **16** (−38.3), **6** (−37.2), **12** (−35.2), **17** (−34.9), **11** (−34.7), **14** (−34.3), **8** (−32.3), **21** (−29.8), **19** (−23.4), **3** (−4.0) kcal/mol with the binding energies in the parenthesis given in units of kcal/mol. Binding energies of these compounds are shown in Figure 4 and Table 3.

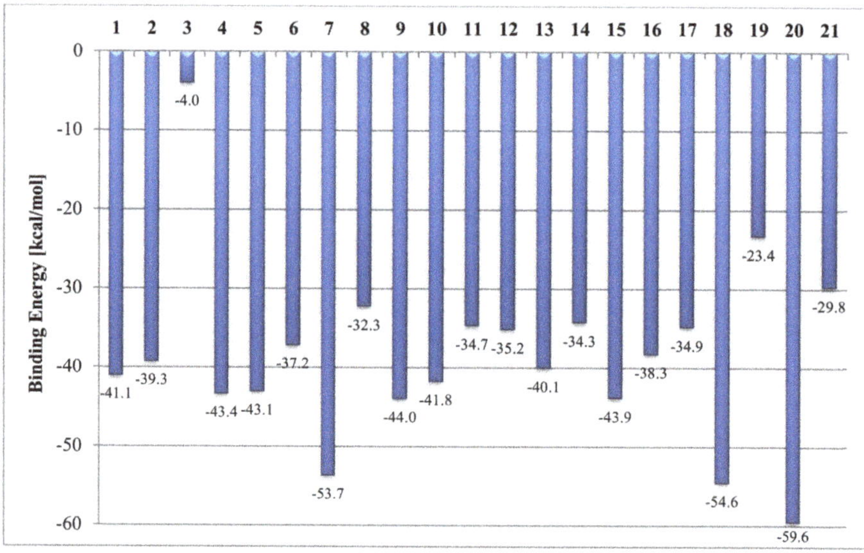

Figure 4. Comparison of binding energies of the tested compounds complexed with tubulin βI. Binding energies have been estimated using the MM/GBSA method.

In view of the calculated binding energies, we can conclude that there is no strong correlation (the lower the binding energy, the more biologically active the chemical compound) between *in silico* computer calculations (BE values, Figure 4) and in vitro activity results (IC_{50} values, Table 2).

The lowest binding energies, −59.6 and −53.7 kcal/mol, were shown by sulfonamide **20** (derivative with the morpholine ring) and amide **7** (derivative of palmitic acid), respectively. However, these compounds showed the weakest antiproliferative activity (highest IC_{50} values) among all compounds tested (**1–21**).

Compound **18** has the third lowest energy (−54.6 kcal/mol) and good cytotoxicity with IC_{50} from 9.3 to 15.5 nM for LoVo, A549 and MCF-7 cancer cells. The molecular-level computations indicate that **18** fits well to βI-tubulin and probably uses this binding site as a target. The majority of the other derivatives **2**, **4–6**, **8–17** exhibited binding energy less than −30.0 kcal/mol, so close to the energy of unmodified colchicine **1** (BE = −41.1 kcal/mol), which is a compound known to inhibit tubulin polymerization. These compounds bind to the active sites of βI-tubulin isotype and may therefore have a mechanism of action similar to **1** and may be colchicine binding site inhibitors, although their in vitro activities towards various cells characterized by an IC_{50} value (Table 2) were lower than that of colchicine **1**.

Derivative **3** showed the highest binding energy value (BE = −4.0 kcal/mol), therefore its antiproliferative activity is not exclusively the result of interaction with tubulin. This is an important finding because compound **3** was the only one which showed any possibility of breaking the drug resistance of the LoVo/DX line (RI = 9.2, see Table 2).

Therefore, we can see that the results only partly correlate with in vitro determined biological activity of these compounds as indicated though the corresponding IC_{50} values. This may be explained by several additional effects taking place in living cells compared to the computational simulations that focus only on the binding mode of the compounds to the target. Primarily off-target interactions involving efflux transporters with different affinities for the individual compounds and differences in solubility of these colchicine derivatives or their membrane permeability. Additionally, the lack of significant correlation may be due to the fact that in various cancer cells the expression of specific β-tubulin isotypes significantly varies [59]. We propose the inclusion of binding affinity calculations for these compounds with regard to not only other tubulin isotypes but also with respect to most important efflux transporters in order to minimize them and hence increase the activity of the drug in vitro and *in vivo*.

Schematic interactions of the compounds with CBS of βI-tubulin residues are shown in Table 3.

In 3D representation, the interacting residues predicted from pairwise per-residue binding free energy decomposition calculations (E < −2 kcal/mol) are shown in stick presentation and their carbons and the ribbon are colored as green. Tubulin is shown in cartoon representation. Hydrogen bonds and their directionality are represented as black dashed arrows. The structures are color-coded as follows: tubulin αI, brown; tubulin βI, beige. Compounds are displayed with sticks and the atoms are colored as O (red), C (gray), N (blue), S (yellow), Cl (green) and F (pink). Binding energy defines the affinity of binding for colchicine derivatives complexed with tubulin βI. Binding energies are predicted by MM/GBSA method. The last column contains information about the active residues with the binding free energy decomposition (E_{decomp}) less than −2 kcal/mol (the residues with E_{decomp} < −3 kcal/mol are highlighted in boldface). The last line contains the graphical key to help interpret the 2D part of the ligand interactions panel.

Derivative compounds are designed with different side chains at C7 position of colchicine **1**. Compounds **2**, **4–8** have alkyl chains of various lengths, straight and branched and compound **19** has an unsaturated alkyl chain. The second lowest binding energy compound **7** within all the compounds is in this group (BE = −53.6 kcal/mol). Compound **7** appears to be engaged in some interactions with α-tubulin (−3 < E_{decomp} < −2 kcal/mol). Most of the compounds in this group are bound through Lys785, Lys687 and Leu688 residues.

Compounds **9–11** were designed with alkyl chains of various length containing halogen atoms side chains at position C7 of colchicine **1**. In this group, the common binding residues with (−3 < E_{decomp} < −2 kcal/mol) are Ala179, Cys674, Asn691, while the strongest binding residues (E_{decomp} < −3 kcal/mol) are Leu688 and Lys785.

Compounds **12–16, 21** were designed with an aromatic group side chain without or with substituents at C7 position of colchicine **1**. The same trend of strong binding of Leu688 and Lys785 residues with the compounds is seen in this group. The binding energies in this group are on the higher side compared to the other compounds.

As the last group, compounds **17–18** and **20** contain the sulfonamide moieties at position C7 of colchicine **1**. The strongest binding residues in this group belong to both α-tubulin (Gln10 and Ser177) in compound **17**, (Gln10, Gly142, Gly143, Thr144 and Ser177) in compound **18** and (Asp68 and Asn100) in compound **20** with (E_{decomp} < −3 kcal/mol) and β-tubulin (Asp684, Asn691, Lys785) in compound **17** and Lys687 in compound **20**. The lowest binding energy between all the compounds characterizes compounds **20** and **18**, which mainly bind to α-tubulin.

In the experimental part of the study, the highest IC_{50} values (the weakest activity) were found for compound **7** from the amides and compound **20** from the sulfonamides studied against all cancer cell lines tested. According to our computational analysis, although these compounds show the lowest binding energies, they do not bind to the CBS, which is located in β-tubulin and has the tendency to go beyond and also bind to α-tubulin.

3. Materials and Methods

3.1. General

All solvents, substrates and reagents were obtained from TriMen Chemicals (Poland) or Sigma Aldrich and were used without further purification. $CDCl_3$ and CD_2Cl_2 spectral grade solvents were stored over 3 Å molecular sieves for several days. TLC analysis was performed using pre-coated glass plates (0.2 mm thickness, GF-254, pore size 60 Å) from Agela Technologies and spots were visualized by UV-light. Products were purified by flash chromatography using high-purity grade silica gel (pore size 60 Å, 230–400 mesh particle size, 40–63 μm particle size) from SiliCycle Inc. Preparative HPLC was performed on LC-20AP Shimadzu with ELSD-LTII detector equipped with Phenomenex Luna C18 250 × 21 mm, 5 μm column eluted with 20 mL/min flow over 20 min of acetonitrile in water. Solvents were removed using a rotary evaporator.

3.2. Spectroscopic Measurements

NMR spectra were recorded on Bruker Avance DRX 500 (^{1}H NMR at 500 MHz and ^{13}C NMR at 126 MHz) magnetic resonance spectrometers. ^{1}H NMR spectra are reported in chemical shifts downfield from TMS using the respective residual solvent peak as internal standard ($CDCl_3$ δ 7.26 ppm, CD_2Cl_2 δ 5.32 ppm, $(CD_3)_2SO$ δ 2.50 ppm). ^{1}H NMR spectra are described as follows: chemical shift (δ, ppm), multiplicity (s = singlet, d = doublet, t = triplet, q = quartet, dd = doublet of doublets, dt = doublet of triplets, dq = doublet of quartets, m = multiplet), coupling constant (*J*) in Hz, and integration. ^{13}C NMR spectra are described in chemical shifts downfield from TMS using the respective residual solvent peak as internal standard ($CDCl_3$ δ 77.16 ppm, CD_2Cl_2 δ 53.84 ppm and $(CD_3)_2SO$ δ 39.52 ppm).

Electrospray ionization (ESI) mass spectra were obtained on a Waters Alliance 2695 separation module with a PDA 2996 UV detector and Waters Micromass ZQ 2000 mass detector equipped with Restek Ultra Biphenyl 50 × 3 mm, 3 μm column eluted with 0.3 mL/min flow of 3–100% gradient (over 6 min) of acetonitrile in water.

3.3. Synthesis

3.3.1. Synthesis of **2**

To a solution of **1** (1.0 equiv.) in EtOH, a methylamine (solution 33% in EtOH, 10.0 equiv.) was added. The mixture was stirred at reflux for 24 h and then concentrated under reduced pressure to dryness. The residue was purified using column flash chromatography (silica gel; DCM/MeOH) and next lyophilized from dioxane to give the pure product **2** as a yellow solid with a yield of 80%.

ESI-MS for $C_{22}H_{26}N_2O_5$ (*m*/*z*): $[M + H]^+$ 399, $[M + Na]^+$ 421, $[2M + H]^+$ 797, $[2M + Na]^+$ 819, $[M - H]^-$ 397, $[M + HCOO^-]^-$ 443.

^{1}H NMR (500 MHz, $CDCl_3$) δ 8.70 (d, *J* = 6.4 Hz, 1H), 7.58 (s, 1H), 7.46 (d, *J* = 11.1 Hz, 1H), 7.28–7.25 (m, 1H), 6.58 (d, *J* = 11.3 Hz, 1H), 6.52 (s, 1H), 4.73–4.64 (m, 1H), 3.93 (s, 3H), 3.88 (s, 3H), 3.61 (s, 3H), 3.08 (d, *J* = 5.4 Hz, 3H), 2.47–2.43 (m, 1H), 2.37–2.31 (m, 1H), 2.29–2.22 (m, 1H), 2.02–1.96 (m, 1H), 1.94 (s, 3H).

^{13}C NMR (126 MHz, $CDCl_3$) δ 175.11, 170.19, 155.23, 152.91, 151.61, 151.10, 141.51, 139.37, 134.66, 130.42, 126.93, 122.81, 108.28, 107.20, 61.46, 61.40, 56.16, 52.72, 37.06, 30.15, 29.53, 22.74.

3.3.2. Synthesis of **3**

To a solution of compound **2** (1.0 equiv.) in dioxane, 2M HCl (10.0 equiv.) was added and the mixture was stirred at reflux. Reaction progress was monitored by LC-MS. Then the reaction mixture was neutralized with 4M NaOH to pH~10 and extracted four times with EtOAc. The organic layers were combined, washed with brine, dried over Na_2SO_4, filtered and evaporated under reduced pressure. The residue was purified using column flash chromatography (silica gel; DCM/MeOH) and next lyophilized from dioxane to give the pure product **3** as a yellow solid with a yield of 73%.

ESI-MS for $C_{20}H_{24}N_2O_4$ (*m/z*): $[M + H]^+$ 357, $[M + Na]^+$ 379, $[2M + Na]^+$ 735.

^{1}H NMR (500 MHz, $CDCl_3$) δ 7.61 (s, 1H), 7.33 (d, *J* = 11.1 Hz, 1H), 7.23–7.21 (m, 1H), 6.50 (s, 1H), 6.50 (d, *J* = 11.4 Hz, 2H), 3.87 (s, 3H), 3.87 (s, 3H), 3.75–3.72 (m, 1H), 3.59 (s, 3H), 3.05 (d, *J* = 5.5 Hz, 3H), 2.41–2.37 (m, 1H), 2.33–2.31 (m, 2H), 2.25 (s, 2H), 1.71–1.61 (m, 1H).

^{13}C NMR (126 MHz, $CDCl_3$) δ 175.57, 154.99, 153.25, 152.76, 150.59, 141.06, 138.73, 135.41, 129.74, 126.63, 123.68, 107.35, 106.94, 61.19, 60.84, 56.06, 54.01, 40.90, 30.69, 29.48.

3.3.3. General Procedure for the Synthesis of Colchicine Derivatives **4, 8, 13, 15–16, 18** and **21**

Compounds **4, 8, 13, 15–16, 18** and **21** were obtained directly from compound **3**. To a solution of compound **3** (1.0 equiv.) and Et_3N (3.0 equiv.) in DCM in an ice bath, the corresponding acid/sulfonyl/sulfamide chloride (1.1 equiv.) diluted with DCM was added slowly. Next the ice bath was removed and the reaction mixture was stirred at RT. Reaction progress was monitored by LC-MS. Then the reaction mixture was diluted with EtOAc, washed with H_2O, 1M K_2CO_3, brine and dried over Na_2SO_4. The residue was purified using column flash chromatography (silica gel; DCM/MeOH) and next lyophilized from dioxane to give respective compound.

Compound **4**

Yellow solid, yield 86%.

ESI-MS for $C_{23}H_{28}N_2O_5$ (*m/z*): $[M + H]^+$ 413, $[M + Na]^+$ 435, $[2M + H]^+$ 825, $[2M + Na]^+$ 847, $[M–H]^-$ 411, $[M + HCOO^-]^-$ 457.

^{1}H NMR (500 MHz, $CDCl_3$) δ 8.46 (s, 1H), 7.53 (s, 1H), 7.44 (d, *J* = 11.1 Hz, 1H), 7.25–7.21 (m, 1H), 6.55 (d, *J* = 11.4 Hz, 1H), 6.50 (s, 1H), 4.72–4.65 (m, 1H), 3.91 (s, 3H), 3.86 (s, 3H), 3.61 (s, 3H), 3.06 (d, *J* = 5.4 Hz, 3H), 2.44–2.40 (m, 1H), 2.33–2.30 (m, 1H), 2.26–2.17 (m, 3H), 1.94–1.88 (m, 1H), 1.05 (t, *J* = 7.6 Hz, 3H).

^{13}C NMR (126 MHz, $CDCl_3$) δ 175.09, 173.89, 155.20, 152.86, 151.64, 151.09, 141.49, 139.23, 134.67, 130.33, 126.95, 122.94, 108.14, 107.20, 61.44, 56.14, 52.37, 37.20, 30.18, 29.53, 29.11, 9.72.

Compound **8**

Yellow solid, yield 96%.

ESI-MS for $C_{24}H_{30}N_2O_5$ (*m/z*): $[M + H]^+$ 427, $[M + Na]^+$ 449, $[2M + H]^+$ 853, $[2M + Na]^+$ 875, $[M–H]^-$ 425, $[M + HCOO^-]^-$ 471.

^{1}H NMR (500 MHz, $CDCl_3$) δ 7.48 (d, *J* = 11.2 Hz, 1H), 7.45 (s, 1H), 7.31–7.28 (m, 1H), 6.67 (d, *J* = 7.3 Hz, 1H), 6.59 (d, *J* = 11.3 Hz, 1H), 6.53 (s, 1H), 4.75–4.63 (m, 1H), 3.94 (s, 3H), 3.89 (s, 3H), 3.63 (s, 3H), 3.10 (d, *J* = 5.4 Hz, 3H), 2.53–2.43 (m, 2H), 2.38–2.32 (m, 1H), 2.28–2.20 (m, 1H), 1.93–1.82 (m, 1H), 1.14 (t, *J* = 6.7 Hz, 6H).

^{13}C NMR (126 MHz, $CDCl_3$) δ 176.86, 175.21, 155.19, 152.85, 151.15, 141.56, 139.08, 134.55, 130.09, 126.97, 123.07, 107.91, 107.22, 61.51, 61.45, 56.13, 51.96, 37.56, 35.21, 30.19, 29.54, 19.70, 19.60.

Compound **13**

Yellow solid, yield 86%.

ESI-MS for $C_{27}H_{27}ClN_2O_5$ (*m/z*): $[M + H]^+$ 495/497, $[M + Na]^+$ 517, $[2M + H]^+$ 989/991, $[M-H]^-$ 493/495, $[M + HCOO^-]^-$ 540.

^{1}H NMR (500 MHz, CD_2Cl_2) δ 8.12 (d, J = 7.5 Hz, 1H), 7.60 (s, 1H), 7.42–7.39 (m, 2H), 7.29–7.22 (m, 2H), 7.19 (t, J = 7.5 Hz, 1H), 7.06 (t, J = 7.4 Hz, 1H), 6.60 (s, 1H), 6.53 (d, J = 11.3 Hz, 1H), 4.88–4.83 (m, 1H), 3.91 (s, 3H), 3.89 (s, 3H), 3.71 (s, 3H), 3.03 (d, J = 5.2 Hz, 3H), 2.52–2,48 (m, 1H), 2.42–2.31 (m, 2H), 2.14–2.04 (m, 1H).

^{13}C NMR (126 MHz, CD_2Cl_2) δ 174.51, 165.99, 155.24, 153.11, 150.94, 150.51, 141.52, 139.19, 135.71, 134.71, 130.64, 130.43, 130.01, 129.60, 129.58, 126.83, 126.79, 123.26, 107.90, 107.46, 61.08, 61.07, 56.02, 52.86, 37.83, 30.11, 29.35.

Compound **15**

Yellow solid, yield 23%.

ESI-MS for $C_{26}H_{27}N_3O_5$ (m/z): $[M + H]^+$ 462, $[M + Na]^+$ 484, $[2M + H]^+$ 923, $[2M + Na]^+$ 945, $[M\text{-}H]^-$ 460, $[M + HCOO^-]^-$ 506.

^{1}H NMR (500 MHz, $CDCl_3$) δ 9.35 (d, J = 7.0 Hz, 1H), 9.07 (d, J = 1.8 Hz, 1H), 8.48 (dd, J = 4.8, 1.5 Hz, 1H), 8.13–8.06 (m, 1H), 7.65 (s, 1H), 7.51 (d, J = 11.2 Hz, 1H), 7.31 (q, J = 5.1 Hz, 1H), 7.05 (dd, J = 7.9, 4.9 Hz, 1H), 6.61 (d, J = 11.4 Hz, 1H), 6.54 (s, 1H), 4.99–4.86 (m, 1H), 3.95 (s, 3H), 3.89 (s, 3H), 3.70 (s, 3H), 3.08 (d, J = 5.4 Hz, 3H), 2.51–2.45 (m, 1H), 2.40–2.34 (m, 1H), 2.33–2.27 (m, 1H), 2.17–2.09 (m, 1H).

^{13}C NMR (126 MHz, $CDCl_3$) δ 174.69, 165.09, 155.37, 153.01, 151.82, 151.42, 151.15, 148.87, 141.59, 139.62, 134.89, 134.61, 130.41, 129.34, 126.86, 123.08, 122.79, 108.49, 107.27, 61.53, 61.48, 56.15, 53.22, 36.83, 30.28, 29.58.

Compound **16**

Yellow solid, yield 39%.

ESI-MS for $C_{26}H_{27}N_3O_5$ (m/z): $[M + H]^+$ 462, $[M + Na]^+$ 484, $[2M + H]^+$ 923, $[2M + Na]^+$ 945, $[M\text{-}H]^-$ 460, $[M + HCOO^-]^-$ 506.

^{1}H NMR (500 MHz, $CDCl_3$) δ 9.71 (d, J = 6.6 Hz, 1H), 8.37 (d, J = 5.8 Hz, 2H), 7.69 (s, 1H), 7.64 (d, J = 5.8 Hz, 2H), 7.54 (d, J = 11.2 Hz, 1H), 7.32–7.28 (m, 1H), 6.65 (d, J = 11.4 Hz, 1H), 6.53 (s, 1H), 4.98–4.81 (m, 1H), 3.95 (s, 3H), 3.87 (s, 3H), 3.71 (s, 3H), 3.10 (d, J = 5.4 Hz, 3H), 2.50–2.41 (m, 1H), 2.41–2.25 (m, 2H), 2.16–2.11 (m, 1H).

^{13}C NMR (126 MHz, $CDCl_3$) δ 174.51, 164.91, 155.37, 153.05, 151.64, 151.17, 150.18, 141.59, 140.46, 139.81, 134.59, 130.64, 126.78, 122.68, 120.99, 108.68, 107.27, 61.55, 61.47, 56.14, 53.46, 36.50, 30.29, 29.60.

Compound **18**

Yellow solid, yield 38%.

ESI-MS for $C_{22}H_{29}N_3O_6S$ (m/z): $[M + H]^+$ 464, $[M + Na]^+$ 486, $[2M + H]^+$ 927, $[2M + Na]^+$ 949, $[M\text{-}H]^-$ 462.

^{1}H NMR (500 MHz, $CDCl_3$) δ 7.85 (s, 1H), 7.45–7.41 (m, 2H), 6.58 (d, J = 11.3 Hz, 1H), 6.54 (s, 1H), 6.49–6.46 (m, 1H), 4.33–4.19 (m, 1H), 3.93–3.89 (m, 6H), 3.57 (s, 3H), 3.10 (d, J = 5.1 Hz, 3H), 2.58 (s, 6H), 2.49–2.39 (m, 2H), 2.35–2.26 (m, 1H), 2.01–1.90 (m, 1H).

^{13}C NMR (126 MHz, $CDCl_3$) δ 174.73, 155.46, 153.08, 150.77, 150.08, 141.39, 139.41, 134.59, 129.64, 126.34, 124.53, 108.22, 107.43, 61.34, 60.80, 56.48, 56.05, 39.91, 37.95, 30.50, 29.57.

Compound **21**

Yellow solid, yield 83%.

ESI-MS for $C_{27}H_{27}F_3N_2O_6S$ (m/z): $[M + H]^+$ 565, $[M + Na]^+$ 587, $[2M + H]^+$ 1129, $[2M + Na]^+$ 1151, $[M\text{-}H]^-$ 563.

^{1}H NMR (500 MHz, $CDCl_3$) δ 8.72 (d, J = 7.5 Hz, 1H), 8.07 (s, 1H), 7.92 (s, 1H), 7.84 (d, J = 8.2 Hz, 2H), 7.53 (d, J = 8.3 Hz, 2H), 7.48 (d, J = 11.5 Hz, 1H), 6.66 (d, J = 11.8 Hz, 1H), 6.46 (s, 1H), 4.16 (q, J = 8.8 Hz, 1H), 3.91 (s, 3H), 3.86 (s, 3H), 3.58 (s, 3H), 3.08 (d, J = 5.2 Hz, 3H), 2.45–2.31 (m, 1H), 2.31–2.18 (m, 2H), 2.16–2.10 (m, 1H).

^{13}C NMR (126 MHz, $CDCl_3$) δ 170.13, 155.43, 153.53, 150.65, 150.15, 144.53, 141.35, 134.75, 133.34, 131.89, 127.57, 125.82, 125.79, 125.49, 124.38, 123.51, 122.21, 111.26, 107.42, 61.29, 60.95, 56.63, 56.04, 38.98, 30.26, 29.78.

3.3.4. General Procedure for the Synthesis of Colchicine Derivatives **5–7**, **9–12** and **14**

Compounds **5–7**, **9–12** and **14** were obtained directly from compound **3**. To a solution of compound **3** (1.0 equiv.) in DCM corresponding carboxylic acid (1.1 equiv.) and 1-(3-dimethylaminopropyl)-3-ethylcarbodiimide hydrochloride (EDCI, 1.1 equiv.) were added. Reaction progress was monitored by LC-MS. Then the reaction mixture was diluted with EtOAc, washed with H_2O, 1M K_2CO_3, brine and dried over Na_2SO_4. The residue was purified using column flash chromatography (silica gel; DCM/MeOH) and next lyophilized from dioxane to give respective compound.

Compound **5**

Yellow solid, yield 93%.

ESI-MS for $C_{24}H_{30}N_2O_5$ (*m/z*): $[M + H]^+$ 427, $[M + Na]^+$ 449, $[2M + H]^+$ 853, $[2M + Na]^+$ 875, $[M\text{-}H]^-$ 425, $[M + HCOO^-]^-$ 471.

^1H NMR (500 MHz, $CDCl_3$) δ 7.88 (s, 1H), 7.51 (s, 1H), 7.45 (d, *J* = 11.1 Hz, 1H), 7.27–7.25 (m, 1H), 6.56 (d, *J* = 11.3 Hz, 1H), 6.51 (s, 1H), 4.76–4.68 (m, 1H), 3.92 (s, 3H), 3.87 (s, 3H), 3.61 (s, 3H), 3.08 (d, *J* = 5.4 Hz, 3H), 2.45–2.41 (m, 1H), 2.35–2.27 (m, 1H), 2.25–2.17 (m, 3H), 1.91 –1.85 (m, 1H), 1.65–1.55 (m, 2H), 0.87 (t, *J* = 7.4 Hz, 3H).

^{13}C NMR (126 MHz, $CDCl_3$) δ 175.10, 172.96, 155.22, 152.87, 151.43, 151.13, 141.52, 139.20, 134.61, 130.31, 126.94, 123.10, 108.13, 107.22, 61.45, 56.13, 52.21, 38.22, 37.45, 30.18, 29.54, 19.09, 13.93.

Compound **6**

Yellow solid, yield 73%.

ESI-MS for $C_{25}H_{32}N_2O_5$ (*m/z*): $[M + H]^+$ 441, $[M + Na]^+$ 463, $[2M + H]^+$ 881, $[2M + Na]^+$ 903, $[M\text{-}H]^-$ 439, $[M + HCOO^-]^-$ 485.

^1H NMR (500 MHz, $CDCl_3$) δ 7.86 (s, 1H), 7.50 (s, 1H), 7.44 (d, *J* = 11.1 Hz, 1H), 7.26–7.21 (m, 1H), 6.55 (d, *J* = 11.3 Hz, 1H), 6.51 (s, 1H), 4.76–4.68 (m, 1H), 3.93 (s, 3H), 3.88 (s, 3H), 3.61 (s, 3H), 3.08 (d, *J* = 5.4 Hz, 3H), 2.45–2.41 (m, 1H), 2.36–2.30 (m, 1H), 2.25–2.18 (m, 3H), 1.93–1.84 (m, 1H), 1.58–1.51 (m, 2H), 1.30–1.22 (m, 2H), 0.81 (t, *J* = 7.3 Hz, 3H).

^{13}C NMR (126 MHz, $CDCl_3$) δ 175.19, 173.02, 155.19, 152.85, 151.32, 151.15, 141.54, 139.11, 134.59, 130.19, 126.98, 123.13, 107.97, 107.20, 61.44, 56.13, 52.20, 37.46, 36.05, 30.19, 29.53, 27.70, 22.46, 13.76.

Compound **7**

Yellow solid, yield 24%.

ESI-MS for $C_{36}H_{54}N_2O_5$ (*m/z*): $[M + H]^+$ 595, $[2M + H]^+$ 1189, $[M\text{-}H]^-$ 593, $[M + HCOO^-]^-$ 639.

^1H NMR (500 MHz, $CDCl_3$) δ 8.18–7.90 (m, 2H), 7.73–7.53 (m, 2H), 6.88 (d, *J* = 10.1 Hz, 1H), 6.55 (s, 1H), 4.74 (s, 1H), 3.93 (s, 3H), 3.89 (s, 3H), 3.62 (s, 3H), 3.19 (s, 3H), 2.47 (d, *J* = 7.4 Hz, 1H), 2.39–2.08 (m, 5H), 1.54–1.49 (m, 2H), 1.28–1.16 (m, 26H), 0.86 (t, *J* = 7.0 Hz, 3H).

^{13}C NMR (126 MHz, $CDCl_3$) δ 175.09, 173.07, 155.23, 152.89, 151.32, 151.14, 141.55, 139.25, 134.58, 130.35, 126.91, 123.12, 108.24, 107.23, 61.45, 56.12, 52.16, 37.56, 36.39, 31.95, 30.18, 29.73, 29.69, 29.54, 29.53, 29.43, 29.39, 25.64, 22.72, 14.16.

Compound **9**

Yellow solid, yield 83%.

ESI-MS for $C_{22}H_{25}ClN_2O_5$ (*m/z*): $[M + H]^+$ 433/435, $[M + Na]^+$ 455/457, $[2M + H]^+$ 865, $[2M + Na]^+$ 887, $[M\text{-}H]^-$ 431.

^{1}H NMR (500 MHz, $CDCl_3$) δ 8.60–8.38 (m, 1H), 7.48–7.39 (m, 2H), 7.29 (q, J = 5.2 Hz, 1H), 6.56 (d, J = 11.4 Hz, 1H), 6.52 (s, 1H), 4.75–4.63 (m, 1H), 4.08–3.95 (m, 2H), 3.92 (s, 3H), 3.87 (s, 3H), 3.60 (s, 3H), 3.07 (d, J = 5.3 Hz, 3H), 2.50–2.43 (m, 1H), 2.40–2.31 (m, 1H), 2.28–2.21 (m, 1H), 2.04–1.93 (m, 1H).

^{13}C NMR (126 MHz, $CDCl_3$) δ 175.04, 166.12, 155.33, 152.97, 151.10, 150.18,141.57, 139.37, 134.41, 129.97, 126.80, 122.73, 108.18, 107.27, 61.45, 61.33, 56.14, 52.91, 42.63, 37.17, 30.02, 29.55.

Compound **10**

Yellow solid, yield 46%.

ESI-MS for $C_{22}H_{24}Cl_2N_2O_5$ (m/z): $[M + H]^+$ 467/469, $[M + Na]^+$ 489/491, $[2M + H]^+$ 933/935, $[2M + Na]^+$ 957/959, $[M-H]^-$ 465/467.

^{1}H NMR (500 MHz, $CDCl_3$) δ 9.53 (d, J = 7.2 Hz, 1H), 7.56 (s, 1H), 7.53 (d, J = 11.2 Hz, 1H), 7.34 (q, J = 5.2 Hz, 1H), 6.64 (d, J = 11.4 Hz, 1H), 6.52 (s, 1H), 6.20 (s, 1H), 4.77–4.69 (m, 1H), 3.94 (s, 3H), 3.89 (s, 3H), 3.63 (s, 3H), 3.12 (d, J = 5.4 Hz, 3H), 2.46–2.44 (m, 1H), 2.38–2.23 (m, 2H), 1.97–1.91 (m, 1H).

^{13}C NMR (126 MHz, $CDCl_3$) δ 174.73, 164.19, 155.51, 153.12, 151.17, 150.51, 141.69, 139.81, 134.31, 130.45, 126.66, 122.71, 108.80, 107.36, 66.56, 61.52, 61.48, 56.17, 53.28, 37.17, 30.06, 29.66.

Compound **11**

Yellow solid, yield 89%.

ESI-MS for $C_{24}H_{27}F_3N_2O_5$ (m/z): $[M + H]^+$ 481, $[M + Na]^+$ 503, $[2M + H]^+$ 961, $[2M + Na]^+$ 983, $[M-H]^-$ 479, $[M + HCOO^-]^-$ 525.

^{1}H NMR (500 MHz, $CDCl_3$) δ 8.77–8.65 (m, 1H), 7.56 (s, 1H), 7.49 (d, J = 11.2 Hz, 1H), 7.35–7.28 (m, 1H), 6.61 (d, J = 11.4 Hz, 1H), 6.51 (s, 1H), 4.75–4.70 (m, 1H), 3.94 (s, 3H), 3.88 (s, 3H), 3.62 (s, 3H), 3.10 (d, J = 5.4 Hz, 3H), 2.56–2.46 (m, 2H), 2.45–2.27 (m, 4H), 2.25–2.20 (m, 1H), 1.90–1.84 (m, 1H).

^{13}C NMR (126 MHz, $CDCl_3$) δ 174.99, 169.79, 155.36, 152.97, 151.33, 151.12, 141.57, 139.53, 134.54, 130.36, 127.98, 126.81, 122.89, 108.41, 107.25, 61.46, 61.34, 56.13, 52.52, 37.37, 30.16, 29.56, 29.33, 28.17.

Compound **12**

Yellow solid, yield 89%.

ESI-MS for $C_{27}H_{28}N_2O_5$ (m/z): $[M + H]^+$ 461, $[M + Na]^+$ 483, $[2M + H]^+$ 921, $[2M + Na]^+$ 943, $[M-H]^-$ 459, $[M + HCOO^-]^-$ 505.

^{1}H NMR (500 MHz, $CDCl_3$) δ 8.36 (d, J = 7.3 Hz, 1H), 7.81 (d, J = 7.2 Hz, 2H), 7.68 (s, 1H), 7.49 (d, J = 11.2 Hz, 1H), 7.29–7.23 (m, 2H), 7.16 (t, J = 7.7 Hz, 2H), 6.57 (d, J = 11.4 Hz, 1H), 6.53 (s, 1H), 4.99–4.93 (m, 1H), 3.96 (s, 3H), 3.89 (s, 3H), 3.70 (s, 3H), 3.06 (d, J = 5.4 Hz, 3H), 2.50–2.45 (m, 1H), 2.41–2.37 (m, 1H), 2.34–2.26 (m, 1H), 2.11–2.06 (m, 1H).

^{13}C NMR (126 MHz, $CDCl_3$) δ 175.02, 167.10, 155.26, 152.91, 151.30, 151.20, 141.57, 139.18, 134.65, 133.84, 131.31, 130.17, 128.28, 127.17, 127.01, 123.23, 108.01, 107.28, 61.53, 61.49, 56.14, 52.85, 37.19, 30.30, 29.53.

Compound **14**

Yellow solid, yield 57%.

ESI-MS for $C_{27}H_{27}FN_2O_5$ (m/z): $[M + H]^+$ 479, $[M + Na]^+$ 501, $[2M + H]^+$ 957, $[2M + Na]^+$ 979, $[M-H]^-$ 477, $[M + HCOO^-]^-$ 523.

^{1}H NMR (500 MHz, $CDCl_3$) δ 8.75 (s, 1H), 7.68 (s, 1H), 7.59 (d, J = 7.5 Hz, 1H), 7.53–7.47 (m, 2H), 7.31–7.26 (m, 1H), 7.10–7.05 (m, 1H), 6.97–6.92 (m, 1H), 6.61 (d, J = 11.4 Hz, 1H), 6.55 (s, 1H), 4.99–4.90 (m, 1H), 3.96 (s, 3H), 3.90 (s, 3H), 3.70 (s, 3H), 3.09 (d, J = 5.4 Hz, 3H), 2.53–2.47 (m, 1H), 2.43–2.37 (m, 1H), 2.35–2.27 (m, 1H), 2.18–2.10 (m, 1H).

^{13}C NMR (126 MHz, $CDCl_3$) δ 174.84, 165.56, 155.31, 152.98, 151.38, 151.20, 141.59, 139.42, 134.63, 130.36, 129.84, 126.92, 123.06, 122.53, 118.29, 118.12, 114.70, 114.52, 108.29, 107.27, 61.52, 61.50, 56.15, 53.09, 37.00, 30.31, 29.56.

3.3.5. Synthesis of **17**

To a solution of compound **3** (1.0 equiv.) in DCM, *N*-(*tert*-Butoxycarbonyl)-*N*-[4-(dimethylazaniumylidene)-1,4-dihydropyridin-1-ylsulfonyl]azanide (4.0 equiv.) was added and the mixture was stirred at RT. Reaction progress was monitored by LC-MS. Then the reaction mixture was diluted with EtOAc, washed with H_2O, 10% citric acid, 1M K_2CO_3, brine and dried over Na_2SO_4. The residue was purified using column flash chromatography (silica gel; EtOAc/hexanes). To the obtained compound, 4M HCl/EtOAc was added and the reaction mixture was stirred at RT overnight. Next the solvent was removed under reduced pressure and the residue was purified using preparative HPLC (MeCN/H_2O) and lyophilized from dioxane to give the pure hydrochloride product **17** as a yellow solid with a yield of 21%.

ESI-MS for $C_{20}H_{25}N_3O_6S$ (*m/z*): $[M + H]^+$ 436, $[M + Na]^+$ 458, $[2M + H]^+$ 871, $[2M + Na]^+$ 893, $[M-H]^-$ 434.

^{1}H NMR (500 MHz, $CDCl_3$) δ 8.19 (s, 2H), 7.50–7.39 (m, 2H), 6.66 (s, 1H), 6.57 (s, 1H), 4.41–4.32 (m, 1H), 3.94 (m, 6H), 3.56 (s, 3H), 3.11 (s, 3H), 2.59–2.46 (m, 2H), 2.56–2.49 (s, 1H), 2.21 (s, 1H).

3.3.6. Synthesis of **19**

To a solution of compound **3** (1.0 equiv.) and Et_3N (3.0 equiv.) in DCM in an ice bath, 2-chloroethanesulfonyl chloride (1.2 equiv.) diluted with DCM was slowly added. Next, the ice bath was removed and the reaction mixture was stirred at RT. Reaction progress was monitored by LC-MS. Then the reaction mixture was diluted with EtOAc, washed with 1M K_2CO_3, brine and dried over Na_2SO_4. The residue was purified using column flash chromatography (silica gel; EtOAc/MeOH) and lyophilized from dioxane to give the pure product **19** as a yellow solid with a yield of 64%.

ESI-MS for $C_{22}H_{26}N_2O_6S$ (*m/z*): $[M + H]^+$ 447, $[2M + H]^+$ 893, $[2M + Na]^+$ 915, $[M-H]^-$ 445.

^{1}H NMR (500 MHz, $(CD_3)_2SO$) δ 8.26 (d, *J* = 7.5 Hz, 1H), 8.04 (s, 1H), 7.41 (s, 1H), 7.23 (d, *J* = 11.2 Hz, 1H), 6.71 (s, 1H), 6.64 (d, *J* = 11.5 Hz, 1H), 6.48 (dd, *J* = 16.4, 9.9 Hz, 1H), 5.71 (dd, *J* = 21.1, 13.1 Hz, 2H), 3.84–3.76 (m, 4H), 3.73 (s, 3H), 3.37 (s, 3H), 2.95 (s, 3H), 2.49 (s, 1H), 2.11–2.01 (m, 2H), 1.88–1.82 (m, 1H).

^{13}C NMR (126 MHz, $(CD_3)_2SO$) δ 173.10, 155.58, 153.04, 150.65, 149.28, 141.12, 139.36, 137.66, 134.78, 128.80, 126.48, 125.64, 123.98, 108.88, 108.07, 61.19, 60.73, 56.26, 55.99, 38.70, 29.82.

3.3.7. Synthesis of **20**

Compound **20** was obtained directly from compound **19**. To **19** in DCM, morpholine was added in excess. Reaction progress was monitored by LC-MS. Then the mixture was diluted with EtOAc, washed with H_2O, brine and dried over Na_2SO_4. The residue was purified using column flash chromatography (silica gel; DCM/MeOH) and subsequently lyophilized from dioxane to give the pure product **20** as a yellow solid with a yield of 63%.

ESI-MS for $C_{26}H_{35}N_3O_7S$ (*m/z*): $[M + H]^+$ 534, $[2M + H]^+$ 1067, $[M-H]^-$ 532.

^{1}H NMR (500 MHz, $CDCl_3$) δ 7.72 (s, 1H), 7.43 (d, *J* = 11.2 Hz, 1H), 7.40–7.38 (m, 1H), 6.84–6.50 (m, 1H), 6.56 (d, *J* = 11.3 Hz, 1H), 6.53 (s, 1H), 4.48–4.35 (m, 1H), 3.93 (s, 3H), 3.90 (s, 3H), 3.63 (t, *J* = 4.5 Hz, 4H), 3.58 (s, 3H), 3.17–3.11 (m, 1H), 3.10 (d, *J* = 5.4 Hz, 3H), 3.07–2.99 (m, 1H), 2.83–2.76 (m, 1H), 2.75–2.69 (m, 1H), 2.51–2.33 (m, 7H), 1.99–1.91 (m, 1H).

^{13}C NMR (126 MHz, $CDCl_3$) δ 175.05, 155.45, 153.09, 150.89, 149.61, 141.54, 139.38, 134.35, 129.35, 129.06, 128.25, 126.38, 124.07, 108.00, 107.38, 61.37, 61.02, 56.09, 55.65, 53.37, 52.68, 51.08, 39.95, 30.38, 29.56.

3.4. *Single Crystal X-ray Measurement*

The single crystals of colchicine derivatives (**6**, **11**, **12**, **14**, **15**, **16**, **18** and **19**) were used for data collection on a four-circle KUMA KM4 diffractometer equipped with two-dimensional CCD area detector at room (295(1) K) and low temperature (100(1) K. The graphite monochromatized Mo-Kα radiation (λ = 0.71073 Å) and the ω-scan technique (Δω = 1°) were used for data collection. Lattice parameters were refined by the least-squares methods at all reflection positions. One image was monitored as a standard after every 40 images for a control of the crystal stability. Data collection and reduction along with absorption correction were performed using the CrysAlis software package [60]. The structures were solved by direct methods using SHELXT [61] giving positions of almost all non-hydrogen atoms. The structures were refined using SHELXL–2018 [62] with the anisotropic thermal displacement parameters. Hydrogen atoms were refined as rigid. Visualizations of the structures were made with the Diamond 3.0 program [63]. Details of the data collection parameters, crystallographic data and final agreement parameters are collected in Supplementary Table S1. The structures have been deposited with the Cambridge Crystallographic Data Center in the CIF format, no. CCDC 1980349–1980354 for **6**, **11**, **12**, CCDC 1980341–1980344 for **14** and **15**, CCDC 1980339–1980340 for **16** and CCDC 1980345–1980348 for **18** and **19** at 100 K and RT, respectively. Copies of this information can be obtained free of charge from The Director, CCDC, 12 Union Road, Cambridge, CB2 1EZ, UK (fax: +44 1223 336 033); email: deposit@ccdc.cam.ac.uk or www:http://www.ccdc.cam.ac.uk).

3.5. DFT Molecular Modeling

Molecular orbital calculations with full geometry optimization of colchicine derivatives (**6**, **11**, **12**, **14**, **15**, **16**, **18** and **19**) were performed with the Gaussian09 program package [52]. All calculations were carried out with the DFT level using the Becke3-Lee–Yang–Parr correlation functional (B3LYP) [53–56] with the 6–31+G basis set assuming the geometry resulting from the X-ray diffraction study as the starting structure. As convergence criteria, the threshold limits of 0.00025 and 0.0012 a.u. were applied for the maximum force and the displacement, respectively. The three-dimensional molecular electrostatic potential (3D MESP) maps are obtained on the basis of the DFT (B3LYP/6–31G) optimized. The calculated 3D MESP is mapped onto the total electron density isosurface (0.008 $eÅ^{-3}$) for each molecule. The color code of MESP maps is in the range of -0.05 $eÅ^{-1}$ (red) to $+0.05$ $eÅ^{-1}$ (blue).

3.6. In Vitro Antiproliferative Activity

3.6.1. Cell Lines and Culturing Conditions

Four human cancer cell lines and one murine normal cell line were used to evaluate antiproliferative activity of colchicine and its derivatives **1**–**21**: human lung adenocarcinoma (A549), human breast adenocarcinoma (MCF-7), human colon adenocarcinoma cell lines sensitive and resistant to doxorubicin (LoVo) and (LoVo/DX) respectively, and normal murine embryonic fibroblast cell line (BALB/3T3). The A549 cell line was purchased from the European Collection of Authenticated Cell Cultures (ECACC, Salisbury, UK). The MCF-7, LoVo and LoVo/DX cell lines was purchased from American Type Culture Collection (ATCC, Manassas, VA, USA). All the cell lines are maintained in the Institute of Immunology and Experimental Therapy (IIET), Wroclaw, Poland.

Human lung adenocarcinoma cell line was cultured in a mixture of OptiMEM and RPMI 1640 (1:1) medium (IIET, Wroclaw, Poland), supplemented with 5% fetal bovine serum HyClone (GE Healthcare, USA) and 2 mM L-glutamine (Sigma-Aldrich, Germany). Human breast adenocarcinoma cell line was cultured in a mixture of Eagle medium (IIET, Wroclaw, Poland), supplemented with 10% fetal bovine serum, 2 mM L-glutamine, 8 μg/mL insulin and 1% amino acids (Sigma-Aldrich, Germany). Human colon adenocarcinoma cell lines were cultured in a mixture of OptiMEM and RPMI 1640 (1:1) medium (IIET, Wroclaw, Poland), supplemented with 5% fetal bovine serum HyClone (GE Healthcare, USA), 2 mM L-glutamine, 1 mM sodium pyruvate (Sigma-Aldrich, Germany) and 10 μg/100 mL doxorubicin (Accord) for LoVo/DX. Murine embryonic fibroblast cells were cultured in Dulbecco medium (Gibco), supplemented with 10% fetal bovine serum (GE Healthcare, USA) and 2 mM L-glutamine (Sigma-Aldrich, Germany). All culture media contained antibiotics: 100 U/mL penicillin (Polfa-Tarchomin, Poland) and 0.1 mg/mL streptomycin (Sigma Aldrich, Germany). All cell lines were cultured during entire experiment in humid atmosphere at 37 °C and 5% CO_2.

3.6.2. Cell Viability Assays

Twenty-four hours before adding the tested compounds, all cell lines were seeded in 96-well plates (Sarstedt, Germany) in appropriate media with 0.5×10^4 cells per well for A549 cell line, 0.75×10^4 cells per well for MCF-7 cell line and 1.0×10^4 cells per well for LoVo, LoVo/DX and BALB/3T3 cell lines. All cell lines were exposed to each tested agent at different concentrations in the range 100–0.001 µg/mL for 72 h. The cells were also exposed to the reference drug cisplatin (Teva Pharmaceuticals, Poland) and doxorubicin (Accord Healthcare Limited, UK). Additionally, all cell lines were exposed to DMSO (solvent used for tested compounds) (POCh, Poland) at concentrations corresponding to those present in dilutions of tested agents. After 72 h sulforhodamine B assay (SRB) was performed [64].

SRB

After 72 h of incubation with the tested compounds, the cells were fixed in situ by gently adding of 50 µL per well of cold 50% trichloroacetic acid TCA (POCh, Poland) and were incubated at room temperature for one hour. Then the wells were washed four times with water and air dried. Next, 50 µL of 0.1% solution of sulforhodamine B (Sigma-Aldrich, Germany) in 1% acetic acid (POCh, Poland) were added to each well and were incubated at room temperature for 0.5 h. After incubation time, unbound dye was removed by washing plates four times with 1% acetic acid, whereas the stain bound to cells was solubilized with 150 µL of 10 mM Tris base (Sigma-Aldrich, Germany). Absorbance of each solution was read from a Synergy H4 Hybrid Multi-Mode Microplate Reader (BioTek Instruments, USA) at the 540 nm wavelength.

Results are presented as mean IC_{50} (concentration of the tested compound that inhibits cell proliferation by 50%) ± standard deviation. IC_{50} values were calculated in Cheburator 0.4, Dmitry Nevozhay software (version 1.2.0 software by Dmitry Nevozhay, 2004–2014, http://www.cheburator.nevozhay.com, freely available for each experiment [65]. Compounds at each concentration were tested in triplicates in a single experiment and each experiment was repeated at least three times independently. Results are summarized in Table 2.

3.7. Molecular Docking Studies

3.7.1. Ligand Preparation

The ligand structures were prepared using Ligprep from the Schrödinger suite [66]. Conformations and tautomeric states were assigned to the ligands by following the ligand preparation protocol implemented in Schrödinger suite with default settings. LigPrep generates variants of the same ligand with different tautomeric, stereochemical, and ionization properties.

3.7.2. Tubulin Model

The tubulin crystal structures available in the PDB are those for bovine protein. The bovine tubulin structure of tubulin (PDB ID: 1SA0) [67] was used as a template to construct the homology model of human αβ-tubulin isotypes (βI (UniProtKb: P07437), which is the most abundant isotype in most tumors using the Molecular Operating Environment (MOE) software package [68]. The sequence corresponding to the gene TUBA1A (UniProt ID: Q71U36) was chosen as a reference sequence for human tubulin, whereas gene TUBB associated to I isoform (UniProt ID: P07437) was chosen for human tubulin. Homology modeling was performed using MOE by setting the number of generated models to 10 and by selecting the final model based on MOE's generalized Born/volume integral (GB/VI) scoring function. The models used in the simulations performed for the present study were developed earlier and described in our previous publications [69]. These earlier investigations can also be considered to be validations of the computational model employed here since they were directly compared to the corresponding experimental data.

3.7.3. Molecular Dynamics Simulations

The missing hydrogens for heavy atoms were added using the tLEAP module of AMBER 14 with the AMBER14SB force field [70]. The protonation states of all ionizable residues were determined at pH = 7 using the MOE program [68]. Each protein model was solvated in a 12 Å box of TIP3P water. In order to bring the salt concentration to the physiological value of 0.15 M, 93 Na^+ ions and 57 Cl^- ions were added. Minimization of the structure was carried out in two steps, using the steepest descent and conjugate gradient methods successively. At first, minimization was made in 2 ps on solvent atoms only, by restraining the protein-ligand complex. Next, minimization was run without the restraint in 10 ps. After minimization, the molecular dynamics (MD) simulations were carried out in three steps: heating, density equilibration, and production. At first, each solvated system was heated to 298 K for 50 ps, with weak restraints on all backbone atoms. Next, density equilibration was carried out for 50 ps of constant pressure equilibration at 298 K, with weak restraints. Finally, MD production runs were performed for all systems for 70 ns. The root-mean-square deviation (RMSD) of both the entire tubulin structure and the colchicine binding site were found to reach a plateau after 40 ns. Clustering analysis of the last 30 ns of the generated MD trajectory was carried out using the Amber's CPPTRAJ program [71] to identify representative conformations of the tubulin dimer. Clustering was made via the hierarchical agglomerative approach using the RMSD of atoms in the colchicine binding site as a metric. An RMSD cutoff of 1.0 Å was set to differentiate the clusters. On the basis of the clustering analysis, three representative structures of the tubulin dimer were found. The docking was performed on all the three representative structures and the one with the highest docking score was selected, which was the largest cluster (about 70% of the simulation) conformation of the tubulin structure. During the modeling, the cofactors including GTP, GDP, colchicine, and the magnesium ion located at the interface between α–and β–monomers were kept as part of the environment and included in the refinement step.

3.7.4. Docking Simulations

We used the AutoDock Vina [72] program to predict the binding pose of the ligands under flexible ligand and rigid receptor conditions. Dockbox package was used to facilitate preparing docking inputs and post-processing of the docking results [73]. Docking simulations performed with a cubic box (size 30.0 Å) were centered at the center of binding pockets and the docking was run separately on tubulin structure. Every generated pose was energy-minimized using Amber14 by keeping the protein fixed and was re-scored using the MOE's GBVI/WSA dG scoring function [68]. No constraints were applied in the docking studies. For each compound/protein-structure pair, the pose with the best score was identified and used as an initial configuration for molecular mechanics Gibbs–Boltzmann surface area MM/GBSA computations.

3.7.5. Binding Energy and Pairwise Per-Residue Free Energy Decomposition Calculations Using MM/GBSA Method

The MM/GBSA technique is used to calculate the free energy associated with the binding of double modified colchicine amides and sulfonamides [74]. This method combines molecular mechanics with continuum solvation models. We performed MM-GBSA integrated in Amber. The binding free energy is estimated as:

$$\Delta G_{bind} = \overline{G}_{complex} - \left[\overline{G}_{protein} + \overline{G}_{ligand}\right] \quad (1)$$

where G is the average free energy of the complex, protein, and ligand, are calculated according to the equation:

$$\overline{G} = \overline{E}_{M+}\overline{G}_{solvation} - T\overline{S} \quad (2)$$

where EMM are determined with the SANDER program and represent the internal energy (bond, angle, and dihedral), van der Waals and electrostatic interactions (see Equation (3)). TS is the entropy contribution estimated using normal mode (nmode) analysis.

$$\overline{E}_M = \overline{E}_{int} + \overline{E}_{elec} + \overline{E}_{vdW} \quad (3)$$

The solvation free energy can be calculated as the sum of polar and nonpolar contributions. The polar parts are obtained by using the generalized-born (GB) model—resulting in the MM/GBSA method, whereas the nonpolar terms are estimated from a linear relation (Equation (4)) to the solvent accessible surface area (SASA).

$$\overline{G}_{non-polar} = \gamma\ SASA + b \quad (4)$$

In the present study, a 2 ns-duration MD trajectory was run in TIP3P water using Amber14, for every top pose generated at the end of the docking step. It is worth noting that to assess the performance of MM/GBSA methodology [75], we evaluated the prediction accuracy of this method by various simulation protocols including 1 ns MD production calculations using PDBbind data set. Too long an MD simulation could be prejudicious for the overall success of the MM/GBSA method. According to this study and the common practice to calculate binding energies using MM/GBSA, we have decided to run MD production simulation for 2 ns. The MM/GBSA calculations were performed on a subset of 200 frames collected at regular time intervals from the trajectory. For PB calculations, an ionic strength of 0.0 nM (istrng = 0.0) and a solvent probe radius of 1.6 Å (prbrad = 1.6) were used. For GB calculations, the igb parameter was set to 5 that corresponds to a modified GB model equivalent to model II in reference. Pairwise free energy decomposition analysis was performed using the MM/GBSA decomposition process by the MM/GBSA program in AMBER 14 to compute the interaction between the inhibitors and each residue. For each of the tested compounds, the active residues estimated from MM/GBSA decomposition process and the best GB score out of the trajectories associated with the representative structures of the tubulin dimer were collected and are reported in Table 3 and Figure 4.

3.8. Calculation clogP

We used the Molinspiration online database (http://www.molinspiration.com, free of charge) to predict the *clogP* values for all synthesized compounds and collected them in Table 3 [76].

4. Conclusions

In an attempt to discover novel potent inhibitors of microtubule dynamics, eighteen novel double modified colchicine analogs comprising methylamine substituent at position C10 of ring C and amide or sulfonamide substituents at position C7 of ring B were successfully synthesized, purified and their structures were confirmed by spectroscopic analyses as well as X-ray measurements. Four human cancer cell lines (A549, MCF-7, LoVo, LoVo/DX) were used to evaluate the anticancer potency of all synthesized compounds.

Compared with unmodified colchicine, the majority of its studied derivatives exhibited excellent potency against A549, MCF-7, and LoVo cell lines. The antiproliferative activity of colchicine derivatives was in the nanomolar range and they also were characterized by lower IC_{50} values also than doxorubicin and cisplatin, commonly used as antitumor agents in cancer chemotherapy. The preliminary SAR revealed that the type of substituent at position C7 in ring B and the presence of $-NHCH_3$ group at position C10 in ring C of colchicine **1** were of cardinal importance to the compounds' cytotoxicity.

The calculated values of the selectivity index (SI) clearly show that it is possible to design more selective compounds than colchicine **1**. The most active double-modified colchicine derivatives were the compounds that included chloroacetamide and dichloroacetamide (**9**, **10**) and 2–chlorobenzamide (**13**) moiety (Table 2). However, in vitro tests showed that they did not have high SI values (except towards the LoVo cells) and *in vivo* testing should be carried out to determine their therapeutic potential.

But of all tested compounds, 4,4,4-trifluorobutyric amide of 10-*N*-methylaminocolchicine **11** was the most prominent. Compound **11** showed high activity towards A549, MCF7 and LoVo cell lines, with antiproliferative IC_{50} values ranging between 10.4 and 14.6 nM as well as SI values higher than 5 for these three cell lines. The most selective towards MCF-7 cell line was compound **17** (SI was almost 10) and towards LoVo cell line the most selective were compounds **7**, **9**, **10**, and **13** (SI were over 6). So we conclude that the appropriate modification of colchicine molecule and synthesis of its analogs might overcome the toxicity, which is a major challenge in designing a potential colchicine-based drug candidate.

Compound **11** was subsequently identified as the that with potentially the best therapeutic index and therefore the most promising candidate for further development, as it showed strong in vitro anticancer activities with high SI against three human cancer cell lines. However, further in vivo studies should be conducted for the successful development of this compound.

Molecular docking study showed the ability of the obtained colchicine derivatives to bind into the active sites of βI-tubulin isotype with the well-defined binding modes. It is worthy to mention that 10-*N*-methylaminocolchicine based compounds serve as useful templates for the further development of the anticancer and antimitotic agents. Further evaluation should help to find more detailed structure-activity relationships of microtubule-targeting drugs and CBS inhibitors, which can help in rational drug design in future.

Supplementary Materials: The following are available online, Table S1: Details of the data collection parameters, crystallographic data and the final agreement parameters. (for compounds **6**, **11**, **12**, **14**, **15**, **16**, **18** and **19**); Table S2: Optimized parameters for colchicine derivatives (**6**, **11**, **12**, **14**, **15**, **16**, **18** and **19**), Figure S1: The LC-MS chromatogram and mass spectra of **2**; Figure S2: The ^{1}H NMR spectrum of **2** in $CDCl_3$; Figure S3: The ^{13}C NMR spectrum of **2** in $CDCl_3$; Figure S4: The LC-MS chromatogram and mass spectra of **3**; Figure S5: The ^{1}H NMR spectrum of **3** in $CDCl_3$; Figure S6: The ^{13}C NMR spectrum of **3** in $CDCl_3$; Figure S7: The LC-MS chromatogram and mass spectra of **4**; Figure S8: The ^{1}H NMR spectrum of **4** in $CDCl_3$, Figure S9: The ^{13}C NMR spectrum of **4** in $CDCl_3$, Figure S10: The LC-MS chromatogram and mass spectra of **5**; Figure S11: The ^{1}H NMR spectrum of **5** in $CDCl_3$, Figure S12: The ^{13}C NMR spectrum of **5** in $CDCl_3$; Figure S13: The LC-MS chromatogram and mass spectra of **6**; Figure S14: The ^{1}H NMR spectrum of **6** in $CDCl_3$; Figure S15: The ^{13}C NMR spectrum of **6** in $CDCl_3$; Figure S16: The LC-MS chromatogram and mass spectra of **7**; Figure S17: The ^{1}H NMR spectrum of **7** in $CDCl_3$; Figure S18: The ^{13}C NMR spectrum of **7** in $CDCl_3$; Figure S19: The LC-MS chromatogram and mass spectra of **8**; Figure S20: The ^{1}H NMR spectrum of **8** in $CDCl_3$; Figure S21:. The ^{13}C NMR spectrum of **8** in $CDCl_3$; Figure S22: The LC-MS chromatogram and mass spectra of **9**; Figure S23: The ^{1}H NMR spectrum of **9** in $CDCl_3$; Figure S24: The ^{13}C NMR spectrum of **9** in $CDCl_3$; Figure S25: The LC-MS chromatogram and mass spectra of **10**; Figure S26: The ^{1}H NMR spectrum of **10** in $CDCl_3$; Figure S27: The ^{13}C NMR spectrum of **10** in $CDCl_3$; Figure S28. The LC-MS chromatogram and mass spectra of **11**; Figure S29. The ^{1}H NMR spectrum of **11** in $CDCl_3$; Figure S30: The ^{13}C NMR spectrum of **11** in $CDCl_3$; Figure S31. The LC-MS chromatogram and mass spectra of **12**; Figure S32: The ^{1}H NMR spectrum of **12** in $CDCl_3$; Figure S33: The ^{13}C NMR spectrum of **12** in $CDCl_3$; Figure S34: The LC-MS chromatogram and mass spectra of **13**; Figure S35: The ^{1}H NMR spectrum of **13** in CD_2Cl_2; Figure S36: The ^{13}C NMR spectrum of **13** in CD_2Cl_2. Figure S37: The LC-MS chromatogram and mass spectra of **14**; Figure S38: The ^{1}H NMR spectrum of **14** in $CDCl_3$; Figure S39: The ^{13}C NMR spectrum of **14** in $CDCl_3$; Figure S40: The LC-MS chromatogram and mass spectra of **15**; Figure S41: The ^{1}H NMR spectrum of **15** in $CDCl_3$; Figure S42: The ^{13}C NMR spectrum of **15** in $CDCl_3$; Figure S43: The LC-MS chromatogram and mass spectra of **16**; Figure S44: The ^{1}H NMR spectrum of **16** in $CDCl_3$. Figure S45: The ^{13}C NMR spectrum of **16** in $CDCl_3$; Figure S46: The LC-MS chromatogram and mass spectra of **17**; Figure S47: The ^{1}H NMR spectrum of **17** in $CDCl_3$; Figure S48: The LC-MS chromatogram and mass spectra of **18**;Figure S49: The ^{1}H NMR spectrum of **18** in $CDCl_3$; Figure S50: The ^{13}C NMR spectrum of **18** in $CDCl_3$; Figure S51: The LC-MS chromatogram and mass spectra of **19**; Figure S52: The ^{1}H NMR spectrum of **19** in $(CD_3)_2SO$; Figure S53: The ^{13}C NMR spectrum of **19** in $(CD_3)_2SO$; Figure S54: The LC-MS chromatogram and mass spectra of **20**; Figure S55: The ^{1}H NMR spectrum of **20** in $CDCl_3$. Figure S56: The ^{13}C NMR spectrum of **20** in $CDCl_3$; Figure S57: The LC-MS chromatogram and mass spectra of **21**; Figure S58: The ^{1}H NMR spectrum of **21** in $CDCl_3$. Figure S59: The ^{13}C NMR spectrum of **21** in $CDCl_3$; Figure S60: Molecular structure of colchicine derivatives (**6**, **11**, **12**, **14**, **15**, **16**, **18** and **19**) at 295 K and 100 K.

Author Contributions: Conceptualization, J.K., and A.H.; methodology, J.K., A.H., J.J., J.W. and J.A.T.; software, J.J.; M.A.; validation, A.H., J.A.T. and J.J.; formal analysis, A.H. and J.K.; investigation, J.K., E.M., J.J. and M.A; resources, A.H.; J.K. and W.M.; data curation, J.K., M.A. and E.M.; writing—original draft preparation, J.K., J.J. and M.A.; writing—review and editing, W.M., A.H. J.W. and J.A.T.; visualization, J.K., J.J. and M.A.; supervision,

A.H.; project administration, A.H.; funding acquisition, A.H. and W.M. All authors have read and agreed to the published version of the manuscript.

Acknowledgments: Financial support by a grant No. 2016/21/B/ST5/00111 of the Polish National Science Centre (NCN) –is gratefully acknowledged. JAT gratefully acknowledges research support from NSERC and the Allard Foundation for his research.

Conflicts of Interest: The authors declare no conflict of interest.

References

1. Amos, L.A. Microtubule structure and its stabilisation. *Org. Biomol. Chem.* **2004**, *2*, 2153–2160. [CrossRef] [PubMed]
2. Wade, R.H. On and around microtubules: An overview. *Mol. Biotechnol.* **2009**, *43*, 177–191. [CrossRef] [PubMed]
3. Hawkins, T.; Mirigian, M.; Selcuk Yasar, M.; Ross, J.L. Mechanics of microtubules. *J. Biomech.* **2010**, *43*, 23–30. [CrossRef] [PubMed]
4. Wittmann, T.; Hyman, A.; Desai, A. The spindle: A dynamic assembly of microtubules and motors. *Nat. Cell Biol.* **2001**, *3*. [CrossRef]
5. Jordan, M.A.; Wilson, L. Microtubules and actin filaments: Dynamic targets for cancer chemotherapy. *Curr. Opin. Cell Biol.* **1998**, *10*, 123–130. [CrossRef]
6. Pellegrini, F.; Budman, D.R. Review: Tubulin function, action of antitubulin drugs, and new drug development. *Cancer Invest.* **2005**, *23*, 264–273. [CrossRef]
7. Kumar, B.; Kumar, R.; Skvortsova, I.; Kumar, V. Mechanisms of Tubulin Binding Ligands to Target Cancer Cells: Updates on their Therapeutic Potential and Clinical Trials. *Curr. Cancer Drug Targets* **2016**, *17*, 357–375. [CrossRef]
8. Capraro, H.G.; Brossi, A. Chapter 1 Tropolonic Colchicum Alkaloids. *Alkaloids Chem. Pharmacol.* **1984**, *23*, 1–70.
9. Boyé, O.; Brossi, A. Tropolonic Colchicum Alkaloids and Allo Congeners. *Alkaloids Chem. Pharmacol.* **1992**, *41*, 125–176.
10. Hastie, S.B. Interactions of colchicine with tubulin. *Pharmacol. Ther.* **1991**, *51*, 377–401. [CrossRef]
11. Sapra, S.; Bhalla, Y.; Nandani Sharma, S.; Singh, G.; Nepali, K.; Budhiraja, A.; Dhar, K.L. Colchicine and its various physicochemical and biological aspects. *Med. Chem. Res.* **2013**, *22*, 531–547. [CrossRef]
12. Skoufias, D.A.; Wilson, L. Mechanism of Inhibition of Microtubule Polymerization by Colchicine: Inhibitory Potencies of Unliganded Colchicine and Tubulin-Colchicine Complexes. *Biochemistry* **1992**, *31*, 738–746. [CrossRef] [PubMed]
13. Bhattacharyya, B.; Panda, D.; Gupta, S.; Banerjee, M. Anti-mitotic activity of colchicine and the structural basis for its interaction with tubulin. *Med. Res. Rev.* **2008**, *28*, 155–183. [CrossRef] [PubMed]
14. Ravelli, R.B.G.; Gigant, B.; Curmi, P.A.; Jourdain, I.; Lachkar, S.; Sobel, A.; Knossow, M. Insight into tubulin regulation from a complex with colchicine and a stathmin-like domain. *Nature* **2004**, *428*, 198–202. [CrossRef]
15. Wiesenfeld, P.L.; Garthoff, L.H.; Sobotka, T.J.; Suagee, J.K.; Barton, C.N. Acute oral toxicity of colchicine in rats: Effects of gender, vehicle matrix and pre-exposure to lipopolysaccharide. *J. Appl. Toxicol.* **2007**, *27*, 421–433. [CrossRef]
16. Spiller, H.A. Colchicine. In *Encyclopedia of Toxicology*, 3rd ed.; Wexler, P., Ed.; Elsevier Inc.: London, UK, 2014; pp. 1007–1008.
17. Roubille, F.; Kritikou, E.; Busseuil, D.; Barrere-Lemaire, S.; Tardif, J.-C. Colchicine: An Old Wine in a New Bottle? *Antiinflamm. Antiallergy. Agents Med. Chem.* **2013**, *12*, 14–23. [CrossRef]
18. Mendis, S. Colchicine cardiotoxicity following ingestion of Gloriosa superba tubers. *Postgrad. Med. J.* **1989**, *65*, 752–755. [CrossRef] [PubMed]
19. Margolis, R.L.; Wilson, L. Addition of colchicine tubulin complex to microtubule ends: The mechanism of substoichiometric colchicine poisoning. *Proc. Natl. Acad. Sci. USA* **1977**, *74*, 3466–3470. [CrossRef]
20. Kuncl, R.W.; Duncan, G.; Watson, D.; Alderson, K.; Rogawski, M.A.; Peper, M. Colchicine Myopathy and Neuropathy. *N. Engl. J. Med.* **1987**, *316*, 1562–1568. [CrossRef]
21. Finkelstein, Y.; Aks, S.E.; Hutson, J.R.; Juurlink, D.N.; Nguyen, P.; Dubnov-Raz, G.; Pollak, U.; Koren, G.; Bentur, Y. Colchicine poisoning: The dark side of an ancient drug. *Clin. Toxicol.* **2010**, *48*, 407–414. [CrossRef]
22. Cocco, G.; Chu, D.C.C.; Pandolfi, S. Colchicine in clinical medicine. A guide for internists. *Eur. J. Intern. Med.* **2010**, *21*, 503–508. [CrossRef] [PubMed]
23. Zemer, D.; Revach, M.; Pras, M.; Modan, B.; Schor, S.; Sohar, E.; Gafni, J. A Controlled Trial of Colchicine in Preventing Attacks of Familial Mediterranean Fever. *N. Engl. J. Med.* **1974**, *291*, 932–934. [CrossRef] [PubMed]

24. Cerquaglia, C.; Diaco, M.; Nucera, G.; La Regina, M.; Montalto, M.; Manna, R. Pharmacological and clinical basis of treatment of Familial Mediterranean Fever (FMF) with colchicine or analogues: An update. *Curr. Drug Targets Inflamm. Allergy* **2005**, *4*, 117–124. [CrossRef] [PubMed]
25. Masuda, K.; Urayama, A.; Kogure, M.; Nakajima, A.; Nakae, K.; Inaba, G. Double-masked trial of cyclosporin versus colchicine and long-term open study of cyclosporin in Behçet's disease. *Lancet* **1989**, *333*, 1093–1096. [CrossRef]
26. Keith, M.P.; Gilliland, W.R. Updates in the Management of Gout. *Am. J. Med.* **2007**, *120*, 221–224. [CrossRef]
27. Hitzeman, N.; Stephens, R. Colchicine for acute gout. *Am. Fam. Physician* **2015**, *91*, 759–760. [PubMed]
28. Kerekes, P.; Sharma, P.N.; Brossi, A.; Chignell, C.F.; Quinn, F.R. Synthesis and Biological Effects of Novel Thiocolchicines. 3. Evaluation of *N*-Acyldeacetylthiocolchicines, *N*-(Alkoxycarbonyl)deacetylthiocolchicines, and O-Ethyldemethylthiocolchicines. New Synthesis of Thiodemecolcine and Antileukemic Effects of 2-Demeth. *J. Med. Chem.* **1985**, *28*, 1204–1208. [CrossRef]
29. Sun, L.; Hamel, E.; Lin, C.M.; Hastie, S.B.; Pyluck, A.; Lee, K.H. Antitumor Agents. 141. Synthesis and Biological Evaluation of Novel Thiocolchicine Analogs: *N*-Acyl-, *N*-Aroyl-, and *N*-(Substituted benzyl)deacetylthiocolchicines as Potent Cytotoxic and Antimitotic Compounds. *J. Med. Chem.* **1993**, *36*, 1474–1479. [CrossRef]
30. Majcher, U.; Urbaniak, A.; Maj, E.; Moshari, M.; Delgado, M.; Wietrzyk, J.; Bartl, F.; Chambers, T.C.; Tuszynski, J.A.; Huczyński, A. Synthesis, antiproliferative activity and molecular docking of thiocolchicine urethanes. *Bioorg. Chem.* **2018**, *81*, 553–566. [CrossRef]
31. Marzo-Mas, A.; Falomir, E.; Murga, J.; Carda, M.; Marco, J.A. Effects on tubulin polymerization and down-regulation of c-Myc, hTERT and VEGF genes by colchicine haloacetyl and haloaroyl derivatives. *Eur. J. Med. Chem.* **2018**, *150*, 591–600. [CrossRef]
32. Shen, L.H.; Li, H.Y.; Shang, H.X.; Tian, S.T.; Lai, Y.S.; Liu, L.J. Synthesis and cytotoxic evaluation of new colchicine derivatives bearing 1,3,4-thiadiazole moieties. *Chinese Chem. Lett.* **2013**, *24*, 299–302. [CrossRef]
33. Shen, L.H.; Li, Y.; Zhang, D.H.; Lai, Y.S.; Liu, L.J. Synthesis and evaluation of nitrate derivatives of colchicine as anticancer agents. *Chinese Chem. Lett.* **2011**, *22*, 768–770. [CrossRef]
34. Shen, L.H.; Wang, S.L.; Li, H.Y.; Lai, Y.S.; Liu, L.J. Synthesis and bioactivity of furoxan-based nitric oxide-releasing colchicine derivatives as anticancer agents. *Asian, J. Chem.* **2013**, *25*, 3294–3296. [CrossRef]
35. Kim, S.K.; Cho, S.M.; Kim, H.; Seok, H.; Kim, S.O.; Kwon, T.K.; Chang, J.S. The colchicine derivative CT20126 shows a novel microtubule-modulating activity with apoptosis. *Exp. Mol. Med.* **2013**, *45*, e19-e7. [CrossRef]
36. Lee, S.H.; Park, S.K.; Kim, J.M.; Kim, M.H.; Kim, K.H.; Chun, K.W.; Cho, K.H.; Youn, J.Y.; Namgoong, S.K. New synthetic thiocolchicine derivatives as low-toxic anticancer agents. *Arch. Pharm. (Weinheim)* **2005**, *338*, 582–589. [CrossRef]
37. Saeedi, M.; Goli, F.; Mahdavi, M.; Dehghan, G.; Faramarzi, M.A.; Foroumadi, A.; Shafiee, A. Synthesis and biological investigation of some novel sulfonamide and amide derivatives containing coumarin moieties. *Iran. J. Pharm. Res.* **2014**, *13*, 881–892.
38. Ashraf, Z.; Mahmood, T.; Hassan, M.; Afzal, S.; Rafique, H.; Afzal, K.; Latip, J. Dexibuprofen amide derivatives as potential anticancer agents: Synthesis, in silico docking, bioevaluation, and molecular dynamic simulation. *Drug Des. Devel. Ther.* **2019**, *13*, 1643–1657. [CrossRef]
39. Ragha Suma, V.; Sreenivasulu, R.; Subramanyam, M.; Rao, K.R.M. Design, Synthesis, and Anticancer Activity of Amide Derivatives of Structurally Modified Combretastatin-A4. *Russ. J. Gen. Chem.* **2019**, *89*, 499–504. [CrossRef]
40. Kachaeva, M.V.; Hodyna, D.M.; Semenyuta, I.V.; Pilyo, S.G.; Prokopenko, V.M.; Kovalishyn, V.V.; Metelytsia, L.O.; Brovarets, V.S. Design, synthesis and evaluation of novel sulfonamides as potential anticancer agents. *Comput. Biol. Chem.* **2018**, *74*, 294–303. [CrossRef]
41. Gul, H.I.; Yamali, C.; Sakagami, H.; Angeli, A.; Leitans, J.; Kazaks, A.; Tars, K.; Ozgun, D.O.; Supuran, C.T. New anticancer drug candidates sulfonamides as selective hCA IX or hCA XII inhibitors. *Bioorg. Chem.* **2018**, *77*, 411–419. [CrossRef]
42. Kiyoshi, A. N-methyldeacetylcolchiceinamide. Patent EP0607647(A1), 27 July 1994.
43. Winum, J.Y.; Toupet, L.; Barragan, V.; Dewynter, G.; Montero, J.L. N-(tert-Butoxycarbonyl)-N-[4-(dimethylazaniumylidene)-1,4-dihydropyridin-1-ylsulfonyl]azanide: A new sulfamoylating agent. Structure and reactivity toward amines. *Org. Lett.* **2001**, *3*, 2241–2243. [CrossRef] [PubMed]

44. Al-Riyami, L.; Pineda, M.A.; Rzepecka, J.; Huggan, J.K.; Khalaf, A.I.; Suckling, C.J.; Scott, F.J.; Rodgers, D.T.; Harnett, M.M.; Harnett, W. Designing anti-inflammatory drugs from parasitic worms: A synthetic small molecule analogue of the acanthocheilonema viteae product ES-62 prevents development of collagen-induced arthritis. *J. Med. Chem.* **2013**, *56*, 9982–10002. [CrossRef] [PubMed]
45. Cruz, C.M.; Ortega-Muñoz, M.; López-Jaramillo, F.J.; Hernández-Mateo, F.; Blanco, V.; Santoyo-González, F. Vinyl Sulfonates: A Click Function for Coupling-and-Decoupling Chemistry and their Applications. *Adv. Synth. Catal.* **2016**, *358*, 3394–3413. [CrossRef]
46. Lessinger, L.; Margulis, T.N. The crystal structure of colchicine. A new application of magic integers to multiple-solution direct methods. *Acta Crystallogr. Sect. B Struct. Crystallogr. Cryst. Chem.* **1978**, *34*, 578–584. [CrossRef]
47. McClure, W.O.; Paulson, J.C. The interaction of colchicine and some related alkaloids with rat brain tubulin. *Mol. Pharmacol.* **1977**, *13*, 560–575. [PubMed]
48. Hastie, S.B.; Williams, R.C.; Puett, D.; Macdonald, T.L. The binding of isocolchicine to tubulin. Mechanisms of ligand association with tubulin. *J. Biol. Chem.* **1989**, *264*, 6682–6688.
49. Politzer, P.; Laurence, P.R.; Jayasuriya, K. Molecular electrostatic potentials: An effective tool for the elucidation of biochemical phenomena. *Environ. Health Perspect.* **1985**, *61*, 191–202. [CrossRef]
50. Chemical Applications of Atomic and Molecular Electrostatic Potentials. Available online: https://www.springer.com/gp/book/9780306406577 (accessed on 13 April 2020).
51. Murray, J.S.; Politzer, P. The electrostatic potential: An overview. *Wiley Interdiscip. Rev. Comput. Mol. Sci.* **2011**, *1*, 153–163. [CrossRef]
52. Frisch, M.J.; Trucks, G.W.; Schlegel, H.B.; Scuseria, G.E.; Robb, M.A.; Cheeseman, J.R.; Scalmani, G.; Barone, V.; Mennucci, B.; Petersson, G.A.; et al. *Gaussian 09, Revision E.01.*; Gaussian, Inc: Wallingford, CT, USA, 2013.
53. Becke, A.D. Density-functional thermochemistry. IV. A new dynamical correlation functional and implications for exact-exchange mixing. *J. Chem. Phys.* **1996**, *104*, 1040–1046. [CrossRef]
54. Lee, C.; Yang, W.; Parr, R.G. Development of the Colle-Salvetti correlation-energy formula into a functional of the electron density. *Phys. Rev. B* **1988**, *37*, 785–789. [CrossRef]
55. Patterson, J.D. Density-functional theory of atoms and molecules. *Ann. Nucl. Energy* **1989**, *16*, 611. [CrossRef]
56. Bai, R.; Pei, X.F.; Boyé, O.; Getahun, Z.; Grover, S.; Bekisz, J.; Nguyen, N.Y.; Brossi, A.; Hamel, E. Identification of cysteine 354 of β-tubulin as part of the binding site for the a ring of colchicine. *J. Biol. Chem.* **1996**, *271*, 12639–12645. [CrossRef] [PubMed]
57. Chaudhuri, A.R.; Seetharamalu, P.; Schwarz, P.M.; Hausheer, F.H.; Ludueña, R.F. The interaction of the B-ring of colchicine with α-Tubulin: A novel footprinting approach. *J. Mol. Biol.* **2000**, *303*, 679–692. [CrossRef] [PubMed]
58. Cheung, C.H.A.; Wu, S.Y.; Lee, T.R.; Chang, C.Y.; Wu, J.S.; Hsieh, H.P.; Chang, J.Y. Cancer cells acquire mitotic drug resistance properties through beta i-tubulin mutations and alterations in the expression of beta-tubulin isotypes. *PLoS ONE* **2010**, *5*, 1–11. [CrossRef]
59. Ravanbakhsh, S.; Gajewski, M.; Greiner, R.; Tuszynski, J.A. Determination of the optimal tubulin isotype target as a method for the development of individualized cancer chemotherapy. *Theor. Biol. Med. Model.* **2013**. [CrossRef] [PubMed]
60. *CrysAlis CCD and CrysAlis RED, version 1171.32.15*; Oxford Diffraction Ltd: Abingdon, Oxford, UK, 2009.
61. Sheldrick, G.M. SHELXT-Integrated space-group and crystal-structure determination. *Acta Crystallogr. Sect. A Found. Crystallogr.* **2015**, *71*, 3–8. [CrossRef]
62. Sheldrick, G.M. Crystal structure refinement with SHELXL. *Acta Crystallogr. Sect. C Struct. Chem.* **2015**, *71*, 3–8. [CrossRef]
63. Brandenburg, K.; Putz, H. *DIAMOND*; Crystal Impact GbR: Bonn, Germany, 2006.
64. Skehan, P.; Storeng, R.; Scudiero, D.; Monks, A.; Mcmahon, J.; Vistica, D.; Warren, J.T.; Bokesch, H.; Kenney, S.; Boyd, M.R. New colorimetric cytotoxicity assay for anticancer-drug screening. *J. Natl. Cancer Inst.* **1990**, *82*, 1107–1112. [CrossRef]
65. Nevozhay, D. Cheburator software for automatically calculating drug inhibitory concentrations from in vitroscreening assays. *PLoS ONE* **2014**, *9*, e106186. [CrossRef]
66. Schrödinger Schrödinger Release 2019–4: LigPrep. 2019. Available online: https://www.schrodinger.com/ligprep (accessed on 13 April 2020).
67. Löwe, J.; Li, H.; Downing, K.H.; Nogales, E. Refined structure of αβ-tubulin at 3.5 Å resolution. *J. Mol. Biol.* **2001**, *313*, 1045–1057. [CrossRef]
68. *Molecular Operating Environment (MOE)*; Chemical Computing Group Inc: Montreal, QC, Canada, 2012.

69. Klejborowska, G.; Urbaniak, A.; Maj, E.; Preto, J.; Moshari, M.; Wietrzyk, J.; Tuszynski, J.A.; Chambers, T.C.; Huczyński, A. Synthesis, biological evaluation and molecular docking studies of new amides of 4-chlorothiocolchicine as anticancer agents. *Bioorg. Chem.* **2020**, *97*. [CrossRef]
70. Case, D.; Babin, V.; Berryman, J.; Betz, R.; Cai, Q.; Cerutti, D.; Cheatham, T., III; Darden, T.; Duke, R.; Gohlke, H.; et al. *Amber 14*; University of California: San Francisco, CA, USA, 2014.
71. Roe, D.R.; Cheatham, T.E. PTRAJ and CPPTRAJ: Software for processing and analysis of molecular dynamics trajectory data. *J. Chem. Theory Comput.* **2013**, *9*, 3084–3095. [CrossRef] [PubMed]
72. Trott, O.; Olson, A.J. Software news and update AutoDock Vina: Improving the speed and accuracy of docking with a new scoring function, efficient optimization, and multithreading. *J. Comput. Chem.* **2010**, *31*, 455–461.
73. Preto, J.; Gentile, F. Assessing and improving the performance of consensus docking strategies using the DockBox package. *J. Comput. Aided. Mol. Des.* **2019**, *33*, 817–829. [CrossRef] [PubMed]
74. Hou, T.; Wang, J.; Li, Y.; Wang, W. Assessing the performance of the MM/PBSA and MM/GBSA methods. 1. The accuracy of binding free energy calculations based on molecular dynamics simulations. *J. Chem. Inf. Model.* **2011**, *51*, 69–82. [CrossRef] [PubMed]
75. Sun, H.; Duan, L.; Chen, F.; Liu, H.; Wang, Z.; Pan, P.; Zhu, F.; Zhang, J.Z.H.; Hou, T. Assessing the performance of MM/PBSA and MM/GBSA methods. 7. Entropy effects on the performance of end-point binding free energy calculation approaches. *Phys. Chem. Chem. Phys.* **2018**, *20*, 14450–14460. [CrossRef]
76. Molinspiration Property Calculation Service. Available online: http://www.molinspiration.com (accessed on 3 April 2020).

Sample Availability: Not available

molecules

MDPI

Article

Overcoming Resistance to Platinum-Based Drugs in Ovarian Cancer by Salinomycin and Its Derivatives—An In Vitro Study

Marcin Michalak [1], Michał Stefan Lach [2,3,4,*], Michał Antoszczak [5], Adam Huczyński [5] and Wiktoria Maria Suchorska [2,4,*]

1 Department of Radiation Therapy and Gynecologic Oncology, Greater Poland Cancer Centre, Garbary 15, 61–866 Poznań, Poland; marcin.michalak@wco.pl
2 Radiobiology Lab, Greater Poland Cancer Centre, Garbary 15, 61–866 Poznań, Poland
3 The Postgraduate School of Molecular Medicine, Medical University of Warsaw, Księcia Trojdena 2a, 02–109 Warsaw, Poland
4 Department of Electroradiology, Poznań University of Medical Sciences, Garbary 15, 61–866 Poznań, Poland
5 Department of Medical Chemistry, Faculty of Chemistry, Adam Mickiewicz University, Uniwersytetu Poznańskiego 8, 61–614 Poznań, Poland; michant@amu.edu.pl (M.A.); adhucz@amu.edu.pl (A.H.)
* Correspondence: michal.lach@wco.pl (M.S.L.); wiktoria.suchorska@wco.pl (W.M.S.); Tel.: +48-61-8850-474 (M.S.L. & W.M.S.)

Received: 12 November 2019; Accepted: 24 January 2020; Published: 26 January 2020

Abstract: Polyether ionophore salinomycin (SAL) and its semi-synthetic derivatives are recognized as very promising anticancer drug candidates due to their activity against various types of cancer cells, including multidrug-resistant populations. Ovarian cancer is the deadliest among gynecologic malignancies, which is connected with the development of chemoresistant forms of the disease in over 70% of patients after initial treatment regimen. Thus, we decided to examine the anticancer properties of SAL and selected SAL derivatives against a series of drug-sensitive (A2780, SK-OV-3) and derived drug-resistant (A2780 CDDP, SK-OV-3 CDDP) ovarian cancer cell lines. Although SAL analogs showed less promising IC_{50} values than SAL, they were identified as the antitumor agents that significantly overcome the resistance to platinum-based drugs in ovarian cancer, more potent than unmodified SAL and commonly used anticancer drugs—5-fluorouracil, gemcitabine, and cisplatin. Moreover, when compared with SAL used alone, our experiments proved for the first time increased selectivity of SAL-based dual therapy with 5-fluorouracil or gemcitabine, especially towards A2780 cell line. Looking closer at the results, SAL acted synergistically with 5-fluorouracil towards the drug-resistant A2780 cell line. Our results suggest that combinations of SAL with other antineoplastics may become a new therapeutic option for patients with ovarian cancer.

Keywords: salinomycin; anticancer activity; overcoming drug resistance; tumor specificity; synergy; 5-fluorouracil; gemcitabine; amides/esters; ovarian cancer

1. Introduction

Despite developing new therapeutic strategies and extensive knowledge about tumor biology, ovarian cancer (OvCa) remains a leading cause of mortality among gynecologic malignancies; asymptomatic early stages and lack of ambiguous biomarkers enabling detection of the disease lead to late diagnosis, mostly at stage III and IV [1,2]. Five-year overall survival for advanced OvCa is approximately 30% [3]. Most of the patients respond well to radical surgery and either neoadjuvant or adjuvant chemotherapy. However, 75% of patients develop recurrence [4]. Prognosis for patients with the recurrent disease is poor, especially for those diagnosed with the recurrence earlier than six months after completion of the initial platinum-based therapy [5]. This state is called platinum-resistance in opposition to platinum-sensitive patients who develop recurrence more than six months after completion of the initial therapy. The intrinsic and acquired resistance to platinum-based chemotherapy is the main reason for OvCa treatment failure [6,7].

A few theories have been proposed to explain the development of chemoresistance in human malignancies. The most likely one is related to cancer stem cell theory [8]. According to this concept, a malignant tumor consists of two populations of cells, namely cancer stem cells (CSCs) and differentiated cells. Self-renewal, repopulation, and resistance to irradiation and cytotoxic drugs are typical of the first narrow population. Contrary to that, differentiated cancer cells are sensitive to treatment and form a bulk population of the tumor cells. CSCs, similarly to pluripotent stem cells, have active developmental signaling pathways, such as Hedgehog, Notch, and Wnt/β-catenin. The latter two seem to be particularly responsible for OvCa platinum resistance [9,10]. Unfortunately, there is no single universal marker capable of distinguishing CSCs from the differentiated cancer cells. Such a marker could help to develop a highly specific targeted therapy against CSCs, which would improve OvCa patient outcome. Therefore, the main focus of OvCa therapies should be the elimination of CSCs. One of the molecules exhibiting anticancer potential and selective properties against CSCs is salinomycin (SAL, **1**, Figure 1).

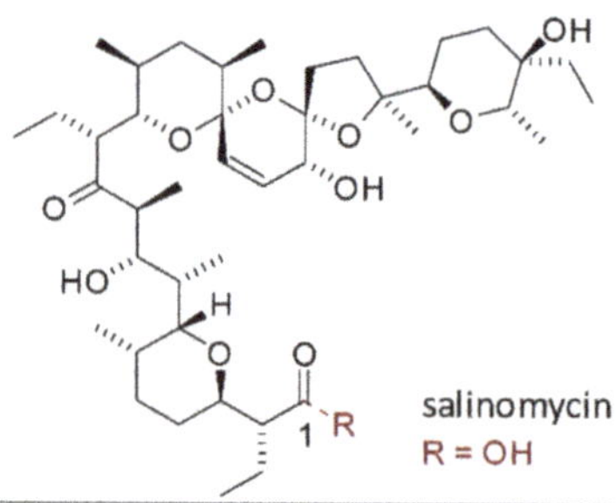

salinomycin (**1**)
R = OH

Amide series		Ester series	
Compound	R =	Compound	R =
2	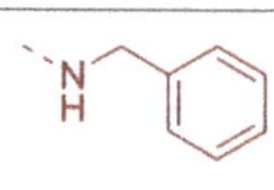	**5**	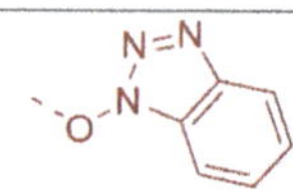
3	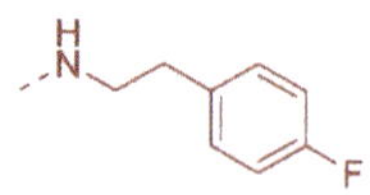	**6**	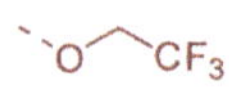
4	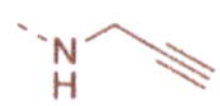	**7**	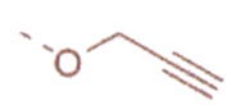

Figure 1. Structure of salinomycin and its derivatives studied in this work.

This is a monocarboxylic polyether antibiotic naturally synthesized by *Streptomyces albus* (strain no. 80614) [11]. SAL was identified in 2009 as the most active agent among 16,000 compounds tested towards breast CSCs [12]. Since then, SAL has been found effective against many other types of cancer cells and CSCs, including those displaying multidrug resistance (MDR) and has been used in a small group of patients with advanced carcinoma of the head, neck, breast, and ovary [13]. SAL acts as a sensitizer of malignant cells to radiotherapy or chemotherapy, i.e., colchicine, doxorubicin, and etoposide [14–17].

2. Results

2.1. Derivation of Cisplatin-Resistant Cell Lines

To test the usefulness of SAL and its derivatives in overcoming cisplatin-resistance, chemoresistant OvCa sub-cell lines were established. MTT and RT-qPCR followed the cell exposure to cisplatin to confirm derivation of stable phenotype of the resistant cell lines. A2780 CDDP and SK-OV-3 CDDP lines responded with morphological changes and increased IC_{50} against cisplatin as compared with their parental population (Figure 2A,B). Both resistant cell lines showed also enhanced expression of ABCB1, ABCG2, and ABCC2 versus control (Figure 2C,D). ABCB4 expression boosted significantly in SK-OV-3 CDDP cell line but only slightly in A2780 CDDP cell line.

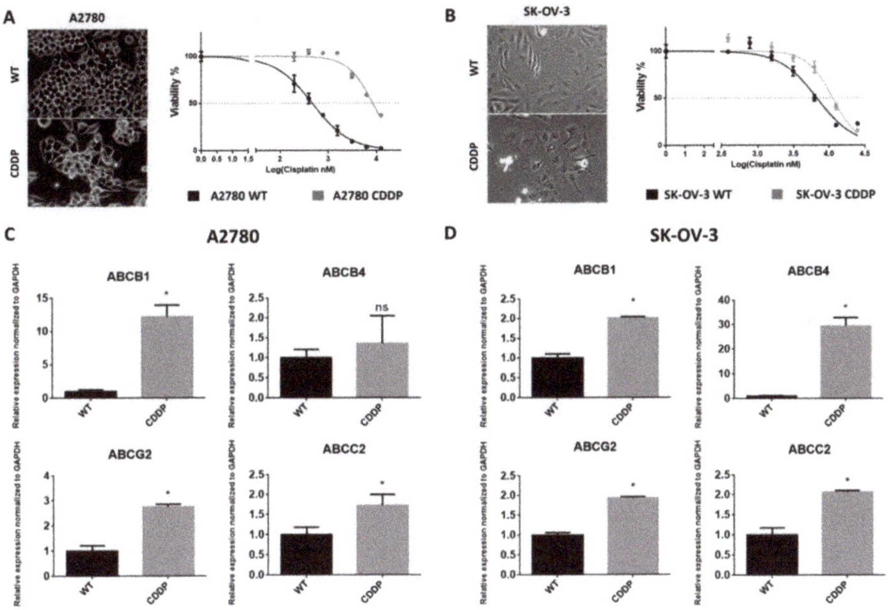

Figure 2. Overview of cisplatin-resistant ovarian cancer cell lines (A2780, SK-OV-3). (**A**,**B**) Morphological changes of both drug-resistant cancer sub-lines represent enlargement and slight spindle-like shape. Survival curves indicate increased IC_{50} for both resistant variants (RI = 18.08 for A2780; RI = 1.56 for SK-OV-3). The pictures were taken under 200× magnification. (**C**,**D**) RT-qPCR analysis of A2780 and SK-OV-3 revealed significantly increased expression of ABC drug transporters in derived resistant variants.

2.2. In Vitro Activity of Cytotoxic Drugs, Salinomycin, and Its Derivatives Against OvCa Cells

It was clearly proven that chemical modification of SAL and other polyether ionophores may not only increase the biological activity of resulting derivatives but also reduce their general toxicity [18–21]. Furthermore, SAL with a modified C1 carboxyl group (amides or esters) transports cations by a biomimetic mechanism, while chemically unmodified SAL transports cations through biological membranes via an electroneutral mechanism [22,23]. This change in ionophoretic properties may result in better biological properties of **SAL** analogs than of those with a native structure.

We devised a library of SAL derivatives based on the most active SAL amides and esters obtained in our previous studies by a chemical modification of C1 carboxyl group, i.e., amides **2** and **3**, as well as esters **5** and **6**, respectively (Figure 1) [18–20]. To expand structural diversity at C1 position and to better determine the structure-activity relationship (SAR), we additionally analyzed propargyl amide **4** and propargyl ester **7** (Figure 1), as these structures had shown promising bioactivity [19].

Data gathered in Table 1 indicate that all tested compounds exhibited biological activity against malignant cells. The effect towards ovarian A2780 cell line was distinctly better than that against metastatic ovarian SK-OV-3 cell line. Briefly, the most effective was chemically unmodified SAL, the activity of which was higher against A2780 cell line and comparable against SK-OV-3 cell line than that of reference anticancer drug—cisplatin (CDDP) (Table 1). In OvCa cell lines A2780, SK-OV-3 as well as their platinum-resistant sub-lines, all semi-synthetic derivatives of SAL (both from amide and ester series) needed significantly higher IC_{50} values to induce comparable biological effects than SAL itself (Table 1). The most active SAL analog was 4-fluorophenethyl amide **3** (Figure 1) but still its activity was one order of magnitude lower than that of unmodified SAL (Table 1). As expected, cisplatin-resistant sub-lines were more resistant to CDDP than both cisplatin-sensitive variants; thus, the anticancer activity of compounds **3** and **5** (Figure 1) was higher than that exhibited by CDDP towards A2780 CDDP cell line (Table 1).

However, to the best of our knowledge, there are no reports describing the effects of a dual therapy using SAL and 5-fluorouracil (5FU) or gemcitabine (GEM) towards OvCa cells. Therefore, we decided to check if SAL shows desired results when combined with these commonly used anticancer drugs. For this purpose, we prepared 1:1 molar mixtures of SAL and 5FU/GEM (**1** + 5FU and **1** + GEM, respectively) and tested their activity towards OvCa cell lines (Table 1). Interestingly, in both cases we witnessed a strong interaction between SAL and either 5FU or GEM. IC_{50} values for **1** + 5FU and **1** + GEM against all OvCa cell lines reached a low micromolar concentration range and were significantly lower than those exhibited by individual components (**1** and 5FU) and reference anticancer drug—CDDP (Table 1). More promising (lower) IC_{50} values were only obtained for GEM (Table 1), which is recommended for treatment of recurrent OvCa.

To determine the real therapeutic potential of novel anticancer drug candidates, it is necessary to check their effects (selectivity) towards normal cells. Judging by IC_{50} values, the tests performed in normal diploid human MRC-5 cell line suggested that all SAL derivatives were significantly less toxic towards non-malignant human cells than the chemically unmodified SAL (Table 1).

Table 1. The IC_{50} values estimated for ovarian cancer cell lines (A2780, SK-OV-3, both drug-sensitive and drug-resistant variants) and normal diploid human MRC-5 cell line after 72 h exposure to salinomycin (**SAL, 1**), its 1:1 molar mixtures with cytotoxic drugs (5-fluorouracil **5FU**, gemcitabine **GEM**), and salinomycin amides and esters (analogs **2–7**).

Compound		A2780		A2780 CDDP		SK-OV-3		SK-OV-3 CDDP		MRC-5	
		IC_{50} (μM)	CI 95%	IC_{50} (μM)	CI 95%	IC_{50} (μM)	CI 95%	IC_{50} (μM)	CI 95%	IC_{50} (μM)	CI 95%
SAL	**1**	0.11	0.08-0.13	0.29	0.27-0.29	4.01	3.13-5.11	3.72	3.24-4.25	10.15	5.14–20.01
salinomycin amides	**2**	27.05	24.25-30.18	24.90	19.98-31.04	183.45	156.43-215.24	140.60	119.40-165.71	213.33	186.19–244.52
	3	8.49	6.74-10.68	6.48	4.71-8.89	79.08	71.25-87.76	69.40	61.88-77.84	66.19	57.31–83.54
	4	14.38	11.99-17.23	12.54	9.58-16.40	91.17	81.42-102.07	58.53	53.22-64.37	98.96	88.13–111.13
salinomycin esters	**5**	25.50	20.44-31.79	7.74	6.04-9.94	205.88	188.71-224.65	103.41	82.63-129.38	58.81	47.05–73.53
	6	13.41	10.58-17.01	50.16	39.26-64.08	125.33	117.36-133.85	91.58	83.78-100.11	110.46	98.87–123.41
	7	37.31	27.95-49.56	45.74	35.49-57.05	179.72	146.77-219.90	94.56	85.65-104.41	160.96	96.41–268.69
1:1 molar mixtures	**1 + 5FU**	0.16	0.14-0.19	0.14	0.14-0.15	3.65	2.96-4.49	3.45	2.91-4.11	1.93	0.83–4.49
	1 + GEM	0.018	0.01-0.03	0.024	0.01-0.04	1.17	1.07-1.29	1.07	1.07-1.29	1.93	1.09–3.43
reference anticancer drugs	**5FU**	3.62	2.15-6.00	1.62	1.23-2.08	20.23	8.85-46.23	36.38	16.85-78.46	13.38	7.23–24.75
	GEM	0.007	0.006-0.007	0.02	0.01-0.02	0.002	0.00007-0.01	0.003	0.00003-0.02	0.04	0.01–0.012
	CDDP	0.47	0.40-0.50	8.33	7.40-9.37	4.03	3.48-4.61	6.72	5.96-7.56	15.7	12.9 –19.27

2.3. Salinomycin and Its Derivatives Overcome Cisplatin Resistance and are More Selective Against Cisplatin-Resistant OvCa Cells

To assess the effectiveness of the studied drugs in overcoming acquired cisplatin resistance, we calculated the resistance index (RI), based on the IC_{50} of derived cell lines (Figure 3A). The RI indicates how many more times a resistant sub-line (either A2780 CDDP or SK-OV-3 CDDP) is chemoresistant as compared with its parental cell line (either A2780 or SK-OV-3, respectively). An RI between 0 and 2 indicates that the cells are sensitive to the tested compound. An RI in the range from 2 to 10 means that the cells show moderate sensitivity to a drug. An RI above 10 indicates strong drug resistance [24]. None of the cancer cell lines developed strong resistance to the tested agents under the combinatory treatment of SAL with either 5FU or GEM (Figure 3A). Contrary to GEM, both **1** + 5FU and **1** + GEM co-treatments were capable of efficiently overcoming the drug resistance of OvCa cells, as manifested by considerably lower values of RI (Figure 3A).

Deeper analysis of RI parameters revealed that cancer cell line A2780, in opposition to SK-OV-3, developed some resistance to SAL (Figure 3A). This finding may indicate possible treatment failure on SAL clinical application. On the other hand, almost no SAL derivatives (except for **6** and **7**) developed even mild resistance during our experiments in both OvCa cell lines (Figure 3A). Generally, A2780 and SK-OV-3 cell lines turned out more sensitive to amide analogs of SAL (compounds **2–4**) than the corresponding ester derivatives (compounds **6–7**). The only exception to this rule was ester **5** (RI = 0.30 and RI = 0.50 for A2780 and SK-OV-3 cell line, respectively) (Figure 3A).

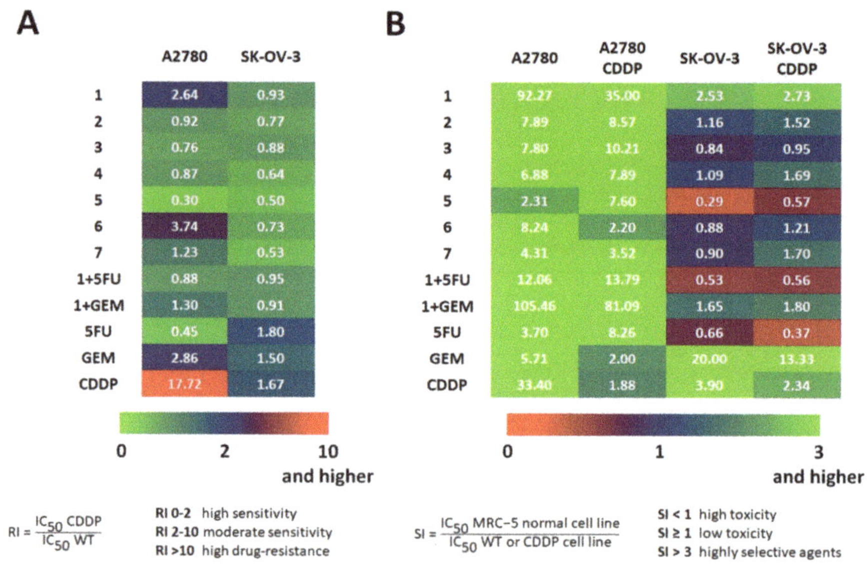

Figure 3. Calculated values of (**A**) the resistance indexes (RI), and (**B**) selectivity indexes (SI) of the tested compounds.

Further, to establish therapeutic potential of the tested anticancer agents, we used the difference in the antiproliferative activity towards the OvCa cell lines and the corresponding normal cell line to calculate the values of the selectivity index (SI) (Figure 3B). The SI is an important pharmaceutical parameter that facilitates the estimation of possible future clinical development; higher values of SI indicate greater anticancer specificity, and the compounds displaying an SI above 3.0 are considered highly selective agents [21,25]. Therefore, our study clearly proved that normal cells were less sensitive to SAL used alone or its combinations with other cytotoxic agents (5FU or GEM) than to amide and ester derivatives of SAL (Figure 3B).

Selectivity of SAL as well as its amide and ester analogs was very promising, especially in non-resistant and resistant to cisplatin A2780 cell lines (Figure 3B). However, the highest values of SI were noted for SAL and its 1:1 molar mixture with GEM (**1** + GEM, Figure 3B), and this effect decreased with time of exposure to the anticancer agents. On the other hand, SAL turned out more selective against SK-OV-3 cell line and its platinum-resistant variant than all analyzed amide and ester derivatives (Figure 3B). A combinatory treatment of OvCa cells involving SAL and GEM (**1** + GEM, Figure 3B) yielded very high SI values. The combination of the cytotoxic agents (regardless of their mechanism of anticancer action), either 5FU or GEM, with SAL was more effective than SAL or its derivatives used alone (Table 1 and Figure 3).

As OvCa cells seemed highly sensitive to the action of both **1** + 5FU and **1** + GEM (Table 1 and Figure 3), we decided to determine the exact effect (addictive, synergistic, or antagonistic) of the specific compound combinations. Using the 1:1 molar mixtures of SAL and 5FU or GEM, we performed standard viability assays and subjected the results to the analysis and determination of values of the combination indexes (CI) (Table 2). As previously described for a pair of drugs [26,27], CI > 1.3 indicates antagonism, CI = 1.1–1.3 indicates moderate antagonism, CI = 0.9–1.1 indicates additive effect, CI = 0.8–0.9 indicates slight synergism, CI = 0.6–0.8 indicates moderate synergism, CI = 0.4–0.6 indicates synergism, and CI = 0.2–0.4 indicates strong synergism. Interestingly, the results presented in Table 2 indicated that SAL in combination with 5FU acted synergistically (CI = 0.56) in A2780 CDDP cell line, whereas in SK-OV-3 and SK-OV-3 CDDP cell lines, they only showed an additive effect (CI = 1.09 and CI = 1.02, respectively).

Table 2. Calculated combination index (CI) values of simultaneously delivered salinomycin (**SAL, 1**) and cytotoxic drugs (5-fluorouracil **5FU**, gemcitabine **GEM**) in the 1:1 molar mixtures.

Combination of Compounds	A2780	A2780 CDDP	SK-OV-3	SK-OV-3 CDDP
1+5FU	1.57	0.56	1.09	1.02
1+GEM	2.86	1.60	691	360

After a primary screening of the compounds, SAL and its amides indicated in both OvCa cell lines variants the most promising response. To confirm their effect, Western blot analysis for B-cell lymphoma 2 (Bcl2), Bcl2 associated X protein (Bax), and caspase-3 (CASP3) was performed (Figure 4).

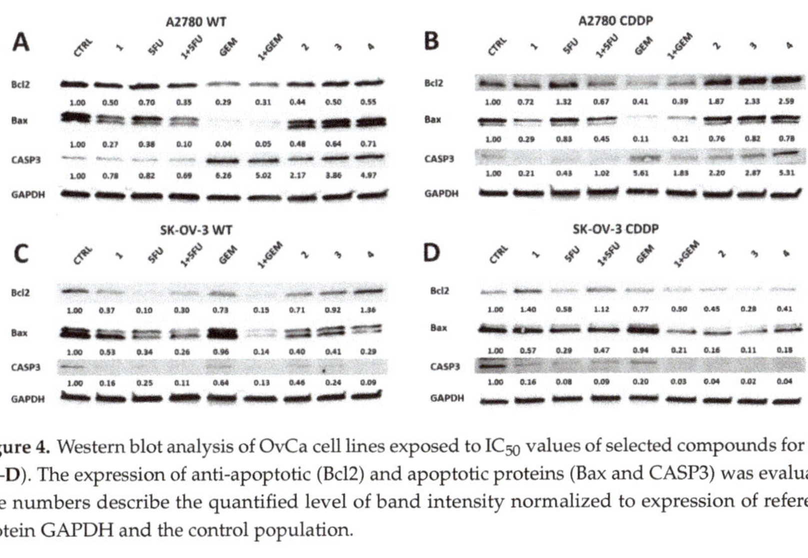

Figure 4. Western blot analysis of OvCa cell lines exposed to IC_{50} values of selected compounds for 72 h (**A–D**). The expression of anti-apoptotic (Bcl2) and apoptotic proteins (Bax and CASP3) was evaluated. The numbers describe the quantified level of band intensity normalized to expression of reference protein GAPDH and the control population.

In A2780 cells, the Bcl2 decreased in all groups in comparison with the control (Figure 4A). The lowest expression was observed in the GEM and 1 + GEM variant, but their effect was similar. The proapoptotic protein Bax also represented similar trends of expression as Bcl2. Interestingly, full form of caspase-3 (CASP3) was decreased in cells treated with SAL, 5FU, and their combination, but GEM and its combination with SAL, as well as amide derivatives of SAL, caused the enhanced expression of that protein. The antagonistic effect of combined SAL with 5FU or GEM was observed by decreasing expression of CASP3. In case of the A2780 CDDP variant, Bcl2 expression in cells treated with SAL, 1 + 5FU, GEM, and 1 + GEM was decreased (Figure 4B). Surprisingly, the SAL amides (**3–5**) caused increased Bcl2 expression. It is worth mentioning that a combination of 5FU with SAL caused downregulation of Bcl2. In all tested compounds the expression of Bax was inhibited in comparison with the control. Among them, a combination of SAL with 5FU caused decreased expression of Bax compared to 5FU alone. A similar effect onto Bax expression was observed in the GEM and its combination with SAL. In A2780 CDDP cell line, CASP3 expression in SAL and 5FU was decreased, and their combination caused a similar effect in comparison to control. However, the expression of that protein in GEM, 1 + GEM, 3, 4, and 5 variants was enhanced in comparison with the control. The combination of SAL with 5FU caused the enhanced expression of the full form of CASP3, which confirmed synergistic action of these compounds. On the other hand, the antagonistic effect was observed in GEM and its combination with SAL, where the cytotoxic effect was enhanced in only GEM-treated cells.

In SK-OV-3 cell line, Bcl2 expression was decreased in all studied compounds, except amide **4**, compared to control (Figure 4C). Among them, SAL, 5FU, and **1**+GEM showed the lowest expression. All tested compounds indicated decreased expression of Bax in comparison with control. The combination of SAL and 5FU did not cause the upregulation of these proteins exciding the level of compounds tested alone. The GEM indicated the highest expression level of Bax among tested molecules. Amide derivatives of SAL did not indicate increased expression of Bax in comparison with SAL. The similar tendencies of CASP3 expression were observed, excluding compound **2** and **3**, which exhibited its higher expression in comparison with SAL. These observations confirmed the antagonistic effect in studied combinations of antineoplastic agents with SAL. In the case of SK-OV-3 CDDP cell line exposed to distinct molecules, the expression of Bcl2 only in SAL and SAL combined with 5FU was upregulated in comparison with the control (Figure 4D). Only the combination of SAL with GEM caused enhanced downregulation of Bcl-2 compared to exposition to them alone. Bax expression in those cells was decreased in comparison with the control. Among tested variants, 1 + 5FU exceeded the level of its expression compared to 5FU, but not to SAL alone. Again, GEM used separately induced its highest expression among all exposed compounds. The amide derivatives of SAL indicated lower expression of Bax in comparison with SAL. The presence of Bax downregulation in cells exposed to a combination of antineoplastics with SAL confirmed their antagonism. The expression of CASP3 and the action of compounds co-cultured with SK-OV-3 CDDP cells was similar to that of Bax. These results confirmed earlier estimated effects of combined SAL with 5FU or GEM in studied cell lines.

3. Discussion

One of the major problems in ovarian cancer (OvCa) treatment is development of chemoresistant residual cancer cells. Cancer stem cell (CSC)-targeted therapies should thus be developed [5]. One of the promising compounds in this respect is salinomycin (SAL). Its short-lasting side effects and low solubility in aqueous solutions may be avoided by some chemical modifications. These modifications provide new SAL molecules with improved stability and unaffected selective properties against CSCs, particularly effective in overcoming chemoresistant forms of the disease [28,29]. However, the synthesis of selective SAL derivatives is complicated due to the presence of multiple functional groups and a sensitive tricyclic 6-6-5 bis-spiroketal ring system in SAL structure [20,29,30].

In this study, we derived cisplatin-resistant cell lines A2780 CDDP and SK-OV-3 CDDP and evaluated the antiproliferative activity of selected amides and esters of SAL, as well as SAL used alone or in combination with other commonly used cytostatic agents, such as 5-fluorouracil (5FU) and gemcitabine (GEM), against these OvCa cells. To confirm the observed effect, Western blot analysis of proteins related to apoptosis (Bcl2, Bax and CASP3) was also performed.

We obtained resistant variants of cancer cell lines, as confirmed by increased IC_{50} against cisplatin estimated by MTT assay. These variants also showed elevated expression of genes related to drug transporters. ABCB1, ABCB4, ABCG2, and ABCC2 are well-described markers of drug resistance development in many cancers [31–35]. These proteins are characteristic of side populations of cells that represent stem-cell-like features, and in some cancers, they are recognized as markers of CSCs. They are responsible for active efflux of many anticancer agents causing treatment failure [35–37].

Our experiments provided interesting data regarding the activity of SAL and its derivatives against platinum resistance developed in OvCa cell lines in vitro. Creation of platinum-resistant OvCa cell line (SK-OV-3) did not induce the resistance of cancer cells to the action of SAL and its derivatives. This indicated that different molecular mechanisms are responsible for either platinum or SAL resistance, and additionally SAL could be identified as an effective agent in overcoming the platinum resistance of OvCa cells. However, A2780 CDDP variant exhibited moderate sensitivity to SAL and its 2,2,2-trifluoroethyl ester derivative (compound **6**, Figure 1). This phenomenon could be related to the increased expression of ABCB1 and ABCG2 in resistant variants of A2780 cancer cell line. A study by the Boesch group revealed that in OvCa cell lines (A2780, IGROV1), selected ABCB1 and ABCG2 positive cells exhibited protective mechanisms against ionophore antibiotics, including SAL [38]. Contrary to that, a study in 2010 demonstrated that SAL treatments restored doxorubicin sensitivity in human doxorubicin-resistant epithelial OvCa cell line (A2780/ADR) exposed to doxorubicin either alone or in combination with SAL by inhibition of ABCB1 functionality [39]. Disparate results of these studies might be related to distinct co-activation of a group of genes in the same chromosomal region, where ABCB1 activation occurs by various cytotoxic agents [31].

Our experiments did not confirm the high anticancer activity of SAL derivatives reported recently in primary acute lymphoblastic leukemia (ALL) cells [20,40], which may be caused by a different type of malignancies and their adverse biology; ALL represents a hematological malignancy, while OvCa represents a malignant solid tumor. Until now, there have been only limited data showing the effects of SAL and its derivatives on OvCa cells. The recent data indicated that SAL itself affects a wide spectrum of mechanisms against OvCa biology, such as inhibition of the epithelial-mesenchymal transition (EMT) process (responsible for the development of metastatic disease), eradication of the CSC population ($CD44^{+}CD117^{+}$), and inhibition of the NF-kB signaling pathway (upregulation of proteins related to that pathway correspond with poor clinical prognosis in OvCa) [41–44]. Our study, for the first time, demonstrates that the combination of SAL with cytostatic agents (5FU and GEM) is more effective than SAL used alone or its amide and ester derivatives. 5FU is not commonly used in OvCa treatment—a few clinical trials revealed no significant improvement in clinical outcomes in advanced OvCa patients receiving 5FU combined with cisplatin or leucovorin [45–47]. Of note is that SAL acted synergistically with 5FU towards drug-resistant A2780 OvCa cell line. A similar effect was presented in studies concerning colorectal and hepatocellular carcinoma, which indicated the neutral or synergistic effect of the combination of SAL and 5FU [48,49]. In case of GEM, which is mostly used as a secondary line of chemotherapy after the development of resistant disease in OvCa, we did not observe the synergistic effect of combined SAL and GEM in both OvCa cell lines, as was found over their action in pancreatic carcinoma cell lines [50,51]. We think that one of the causes was their high molar ratio 1:1 used in our study versus 5 μM concentration of SAL and 5 $\mu g \cdot mL^{-1}$ applied in the pancreatic cancer cell lines [51]. The differences between the observed effects of these two nucleoside analogs in combination with SAL might be related to a disturbance of their cellular uptake by an ion imbalance caused by SAL. The concentrative nucleoside transporters (CNT) and equilibrative nucleoside transporters (ENT) are mostly engaged in the transport of GEM, while for 5FU, only ENT proteins are involved [52–55]. The mechanism of nucleoside transport by CNT proteins is Na^{+}-dependent, whereas in the case of ENT, they are mediated by facilitated diffusion [53,54]. SAL is responsible for the transport of potassium and sodium cations, which could lead to disturbance of the GEM uptake through CNT transporters (indicating high affinity to GEM), decreasing its activity against cancer cells [29,54,55].

The effect of combination of SAL with GEM or 5FU was confirmed by Western blot analysis of proteins related to apoptosis (Bcl2, Bax, and CASP3). Besides the same IC_{50} effect at distinct concentrations of studied compounds, SAL amide derivatives (3–5) caused enhanced expression of CASP3 in A2780 and A2780 CDDP cell lines, which could suggest different or more effective induction of apoptosis by these molecules. We did not observe a similar effect in SK-OV-3 cells, which could be related to intrinsic resistance mechanisms due to their metastatic origin. However, there is a lack of detailed mechanistic studies explaining the differences between SAL and amide derivatives against OvCa cell biology; thus, their further detailed characterization of action should be performed. On the other hand, for SAL used alone, we obtained similar findings as the Parajuli group, where the A2780 CDDP variant was tested, and a decrease of the Bcl2, Bax, and CASP3 was noted at similar doses that we used in our study; however, in their study, only after 1 μM of SAL, caspases were significantly increased [44,56]. They also indicated that the cause of apoptosis is related to activation of death receptor 5 (DR5) pathway, which was observed even at low doses of SAL (0.5 μM) [56]. In contrast, the Kaplan group observed induction of apoptosis by upregulation of CASP3 in OVCAR3 cell line even at 0.1 μM of SAL [57].

In summary, all findings mentioned above corresponded well with our results. Potent anticancer activity of SAL, lack of SAL resistance in platinum-resistant OvCa cell lines, and reversible SAL resistance imply the possible application of SAL in overcoming either primary or acquired platinum resistance (in platinum-resistant cell lines/patients). Further analyses of the SAL treatment used alone or in combination with other anticancer drugs, such as 5FU and GEM, will require identification of the most effective combination of SAL and the cytotoxic agent, and the mode of their administration (synchronous or sequential). Our results may contribute to the development of anticancer therapy based on SAL, which may give hope for heavily treated OvCa patients. Further studies should focus on discovering the mechanisms of action for SAL and its derivatives.

4. Materials and Methods

4.1. Chemical Part

4.1.1. Isolation of Salinomycin

Salinomycin sodium salt was isolated from commercially available veterinary premix SACOX® following acidic extraction, using the previously described procedure [18,19]. Briefly, isolated sodium salt of salinomycin was dissolved in CH_2Cl_2 and stirred vigorously with a layer of aqueous sulfuric acid (pH = 1.0). The organic layer containing salinomycin (SAL, **1**, Figure 1) was washed with distilled water. Then, CH_2Cl_2 was evaporated under reduced pressure to dryness giving SAL as clear oil. After three cycles of evaporation with *n*-pentane, this oil was transformed into white amorphous solid. Spectroscopic data for SAL were closely matched previously published data [22].

4.1.2. Synthesis of Salinomycin Derivatives

All SAL amides and esters (compounds **2–7**, Figure 1) obtained by a chemical modification of the C1 carboxyl group were prepared according to the procedures we described previously [18,19]. Spectroscopic data of all the compounds matched those found in the reference literature [18,19].

4.2. Biological Part

4.2.1. Cell Culture and Derivation of Cisplatin-Resistant Cell Lines

In this study, OvCa cell lines A2780 and SK-OV-3 (ATCC, Manassas, VA, USA) and human fetal lung fibroblasts cell line (MRC-5 pd19; ECACC, Salisbury, United Kingdom) were used to evaluate the antiproliferative activity of the tested compounds. OvCa cell lines were cultivated in RPMI 1640 containing 25 mM HEPES and 5 mM L-glutamine with 10% fetal bovine serum (FBS) (all provided from Biowest, Nuaillé, France) and 1% penicillin-streptomycin (Merck KGaA, Darmstadt, Germany). MRC-5 pd19 was cultured in DMEM supplemented with 10% FBS, 2 mM L-glutamine (all provided from Biowest, Nuaillé, France), 1% penicillin-streptomycin and 1% non-essential amino acids (NEAA) (both provided from Merck KGa, Darmstadt, Germany). To generate the cisplatin-resistant cell lines (A2780 CDDP; SK-OV-3 CDDP), increasing doses of cisplatin (CDDP) (Teva Pharmaceutical Industries Ltd. Petach Tikwa, Israel) were added to the culture medium, starting from the concentration of 100 ng mL^{-1}. Then, the cells were exposed to CDDP (3 cycles of 3 days each). After that, the cell culture medium was replaced with the fresh one without drugs for the next 3 days or one week until the cells recovered. After the 3 cycles, the dose of cisplatin was doubled until the concentration of 1000 ng· mL^{-1} was achieved. Then, to maintain a resistant phenotype, 1000 ng·mL^{-1} of **CDDP** was added once per 2 weeks for 3 days.

4.2.2. Isolation of RNA and RT-qPCR

The cells (2.5×10^5) were washed twice in Dulbecco's phosphate buffered saline (DPBS, Biowest, Nuaillé, France) and suspended in TRI reagent (Sigma-Aldrich, St. Louis, MO, USA). Next, RNA was isolated using Direct-zol RNA MiniPrep (Zymoresearch, Irvine, CA, USA) according to the manufacturer's instructions. Then 1 µg of RNA was collected to synthesize cDNA using iScript kit (BioRAD, Hercules, CA, USA). The cDNA was diluted 20 times, and 2.5 µL was added to the reaction mix composed of FastStart Essential DNA Probes Mix and specific probes (both provided by Roche Molecular Systems, Inc, Basel, Switzerland). The RT-qPCR reaction was performed as previously described [58]. The tested genes related to drug resistance included: ATP-binding cassette subfamily B member 1 (ABCB1), ATP-binding cassette subfamily B member 4 (ABCB4), ATP-binding cassette subfamily G member 2 (ABCG2), and ATP-binding cassette subfamily C member 2 (ABCC2). Relative gene expression level was determined using reference gene glyceraldehyde 3-phosphate dehydrogenase (GAPDH). The primers and molecular probes used in this study are listed in Table S1 (Supplementary Material).

4.2.3. Cell Viability Assay

For the evaluation of cell proliferation inhibition, we used the MTT (3-(4,5-dimethylthiazol-2-yl)-2,5-diphenyltetrazolium bromide) assay as previously described [59]. Briefly, A2780 WT and CDDP (2000 cells/well), SK-OV-3 WT and CDDP (800 cells/well), and MRC-5 pd19 (3000 cells/well) were seeded onto a 96-well plate for overnight until the cells attached. Next, the cells were exposed to the estimated concentrations of SAL, its derivatives, and anticancer drugs for 72 h (Table S2, Supplementary Material). Then the cell culture medium was replaced with the fresh one containing 0.5 mg·mL^{-1} of MTT (Affymetrix, Santa Clara, MA, USA) and left for 2 h at 37 °C. After that, the medium was replaced with DMSO (VWR, Darmstadt, Germany) and left at 37 °C for 10 min until the crystals were dissolved. The measurement was performed with a plate reader, Multiskan FC (Thermofisher, San Jose CA, USA) at 570 and 690 nm. Then, IC_{50} and mean 95% CI were determined using GraphPad Prism 6 (Graph Pad Software, San Diego, CA, USA). The values of resistance index (RI), selectivity index (SI), and combination index (CI) were calculated as described previously [20,60].

4.2.4. Western Blot Analysis

After 72 h of exposure to IC_{50} concentration of selected compounds, the OvCa cell lines were lysed using RIPA lysing buffer (Sigma Aldrich, St. Louis, MO, USA). For analysis, 10 µg of protein was used, calculated using Pierce™ BCA Protein Assay Kit (Thermofisher, San Jose, CA, USA) according to the manufacturer's instructions. The procedure was performed as previously described [52]. Briefly, after electrophoresis, proteins were transferred onto polyvinylidene difluoride (PVDF) membrane. After 2 h of blocking with non-fat milk (Sigma Aldrich, St. Louis, MO, USA), the membrane was incubated overnight at 4 °C with primary antibodies: anti-Bcl-2 (dilution 1:500; sc-509, Santa Cruz, Dallas, TX,

USA), anti-Bax (dilution 1:500; sc-7480, Santa Cruz, Dallas, TX, USA), anti-CASP3 (full-form)(dilution 1:1000; no. ab49822, Abcam, Cambridge, UK), and reference protein GAPDH (dilution 1:500; no. sc-47724, Santa Cruz, Dallas, TX, USA). On the next day, after washes, the membranes were incubated with appropriate secondary antibodies conjugated with horseradish peroxidase (HRP) (dilution 1:1000; no. 7076 and 7074, Cell Signaling Technology, Leiden, Netherlands). Then the protein bands were visualized using WesternBright™ Quantum kit (Advansta, San Jose, CA, USA) and documented using the ChemiDoc Touch Imaging System (Bio-Rad Laboratories Ltd., Hercules, CA, USA). The intensity was measured using Image Lab Software (ver 6.0.1, Bio-Rad Laboratories Ltd., CA, USA). All buffers and equipment used during Western blot analysis were provided from Bio-Rad Laboratories Ltd., CA, USA.

4.2.5. Statistical Analysis

The statistical analysis of genes expression (Student's *t*-test) was performed using GraphPadPrism 6 package (Graph Pad Software, San Diego, CA, USA). The data were deemed significant at $p < 0.05$. All experiments were repeated at least three times.

Supplementary Materials: The following are available online, Table S1: List of primers used in this study, Table S2: Concentration of drugs, dilution range, and serial dilution factors used in this study.

Author Contributions: Conceptualization, A.H., M.A. and M.M.; methodology, M.A., M.S.L; validation, A.H., M.S.L, M.A., M.M. and W.M.S.; formal analysis, M.M., M.A., A.H, M.S.L., W.M.S.; investigation, M.A, M.S.L and M.M.; resources, A.H., M.A. and M.M., M.S.L.; writing—original draft preparation, M.M, M.A. and M.S.L.; writing—review and editing, M.A, A.H, M.M, M.S.L., W.M.S; supervision, M.M., A.H., W.M.S.; funding acquisition, M.A., M.M. All authors have read and agreed to the published version of the manuscript.

Funding: M.A. wishes to acknowledge the National Science Centre (NCN) for financial support under SONATA grant (2016/23/D/ST5/00242). M.M. wishes to acknowledge the Greater Poland Cancer Center for financial support under the internal WCO grant 5/2018/183.

Conflicts of Interest: The authors declare no conflict of interest.

Abbreviations

5FU	5-fluorouracil
ABCB1	ATP-binding cassette subfamily B member 1
ABCB4	ATP-binding cassette subfamily B member 4
ABCC2	ATP-binding cassette subfamily C member 2
ABCG2	ATP-binding cassette subfamily G member 2
ALL	Acute lymphoblastic leukemia
Bax	Bcl2 associated X protein
Bcl-2	B-cell lymphoma 2
CASP3	Caspase 3
CDDP	Cisplatin
CI	Combination index
CNT	Concentrative nucleoside transporters
CSCs	Cancer stem cells
DMEM	Dulbecco modified eagle medium
EMT	Epithelial-mesenchymal transition
ENT	Equilibrative nucleoside transporters
FBS	Fetal bovine serum
GAPDH	Glyceraldehyde 3-phosphate dehydrogenase
GEM	Gemcitabine
HRP	Horseradish peroxidase
MDR	Multidrug resistance

MTT	3-(4,5-dimethylthiazol-2-yl)-2,5-diphenyltetrazolium bromide
NEAA	Non-essential amino acids
OvCa	Ovarian cancer
P-gp	P-glycoprotein
PVDF	Polyvinylidene difluoride
RI	Resistance indexes
RT-qPCR	Reverse transcriptase quantitative polymerase chain reaction
SAR	Structure-activity relationship
SI	Selectivity indexes

References

1. Siegel, R.L.; Miller, K.D.; Jemal, A. Cancer statistics, 2017. *CA Cancer J. Clin.* **2017**, *67*, 7–30. [CrossRef]
2. Rosenthal, A.N.; Menon, U.; Jacobs, I.J. Screening for ovarian cancer. *Clin. Obstet. Gynecol.* **2006**, *49*, 433–447. [CrossRef]
3. Marcus, C.S.; Maxwell, G.L.; Darcy, K.M.; Hamilton, C.A.; McGuire, W.P. Current Approaches and Challenges in Managing and Monitoring Treatment Response in Ovarian Cancer. *J. Cancer.* **2014**, *5*, 25–30.
4. Cooke, S.L.; Brenton, J.D. Evolution of platinum resistance in high-grade serous ovarian cancer. *Lancet Oncol.* **2011**, *12*, 1169–1174. [CrossRef]
5. Rocconi, R.P.; Case, A.S.; Straughn, J.M.; Estes, J.M.; Partridge, E.E. Role of chemotherapy for patients with recurrent platinum-resistant advanced epithelial ovarian cancer: A cost-effectiveness analysis. *Cancer* **2006**, *107*, 536–543. [CrossRef]
6. Au, K.K.; Josahkian, J.A.; Francis, J.A.; Squire, J.A.; Koti, M. Current state of biomarkers in ovarian cancer prognosis. *Futur. Oncol.* **2015**, *11*, 3187–3195. [CrossRef] [PubMed]
7. Kurman, R.J.; Shih, I.M. The Dualistic Model of Ovarian Carcinogenesis. *Am. J. Pathol.* **2016**, *186*, 733–747. [CrossRef] [PubMed]
8. Zhan, Q.; Wang, C.; Ngai, S. Ovarian Cancer Stem Cells: A New Target for Cancer. *Therapy* **2013**, *2013*, 916819. [CrossRef] [PubMed]
9. Nagaraj, A.B.; Joseph, P.; Kovalenko, O.; Singh, S.; Armstrong, A.; Redline, R.; Resnick, K.; Zanotti, K.; Waggoner, S.; DiFeo, A. Critical role of Wnt/β-catenin signaling in driving epithelial ovarian cancer platinum resistance. *Oncotarget* **2015**, *6*, 23720–23734. [CrossRef] [PubMed]
10. McAuliffe, S.M.; Morgan, S.L.; Wyant, G.A.; Tran, L.T.; Muto, K.W.; Chen, Y.S.; Chin, K.T.; Partridge, J.C.; Poole, B.B.; Cheng, K.H.; et al. Targeting Notch, a key pathway for ovarian cancer stem cells, sensitizes tumors to platinum therapy. *Proc. Natl. Acad. Sci.* **2012**, *109*, E2939–E2948. [CrossRef] [PubMed]
11. Miyazaki, Y.; Shibuya, M.; Sugawara, H.; Kawaguchi, O.; Hirsoe, C. Salinomycin, a new polyether antibiotic. *J. Antibiot. (Tokyo).* **1974**, *27*, 814–821. [CrossRef] [PubMed]
12. Gupta, P.B.; Onder, T.T.; Jiang, G.; Tao, K.; Kuperwasser, C.; Weinberg, R.A.; Lander, E.S. Identification of Selective Inhibitors of Cancer Stem Cells by High-Throughput Screening. *Cell* **2009**, *138*, 645–659. [CrossRef] [PubMed]
13. Naujokat, C.; Steinhart, R. Salinomycin as a Drug for Targeting Human Cancer Stem Cells. *J. Biomed. Biotechnol.* **2012**, *2012*, 950658. [CrossRef] [PubMed]
14. Antoszczak, M. A medicinal chemistry perspective on salinomycin as a potent anticancer and anti-CSCs agent. *Eur. J. Med. Chem.* **2019**, *164*, 366–377. [CrossRef]
15. Antoszczak, M.; Huczyński, A. Salinomycin and its derivatives–A new class of multiple-targeted "magic bullets". *Eur. J. Med. Chem.* **2019**, *176*, 208–227. [CrossRef]
16. Kaushik, V.; Yakisich, J.; Kumar, A.; Azad, N.; Iyer, A. Ionophores: Potential Use as Anticancer Drugs and Chemosensitizers. *Cancers* **2018**, *10*, 360. [CrossRef]
17. Versini, A.; Saier, L.; Sindikubwabo, F.; Müller, S.; Cañeque, T.; Rodriguez, R. Chemical biology of salinomycin. *Tetrahedron* **2018**, *74*, 5585–5614. [CrossRef]
18. Antoszczak, M.; Maj, E.; Stefańska, J.; Wietrzyk, J.; Janczak, J.; Brzezinski, B.; Huczyński, A. Synthesis, antiproliferative and antibacterial activity of new amides of salinomycin. *Bioorg. Med. Chem. Lett.* **2014**, *24*, 1724–1729. [CrossRef]

19. Antoszczak, M.; Popiel, K.; Stefańska, J.; Wietrzyk, J.; Maj, E.; Janczak, J.; Michalska, G.; Brzezinski, B.; Huczyński, A. Synthesis, cytotoxicity and antibacterial activity of new esters of polyether antibiotic – salinomycin. *Eur. J. Med. Chem.* **2014**, *76*, 435–444. [CrossRef]
20. Urbaniak, A.; Delgado, M.; Antoszczak, M.; Huczyński, A.; Chambers, T.C. Salinomycin derivatives exhibit activity against primary acute lymphoblastic leukemia (ALL) cells in vitro. *Biomed. Pharmacother.* **2018**, *99*, 384–390. [CrossRef]
21. Huczyński, A.; Rutkowski, J.; Popiel, K.; Maj, E.; Wietrzyk, J.; Stefańska, J.; Majcher, U.; Bartl, F. Synthesis, antiproliferative and antibacterial evaluation of C-ring modified colchicine analogues. *Eur. J. Med. Chem.* **2015**, *90*, 296–301. [CrossRef] [PubMed]
22. Huczyński, A.; Janczak, J.; Antoszczak, M.; Wietrzyk, J.; Maj, E.; Brzezinski, B. Antiproliferative activity of salinomycin and its derivatives. *Bioorg. Med. Chem. Lett.* **2012**, *22*, 7146–7150. [CrossRef] [PubMed]
23. Antonenko, Y.N.; Rokitskaya, T.I.; Huczyński, A. Electrogenic and nonelectrogenic ion fluxes across lipid and mitochondrial membranes mediated by monensin and monensin ethyl ester. *Biochim. Biophys. Acta - Biomembr.* **2015**, *1848*, 995–1004. [CrossRef] [PubMed]
24. Harker, W.G.; Slade, D.L.; Dalton, W.S.; Meltzer, P.S.; Trent, J.M. Multidrug resistance in mitoxantrone-selected HL-60 leukemia cells in the absence of P-glycoprotein overexpression. *Cancer Res.* **1989**, *49*, 4542–4549. [PubMed]
25. Badisa, R.B.; Darling-Reed, S.F.; Joseph, P.; Cooperwood, J.S.; Latinwo, L.M.; Goodman, C.B. Selective cytotoxic activities of two novel synthetic drugs on human breast carcinoma MCF-7 cells. *Anticancer Res.* **2009**, *29*, 2993–2996.
26. Chou, T.C. Drug combination studies and their synergy quantification using the Chou-Talalay method. *Cancer Res.* **2010**, *70*, 440–446. [CrossRef]
27. Ichite, N.; Chougule, M.B.; Jackson, T.; Fulzele, S.V.; Safe, S.; Singh, M. Enhancement of Docetaxel Anticancer Activity by a Novel Diindolylmethane Compound in Human Non-Small Cell Lung Cancer. *Clin. Cancer Res.* **2009**, *15*, 543–552. [CrossRef]
28. Dewangan, J.; Srivastava, S.; Rath, S.K. Salinomycin: A new paradigm in cancer therapy. *Tumor Biol.* **2017**, *39*, 101042831769503. [CrossRef]
29. Piperno, A.; Marrazzo, A.; Scala, A.; Rescifina, A. Chemistry and biology of salinomycin and its analogues. salinomycin and its analogues. In *Targets In Heterocyclic Systems*; Attanasi, O.A., Merino, P., Spinelli, D., Eds.; Società Chimica Italiana: Rome, Italy, 2015; Volume 19, pp. 177–213.
30. Kocieński, P.J.; Brown, R.C.D.; Pommier, A.; Procter, M.; Schmidt, B. Synthesis of salinomycin. *J. Chem. Soc. Perkin Trans.* **1998**, *1*, 9–40. [CrossRef]
31. Genovese, I.; Ilari, A.; Assaraf, Y.G.; Fazi, F.; Colotti, G. Not only P-glycoprotein: Amplification of the ABCB1- containing chromosome region 7q21 confers multidrug resistance upon cancer cells by coordinated overexpression of an assortment of resistance-related proteins. *Drug Resist. Updat.* **2017**, *32*, 23–46. [CrossRef]
32. Comsa, E.; Nguyen, K.; Loghin, F.; Boumendjel, A.; Peuchmaur, M.; Andrieu, T.; Falson, P. Ovarian cancer cells cisplatin sensitization agents selected by mass cytometry target ABCC2 inhibition. *Future Med. Chem.* **2018**, *10*, 1349–1360. [CrossRef] [PubMed]
33. Rubiś, B.; Hołysz, H.; Barczak, W.; Gryczka, R.; Łaciński, M.; Jagielski, P.; Czernikiewicz, A.; Półrolniczak, A.; Wojewoda, A.; Perz, K.; et al. Study of ABCB1 polymorphism frequency in breast cancer patients from Poland. *Pharmacol. Reports* **2012**, *64*, 1560–1566. [CrossRef]
34. Duan, Z.; Brakora, K.A.; Seiden, M.V. Inhibition of ABCB1 (MDR1) and ABCB4 (MDR3) expression by small interfering RNA and reversal of paclitaxel resistance in human ovarian cancer cells. *Mol. Cancer Ther.* **2004**, *3*, 833–838. [PubMed]
35. Luqmani, Y.A. Mechanisms of drug resistance in cancer chemotherapy. *Med. Princ. Pract.* **2005**, *14* (Suppl. 1), 35–48. [CrossRef]
36. Januchowski, R.; Wojtowicz, K.; Sujka-kordowska, P.; Andrzejewska, M.; Zabel, M. MDR Gene Expression Analysis of Six Drug-Resistant Ovarian Cancer Cell Lines. *Biomed. Res. Int.* **2013**, *2013*, 241763. [CrossRef] [PubMed]
37. Eckford, P.D.; Sharom, F.J. ABC Efflux Pump-Based Resistance to Chemotherapy Drugs. *Chem. Rev.* **2009**, 2989–3011. [CrossRef] [PubMed]
38. Boesch, M.; Zeimet, A.G.; Rumpold, H.; Gastl, G.; Sopper, S.; Wolf, D. Drug Transporter-Mediated Protection of Cancer Stem Cells From Ionophore Antibiotics. *Stem Cells Transl. Med.* **2015**, *4*, 1028–1032. [CrossRef]

39. Riccioni, R.; Dupuis, M.L.; Bernabei, M.; Petrucci, E.; Pasquini, L.; Mariani, G.; Cianfriglia, M.; Testa, U. The cancer stem cell selective inhibitor salinomycin is a p-glycoprotein inhibitor. *Blood Cells Mol. Dis.* **2010**, *45*, 86–92. [CrossRef]
40. Antoszczak, M.; Urbaniak, A.; Delgado, M.; Maj, E.; Borgström, B.; Wietrzyk, J.; Huczyński, A.; Yuan, Y.; Chambers, T.C.; Strand, D. Biological activity of doubly modified salinomycin analogs – Evaluation in vitro and ex vivo. *Eur. J. Med. Chem.* **2018**, *156*, 510–523. [CrossRef]
41. Li, R.; Dong, T.; Hu, C.; Lu, J.; Dai, J.; Liu, P. Salinomycin repressed the epithelial-mesenchymal transition of epithelial ovarian cancer cells via downregulating Wnt/β-catenin pathway. *Onco. Targets. Ther.* **2017**, *10*, 1317–1325. [CrossRef]
42. Chung, H.; Kim, Y.H.; Kwon, M.; Shin, S.J.; Kwon, S.H.; Cha, S.D.; Cho, C.H. The effect of salinomycin on ovarian cancer stem-like cells. *Obstet. Gynecol. Sci.* **2016**, *59*, 261–268. [CrossRef] [PubMed]
43. Lee, H.; Shin, S.; Chung, H.; Kwon, S.; Cha, S.; Lee, J.; Cho, C.; Lee, J. Salinomycin reduces stemness and induces apoptosis on human ovarian cancer stem cell. *J. Gynecol. Oncol.* **2017**, *28*, e14. [CrossRef] [PubMed]
44. Parajuli, B.; Lee, H.G.; Kwon, S.; Cha, S.; Shin, S.; Lee, G.; Bae, I.; Cho, C. Salinomycin inhibits Akt/NF-κB and induces apoptosis in cisplatin resistant ovarian cancer cells. *Cancer Epidemiol.* **2013**, *37*, 512–517. [CrossRef] [PubMed]
45. Préfontaine, M.; Donovan, J.T.; Powell, J.L.; Buley, L. Treatment of Refractory Ovarian Cancer with 5-Fluorouracil and Leucovorin. *Gynecol. Oncol.* **1996**, *61*, 249–252. [CrossRef] [PubMed]
46. Burnett, A.F.; Barter, J.F.; Potkul, R.K.; Jarvis, T.; Barnes, W.A. Ineffectiveness of continuous 5-fluorouracil as salvage therapy for ovarian cancer. *Am. J. Clin. Oncol.* **1994**, *17*, 490–493. [CrossRef]
47. Braly, P.S.; Berek, J.S.; Blessing, J.A.; Homesley, H.D.; Averette, H. Intraperitoneal Administration of Cisplatin and 5-Fluorouracil in Residual Ovarian Cancer: A Phase II Gynecologic Oncology Group Trial. *Gynecol. Oncol.* **1995**, *56*, 164–168. [CrossRef]
48. Wang, F.; Dai, W.; Wang, Y.; Shen, M.; Chen, K.; Cheng, P.; Zhang, Y.; Wang, C.; Li, J.; Zheng, Y.; et al. The synergistic in vitro and in vivo antitumor effect of combination therapy with salinomycin and 5-fluorouracil against hepatocellular carcinoma. *PLoS ONE* **2014**, *9*, e97414. [CrossRef]
49. Klose, J.; Eissele, J.; Volz, C.; Schmitt, S.; Ritter, A.; Ying, S.; Schmidt, T.; Heger, U.; Schneider, M.; Ulrich, A. Salinomycin inhibits metastatic colorectal cancer growth and interferes with Wnt/β-catenin signaling in CD133+ human colorectal cancer cells. *BMC Cancer* **2016**, *16*, 896. [CrossRef]
50. Berg, T.; Nøttrup, T.J.; Roed, H. Gemcitabine for recurrent ovarian cancer—A systematic review and meta-analysis. *Gynecol Oncol.* **2019**, *155*, 530–537. [CrossRef]
51. Zhang, G.N.; Liang, Y.; Zhou, L.J.; Chen, S.P.; Chen, G.; Zhang, T.P.; Kang, T.; Zhao, Y.P. Combination of salinomycin and gemcitabine eliminates pancreatic cancer cells. *Cancer Lett.* **2011**, *313*, 137–144. [CrossRef]
52. Hagmann, W.; Jesnowski, R.; Löhr, J.M. Interdependence of gemcitabine treatment, ransporter expression, and resistance in human pancreatic carcinoma cells. *Neoplasia.* **2010**, *12*, 740–747. [CrossRef] [PubMed]
53. Pastor-Anglada, M.; Pérez-Torras, S. Emerging Roles of Nucleoside Transporters. *Front Pharmacol.* **2018**, *9*, 606. [CrossRef] [PubMed]
54. Mackey, J.R.; Yao, S.Y.; Smith, K.M.; Karpinski, E.; Baldwin, S.A.; Cass, C.E.; Young, J.D. Gemcitabine transport in xenopus oocytes expressing recombinant plasma membrane mammalian nucleoside transporters. *J Natl Cancer Inst.* **1999**, *91*, 1876–1881. [CrossRef] [PubMed]
55. Hung, S.W.; Marrache, S.; Cummins, S.; Bhutia, Y.D.; Mody, H.; Hooks, S.B.; Dhar, S.; Govindarajan, R. Defective hCNT1 transport contributes to gemcitabine chemoresistance in ovarian cancer subtypes: Overcoming transport defects using a nanoparticle approach. *Cancer Lett.* **2015**, *359*, 233–240. [CrossRef]
56. Parajuli, B.; Shin, S.J.; Kwon, S.H.; Cha, S.D.; Chung, R.; Park, W.J.; Lee, H.G.; Cho, C.H. Salinomycin induces apoptosis via death receptor-5 up-regulation in cisplatin-resistant ovarian cancer cells. *Anticancer Res.* **2013**, *33*, 1457–1462.
57. Kaplan, F.; Teksen, F. Apoptotic effects of salinomycin on human ovarian cancer cell line (OVCAR-3). *Tumour Biol.* **2016**, *37*, 3897–3903. [CrossRef]
58. Lach, M.S.; Kulcenty, K.; Jankowska, K.; Trzeciak, T.; Richter, M.; Suchorska, W.M. Effect of cellular mass on chondrogenic differentiation during embryoid body formation. *Mol. Med. Rep.* **2018**, *18*, 2705–2714. [CrossRef]

59. Blaszczak, W.; Lach, M.; Barczak, W.; Suchorska, W. Fucoidan Exerts Anticancer Effects Against Head and Neck Squamous Cell Carcinoma In Vitro. *Molecules* **2018**, *23*, 3302. [CrossRef]
60. Chou, T.C. Theoretical Basis, Experimental Design, and Computerized Simulation of Synergism and Antagonism in Drug Combination Studies. *Pharmacol. Rev.* **2006**, *58*, 621–681. [CrossRef]

Sample Availability: Samples of the all compounds are available from the authors.

molecules

MDPI

Article

Organosilicon Compounds, SILA-409 and SILA-421, as Doxorubicin Resistance-Reversing Agents in Human Colon Cancer Cells

Olga Wesołowska [1,*], Krystyna Michalak [1], Maria Błaszczyk [1], Joseph Molnár [2] and Kamila Środa-Pomianek [1]

1 Department of Biophysics and Neuroscience, Wroclaw Medical University, 50-367 Wroclaw, Poland; krystyna.michalak@umed.wroc.pl (K.M.); maria.blaszczyk@student.umed.wroc.pl (M.B.); kamila.sroda-pomianek@umed.wroc.pl (K.Ś.-P.)

2 Institute of Medical Microbiology and Immunobiology, University of Szeged, 6720 Szeged, Hungary; molnar.jozsef@med.u-szeged.hu

* Correspondence: olga.wesolowska@umed.wroc.pl; Tel.: +48-71-784-14-15

Received: 18 March 2020; Accepted: 1 April 2020; Published: 3 April 2020

Abstract: Multidrug resistance (MDR) that occurs in cancer cells constitutes one of the major reasons for chemotherapy failure. The main molecular mechanism of MDR is overexpression of protein transporters from the ATP-binding cassette (ABC) superfamily, such as ABCB1 (multidrug resistance protein 1 (MDR1), P-glycoprotein). At the expense of ATP hydrolysis, ABCB1 pumps a diverse range of substrates (including anticancer drugs) out of the cell, thereby reducing their intracellular concentration. In the present study, the ability of two patented disiloxanes (SILA-409 and SILA-421) to reverse drug resistance in human colon adenocarcinoma cell lines LoVo and LoVo/Dx was investigated. It was demonstrated that both compounds in concentrations of 0.5–1 μM strongly increased the sensitivity of LoVo/Dx cells to doxorubicin. By means of an accumulation test in which rhodamine 123 was used as an ABCB1 substrate analogue, both organosilicon compounds were also shown to inhibit ABCB1 transport activity. The intracellular accumulation of doxorubicin was also increased, and more drug entered the cellular nuclei of resistant cells in the presence of the studied compounds. In conclusion, both SILA-409 and SILA-421 were demonstrated to be effective MDR reversal agents in resistant human colon cancer cells.

Keywords: organosilicon compounds; SILA-409 (Alis-409); SILA-421 (Alis-421); multidrug resistance (MDR) reversal; ABCB1 (P-glycoprotein); colon cancer

1. Introduction

Since chemotherapy continues to be a method of choice for the treatment of various types of cancer, any factors that undermine its effectiveness constitute a serious therapeutic issue. In the majority of patients, the initial response to chemotherapy is satisfactory; however, the occurrence of multidrug resistance (MDR) during treatment results in a development of progressive disease [1,2]. Cells displaying the MDR phenotype are no longer vulnerable to cytotoxic actions of many functionally and structurally dissimilar anti-cancer drugs.

Among several mechanisms that may lead to the development of MDR, the overexpression of ATP-binding cassette (ABC) transporters such as ABCB1 (P-glycoprotein, MDR1: multidrug resistance protein 1), ABCC1 (MRP1: multidrug resistance-associated protein 1), and ABCG2 (BCRP: breast cancer resistance protein) proteins seems to prevail [3,4]. It was recently reported that non-ABC transporters such as Hedgehog receptor Patched were also engaged in doxorubicin (Dox) efflux and conferred Dox resistance to cancer cells [5,6]. ABCB1 is a transporter that utilizes the energy gained from the hydrolysis of ATP to pump many structurally variable substrates (including xenobiotics and chemotherapeutics) out of the cell [7]. Among the numerous strategies proposed to overcome MDR, the most basic approach is the idea to use the inhibitor of a multidrug transporter (MDR modulator) along with chemotherapy in hopes to increase the intracellular accumulation of an anti-cancer drug and to improve the outcome of the treatment. Although this approach is yet to result in any clinical success [8–10], the search for new substances that could serve as clinically applicable MDR modulators is continuously ongoing.

Silicon is a metalloid, which is a group of chemical elements also called semi-metals [11]. It can form chemical bonds with carbon and oxygen, and silicon-containing compounds are widely used in medicine and engineering. Silicone is a synthetic polymer composed of repeating siloxane units. Due to its high biocompatibility and favorable mechanical properties, silicone is used for the production of various medical implants (e.g., breast or testicle), as well as contact lenses [11]. On the other hand, silica materials are applied as controlled drug delivery systems and three-dimensional scaffolds for tissue engineering [11]. The introduction of a silicon atom to a structure usually yields a molecule of higher lipophilicity than its carbon analogue. The increased anti-cancer activity of silicon–indomethacin derivatives was recorded, and it was claimed that the higher lipophilicity of silicon derivatives resulted in their increased uptake by cancer cells [12]. New sila-organosulfur compounds were recently synthesized that were reported to be effective anti-cancer and antibacterial agents [13].

SILA-409 and SILA-421 are water-soluble disiloxanes that were synthesized and patented as putative MDR modulators [14]. They were previously demonstrated to increase fluorescent dye accumulation in human *ABCB1* gene-transfected mouse lymphoma cells and, to much lesser extent, in colon carcinoma Colo320/MDR1-LRP cells, but not in ABCC1 expressing breast cancer (HTB-26/MRP1) and stomach cancer (257P/MDR) cells, which was attributed to their specific interactions with the ABCB1 transporter [15]. The specificity of disiloxanes toward ABCB1 was corroborated in a study by Kars et al. conducted in a model system of breast cancer cells [16]. Recently, the synergism between disiloxanes and amyloid β-protein in the inhibition of ABCB1 transporter activity was reported [17]. In an in vivo study on mice bearing human pancreatic cancer xenografts, the application of SILA-409 resulted in the reduction of tumor growth that was accompanied by increased apoptosis and a reduced level of ABCB1 protein in cancer cells [18]. SILA-421 was found to cause cell-cycle arrest and apoptosis in several non-MDR cancer cell lines [19]. The analysis of the global gene expression profile of HL-60 leukemia cells treated with this compound revealed multiple cellular pathways affected by SILA-421, including DNA replication and transcription processes. Interference with these processes was also attributed to the antimicrobial activity of SILA-409 and SILA-421 compounds [20–22], as well as their ability to eliminate resistance-bearing plasmids from *Escherichia coli* strains [23]. Additionally, the weak chemopreventive activity of disiloxanes was reported both in vitro and in vivo [24].

In the present work, the ability of SILA-409 and SILA-421 to reverse Dox resistance in human adenocarcinoma cells LoVo/Dx was demonstrated. The disiloxanes inhibited the transport function of ABCB1 protein both in LoVo/Dx cells and in Madin-Darby Canine Kidney (MDCK) cells expressing human ABCB1 (MDCK-MDR1). The amount of Dox accumulated inside LoVo/Dx cells was also elevated in the presence of studied compounds, and its distribution pattern was changed.

2. Results and Discussion

2.1. Cytotoxicity of Disiloxanes

A human adenocarcinoma cell line sensitive to Dox (LoVo) and its Dox-resistant counterpart (LoVo/Dx) were employed as a model system. It was previously demonstrated that the increased expression of ABCB1 transporter is mainly responsible for the resistance of LoVo/Dx cells [25]. The cytotoxicity of both SILA-409 and SILA-421 to LoVo and LoVo/Dx cells was comparable (Figure 1). Both compounds were strongly cytotoxic to the cells in concentrations above 10 μM. The half maximal inhibitory concentration (IC_{50}) values of SILA-409 were 15.6 μM and 24.6 μM for LoVo and LoVo/Dx cells, respectively. For SILA-421, IC_{50} values were 8.4 μM in LoVo cells and 9.2 μM in LoVo/Dx cells. SILA-421 was more toxic than SILA-409, which might be the result of the higher lipophilicity of this compound.

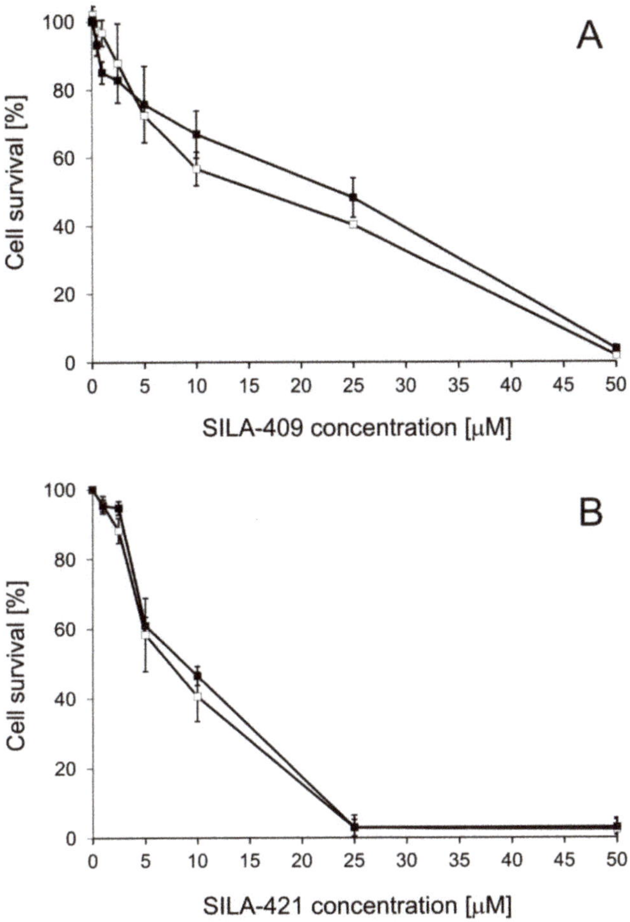

Figure 1. Cytotoxicity of SILA-409 (**A**) and SILA-421 (**B**) to LoVo (open symbols) and LoVo/Dx cells (full symbols). Means of three experiments ± SD are presented.

The cytotoxicity of both disiloxanes to MDCK cells and MDCK transfected with human *ABCB1* gene (MDCK-MDR1) was similar (Figure S1, Supplementary Materials). Both compounds in concentrations below 5 μM slightly stimulated cell growth, whereas, in concentrations of 25 μM and higher, <10% of cells survived. IC_{50} values of SILA-409 in MDCK and MDCK-MDR1 cells were 14.2 μM and 13.9 μM, respectively. For SILA-421, the values of 11.6 μM and 12.1 μM were analogously recorded. Similarly to the findings in colon cancer cells, IC_{50} values for SILA-421 were slightly lower than those for SILA-409.

The cytotoxicity of the studied disiloxanes to various cancer cell lines reported previously [15,19] was similar to the results of the present study. The IC_{50} values of SILA-421 analyzed in several various cancer cell lines, as well as in normal cells HEK-293, lay within the range 5–35 μM [19]. In another study, the cytotoxicity of both SILA-409 and SILA-421 was assessed in a panel of multidrug resistant cancer cell lines of different patterns of expression of MDR-associated transporters [15]. IC_{50} values varied from 8–80 μM depending on cell line. In three out of five cell lines studied, SILA-421 was found to be slightly more cytotoxic than SILA-409.

The analysis of the disiloxanes' chemical structures (Figure S3, Supplementary Materials) and the calculation of their theoretical logP values, performed using the free web tool Molinspiration (https://www.molinspiration.com/cgi-bin/properties), demonstrated that SILA-421 was more lipophilic than SILA-409 (logP values were 5.83 and 9.60 for SILA-409 and SILA-421, respectively). Lipophilicity was observed to positively correlate with the antiproliferative activity of various compounds toward cancer cells [26,27]. However, in other experimental settings, molecular parameters other than lipophilicity were found to affect cytotoxicity to the highest extent [28,29]. Therefore, a larger series of disiloxanes and a characterization of more of their molecular descriptors would be required to determine the effect of lipophilicity on the biological activity of these compounds.

2.2. Influence of Disiloxanes on Doxorubicin Cytotoxicity

Next, the influence of the studied modulators on Dox cytotoxicity was investigated (Figure 2). SILA-409 and SILA-421 were applied in concentrations in which they killed <10% of LoVo/Dx cells. The treatment of cells with a combination of either SILA-409 or SILA-421 with Dox significantly reduced the survival rate of resistant colon cancer cells, i.e., the disiloxanes partially reversed Dox resistance. Non-toxic concentrations of SILA-409 and SILA-421 were applied together with doxorubicin. Sensitive LoVo cells were more vulnerable to this anticancer drug (IC_{50} Dox = 4.0 μM) than ABCB1-overexpressing LoVo/Dx cells (IC_{50} Dox = 30.0 μM) [30]. It was demonstrated that both compounds strongly increased the sensitivity of LoVo/Dx cells to doxorubicin without changing the sensitivity of LoVo cells to this drug. The value of IC_{50} for Dox was reduced to 5.7 μM in the presence of SILA-409 at 0.5 μM concentration, and to 6.1 μM in the presence of SILA-421 (1 μM). The isobolographic analysis applied to the obtained results revealed the existence of synergism between Dox and each of the studied disiloxanes (Table 1).

Table 1. Combination of disiloxanes with Dox against LoVo/Dx cell growth.

Concentration (μM)		**Ratio**	**Combination Index**
Dox	SILA-409		
8.62	0.5	17.24:1	0.7772
17.24	0.5	34.48:1	0.6136
	SILA-421		
8.62	1	8.62:1	0.6467
17.24	1	17.24:1	0.5632

Dose and effect data were obtained from the sulforhodamine B (SRB) assay (mean values of three experiments) and subjected to CompuSyn analysis. CI (combination index) values were generated by CompuSyn software. CI = 1 indicates additive effect, CI < 1 indicates synergism, and CI > 1 indicates antagonism.

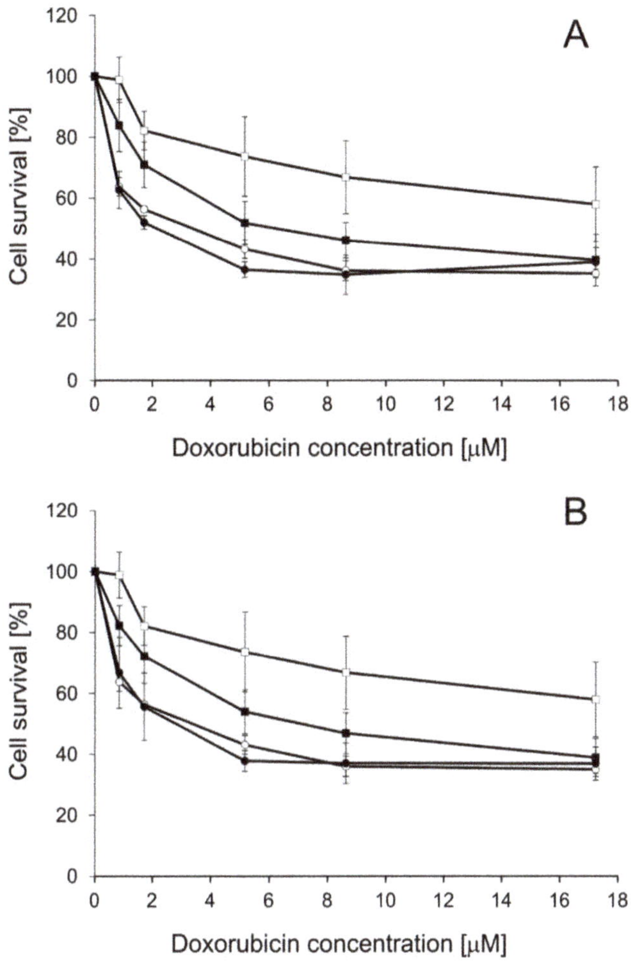

Figure 2. The changes in doxorubicin (Dox) cytotoxicity in LoVo (circles) and LoVo/Dx cells (squares) caused by SILA-409 at 0.5 μM (**A**) and SILA-421 at 1 μM (**B**). Open symbols represent cells treated with Dox only, whereas full symbols represent cells treated with Dox and the modulator. Means of three experiments ± SD are presented.

The reduction of Dox cytotoxicity by SILA-409 and SILA 421 was previously observed in human *ABCB1* gene-transfected mouse lymphoma cells (L5718/MDR) and the resistant colon cancer cell line (Colo320/MDR1-LRP) [15]. Synergism between disiloxanes and Dox was observed in these cell lines but not in breast cancer cell lines MCF-7, T47-D, and HTB-26/MRP1. The authors concluded that the presence of a functional ABCB1 transporter was essential for disiloxanes to be able to revert Dox resistance [15]. This pointed to the specific interactions between SILA-409 and SILA-421 and ABCB1 protein. Similar synergistic interactions with appropriate anticancer drugs were also observed for SILA-409 and SILA-421 in MCF-7 cell lines resistant to paclitaxel and docetaxel, but not in the sublines resistant to Dox and vincristine [16].

Dox cytotoxicity was significantly lower ($p < 0.05$) in LoVo/Dx than in LoVo cells as determined by Student's t-test. Significant enhancement ($p < 0.05$) of Dox cytotoxicity was recorded for both SILA-409 and SILA-421in LoVo/Dx cells in the whole concentration range

2.3. *Intracellular Accumulation of Rhodamine 123 (R123)*

Rhodamine 123 (R123) is popularly used as a fluorescent reporter substrate of the ABCB1 transporter. Both SILA-409 and SILA-421 caused an increase in R123 accumulation in LoVo/Dx and MDCK-MDR1 cells (Figure 3) in a concentration-dependent manner, which suggested that both compounds were inhibitors of ABCB1 transport activity. SILA-421 seemed to exert its inhibitory action in lower concentrations than SILA-409, which significantly elevated fluorescence intensity ratio (FIR) values only in concentrations above 10 μM in Dox-resistant colon cancer cells.

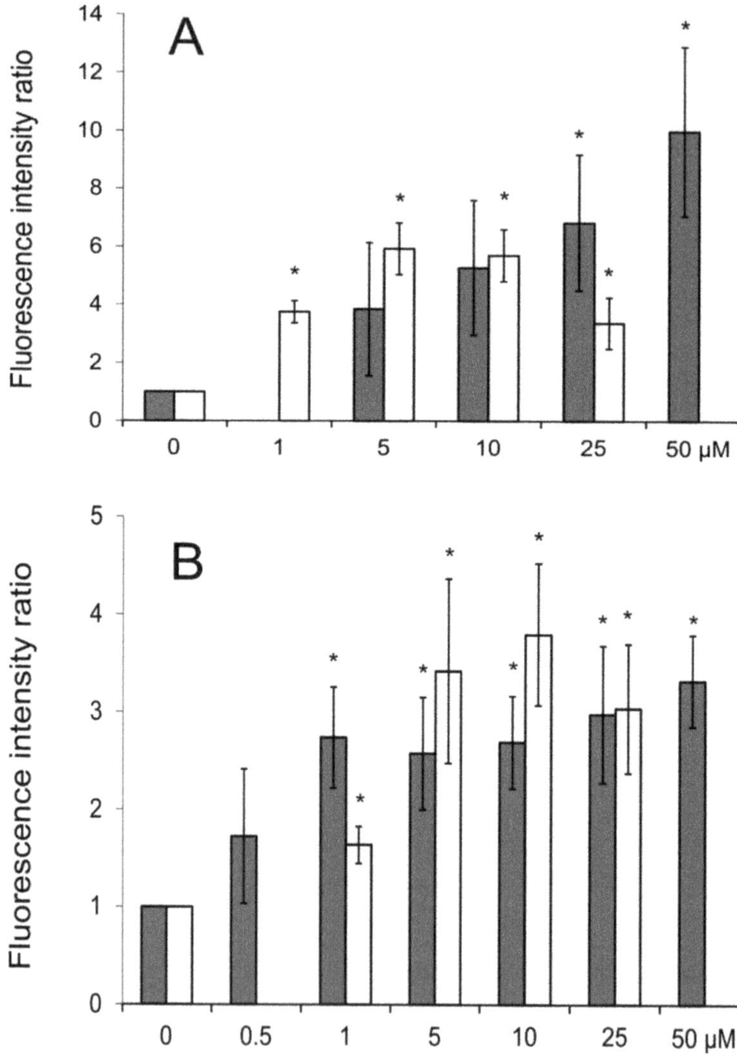

Figure 3. The influence of SILA-409 (gray) and SILA-421 (white) on R123 intracellular accumulation in LoVo/Dx (**A**) and Madin-Darby Canine Kidney-multidrug resistance protein 1 (MDCK-MDR1) cells (**B**). Means ± SD of three experiments are presented. The statistically significant differences from the untreated cells were determined using Student's *t*-test (* $p < 0.05$).

Molnar et al. [15] also observed increased R123 accumulation in human *ABCB1* gene-transfected mouse lymphoma cells (L5718/MDR) treated with SILA-409 and SILA-421 in concentrations up to 2 µg/mL. Both compounds demonstrated similar activity in this respect. They were, however, unable to affect R123 accumulation in sensitive breast and prostate cancer cells and it was again concluded that the activity of disiloxanes can only be observed in cell lines that express a functional ABCB1 transporter [15]. In the study of Kars et al. [16], both disiloxanes were demonstrated to increase R123 accumulation in a series of breast cancer cell lines resistant to paclitaxel, docetaxel, Dox, and vincristine. In contrast to our findings, SILA-409 was observed to be more active then SILA-421 in this experimental setting.

2.4. *Intracellular Accumulation of Doxorubicin*

Accumulation of Dox itself by human colon cancer cells was also investigated. As presented in Figure 4, drug-sensitive LoVo cells accumulated more drug than Dox-resistant LoVo/Dx cells. The treatment of cells by disiloxanes at a concentration of 5 µM resulted in a significant increase in Dox accumulation by LoVo/Dx cells with apparently no effect observed in LoVo cells.

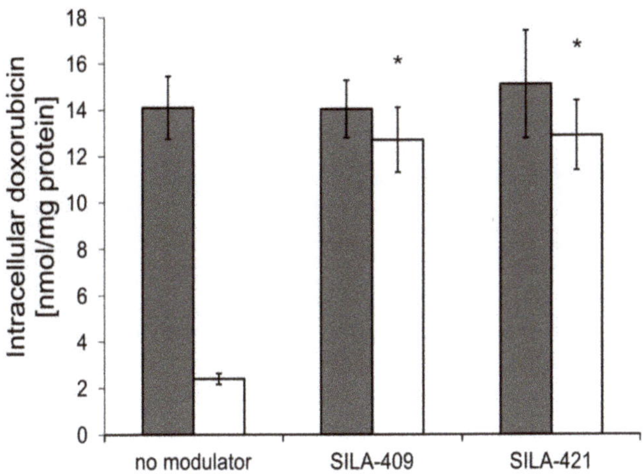

Figure 4. Intracellular doxorubicin (Dox) accumulation in LoVo (gray bars) and LoVo/Dx cells (white bars) treated with SILA-409 and SILA-421 at 5 µM concentration. Means ± SD of three experiments are presented. The statistically significant differences between untreated and disiloxane-treated cells were determined using Student's *t*-test (* $p < 0.05$).

Since Dox is characterized by strong intrinsic fluorescence, its intracellular accumulation may also be examined directly by means of fluorescence microscopy. Again, LoVo cells accumulated more Dox than LoVo/Dx cells (Figure 5 and Figure S2, Supplementary Materials), and the application of disiloxanes at a concentration of 5 µM resulted in an increase in accumulation of the drug in Dox-resistant cells but not in the sensitive ones. SILA-421 was more effective in this respect than SILA-409. The intracellular distribution of Dox was also affected by organosilicon compounds. Dox that was excluded from the nuclei of untreated resistant cells was demonstrated to localize within these organelles in modulator-treated LoVo/Dx cells.

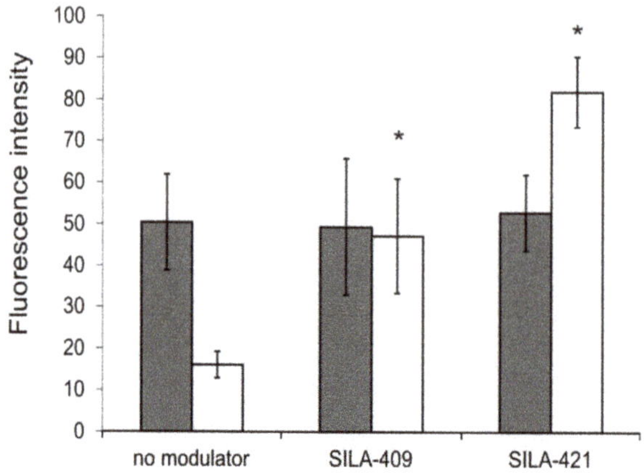

Figure 5. Intensity of intracellular fluorescence of Dox, measured by ImageJ software, in LoVo (gray bars) and LoVo/Dx cells (white bars) treated with 5 μM of SILA-409 and SILA-421 is presented as the mean fluorescence values ± SD measured in 20 representative cells. The statistically significant differences from the untreated cells were determined using Student's *t*-test (* $p < 0.05$).

According to our best knowledge, the influence of SILA-409 and SILA-421 on Dox accumulation and cellular localization was not previously studied. The pattern of changes in Dox accumulation caused by disiloxanes was similar to the changes caused by verapamil (a well-known inhibitor of ABCB1 protein) observed previously in the same colon cancer cell lines as those used in the present work [25].

2.5. Expression of ABCB1 Transporter

Additionally, the influence of disiloxanes on ABCB1 transporter expression was analyzed by Western blotting (Figure 6). Both SILA-409 and SILA-421 significantly decreased ABCB1 protein level in LoVo/Dx cells during 48 h of treatment. SILA-421 turned out to be more active in this respect in comparison with SILA-409. No effect of organosilicon compounds on ABCB1 protein level was noted during 60 min of treatment with modulators (data not shown).

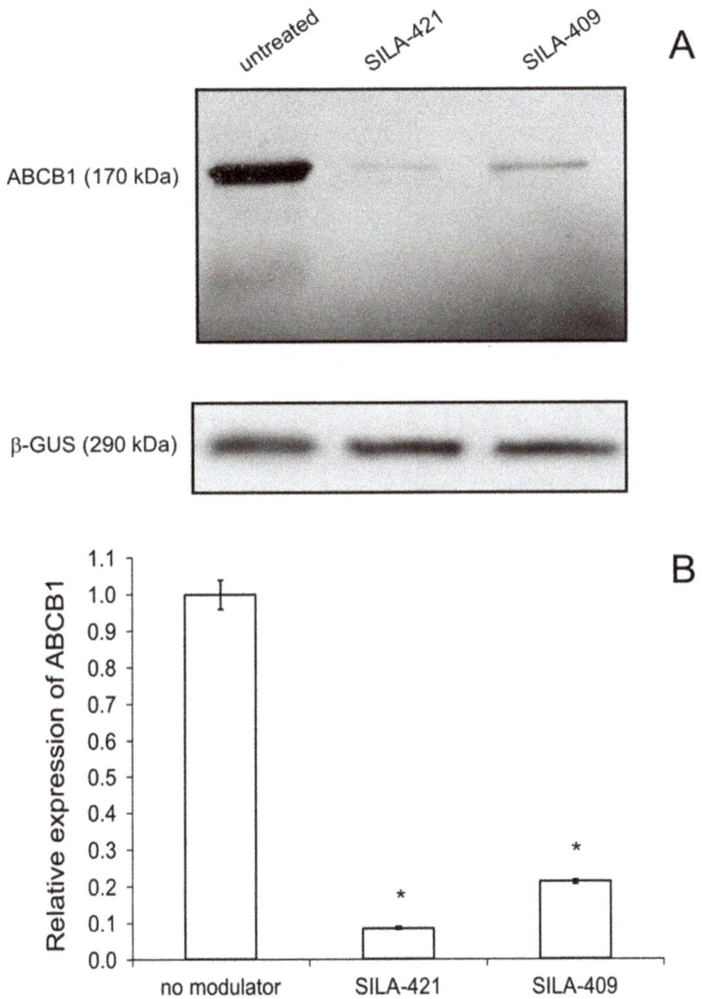

Figure 6. Western blot analysis of ATP-binding cassette B1 (ABCB1) protein level (**A**) in LoVo/Dx cells cultured with 0.5 μM SILA-409 and SILA-421 for 48 h. The molecular masses of the proteins are indicated on the left side of the gel. β-Glucuronidase (β-GUS) was used as a reference protein. The relative level of ABCB1 expression (**B**) was normalized to the control derived from non-treated LoVo/Dx cells. The results of three experiments ± SD are presented. The statistically significant differences from the untreated controls were determined using Student's *t*-test (* $p < 0.05$).

The downregulation of ABCB1 expression was previously demonstrated using immunohistochemical methods in pancreatic tumor samples isolated from mice treated with SILA-409 [18]. On the other hand, no influence of disiloxanes (tested in concentrations of 380–500 μg/mL) on *ABCB1* expression level was detected in mouse T-lymphoma cells transfected with human *ABCB1* [15].

3. Materials and Methods

3.1. Chemicals

Orgasnosilicon compounds 1,3-dimethyl-1,3-bis(4-fluorophenyl)-1,3-bis(3-morpholino-propyl)disiloxan dihydrochloride (SILA-409) and 1,3-dimethyl-1,3-bis(4-fluorophenyl)-1,3-bis{3-[1(4-butylpiperazinyl)]-propyl}-disiloxan tetrahydrochloride (SILA-421) were synthesized and patented [14]. Their chemical structures are presented in Figure S3 (Supplementary Materials). Stock solutions of organosilicon compounds were prepared in dimethyl sulfoxide (DMSO). Sulforhodamine B (SRB), rhodamine 123 (R123), and doxorubicin (Dox) were obtained from Sigma-Aldrich (Poznan, Poland) and dissolved in water.

3.2. Cell Culture

Human colorectal adenocarcinoma cell line, LoVo, and its resistant subline, LoVo/Dx, obtained by prolonged exposure to Dox [31], were obtained from the Institute of Immunology and Experimental Therapy of Polish Academy of Science (Wroclaw, Poland). Cultivation conditions were Ham's F12 medium (with the addition of 10% fetal bovine serum, L-glutamine, antibiotics, and, in the case of LoVo/Dx cells, Dox at 100 ng/mL), at 37 °C and 5% CO_2.

Madin-Darby Canine Kidney cells (MDCK) and MDCK cells expressing human ABCB1 (MDCK-MDR1) [32] were purchased from the Netherlands Cancer Institute (NKI-AVL, Amsterdam, the Netherlands). The cells were cultured in DMEM medium supplemented with 10% fetal bovine serum, L-glutamine, and antibiotics at 37 °C and 5% CO_2.

3.3. Cell Viability Assay

The SRB assay [33] with minor modifications was used for the estimation of the effect of the studied compounds on cell growth. Cells were seeded in 96-well flat-bottom microtiter plates in 75 µL of medium and allowed to attach (60 min, 37 °C). Then, 75 µL of medium containing an amount of the studied compounds (such that a desired compound concentration was obtained in a final sample volume) was added to each well, with the exception of the control wells, which contained medium only. The culture plates were then incubated for 48 h at 37 °C. The further procedure was carried out as previously described [34]. Cytotoxicity of DMSO to LoVo and LoVo/Dx cells was negligible.

3.4. Isobolographic Analysis

Combination index (CI) values were calculated using the CompuSyn software (www.combosyn.com, ComboSyn, Inc., Paramus, USA) according to the classic median-effect equation as described by Chou and Martin [35].

$$CI = \frac{(D)_1}{(Dx)_1} + \frac{(D)_2}{(Dx)_2}, \tag{1}$$

where $(Dx)_1$ is the dose of drug 1 alone that inhibits a system by x%, $(Dx)_2$ is the dose of drug 2 alone that inhibits a system by x%, and $(D)_1 + (D)_2$ are doses of drugs 1 and 2 in combination that also inhibit a system by x%.

3.5. Accumulation of Rhodamine 123 in Cancer Cells

In order to determine R123 accumulation, the cells were harvested and incubated (300,000 cells/mL) with the appropriate concentration of the studied compound (15 min; 25 °C). Next, R123 (10 µM) was added, and the cells were incubated for 60 min at 37 °C. After centrifugation, the samples were washed twice with ice-cold phosphate-buffered saline (PBS) and dissolved in lysis buffer (20 mM Tris-HCl, 0.2% SDS, pH = 7.7). Intracellular fluorescence (λ_{ex} = 485 nm, λ_{em} = 538 nm) was collected with the use of an Infinite M200Pro plate reader (Tecan Instruments, Maennedorf, Switzerland). Based on measured the fluorescence intensity (FL) of the treated and control samples (without modulator), the fluorescence intensity ratio (FIR) was calculated according to the following equation:

$$FIR = \frac{(FL_{LoVoDx \text{ or } MDCK-MDR1 \text{ treated}})/(FL_{LoVoDx \text{ or } MDCK-MDR1 \text{ control}})}{(FL_{LoVo \text{ or } MDCK \text{ treated}})/(FL_{LoVo \text{ or } MDCK \text{ control}})}. \quad (2)$$

3.6. Intracellular Accumulation of Doxorubicin

Intracellular Dox accumulation was detected with a fluorimetry based assay as described previously [36]. Briefly, cells were seeded (800,000/well) onto a six-well plate and incubated for 24 h at 37 °C. Then, the cells were incubated in PBS containing Dox (4 μM) and treated with the modulators. After 48 h of incubation, cells were washed twice in ice-cold PBS and detached. Next, cells were centrifuged and lysed. The cellular protein content was determined using the standard method of Bradford reaction [37]. Dox content was measured using an LS-5 spectrofluorimeter (Perkin-Elmer, Beaconsfield, UK). Excitation and emission wavelengths were 475 and 553 nm, respectively. Fluorescence was expressed in ng of Dox per mg of cellular protein with the use of the calibration curve prepared previously.

For fluorescence microscopic experiments, LoVo and LoVo/Dx cells were cultivated on eight-well μ-Slide microscopy chambers (Ibidi, Munich, Germany) for 48 h. For the experiment, a fresh portion of F12 medium was added containing 50 μM Dox (plus 5 μM of the studied compounds in treated samples), and cells were incubated for 60 min at 37 °C. After incubation, the chambers were washed with PBS and with serum- and phenol red-free F12 medium. The images were collected with a Nikon Eclipse TE2000-E microscope. Fluorescence was excited in the range 528–553 nm and collected in the range 578–633 nm.

3.7. Expression of ABCB1 Protein

Cell lysates were prepared in ice-cold lysis buffer (1% Triton X-100, 50 mM Hepes, 150 mM NaCl, 1.5 mM $MgCl_2$, 1 mM ethylene glycol-bis(β-aminoethyl ether)-*N,N,N′,N′*-tetraacetic acid (EGTA), 1 mM phenylmethylsulfonyl fluoride (PMSF), 100 mM NaF, 10 mM sodium pyrophosphate, 10 μg/mL aprotinin, and 10% glycerol, pH 7.4). After centrifugation of whole-cell lysates (13,000× *g*, 10 min, 4 °C), the supernatants were taken for analysis. The standard method of Bradford reaction was used to measure protein content (Bradford, 1976). The proteins were subjected to SDS-PAGE, transferred to polyvinylidene difluoride (PVDF) membranes, and detected using primary antibodies in tris-buffered saline with Tween (TBS-T) buffer (0.1% Triton X-100, 50 mM Tris-HCl, 150 mM NaCl, 1, pH 7.4) with 5% bovine serum albumin (BSA). The anti-ABCB1 mouse monoclonal primary antibodies (C494) (Alexis) were used at dilution 1:1000. The level of β-glucuronidase (β-GUS) was also determined as a reference protein (anti-glucuronidase mouse monoclonal antibody, diluted 1:1000, Thermo Scientific). After incubation (overnight at 4 °C), the membranes were washed in TBS-T and incubated with rabbit anti-mouse immunoglobulin G (IgG) secondary antibody conjugated to horseradish peroxidase (HRP) (dilution 1:1000, Thermo Scientific) for 30 min at 4 °C. The membranes were then washed with TBS-T, and the proteins were visualized. The relative amount of protein normalized to the control (non-treated cells) was determined. The optical density of the bands on the electrophoregram was detected with the Image J softwar version 1.43m.

3.8. Statistical Analysis

Data represent the means ± standard deviation (SD) of at least three replications. Student's *t*-test was applied, and *p*-values less than 0.05 were considered to be statistically significant.

4. Conclusions

Organosilicon compounds, SILA-409 and SILA-421, were demonstrated to reverse doxorubicin resistance in a human colon cancer cell line. Both compounds were inhibitors of the transport function of ABCB1 protein judging from the increased accumulation of R123 by modulator-treated cells. Intracellular accumulation of Dox was also increased, and more drug entered cellular nuclei in the presence of the studied compounds. SILA-421 demonstrated slightly higher activity than SILA-409. Additionally, the decreased expression of ABCB1 protein after treatment with disiloxanes was recorded. Therefore, the studied compounds acted as resistance-reversing agents via two mechanisms. They were effective inhibitors of the ABCB1 transport function, and its reduction was easily observed after 60 min of disiloxane treatment (e.g., in fluorescence microscopy and R123 accumulation experiments). Moreover, after prolonged treatment with SILA-409 and SILA-421, the reduction of ABCB1 protein level that occurred certainly increased the MDR-reversing potency of these compounds. In conclusion, both SILA-409 and SILA-421 were demonstrated to be effective anti-MDR agents in resistant human colon cancer cells.

Supplementary Materials: The following are available online at http://www.mdpi.com/1420-3049/25/7/1654/s1: Figure S1: Cytotoxicity of SILA-409 (A) and SILA-421 (B) to MDCK (full symbols) and MDCK-MDR1 cells (open symbols). Means of three experiments ± SD are presented; Figure S2: Fluorescence microscopy images illustrating doxorubicin accumulation in LoVo (A) and LoVo/Dx (B) cells treated with 5 μM SILA-409 (C and D for LoVo and LoVo/Dx, respectively) and with 5 μM SILA-421 (E and F). Scale bar is 50 μm. Illumination conditions were the same for all images; Figure S3: Chemical structures of SILA-409 and SILA-421.

Author Contributions: Conceptualization, O.W. and K.M.; Validation, O.W.; Formal analysis, O.W. and K.Ś.-P.; Investigation, O.W., K.Ś.-P., and M.B.; Resources, J.M.; Writing—Original draft preparation, O.W.; Writing—Review and editing, O.W., K.Ś.-P., J.M. and K.M.; Visualization, O.W.; Supervision, K.M.; Funding acquisition, K.M. All authors have read and approved the final version of the manuscript.

Funding: This work was financed by Wroclaw Medical University, subject Simple No. SUB.A050.20.018. J.M. was supported by the Szeged Foundation for Cancer Research.

Conflicts of Interest: The authors declare no conflicts of interest.

References

1. Gottesman, M.M. Mechanisms of cancer drug resistance. *Ann. Rev. Med.* **2002**, *53*, 615–627. [CrossRef] [PubMed]
2. Li, W.; Zhang, H.; Assaraf, Y.G.; Zhao, K.; Xu, X.; Xie, J.; Yang, D.H.; Chen, Z.S. Overcoming ABC transporter-mediated multidrug resistance: Molecular mechanisms and novel therapeutic drug strategies. *Drug Resist. Updat.* **2016**, *27*, 14–29. [CrossRef] [PubMed]
3. Szakacs, G.; Paterson, J.K.; Ludwig, J.A.; Booth-Genthe, C.; Gottesman, M.M. Targeting multidrug resistance in cancer. *Nat. Rev. Drug Discov.* **2006**, *5*, 219–234. [CrossRef] [PubMed]
4. Choi, Y.H.; Yu, A.M. ABC transporters in multidrug resistance and pharmacokinetics, and strategies for drug development. *Curr. Pharm. Des.* **2014**, *20*, 793–807. [CrossRef] [PubMed]
5. Bidet, M.; Tomico, A.; Martin, P.; Guizouarn, H.; Mollat, P.; Mus-Veteau, I. The Hedgehog receptor patched functions in multidrug transport and chemotherapy resistance. *Mol. Cancer Res.* **2012**, *10*, 1496–1508. [CrossRef]
6. Hasanovic, A.; Ruggiero, C.; Jung, S.; Rapa, I.; Signetti, L.; Ben Hadj, M.; Terzolo, M.; Beuschlein, F.; Volante, M.; Hantel, C.; et al. Targeting the multidrug transporter Patched potentiates chemotherapy efficiency on adrenocortical carcinoma in vitro and in vivo. *Int. J. Cancer* **2018**, *143*, 199–211. [CrossRef]
7. Sharom, F.J. ABC multidrug transporters: Structure, function and role in chemoresistance. *Pharmacogenomics* **2008**, *9*, 105–127. [CrossRef]
8. Shukla, S.; Wu, C.P.; Ambudkar, S.V. Development of inhibitors of ATP-binding cassette drug transporters: Present status and challenges. *Expert Opin. Drug Metab. Toxicol.* **2008**, *4*, 205–223. [CrossRef]
9. Kelly, R.J.; Draper, D.; Chen, C.C.; Robey, R.W.; Figg, W.D.; Piekarz, R.L.; Chen, X.; Gardner, E.R.; Balis, F.M.; Venkatesan, A.M.; et al. A pharmacodynamic study of docetaxel in combination with the P-glycoprotein antagonist tariquidar (XR9576) in patients with lung, ovarian, and cervical cancer. *Clin. Cancer Res.* **2011**, *17*, 569–580. [CrossRef]

10. Cripe, L.D.; Uno, H.; Paietta, E.M.; Litzow, M.R.; Ketterling, R.P.; Bennett, J.M.; Rowe, J.M.; Lazarus, H.M.; Luger, S.; Tallman, M.S. Zosuquidar, a novel modulator of P-glycoprotein, does not improve the outcome of older patients with newly diagnosed acute myeloid leukemia: A randomized, placebo-controlled trial of the Eastern Cooperative Oncology Group 3999. *Blood* **2010**, *116*, 4077–4085. [CrossRef]
11. Sekhon, B.S. Metalloid compounds as drugs. *Res. Pharm. Sci.* **2013**, *8*, 145–158. [PubMed]
12. Gately, S.; West, R. Novel therapeutics with enhanced biological activity generated by the strategic introduction of silicon isosteres into known drug scaffolds. *Drug Develop. Res.* **2007**, *68*, 156–163. [CrossRef]
13. Mousazadeh, H.; Milani, M.; Zarghami, N.; Alizadeh, E.; Safa, K.D. Study of the cytotoxic and bactericidal effects of sila-substituted thioalkyne and mercapto-thione compounds based on 1,2,3-triazole scaffold. *Basic Clin. Pharmacol Toxicol.* **2017**, *121*, 390–393. [CrossRef] [PubMed]
14. Varga, A.; Hegyes, P.; Molnar, J.; Mucsi, I.; Hever, A.; Szabo, D.; Kiesig, S.; Lage, H.; Gaal, D.; Nacsa, J. Substituted Disiloxanes, Method for the Production Thereof and the Use Thereof for Reversal of Multidrug Resistance (MDR). EP Patent 1 432 717 B1, 19 May 1999.
15. Molnar, J.; Mucsi, I.; Nacsa, J.; Hever, A.; Gyemánt, N.; Ugocsai, K.; Hegye, P.; Kiessig, S.T.; Gaal, D.; Lage, H.; et al. New silicon compounds as resistance modifiers against multidrug-resistant cancer cells. *Anticancer Res.* **2004**, *24*, 865–872. [PubMed]
16. Kars, M.D.; Iseri, O.D.; Gunduz, U.; Ural, A.U.; Arpaci, F.; Molnar, J. Development of rational in vitro models for drug resistance in breast cancer and modulation of MDR by selected compounds. *Anticancer Res.* **2006**, *26*, 4559–4568.
17. Molnar, J.; Ocsovszki, I.; Pusztai, R. Amyloid-beta interactions with ABC transporters and resistance modifiers. *Anticancer Res.* **2018**, *38*, 3407–3410. [CrossRef]
18. Zalatnai, A.; Molnar, J. Effect of SILA-409, a new organosilicon multidrug- resistance modifier, on human pancreatic cancer xenografts. *In Vivo* **2006**, *20*, 137–140.
19. Olszewski, U.; Zeillinger, R.; Kars, M.D.; Zalatnai, A.; Molnar, J.; Hamilton, G. Anticancer effects of the organosilicon multidrug-resistance modulator SILA 421. *Anticancer Agents Med. Chem.* **2012**, *12*, 663–671. [CrossRef]
20. Martins, M.; Viveiros, M.; Ramos, J.; Couto, I.; Molnar, J.; Boeree, M.; Amaral, L. SILA-421, an inhibitor of efflux pumps of cancer cells, enhances the killing of intracellular extensively drug-resistant tuberculosis (XDR-TB). *Int. J. Antimicrob. Ag.* **2009**, *33*, 479–482. [CrossRef]
21. Simons, S.O.; Kristiansen, J.E.; Hajos, G.; van der Laan, T.; Molnár, J.; Boeree, M.J.; van Ingen, J.; Christensen, J.B.; Viveiros, M.; Riedl, Z.; et al. Activity of the efflux pump inhibitor SILA 421 against drug-resistant tuberculosis. *Int. J. Antimicrob. Ag.* **2013**, *41*, 488–489. [CrossRef]
22. De Knegt, G.J.; Bakker-Woudenberg, I.A.; van Soolingen, D.; Aarnoutse, R.; Boeree, M.J.; de Steenwinkel, J.E. SILA-421 activity in vitro against rifampicin-susceptible and rifampicin-resistant Mycobacterium tuberculosis, and in vivo in a murine tuberculosis model. *Int. J. Antimicrob. Ag.* **2015**, *46*, 66–72. [CrossRef] [PubMed]
23. Schelz, Z.; Martins, M.; Martins, A.; Viveiros, M.; Molnar, J.; Amaral, L. Elimination of plasmids by SILA compounds that inhibit efflux pumps of bacteria and cancer cells. *In Vivo* **2007**, *21*, 635–639.
24. Tokuda, H.; Maoka, T.; Suzuiki, N.; Hohmann, J.; Vasas, A.; Engi, H.; Mucsi, I.; Olszewski, U.; Hamilton, G.; Amaral, L.; et al. Effects of two disiloxanes ALIS-409 and ALIS-421 on chemoprevention in model experiments. *Anticancer Res.* **2013**, *33*, 2021–2027. [PubMed]
25. Wesołowska, O.; Wiśniewski, J.; Środa, K.; Krawczenko, A.; Bielawska-Pohl, A.; Paprocka, M.; Duś, D.; Michalak, K. 8-Prenylnaringenin is an inhibitor of multidrug resistance associated transporters, P-glycoprotein and MRP1. *Eur. J. Pharmacol.* **2010**, *644*, 32–40. [CrossRef] [PubMed]
26. Dobhal, M.P.; Li, G.; Gryshuk, A.; Graham, A.; Bhatanager, A.K.; Khaja, S.D.; Joshi, Y.C.; Sharma, M.C.; Oseroff, A.; Pandey, R.K. Structural modifications of plumieride isolated from *Plumeria bicolor* and the effect of these modifications on in vitro anticancer activity. *J. Org. Chem.* **2004**, *69*, 6165–6172. [CrossRef] [PubMed]
27. Carella, A.; Roviello, V.; Iannitti, R.; Palumbo, R.; La Manna, S.; Marasco, D.; Trifuoggi, M.; Diana, R.; Roviello, G.N. Evaluating the biological properties of synthetic 4-nitrophenyl functionalized benzofuran derivatives with telomeric DNA binding and antiproliferative activities. *Int. J. Biol. Macromol.* **2019**, *121*, 77–88. [CrossRef]

28. Środa-Pomianek, K.; Michalak, K.; Świątek, P.; Poła, A.; Palko-Łabuz, A.; Wesołowska, O. Increased lipid peroxidation, apoptosis and selective cytotoxicity in colon cancer cell line LoVo and its doxorubicin-resistant subline LoVo/Dx in the presence of newly synthesized phenothiazine derivatives. *Biomed. Pharmacother.* **2018**, *106*, 624–636. [CrossRef]
29. Deo, K.M.; Sakoff, J.; Gilbert, J.; Zhang, Y.; Aldrich Wright, J.R. Synthesis, characterisation and influence of lipophilicity on cellular accumulation and cytotoxicity of unconventional platinum(iv) prodrugs as potent anticancer agents. *Dalton Trans.* **2019**, *48*, 17228–17240. [CrossRef]
30. Środa-Pomianek, K.; Michalak, K.; Palko-Łabuz, A.; Poła, A.; Dzięgiel, P.; Puła, B.; Świątek, P.; Wesołowska, O. Cytotoxic and multidrug resistance reversal activity of phenothiazine derivative is strongly enhanced by theobromine, a phytochemical from cocoa. *Eur. J. Pharmacol.* **2019**, *849*, 124–134. [CrossRef]
31. Grandi, M.; Geroni, C.; Giuliani, F.C. Isolation and characterization of a human colon adenocarcinoma cell line resistant to doxorubicin. *Br. J. Cancer* **1986**, *54*, 515–518. [CrossRef]
32. Pastan, I.; Gottesman, M.M.; Ueda, K.; Lovelace, E.; Rutherford, A.V.; Willingham, M.C. A retrovirus carrying an MDR1 cDNA confers multidrug resistance and polarized expression of P-glycoprotein in MDCK cells. *Proc. Natl. Acad. Sci. USA* **1988**, *85*, 4486–4490. [CrossRef] [PubMed]
33. Skehan, P.; Storeng, R.; Scudiero, D.; Monks, A.; McMahon, J.; Vistica, D.; Warren, J.T.; Bokesch, H.; Kenney, S.; Boyd, M.R. New colorimetric cytotoxicity assay for anticancer-drug screening. *J. Natl. Cancer Inst.* **1990**, *82*, 1107–1112. [CrossRef] [PubMed]
34. Palko-Łabuz, A.; Środa-Pomianek, K.; Uryga, A.; Kostrzewa-Susłow, E.; Michalak, K. Anticancer activity of baicalein and luteolin studied in colorectal adenocarcinoma LoVo cells and in drug-resistant LoVo/Dx cells. *Biomed. Pharmacother.* **2017**, *88*, 232–241. [CrossRef]
35. Chou, T.C.; Martin, N. *CompuSyn for Drug Combinations: PC Software and User's Guide: A Computer Program for Quantitation of Synergism and Antagonism in Drug Combinations, and the Determination of IC50 and ED50 and LD50 Values*; ComboSyn Inc.: Paramus, NJ, USA, 2005.
36. Riganti, C.; Miraglia, E.; Viarisio, D.; Costamagna, C.; Pescarmona, G. Nitric oxide reverts the resistance to doxorubicin in human colon cancer cells by inhibiting the drug efflux. *Cancer Res.* **2005**, *65*, 516–525.
37. Bradford, M.M. A rapid and sensitive method for the quantitation of microgram quantities of protein utilizing the principle of protein-dye binding. *Anal. Biochem.* **1976**, *72*, 248–254. [CrossRef]

Sample Availability: Samples of the compounds are not available from the authors.

molecules

MDPI

Article

Synthesis, Anti-Cancer and Anti-Migratory Evaluation of 3,6-Dibromocarbazole and 5-Bromoindole Derivatives

Krystal M. Butler-Fernández [1], Zulma Ramos [1], Adela M. Francis-Malavé [2], Joseph Bloom [1], Suranganie Dharmawardhane [3] and Eliud Hernández [1,*]

1 Department of Pharmaceutical Sciences, University of Puerto Rico, School of Pharmacy, San Juan 00936, Puerto Rico
2 Department of Biology, College of Natural Sciences, University of Puerto Rico, San Juan 00931, Puerto Rico
3 Department of Biochemistry, University of Puerto Rico, School of Medicine, San Juan 00936, Puerto Rico
* Correspondence: eliud.hernandez@upr.edu; Tel.: +1-(787)-758-2525 (ext. 5436)

Academic Editor: Qiao-Hong Chen
Received: 2 July 2019; Accepted: 19 July 2019; Published: 24 July 2019

Abstract: In this study, a new series of *N*-alkyl-3,6-dibromocarbazole and *N*-alkyl-5-bromoindole derivatives have been synthesized and evaluated in vitro as anti-cancer and anti-migration agents. Cytotoxic and anti-migratory effects of these compounds were evaluated in MCF-7 and MDA-MB-231 breast cancer cell lines and an insight on the structure-activity relationship was developed. Preliminary investigations of their anti-cancer activity demonstrated that several compounds have moderate antiproliferative effects on cancer cell lines with GI_{50} values in the range of 4.7–32.2 μM. Moreover, carbazole derivatives **10**, **14**, **15**, **23**, and **24** inhibit migration activity of metastatic cell line MDA-MB-231 in the range of 18–20%. The effect of compounds **10**, **14**, and **15** in extension of invadopodia and filopodia was evaluated by fluorescence microscopy and results demonstrated a reduction in actin-based cell extensions by compounds **10** and **15**.

Keywords: 3,6-dibromocarbazole; 5-bromoindole; carbazole; actin; breast cancer; migration

1. Introduction

In women, breast cancer is the leading cause of death, mainly due to metastasis [1]. If breast cancer is detected and treated prior to metastasis, the patient has a higher probability of being cured of their disease. Cancer cell invasion involves cell migration through the extracellular matrix (ECM) and the accompanying degradation of the ECM [2]. Several proteins play a key role in this process, by the extension of structures known as invadopodia. Invadopodia are actin-rich protrusive structures with associated matrix degradation activity and are believed to be important for tumor cells to penetrate the basement membrane of epithelia and blood vessels [3]. In cell migration, the reorganization of the actin cytoskeleton produces the force necessary for cell migration [4]. The Rho GTPases, Rac, and Cdc42 are key molecular switches activated by a myriad of cell surface receptors to promote breast cancer cell migration/invasion, proliferation, and survival [5]. Unlike Ras, Rac and Cdc42 are not mutated in breast cancer, but activated via the deregulation of expression and/or activity of their upstream regulators, guanine nucleotide exchange factors (GEFs) [6]. The WASP family proteins are key regulators of the actin cytoskeleton and cell migration through induction of membrane protrusions at the leading edge [7]. In cancer cells, when N-WASP interacts and activates the Arp2/3 complex, it catalyzes actin polymerization and assembly into filopodia and invadopodia [7,8]. To initiate this process, the Rho GTPase Cdc42, in its GTP-activated form, binds and activates N-WASP by inducing a conformational change that liberates the autoinhibited structure, thereby interacting with Arp2/3 complex, and regulating the protrusive formation in membrane structures promoting extracellular matrix (ECM) degradation [8]. Therefore, inhibition of these processes decreases cell motility and invasion, and may greatly improve the potential therapeutic applications of such inhibitors against cancer metastasis.

Natural and synthetic carbazole derivatives comprise a wide variety of biologically active agents with diverse pharmacological activities, including antitumoral, antioxidant, anti-inflammatory, antibacterial, anticonvulsant, antipsychotic, antidiabetic, and larvicidal properties [9–28]. Carbazoles are tricyclic aromatic compounds with a benzene ring fused to the 2,3-positions of an indole ring [29]. The antitumor properties of carbazole derivatives have been correlated to their polycyclic, planar aromatic structure, and large π-conjugated backbone that noncovalently bind with DNA base pairs, hydrophobic pockets, and forms electrostatic interactions to intercalate into DNA [9,30]. In particular, among a wide variety of carbazoles, a series of *N*-alkyl-3,6-disubstituted carbazole derivatives has been discovered and evaluated for their potential as neuroprotective agents [31], antimalarial [32], antitumoral [33,34], anti-apoptotic [35], and antibacterial activities [36]. Selected examples of bioactive *N*-alkyl-3,6-disubstituted carbazole derivatives are represented in Figure 1.

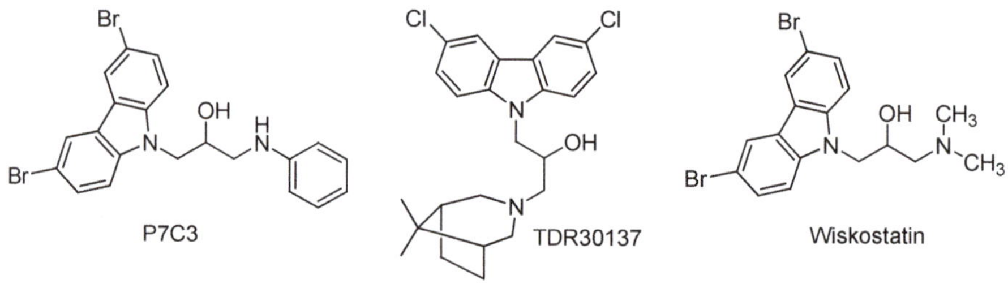

Figure 1. Structure of representative *N*-alkyl-3,6-dihalogencarbazole derivatives.

The compound P7C3 (Figure 1) was discovered from a library of 200,000 drug-like molecules, and showed proneurogenic and neuroprotective properties, stabilized mitochondrial membrane potential, and inhibits neuronal apoptosis [37]. Several derivatives of P7C3 have been synthesized with modifications at the linker chain. Replacement of the hydroxyl group with a fluorine atom, and an additional methylene group between the hydroxyl group and the aniline, increases activity [37]. The aromatic ring was replaced with heteroaromatic groups, but activity was found to be less effective. The commercially available TDR30137 (Figure 1) was discovered and characterized as an inhibitor of P. *falciparum* K1 (Pf-K1) in human red blood cells with an IC_{50} of 57 nM [32]. However, TDR30137 was not active in in vivo studies with the *Plasmodium berghei* mouse model. In structure-activity relationship (SAR) studies, the importance of 3,6-halogen substitution, hydroxyl group, and the tertiary amine correlated with improved activity on Pf-K1 strains [32]. A carbazole derivative named Wiskostatin (Figure 1) was identified to bind within a pocket in the GBD regulatory module that maintains N-WASP in an inactive, autoinhibited conformation [38]. In a pyrene-actin polymerization assay, using purified proteins, it was demonstrated that Wiskostatin inhibited full-length N-WASP activation of the Arp2/3 complex at IC_{50} = 10 μM [38]. The specific binding site of Wiskostatin was determined to be within the GBD of the autoinhibited conformation of N-WASP after performing the experiment with activated Cdc42-GTP. Unfortunately, a recent report described that Wiskostatin inhibited other cellular functions that are not believed to be N-WASP dependent [39]. These studies revealed that Wiskostatin caused an irreversible decrease in cellular ATP levels, and that it does not function as a selective inhibitor of N-WASP dependent functions in intact cells, and caused an overall change in the energy status of cells; thus, inhibiting normal transport processes [39]. Herein, we designed and synthesized a new series of *N*-alkyl-3,6-dibromocarbazole and 5-bromoindole derivatives, tested for their antiproliferative and antimigratory activities in MCF-7 and MDA-MB-231 breast cancer cell lines, and analyzed the effect of the most active migration inhibitor on actin dynamics and actin cytoskeleton rearrangement.

2. Results and Discussion

The aim of this study is to design and synthesize a new series of *N*-alkyl-3,6-dibromocarbazole and *N*-alkyl-5-bromoindole derivatives and analyze their cytotoxic effect and potential to inhibit actin cytoskeleton rearrangement and cancer cell migration. The structural elements of Wiskostatin and derivatives identified as pharmacophoric unit are a 3,6-dihalogen carbazole and a dialkylamino-2-propanol chain. Our strategy was to design and synthesize a new series of compounds with a 3,6-dibromocarbazole or 5-bromoindole ring connected, via a three-carbon atom aliphatic chain, to an amide group. The influence of different N-alkyl or aromatic substituents at the amide group was examined.

We screened all compounds to determine their cytotoxic effect against MCF-7 and MDA-MB-231 breast cancer cells using the Sulforhodamine B (SRB) assay [40] (Figure 2). In addition, anti-migratory activity was determined using the wound healing assay (scratch method) [41] on the metastatic MDA-MB-231 cancer cells. In this assay, the relative migration of MDA-MB-231 breast cancer cells in the presence of carbazole or indole derivatives at a concentration of 10 μM (or at concentrations that do not affect cell viability) was compared to the migration in the presence of vehicle (0.02% DMSO). Representative photomicrographs of the migration inhibition of compounds **10, 14, 15,** and Wiskostatin are represented in Figure 3. Results show that in the vehicle-treated control experiment, wound healing is progressing considerably, and after 24 h, the wound is completely healed. When cells are incubated with compounds **10, 14,** and **15** after 24 h, the wound healing is inhibited. However, Wiskostatin did not elicit an inhibitory effect on wound healing when incubated with MDA-MB-231 cells after 24 h at a concentration of 2 μM. Actin and Arp2/3 regulation by active WASP induce de novo actin polymerization and assembly to generate the F-actin structures filopodia and invadopodia used for cell migration [42]. Therefore, to investigate the effect of compounds **10, 14, 15,** and Wiskostatin on actin dynamics, we performed immunofluorescence microscopy to detect polymerized actin on MDA-MB-231 cancer cells (Figure 4). The structure and biological activities of new compounds are summarized in Tables 1 and 2.

2.1. *N-Alkyl-3,6-Dibromocarbazole Derivatives*

The synthetic method to construct the 3,6-dibromocarbazole derivatives library is described in Scheme 1 (see the Supplementary Materials for representative ^{1}H and ^{13}C NMR spectral data). The *N*-alkyl-3,6-dibromocarbazole derivatives were generated in a three-step synthesis using 3,6-dibromocarbazole **1** as origin of the carbazole derivatives core. Compound **1** was reacted with ethyl 4-bromobutyrate to introduce the aliphatic side chain by nucleophilic substitution (Scheme 1), followed by hydrolysis to afford the corresponding 3,6-diromocarbazole-4-butyric acid **2**. For the generation of 3,6-dibromocarbazole-4-butyramide derivatives **3**, compound **2** was therefore used as starting material, which reacted with different amines via an amide coupling reaction using N-(3-Dimethylaminopropyl)-N′-ethylcarbonate (EDAC) with Hydroxybenzotriazole (HOBt) as an additive dissolved in methylene chloride (CH_2Cl_2).

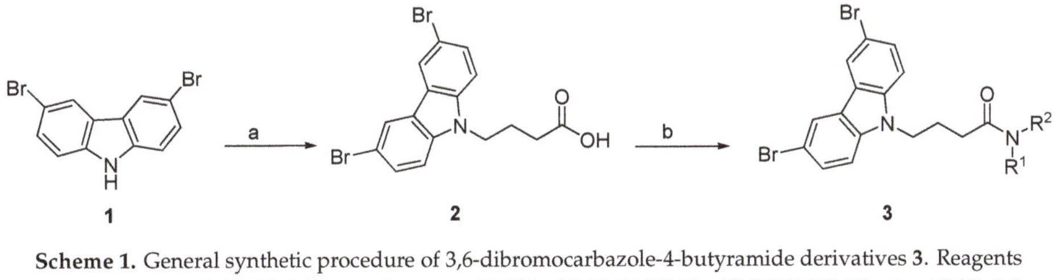

Scheme 1. General synthetic procedure of 3,6-dibromocarbazole-4-butyramide derivatives **3**. Reagents and conditions: (**a**) (i) Ethyl 4-bromobutyrate, K_2CO_3, DMF, 80 °C, 2h; (ii) KOH, DMF/water, 80 °C, 2-6 h, 86%; (**b**) HOBt, EDAC, CH_2Cl_2, Et_3N, rt, amine: R-NH_2 or HNR^1R^2, 2-8 h.

The in vitro anti-proliferative and anti-migratory activities of compounds **4–27**, and Wiskostatin are represented in Table 1. From the twenty-four compound derivatives of 3,6-dibromocarbazole, it can be observed that in the MCF-7 (ER+) cancer cell line, compounds **6–10**, **14**, **16–21**, and **32** showed good to moderate antiproliferative activity with a GI_{50} in the range of 6.8–32.2 μM. In the MDA-MB-231 cell line, compounds **6–10**, **14**, **16**, **18**, **20–21**, and **23** inhibited cell proliferation with a GI_{50} in the range of 4.7–23 μM. The remaining compounds in that series had a GI_{50} above 50 μM in both breast cancer cell lines. Compound **8** with a 2-piperazinyl ethyl butyramide chain showed very good anticancer activity against both cancer cell lines MCF-7 and MDA-MB-231 with GI_{50} values of 8 and 4.7 μM, respectively. Also, compound **18** with a piperazinyl amide showed significant anticancer activity against both cancer cell lines with GI_{50} values of 7.5 and 6.7 μM, respectively. Similarly, compound **21**, another piperazinyl amide derivative, showed very good in vitro anticancer activity against both cancer cell lines with GI_{50} values of 6.5 and 8 μM, respectively. Shortening the aliphatic chain between the N-atom of the amide group and the morpholine from C3 (**9**), over C2 (**4**), to C0 (**12**) led to a complete loss of antiproliferative activity on both cancer cell lines. On the other hand, introduction of an aromatic ring or aromatic heterocycle (**22–27**, Table 1) in the amide group led to lack of antiproliferative activity with GI_{50} above 50 μM on both cancer cell lines. Thus, in general, compounds with a piperazinyl butyramide group attached to the N-atom of the carbazole appear to be more cytotoxic than compounds with other butyramide group in this series of compounds. In addition, three compounds—**8**, **18**, and **21**—were found to be more cytotoxic against both cancer cell lines MCF-7 and MDA-MB-231 than Wiskostatin, which in this assay showed GI_{50} values of 9.7 and 8.3 μM, respectively (Table 1, Figure 2).

To further assess the anti-migratory activity of carbazole derivatives in vitro, we examined its inhibitory effects on the migration of the metastatic breast cancer cell line MDA-MB-231 using the wound-healing assay at concentrations that do not affect cell viability. We chose the MDA-MB-231 breast cancer cells over MCF-7 due to its enhanced metastatic and migratory properties, with concomitant Rac and Cdc42 expression, compared to the non-metastatic and poorly migrating MCF-7 cells. The relative migration of treated cells with 3,6-dibromocarbazole derivatives compared with control (MDA-MB-231 cells) are summarized in Table 1.

Table 1. Cell growth inhibition and anti-migration activity of 3,6-dibromocarbazole derivatives.

Comp.	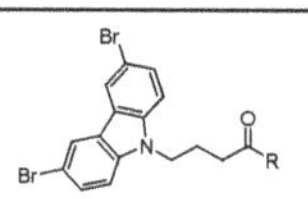 R =	GI_{50} (μM)[a] MCF-7	MDA-MB-231	Migration (%)[b,c]
4	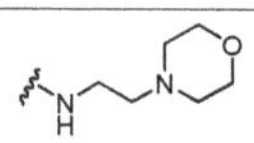	>50	>50	99 ± 6.03
5	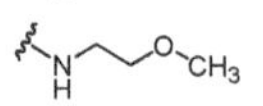	>50	>50	99 ± 5.98
6	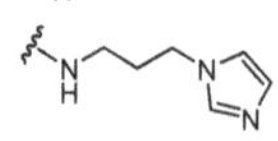	16.8	16	94 ± 3.93
7	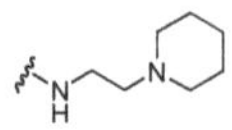	6.8	10	99 ± 0.03 (at 2 μM)
8	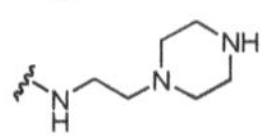	8	4.7	97 ± 4.90 (at 1 μM)
9	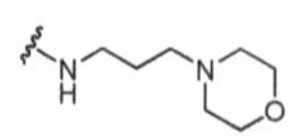	13.4	15.4	99 ± 1.58 (at 3.1 μM)
10	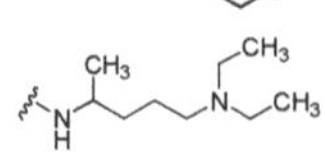	8.1	10.5	87 ± 4.65 (at 2.1 μM)

Table 1. *Cont.*

Comp.	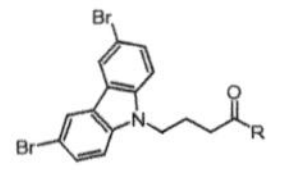 R =	GI_{50} (μM)[a] MCF-7	GI_{50} (μM)[a] MDA-MB-231	Migration (%)[b,c]
11	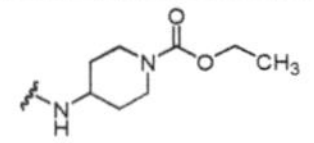	>50	>50	99 ± 0.02
12	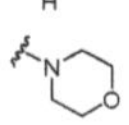	>50	>50	97 ± 6.41
13	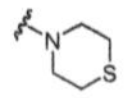	>50	25	99 ± 0.03
14	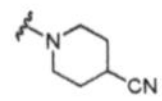	11.8	16.7	81 ± 8.96
15	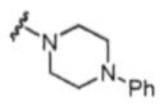	>50	>50	80 ± 5.87
16	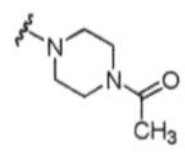	18.2	23	82 ± 7.52
17	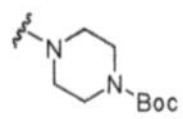	17.5	>50	99 ± 2.09
18	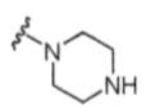	7.5	6.7	99 ± 0.02
19	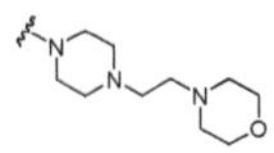	12.4	>50	99 ± 0.97
20	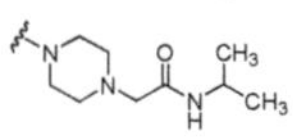	9.1	13.4	99 ± 0.05 (at 2.7 μM)
21	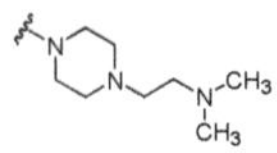	6.5	8	99 ± 0.48 (at 1.6 μM)
22	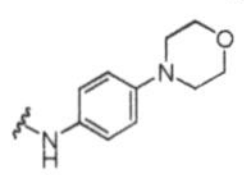	>50	>50	97 ± 4.19
23	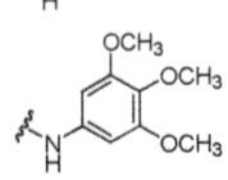	>50	19	90 ± 6.60
24	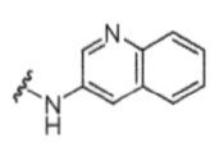	32.2	>50	82 ± 5.19
25	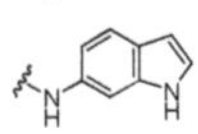	>50	>50	96 ± 4.69
26	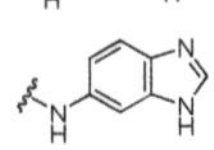	>50	>50	99 ± 6.52
27	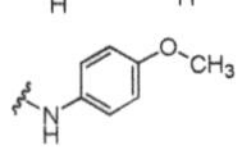	>50	>50	99 ± 0.05
Wiskostatin		9.7	8.3	95 ± 6.79 (at 2 μM)

[a] GI_{50} = compound concentration required to inhibit MDA-MB-231 proliferation by 50% after 48 h treatment. Values are expressed as the mean of triplicate experiments, and standard deviation (SD) is <10%. [b] After 24 h, MDA-MB-231 cellular migration was determined by measuring the distance traveled from the edge of the scratch toward the center of the scratch, relative to control. [c] Percent relative migration values at 10 μM (or at concentrations that do not affect cell viability). Results are presented as means ± SD of three independent experiments.

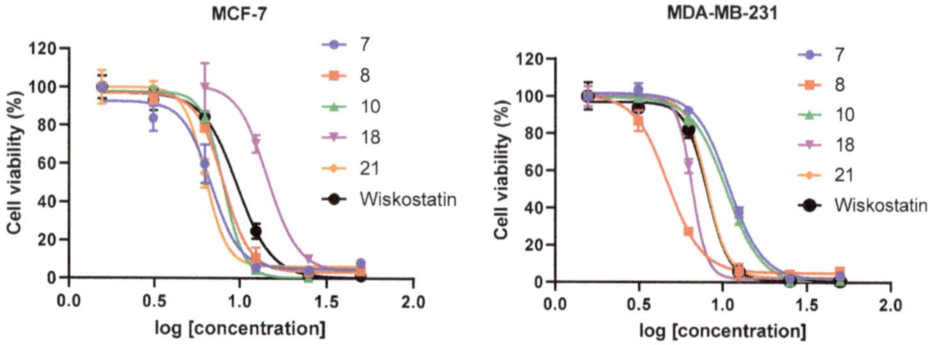

Figure 2. Log-dose response curve for compounds **7**, **8**, **10**, **18**, **21**, and Wiskostatin on MCF-7 and MDA-MB-231 breast cancer cell lines. Each data point represents the mean of three replicates and error bars represent ± SD. Each GI_{50} value was calculated based on sigmoidal curve fitting to the respective data set.

Among the twenty-four compounds tested for their anti-migratory effect, five compounds (**10**, **14**, **15**, **23**, **24**) inhibited migration in the range of 10–20%. While compounds **7**, **8**, **18**, and **21** were among the most cytotoxic compounds tested against MDA-MB-231 and MCF-7 cancer cell lines, they did not show significant anti-migratory effect. In contrast, compounds **14–16** and **24** inhibited migration in the range of 18–20%, compared to Wiskostatin that inhibit 5% of migration at 2 μM. Compound **14**, a carbazole derivative with a piperidine-4-carbonitrile amide group that showed moderate anti-proliferative activity on both MCF-7 and MDA-MB-231 cell lines, inhibit 19% of migration. Both compounds **15** and **16**, with phenyl- and acetyl-piperazine amide group, respectively, showed comparable anti-migratory activity with 20% and 18%, respectively. The anti-proliferative effect of **16** on both cancer cell lines was moderate, compared to **15**, which lacks cytotoxic activity. On the other hand, the 3-aminoquinoline amide **24**, showed anti-migratory activity of 18% with GI_{50} above 50 μM on MDA-MB-231 cell line. When comparing Wiskostatin and carbazole derivatives from Table 1, compound **10** exhibited anti-proliferative activity with GI_{50} values comparable with Wiskostatin on both cancer cell lines. However, compound **10** showed higher anti-migratory potency with 13% at 2.1 μM, compared with 5% anti-migratory effect of Wiskostatin at 2 μM on MDA-MB-231 breast cancer cells. Therefore, compound **10** exhibits similar cytotoxicity with improved anti-migratory potential compared to Wiskostatin.

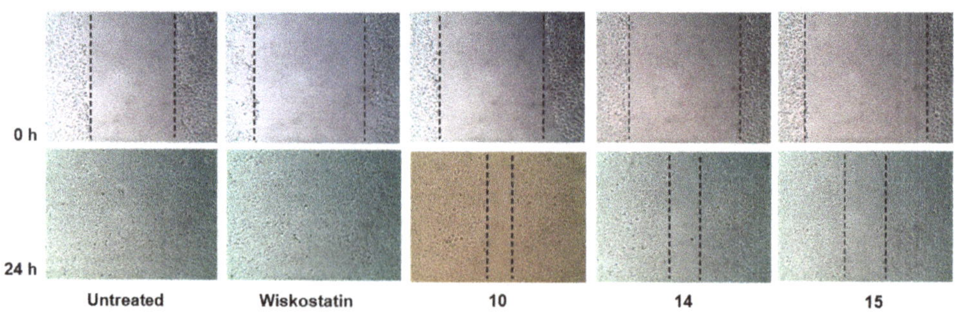

Figure 3. Inhibitory effect of compounds **10**, **14**, **15**, and Wiskostatin on MDA-MB-231 cells migration detected by wound-healing assay. MDA-MB-231 cells were treated with vehicle or with compounds **10**, **14**, **15**, and Wiskostatin. The photomicrographs were obtained at 0 and 24 h. Percent relative migration values are the average of three independent experiments. Dotted lines show the area occupied by the initial scraping for 0 h, and the wound edge for 24 h.

The Rho GTPases are believed to stimulate plasma membrane protrusion by inducing actin filament nucleation and polymerization on or close to membranes [43]. In particular, the Rho GTPase protein Cdc42, through activation of N-WASP/Arp2/3 pathway, is an important mediator of actin polymerization and filopodium extension [44,45]. Therefore, compounds that interfere with this process might be potentially useful molecular probes for the study of cell migration and invasion. To determine changes in actin cytoskeletal structures, we treated MDA-MB-231 breast cancer cells with vehicle or compounds **10**, **14**, **15**, and Wiskostatin at 10 μM for 24 h (Figure 4).

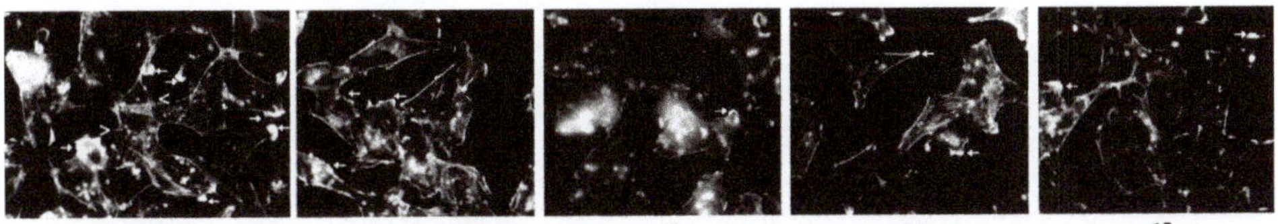

Figure 4. Effect of Wiskostatin and compounds **10**, **14**, and **15** on actin cytoskeleton of metastatic cancer cell MDA-MB-231. MDA-MB-231 metastatic breast cancer cells were treated with vehicle or Wiskostatin (2 μM) and compounds **10**, **14**, or **15** at 10 μM for 24 h to determine changes in actin cytoskeletal structures. Cells were fixed, permeabilized, and stained with rhodamine phalloidin to visualize F-actin. Arrows, lamellipodia; arrowheads, filopodia.

To identify F-actin based cell surface extensions, cells were stained with rhodamine phalloidin to localize F-actin. The results showed that untreated cells (control) demonstrated a strong formation of lamellipodia extensions, membrane ruffles, and stress fibers, with few filopodia. Wiskostatin and compounds **14** and **15** moderately reduced lamellipodia extensions when compared with control cells at concentrations that do not affect cell viability. In addition, compound **10**, at concentrations that inhibit 13% cell migration (2 μM), exhibited a marked reduction in lamellipodia formation when compared to vehicle, and in particular with Wiskostatin, which inhibits cell migration in 5% at 2 μM (Table 1). Compound **15** demonstrates a marked reduction in polymerized actin indicating inhibition of Arp2/3 mediated actin nucleation. Specific inhibition of filopodia, as would be predicted by WASP inhibition, could not be determined since the vehicle control cells exhibited more invadopodia and lamellipodia than filopodia. In general, these results suggest that new N-alkyl-3,6-dibromocarbazoles and compounds derivatives of Wiskostatin can be explored as new probes to study actin dynamics in cancer cells, or to further develop new anti-cancer and anti-metastatic drugs.

2.2. *N-alkyl-5-Bromoindole Derivatives*

To further explore the N-alkyl-5-bromoindole butyramide derivative series, we synthesized several compounds in which the carbazole core was replaced by a 5-bromoindole ring (Scheme 2). The strategy is to analyze the effect of using a smaller ring system as a core connected to the C3 linker side chain and the amide group. The synthesis of N-alkyl-5-bromoindole derivatives is described in Scheme 2. The 5-bromoindole **28** was reacted with ethyl 4-bromobutyrate, followed by hydrolysis to yield the corresponding 5-bromoindole-4-butyric acid **29**. Since N-alkylation in indoles is more difficult than in carbazoles, the reaction rate to obtain **29** was improved by using Cs_2CO_3 as a base over K_2CO_3, where Cs_2CO_3 solubility is ten times higher in organic solvents than K_2CO_3. For the generation of 5-bromoindole-4-butyramide derivative **30**, carboxylic acid **29** was therefore used as starting material, which reacted with different amines via an amide coupling reaction using reaction conditions similar as described in Scheme 1 (see the Supplementary Materials for representative ^{1}H and ^{13}C NMR spectral data).

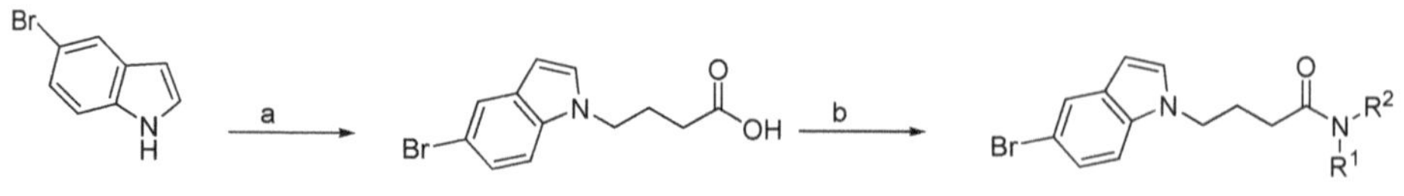

28 29 30

Scheme 2. General synthetic procedure of 5-bromoindole-4-butyramide derivative **30**. Reagents and conditions: (**a**) (i) Ethyl 4-bromobutyrate, Cs_2CO_3, DMF, 100 °C, 16 h; (ii) KOH, DMF/water, 80 °C, 2–6 h, 80%; (**b**) HOBt, EDAC, CH_2Cl_2, Et_3N, rt, amine: R-NH_2 or HNR^1R^2, 2-8 h.

The in vitro anti-proliferative and anti-migratory activities of compounds **31–34** are represented in Table 2. In this assay, the replacement of the rigid carbazole ring core by an indole resulted in loss of cytotoxic activity on both MCF-7 and MDA-MB-231 cell lines. For example, from the four representative 5-bromoindole derivatives synthesized, it can be observed that only compound **34** showed moderate cytotoxic effect on MCF-7 cells with GI_{50} of 18.4 μM, while GI_{50} value on MDA-MB-231 breast cancer cells was above 50 μM. Furthermore, the remaining compounds in that series had GI_{50}s above 50 μM in both breast cancer cell lines. Additionally, after 24 h treatment at 10 μM using the wound-healing assay in the MDA-MB-231 cell line, no migration inhibition could be observed. Hence, the absence of any activity of 5-bromoindole derivative series, together with the fact that several carbazole derivatives show promising activity, a structure-activity relationship (SAR) can be established. For example, it appears that the presence of a carbazole ring core, the C3 linker region, and amide group improve both anti-proliferative and anti-migratory activity.

Table 2. Cell growth inhibition and anti-migration activity of 5-bromoindole derivatives.

Comp.	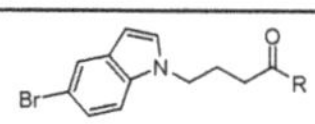 R =	GI_{50} (μM)[a] MCF-7	GI_{50} (μM)[a] MDA-MB-231	Migration (%)[b,c]
31	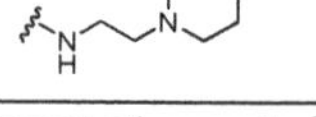	>50	>50	99 ± 0.05
32	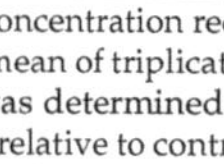	>50	>50	99 ± 7.78
33	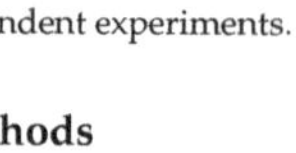	>50	>50	99 ± 0.02
34	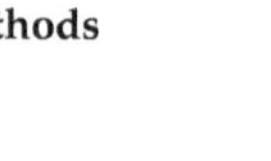	18.4	>50	99 ± 6.60

[a] GI_{50} = compound concentration required to inhibit MDA-MB-231 proliferation by 50% after 48 h treatment. Values are expressed as the mean of triplicate experiments, and standard deviation (SD) is <10%. [b] After 24 h, MDA-MB-231 cellular migration was determined by measuring the distance traveled from the edge of the scratch toward the center of the scratch, relative to control. [c] Percent relative migration values at 10 μM. Results are presented as means ± SD of three independent experiments.

3. Materials and Methods

3.1. General Methods

All experiments were carried out in pre-dried glassware (≥1 h, 80–90 °C) under a nitrogen atmosphere. Nuclear magnetic resonance (NMR) spectra were obtained using a 400 MHz Bruker Avance UltraShield™ spectrometer. ^1H (400 MHz) and ^{13}C (100 MHz) NMR were recorded in $CDCl_3$ or DMSO-d_6, unless otherwise used, and the chemical shift was expressed in parts per million (ppm) relative to CDCl3 (δ 7.26 for ^1H and δ 77.0 for ^{13}C) or DMSO-d_6 (δ 2.50 for ^1H and δ 39.5 for ^{13}C) as the internal standard. ^1H NMR data is reported as position (δ), relative integral, multiplicity (s, singlet; d, doublet; t, triplet; q, quartet; dt, doublet of triplets; dd, doublet of doublets; dq, doublet of quartets; m, multiplet; br, broad peak), coupling constant (*J*) in hertz (Hz), and the assignment of the atom. The shift in ppm for multiplets correspond to the centermost value of the entire splitting pattern. ^{13}C NMR data are reported as position (δ) and assignment of the atom. Microwave reactions were conducted in a CEM Discovery Microwave for Drug Discovery, SP- 1445. High resolution electrospray ionization mass spectrometry (ESI-HRMS) data were obtained on a Thermo Scientific™ Q Exactive™ Hybrid Quadrupole-Orbitrap Mass Spectrometer with high performance liquid chromatography (HPLC) Agilent 1200 utilizing a Zorbax SB-C18 column (2.1 mm × 50 mm, 1.8μm) at 40 °C, and a mobile phase of acetonitrile containing 5% Milli Q water at a flow rate of 0.35 mL/min (run time: 6.5 min), and 1 μL injection volume.

3.2. *Synthesis Methods*

Progress of the reaction was monitored via TLC analysis using general purpose silica gel on glass 5 × 20 cm with UV indicator, 250 μm, 60 Å medium pore diameter, UV indicator, and visualized by UV fluorescent Spectroline E Series Ultraviolet lamps, in most cases followed by staining with I2. The compounds were purified via column chromatography over silica gel (70–230 mesh, 60 Å) with the appropriate size column (24/40, 12 in. × 0.5 in.) or (24/40, 12 in. × 0.72 in.). Wiskostatin compound was obtained from MilliporeSigma.

3.2.1. General Procedure for the Synthesis of 4-(3,6-Dibromo-Carbazol-9-yl)-Butyric Acid (**2**)

A 50 mL three-neck round-bottom flask, equipped with a reflux condenser, was charged with 3,6-dibromocarbazole **1** (0.325 g, 1.0 mmol), K_2CO_3 (0.1382 g, 1 mmol), and ethyl 4-bromobutyrate 2 (0.4436 mL, 3.1 mmol), dissolved in DMF (5 mL). After 15 min of stirring at room temperature, the reaction mixture was refluxed at 80 °C for 2 h. After completion of the reaction (analyzed by TLC), water (1 mL) and KOH (1.0 mmol) was added and the reaction mixture, refluxed at 80 °C for 2 h. After the reaction was completed (analyzed by TLC), the mixture was allowed to reach room temperature. The mixture was washed with water (20 mL) and the product was extracted using dichloromethane (3 × 10 mL). The organic layer was washed with brine and dried with Na2SO4, and filtered and concentrated under reduced pressure. The crude oil was purified via column chromatography over silica gel and 50% ethyl acetate in hexane, and the product obtained as a white solid for the precursor 4-(3,6-Dibromo-carbazol-9-yl)-butyric acid **2** (0.3535 g, 0.86 mmol, 86%). TLC analysis in ethyl acetate-hexane (1:1), R_f = 0.19. ^{1}H NMR (400 MHz, $CDCl_3$) δ 1.98 (2H, m), 2.27 (2H, t, *J* = 7.2 Hz), 4.41 (2H, t, *J* = 7.2 Hz), 7.30 (2H, d, *J* = 8.9 Hz), 7.56 (2H, dd, *J* = 2.0, 8.8 Hz), 8.14 (1H, d, *J* = 2.0 Hz); ^{13}C NMR (100 MHz, $CDCl_3$) 24.2, 31.1, 42.2, 111.8, 112.0, 123.4, 123.9, 139.5, 174.3. HR-FTMS (ESI) *m/z* calcd. for $C_{16}H_{13}Br_2NO_2$, $[M + H]^+$ 411.9365, found 411.9365.

3.2.2. Synthesis of 3,6-Dibromocarbazole-4-butyramide Derivatives (**4–27**)

3.2.3. General Procedure for the Synthesis of 4-(3,6-Dibromocarbazol-9-yl)-N-(2-Morpholin-4-Ylethyl)Butyramide (**4**), and for Compounds **5–27**

A 50 mL three-neck round-bottom flask was charged with 4-(3,6-Dibromo-carbazol-9-yl)-butyric acid **2** (0.4111 g, 1.0 mmol), HOBT (0.2027 g, 1.5 mmol), and EDAC (0.2876 g, 1.5 mmol). The mixture was dissolved in CH_2Cl_2 (10 mL), stirred for 30 min, and 2-(4-morpholinyl)ethanamine **2** (0.133 g, 1.0 mmol) was added. After 15 min, Et_3N (0.43 mL, 3.0 mmol) was added and the mixture was stirred at room temperature for 16 h. After completion of the reaction (analyzed by TLC), water was added (30 mL) and the product was extracted using dichloromethane (3 × 10 mL). The organic layer was washed with brine and dried with Na_2SO_4, and filtered and concentrated under reduced pressure. The crude oil was purified via column chromatography over silica gel and 10% methanol in dichloromethane, and the product obtained as a white solid (0.382 g, 0.73 mmol, 73%). TLC analysis in CH_2Cl_2-MeOH (9:1), R_f = 0.26. ^{1}H NMR (400 MHz, $CDCl_3$) δ 2.0 (2H, m), 2.22 (2H, t, *J* = 6.8 Hz), 2.35 (2H, t, *J* = 4 Hz), 2.50 (4H, t, *J* = 1.6 Hz), 3.19 (2H, m), 3.56 (4H, t, *J* = 4.4 Hz), 4.39 (2H, t, *J* = 6.8 Hz),

7.60 (2H, d, J = 1.6 Hz), 8.0 (2H, bs), 8.46 (2H, bs); ^{13}C NMR (100 MHz, $CDCl_3$) 24.0, 31.2, 34.3, 41.8, 53.15, 53.2, 54.9, 57.2, 66.1, 111.3, 111.5, 122.9, 123.4, 128.8, 139.0, 161.0. HR-FTMS (ESI) m/z calcd. for $C_{22}H_{25}Br_2N_3O_2$, $[M + H]^+$ 524.0366, found 524.0367.

Synthesis of 4-(3,6-Dibromocarbazol-9-yl)-*N*-(2-methoxyethyl)butyramide (**5**)

The crude oil was purified via column chromatography over silica gel and 10% methanol in dichloromethane, and the product obtained as a white solid (0.096 g, 0.21 mmol, 63%). TLC analysis in CH_2Cl_2-MeOH (9:1), R_f = 0.56. ^{1}H NMR (400 MHz, $CDCl_3$) δ 1.63 (2H, bs), 2.15 (2H, t, J = 6.0 Hz), 2.21 (2H, m), 3.63 (3H, s), 3.46 (2H, d, J = 2.0 Hz), 4.39 (2H, t, J = 6.4 Hz), 7.35 (2H, d, J = 8.8 Hz), 7.57 (2H, dd, J = 1.6, 8.8 Hz), 8.16 (2H, *d*, J = 1.6 Hz); ^{13}C NMR (100 MHz, $CDCl_3$) 24.1, 32.4, 39.2, 42.3, 58.7, 71.0, 110.5, 112.1, 123.2, 123.4, 129.1, 139.2, 171.6. HR-FTMS (ESI) m/z calcd. for $C_{19}H_{20}Br_2N2O_2$, $[M + H]^+$ 468.9944, found 468.9947.

Synthesis of 4-(3,6-Dibromocarbazol-9-yl)-*N*-(3-imidazol-1-yl-propyl)butyramide (**6**)

The crude oil was purified via column chromatography over silica gel and 10% methanol in dichloromethane, and the product obtained as a white solid (0.078 g, 0.15 mmol, 49%). TLC analysis in CH_2Cl_2-MeOH (9:1), R_f = 0.22. ^{1}H NMR (400 MHz, $CDCl_3$) δ 1.96 (2H, t, J = 6.8 Hz), 2.07 (2H, t, J = 6.4 Hz), 2.20 (2H, m), 3.23 (2H, q, J = 6.4 Hz), 3.98 (2H, t, J = 6.8 Hz), 4.38 (2H, t, J = 6.8 Hz), 6.93 (1H, bs), 7.05 (1H, Bs), 7.33 (2H, d, J = 8.4 Hz), 7.51 (1H, bs), 7.56 (2H, dd, J = 2.0, 8.8 Hz), 8.15 (2H, d, J = 1.6 Hz); ^{13}C NMR (100 MHz, $CDCl_3$) 24.0, 31.0, 32.3, 36.9, 42.2, 44.8, 110.5, 112.2, 112.3, 123.3, 123.4, 129.1, 129.3, 129.4, 139.3, 171.9. HR-FTMS (ESI) m/z calcd. for $C_{22}H_{22}Br_2N_4O$, $[M + H]^+$ 519.0213, found 519.0211.

Synthesis of 4-(3,6-Dibromocarbazol-9-yl)-*N*-(2-piperidin-1-ylethyl)butyramide (**7**)

The crude oil was purified via column chromatography over silica gel and 10% methanol in dichloromethane, and the product obtained as a white solid (0.1033 g, 0.2 mmol, 59%). TLC analysis in CH_2Cl_2-MeOH (9:1), R_f = 0.47. ^{1}H NMR (400 MHz, $CDCl_3$) δ 1.43 (2H, q, J = 4. 9 Hz), 1.52 (4H, m), 2.11 (4H, dt, J = 3.3, 11.7 Hz), 2.34 (3H, bs), 2.38 (3H, t, J = 6.0 Hz), 3.31 (2H, q, J = 5.5 Hz), 4.29 (2H, t, J = 6.4 Hz), 6.05 (1H, bs), 7.28 (2H, d, J = 8.7 Hz), 7.5 (2H, dd, J = 1.9, 8.7 Hz), 8.06 (2H, d, J = 1.9 Hz); ^{13}C NMR (100 MHz, $CDCl_3$) 24.0, 24.2, 32.2, 35.9, 42.2, 54.2, 57.0, 110.5, 112.0, 123.1, 123.2, 128.9, 139.2, 171.4. HR-FTMS (ESI) m/z calcd. for $C_{23}H_{27}Br_2N_3O$, $[M + H]^+$ 522.0573, found 522.0572.

Synthesis of 4-(3,6-Dibromocarbazol-9-yl)-*N*-(2-piperazin-1-ylethyl)butyramide (**8**)

The crude oil was purified via column chromatography over silica gel and 10% methanol in dichloromethane, and the product obtained as a white solid (0.1425 g, 0.27 mmol, 71%). TLC analysis in CH_2Cl_2-MeOH (9:1), R_f = 0.23. ^{1}H NMR (400 MHz, $CDCl_3$) δ 1.9 (1H, bs), 2.11 (2H, t, J = 6.4 Hz), 2.20 (2H, m), 2.38 (3H, bs), 2.42 (4H, t, J = 5.9 Hz), 2.84 (4H, t, J = 4.7 Hz), 3.32 (2H, q, J = 5.4 Hz), 4.38 (2H, t, J = 6.7 Hz), 7.33 (2H, d, J = 8.7 Hz), 7.54 (2H, dd, J = 1.9, 10.6 Hz), 8.14 (2H, s); ^{13}C NMR (100 MHz, $CDCl_3$) 24.0, 32.2, 35.6, 42.4, 45.9, 54.1, 57.0, 110.6, 112.1, 123.2, 123.5, 139.4, 171.4. HR-FTMS (ESI) m/z calcd. for $C_{23}H_{27}Br_2N_3O$, $[M + H]^+$ 523.0526, found 523.0526.

Synthesis of 4-(3,6-Dibromocarbazol-9-yl)-*N*-(3-morpholin-4-ylpropyl)butyramide (**9**)

The crude oil was purified via column chromatography over silica gel and 10% methanol in dichloromethane, and the product obtained as a white solid (0.1496 g, 0.28 mmol, 69%). TLC analysis in CH_2Cl_2-MeOH (9:1), R_f = 0.59. ^{1}H NMR (400 MHz, $CDCl_3$) δ 1.56 (2H, m, J = 6.0 Hz), 1.95 (2H, t, J = 6.8 Hz), 2.14 (4H, m), 2.23 (2H, bs), 2.36 (2H, t, J = 6.4 Hz), 3.25 (2H, q, J = 5.6 Hz), 3.42 (1H, bs), 4.31 (2H, t, J = 6.8 Hz), 7.31 (2H, d, J = 8.8 Hz), 7.54 (2H, dd, J = 2.0, 8.8 Hz), 8.12 (2H, d, J = 1.6 Hz); ^{13}C NMR (100 MHz, $CDCl_3$) 24.0, 24.4, 32.3, 39.6, 42.1, 53.5, 58.0, 66.8, 110.6, 112.1, 123.2, 123.4, 129.1, 139.3, 171.1. HR-FTMS (ESI) m/z calcd. for $C_{23}H_{27}Br_2N_3O_2$, $[M + H]^+$ 538.0522, found 538.0521.

Synthesis of 4-(3,6-Dibromocarbazol-9-yl)-*N*-(4-diethylamino-1-methylbutyl)butyramide (**10**)

The crude oil was purified via column chromatography over silica gel and 10% methanol in dichloromethane, and the product obtained as a white solid (0.0063 g, 0.040 mmol, 9.1%). TLC analysis in CH_2Cl_2-MeOH (9:1), $R_f = 0.21$. ^{1}H NMR (400 MHz, $CDCl_3$) δ 0.89 (2H, m), 1.19 (6H, t, *J* = 7.6 Hz), 1.64 (2H, m), 2.20 (3H, bs), 2.25 (2H, t, *J* = 6.8 Hz), 2.62 (2H, t, *J* = 6.4 Hz), 3.29 (4H, m), 3.60 (2H, t, *J* = 7.20 Hz), 4.37 (2H, t, *J* = 7.20 Hz), 7.33 (2H, d, *J* = 8.8 Hz), 7.55 (2H, dd, *J* = 2.0, 8.8 Hz), 8.13 (2H, d, *J* = 2.0 Hz), 9.28 (1H, bs); ^{13}C NMR (100 MHz, $CDCl_3$) 8.5, 21.2, 21.3, 24.4, 29.7, 32.7, 33.6, 42.6, 44.6, 47.0, 52.3, 110.7, 112.0, 123.2, 123.5, 129.1, 139.4, 172.0. HR-FTMS (ESI) *m*/*z* calcd. for $C_{25}H_{33}Br_2N_3O_2$, $[M + H]^+$ 552.1043, found 552.1044.

Synthesis of 4-[4-(3,6-Dibromocarbazol-9-yl)-butyrylamino]piperidine-1-carboxylic acid ethyl ester (**11**)

The crude oil was purified via column chromatography over silica gel and 10% methanol in dichloromethane, and the product obtained as a white solid (0.1254 g, 0.22 mmol, 85.3%). TLC analysis in CH_2Cl_2-MeOH (9:1), $R_f = 0.63$. ^{1}H NMR (400 MHz, $CDCl_3$) δ 1.25 (3H, t, *J* = 7.2 Hz), 1.88 (2H, dd, *J* = 2.8, 12.4 Hz), 2.08 (2H, t, *J* = 6.4 Hz), 2.19 (2H, m, *J* = 6.8 Hz), 2.88 (2H, t, *J* = 12.0 Hz), 3.92 (1H, m, *J* = 3.6 Hz), 4.12 (4H, q, *J* = 6.8 Hz), 4.37 (2H, t, *J* = 6.8 Hz), 5.16 (1H, d, *J* = 7.6 Hz), 7.32 (2H, d, *J* = 8.8 Hz), 7.55 (2H, dd, *J* = 2.0, 8.8 Hz), 8.14 (2H, d, *J* = 1.6 Hz); ^{13}C NMR (100 MHz, $CDCl_3$) 14.7, 24.0, 32.0, 32.4, 42.2, 42.7, 46.8, 61.4, 110.5, 112.2, 123.3, 123.5, 129.2, 139.3, 155.4, 170.1. HR-FTMS (ESI) *m*/*z* calcd. for $C_{24}H_{27}Br_2N_3O_3$, $[M + H]^+$ 566.0471, found 566.0470.

Synthesis of 4-(3,6-Dibromocarbazol-9-yl)-1-morpholin-4-ylbutan-1-one (**12**)

The crude oil was purified via column chromatography over silica gel and 10% methanol in dichloromethane, and the product obtained as a white solid (0.0768 g, 0.16 mmol, 52%). TLC analysis in CH_2Cl_2-MeOH (9:1), $R_f = 0.94$. ^{1}H NMR (400 MHz, $CDCl_3$) δ 2.15 (4H, t, *J* = 6.0 Hz), 2.21 (2H, m, *J* = 6.8 Hz), 3.16 (2H, t, *J* = 4.8 Hz), 3.50 (2H, t, *J* = 4.4 Hz), 3.64 (4H, dt, *J* = 2.8, 6.4 Hz), 7.31 (2H, d, *J* = 8.8 Hz), 7.55 (2H, dd, *J* = 1.6, 8.4 Hz), 8.14 (2H, d, *J* = 1.6 Hz); ^{13}C NMR (100 MHz, $CDCl_3$) 23.6, 28.6, 41.5, 41.9, 45.1, 65.9, 66.0, 111.3, 111.5, 122.9, 123.41, 128.8, 139.0, 170.0. HR-FTMS (ESI) *m*/*z* calcd. for $C_{20}H_{20}Br_2N_2O_2$, $[M + H]^+$ 480.9944, found 480.9945.

Synthesis of 4-(3,6-Dibromocarbazol-9-yl)-1-thiomorpholin-4-ylbutan-1-one (**13**)

The crude oil was purified via column chromatography over silica gel and 10% methanol in dichloromethane, and the product obtained as a white solid (0.0712 g, 0.41 mmol, 35%). TLC analysis in CH_2Cl_2-MeOH (9:1), $R_f = 0.60$. ^{1}H NMR (400 MHz, $CDCl_3$) δ 2.11 (2H, t, *J* = 6.3 Hz), 2.21 (2H, m), 2.34 (2H, t, *J* = 5.0 Hz), 2.62 (2H, t, *J* = 5.2 Hz), 3.46 (2H, t, *J* = 5.0 Hz), 3.89 (2H, t, *J* = 5.0 Hz), 4.41 (2H, t, *J* = 6.7 Hz), 7.32 (2H, d, *J* = 8.6 Hz), 7.56 (2H, dd, *J* = 1.9, 8.7 Hz), 8.15 (2H, d, *J* = 1.7 Hz); ^{13}C NMR (100 MHz, $CDCl_3$) 23.5, 27.3, 27.4, 29.0, 42.1, 44.3, 47.8, 110.6, 112.2, 123.3, 123.5, 129.1, 139.4, 169.9. HR-FTMS (ESI) *m*/*z* calcd. for $C_{20}H_{20}Br_2N_3OS$, $[M + H]^+$ 496.9715, found 496.9713.

Synthesis of 1-[4-(3,6-Dibromocarbazol-9-yl)butyryl]piperidine-4-carbonitrile (**14**)

The crude oil was purified via column chromatography over silica gel and 10% methanol in dichloromethane, and the product obtained as a white solid (0.0775 g, 0.16 mmol, 44%). TLC analysis in CH_2Cl_2-MeOH (9:1), $R_f = 0.97$. ^{1}H NMR (400 MHz, $CDCl_3$) δ 1.63 (2H, t, *J* = 5.6 Hz), 1.85 (1H, m), 2.15 (2H, m), 2.84 (2H, m), 3.14 (2H, dt, *J* = 5.2, 13.6 Hz), 3.35 (2H, dt, *J* = 6.0, 14.4 Hz), 3.63 (2H, dq, *J* = 4.4, 13.6 Hz), 3.76 (2H, dq, *J* = 3.2, 13.6 Hz), 4.41 (2H, m), 7.31 (2H, d, *J* = 8.4 Hz), 7.54 (2H, dd, *J* = 1.6, 8.4 Hz), 8.14 (2H, d, *J* = 1.6 Hz); ^{13}C NMR (100 MHz, $CDCl_3$) 23.4, 26.2, 28.1, 28.6, 28.7, 39.5, 42.1, 43.0, 110.6, 112.2, 120.5, 123.3, 123.5, 129.1, 139.4, 169.8. HR-FTMS (ESI) *m*/*z* calcd. for $C_{22}H_{21}Br_2N_3O$, $[M + H]^+$ 504.0104, found 504.0104.

Synthesis of 4-(3,6-Dibromocarbazol-9-yl)-1-(4-phenylpiperazin-1-yl)butan-1-one (**15**)

The crude oil was purified via column chromatography over silica gel and 10% methanol in dichloromethane, and the product obtained as a white solid (0.2658 g, 0.27 mmol, 69%). TLC analysis in CH_2Cl_2-MeOH (9:1), $R_f = 0.53$. ^1H NMR (400 MHz, $CDCl_3$) δ 1.55 (2H, bs), 2.22 (2H, m), 2.97 (2H, t, $J = 5.3$ Hz), 3.15 (2H, t, $J = 4.9$ Hz), 3.34 (2H, t, $J = 4.5$ Hz), 3.30 (2H, t, $J = 4.7$ Hz), 4.43 (2H, t, $J = 3.4$ Hz), 6.92 (2H, t, $J = 7.9$ Hz), 7.29 (3H, t, $J = 7.9$ Hz), 7.34 (2H, d, $J = 8.7$ Hz), 7.54 (2H, dd, $J = 1.8$, 8.6 Hz), 8.15 (2H, d, $J = 1.7$ Hz); ^{13}C NMR (100 MHz, $CDCl_3$) 23.6, 28.9, 41.6, 42.2, 45.1, 49.4, 49.5, 110.6, 112.1, 116.8, 120.7, 123.3, 123.5, 129.2, 129.3, 139.4, 150.9, 170.0. HR-FTMS (ESI) m/z calcd. for $C_{26}H_{25}Br_2N_3O$, $[M + H]^+$ 556.0417, found 556.0417.

Synthesis of 1-(4-Acetylpiperazin-1-yl)-4-(3,6-dibromocarbazol-9-yl)butan-1-one (**16**)

The crude oil was purified via column chromatography over silica gel and 10% methanol in dichloromethane, and the product obtained as a white solid (0.0775 g, 0.15 mmol, 62%). TLC analysis in CH_2Cl_2-MeOH (9:1), $R_f = 0.67$. ^1H NMR (400 MHz, $CDCl_3$) δ 1.57 (3H, s), 2.08 (2H, bs), 2.12 (2H, bs), 2.21 (2H, bs), 3.19 (2H, t, $J = 5.3$ Hz), 3.45 (2H, t, $J = 6.2$), 3.64 (2H, t, $J = 5.0$ Hz), 4.42 (2H, t, $J = 6.6$ Hz), 7.32 (2H, dd, $J = 4.2$, 8.7 Hz), 7.54 (2H, dd, $J = 1.9$, 8.7 Hz), 8.14 (2H, d, $J = 1.8$ Hz); ^{13}C NMR (100 MHz, $CDCl_3$) 21.4, 28.8, 31.0, 41.5, 42.0, 42.2, 44.8, 45.9, 110.5, 112.2, 123.4, 129.1, 139.3, 169.3, 170.4. HR-FTMS (ESI) m/z calcd. for $C_{22}H_{23}Br_2N_3O_2$, $[M + H]^+$ 522.0209, found 522.0209.

Synthesis of 4-[4-(3,6-Dibromocarbazol-9-yl)butyryl]piperazine-1-carboxylic acid tert-butyl ester (**17**)

The crude oil was purified via column chromatography over silica gel and hexane-ethyl acetate (1:1) as the mobile phase, and the product obtained as a white solid (0.1977 g, 0.4 mmol, 80%). TLC analysis in hexane-ethyl acetate (1:1), $R_f = 0.35$. ^1H NMR (400 MHz, $CDCl_3$) δ 1.47 (9H, s), 2.20 (4H, m), 3.16 (2H, bs), 3.26 (2H, bs), 3.40 (2H, t, $J = 5.2$ Hz), 3.60 (2H, t, $J = 4.4$ Hz), 4.41 (2H, t, $J = 6.4$ Hz), 7.32 (2H, d, $J = 8.4$ Hz), 7.54 (2H, dd, $J = 1.6$, 8.4 Hz), 8.14 (2H, d, $J = 2.0$ Hz); ^{13}C NMR (100 MHz, $CDCl_3$) 23.5, 28.4, 29.0, 41.4, 42.2, 45.0, 80.4, 110.5, 112.2, 123.3, 123.5, 129.1, 139.4, 154.5, 170.2. HR-FTMS (ESI) m/z calcd. for $C_{25}H_{29}Br_2N_3O_3$, $[M + Na]^+$ 602.0447, found 602.0446.

Synthesis of 4-(3,6-Dibromocarbazol-9-yl)-1-piperazin-1-ylbutan-1-one (**18**)

The crude oil was purified via column chromatography over silica gel and 10% methanol in dichloromethane, and the product obtained as a white solid (0.0383 g, 0.080 mmol, 80%). TLC analysis in CH_2Cl_2-MeOH (9:1), $R_f = 0.38$. ^1H NMR (400 MHz, $CDCl_3$) δ 1.25 (1H, s), 2.18 (4H, m), 2.68 (2H, t, $J = 4.8$ Hz), 2.84 (2H, t, $J = 5.2$ Hz), 3.16 (2H, t, $J = 4.8$ Hz), 3.61 (2H, t, $J = 5.2$ Hz), 4.41 (2H, t, $J = 6.4$ Hz), 7.32 (2H, d, $J = 8.4$ Hz), 7.54 (2H, dd, $J = 2.0$, 8.8 Hz), 8.14 (2H, d, $J = 1.6$ Hz); ^{13}C NMR (100 MHz, $CDCl_3$) 22.6, 23.6, 42.2, 42.7, 45.8, 46.0, 46.3, 110.6, 112.1, 123.3, 123.5, 129.1, 139.4, 170.0. HR-FTMS (ESI) m/z calcd. for $C_{20}H_{21}Br_2N_3O$, $[M + H]^+$ 480.0104, found 480.0101.

Synthesis of 4-(3,6-Dibromocarbazol-9-yl)-1-[4-(2-morpholin-4-ylethyl)piperazin-1-yl]butan-1-one (**19**)

The crude oil was purified via column chromatography over silica gel and 10% methanol in dichloromethane, and the product obtained as a white solid (0.2036 g, 0.34 mmol, 76.4%). TLC analysis in CH_2Cl_2-MeOH (9:1), $R_f = 0.52$. ^1H NMR (400 MHz, $CDCl_3$) δ 2.12 (2H, t, $J = 6.0$ Hz), 2.18 (2H, t, $J = 7.2$ Hz), 2.24 (2H, m), 2.44 (2H, t, $J = 5.2$ Hz), 2.48 (4H, t, $J = 4.4$ Hz), 3.17 (2H, t, $J = 4.8$ Hz), 3.63 (2H, t, $J = 5.2$ Hz), 3.70 (4H, t, $J = 4.8$ Hz), 4.41 (2H, t, $J = 6.4$ Hz), 7.28 (2H, d, $J = 6.0$ Hz), 7.37 (2H, dd, $J = 6.4$ Hz, 8.8 Hz), 8.15 (2H, d, $J = 2.1$ Hz); ^{13}C NMR (100 MHz, $CDCl_3$) 23.5, 28.7, 41.6, 42.1, 45.0, 53.2, 53.3, 54.1, 55.4, 56.3, 66.9, 110.7, 112.1, 123.3, 123.4, 129.2, 139.4, 169.8. HR-FTMS (ESI) m/z calcd. for $C_{26}H_{32}Br_2N_4O_2$, $[M + H]^+$ 593.0944, found 593.0945.

Synthesis of 2-{4-[4-(3,6-Dibromocarbazol-9-yl)-butyryl]piperazin-1-yl}-*N*-isopropylacetamide (**20**)

The crude oil was purified via column chromatography over silica gel and 10% methanol in dichloromethane, and the product obtained as a white solid (0.2273 g, 0.39 mmol, 87.3%). TLC analysis in CH_2Cl_2-MeOH (9:1), R_f = 0.68. ^{1}H NMR (400 MHz, $CDCl_3$) δ 1.17 (6H, d, *J* = 6.6 Hz), 2.10 (2H, t, *J* = 6.3 Hz), 2.21 (2H, m), 2.26 (2H, t, *J* = 4.7 Hz), 2.47 (2H, t, *J* = 4.5 Hz), 3.15 (2H, t, *J* = 4.5 Hz), 3.64 (2H, t, *J* = 4.5 Hz), 4.10 (1H, m), 4.43 (2H, t, *J* = 6.6 Hz), 6.73 (1H, bs), 7.31 (2H, d, *J* = 8.7 Hz), 7.54 (2H, dd, *J* = 1.9, 8.7 Hz), 8.14 (2H, d, *J* = 1.9 Hz); ^{13}C NMR (100 MHz, $CDCl_3$) 22.8, 23.4, 28.7, 40.8, 41.6, 42.0, 45.0, 53.0, 53.1, 61.5, 110.64, 112.1, 123.3, 123.5, 129.2, 139.4, 168.4, 170.0. HR-FTMS (ESI) *m*/*z* calcd. for $C_{25}H_{30}Br_2N_4O_2$, $[M + H]^+$ 579.0788, found 579.0790.

Synthesis of 4-(3,6-Dibromocarbazol-9-yl)-1-[4-(2-dimethylaminoethyl)piperazin-1-yl]butan-1-one (**21**)

The crude oil was purified via column chromatography over silica gel and 10% methanol in dichloromethane, and the product obtained as a white solid (0.0228 g, 0.04 mmol, 7%). TLC analysis in CH_2Cl_2-MeOH (9:1), R_f = 0.50. ^{1}H NMR (400 MHz, $CDCl_3$) δ 1.25 (6H, s), 2.12 (2H, t, *J* = 6.0 Hz), 2.19 (2H, m), 2.24 (4H, t, *J* = 5.6 Hz), 2.43 (4H, t, *J* = 4.8 Hz), 3.19 (2H, t, *J* = 4.4 Hz), 3.64 (2H, t, *J* = 4.4 Hz), 4.40 (2H, t, *J* = 6.4 Hz), 7.31 (2H, d, *J* = 8.8 Hz), 7.53 (2H, dd, *J* = 1.6, 8.4 Hz,), 8.21 (2H, d, *J* = 2.0 Hz); ^{13}C NMR (100 MHz, $CDCl_3$) 23.5, 28.7, 41.5, 42.1, 45.0, 45.6, 53.1, 53.3, 56.1, 56.5, 110.6, 112.1, 123.2, 123.4, 129.2, 139.4, 170.0. HR-FTMS (ESI) *m*/*z* calcd. for $C_{24}H_{30}Br_2N_4O$, $[M + H]^+$ 551.0839, found 551.0842.

Synthesis of 4-(3,6-Dibromocarbazol-9-yl)-*N*-(4-morpholin-4-ylphenyl)butyramide (**22**)

The crude oil was purified via column chromatography over silica gel and 10% methanol in dichloromethane, and the product obtained as a white solid (0.0689 g, 0.12 mmol, 40%). TLC analysis in CH_2Cl_2-MeOH (9:1), R_f = 0.80. ^{1}H NMR (400 MHz, DMSO-d_6) δ 2.05 (2H, t, *J* = 6.8 Hz), 2.30 (2H, m), 3.02 (4H, t, *J* = 4.8 Hz), 3.71 (4H, t, *J* = 4.4 Hz), 4.44 (2H, t, *J* = 6.8 Hz), 6.86 (2H, d, *J* = 8.8 Hz), 7.41 (2H, d, *J* = 8.8 Hz), 7.61 (2H, dd, *J* = 0.8, 8.8 Hz), 7.64 (2H, d, *J* = 8.4 Hz), 8.48 (2H, s), 9.62 (1H, s); ^{13}C NMR (100 MHz, DMSO-d_6) 24.1, 32.7, 42.0, 48.9, 66.1, 111.3, 111.6, 115.4, 120.3, 122.9, 123.4,128.8, 131.5, 139.0, 147.0, 169.7. HR-FTMS (ESI) *m*/*z* calcd. for $C_{26}H_{25}Br_2N_3O_2$, $[M + H]^+$ 572.0366, found 572.0365.

Synthesis of 4-(3,6-Dibromocarbazol-9-yl)-*N*-(3,4,5-trimethoxyphenyl)butyramide (**23**)

The crude oil was purified via column chromatography over silica gel and 10% methanol in dichloromethane, and the product obtained as a white solid (0.051 g, 0.10 mmol, 30%). TLC analysis in CH_2Cl_2-MeOH (9:1), R_f = 0.17. ^{1}H NMR (400 MHz, DMSO-d_6) δ 2.08 (2H, m), 2.28 (2H, t, *J* = 7.2 Hz), 3.60 (3H, s), 3.71 (3H, s), 3.72 (3H, s), 4.46 (2H, t, *J* = 6.8 Hz), 6.90 (2H, s), 7.60 (2H, dd, *J* = 1.6, 8.4 Hz), 7.64 (2H, d, *J* = 8.8 Hz), 8.47 (2H, d, *J* = 1.6 Hz), 9.71 (1H, s); ^{13}C NMR (100 MHz, DMSO-d_6) 6.96, 24.0, 32.0, 42.0, 55.6, 60.0, 96.9, 111.3, 111.6, 122.9, 123.4, 128.8, 133.3, 135.2, 139.1, 152.6, 170.1. HR-FTMS (ESI) *m*/*z* calcd. for $C_{25}H_{24}Br_2N_2O_4$, $[M + H]^+$ 577.0155, found 577.0142.

Synthesis of 4-(3,6-Dibromocarbazol-9-yl)-*N*-quinolin-3-ylbutyramide (**24**)

The crude oil was purified via column chromatography over silica gel and 10% methanol in dichloromethane, and the product obtained as a white solid (0.0275 g, 0.052 mmol, 15%). TLC analysis in hexane-ethyl acetate (1:1), R_f = 0.20. ^{1}H NMR (400 MHz, DMSO-d_6) δ 2.13 (2H, m), 2.44 (2H, t, *J* = 6.8 Hz), 4.50 (2H, t, *J* = 6.5 Hz), 7.41 (1H, t, *J* = 7.4 Hz), 7.54 (1H, t, *J* = 8.0 Hz), 7.62 (1H, t, *J* = 7.9 Hz), 7.67 (1H, d, *J* = 8.6 Hz), 7.71 (1H, d, *J* = 8.3 Hz), 7.92 (2H, t, *J* = 8.4 Hz), 7.98 (2H, d, *J* = 8.4 Hz), 8.47 (2H, s), 8.64 (1H, s), 8.82 (1H, s), 10.3 (1H, s); ^{13}C NMR (100 MHz, DMSO-d_6) 23.9. 32.9, 42.0, 109.6, 111.4, 111.7, 119.2, 122.0, 123.0, 123.5, 124.5, 127.0, 127.4, 127.6, 127.7, 127.8, 128.5, 128.9, 132.8, 139.1, 144.1, 144.5, 171.3. HR-FTMS (ESI) *m*/*z* calcd. for $C_{25}H_{19}Br_2N_3O$, $[M + H]^+$ 537.9947, found 537.9946.

Synthesis of 4-(3,6-Dibromocarbazol-9-yl)-*N*-(1H-indol-6-yl)butyramide (**25**)

The crude oil was purified via column chromatography over silica gel and 10% methanol in dichloromethane, and the product obtained as a white solid (0.1152 g, 0.22 mmol, 38%). TLC analysis in hexane-ethyl acetate (1:1), R_f = 0.50. ^{1}H NMR (400 MHz, DMSO-d_6) δ 2.08 (2H, m), 2.35 (2H, t, *J* = 7.1 Hz), 4.47 (2H, t, *J* = 7.0 Hz), 6.33 (1H, s), 6.97, (1H, d, *J* = 9.1 Hz), 7.24 (1H, s), 7.40 (1H, d, *J* = 8.4 Hz), 7.61 (2H, d, *J* = 7.2 Hz), 7.66 (2H, d, *J* = 8.7 Hz), 7.95 (1H, s), 8.49 (2H, s), 9.75 (1H, s); ^{13}C NMR (100 MHz, DMSO-d_6) 24.2, 32.9, 42.1, 100.9, 102.2, 111.3, 111.6, 112.3, 119.7, 123.0, 123.5, 123.7, 124.8, 128.9, 133.3, 135.9, 139.1. HR-FTMS (ESI) *m*/*z* calcd. for $C_{24}H_{19}Br_2N_3O$, $[M + H]^+$ 525.9947, found 9946.

Synthesis of *N*-(3H-Benzoimidazol-5-yl)-4-(3,6-dibromocarbazol-9-yl)butyramide (**26**)

The crude oil was purified via column chromatography over silica gel and 10% methanol in dichloromethane, and the product obtained as a white solid (0.100 g, 0.20 mmol, 44%). TLC analysis in hexane-ethyl acetate (1:1), R_f = 0.70. ^{1}H NMR (400 MHz, DMSO-d_6) δ 2.16 (2H, m, *J* = 7.2 Hz), 3.18 (2H, t, *J* = 7.6 Hz), 4.52 (2H, t, *J* = 7.2 Hz), 6.66 (1H, dd, *J* = 2.0, 8.8 Hz), 7.60 (1H, dd, *J* = 2.0, 8.8 Hz), 7.68 (1H, d, *J* = 8.8 Hz), 8.05 (1H, s), 8.47 (1H, dd, *J* = 1.6, 8.0 Hz); ^{13}C NMR (100 MHz, DMSO-d_6) 23.6, 32.0, 42.3, 97.2, 111.8, 112.0, 114.3, 117.2, 122.3, 123.5, 124.0, 129.4, 139.5, 141.0, 141.2, 151.7, 173.0. HR-FTMS (ESI) *m*/*z* calcd. for $C_{23}H_{18}Br_2N_4O$, $[M + H]^+$ 526.9900, found 526.9904.

Synthesis of 4-(3,6-Dibromocarbazol-9-yl)-*N*-(4-methoxyphenyl)butyramide (**27**)

The crude oil was purified via column chromatography over silica gel and 10% methanol in dichloromethane, and the product obtained as a white solid (0.1830 g, 0.35 mmol, 94%). TLC analysis in hexane-ethyl acetate (1:1), R_f = 0.64. ^{1}H NMR (400 MHz, DMSO-d_6) δ 2.05 (2H, m), 2.30 (2H, t, *J* = 7.2 Hz), 3.70 (3H, s), 4.45 (2H, t, *J* = 7.2 Hz), 6.84 (2H, d, *J* = 9.2 Hz), 7.44 (2H, d, *J* = 9.2 Hz), 7.60 (2H, dd, *J* = 2.0, 8.8 Hz), 7.65 (2H, d, *J* = 8.8 Hz), 8.48 (2H, d, *J* = 2.0 Hz), 9.68 (1H, s); ^{13}C NMR (100 MHz, DMSO-d_6) 24.1, 32.7, 42.0, 55.1, 111.3, 111.6, 113.8, 120.7, 123.0, 123.5, 128.7, 132.3, 139.1, 155.1, 169.9. HR-FTMS (ESI) *m*/*z* calcd. for $C_{23}H_{20}Br_2N_2O_2$, $[M + H]^+$ 516.9944, found 516.9941.

3.2.4. Synthesis of N-Alkyl-5-Bromoindole Derivatives (**31–34**)

3.2.5. General Procedure for the Synthesis of 4-(5-Bromoindol-1-yl)Butyric Acid (**29**)

A 50 mL three-neck round-bottom flask, equipped with a reflux condenser, was charged with 5-bromoindole **28** (0.1960 g, 1.0 mmol), Cs_2CO_3 (0.9770 g, 3 mmol) and ethyl 4-bromobutyrate (0.43 mL, 3.0 mmol), dissolved in DMF (3 mL). After 15 min of stirring at room temperature, the reaction mixture was refluxed at 100 °C for 16 h. After completion of the reaction (analyzed by TLC), water (1 mL) and KOH (1.0 mmol) were added and the reaction mixture refluxed at 80 °C for 2 h. After the reaction was completed (analyzed by TLC), the mixture was allowed to reach room temperature and 1N HCl solution was added until reach neutral pH. The mixture was washed with water (20 mL) and the product was extracted using dichloromethane (3 × 10 mL). The organic layer was washed with brine and dried with Na_2SO_4, and filtered and concentrated under reduced pressure. The crude oil was purified via column chromatography over silica gel and 10% CH_2Cl_2 in MeOH, and the product obtained as a white solid for the precursor 4-(5-Bromoindol-1-yl)Butyric acid **29** (0.2260 g, 0.801 mmol, 80%). TLC analysis in CH_2Cl_2-MeOH (9:1), R_f = 0.25. ^{1}H NMR (400 MHz, $CDCl_3$) δ 2.16 (2H, m), 2.34 (2H, t, *J* = 7.2 Hz), 4.20 (2H, t, *J* = 6.80 Hz), 6.44 (1H, d, *J* = 2.4 Hz), 7.08 (1H, 2, *J* = 3.2 Hz), 7.22 (1H, d, *J* = 6.4 Hz), 7.29 (1H, dd, *J* = 2.0, 8.8 Hz), 7.74 (1H, d, *J* = 1.6 Hz); ^{13}C NMR (100 MHz, $CDCl_3$) 25.1, 30.5, 45.3, 101.1, 110.7, 112.8, 123.5, 124.5, 128.9, 130.3, 134.6, 177.4. HR-FTMS (ESI) *m*/*z* calcd. for $C_{12}H_{12}BrNO_2$, $[M + H]^+$ 284.0104, found 284.0102.

3.2.6. General Procedure for the Synthesis of 4-(5-Bromoindol-1-yl)-N-(3-Morpholin-4-ylpropyl)Butyramide (**31**), and for Compounds **32**–**34**

A 50 mL three-neck round-bottom flask was charged with 4-(5-Bromoindol-1-yl)Butyric acid **29** (0.098 g, 0.35 mmol), HOBT (0.2027 g, 1.5 mmol), and EDAC (0.2876 g, 1.5 mmol). The mixture was dissolved in DMF (5 mL), stirred for 30 min, and 3-morpholinopropylamine (0.0512 mL, 0.35 mmol) was added. After 15 min, Et_3N (0.43 mL, 3.0 mmol) was added and the mixture stirred at room temperature for 16 h. After the reaction was completed (analyzed by TLC), water was added (30 mL) and the product was extracted using dichloromethane (3 × 10 mL). The organic layer was washed with brine and dried with Na_2SO_4, and filtered and concentrated under reduced pressure. The crude oil was purified via column chromatography over silica gel and 10% methanol in dichloromethane, and the product obtained as a white solid (0.0748 g, 0.18 mmol, 53%). TLC analysis in hexane-ethyl acetate (1:1), $R_f = 0.36$. ^{1}H NMR (400 MHz, $CDCl_3$) δ 1.62 (2H, m), 2.01 (2H, t, $J = 6.8$ Hz), 2.21 (2H, m), 2.35 (4H, bs), 2.42 (2H, t, $J = 6.4$ Hz), 3.32 (2H, q, $J = 5.6$ Hz), 3.47 (4H, bs), 4.39 (2H, t, $J = 6.8$ Hz), 7.0 (1H, bs), 7.26 (1H, d, $J = 1.2$ Hz), 7.32 (1H, d, $J = 8.8$ Hz), 7.55 (1H, dd, $J = 2.0$, 8.8 Hz), 8.14 (1H, d, $J = 1.6$ Hz); ^{13}C NMR (100 MHz, $CDCl_3$) 24.5, 25.8, 32.6, 39.6, 45.2, 53.6, 58.0, 67.0, 101.1, 110.9, 112.6, 123.4, 124.3, 128.8, 130.2, 134.9, 171.2. HR-FTMS (ESI) *m/z* calcd. for $C_{19}H_{26}BrN_3O_2$, $[M + H]^+$ 410.1261, found 410.1257.

Synthesis of 1-[4-(5-Bromoindol-1-yl)butyryl]piperidine-4-carbonitrile (**32**)

The crude oil was purified via column chromatography over silica gel and 10% methanol in dichloromethane, and the product obtained as a white solid (0.0356 g, 0.10 mmol, 24.4%). TLC analysis in CH_2Cl_2-MeOH (9:1), $R_f = 0.76$. ^{1}H NMR (400 MHz, DMSO-d_6) δ 1.58 (4H, m), 1.81 (2H, bs), 1.94 (2H, t, $J = 7.2$ Hz), 2.26 (2H, t, $J = 7.2$ Hz), 3.07 (1H, m), 3.50 (2H, dt, $J = 4.8$, 15.2 Hz), 3.78 (2H, dt, $J = 4.8$, 13.6Hz), 4.18 (2H, t, $J = 6.8$Hz), 6.42 (1H, d, $J = 3.2$ Hz), 7.24 (1H, dd, $J = 2.0$, 8.4 Hz), 7.41 (1H, d, $J = 3.2$ Hz), 7.47 (1H, d, $J = 8.8$ Hz), 7.73 (1H, d, $J = 2.0$ Hz); ^{13}C NMR (100 MHz, DMSO-d_6) 22.7, 25.3, 28.2, 29.4, 29.7, 39.5, 43.1, 45.3, 101.0, 111.0, 112.7, 120.6, 123.5, 124.4, 128.9, 130.2, 134.9, 169.9. HR-FTMS (ESI) *m/z* calcd. for $C_{18}H_{20}BrN_3O$, $[M + H]^+$ 376.0842, found 376.0837.

Synthesis of 4-(5-Bromoindol-1-yl)-N-(3-imidazol-1-yl-propyl)butyramide (**33**)

The crude oil was purified via column chromatography over silica gel and 10% methanol in dichloromethane, and the product obtained as a white solid (0.1255 g, 0.32 mmol, 57%). TLC analysis in CH_2Cl_2-MeOH (9:1), $R_f = 0.44$. ^{1}H NMR (400 MHz, $CDCl_3$) δ 1.81 (2H, m, $J = 6.8$ Hz), 1.98 (2H, m, $J = 6.8$ Hz), 2.06 (2H, t, $J = 6.4$ Hz), 3.01 (2H, q, $J = 5.6$ Hz), 3.95 (2H, t, $J = 6.8$ Hz), 4.17 (2H, t, $J = 7.2$ Hz), 6.42 (1H, d, $J = 2.8$ Hz), 6.95 (1H, bs), 7.23 (2H, dd, $J = 1.6$, 8.4 Hz), 7.40 (1H, d, $J = 2.8$ Hz), 7.45 (1H, d, $J = 8.8$ Hz), 7.72 (1H, d, $J = 2.0$ Hz), 7.90 (1H, t, $J = 5.2$ Hz); ^{13}C NMR (100 MHz, $CDCl_3$) 25.7, 31.0, 32.2, 36.5, 44.2, 45.6, 101.0, 111.0, 112.5, 119.1, 123.3, 124.4, 128.7, 128.8, 130.2, 134.7, 136.9, 172.4. HR-FTMS (ESI) *m/z* calcd. for $C_{18}H_{21}BrN_4O$, $[M + H]^+$ 391.0951, found 391.0956.

Synthesis of 4-(5-Bromoindol-1-yl)-N-(2-piperidin-1-ylethyl)butyramide (**34**)

The crude oil was purified via column chromatography over silica gel and 10% methanol in dichloromethane, and the product obtained as a white solid (0.1967 g, 0.50 mmol, 50%). TLC analysis in CH_2Cl_2-MeOH (9:1), $R_f = 0.47$. ^{1}H NMR (400 MHz, DMSO-d_6) δ 1.35 (2H, m, $J = 5.2$ Hz), 1.47 (4H, m, $J = 5.6$ Hz), 1.96 (2H, m, $J = 6.4$ Hz), 2.01 (2H, t, $J = 6.0$ Hz), 2.30 (2H, t, $J = 6.8$ Hz), 2.35 (2H, bs), 3.13 (2H, q, $J = 6.4$ Hz), 4.18 (2H, t, $J = 6.4$ Hz) 7.35 (1H, dd, $J = 2.0$, 8.8 Hz), 7.54 (2H, d, $J = 2.4$ Hz), 7.56 (1H, s), 7.68 (1H, s), 7.71 (1H, t, $J = 5.6$ Hz); ^{13}C NMR (100 MHz, DMSO-d_6) 24.1, 25.5, 25.7, 32.4, 35.7, 45.8, 54.3, 57.2, 100.8, 109.4, 111.0, 118.5, 120.3, 128.9, 129.0, 134.7, 171.7. HR-FTMS (ESI) *m/z* calcd. for $C_{25}H_{30}Br_2N_4O_2$, $[M + H]^+$ 394.1312, found 394.1313.

3.3. Biological Evaluation

3.3.1. Cell Culture

MCF-7 and MDA-MB-231 cells were cultured in Minimum Essential Medium Eagle (MEME) 10% FBS supplemented with Earle's Balanced Salt Solution (EBSS), Non-essential Amino Acids (NEAA), Sodium Pyruvate, Pen/Strep, and L-glutamine 37 °C in 5% CO_2.

3.3.2. Sulforhodamine B (SRB) Assay

A stock solution of compounds was prepared at 50 mM in 100% DMSO. For cell preparation, a flask of 75 cm^2 or 25 cm^2 was used for 2.6×10^5 cells/mL or 1.44×10^5 cells/mL, respectively, with an 80–90% confluence. Cells were washed with PBS and trypsinized. The concentration of cells was determined using a 1:2 dilution with Trypan Blue and a hemocytometer. After cell count, the concentration was adjusted to have a $7.0–10.0 \times 10^4$ cells/mL. Approximately 100 µL of cells suspension, compounds, control positive and control negative were added in triplicates to a 96 well plate. The positive control used was doxorubicin, and the negative control was DMSO 0.1%. All compounds at 50, 25, 12.5, 6.3, and 1.6 µM were incubated with cells at 37 °C for 48 hrs. For fixation, cold TCA 50% was used and incubated at 4 °C for 1 hr. Wells were washed and dried prior to tincture with 100 µL of SRB 0.4%. To remove excess SRB, acetic acid was used. For analysis, TRIS-Base Solution (pH = 10.5) was used and shaken prior to reading using an ELISA reader at 540 nm and the software SoftMax Pro 4.8. For each compound, 50% growth inhibition (GI_{50}) was calculated from sigmoidal dose-response curves (variable-slope) that were generated with data obtained from experiments carried out in triplicates (GI_{50} values were generated with GraphPad Prism V. 6.02, GraphPad Software, Inc.).

3.3.3. Wound Healing Assay (Scratch Method) Using MDA-MB-231 Cancer Cells

Prior to assays, cells were grown until 80–90% confluence was observed. We used a 75 cm^2 flask for 2.6×10^5 cells/mL in 10 mL, and for a 25 cm^2 flask 1.44×10^5 cells/mL in 5 mL. The cells were washed with PBS to remove all traces of FBS. We added trypsin at 2 mL for a 25 cm^2 flask or 4 mL for a 75 cm^2 flask, and incubated 5–10 min at 37 °C. At the end of the incubation time, cells were re-suspended and counted with hemocytometer using 1:2 dilutions with Trypan Blue. Subsequently, cell viability was calculated. In a 12 multiwell plate. Cells were seeded at $1.5–2.2 \times 10^5$ cells/mL in 1 mL and incubated for 24 h. Cells were then rinsed with PBS and incubated in starving media (0.5% FBS) overnight. All controls and drugs were tested in triplicate. The vehicle control for each drug was prepared according to the drug's DMSO concentration. Drugs were diluted and the final concentration at each well was 10 µM (or $GI_{50}/5$ on MDA-MB-231 cells). The wound was made using a sterile pipette tip of 200 µL. Cells were then rinsed very gently with media without FBS and media with vehicle controls or drugs were added. After a 24 h incubation, the gap distance was evaluated using the software Lumera Infinity Analyze 6.4.0. Pictures were taken at 0, 8, 12, and 24 h using a 10X objective in an Inverted Laboratory Microscope Leica DM IL LED, and an Infinity1-3 3.1 Megapixel USB 2.0 camera CMOS. The percentage of migration was calculated using the following formula:

$100 - [\,(X_0/\ddot{X}_0)]*100$ for time 0 h measurements

$100 - [\,(X_{24}/\ddot{X}_0)]*100$ for time 24 h measurements

3.3.4. Actin Polymerization Assay

MDA-MB-231 cells were treated with vehicle or compound derivatives at 10 µM (or at concentrations that do not affect cell viability) for 24 h at 37 °C in 5% CO_2. Cells were fixed in 3.7% of formaldehyde, permeabilized using 0.2% Triton, and stained with Rhodamine Phalloidin to visualize F-actin. Fluorescence micrographs were acquired at 60x in an Eclipse E400 fluorescence microscope using a DS-Qi2 monochrome digital camera from Nikon for fluorescence imaging.

4. Conclusions

In this study, a new series of *N*-alkyl-3,6-dibromocarbazole and *N*-alkyl-5-bromoindole derivatives were designed, synthesized, and biologically evaluated for their anti-cancer and anti-migration effect on MCF-7 and MDA-MB-231 cancer cells. In addition, the effect of compounds on the actin cytoskeleton of MDA-MB-231 cancer cells was explored. From the results, we have established the Structure-Activity Relationships of novel derivatives of the lead compound Wiskostatin. We found that the carbazole moiety is needed for in vitro anti-cancer and anti-migratory potency. The replacement of the carbazole by an indole ring resulted in loss of activity. Moreover, the aliphatic or aromatic amide group was extended 3-carbon atoms away from the carbazole moiety. The most potent anti-proliferative compounds were those bearing a 3,6-dibromocarbazole group with GI_{50} values between 7–32 μM and 4.7–23 μM on MCF-7 and MDA-MB-231 cancer cells, respectively. The most promising results in terms of anti-migratory effect was exhibited by carbazole derivatives **10**, **23**, **14–16**, and **24** with migration inhibition in the range of 10–20% on the highly metastatic breast cancer cells MDA-MB-231. Future studies will improve these derivatives and also test their effects at higher concentrations and shorter times of migration to reduce potential cytotoxic effects, which may confound inhibition of cell migration. The carbazole derivatives **10**, **14**, and **15** were further examined as actin polymerization inhibitors and results demonstrated reduction in actin polymerization and extension of F-actin based structures. Further studies of mechanism of actions focused on the effect of these novel compounds in the Cdc42/N-WASP/Arp2/3 pathway is needed to fully characterize and analyze the potential of this new series of compounds as in vitro and in vivo anti-metastatic drugs.

Supplementary Materials: The following are available online. ^{1}H and ^{13}C NMR spectral data for representative compounds. Figure S1: ^{1}H NMR Spectral Data of 2; Figure S2: ^{13}C NMR Spectral Data of 2; Figure S3: ^{1}H NMR Spectral Data of 7; Figure S4: ^{13}C NMR Spectral Data of 7; Figure S5: ^{1}H NMR Spectral Data of 12; Figure S6: ^{13}C NMR Spectral Data of 12; Figure S7: ^{1}H NMR Spectral Data of 14; Figure S8: ^{13}C NMR Spectral Data of 14; Figure S9: ^{1}H NMR Spectral Data of 16; Figure S10: ^{1}H NMR Spectral Data of 22; Figure S11: ^{13}C NMR Spectral Data of 22; Figure S12: ^{1}H NMR Spectral Data of 24; Figure S13: ^{13}C NMR Spectral Data of 24; Figure S14: ^{1}H NMR Spectral Data of 29; Figure S15: ^{13}C NMR Spectral Data of 29; Figure S16: ^{1}H NMR Spectral Data of 33; Figure S17: ^{13}C NMR Spectral Data of 33.

Author Contributions: K.B., Z.R., and A.F. performed the experiments and data collection; J.B. performed data analysis of GCMS; S.D. developed a methodology for actin assay experiments; and E.H. supervised, administrated, and was in charge of funding acquisition of the project. All authors read and approved the final manuscript.

Funding: This research was funded by the National Institutes of Health (MBRS-SCORE NIH/NIGMS SC2GM116712).

Acknowledgments: We thank Fernando González-Illán from the US FDA for assisting with the high-resolution electrospray ionization mass spectrometry data and analysis.

Conflicts of Interest: The authors declare no conflict of interest.

References

1. Gupta, G.P.; Massagué, J. Cancer Metastasis: Building a Framework. *Cell* **2006**, *127*, 679–695. [CrossRef] [PubMed]
2. Walker, C.; Mojares, E.; Hernández, A.D.R. Role of Extracellular Matrix in Development and Cancer Progression. *Int. J. Mol. Sci.* **2018**, *19*, 3028. [CrossRef] [PubMed]
3. Chen, W.T. Proteolytic activity of specialized surface protrusions formed at rosette contact sites of transformed cells. *J. Exp. Zool.* **1989**, *251*, 167–185. [CrossRef] [PubMed]
4. Pollard, T.D.; Borisy, G.G. Cellular Motility Driven by Assembly and Disassembly of Actin Filaments. *Cell* **2003**, *113*, 549. [CrossRef]
5. Wertheimer, E.; Gutierrez-Uzquiza, A.; Rosemblit, C.; Lopez-Haber, C.; Sosa, M.S.; Kazanietz, M.G. Rac signaling in breast cancer: A tale of GEFs and GAPs. *Cell. Signal.* **2012**, *24*, 353–362. [CrossRef] [PubMed]

6. Muise, A.M.; Walters, T.; Xu, W.; Shen-Tu, G.; Guo, C.H.; Fattouh, R.; Lam, G.Y.; Wolters, V.M.; Bennitz, J.; Van Limbergen, J.; et al. Single nucleotide polymorphisms that increase expression of the guanosine triphosphatase RAC1 are associated with ulcerative colitis. *Gastroenterology* **2011**, *141*, 633–641.
7. (a) Worthylake, R.A.; Lemoine, S.; Watson, J.M.; Burridge, K. RhoA is required for monocyte tail retraction during transendothelial migration. *J. Cell Biol.* **2001**, *154*, 147–160, (b) Takenawa, T.; Miki, H. WASP and WAVE family proteins: key molecules for rapid rearrangement of cortical actin filaments and cell movement. *J. Cell Sci.* **2001**, *114*, 1801–1809. [CrossRef]
8. Rohatgi, R.; Ma, L.; Miki, H.; Lopez, M.; Kirchhausen, T.; Takenawa, T.; Kirschner, M.W. The Interaction between N-WASP and the Arp2/3 Complex Links Cdc42-Dependent Signals to Actin Assembly. *Cell* **1999**, *97*, 221–231. [CrossRef]
9. Vlaar, C.P.; Castillo-Pichardo, L.; Medina, J.I.; Marrero-Serra, C.M.; Velez, E.; Ramos, Z.; Hernández, E. Design, synthesis and biological evaluation of new carbazole derivatives as anti-cancer and anti-migratory agents. *Biorganic. Med. Chem.* **2018**, *26*, 884–890. [CrossRef]
10. Montalvo-Ortiz, B.L.; Castillo-Pichardo, L.; Hernández, E.; Humphries-Bickley, T.; De La Mota-Peynado, A.; Cubano, L.A.; Vlaar, C.P.; Dharmawardhane, S. Characterization of EHop-016, novel small molecule inhibitor of Rac GTPase. *J. Biol. Chem.* **2012**, *287*, 13228–13238. [CrossRef]
11. Castillo-Pichardo, L.; Humphries-Bickley, T.; De La Parra, C.; Forestier-Roman, I.; Martinez-Ferrer, M.; Hernandez, E.; Vlaar, C.; Ferrer-Acosta, Y.; Washington, A.V.; Cubano, L.A.; et al. The Rac inhibitor EHop-016 inhibits mammary tumor growth and metastasis in a nude mouse model. *Transl. Oncol.* **2014**, *7*, 546–555. [CrossRef] [PubMed]
12. Dharmawardhane, S.; Hernandez, E.; Vlaar, C. Development of EHop-016: a small molecule inhibitor of Rac. *Enzymes* **2013**, *33*, 117–146. [PubMed]
13. Humphries-Bickley, T.; Castillo-Pichardo, L.; Corujo-Carro, F.; Duconge, J.; Hernandez-O'Farrill, E.; Vlaar, C.; Rodriguez-Orengo, J.F.; Cubano, L.; Dharmawardhane, S. Pharmacokinetics of Rac inhibitor EHop-016 in mice by ultra-performance liquid chromatography tandem mass spectrometry. *J. Chromatogr. B* **2015**, *981*, 19–26. [CrossRef] [PubMed]
14. Głuszyńska, A. Biological potential of carbazole derivatives. *Eur. J. Med. Chem.* **2015**, *94*, 405–426. [CrossRef] [PubMed]
15. Guillonneau, C.; Pierré, A.; Charton, Y.; Guilbaud, N.; Kraus-Berthier, L.; Léonce, S.; Michel, A.; Bisagni, E.; Atassi, G. Synthesis of 9-*O*-substituted derivatives of 9-hydroxy-5,6-dimethyl-6*H*-pyrido[4,3-*b*]carbazole-1-carboxylic acid (2-(Dimethylamino)-ethyl) amide and their 10-and 11-methyl analogues with improved antitumor activity. *J. Med. Chem.* **1999**, *42*, 2191–2203. [CrossRef] [PubMed]
16. Saturnino, C.; Iacopetta, D.; Sinicropi, M.; Rosano, C.; Caruso, A.; Caporale, A.; Marra, N.; Marengo, B.; Pronzato, M.; Parisi, O.; et al. N-alkyl carbazole derivatives as new tools for Alzheimer's disease: preliminary studies. *Molecules* **2014**, *19*, 9307–9317. [CrossRef] [PubMed]
17. Bandgar, B.P.; Adsul, L.K.; Chavan, H.V.; Jalde, S.S.; Shringare, S.N.; Shaikh, R.; Meshram, R.J.; Gacche, R.N.; Masand, V. Synthesis, biological evaluation, and docking studies of 3-(substituted)-aryl-5-(9-methyl-3-carbazole)-1H-2-pyrazolines as potent anti-inflammatory and antioxidant agents. *Bioorganic Med. Chem. Lett.* **2012**, *22*, 5839–5844. [CrossRef] [PubMed]
18. Biamonte, M.A.; Wanner, J.; Le Roch, K.G. Recent advances in malaria drug discovery. *Bioorganic Med. Chem. Lett.* **2013**, *23*, 2829–2843. [CrossRef]
19. Caruso, A.; Voisin-Chiret, A.S.; Lancelot, J.-C.; Sinicropi, M.S.; Garofalo, A.; Rault, S. Efficient and Simple Synthesis of 6-Aryl-1,4-dimethyl-9H-carbazoles. *Molecules* **2008**, *13*, 1312–1320. [CrossRef] [PubMed]
20. Chakrabarty, M.; Ghosh, N.; Harigaya, Y. A clay-mediated, regioselective synthesis of 2-(aryl/alkyl) amino-thiazolo [4, 5-c] carbazoles. *Tetrahedron Lett.* **2004**, *45*, 4955–4957. [CrossRef]
21. Caruso, A.; Sinicropi, M.S.; Lancelot, J.C.; El-Kashef, H.; Saturnino, C.; Aubert, G.; Ballandonne, C.; Lesnard, A.; Cresteil, T.; Dallemagne, P.; et al. Synthesis and evaluation of cytotoxic activities of new guanidines derived from carbazoles. *Bioorganic Med. Chem. Lett.* **2014**, *24*, 467–472. [CrossRef] [PubMed]
22. Iacopetta, D.; Rosano, C.; Puoci, F.; Parisi, O.I.; Saturnino, C.; Caruso, A.; Longo, P.; Ceramella, J.; Malzert-Fréon, A.; Dallemagne, P.; et al. Multifaceted properties of 1, 4-dimethylcarbazoles: Focus on trimethoxybenzamide and trimethoxyphenylurea derivatives as novel human topoisomerase II inhibitors. *Eur. J. Pharm. Sci.* **2017**, *96*, 263–272. [CrossRef] [PubMed]

23. Saturnino, C.; Palladino, C.; Napoli, M.; Sinicropi, M.S.; Botta, A.; Sala, M.; Carcereri de Prati, A.; Novellino, E.; Suzuki, H. Synthesis and biological evaluation of new N-alkylcarbazole derivatives as STAT3 inhibitors: Preliminary study. *Eur. J. Pharm. Sci.* **2013**, *60*, 112–119. [CrossRef] [PubMed]
24. Rizza, P.; Pellegrino, M.; Caruso, A.; Iacopetta, D.; Sinicropi, M.S.; Rault, S.; Lancelot, J.C.; El-Kashef, H.; Lesnard, A.; Rochais, C.; et al. 3-(Dipropylamino)-5-hydroxybenzofuro [2, 3-f] quinazolin-1 (2H)-one (DPA-HBFQ-1) plays an inhibitory role on breast cancer cell growth and progression. *Eur. J. Pharm. Sci.* **2016**, *107*, 275–287. [CrossRef] [PubMed]
25. Issa, S.; Walchshofer, N.; Kassab, I.; Termoss, H.; Chamat, S.; Geahchan, A.; Bouaziz, Z. Synthesis and antiproliferative activity of oxazinocarbazole and N,N-bis(carbazolylmethyl)amine derivatives. *Eur. J. Med. Chem.* **2010**, *45*, 2567–2577. [CrossRef] [PubMed]
26. Danish, I.A.; Prasad, K.J.R. A one-pot synthesis of 1, 2, 4, 5-tetraazaspiro [5.5]-6, 7, 8, 9-tetrahydrocarbazol-3-thiones and their antibacterial activities. *Indian J. Heterocycl. Chemstry* **2004**, *14*, 19–22.
27. Indumathi, T.; Fronczek, F.R.; Prasad, K.R. Synthesis of 2-amino-8-chloro-4-phenyl-5, 11-dihydro-6H-pyrido[2,3-a]carbazole-3-carbonitrile: Structural and biological evaluation. *J. Mol. Struct.* **2012**, *1016*, 134–139. [CrossRef]
28. Kantevari, S.; Yempala, T.; Surineni, G.; Sridhar, B.; Yogeeswari, P.; Sriram, D. Synthesis and antitubercular evaluation of novel dibenzo[b,d]furan and 9-methyl-9H-carbazole derived hexahydro-2H-pyrano[3,2-c]quinolines via Povarov reaction. *Eur. J. Med. Chem.* **2011**, *46*, 4827–4833. [CrossRef] [PubMed]
29. Woon, K.L.; Ariffin, A.; Ho, K.W.; Chen, S.-A. Effect of conjugation and aromaticity of 3,6 di-substituted carbazoles on triplet energy and the implication of triplet energy in multiple-cyclic aromatic compounds. *RSC Adv.* **2018**, *8*, 9850–9857. [CrossRef]
30. Bashir, M.; Bano, A.; Ijaz, A.S.; Chaudhary, B.A. Recent Developments and Biological Activities of N-Substituted Carbazole Derivatives: A Review. *Molecules* **2015**, *20*, 13496–13517. [CrossRef]
31. Mac Millan, K.S.; Naidoo, J.; Liang, J.; Melito, L.; Williams, L.S.; Morlock, L.; Huntington, P.J.; Estill, S.J.; Longood, J.; Becker, G.; et al. Development of Proneurogenic, Neuroprotective Small Molecules. *J. Am. Chem. Soc.* **2011**, *133*, 1428–1437. [CrossRef] [PubMed]
32. Molette, J.; Routier, J.; Abla, N.; Besson, D.; Bombrun, A.; Brun, R.; Burt, H.; Georgi, K.; Kaiser, M.; Nwaka, S.; et al. Identification and Optimization of an Aminoalcohol-Carbazole Series with Antimalarial Properties. ACS Med. *Chem. Lett.* **2013**, *4*, 1037–1041.
33. Saturnino, C.; Caruso, A.; Iacopetta, D.; Rosano, C.; Caramella, J.; Muia, N.; Mariconda, A.; Grazia Bonomo, M.; Ponassi, M.; Rosace, G.; et al. Inhibition of Human Topoisomerase II by N,N,N-Trimethylethanammonium Iodide Alkylcarbazole Derivatives. *Chem. Med. Chem.* **2018**, *13*, 2635–2643. [CrossRef] [PubMed]
34. Caruso, A.; Iacopetta, D.; Pouci, F.; Cappello, A.R.; Saturnino, C.; Sinicropi, M.S. Carbazole derivatives: A promising scenario for breast cancer treatment. *Mini Rev. Med. Chem.* **2016**, *16*, 630. [CrossRef] [PubMed]
35. Bombrun, A.; Gerber, P.; Casi, G.; Terradillos, O.; Antonsson, B.; Halazy, S. 3,6-dibromocarbazole piperazine derivatives of 2-propanol as first inhibitors of cytochrome c release via Bax channel modulation. *J. Med. Chem.* **2003**, *46*, 4365–4368. [CrossRef] [PubMed]
36. Zhang, Y.; Tangadanchu, V.K.R.; Cheng, Y.; Yang, R.G.; Lin, J.M.; Zhou, C.H. Potential Antimicrobial Isopropanol-Conjugated Carbazole Azoles as Dual Targeting Inhibitors of Enterococcus faecalis. *ACS Med. Chem. Lett.* **2018**, *9*, 244–249. [CrossRef]
37. Pieper, A.A.; Xie, S.; Capota, E.; Estill, S.J.; Zhong, J.; Long, J.M.; Becker, G.L.; Huntington, P.; Goldman, S.E.; Shen, C.-H.; et al. Discovery of a proneurogenic, neuroprotective chemical. *Cell* **2010**, *142*, 39. [CrossRef]
38. Peterson, J.R.; Bickford, L.C.; Morgan, D.; Kim, A.S.; Ouerfelli, O.; Kirschner, M.W.; Rosen, M.K. Chemical inhibition of N-WASP by stabilization of a native autoinhibited conformation. *Nat. Struct. Mol. Boil.* **2004**, *11*, 747–755. [CrossRef]
39. Guerriero, C.J.; Weisz, O.A. N-WASP inhibitor wiskostatin non-selectively perturbs membrane transport by decreasing cellular ATP levels. *Am. J. Physiol. Cell Physiol.* **2007**, *292*, C1562–C1566. [CrossRef]
40. Orellana, E.A.; Kasinski, A.L. Sulforhodamine B (SRB) Assay in Cell Culture to Investigate Cell Proliferation. *Bio-protocol* **2016**, *6*, e1984. [CrossRef]
41. Liang, C.C.; Park, A.Y.; Guan, J.L. In vitro scratch assay: A convenient and inexpensive method for analysis of cell migration in vitro. *Nat. Protoc.* **2007**, *2*, 329–333. [CrossRef] [PubMed]

42. Olson, M.F.; Sahai, E. The actin cytoskeleton in cancer cell motility. *Clin. Exp. Metastasis* **2009**, *26*, 273. [CrossRef] [PubMed]
43. Ridley, A.J. Rho GTPases and actin dynamics in membrane protrusions and vesicle trafficking. *Trends Cell Boil.* **2006**, *16*, 522–529. [CrossRef] [PubMed]
44. Takenawa, T.; Suetsugu, S. The WASP–WAVE protein network: Connecting the membrane to the cytoskeleton. *Nat. Rev. Mol. Cell Boil.* **2007**, *8*, 37–48. [CrossRef]
45. Frugtniet, B.; Jiang, W.G.; Martin, T.A.; Martin, T. Role of the WASP and WAVE family proteins in breast cancer invasion and metastasis. *Breast Cancer: Targets Ther.* **2015**, *7*, 99–109.

Sample Availability: Not available.

molecules

MDPI

Article

Novel Homo-Bivalent and Polyvalent Compounds Based on Ligustrazine and Heterocyclic Ring as Anticancer Agents

Jiawen Wang [1,†], Ge Hong [2,3,†], Guoliang Li [2], Wenzhi Wang [2] and Tianjun Liu [1,2,3,*]

1 Graduate Institute, Tianjin University of Traditional Chinese Medicine, Tianjin 301617, China; m13260192393@163.com
2 Tianjin Key Laboratory of Biomedical Materials, Institute of Biomedical Engineering, Chinese Academy of Medical Sciences & Peking Union Medical College, Tianjin 300192, China; hongge6688@aliyun.com (G.H.); liguoliangsx@163.com (G.L.); wxwnx123@163.com (W.W.)
3 State Key Laboratory of Bioactive Substances and Functions of Natural Medicines, Institute of Materia Medica, Chinese Academy of Medical Sciences and Peking Union Medical College, Beijing 100050, China
* Correspondence: Liutj@bme.org.cn
† These authors contributed equally to this work.

Academic Editor: Qiao-Hong Chen
Received: 7 November 2019; Accepted: 6 December 2019; Published: 9 December 2019

Abstract: Bivalent and polyvalent inhibitors can be used as antitumor agents. In this experiment, eight ligustrazine dimers and seven ligustrazine tetramers linked by alkane diamine with different lengths of carbon chain lengths were synthesized. After screening their antiproliferation activities against five cancer cell lines, most ligustrazine derivatives showed better cytotoxicity than the ligustrazine monomer. In particular, ligustrazine dimer **8e** linked with decane-1,10-diamine exhibited the highest cytotoxicity in FaDu cells with an IC_{50} (50% inhibiting concentration) value of 1.36 nM. Further mechanism studies suggested that **8e** could induce apoptosis of FaDu cells through the depolarization of mitochondrial membrane potential and S-phase cell cycle arrest. Inspired by these results, twenty-seven additional small molecule heterocyclic dimers linked with decane-1,10-diamine and nine cinnamic acid dimers bearing ether chain were synthesized and screened. Most monocyclic and bicyclic aromatic systems showed highly selective anti-proliferation activity to FaDu cells and low toxicity to normal MCF 10A cells. The structure-activity relationship revealed that the two terminal amide bonds and the alkyl linker with a chain length of 8–12 carbon were two important factors to maintain its antitumor activity. In addition, the ADMET calculation predicted that most of the potent compounds had good oral bioavailability.

Keywords: bivalency; polyvalency; antitumor; apoptosis; cell cycle

1. Introduction

Natural products play a vital role in the development of the drug, especially anticancer drugs [1]. Ligustrazine (2,3,5,6-tetramethylpyrazine, TMP), an important component of the Chinese traditional medicinal herb Chuanxiong (*Ligusticum chuanxiong Hort*), has been of wide clinical use for cardiovascular and cerebrovascular diseases [2]. Recently, TMP has been reported to possess anticancer activity in vitro and in vivo, inducing cancer cell apoptosis and cell cycle modulation [3,4]. More importantly, the introduction of different substituted groups into ligustrazine has helped to improve the antitumor activity. Many ligustrazine derivatives with potent antitumor activity have been developed in the past few years, like monocarbonyl ligustrazine-curcumin hybrids [5], ligustrazine-betulinic acid hybrids [6], and ligustrazine-rhein derivatives [7]. This advancement stimulated our interest in using TMP as the scaffold to synthesize new antitumor agents.

In the interaction between host and guest molecules, both bivalency and polyvalency could enhance the affinity and activity of monovalent ligand [8,9]. This phenomenon has attracted attention in drug design. Many effective bivalent anti-cancer drugs have been found, such as artemisinin-derivative dimers [10], jesterone dimer [11], indole-3-carbinol dimer [12], bis-daunorubicin [13]. Previous work in this field has designed and synthesized several ligustrazine dimers linked by cyclohexanone and oxime [14], curcumin [15], or triterpenes [16], which had a good cytotoxic effect on human cancer cells. The result showed that the dimerization of ligustrazine could obviously improve the antitumor potency of its monomer.

With an effort to developing new antitumor agents, we designed and synthesized a series of novel TMP dimers and tetramers linked with different alkyl diamines and screened their anti-proliferation potential on a panel of human cancer cell lines, including HeLa, Hep G2, MCF-7, FaDu, and A549. Based on these experimental results, according to the importance of small molecular heterocyclic rings in drug discovery [17], additional dimers series of aromatic rings instead of ligustrazine, a total of 51 new compounds were synthesized, screened, and their structure-activity relationship was briefly discussed. Meanwhile, through morphological observation and flow cytometric analysis, the antitumor mechanisms of the most potent one were preliminarily discussed in this study. ADMET properties of all compounds were also evaluated to explore the drug-likeness.

2. Results and Discussion

2.1. Chemistry

In this study, 51 novel designed compounds were synthesized. Series **6a–g** and **8a–f** were obtained according to the synthetic method described in Schemes 1 and 2. The important intermediate 2-chloromethyl-3,5,6-trimethyl-pyrazine **5** was prepared from ligustrazine by the tandem reaction: Boekelheide reaction [18] and deprotection and the chlorination reaction [19]. The key intermediate 2-carboxylic acid-3,5,6-trimethyl-pyrazine **7** was synthesized by the one-pot reaction, as previously reported [20]. To explore the length effect, the TMP moieties, with 2–12 methylene alkyl chain as a linker, were synthesized.

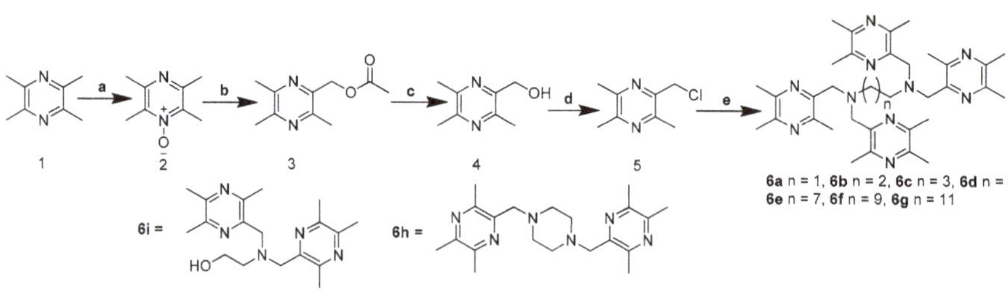

Scheme 1. Synthesis of the TMP complexes **6a–6i**. *Reagents and conditions:* (a) 30% H_2O_2, CH_3COOH, 95 °C, 2 h; (b) $(CH_3CO)_2O$, 140 °C, 2.5 h; (c) CH_3ONa, CH_3OH, r.t., 0.5 h; (d) $SOCl_2$, CH_2Cl_2, r.t., 2.5 h; (e) n-diaminoalkane (piperazine and monoethanolamine), K_2CO_3, CH_3CN, 95 °C, 2 h.

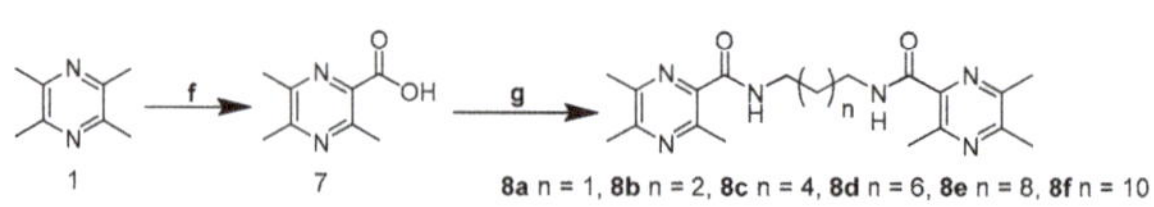

Scheme 2. Synthesis of the Bis-TMP hybrids **8a–8f**. *Reagents and conditions:* (f) $KMnO_4$, H_2O, 37 °C, 24 h; (g) n-diamino-alkane, EDCI/DMAP, r.t., 12 h.

Using heteroaromatic acids with decane-1,10-diamine as raw materials, the target compounds **9e–35e** (outlined in Scheme 3) linked by amide chain were synthesized with EDCI (1-(3-Dimethylaminopropyl)-3-ethylcarbodiimide hydrochloride) and DMAP

(4-Dimethylaminopyridine) in anhydrous CH_2Cl_2 at room temperature. Series **9d**, **9f–l** (shown in Scheme 4) linked by ether chain or amide chain were synthesized by the above method. All the newly synthesized compounds were characterized by ^{1}H-NMR, ^{13}C-NMR, and high-resolution mass spectra (HRMS). Details were provided in the experimental part. The purity of the compounds was over 95% measured by HPLC (Figure 1).

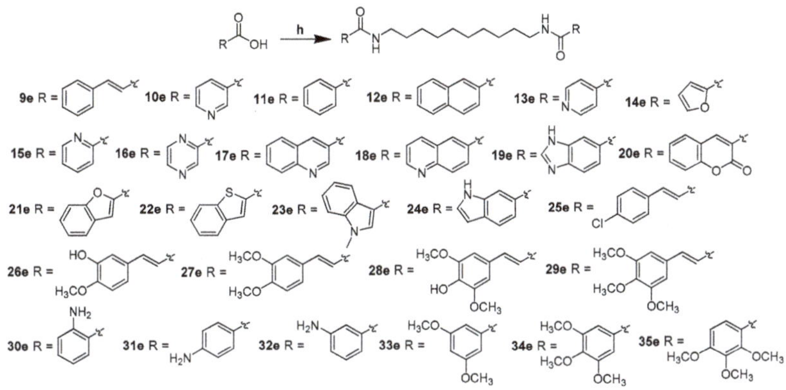

Scheme 3. Synthesis of compounds **9e–35e**. *Reagents and conditions*: (h) decane-1,10-diamine, EDCI/DMAP, r.t., 12 h.

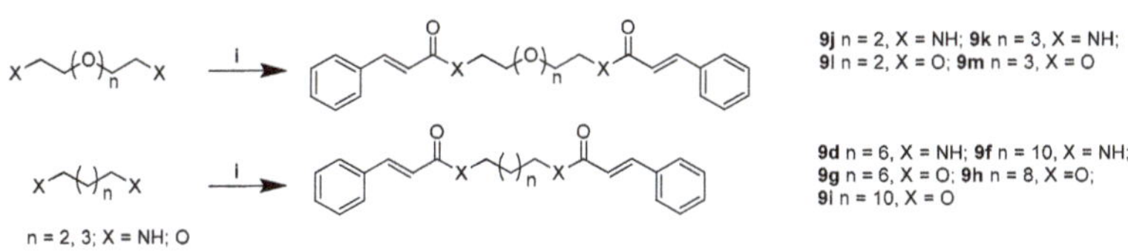

Scheme 4. Synthesis of compounds **9d**, **9f–9m**. *Reagents and conditions*: (i) cinnamic acid, EDCI/DMAP, r.t., 12 h.

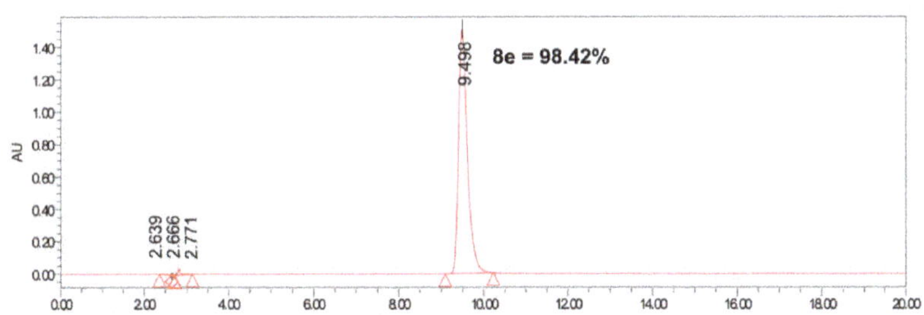

Figure 1. The purity of compound **8e** as a representative analyzed by HPLC (Kromasil C18 column, eluted by methanol/water (80/20) containing 0.1% trifluoroacetic acid at a flow rate of 1 mL/min).

2.2. Anti-Proliferative Activity In Vitro

For the newly synthesized compounds, their anti-proliferative activity on human cancer cell lines, HeLa (cervical carcinoma), Hep G2 (hepatoma carcinoma), MCF-7 (breast carcinoma), FaDu (head and neck carcinoma), A549 (lung carcinoma), and normal mammary epithelial cell line MCF 10A, was screened by MTT assay [21] with doxorubicin (DOX) as the positive control. The IC_{50} values of these compounds are summarized in Table 1. Among the ligustrazine derivatives, **6a–g** and **8a–f**, the tetramers **6f** and **6g** had broad-spectrum cytotoxic activities in all cell lines (IC_{50}

6.57–20.83 μM), and the cytotoxicity activities increased with the increase of carbon chain length. The dimeric ligustrazine **8d, 8e, 8f** showed the most promising anticancer activity in most tested tumor cell lines with IC_{50} values between 0.00136 and 6.35 μM, a much better result than DOX and TMP. In particular, compound **8e**, two ligustrazine rings linked with decane-1,10-diamine, exhibited the best anti-proliferative ability in cells (except Hep G2), and compared with other linkers, its IC_{50} values were 1.42 ± 0.71 μM, 0.037 ± 0.001 μM, 0.00136 ± 0.00035 μM, 1.05 ± 0.05 μM, and 0.047 ± 0.008 μM against HeLa, MCF-7, FaDu, A549, and MCF 10A, respectively. In light of these results, we replaced TMP with aromatic heterocycles similar to ligustrazine in electronic space. The novel small aromatic molecule and heterocyclic dimers **9e–35e** were synthesized, and their anti-proliferative ability was evaluated. Compounds **9e, 10e, 11e, 17e, 18e, 21e, 22e, 23e,** and **25e,** aromatic acid dimers (cinnamoyl, nicotinoyl, benzoyl, quinoline-3-carboxyl, quinoline-6-carboxyl, benzofuran-2-carboxyl, benzothiophene-2-carboxyl, indol-3-carboxyl, chlorinated cinnamoyl), were linked by decane-1,10-diamine, which had potent anti-proliferative ability in FaDu or A549 cell lines. Their IC_{50} in FaDu cell lines were less than 1 μM, in the range of 20 nM (benzothiophene-2-carboxyl) and 697 nM (benzofuran-2-carboxyl). Also, they had nearly no toxicity in normal cells like MCF 10A. In series **9d–n**, compounds **9d–f** (IC_{50} < 1 μM), two cinnamic acids linked by C8, C10, C12 chain with two terminal amide bonds, were more effective than compounds **9g–i** (IC_{50} > 20 μM), two cinnamic acids linked by the same alkyl chain with two terminal ester bonds instead of amide bonds. This demonstrated the vital role of two-terminal amide bonds in antitumor activity. Compared with compounds **9d–f**, the inhibition of compounds **9j–m**, two cinnamic acids linked by the similar length ether chain instead of alky chain, was weaker in tumor cells (IC_{50} > 20 μM), which confirmed that the alkyl chain played an important role in the structure. Then, we evaluated the position effect of the substitution at the ortho, meta, or para positions of the same aromatic ring. Compounds **25–35e** and the unsubstituted compounds **9e** and **11e** were all derivatives of cinnamic acid or benzoic acid with different substituents and electronic effects. The results of the compounds **26–27e** or **28–29e** confirmed that the substituents had a general effect on the activity, -OH, -OCH_3, -NH_2, and other electron donor groups could significantly reduce the activity, with the influence of -OH greater than that of -OCH_3. However, the electron attraction group like -Cl (**25e**) had no obvious effect. The compounds with para-substituted analogs (**31e**, para position, IC_{50} = 5.594 μM) exhibited better cell growth inhibitory activities in FaDu cells than ortho- and meta- substituted analogs (**30e, 32e**, ortho and meta position, IC_{50} > 20 μM). It is worth noting that para -OCH_3 substitution could enhance anticancer activity. The IC_{50} value of compound **34e** was 5.853 ± 0.408 μM, the IC_{50} value of para- OCH_3 was half that of the parent compound **33e**, and the IC_{50} value of compound **33e** was 10.393 ± 0.949 μM. Generally, there were three crucial elements in the structure-activity relationship of these systems: alkyl chain linker, two-terminal amide bonds, and heteroaromatic substituents. This SAR (structure-activity relationship) study would help to discover more effective compounds in the future.

To study the selective antiproliferative activities of bivalent and polyvalent inhibitors in normal cells and cancer cell lines, the cytotoxicity of compounds in FaDu cells and normal mammary epithelial MCF 10A cells was measured. The results listed in Table 1 showed that although the ligustrazine dimers **8d** and **8e** had high cytotoxicity in MCF 10A, their IC_{50} values were 2.69 ± 0.46 and 0.047 ± 0.008 μM, while the IC_{50} values in FaDu cells were 110 ± 30 and 1.36 ± 0.035 nM, respectively, which were far lower than that in MCF 10A. The selective index (SI) between MCF10A and Fadu ($IC_{50}^{MCF\ 10A}/IC_{50}^{FaDu}$) was 24.45 and 34.56, respectively. In addition, the heteroaromatic acid dimers **9e–12e, 21e–23e,** and **25e** had the similar activity, which was stronger than doxorubicin in FaDu cells, and had high selectivity in FaDu cells and MCF 10A cells with SI ($IC_{50}^{MCF\ 10A}/IC_{50}^{FaDu}$) values over 28.69. In contrast, the SI ($IC_{50}^{MCF\ 10A}/IC_{50}^{FaDu}$) value of doxorubicin was 0.43. These results encouraged us to further investigate the possible cellular mechanisms.

Table 1. Inhibitory effects of synthetic compounds on the growth of different types of human cancer cells and normal mammary epithelial cells.

Comp.	Antiproliferative Activity IC_{50} ± SEM (μM)						
	HeLa[a]	Hep G2[b]	MCF-7[c]	FaDu[d]	A549[e]	MCF 10A[f]	SI[g]
6a	>100	>100	>100	>100	>100	90.29 ± 3.41	NC[h]
6b	>100	>100	>100	>100	>100	>100	NC[h]
6c	>100	>100	>100	>100	>100	>100	NC[h]
6d	>100	>100	>100	>100	>100	>100	NC[h]
6e	62.67 ± 4.19	50.77 ± 1.35	66.36 ± 0.05	49.50 ± 1.61	>100	85.44 ± 2.28	1.73
6f	10.16 ± 0.55	10.72 ± 0.22	20.83 ± 0.14	10.94 ± 0.12	20.05 ± 0.41	12.97 ± 0.55	1.19
6g	7.89 ± 0.86	9.62 ± 0.11	9.83 ± 0.17	6.80 ± 0.05	9.23 ± 0.16	6.57 ± 0.30	0.97
6h	>100	>100	>100	>100	>100	>100	NC[h]
6i	>100	>100	>100	>100	>100	>100	NC[h]
8a	>100	>100	>100	>100	>100	>100	NC[h]
8b	>100	>100	>100	>100	>100	>100	NC[h]
8c	>100	>100	>100	80.41 ± 1.36	>100	46.59 ± 0.65	NC[h]
8d	3.31 ± 0.14	>20	0.480 ± 0.003	0.11 ± 0.03	6.35 ± 0.05	2.69 ± 0.46	24.45
8e	1.42 ± 0.71	>20	0.037 ± 0.001	0.00136 ± 0.00035	1.05 ± 0.05	0.047 ± 0.008	34.56
8f	4.96 ± 1.62	>20	0.158 ± 0.009	0.174 ± 0.010	2.46 ± 0.05	0.051 ± 0.021	0.29
9e	>100	>100	>100	0.054 ± 0.002	11.27 ± 0.81	>100	>1851.85
10e	>100	>100	>100	0.25 ± 0.02	2.94 ± 0.25	38.60 ± 2.48	154.40
11e	>100	>100	>100	0.50 ± 0.06	64.30 ± 3.46	80.54 ± 7.60	161.08
12e	>100	>100	>100	1.33 ± 0.07	8.77 ± 0.47	>100	>75.19
13e	>100	>100	>100	48.31 ± 3.17	>100	>100	>2.07
14e	>100	97.75 ± 1.55	>100	6.33 ± 0.65	44.37 ± 0.29	19.82 ± 1.41	3.13
15e	37.74 ± 4.32	26.34 ± 5.36	21.48 ± 1.47	8.85 ± 0.45	23.08 ± 0.12	54.65 ± 5.92	6.18
16e	>100	>100	>100	88.11 ± 1.37	>100	>100	NC[h]
17e	>20	>20	>20	0.236 ± 0.005	>20	>20	>84.75
18e	>20	>20	>20	0.697 ± 0.021	>20	>20	>28.69
19e	>20	>20	>20	8.74 ± 0.44	>20	>20	>2.29
20e	>20	>20	>20	>20	>20	>20	NC[h]
21e	>20	>20	>20	0.665 ± 0.028	>20	>20	>30.08
22e	>20	>20	>20	0.020 ± 0.002	>20	>20	>1000
23e	>20	>20	>20	0.638 ± 0.089	>20	>20	>31.35
24e	>20	>20	>20	5.296 ± 0.366	>20	>20	>3.78
25e	>20	>20	>20	0.056 ± 0.016	>20	>20	>357.14
26e	>20	>20	>20	>20	>20	>20	NC[h]
27e	>20	>20	>20	4.621 ± 0.539	>20	>20	>4.33
28e	>20	>20	>20	>20	>20	>20	NC[h]
29e	>20	>20	>20	5.067 ± 0.461	>20	>20	>3.95
30e	>20	>20	>20	>20	>20	>20	NC[h]
31e	>20	>20	>20	5.594 ± 0.628	>20	>20	>3.58
32e	>20	>20	>20	>20	>20	>20	NC[h]
33e	>20	>20	>20	10.393 ± 0.949	>20	>20	>1.92
34e	>20	>20	>20	5.853 ± 0.408	>20	>20	>3.42
35e	>20	>20	>20	>20	>20	>20	NC[h]
9d	>20	>20	>20	1.054 ± 0.091	>20	>20	>18.98
9f	>20	>20	>20	0.027 ± 0.002	>20	>20	>740.74
9g	>20	>20	>20	>20	>20	>20	NC[h]
9h	>20	>20	>20	>20	>20	>20	NC[h]
9i	>20	>20	>20	>20	>20	>20	NC[h]
9j	>20	>20	>20	>20	>20	>20	NC[h]
9k	>20	>20	>20	4.447 ± 0.208	>20	>20	>4.50
9l	>20	>20	>20	>20	>20	>20	NC[h]
9m	>20	>20	>20	>20	>20	>20	NC[h]
TMP	>100	>100	>100	>100	>100	>100	NC[h]
DOX	11.39 ± 0.48	28.04 ± 1.09	6 ± 0.07	1.27 ± 0.13	>100	0.55 ± 0.03	0.43

[a] HeLa (cervical cancer cell line); [b] Hep G2 (hepatocarcinoma cell line); [c] MCF-7 (breast cancer cell line); [d] FaDu (head and neck squamous carcinoma cell line); [e] A549 (epithelial cancer cell line); [f] MCF 10A (normal mammary epithelial cell); [g] SI: selectivity index. It was calculated as: SI = $IC_{50\,(MCF\,10A)}/IC_{50\,(FaDu)}$; [h] NC: not calculated.

2.3. Colony Formation Assay

As ligustrazine dimer **8e** had the most potent antiproliferative activity in all synthesized compounds, the colony formation assay in FaDu cells was conducted. As shown in Figure 2, FaDu cells treated with compound **8e** at concentrations 0.75 nM, 1.50 nM, 3 nM, 6 nM for 10 days formed smaller and fewer colonies compared to untreated control group, indicating that compound **8e** had a dose-dependent inhibition on the proliferation of FaDu cells, and the colony inhibition rate reached around 85.4% at 6 nM.

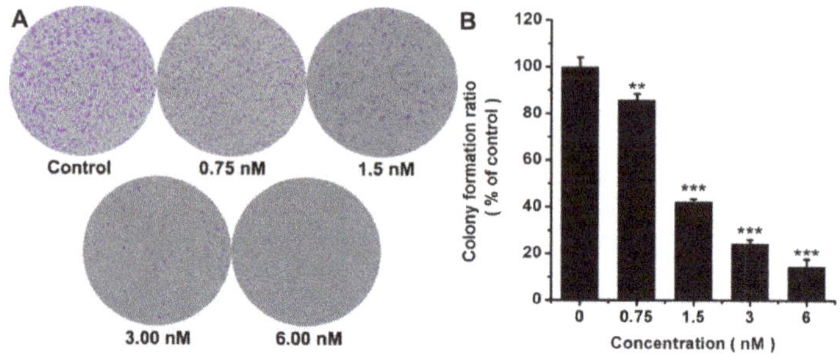

Figure 2. Effect of **8e** on the colony formation in FaDu cells. (**A**) Representative images of FaDu colonies after treatment at the indicated concentrations for 10 days; (**B**) The percentage of colonies compared with control group, $n = 3$. **: $p < 0.01$; ***: $p < 0.001$ versus control.

2.4. *Live/Dead Staining*

Live-dead double staining experiment was conducted to visually evaluate the cell toxicity of compound **8e**, the most potent one obtained by MTT assay. Propidium iodide (PI)-stained dead cells in red and calcein AM-stained living cells in green. The number of dead cells increased with the dose of **8e** while living cells decreased. Simultaneously, the densities of **8e**-treated cells were much lower than that of the control group. The concentration-dependent loss of FaDu cell viability was consistent with the MTT results (Figure 3).

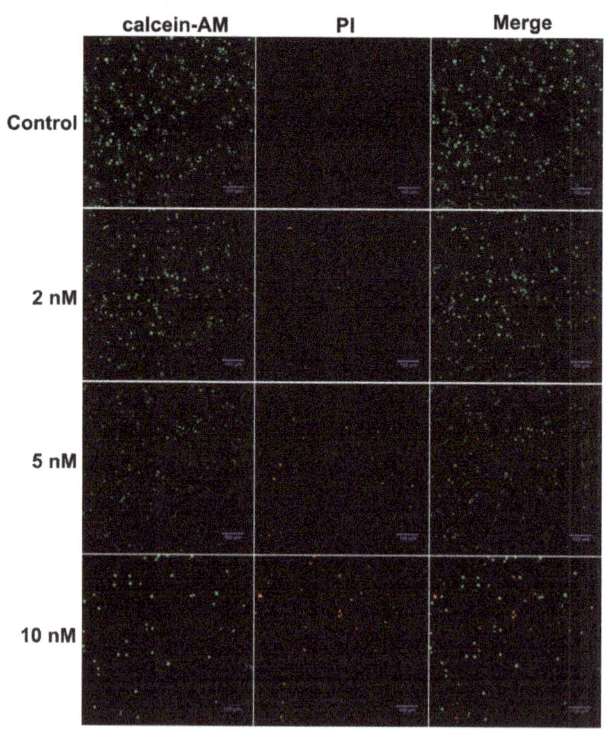

Figure 3. The confocal images of FaDu cells after incubation with compound **8e** at concentrations of 0, 2, 5, and 10 nM for 24 h, respectively. Viable cells were stained in green with Calcein-AM, and dead cells were stained in red with PI. The scale bar was 100 μm.

2.5. Morphological Observation by Hoechst 33,342 Staining

To investigate whether the anti-proliferation behavior of **8e** was related to the apoptosis pathway, the interaction between **8e**- and FaDu cells was analyzed through Hoechst 33,342 staining with a laser scanning confocal microscope. As shown in Figure 4, cells without treatment as the control group exhibited almost negligible apoptotic characteristics with homogenous and round blue-stained nuclei. On the contrary, the typical apoptotic nuclei with irregular nuclear morphology and condensation of chromatin (much brighter stained cells) were observed, and most FaDu cells were shrunken and rounded up from the culture dish after exposure to **8e**. The result demonstrated that inducing apoptosis in FaDu cells might be one cause of cell growth inhibition by compound **8e**.

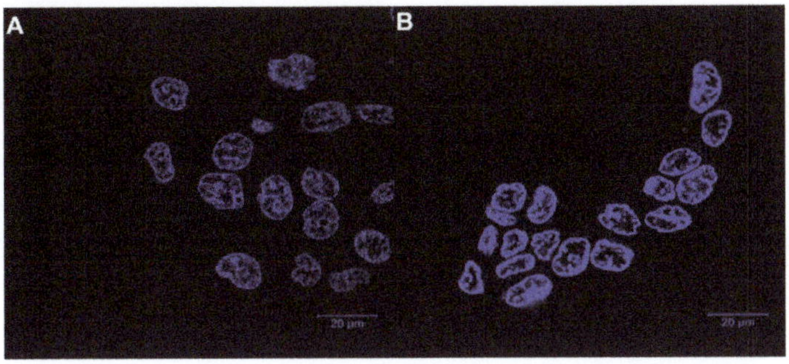

Figure 4. Hoechst staining of FaDu cells treated with compound **8e**, (**A**) Control group; (**B**) 20 nM group.

2.6. Apoptosis Analysis by Annexin V-FITC/PI Staining

To substantiate whether the cell death induced by the ligustrazine dimer **8e** was associated with apoptosis, the interaction of FaDu cells with **8e** was further analyzed by an annexin V-FITC/PI staining, and the apoptosis ratios were quantitated by flow cytometry. The cells were divided into four quadrants: Q1 represented necrotic cells (annexin V^-/PI^+), Q2 represented late apoptotic cells (annexin V^+/PI^+), Q3 represented early apoptotic cells (annexin V^+/PI^-), Q4 represented living cells (annexin V^-/PI^-). As shown in Figure 5, after being exposed to different concentrations of **8e** (2, 5, 10 nM) for 24 h in FaDu cells, the apoptotic cells (including the early and late apoptosis ratios) increased gradually from 8.23% of the control to 34.2%, 57.7%, 79.5%, respectively. The results revealed that **8e** could induce FaDu cells' apoptosis in a dose-dependent manner. This was consistent with other reports showing TMP and its derivatives could induce apoptosis of cancer cells [22–24].

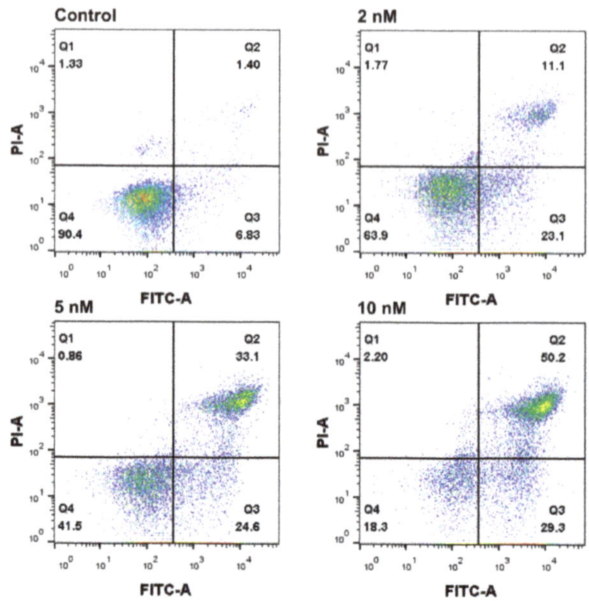

Figure 5. Flow cytometry analysis of apoptosis using annexin V-FITC/PI double staining in FaDu cells treated with compound **8e** at the indicated concentrations for 24 h. The percentage of cells was given in the respective quadrants.

2.7. *Mitochondrial Membrane Potential (ΔΨm) Analysis*

Mitochondria play an essential role in cell apoptotic progression by regulating mitochondrial membrane potential (ΔΨm). Depolarization of ΔΨm is considered an indicator of cell apoptosis [25]. To better understand the mechanism of **8e**-induced FaDu cells apoptosis, the depolarization of ΔΨm was quantitated by JC-1 (tetraethylbenzimidazolylcarbocyanine iodide) dye. As a mitochondrial-specific dual-fluorescence probe, JC-1 selectively entered the mitochondria. In healthy cells with high ΔΨm, it accumulated in the mitochondrial matrix as J-aggregates with red fluorescence, while in the reduced ΔΨm cells, it remained in the cytoplasm as a monomer with green fluorescence. The change of ΔΨm could be easily detected by the change of fluorescence color. Flow cytometric analysis of FaDu cells treated with different concentrations of **8e** (2, 5, 10 nM) for 24 h revealed that the ratio of green to red fluorescence was significantly higher than that of the control group in a concentration-dependent manner, indicating that the number of lower ΔΨm cells increased (Figure 6). These results suggested that **8e** could induce apoptosis of FaDu cells by decreasing ΔΨm.

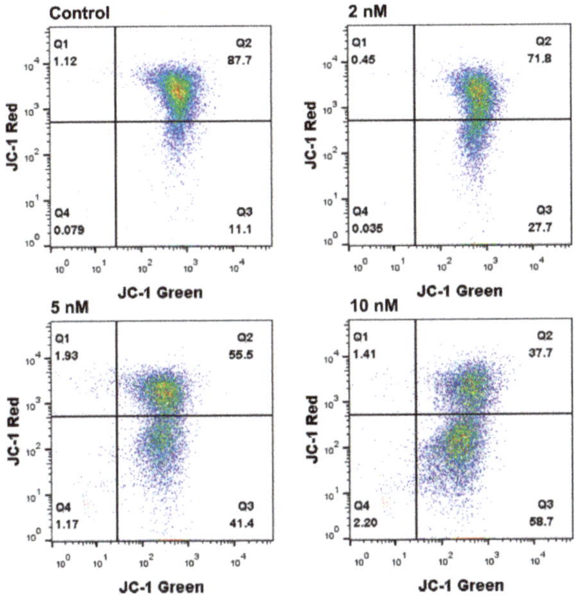

Figure 6. Flow cytometry analysis of the mitochondrial membrane potential using the JC-1 (tetraethylbenzimidazolylcarbocyanine iodide) dye in FaDu cells treated with compound **8e** at the indicated concentrations for 24 h. The percentage of cells was given in the respective quadrants.

2.8. Cell Cycle Analysis

In order to investigate whether **8e** induced cell cycle disturbances in FaDu cells, the flow cytometric analysis was performed with PI staining. The fluorescence intensity was proportional to the content of double-stranded DNA. The separation of cells in G0/G1, S, and G2/M was based upon the distribution of DNA content. Cytometric profiles of the PI-stained DNA showed that after being treated with **8e** at different concentrations (2, 5, 10 nM) for 24 h, the cell cycle of FaDu cells was arrested. As shown in Figure 7, the percentage of cells in the S phase (33.7%, 44.3%, and 54.7%) was markedly improved compared with the control group (28.1%), and this effect was concentration-dependent in FaDu cells. The population of the G0/G1 phase decreased from 51.9% to 41.8%, 44.2%, and 32.4%, respectively. These data indicated that **8e** significantly arrested cell cycle at S phase. This was different from the previously reported cell cycle arrest in the G0/G1 phase induced by TMP [4], which revealed that the dimerization of TMP could change the modulation of the cell cycle of its monomer.

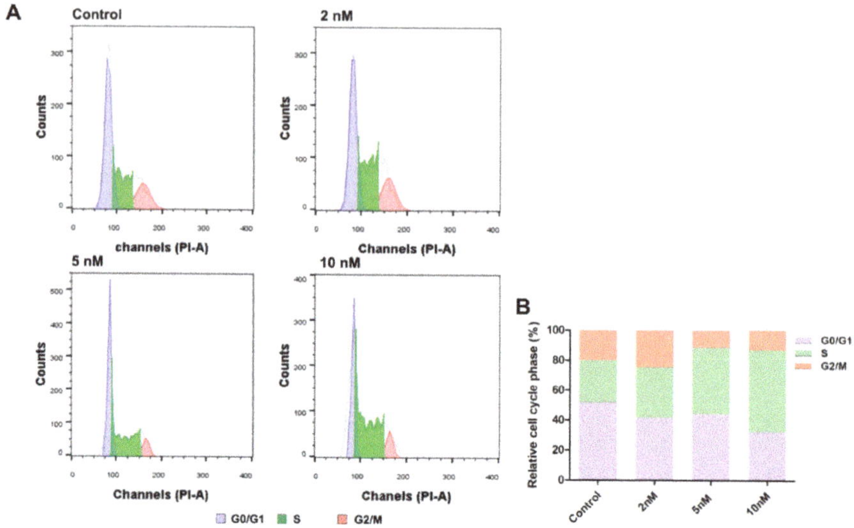

Figure 7. Flow cytometry analysis for cell cycle distribution of FaDu cells. (**A**) Representative cell cycle distribution of FaDu cells with compound 8e treatment (0, 2, 5, and 10 nM) for 24 h. The tall peak (**left**) represents cells in the G0/G1 phase, the small peak (**right**) represents cells in the G2/M phase, and the middle area represents cells in the S phase. (**B**) Quantification of the percentage of cell cycle distribution.

2.9. *In Silico ADMET Prediction*

ADMET prediction is becoming increasingly crucial as most drugs fail in clinical trials owing to poor pharmacokinetic parameters [26,27]. Table 2 shows the ADMET calculated descriptors for our synthesized compounds and two biplots shown in Figure 8. All compounds had 0–4 HBD (hydrogen bond donor) and 4–10 HBA (hydrogen bond acceptor), which were under Lipinski's rule of five (HBD < 5, HBA < 10). PPB (plasma protein binding) was one of the key properties related to drug efficacy. Except for compounds **10–15e**, **17–24e**, and **9d**, most of the compounds had weak (<90%) binding with plasma proteins in the blood, which were predicted to be non-inhibitors of cytochrome P450 2D6, and participated in the good- metabolism of phase I metabolism. $T_{1/2}$ of the target molecules was in the range of 1.63–2.29 h, showing the characteristic of rapid metabolism. The HT (hepatotoxicity) values estimated the hepatoxicity of the chemical compounds. HT values for series **6a–i**, **13–14e**, **20e**, **29e**, **31–35e**, **9f**, **9i**, **9k**, and **9m** were zero, and there was no hepatoxicity, while other compounds might be hepatotoxic. Moreover, the LD_{50} (median lethal dose) predicted that series **8a–f**, **9–35e**, and **9d–m** were over 500 mg/kg, implying they were less toxic. In addition, an ADMET model formed with descriptors 2D polar surface area (PSA) and AlogP98 could predict human intestinal absorption and the blood-brain barrier penetration (BBB) at 95% and 99% confidence level. In the absorption plot, compounds **6a–f**, **6h–i**, **8a–f**, **9–11e**, **13–19e**, **23e**, **30–33e**, **9d**, **9g**, and **9j–m** were predicted to be easily absorbed by the intestine at 99% confidence level. While in the BBB plot, the most potent compounds **8e** and **8f** were fallen out of the 99% ellipse (undefined), suggesting its poor blood-brain barrier penetration ability. Therefore, these molecules might possess low or no side effects of the central nervous system (CNS). In conclusion, ADMET prediction of the compounds might be helpful for further designing new drugs with favorable oral bioavailability.

Table 2. The ADMET properties of all synthetic compounds.

Comp.	HBD[a]	HBA[b]	RBN[c]	logP[d]	logS[e]	PSA[f]	HIA[g]	PPB[h]	BBB[i]	CYP3A4[j]	$T_{1/2}$ (h)[k]	HT[l]	LD_{50}(mg/kg)[m]
6a	0	10	11	1.84	−2.23	96.79	0.81	0.68	0.94	0	2.02	0	459.04
6b	0	10	12	1.90	−1.93	96.79	0.80	0.67	0.91	0	2.13	0	429.48
6c	0	10	13	2.48	−2.05	96.79	0.80	0.68	0.91	0	2.14	0	462.17
6d	0	10	15	3.39	−2.02	96.79	0.80	0.65	0.91	0	2.12	0	447.58
6e	0	10	17	4.31	−1.90	96.79	0.80	0.65	0.91	0	2.14	0	425.74
6f	0	10	19	5.22	−1.67	96.79	0.80	0.66	0.91	0	2.18	0	460.97
6g	0	10	21	6.13	−1.35	96.79	0.80	0.67	0.91	0	2.23	0	508.77
6h	0	6	4	0.97	−2.49	51.75	0.79	0.67	0.98	0	2.00	0	664.69
6i	1	6	6	0.47	−1.52	69.21	0.78	0.70	0.75	0	1.77	0	1011.08
8a	2	6	6	−0.09	−1.53	105.27	0.69	0.78	0.98	0	1.81	1	1027.40
8b	2	6	7	0.49	−1.87	105.27	0.72	0.79	0.98	0	1.88	1	988.28
8c	2	6	9	1.40	−2.30	105.27	0.72	0.80	0.98	0	1.89	1	1033.87
8d	2	6	11	2.31	−2.67	105.27	0.72	0.83	0.98	0	1.92	1	1099.10
8e	2	6	13	3.22	−2.97	105.27	0.72	0.85	0.98	0	2.03	1	1278.93
8f	2	6	15	4.14	−3.21	105.27	0.72	0.85	0.98	0	2.01	1	1318.54
9e	2	2	15	6.21	−4.45	60.22	0.69	0.89	0.99	0	1.93	1	961.82
10e	2	4	13	2.97	−2.60	82.74	0.70	0.91	0.99	0	1.85	1	1075.58
11e	2	2	13	5.27	−4.27	60.22	0.68	0.91	1.00	0	1.96	1	1653.45
12e	2	2	13	7.09	−6.11	60.22	0.69	0.92	0.99	0	2.12	1	1818.99
13e	2	4	13	2.97	−2.60	82.74	0.72	0.91	0.99	0	1.89	0	1070.63
14e	2	2	13	4.06	−3.66	85.33	0.41	0.90	1.00	0	1.78	0	1145.12
15e	2	4	13	3.83	−3.35	82.74	0.70	0.91	0.99	0	1.89	1	1128.86
16e	2	6	13	1.53	−1.68	105.27	0.68	0.85	0.99	0	1.82	1	1461.77
17e	2	4	13	5.65	−5.10	82.74	0.70	0.95	0.98	0	2.22	1	1217.90
18e	2	4	13	5.65	−5.10	82.74	0.72	0.96	0.95	0	1.99	1	1254.91
19e	4	4	13	4.31	−4.38	112.85	0.69	0.90	0.94	0	1.91	1	1167.64
20e	2	6	13	5.33	−4.57	112.68	0.43	0.93	0.98	0	2.29	0	973.08
21e	2	2	13	6.46	−6.02	85.33	0.47	0.94	0.99	0	2.00	1	966.72
22e	2	2	13	7.40	−6.99	60.22	0.69	0.91	0.99	0	2.07	1	904.88
23e	2	2	13	6.27	−5.55	70.92	0.75	0.95	0.99	0	2.27	1	995.92
24e	4	2	13	5.86	−5.15	90.33	0.72	0.95	0.96	0	2.01	1	1072.61
25e	2	2	15	7.54	−5.78	60.22	0.67	0.89	0.99	0	1.98	1	1322.11
26e	4	6	17	5.69	−3.28	119.71	0.45	0.87	0.85	0	1.93	1	1249.90
27e	2	6	19	6.14	−3.64	95.94	0.54	0.82	0.98	0	1.82	1	1217.58
28e	4	8	19	5.66	−3.13	137.57	0.46	0.77	0.94	0	2.02	1	1163.97
29e	2	8	21	6.11	−3.08	113.80	0.54	0.73	0.96	0	1.95	0	927.46
30e	4	4	13	3.78	−2.74	113.30	0.59	0.90	0.99	0	1.96	1	849.92
31e	4	4	13	3.78	−2.69	113.30	0.64	0.90	0.97	0	1.93	0	951.43
32e	4	4	13	3.78	−2.72	113.30	0.64	0.90	0.98	0	1.94	0	853.84
33e	2	6	17	5.21	−3.97	95.94	0.53	0.81	0.99	0	1.76	0	1184.47
34e	2	8	19	5.18	−3.62	113.80	0.54	0.76	0.98	0	1.63	0	1073.30
35e	2	8	19	5.18	−3.67	113.80	0.53	0.76	0.97	0	1.72	0	1061.01
9d	2	2	13	5.30	−4.11	60.22	0.69	0.91	0.99	0	1.92	1	1523.97
9f	2	2	17	7.12	−4.73	60.22	0.69	0.87	0.99	0	1.95	0	1003.19
9g	0	4	15	6.59	−5.34	52.46	0.55	0.88	0.98	0	1.96	1	6181.36
9h	0	4	17	7.50	−5.69	52.46	0.55	0.86	0.98	0	1.96	1	4624.51
9i	0	4	19	8.42	−5.96	52.46	0.55	0.85	0.98	0	1.96	0	3127.76
9j	2	4	13	2.57	−2.06	78.08	0.37	0.86	0.99	0	1.97	1	1574.67
9k	2	5	16	2.44	−1.41	87.01	0.37	0.85	0.99	0	1.90	0	1693.04
9l	0	6	15	3.86	−2.96	70.32	0.50	0.88	0.98	0	1.89	1	4511.05
9m	0	7	18	3.73	−2.14	79.25	0.50	0.86	0.98	0	1.83	0	4493.16
DOX	6	12	5	−0.04	−4.80	209.31	0.02	0.78	0.02	0	2.71	1	324.50
TMP	0	2	0	0.66	−1.51	22.52	0.93	0.49	0.99	0	1.77	0	1194.46

[a] HBD (hydrogen bond donor), [b] HBA (hydrogen bond acceptor), [c] RBN (number of rotatable bonds), [d] logP (log of the octanol/water partition coefficient), [e] log S (log of the aqueous solubility), and [f] PSA (polar surface area) were predicted using Discovery Studio 2.0 software. [g] HIA (human intestinal absorption), [h] PPB (plasma protein binding), [I] CYP3D4 (CYP3D4 inhibition), [j] T1/2 (half lifetime), [k] HT (human hepatoxicity), and [l] LD50 (median lethal dose) were calculated via http://admet.scbdd.com/home/index/

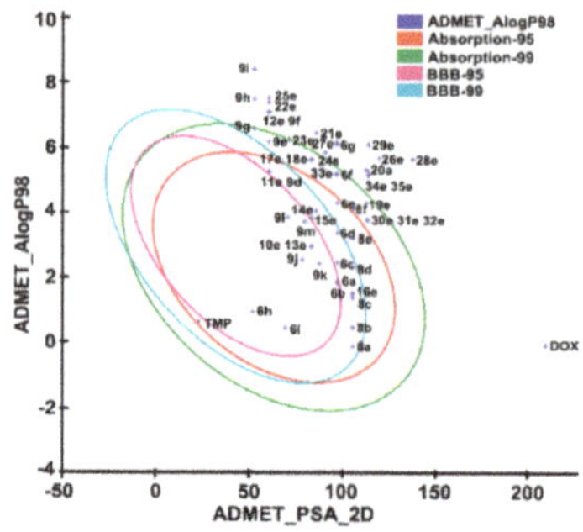

Figure 8. The plot of PSA (polar surface area) versus AlogP98 for the newly synthesized compounds showing the 95% and 99% confidence limit ellipses corresponding to the intestinal absorption and blood-brain barrier models.

3. Conclusions

Using ligustrazine, aromatic, or heteroaromatic acids as the main raw materials and linked by alkyl or ether chain, bivalent antitumor agents were synthesized and screened from five different human cancer cell lines and one normal mammary epithelial cell line. SAR revealed that the two terminal amide bonds and the alky chain were the dominant factors with 10 C atom chain showing the most potent antitumor effect. Among different aromatic moieties, the ligustrazine dimer **8e** was the best candidate; its IC_{50} was 1.36 nM in FaDu cell, it showed a broad-spectrum antitumor activity with IC_{50} in the range of 0.00136–1.42 μM, and the selective ratio MCF 10A/FaDu was 34.56. The subsequent fluorescence staining and flow cytometry analysis indicated that **8e** could induce apoptosis through depolarization of the mitochondrial membrane potential in FaDu cells. Further mechanism investigation showed that **8e** could arrest cell cycle at the S phase in FaDu cells. Furthermore, ADMET predicted that most of the potent compounds followed Lipinski's law and became 'drug-like' molecules, further confirming that the dimerization of ligustrazine could improve the antitumor activity of its monomer. The highly selective inhibition of these dimers on the proliferation of FaDu cells might be related to the effect on a specific target in FaDu cells. Based on the characteristics of FaDu cells, further targeted screening would give insight into the selectivity of such potent compounds.

4. Materials and Methods

4.1. Chemistry

^{1}H-NMR and ^{13}C-NMR spectra were recorded on a Mercury Vx-300 (300 MHz) or AVANCE III (400 MHz). Chemical shifts were reported in ppm (δ) using the residue solvent line as the internal standard (for TMS: 0 ppm, ^{1}H and ^{13}C; for $CHCl_3$-*d*: 7.26 ppm, ^{1}H and 77.16 ppm, ^{13}C). Coupling constants were given in Hertz (*J*). High-resolution MS (HRMS) were recorded on an Agilent 6520 Q-TOF LC/MS. Melting points were uncorrected and were determined on a digital melting point apparatus (Shenguang WRS-1B, shanghai, China). Flash column chromatography was carried out by using silica gel (200–300 mesh). Reactions were monitored by thin-layer chromatography (TLC) on silica gel GF254 plates (Qingdao Haiyang Chemical Plant, Qingdao, China). Reagents and solvents were used as purchased from commercial sources without further purification. The purity of the synthesized compounds was over 95% analyzed by HPLC (Waters 2695 Alliance system, Waters Corp., Milford, MA, USA), with the Kromasil C18 column eluted by methanol/water (80/20) containing 0.1% trifluoroacetic acid at a flow rate of 1 mL/min. Compounds **4** and **5** were prepared, as reported previously [19]. ^{1}H-NMR, ^{13}C-NMR and HR-MS spectra of compounds **6a**–**9m** can be seen in supplementary materials.

4.2. *General Synthetic Procedure for* **6a–g**

A mixture of alkane-diamine (10 mmol), TMP-Cl (50 mmol), KOH (60 mmol), and dimethylformamide (35 mL) was heated to reflux. The reaction progress was monitored via TLC. After 2 h, the reaction mixture was cooled to room temperature. Subsequently, the solid was filtered off, and the filtrate was added with H_2O (100 mL) and extracted with ethyl acetic acid three times. The organic layers were combined and washed with H_2O and brine, and then separated and dried over anhydrous Na_2SO_4 for 8 h. The solvent was removed under reduced pressure; the resulting residue was separated on flash column chromatography eluted by a mixture of petroleum ether/acetone in a volume ratio of 7:1–3:1, and further recrystallized from acetone to give pale white solid.

4.2.1. N^1,N^1,N^2,N^2-Tetrakis((3,5,6-Trimethylpyrazin-2-yl)Methyl)Ethane-1,2-Diamine (**6a**)

Pale white solid, yield 28%, m.p. 207.6–208.3 °C; ^{1}H-NMR (300 MHz, $CDCl_3$) δ: 3.60 (s, 8H), 2.67 (s, 4H), 2.43 (s, 12H), 2.41 (s, 12H), 2.23 (s, 12H); ^{13}C-NMR (101 MHz, DMSO) δ: 149.91, 149.63, 148.37, 147.85, 58.75, 52.14, 50.83, 21.61, 21.42, 20.65; HRMS (ESI) *m/z*: 597.4134 $[M + H]^+$, calcd. for $[C_{34}H_{49}N_{10}]^+$ 597.4142.

4.2.2. N^1,N^1,N^3,N^3-Tetrakis((3,5,6-Trimethylpyrazin-2-yl)Methyl)Propane-1,3-Diamine (**6b**)

Pale white solid, yield 27%, m.p. 113–114.3 °C; ^{1}H-NMR (300 MHz, $CDCl_3$) δ: 3.65 (s, 8H), 2.46 (s, 12H), 2.43 (s, 12H), 2.41–2.38 (m, 4H), 2.32 (s, 12H), 1.81–1.71 (m, 2H). ^{13}C-NMR (101 MHz, DMSO) δ: 149.93, 149.53, 148.51, 147.82, 58.63, 53.36, 21.61, 21.44, 20.70; HRMS (ESI) *m/z*: 611.4286 $[M + H]^+$, calcd. for $[C_{35}H_{51}N_{10}]^+$ 611.4298.

4.2.3. N^1,N^1,N^4,N^4-Tetrakis((3,5,6-Trimethylpyrazin-2-yl)Methyl)Butane-1,4-Diamine (**6c**)

Pale white solid, yield 37%, m.p. 129.2–129.5 °C; ^{1}H-NMR (300 MHz, $CDCl_3$) δ: 3.62 (s, 8H), 2.44 (s, 24H), 2.40–2.37 (m, 4H), 2.30 (s, 12H), 1.37 (s, 4H); ^{13}C-NMR (101 MHz, DMSO) δ: 150, 149.53, 148.60, 147.79, 58.54, 54.85, 24.39, 21.64, 21.47, 20.71; HRMS (ESI) *m/z*: 625.4451 $[M + H]^+$, calcd. for $[C_{36}H_{53}N_{10}]^+$ 625.4455.

4.2.4. N^1,N^1,N^6,N^6-Tetrakis((3,5,6-Trimethylpyrazin-2-yl)Methyl)Hexane-1,6-Diamine (**6d**)

Pale white solid, yield 43%, m.p. 146.7–147.9 °C; ^{1}H-NMR (300 MHz, $CDCl_3$) δ: 3.67 (s, 8H), 2.46–2.45 (m, 24H), 2.43–2.40 (m, 4H), 2.34 (s, 12H), 1.43 (br, 4H), 1.04 (br, 4H); ^{13}C-NMR (101 MHz, DMSO) δ: 150.05, 149.48, 148.71, 147.77, 58.64, 54.93, 27.34, 26.56, 21.65, 21.48, 20.74; HRMS (ESI) *m/z*: 653.4765 $[M + H]^+$, calcd. for $[C_{38}H_{57}N_{10}]^+$ 653.4768.

4.2.5. N^1,N^1,N^8,N^8-Tetrakis((3,5,6-Trimethylpyrazin-2-yl)Methyl)Octane-1,8-Diamine (**6e**)

Pale white solid, yield 48%, m.p. 107.8–108.6 °C; ^{1}H-NMR (300 MHz, $CDCl_3$) δ: 3.67 (s, 8H), 2.45 (br, 24H), 2.42–2.38 (m, 4H), 2.34 (s, 12H), 1.48–1.40 (m, 4H), 1.05 (br, 8H); ^{13}C-NMR (101 MHz, $CDCl_3$) δ: 150.09, 149.47, 148.75, 147.76, 58.69, 54.90, 29.52, 27.46, 26.55, 21.65, 21.47, 20.73; HRMS (ESI) *m/z*: 681.5076 $[M + H]^+$, calcd. for $[C_{40}H_{61}N_{10}]^+$ 681.5081.

4.2.6. N^1,N^1,N^{10},N^{10}-Tetrakis((3,5,6-Trimethylpyrazin-2-yl)Methyl)Decane-1,10-Diamine (**6f**)

Pale white solid, yield 76%, m.p. 67.4–68 °C; ^{1}H-NMR (300 MHz, $CDCl_3$) δ: 3.69 (s, 8H), 2.46 (br, 24H), 2.41–2.39 (m, 4H), 2.35 (s, 12H), 1.47 (br, 4H), 1.11 (br, 12H); ^{13}C-NMR (101 MHz, DMSO) δ: 150.10, 149.45, 148.78, 147.76, 58.71, 54.92, 29.73, 29.52, 27.48, 26.57, 21.64, 21.47, 20.74; HRMS (ESI) *m/z*: 709.5378 $[M + H]^+$, calcd. for $[C_{42}H_{65}N_{10}]^+$ 709.5394.

4.2.7. N^1,N^1,N^{12},N^{12}-Tetrakis((3,5,6-Trimethylpyrazin-2-yl)Methyl)Dodecane-1,12-Diamine (**6g**)

Pale white solid, yield 76%, m.p. 84.7–85.3 °C; ^{1}H-NMR (300 MHz, $CDCl_3$) δ: 3.69 (s, 8H), 2.46 (br, 24H), 2.44 (br, 4H), 2.35 (s, 12H), 1.47 (br, 4H), 1.15–1.12 (br, 16H); ^{13}C-NMR (101 MHz, DMSO) δ:

150.10, 149.44, 148.78, 147.74, 58.72, 54.89, 29.75, 29.53, 27.46, 26.56, 21.64, 21.47, 20.73; HRMS (ESI) *m/z*: 737.5689 [M + H]$^+$, calcd. for $[C_{44}H_{69}N_{10}]^+$ 737.5707.

4.3. *1,4-Bis((3,5,6-Trimethylpyrazin-2-yl)Methyl)Piperazine* (**6h**)

A mixture of piperazine (0.800 g, 9.29 mmol), TMP-Cl (3.80 g, 22.29 mmol), KOH (1.56 g, 27.66 mmol), and dimethylformamide (20 mL) was heated under reflux for 2 h. The reaction was monitored by TLC. The reaction was quenched, filtered, and the filtrate was added with 100 mL H_2O and extracted with ethyl acetate three times. The organic layers were combined, washed with H_2O and brine, and then dried over anhydrous Na_2SO_4 for 8 h. The solvent was evaporated in vacuo. The resulting residue was separated on flash column chromatography with a mixture of petroleum ether/acetone 7:1–3:1(volume ratio) as eluent, and then further recrystallized from acetone to afford compound **6h**.

Pale white solid, yield 62%, m.p. 155.8–156.3 °C; ^{1}H-NMR (300 MHz, $CDCl_3$) δ: 3.58 (s, 4H), 2.55 (s, 8H), 2.47 (br, 18H); ^{13}C-NMR (101 MHz, DMSO) δ: 150.01, 149.57, 148.10, 147.98, 61.88, 53.26, 50.70, 21.61, 21.51, 21.04; HRMS (ESI) *m/z*: 355.2610 [M + H]$^+$, calcd. for $[C_{20}H_{31}N_6]^+$ 355.2610.

4.4. *2-(Bis((3,5,6-Trimethylpyrazin-2-yl)Methyl)Amino)Ethanol* (**6i**)

A mixture of ethanolamine (0.500 g, 8.19 mmol), TMP-Cl (3.35 g, 19.65 mmol), K_2CO_3 (3.39 g, 24.56 mmol), and acetonitrile (20 mL) was heated under reflux for 3 h. The product formation was monitored via TLC. After cooling, the mixture was filtered, and the filtrate was evaporated in vacuo. The residue was purified by flash column chromatography with an eluent of petroleum ether/acetone = 10:1–3:1 to afford compound **6i**.

Light yellow oil, yield 72%; ^{1}H-NMR (300 MHz, $CDCl_3$) δ: 3.82 (13s, 4H), 3.66 (t, J = 5 Hz, 2H), 2.87 (t, J = 5.1 Hz, 2H), 2.41 (s, 6H), 2.37 (s, 6H), 2.35 (s, 6H); ^{13}C-NMR (101 MHz, DMSO) δ: 149.54, 148.94, 148.27, 147.87, 59.67, 58.15, 57.36, 21.41, 21.21, 20.52; HRMS (ESI) *m/z*: 330.2290 [M + H]$^+$, calcd. for $[C_{18}H_{28}N_5O]^+$ 330.2294.

4.5. *General Synthetic Procedure for* **8a–f**

Compound **7** was gained according to the method described by Wu [20]. A mixture of tetramethylpyrazine acid (4.40 mmol), EDCI (4.72 mmol), triethylamine (12 mmol), DMAP (2.40 mmol), and anhydrous dichloromethane (10 mL) was stirred to dissolve, then diamino-alkane (2 mmol) was added and stirred at room temperature until the reaction was finished (monitored by TLC). The reaction mixture was washed with brine and water, extracted with dichloromethane (20 mL), dried over anhydrous sodium sulfate for 8 h, filtered, and the solvent was evaporated. The resulting residue was purified by flash column chromatography with an eluent of petroleum ether/acetone = 15:1–3:1(volume ratio) to give pale white solid.

4.5.1. N,N′-(Propane-1,3-Diyl)Bis(3,5,6-Trimethylpyrazine-2-Carboxamide) (**8a**)

Pale white solid, yield 16%, m.p. 125.4–126.4 °C; ^{1}H-NMR (300 MHz, $CDCl_3$) δ: 8.30 (t, J = 5.9 Hz, 2H), 3.58–3.52 (m, 4H), 2.92 (s, 6H), 2.56 (s, 6H), 2.50 (s, 6H), 1.99–1.90 (m, 2H); ^{13}C-NMR (101 MHz, CDC13) δ: 165.57, 154.09, 151.29, 147.80, 139.09, 36.89, 29.87, 22.94, 22.07, 21.47; HRMS (ESI) *m/z*: 371.2189 [M + H]$^+$, calcd. for $[C_{19}H_{27}N_6O_2]^+$ 371.2195.

4.5.2. N,N′-(Butane-1,4-Diyl)Bis(3,5,6-Trimethylpyrazine-2-Carboxamide) (**8b**)

Pale white solid, yield 30%, m.p. 168.4–168.6 °C; ^{1}H-NMR (300 MHz, $CDCl_3$) δ: 8.07 (t, J = 5.5 Hz, 2H), 3.50–3.48 (m, 4H), 2.91 (s, 6H), 2.56 (s, 6H), 2.52 (s, 6H), 1.75–1.73 (m, 4H); ^{13}C-NMR (101 MHz, $CDCl_3$) δ: 165.25, 154.15, 151.38, 147.75, 139.07, 50.90, 39.13, 27.49, 22.96, 22.06, 21.48; HRMS (ESI) *m/z*: 385.2352 [M + H]$^+$, calcd. for $[C_{20}H_{29}N_6O_2]^+$ 385.2352.

4.5.3. N,N′-(Hexane-1,6-Diyl)Bis(3,5,6-Trimethylpyrazine-2-Carboxamide) (**8c**)

Pale white solid, yield 47%, m.p. 114.2–114.7 °C; ^{1}H-NMR (300 MHz, $CDCl_3$) δ: 8.02 (t, *J* = 5.4 Hz, 2H), 3.45–3.38 (m, 4H), 2.90 (s, 6H), 2.55 (s, 6H), 2.51 (s, 6H), 1.67–1.63 (m, 4H), 1.47–1.43 (m, 4H); ^{13}C-NMR (101 MHz, $CDCl_3$) δ: 165.12, 154.03, 151.35, 147.63, 139.11, 39.33, 29.74, 26.82, 22.98, 22.06, 21.48; HRMS (ESI) *m/z*: 413.2662 [M + H]$^+$, calcd. for $[C_{22}H_{33}N_6O_2]^+$ 413.2665.

4.5.4. N,N′-(Octane-1,8-Diyl)Bis(3,5,6-Trimethylpyrazine-2-Carboxamide) (**8d**)

Pale white solid, yield 68%, m.p. 113.6–113.8 °C; ^{1}H-NMR (300 MHz, $CDCl_3$) δ: 8 (t, *J* = 5.3 Hz, 2H), 3.45–3.38 (m, 4H), 2.91 (s, 6H), 2.56 (s, 6H), 2.52 (s, 6H), 1.65–1.60 (m, 4H), 1.37–1.37 (m, 8H); ^{13}C-NMR (101 MHz, $CDCl_3$) δ: 165.10, 154.02, 151.40, 147.65, 139.20, 39.45, 29.81, 29.34, 27.11, 23.01, 22.08, 21.53; HRMS (ESI) *m/z*: 441.2975 [M + H]$^+$, calcd. for $[C_{24}H_{37}N_6O_2]^+$ 441.2978.

4.5.5. N,N′-(Decane-1,10-Diyl)Bis(3,5,6-Trimethylpyrazine-2-Carboxamide) (**8e**)

Pale white solid, yield 66%, m.p. 110.3–110.6 °C; ^{1}H-NMR (300 MHz, $CDCl_3$) δ: 8 (t, *J* = 5.2 Hz, 2H), 3.44–3.37 (m, 4H), 2.91 (s, 6H), 2.55 (s, 6H), 2.51 (s, 6H), 1.64–1.57 (m, 4H), 1.34–1.30 (m, 12H); ^{13}C-NMR (101 MHz, $CDCl_3$) δ: 165.07, 153.97, 151.33, 147.66, 139.21, 39.47, 29.80, 29.56, 29.39, 27.14, 22.94, 22.02, 21.49; HRMS (ESI) *m/z*: 469.3287 [M + H]$^+$, calcd. for $[C_{26}H_{41}N_6O_2]^+$ 469.3291.

4.5.6. N,N′-(Dodecane-1,12-Diyl)Bis(3,5,6-Trimethylpyrazine-2-Carboxamide) (**8f**)

Pale white solid, yield 72%, m.p. 98.3–99.1 °C; ^{1}H-NMR (300 MHz, $CDCl_3$) δ: 8 (t, *J* = 4.9 Hz, 2H), 3.45–3.38 (m, 4H), 2.91 (s, 6H), 2.56 (s, 6H), 2.52 (s, 6H), 1.67–1.57 (m, 4H), 1.34–1.27 (m, 16H); ^{13}C-NMR (101 MHz, $CDCl_3$) δ: 165.07, 153.98, 151.37, 147.62, 139.22, 39.49, 29.83, 29.66, 29.44, 27.18, 22.99, 22.07, 21.51; HRMS (ESI) *m/z*: 497.3602 [M + H]$^+$, calcd. for $[C_{28}H_{45}N_6O_2]^+$ 497.3604.

4.6. *General Synthetic Procedure for* **9e–35e**

Compounds **9e–35e** were obtained by using one-pot reaction. A mixture of aromatic acid (6.30 mmol), EDCI (7.50 mmol), DMAP (0.60 mmol), and anhydrous dichloromethane (20 mL) was stirred to dissolve, then decane-diamine (3 mmol) was added and stirred at room temperature for 12 h. The mixture solution was filtered under reduced pressure. After that, the residue was washed with little amount of CH_2Cl_2 and water successively, and dried to give the solid. Then, the residue was purified on preparative TLC eluted with chloroform/methanol = 40:1–7:1 to yield compounds **26e**, **28e, 30e,** and **31e**.

4.6.1. (2E,2′E)-N,N′-(Decane-1,10-Diyl)Bis(3-Phenylacrylamide) (**9e**)

Pale white solid, yield 62%, m.p. 169.8–170.5 °C; ^{1}H-NMR (300 MHz, $CDCl_3$+CD_3OD) δ: 7.54 (d, *J* = 15.7 Hz, 2H), 7.49–7.46 (m, 4H), 7.36–7.31 (m, 6H), 6.47 (d, *J* = 15.6 Hz, 2H), 3.33–3.28 (m, 4H), 1.57–1.54 (m, 4H), 1.52–1.28 (m, 12H); ^{13}C-NMR (101 MHz, $CDCl_3$+CD_3OD) δ: 150.10, 149.45, 148.78, 147.76, 58.71, 54.92, 29.73, 29.52, 27.48, 26.57, 21.64, 21.47, 20.74; HRMS (ESI) *m/z*: 433.2851 [M + H]$^+$, calcd. for $[C_{28}H_{45}N_6O_2]^+$ 433.2855

4.6.2. N,N′-(Decane-1,10-Diyl)Dinicotinamide (**10e**)

Pale white solid, yield 67%, m.p. 167.4–167.8 °C; ^{1}H-NMR (300 MHz, $CDCl_3$+CD_3OD) δ: 8.84 (s, 2H), 8.55 (d, *J* = 3.9 Hz, 2H), 8.11 (dt, *J* = 8, 1.7 Hz, 2H), 7.35 (dd, *J* = 7.9, 4.9 Hz, 2H), 3.34 (t, *J* = 7.2 Hz, 4H), 1.58–1.51 (m, 4H), 1.27–1.24 (m, 12H); ^{13}C-NMR (101 MHz, $CDCl_3$+CD_3OD) δ: 165.85, 151.29, 147.53, 135.93, 130.87, 123.79, 40.16, 29.28, 29.12, 26.86; HRMS (ESI) *m/z*: 383.2441 [M + H]$^+$, calcd. for $[C_{28}H_{45}N_6O_2]^+$ 383.2447.

4.6.3. N,N′-(Decane-1,10-Diyl)Dibenzamide (**11e**)

Pale white solid, yield 70%, m.p. 154.3–154.6 °C; ^{1}H-NMR (300 MHz, $CDCl_3$+CD_3OD) δ: 7.77–7.73 (m, 4H), 7.51–7.33 (m, 6H), 3.42–3.35 (m, 4H), 1.63–1.56 (m, 4H), 1.34–1.30 (m, 12H); ^{13}C-NMR (101 MHz, $CDCl_3$+CD_3OD) δ: 168.39, 134.55, 131.36, 128.45, 126.86, 40.02, 29.36, 29.27, 29.13, 26.84. HRMS (ESI) *m/z*: 381.2702 [M + H]$^+$, calcd. for $[C_{24}H_{33}N_2O_2]^+$ 381.2542.

4.6.4. N,N′-(Decane-1,10-Diyl)Bis(2-Naphthamide) (**12e**)

Pale white solid, yield 64%, m.p. 163.9–164 °C; ^{1}H-NMR (300 MHz, $CDCl_3$+CD_3OD) δ: 8.22–8.17 (m, 2H), 7.89–7.82 (m, 4H), 7.54–7.39 (m, 8H), 3.49–3.44 (m, 4H), 1.67–1.60 (m, 4H), 1.38–1.34 (m, 12H); ^{13}C-NMR (101 MHz, $CDCl_3$ + CD_3OD) δ: 170.38, 134.50, 133.56, 130.33, 129.96, 128.22, 126.89, 126.29, 125.10, 124.77, 124.65, 39.94, 29.36, 29.30, 29.11, 26.85. HRMS (ESI) *m/z*: 481.2853 [M + H]+, calcd. for $[C_{32}H_{37}N_2O_2]^+$ 481.2855.

4.6.5. N,N′-(Decane-1,10-Diyl)Diisonicotinamide (**13e**)

Pale white solid, yield 60%, m.p. 175.6–176.3 °C; ^{1}H-NMR (300 MHz, $CDCl_3$+CD_3OD) δ: 8.62 (d, *J* = 5.6 Hz, 4H), 7.71 (dd, *J* = 6.1, 2.8 Hz, 4H), 3.41–3.33 (m, 4H), 1.64–1.57 (m, 4H), 1.33–1.31 (m, 12H); ^{13}C-NMR (101 MHz, $CDCl_3$+CD_3OD) δ: 165.88, 149.48, 142.45, 121.46, 40.04, 29.16, 28.99, 26.71. HRMS (ESI) *m/z*: 383.2445 [M + H]$^+$, calcd. for $[C_{22}H_{31}N_4O_2]^+$ 383.2447.

4.6.6. N,N′-(Decane-1,10-Diyl)Bis(Furan-2-Carboxamide) (**14e**)

Pale white solid, yield 62%, m.p. 132.6–133.3 °C; ^{1}H-NMR (300 MHz, $CDCl_3$) δ: 7.41 (dd, *J* = 1.7, 0.8 Hz, 2H), 7.09 (dd, *J* = 3.5, 0.7 Hz, 2H), 6.48 (dd, *J* = 3.5, 1.7 Hz, 2H), 6.37 (br, 2H), 3.45–3.38 (m, 4H), 1.65–1.55 (m, 4H), 1.36–1.30 (m, 12H); ^{13}C-NMR (101 MHz, $CDCl_3$) δ: 158.53, 148.38, 143.77, 114.02, 112.22, 39.29, 29.80, 29.48, 29.33, 26.98. HRMS (ESI) *m/z*: 383.1944 [M + Na]$^+$, calcd. for $[C_{20}H_{28}N_2NaO_4]^+$ 383.1947.

4.6.7. N,N′-(Decane-1,10-Diyl)Dipicolinamide (**15e**)

Pale white solid, yield 68%, m.p. 156.6–156.9 °C; ^{1}H-NMR (300 MHz, $CDCl_3$) δ: 9.35 (d, *J* = 1.4 Hz, 2H), 8.69 (d, *J* = 2.5 Hz, 2H),.8.47–8.46 (m, 2H), 7.77 (br, 2H), 3.47–3.40 (m, 4H), 1.65–1.55 (m, 4H), 1.34–1.26 (m, 12H); ^{13}C-NMR (101 MHz, $CDCl_3$) δ: 163.01, 147.26, 144.76, 144.55, 142.58, 39.61, 29.68, 29.51, 29.34, 27.03. HRMS (ESI) *m/z*: 383.2441 [M + H]$^+$, calcd. for $[C_{22}H_{31}N_4O_2]^+$ 383.2447

4.6.8. N,N′-(Decane-1,10-Diyl)Bis(Pyrazine-2-Carboxamide) (**16e**)

Pale white solid, yield 70%, m.p. 77.6–80.1 °C; ^{1}H-NMR (300 MHz, $CDCl_3$) δ: 8.54–8.51 (m, 2H), 8.20–8.17 (m, 2H), 8.05 (br, 2H), 7.85–7.80 (m, 2H), 7.42–7.38 (m, 2H), 3.49–3.43 (m, 4H), 1.68–1.58 (m, 4H), 1.38–1.26 (m, 12H); ^{13}C-NMR (101 MHz, $CDCl_3$) δ: 164.31, 150.25, 148.09, 137.49, 126.13, 122.34, 39.61, 29.77, 29.56, 29.41, 27.11. HRMS (ESI) *m/z*: 385.2350 [M + H]$^+$, calcd. for $[C_{20}H_{29}N_6O_2]^+$ 385.2352.

4.6.9. N,N′-(Decane-1,10-Diyl)Bis(Quinoline-3-Carboxamide) (**17e**)

Pale white solid, yield 59%, m.p. 206.7–207.1 °C; ^{1}H-NMR (300 MHz, DMSO-d_6 + CD_3OD) δ: 8.57 (d, *J* = 1.8 Hz, 2H), 8.09 (s, 2H), 7.39 (dd, *J* = 8.3, 3.1 Hz, 4H), 7.17 (t, *J* = 7.6 Hz, 2H), 7 (t, *J* = 7.4 Hz, 2H), 2.68 (t, *J* = 7 Hz, 4H), 0.99–0.88 (m, 4H), 0.76–0.62 (m, 12H). ^{13}C-NMR (101 MHz, $CDCl_3$) δ: 165.92, 148.01, 136.52, 131.47, 128.81, 127.93, 127.56, 127.35, 127.06, 40.11, 29.20, 29.15, 29.04, 26.78. HRMS (ESI) *m/z*: 483.2756 [M + H]$^+$, calcd. for $[C_{30}H_{35}N_4O_2]^+$ 483.2760.

4.6.10. N,N′-(Decane-1,10-Diyl)Bis(Quinoline-6-Carboxamide) (**18e**)

Pale yellow solid, yield 73%, m.p. 197.7–198.3 °C; ^{1}H-NMR (300 MHz, $CDCl_3$ + CD_3OD) δ: 8.71 (dd, *J* = 4.3, 1.6 Hz, 2H), 8.19 (d, *J* = 1.6 Hz, 2H), 8.16 (dd, *J* = 8.3, 1.3 Hz, 2H), 7.95 (dd, *J* = 8.8, 1.9 Hz, 2H), 7.91 (s, 2H), 7.35 (dd, *J* = 8.3, 4.3 Hz, 2H), 3.28 (t, *J* = 7.2 Hz, 4H), 1.53–1.45 (m, 5H), 1.22–1.13

(m, 12H). ^{13}C-NMR (101 MHz, $CDCl_3$ + CD_3OD) δ: 167.43, 151.15, 148.21, 137.99, 132.82, 128.38, 127.79, 127.71, 127.64, 121.81, 40.14, 29.19, 29.04, 26.78. HRMS (ESI) *m/z*: 483.2758 $[M + H]^+$, calcd. for $[C_{30}H_{35}N_4O_2]^+$ 483.2760.

4.6.11. N,N′-(Decane-1,10-Diyl)Bis(1H-Benzo[d]Imidazole-6-Carboxamide) (**19e**)

Brick red solid, yield 75%, m.p. 229.7–230.3 °C; ^{1}H-NMR (300 MHz, $CDCl_3$+ CD_3OD) δ: 8.11 (s, 2H), 8.07 (s, 2H), 7.73 (dd, *J* = 8.5, 1.6 Hz, 2H), 7.61 (d, *J* = 8.5 Hz, 2H), 3.42 (t, *J* = 7.1 Hz, 4H), 1.70–1.56 (m, 4H), 1.42–1.25 (m, 12H). ^{13}C-NMR (101 MHz, $CDCl_3$+ CD_3OD) δ: 168.61, 142.46, 128.70, 121.15, 39.32, 28.66, 28.62, 28.50, 26.19. HRMS (ESI) *m/z*: 461.2662 $[M + H]^+$, calcd. for $[C_{26}H_{33}N_6O_2]^+$ 461.2665.

4.6.12. N,N′-(Decane-1,10-Diyl)Bis(2-Oxo-2H-Chromene-3-Carboxamide) (**20e**)

Pale white solid, yield 60%, m.p. 208.9–209.3 °C; ^{1}H-NMR (300 MHz, $CDCl_3$) δ: 8.90 (s, 2H), 8.80 (s, 2H), 7.71–7.61 (m, 4H), 7.43–7.32 (m, 4H), 3.45 (dd, *J* = 13, 7 Hz, 4H), 1.63 (dt, *J* = 14.4, 7.2 Hz, 4H), 1.44–1.26 (m, 12H). ^{13}C-NMR (101 MHz, $CDCl_3$ + CD_3OD) δ: 161.74, 161.44, 154.23, 148.38, 134.16, 129.80, 125.30, 118.46, 117.97, 116.38, 39.69, 29.20, 29.02, 29.01, 26.77. HRMS (ESI) *m/z*: 517.2338 $[M + H]^+$, calcd. for $[C_{30}H_{33}N_2O_6]^+$ 517.2339.

4.6.13. N,N′-(Decane-1,10-Diyl)Bis(Benzofuran-2-Carboxamide) (**21e**)

Pale white solid, yield 43%, m.p. 135.8–136.3 °C; ^{1}H-NMR (300 MHz, DMSO-d_6) δ: 8.64 (s, 2H), 7.74 (d, *J* = 7.7 Hz, 2H), 7.62 (d, *J* = 8.2 Hz, 2H), 7.49 (s, 2H), 7.43 (t, *J* = 7.5 Hz, 2H), 7.30 (t, *J* = 7.4 Hz, 2H), 3.25 (dd, *J* = 13.1, 6.6 Hz, 4H), 1.58–1.43 (m, 4H), 1.37–1.14 (m, 12H). ^{13}C-NMR (101 MHz, DMSO-d_6) δ: 157.94, 154.13, 149.37, 127.17, 126.61, 123.59, 122.63, 111.70, 109.02, 38.68, 29.01, 28.91, 28.71, 26.39. HRMS (ESI) *m/z*: 461.2438 $[M + H]^+$, calcd. for $[C_{28}H_{33}N_2O_4]^+$ 461.2430.

4.6.14. N,N′-(Decane-1,10-Diyl)Bis(Benzo[b]Thiophene-2-Carboxamide) (**22e**)

Pale yellow solid, yield 46%, m.p. 175–175.7 °C; ^{1}H-NMR (300 MHz, DMSO-d_6) δ: 8.68 (s, 2H), 8.04 (s, 2H), 8.01–7.95 (m, 2H), 7.93–7.87 (m, 2H), 7.41 (p, *J* = 7 Hz, 4H), 3.25 (dd, *J* = 12.8, 6.6 Hz, 4H), 1.58–1.44 (m, 4H), 1.37–1.21 (m, 12H). ^{13}C-NMR (101 MHz, DMSO-d_6) δ: 161.28, 140.28, 140.07, 139.16, 126, 125.02, 124.80, 124.33, 122.72, 28.99, 28.92, 28.72, 26.43. HRMS (ESI) *m/z*: 493.1976 $[M + H]^+$, calcd. for $[C_{28}H_{33}N_2O_2S_2]^+$ 493.1983.

4.6.15. N,N′-(Decane-1,10-Diyl)Bis(1-Methyl-1H-Indole-3-Carboxamide) (**23e**)

Pale white solid, yield 43%, m.p. 192.8–193.2 °C; ^{1}H-NMR (300 MHz, DMSO-d_6 + CD_3OD) δ: 8.08 (d, *J* = 7.7 Hz, 2H), 7.86 (s, 2H), 7.41 (d, *J* = 8 Hz, 2H), 7.20–7.13 (m, 2H), 7.13–7.06 (m, 2H), 3.78 (s, 6H), 3.22 (t, *J* = 7.1 Hz, 4H), 1.55–1.43 (m, 4H), 1.32–1.22 (m, 12H). ^{13}C-NMR (101 MHz, $CDCl_3$ + CD_3OD) δ: 166.26, 137.01, 131.75, 125.56, 122.27, 121.03, 120.13, 109.63, 39.26, 32.62, 29.33, 29.07, 28.94, 26.66. HRMS (ESI) *m/z*: 487.3064 $[M + H]^+$, calcd. for $[C_{30}H_{39}N_4O_2]^+$ 487.3073.

4.6.16. N,N′-(Decane-1,10-Diyl)Bis(1H-Indole-6-Carboxamide) (**24e**)

Pale white solid, yield 47%, m.p. 168.4–169.2 °C; ^{1}H-NMR (300 MHz, DMSO-d_6) δ: 11.32 (s, 2H), 8.30 (s, 2H), 7.92 (s, 2H), 7.59–7.41 (m, 6H), 6.46 (s, 2H), 3.25 (dd, *J* = 12.7, 6.4 Hz, 4H), 1.61–1.43 (m, 4H), 1.38–1.21 (m, 12H). ^{13}C-NMR (101 MHz, DMSO) δ: 167.04, 135.24, 129.61, 127.74, 127.66, 119.27, 117.90, 111.07, 101.14, 39.21, 29.27, 29, 28.83, 26.55. HRMS (ESI) *m/z*: 459.2760 $[M + H]^+$, calcd. for $[C_{28}H_{35}N_4O_2]^+$ 459.2760.

4.6.17. (2E,2′E)-N,N′-(Decane-1,10-Diyl)Bis(3-(4-Chlorophenyl)Acrylamide) (**25e**)

Pale white solid, yield 64%, m.p. 230.3–230.9 °C; ^{1}H-NMR (300 MHz, $CDCl_3$ +CF_3COOD) δ: 7.64 (d, *J* = 13 Hz, 2H), 7.54–7.38 (m, 8H), 6.51 (d, *J* = 11.9 Hz, 2H), 3.62–3.37 (m, 4H), 1.73–1.54 (m, 4H),

1.46–1.18 (m, 12H). ^{13}C-NMR (101 MHz, $CDCl_3$ + CF_3COOD) δ: 129.71, 118.78, 115.96, 113.13, 110.30, 29.22, 28.99, 26.64. HRMS (ESI) *m/z*: 501.2075 $[M + H]^+$, calcd. for $[C_{28}H_{35}Cl_2N_2O_2]^+$ 501.2076.

4.6.18. (2E,2′E)-N,N′-(Decane-1,10-Diyl)Bis(3-(3-Hydroxy-4-Methoxyphenyl)Acrylamide) (**26e**)

Pale yellow solid, yield 35%, m.p. 192.9–195.3 °C; ^{1}H-NMR (300 MHz, $CDCl_3$ + CD_3OD) δ: 7.42 (d, *J* = 15.3 Hz, 2H), 7.05 (s, 2H), 6.98 (d, *J* = 8.1 Hz, 2H), 6.83 (d, *J* = 8.3 Hz, 2H), 6.33 (d, *J* = 15.6 Hz, 2H), 3.89 (s, 6H), 3.29 (t, *J* = 7 Hz, 4H), 1.55–1.50 (m, 4H), 1.31–1.27 (m, 12H). ^{13}C-NMR (101 MHz, $CDCl_3$ + CD_3OD) δ: 167.37, 148.94, 146.05, 140.42, 128.11, 121.06, 118.25, 113.07, 111, 55.57, 39.50, 29.13, 28.98, 26.69. HRMS (ESI) *m/z*: 525.2951 $[M + H]^+$, calcd. for $[C_{30}H_{41}N_2O_6]^+$ 525.2965.

4.6.19. (2E,2′E)-N,N′-(Decane-1,10-Diyl)Bis(3-(3,4-Dimethoxyphenyl)Acrylamide) (**27e**)

Pale white solid, yield 59%, m.p. 168.9–169.9 °C; ^{1}H-NMR (300 MHz, DMSO-d_6) δ: 7.95 (br, 2H), 7.30 (br, 2H), 7.11 (br, 4H), 6.97 (br, 2H), 6.50 (br, 2H), 3.78 (br, 12H), 3.14 (br, 4H), 1.42 (br, 4H), 1.27 (br, 12H). ^{13}C-NMR (101 MHz, $CDCl_3$+ CD_3OD) δ: 167.15, 150.31, 148.90, 140.25, 127.89, 121.77, 118.56, 111.04, 109.74, 55.66, 55.58, 39.47, 29.16, 29.14, 28.99, 26.69. HRMS (ESI) *m/z:* 553.3272 $[M + H]^+$, calcd. for $[C_{32}H_{45}N_2O_6]^+$ 553.3278.

4.6.20. (2E,2′E)-N,N′-(Decane-1,10-Diyl)Bis(3-(4-Hydroxy-3,5-Dimethoxyphenyl)Acrylamide) (**28e**)

Pale yellow solid, yield 33%, m.p. 179.8–180.5 °C; ^{1}H-NMR (300 MHz, $CDCl_3$ + CD_3OD) δ: 7.44 (d, *J* = 15.5 Hz, 3H), 6.76 (s, 4H), 6.37 (d, *J* = 15.6 Hz, 2H), 3.88 (s, 12H), 3.30 (t, *J* = 7.1 Hz, 4H), 1.61–1.49 (m, 4H), 1.38–1.24 (m, 12H). ^{13}C-NMR (101 MHz, $CDCl_3$ + CD_3OD) δ: 166.94, 147.48, 141.03, 136.87, 126.16, 118.46, 104.99, 56.23, 39.63, 29.39, 29.21, 29.08, 26.79. HRMS (ESI) *m/z*: 585.3164 $[M+H]^+$, calcd. for $[C_{32}H_{45}N_2O_8]^+$ 585.3176

4.6.21. (2E,2′E)-N,N′-(Decane-1,10-Diyl)Bis(3-(3,4,5-Trimethoxyphenyl)Acrylamide) (**29e**)

Pale white solid, yield 67%, m.p. 193.4–194.3 °C; ^{1}H-NMR (300 MHz, $CDCl_3$ + CD_3OD) δ: 7.45 (d, *J* = 15.4 Hz, 2H), 6.76 (s, 4H), 6.44 (d, *J* = 15.6 Hz, 2H), 3.88 (s, 12H), 3.85 (s, 6H), 3.31 (t, *J* = 7.1 Hz, 4H), 1.63–1.47 (m, 4H), 1.40–1.23 (m, 12H). ^{13}C-NMR (101 MHz, $CDCl_3$ + CD_3OD) δ: 166.73, 153.26, 140.53, 139.33, 130.65, 120.18, 104.99, 60.81, 56, 39.63, 29.28, 29.21, 29.05, 26.76. HRMS (ESI) *m/z*:613.3472 $[M + H]^+$, calcd. for $[C_{34}H_{49}N_2O_8]^+$ 613.3489.

4.6.22. N,N′-(Decane-1,10-Diyl)Bis(2-Aminobenzamide) (**30e**)

Pale white solid, yield 67%, m.p. 90.2–91 °C; ^{1}H-NMR (300 MHz, $CDCl_3$ + CD_3OD) δ: 7.36 (dd, *J* = 7.8, 1.2 Hz, 2H), 7.22–7.15 (m, 2H), 6.79–6.60 (m, 4H), 3.35 (dt, *J* = 9.7, 5.5 Hz, 4H), 1.66–1.49 (m, 4H), 1.41–1.24 (m, 12H). ^{13}C-NMR (101 MHz, $CDCl_3$ + CD_3OD) δ: 173.92, 151.77, 135.96, 131.40, 121.48, 121.28, 120.96, 43.54, 33.31, 33.26, 33.11, 30.83. HRMS (ESI) *m/z*:411.2759 $[M + H]^+$, calcd. for $[C_{24}H_{35}N_4O_2]^+$ 411.2760.

4.6.23. N,N′-(Decane-1,10-Diyl)Bis(4-Aminobenzamide) (**31e**)

Pale yellow solid, yield 31%, m.p. 186.7–187.7 °C; ^{1}H-NMR (300 MHz, $CDCl_3$ + CD_3OD) δ: 7.57 (d, *J* = 8.6 Hz, 4H), 6.66 (d, *J* = 8.6 Hz, 4H), 3.34 (t, *J* = 7.2 Hz, 4H), 1.63–1.53 (m, 4H), 1.31–1.26 (m, 12H). ^{13}C-NMR (101 MHz, $CDCl_3$ + CD_3OD) δ: 168.44, 150.01, 128.49, 123.39, 114.04, 39.77, 29.33, 29.18, 29.06, 26.76. HRMS (ESI) *m/z*: 411.2755 $[M + H]^+$, calcd. for $[C_{24}H_{35}N_4O_2]^+$ 411.2760.

4.6.24. N,N′-(Decane-1,10-Diyl)bis(3-Aminobenzamide) (**32e**)

Pale white solid, yield 57%, m.p. 135.7–136.3 °C; ^{1}H-NMR (300 MHz, $CDCl_3$ + CD_3OD) δ: 7.30–6.97 (m, 6H), 6.83 (dd, *J* = 20.8, 7.2 Hz, 2H), 3.36 (t, *J* = 6.8 Hz, 4H), 1.67–1.47 (m, 4H), 1.46–1.06 (m, 12H). ^{13}C-NMR (101 MHz, $CDCl_3$ + CD_3OD) δ: 168.75, 146.84, 135.56, 129.27, 118.09, 116.55, 113.73,

77.48, 77.16, 76.84, 49.31, 49.09, 48.88, 48.67, 48.45, 39.93, 29.29, 29.22, 29.09, 26.79. HRMS (ESI) *m/z*: 411.2758 [M + H]$^+$, calcd. for $[C_{24}H_{35}N_4O_2]^+$ 411.2760

4.6.25. N,N′-(Decane-1,10-Diyl)Bis(3,5-Dimethoxybenzamide) (**33e**)

Pale white solid, yield 56%, m.p. 143.4–144.2 °C; ^{1}H-NMR (300 MHz, $CDCl_3$ + CD_3OD) δ: 6.79 (d, *J* = 2.1 Hz, 4H), 6.43 (t, *J* = 1.9 Hz, 2H), 3.69 (s, 12H), 3.25 (t, *J* = 7.2 Hz, 4H), 1.50–1.45 (m, 4H), 1.25–1.15 (m, 12H). ^{13}C-NMR (101 MHz, $CDCl_3$ + CD_3OD) δ: 168.01, 160.73, 136.74, 104.94, 103.34, 55.40, 40.03, 29.28, 29.26, 29.11, 26.82. HRMS (ESI) *m/z:* 501.2959 [M + H]$^+$, calcd. for $[C_{28}H_{41}N_2O_6]^+$ 501.2965.

4.6.26. N,N′-(Decane-1,10-Diyl)Bis(3,4,5-Trimethoxybenzamide) (**34e**)

Pale white solid, yield 63%, m.p. 194–194.9 °C; ^{1}H-NMR (300 MHz, $CDCl_3$ + CD_3OD) δ: 6.91 (s, 4H), 3.72 (s, 12H), 3.67 (s, 6H), 3.22–3.16 (m, 4H), 1.50–1.36 (m, 4H), 1.22–1.08 (m, 12H). ^{1}H-NMR (300 MHz, $CDCl_3$ + CD_3OD). δ: 6.91 (s, 4H), 3.72 (s, 12H), 3.67 (s, 6H), 3.22–3.16 (m, 4H), 1.50–1.36 (m, 4H), 1.22–1.08 (m, 12H). ^{13}C-NMR (101 MHz, $CDCl_3$ + CD_3OD) δ: 167.81, 152.77, 129.84, 104.42, 60.53, 55.85, 40.01, 29.17, 29.03, 26.73. HRMS (ESI) *m/z:* 561.3169 [M + H]$^+$, calcd. for $[C_{30}H_{45}N_2O_8]^+$ 561.3176.

4.6.27. N,N′-(Decane-1,10-Diyl)Bis(2,3,4-Trimethoxybenzamide) (**35e**)

Pale white solid, yield 26%, m.p. 112.3–112.5 °C; ^{1}H-NMR (300 MHz, $CDCl_3$) δ: 7.94 (s, 2H), 7.89 (d, *J* = 8.9 Hz, 2H), 6.76 (d, *J* = 9 Hz, 2H), 3.96 (s, 6H), 3.90 (s, 6H), 3.87 (s, 6H), 3.44 (dd, *J* = 12.7, 6.9 Hz, 4H), 1.62 (dt, *J* = 14.3, 7.1 Hz, 4H), 1.41–1.29 (m, 12H). ^{13}C-NMR (101 MHz, $CDCl_3$) δ: 164.90, 156.35, 152.42, 141.83, 126.76, 119.31, 107.67, 61.71, 61.08, 56.15, 39.71, 29.78, 29.65, 29.43, 27.24. HRMS (ESI) *m/z:* 561.3172 [M + H]$^+$, calcd. for $[C_{30}H_{45}N_2O_8]^+$ 561.3176.

4.7. General Synthetic Procedure for **9d**, **9f**

A mixture of cinnamic acid (6.30 mmol), EDCI (7.50 mmol), DMAP (0.60 mmol), and anhydrous dichloromethane (20 mL) was stirred to dissolve, then diamino-alkane (3 mmol) was added and stirred at room temperature for 12 h. The mixture solution was filtered under reduced pressure. After that, the residue was washed with dichloromethane and water successively, and then dried to give a pale white solid. TLC indicated that it was a single point.

4.7.1. (2E,2′E)-N,N′-(Octane-1,8-Diyl)Bis(3-Phenylacrylamide) (**9d**)

Pale white solid, yield 63%, m.p. 186–186.4 °C; ^{1}H-NMR (300 MHz, $CDCl_3$ + CD_3OD) δ: 7.58–7.29 (m, 12H), 6.53 (d, *J* = 15.7 Hz, 2H), 3.31 (t, *J* = 7.1 Hz, 4H), 1.59–1.55 (m, 4H), 1.35 (s, 8H). ^{13}C-NMR (101 MHz, $CDCl_3$ + CD_3OD) δ: 166.96, 140.39, 134.78, 129.42, 128.59, 127.54, 120.60, 39.43, 29.04, 28.85, 26.57. HRMS (ESI) *m/z:* 405.2537 [M + H]$^+$, calcd. for $[C_{26}H_{33}N_2O_2]^+$ 405.2542.

4.7.2. (2E,2′E)-N,N′-(Dodecane-1,12-Diyl)Bis(3-Phenylacrylamide) (**9f**)

Pale white solid, yield 49%, m.p. 164.7–165 °C; ^{1}H-NMR (300 MHz, $CDCl_3$ + CD_3OD) δ: 7.56–7.49 (m, 6H), 7.40–7.28 (m, 6H), 6.53 (d, *J* = 15.7 Hz, 2H), 3.30 (t, *J* = 7.1 Hz, 4H), 1.62–1.51 (m, 4H), 1.38–1.23 (m, 16H). ^{13}C-NMR (101 MHz, $CDCl_3$ + CD_3OD) δ: 166.94, 140.22, 134.73, 129.29, 128.47, 127.42, 120.54, 39.42, 29.19, 29.03, 28.99, 26.66. HRMS (ESI) *m/z:* 461.3166 [M + H]$^+$, calcd. for $[C_{30}H_{41}N_2O_2]^+$ 461.3168.

4.8. General Synthetic Procedure for **9g–9i**

A mixture of cinnamic acid (6.30 mmol), EDCI (7.50 mmol), DMAP (0.60 mmol), and anhydrous dichloromethane (20 mL) was stirred to dissolve, then alkane-diol (3 mmol) was added and stirred at room temperature for 12 h. The mixture solution was filtered under reduced pressure. After that, the residue was washed with dichloromethane and water successively, subsequently, purified by preparative TLC eluted with petroleum ether/ethyl acetate = 5:1 to give pale white solid.

4.8.1. Octane-1,8-Diyl (2E,2′E)-Bis(3-Phenylacrylate) (**9g**)

Pale white solid, yield 35%, m.p. 61.1–62.5 °C; ^{1}H-NMR (300 MHz, $CDCl_3$) δ: 7.68 (d, J = 16 Hz, 2H), 7.58–7.46 (m, 4H), 7.43–7.30 (m, 6H), 6.45 (d, J = 16 Hz, 2H), 4.21 (t, J = 6.7 Hz, 4H), 1.77–1.68 (m, 4H), 1.46–1.40 (m, 8H). ^{13}C-NMR (101 MHz, $CDCl_3$) δ: 167.22, 144.72, 134.62, 130.35, 129.01, 128.19, 118.43, 64.79, 29.31, 28.85, 26.05. HRMS (ESI) *m/z:* 407.2223 $[M + H]^+$, calcd. for $[C_{26}H_{31}O_4]^+$ 407.2222.

4.8.2. Decane-1,10-Diyl (2E,2′E)-Bis(3-Phenylacrylate) (**9h**)

Pale white solid, yield 33%, m.p. 118.6–119.2 °C; ^{1}H-NMR (300 MHz, $CDCl_3$) δ: 7.68 (d, J = 16 Hz, 2H), 7.57–7.48 (m, 4H), 7.38 (dd, J = 6.6, 3.6 Hz, 6H), 6.45 (d, J = 16 Hz, 2H), 4.21 (t, J = 6.7 Hz, 4H), 1.77–1.62 (m, 4H), 1.48–1.25 (m, 12H). ^{13}C-NMR (101 MHz, $CDCl_3$) δ: 167.23, 144.69, 134.64, 130.35, 129.01, 128.19, 118.46, 64.85, 29.58, 29.40, 28.88, 26.12. HRMS (ESI) *m/z:* 435.2534 $[M + H]^+$, calcd. for $[C_{28}H_{35}O_4]^+$ 435.2535.

4.8.3. Dodecane-1,12-Diyl (2E,2′E)-Bis(3-Phenylacrylate) (**9i**)

Pale white solid, yield 28%, m.p. 63.1–64 °C; ^{1}H-NMR (300 MHz, $CDCl_3$) δ: 7.68 (d, J = 16 Hz, 2H), 7.52 (dt, J = 4.6, 3.2 Hz, 4H), 7.42–7.33 (m, 6H), 6.45 (d, J = 16 Hz, 2H), 4.21 (t, J = 6.7 Hz, 4H), 1.77–1.65 (m, 4H), 1.43–1.25 (m, 16H). ^{13}C-NMR (101 MHz, $CDCl_3$) δ: 167.22, 144.68, 134.64, 130.34, 129.01, 128.18, 118.47, 64.87, 29.68, 29.66, 29.42, 28.87, 26.12. HRMS (ESI) *m/z:* 463.2851 $[M + H]^+$, calcd. for $[C_{30}H_{39}O_4]^+$ 463.2828.

4.9. General Synthetic Procedure for **9j–9m**

A mixture of cinnamic acid (6.30 mmol), EDCI (7.50 mmol), DMAP (0.60 mmol), and anhydrous dichloromethane (20 mL) was stirred to dissolve, then diamino-ether (3 mmol) was added and stirred at room temperature for 12 h. Then, the solid was filtered off, the filtrate was added with H_2O (50 mL) and extracted by dichloromethane three times. The combined organic layers were washed with H_2O and brine, dried with anhydrous sodium sulfate for 8 h, filtered, and evaporated. The resulting residue was purified by preparative TLC with petroleum ether/ethyl acetate = 2:1–1:1 to give pale white solid or light yellow oil.

4.9.1. (2E,2′E)-N,N′-((Ethane-1,2-Diylbis(Oxy))Bis(Ethane-2,1-Diyl))Bis(3-Phenylacrylamide) (**9j**)

Pale white solid, yield 78%, m.p. 117.9–118.5 °C; ^{1}H-NMR (300 MHz, $CDCl_3$) δ: 7.62 (d, J = 15.6 Hz, 2H), 7.51–7.41 (m, 4H), 7.37–7.27 (m, 6H), 6.48 (d, J = 15.6 Hz, 2H), 3.65–3.60 (m, 12H). ^{13}C-NMR (101 MHz, $CDCl_3$) δ: 166.26, 141.19, 134.95, 129.77, 128.92, 127.92, 120.82, 70.50, 70.05, 39.63. HRMS (ESI) *m/z*: 409.2121 $[M + H]^+$, calcd. for $[C_{24}H_{29}N_2O_4]^+$ 409.2127.

4.9.2. (2E,2′E)-N,N′-(((Oxybis(Ethane-2,1-Diyl))Bis(Oxy))Bis(Ethane-2,1-Diyl))Bis(3-Phenylacrylamide) (**9k**)

Light yellow oil, yield 28%; ^{1}H-NMR (300 MHz, $CDCl_3$) δ: 7.60 (d, J = 15.6 Hz, 2H), 7.45 (dd, J = 6.5, 3.1 Hz, 4H), 7.32–7.30 (m, 4H), 6.71 (t, J = 5.7 Hz, 2H), 6.47 (d, J = 15.6 Hz, 2H), 3.65 (s, 8H), 3.63–3.54 (m, 8H). ^{13}C-NMR (101 MHz, $CDCl_3$) δ: 166.17, 140.96, 134.98, 129.70, 128.89, 127.86, 120.93, 70.49, 70.27, 70, 39.59. HRMS (ESI) *m/z:* 453.2387 $[M + H]^+$, calcd. for $[C_{26}H_{33}N_2O_5]^+$ 453.2389.

4.9.3. (Ethane-1,2-Diylbis(Oxy))Bis(Ethane-2,1-Diyl) (2E,2′E)-Bis(3-Phenylacrylate) (**9l**)

Light yellow oil, yield 65%; ^{1}H-NMR (300 MHz, $CDCl_3$) δ: 7.70 (d, J = 16 Hz, 2H), 7.54–7.48 (m, 4H), 7.40–7.34 (m, 6H), 6.48 (d, J = 16 Hz, 2H), 4.42–4.36 (m, 4H), 3.84–3.77 (m, 4H), 3.73 (s, 4H). ^{13}C-NMR (101 MHz, $CDCl_3$) δ: 167.03, 145.21, 134.50, 130.44, 129.01, 128.23, 118, 70.79, 69.48, 63.78. HRMS (ESI) *m/z:* 411.1805 $[M + H]^+$, calcd. for $[C_{24}H_{27}O_6]^+$ 411.1808.

4.9.4. ((Oxybis(Ethane-2,1-Diyl))Bis(Oxy))Bis(Ethane-2,1-Diyl) (2E,2′E)-bis(3-Phenylacrylate) (**9m**)

Light yellow oil, yield 87%; ^{1}H-NMR (300 MHz, $CDCl_3$) δ: 7.70 (d, J = 16 Hz, 2H), 7.55–7.48 (m, 4H), 7.38 (dd, J = 3.8, 2.7 Hz, 6H), 6.48 (d, J = 16 Hz, 2H), 4.37 (dd, J = 5.5, 4.1 Hz, 4H), 3.81–3.74 (m, 4H), 3.70 (s, 8H). ^{13}C-NMR (101 MHz, $CDCl_3$) δ: 167.03, 145.19, 134.52, 130.45, 129.02, 128.23, 118.04, 77.48, 77.36, 77.16, 76.84, 70.82, 70.79, 69.42, 63.80. HRMS (ESI) *m/z*: 472.2337 [M + NH_4]$^+$, calcd. for [$C_{26}H_{34}NO_7$]$^+$ 472.2335.

4.10. Biological Assays

4.10.1. Cell Culture

The tested cells were obtained from Shanghai Institute of Biochemistry and Cell Biology of the Chinese Academy of Sciences (Shanghai, China). HeLa and Hep G2 cell lines were cultured in Dulbecco's modified Eagle's medium (DMEM; gibco, Life Technologies, Carlsbad, CA, USA) supplemented with 10% fetal bovine serum (FBS; Biological Industries), 100 U/mL penicillin-streptomycin (PS; gibco, Life Technologies, Carlsbad, CA, USA). MCF-7 and A549 cell lines were maintained in RPMI-1640 media (gibco, Life Technologies, Carlsbad, CA, USA) supplemented with 10% FBS and 100 U/mL PS. FaDu cell lines were cultured in minimum essential medium (MEM; Gibco, Life Technologies, Carlsbad, CA, USA) supplemented with 10% FBS and 100 U/mL PS. MCF 10A cell lines were maintained in Mammary MEGM kit (Lonza/Clonetics) supplemented with 100 ng/mL cholera toxin (Sigma, Shanghai, China). Cell lines were grown at 37 °C in a humidified atmosphere of 5% CO_2.

4.10.2. Cell Viability Assay

The growth-inhibitory effects against HeLa, Hep G2, MCF-7, FaDu, and A549 cancer cells and normal cell lines MCF 10A were determined by MTT assay [21]. All of the synthesized compounds and the positive control drug doxorubicin were dissolved in 0.1% DMSO. Cells were seeded in 96 well plates at a density of 1 × 10^4 cells per well and incubated for 24 h at 37 °C in a humidified atmosphere of 5% CO_2. The cells were then incubated with various concentrations of drugs for 48 h in a 5% CO_2 incubator at 37 °C. After treatment with 1 mg/mL 3-(4,5-dimethylthiazol-2-yl)-2,5-diphenyltetrazolium bromide (MTT) solution for 4 h, the formazan crystals were dissolved in 100 μL DMSO in each well. Plates were read on a microplate reader (Thermo Varioskan Flash 3001) at 490 nm. The experiment was performed in triplicate. The inhibitory concentration at 50% (IC_{50}) was calculated based on concentration-inhibition relationships via regression using SPSS software (Version 17.0).

4.10.3. Colony Formation Assay

FaDu cells were seeded in a 6-well plate with 500 cells per well and incubated for 24 h. Then, the cells were treated with compound **8e** at various final concentrations of 0, 0.75, 1.50, 3 nM. Following treatment for 10 days, the cells were washed with PBS twice and fixed with 4% paraformaldehyde for 10 min at room temperature. Then, the cell colonies were visualized by staining with 0.1% crystal violet for 10 min. The image was photographed with Handy camera, and the numbers of cell colonies were analyzed using the open Image J software (Developed by National Institutes of Health). A group of >50 cells was defined as one colony. Triplicate wells were set up for each concentration.

4.10.4. Live/Dead Staining

The Calcein AM/propidium iodide (PI) double staining was performed following the manufacturer's instructions (Dojindo Laboratory, Kumamoto, Japan). Briefly, FaDu cells were seeded in 6-well plates overnight. Then, the **8e** solutions at final concentrations of 2.5 nM, 5 nM, and 10 nM were added. After incubation for 24 h, the cells were collected, washed with PBS, and stained by a mixture of 2 μM Calcein-AM (live cells, green) and 4.5 μM PI (dead cells, red) solution in the dark for 30 min at 37 °C (excitation 490 nm). Then, the cells were rinsed with PBS twice and re-suspended in the cell medium. Confocal fluorescence images were acquired using a laser scanning confocal microscope (LSCM, Carl-Zeiss LSM 710).

4.10.5. Hoechst 33,342 Staining

For Hoechst staining, FaDu cells were seeded onto a glass-bottom of cell culture dish at a density of 1×10^5 cells. After incubation for 24 h, the media containing 20 nM of the compound **8e** was used to replace the culture medium. Then, the cells were stained with Hoechst 33,342 solution (10 μg/mL in the culture medium, Beyotime Institute of Biotechnology, Shanghai, China) at 37 °C in the dark for 20 min after treatment with **8e**. Then, the cells were washed with the serum-free medium to remove excess dye. LSCM (Carl-Zeiss LSM 710) was used to capture the images of nuclear morphological changes to find apoptotic cells.

4.10.6. Flow Cytometric Analysis of Apoptosis by Annexin V-FITC/PI Staining

Apoptosis in FaDu cells was evaluated by an annexin V-FITC/PI apoptosis detection kit (Beyotime Institute of Biotechnology, Shanghai, China). Briefly, FaDu cells were treated with various concentrations of compound **8e** (2, 5, 10 nM) or DMSO as vehicle control for 24 h at 37 °C; then, the cells were washed twice with cold 1× PBS and centrifuged at 1000 rpm for 5 min. The harvested cells were resuspended gently in 400 μL binding buffer, containing 5 μL annexin V-FITC and 10 μL PI. After incubating for 15 min in the dark at room temperature, the cells were analyzed with flow cytometry (CyFlow® Cube 6, Sysmex). Data were shown as pseudo color graphs and analyzed using FlowJo Software (Tree Star Inc, Ashland, OR).

4.10.7. Mitochondrial Membrane Potential (ΔΨm) Analysis

The mitochondrial membrane potential (ΔΨm) was detected by a mitochondrial membrane potential assay kit with JC-1 (Beyotime Institute of Biotechnology, Shanghai, China). Briefly, after treatment with various concentrations of compound **8e** (2, 5, 10 nM) for 24 h, FaDu cells were harvested and stained with 500 μL 1× JC-1 dye solution at 37 °C for 20 min in the dark. Then, the treated cells were washed twice and resuspended by 1× JC-1 staining buffer. The fluorescence of approximately 1×10^4 cells was analyzed using flow cytometry (CyFlow® Cube 6, Sysmex).

4.10.8. Cell Cycle Analysis

The cell cycle analysis was carried out by a cell cycle and apoptosis analysis kit with a propidium iodide (PI) staining method (Beyotime Institute of Biotechnology, Shanghai, China). Briefly, FaDu cells were incubated with the above-mentioned doses of compound **8e** for 24 h; all samples were collected, washed once with cold 1× PBS, and fixed by 70% ice-cold ethanol at 4 °C for 12 h. Then, the fixed cells were washed once with cold 1× PBS and stained with 500 μL 1× PI dye solution (containing 10 μL RNase A) at 37 °C for 30 min in the dark. The red fluorescence was detected using a flow cytometer (CyFlow® Cube 6, Sysmex). The data were analyzed using FlowJo Software (Tree Star Inc, Ashland, OR, USA).

4.10.9. In Silico ADMET Prediction

A computational study of all synthesized compounds was carried out for the prediction of ADMET (absorption, distribution, metabolism, excretion, and toxicity) properties. In this module, thirteen mathematical models, such as HBD (hydrogen bond donor), HBA (hydrogen bond acceptor), RBN (number of rotatable bonds), logP (log of the octanol/water partition coefficient), log S (log of the aqueous solubility), and PSA (polar surface area) were predicted via Discovery Studio 2.0 Software (Studio 2.5, Accelrys, Co. Ltd., San Diego, CA, USA) and HIA (human intestinal absorption), PPB (plasma protein binding), CYP3D4 (CYP3D4 inhibition), $T_{1/2}$ (half lifetime), HT (human hepatotoxicity), and LD_{50} (median lethal dose) were calculated using web-based applications and then analyzed to predict the drug likeliness profile (Xiangya School of Pharmaceutical Sciences and Central South University, http://admet.scbdd.com/home/index/) [28]. We also screened our novel derivatives through the prediction model by Egan et al. [29,30]. Two molecular descriptors, AlogP98 and PSA, were computed and plotted in a 2D plane to comprehensively evaluate the absorption and blood-brain penetration of the compounds.

Supplementary Materials: The following are available online at http://www.mdpi.com/1420-3049/24/24/4505/s1, ^{1}H-NMR, ^{13}C-NMR and HR-MS spectra of compounds.

Author Contributions: Ideas and experiment design: J.W., G.H., and T.L.; Chemistry and Biology: J.W., G.H., G.L., and W.W.; Analysis and interpretation of data: J.W., G.H., G.L., and W.W.; Writing and review of the manuscript: J.W., G.H., G.L., W.W., and T.L.; Study supervision: T.L. and G.H.

Funding: This research was funded by the national major science and technology special project for "significant new drugs development" (2018ZX09711001-005-018), "the medical and health science and technology innovation project of Chinese Academy of Medical Science" (2017-I2M-3-021/2019-I2M-1-005), "the Tianjin special support program for talent development" (TJTZJH-GCCCXCYTD-1-30).

Acknowledgments: The authors gratefully acknowledge the Institute of Materia Medica, Chinese Academy of Medical Sciences and Peking Union Medical College and information technology center for affording the Discovery Studio 2.0 Software.

Conflicts of Interest: The authors declare that they have no competing interests.

References

1. Cragg, G.M.; Newman, D.J. Natural products: A continuing source of novel drug leads. *Biochim. Et Biophys. Acta (Bba) - Gen. Subj.* **2013**, *1830*, 3670–3695. [CrossRef] [PubMed]
2. Chang, C.-Y.; Kao, T.-K.; Chen, W.-Y.; Ou, Y.-C.; Li, J.-R.; Liao, S.-L.; Raung, S.-L.; Chen, C.-J. Tetramethylpyrazine inhibits neutrophil activation following permanent cerebral ischemia in rats. *Biochem. Biophys. Res. Commun.* **2015**, *463*, 421–427. [CrossRef] [PubMed]
3. Cao, J.; Miao, Q.; Miao, S.; Bi, L.; Zhang, S.; Yang, Q.; Zhou, X.; Zhang, M.; Xie, Y.; Zhang, J.; et al. Tetramethylpyrazine (TMP) exerts antitumor effects by inducing apoptosis and autophagy in hepatocellular carcinoma. *Int. Immunopharmacol.* **2015**, *26*, 212–220. [CrossRef] [PubMed]
4. Bi, L.; Yan, X.; Chen, W.; Gao, J.; Qian, L.; Qiu, S. Antihepatocellular Carcinoma Potential of Tetramethylpyrazine Induces Cell Cycle Modulation and Mitochondrial-Dependent Apoptosis: Regulation of p53 Signaling Pathway in HepG2 Cells In Vitro. *Integr. Cancer Ther.* **2016**, *15*, 226–236. [CrossRef]
5. Ai, Y.; Zhu, B.; Ren, C.; Kang, F.; Li, J.; Huang, Z.; Lai, Y.; Peng, S.; Ding, K.; Tian, J.; et al. Discovery of New Monocarbonyl Ligustrazine–Curcumin Hybrids for Intervention of Drug-Sensitive and Drug-Resistant Lung Cancer. *J. Med. Chem.* **2016**, *59*, 1747–1760. [CrossRef]
6. Xu, B.; Yan, W.-Q.; Xu, X.; Wu, G.-R.; Zhang, C.-Z.; Han, Y.-T.; Chu, F.-H.; Zhao, R.; Wang, P.-L.; Lei, H.-M. Combination of amino acid/dipeptide with ligustrazine-betulinic acid as antitumor agents. *Eur. J. Med. Chem.* **2017**, *130*, 26–38. [CrossRef]
7. Wang, P.-L.; Cheng, Y.-T.; Xu, K.; An, Y.-W.; Wang, W.; Li, Q.-S.; Han, Q.-J.; Li, Q.; Zhang, H.-G.; Lei, H.-M. Synthesis and Antitumor Evaluation of One Novel Tetramethylpyrazine-Rhein Derivative. *Asian J. Chem.* **2013**, *25*, 4885–4888. [CrossRef]
8. Chow, L.M.C.; Chan, T.H. Novel Classes of Dimer Antitumour Drug Candidates. *Curr. Pharm. Des.* **2009**, *15*, 659–674. [CrossRef]
9. Joshi, A.; Vance, D.; Rai, P.; Thiyagarajan, A.; Kane, R.S. The Design of Polyvalent Therapeutics. *Chem. –A Eur. J.* **2008**, *14*, 7738–7747. [CrossRef]
10. Beekman, A.C.; Barentsen, A.R.W.; Woerdenbag, H.J.; Van Uden, W.; Pras, N.; Konings, A.W.T.; El-Feraly, F.S.; Galal, A.M.; Wikström, H.V. Stereochemistry-Dependent Cytotoxicity of Some Artemisinin Derivatives. *J. Nat. Prod.* **1997**, *60*, 325–330. [CrossRef]
11. Hu, Y.; Li, C.; Kulkarni, B.A.; Strobel, G.; Lobkovsky, E.; Torczynski, R.M.; Porco, J.A. Exploring Chemical Diversity of Epoxyquinoid Natural Products: Synthesis and Biological Activity of (−)-Jesterone and Related Molecules. *Org. Lett.* **2001**, *3*, 1649–1652. [CrossRef] [PubMed]
12. Verhoeven, D.T.; Goldbohm, R.A.; van Poppel, G.; Verhagen, H.; van den Brandt, P.A. Epidemiological studies on brassica vegetables and cancer risk. *Cancer Epidemiol. Biomark. Amp; Prev.* **1996**, *5*, 733–748.

13. Chaires, J.B.; Leng, F.; Przewloka, T.; Fokt, I.; Ling, Y.H.; Perezsoler, R.; Priebe, W. Structure-based design of a new bisintercalating anthracycline antibiotic. *J. Med. Chem.* **1997**, *40*, 261–266. [CrossRef] [PubMed]
14. Zha, G.-F.; Qin, H.-L.; Youssif, B.G.M.; Amjad, M.W.; Raja, M.A.G.; Abdelazeem, A.H.; Bukhari, S.N.A. Discovery of potential anticancer multi-targeted ligustrazine based cyclohexanone and oxime analogs overcoming the cancer multidrug resistance. *Eur. J. Med. Chem.* **2017**, *135*, 34–48. [CrossRef]
15. Wang, P.; She, G.; Yang, Y.; Li, Q.; Zhang, H.; Liu, J.; Cao, Y.; Xu, X.; Lei, H. Synthesis and Biological Evaluation of New Ligustrazine Derivatives as Anti-Tumor Agents. *Molecules* **2012**, *17*, 4972–4985. [CrossRef]
16. Xu, B.; Chu, F.; Zhang, Y.; Wang, X.; Li, Q.; Liu, W.; Xu, X.; Xing, Y.; Chen, J.; Wang, P.; et al. A Series of New Ligustrazine-Triterpenes Derivatives as Anti-Tumor Agents: Design, Synthesis, and Biological Evaluation. *Int. J. Mol. Sci.* **2015**, *16*, 21035–21055. [CrossRef]
17. Taylor, A.P.; Robinson, R.P.; Fobian, Y.M.; Blakemore, D.C.; Jones, L.H.; Fadeyi, O. Modern advances in heterocyclic chemistry in drug discovery. *Org. Biomol. Chem.* **2016**, *14*, 6611–6637. [CrossRef]
18. Klein, B.; Berkowitz, J. Pyrazines. I. Pyrazine-N-oxides. Preparation and Spectral Characteristics1. *J. Am. Chem. Soc.* **1959**, *81*, 5160–5166. [CrossRef]
19. Cheng, X.-C.; Liu, X.-Y.; Xu, W.-F.; Guo, X.-L.; Zhang, N.; Song, Y.-N. Ligustrazine derivatives. Part 3: Design, synthesis and evaluation of novel acylpiperazinyl derivatives as potential cerebrocardiac vascular agents. *Bioorganic Med. Chem.* **2009**, *17*, 3018–3024. [CrossRef]
20. Wu, G.-R.; Xu, B.; Yang, Y.-Q.; Zhang, X.-Y.; Fang, K.; Ma, T.; Wang, H.; Xue, N.-N.; Chen, M.; Guo, W.-B.; et al. Synthesis and biological evaluation of podophyllotoxin derivatives as selective antitumor agents. *Eur. J. Med. Chem.* **2018**, *155*, 183–196. [CrossRef]
21. van Meerloo, J.; Kaspers, G.J.L.; Cloos, J. Cell Sensitivity Assays: The MTT Assay. In *Cancer Cell Culture: Methods and Protocols*; Cree, I.A., Ed.; Humana Press: Totowa, NJ, USA, 2011; pp. 237–245.
22. Yi, B.; Liu, D.; He, M.; Li, Q.; Liu, T.; Shao, J. Role of the ROS/AMPK signaling pathway in tetramethylpyrazine-induced apoptosis in gastric cancer cells. *Oncol. Lett.* **2013**, *6*, 583–589. [CrossRef] [PubMed]
23. Shen, J.; Zeng, L.; Pan, L.; Yuan, S.; Wu, M.; Kong, X. Tetramethylpyrazine regulates breast cancer cell viability, migration, invasion and apoptosis by affecting the activity of Akt and caspase-3. *Oncol. Lett.* **2018**, *15*, 4557–4563. [CrossRef] [PubMed]
24. Chu, F.; Xu, X.; Li, G.; Gu, S.; Xu, K.; Gong, Y.; Xu, B.; Wang, M.; Zhang, H.; Zhang, Y.; et al. Amino acid derivatives of ligustrazine-oleanolic acid as new cytotoxic agents. *Molecules* **2014**, *19*, 18215–18231. [CrossRef] [PubMed]
25. Song, F.; Zhang, L.; Yu, H.-X.; Lu, R.-R.; Bao, J.-D.; Tan, C.; Sun, Z. The mechanism underlying proliferation-inhibitory and apoptosis-inducing effects of curcumin on papillary thyroid cancer cells. *Food Chem.* **2012**, *132*, 43–50. [CrossRef] [PubMed]
26. Lipinski, C.A.; Lombardo, F.; Dominy, B.W.; Feeney, P.J. Experimental and computational approaches to estimate solubility and permeability in drug discovery and development settings. *Adv. Drug Deliv. Rev.* **2012**, *64*, 4–17. [CrossRef]
27. Meena, A.; Yadav, D.K.; Srivastava, A.; Khan, F.; Chanda, D.; Chattopadhyay, S.K. In Silico Exploration of Anti-Inflammatory Activity of Natural Coumarinolignoids. *Chem. Biol. Drug Des.* **2011**, *78*, 567–579. [CrossRef]
28. Dong, J.; Wang, N.-N.; Yao, Z.-J.; Zhang, L.; Cheng, Y.; Ouyang, D.; Lu, A.-P.; Cao, D.-S. ADMETlab: A platform for systematic ADMET evaluation based on a comprehensively collected ADMET database. *J. Cheminformatics* **2018**, *10*, 29. [CrossRef]
29. Egan, W.J.; Lauri, G. Prediction of intestinal permeability. *Adv. Drug Deliv. Rev.* **2002**, *54*, 273–289. [CrossRef]
30. Egan, W.J.; Merz, K.M.; Baldwin, J.J. Prediction of Drug Absorption Using Multivariate Statistics. *J. Med. Chem.* **2000**, *43*, 3867–3877. [CrossRef]

Sample Availability: Samples of all compounds are available from the authors.

molecules

MDPI

Article

Novel Chrysin-De-Allyl PAC-1 Hybrid Analogues as Anticancer Compounds: Design, Synthesis, and Biological Evaluation

Buthina A. Al-Oudat [1,†], Hariteja Ramapuram [2,†], Saloni Malla [2], Suaad A. Audat [3], Noor Hussein [2], Jenna M. Len [2], Shikha Kumari [4], Mel F. Bedi [5], Charles R. Ashby, Jr. [6] and Amit K. Tiwari [2,*]

1. Department of Medicinal Chemistry and Pharmacognosy, Faculty of Pharmacy, Jordan University of Science and Technology, P.O. Box 3030, Irbid 22110, Jordan; baoudat@just.edu.jo
2. Department of Pharmacology and Experimental Therapeutics, College of Pharmacy & Pharmaceutical Sciences, University of Toledo, Toledo, OH 43614, USA; hzr0030@tigermail.auburn.edu (H.R.); saloni.malla@rockets.utoledo.edu (S.M.); noor.hussein@rockets.utoledo.edu (N.H.); jenna.len@rockets.utoledo.edu (J.M.L.)
3. Department of Chemistry, College of Science and Arts, Jordan University of Science and Technology, P.O. Box 3030, Irbid 22110, Jordan; saaudat@just.edu.jo
4. Department of Pharmaceutical Sciences, College of Pharmacy, University of Nebraska Medical Center, Omaha, NE 68198, USA; fnu.shikha@unmc.edu
5. Department of Medicinal and Biological Chemistry, College of Pharmacy & Pharmaceutical Sciences, University of Toledo, Toledo, OH 43614, USA; Fernand.Bedi@utoledo.edu
6. Department of Pharmaceutical Sciences, College of Pharmacy & Pharmaceutical Sciences, St. John's University, Queens, NY 11439, USA; cnsratdoc@optonline.net

* Correspondence: Amit.Tiwari@UToledo.edu; Tel.: +1-419-383-1913; Fax: +1-419-383-1909

† These authors contributed equally to this work.

Academic Editor: Qiao-Hong Chen

Received: 2 June 2020; Accepted: 30 June 2020; Published: 4 July 2020

Abstract: New chrysin-De-allyl-Pac-1 hybrid analogues, tethered with variable heterocyclic systems (**4a–4o**), were rationally designed and synthesized. The target compounds were screened for in vitro antiproliferative efficacy in the triple-negative breast cancer (TNBC) cell line, MDA-MB-231, and normal human mammary epithelial cells (HMECs). Two compounds, **4g** and **4i**, had the highest efficacy and selectivity towards MDA-MB-231 cells, and thus, were further evaluated by mechanistic experiments. The results indicated that both compounds **4g** and **4i** induced apoptosis by (1) inducing cell cycle arrest at the G2 phase in MDA-MB-231 cells, and (2) activating the intrinsic apoptotic pathways in a concentration-dependent manner. Physicochemical characterizations of these compounds suggested that they can be further optimized as potential anticancer compounds for TNBC cells. Overall, our results suggest that **4g** and **4i** could be suitable leads for developing novel compounds to treat TNBC.

Keywords: triple-negative breast cancer; cytotoxicity; chrysin analogues; flavonoid; anticancer compounds

---

1. Introduction

Breast cancer is the second leading cause of death among all cancers affecting women [1]. Triple-negative breast cancer (TNBC) lacks the expression of hormone receptors (estrogen (ER) or progesterone (PR)) and/or human epidermal growth factor receptor 2 (HER2), which are more amenable to targeted therapy [2]. TNBC often presents as a high-grade invasive ductal carcinoma (IDC) in patients, accounting for one-fourth of all breast cancer deaths. Consequently, there is an urgent need for the development of compounds that are efficacious and safe for the treatment of breast cancer. Flavonoids are ubiquitous naturally occurring polyphenolic compounds that are commonly found in fruits and vegetables [3]. Flavonoids comprise several classes of low molecular weight compounds, including flavanones, anthocyanidins, flavonols, flavanols, isoflavones, dihydroflavonols, and flavones [4–6]. Chrysin (5, 7-dihydroxyflavone, Figure 1) is a natural flavone found in many plant extracts, such as the blue passionflower, as well as in honey and propolis [7,8]. Chrysin has been reported to have properties, such as antioxidant [9], antihypertensive [10], antibacterial [11], anti-inflammatory [12], antiviral [13], antiallergic [14], antidiabetic [15], anxiolytic [16], and anticancer efficacy [17,18]. The activation of apoptosis plays a major role in producing the anticancer efficacy of chrysin [19–21]. Mechanistically, apoptosis involves a cascade of initiator and effector caspases [22]. Among these caspases, caspase-3 and caspase-7 are downstream executioner caspases that play an essential role in inducing apoptosis by cleaving a variety of cellular substrates [23]. Therefore, caspase-dependent apoptosis pathways represent targets for the development of efficacious anticancer drugs. Recently, a number of studies have been done to augment the pharmacological activity of chrysin by producing synthetic analogues [24–29]. Moreover, there are studies indicating that chrysin-based compounds have in vitro efficacy in breast cancer cells [30–32]. The compound, de-allyl procaspase-activating compound 1 (PAC-1), induces apoptosis in different types of cancer cells by activating caspase-3 and/or caspase-7 [33–36]. Previously, we reported that molecular hybridization between chrysin and de-allyl PAC-1 can be used to produce novel hybrid molecules with cytotoxic efficacy [29]. Molecular hybridization is a process that comprises the amalgamation of two or more pharmacophoric moieties of different bioactive molecules into a single molecular framework [37,38].

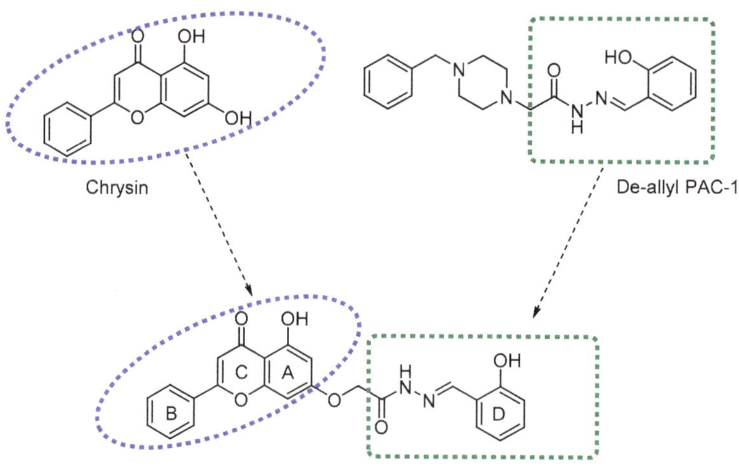

Figure 1. Chemical structures of chrysin, de-allyl PAC-1, and a representative designed hybrid molecule **4a**.

In this study, new chrysin-de-allyl PAC-1 hybrid analogues, substituted with variable aromatic heterocyclic cores, were synthesized and evaluated to identify a more potent bioactive hybrid against breast cancer cells (Figure 1). The in silico parameters of the synthesized compounds were calculated to predict their pharmacokinetic profile and drug-likeness using SwissSimilarity ADME, a web tool [39]. Subsequently, the target compounds were screened for antiproliferative efficacy in the human breast cancer cell line MDA-MB-231, using the MTT 3-(4,5-Dimethylthiazol-2-yl)-2,5-Diphenyltetrazolium

Bromide) colorimetric assay. Finally, we determined the effects of the most potent compounds on the cell cycle.

2. Results and Discussions

2.1. Chemistry

The target compounds (**4a–4o**) were prepared according to Scheme 1, starting from the commercially available chrysin, using previously published synthetic procedures [29]. Briefly, chrysin was added to methyl 2-bromoacetate at a low temperature in the presence of K_2CO_3, yielding the desired alkylation product **2**. The conversion of ester **2** into hydrazide **3** was accomplished using 80% hydrazine hydrate and a few drops of hydrochloric acid at low temperature. ^{1}H and ^{13}C NMR data confirmed the formation of hydrazide **3** as a pure single product. Target compounds (**4a–4o**) were obtained by adding hydrazide **3** to an appropriate aldehyde in the presence of a catalytic amount of hydrochloric acid at room temperature. All analogues gave adequate analytical and spectroscopic data, which were in full accordance with their structures. ^{1}H and ^{13}C NMR spectra showed that compounds **4a–4o** existed as geometrical isomers (E/Z isomers). The E:Z ratio for each compound was determined from ^{1}H NMR spectra utilizing the integration of the neat methylene group peaks that appeared as two separated singlets for each isomer. Target compounds were analyzed using SwissSimilarity (Swiss Institute of Bioinformatics, Lausanne, Switzerland). Compounds **4a–4j** and **4n–4o** were the most structurally similar to apigenin, a flavonoid similar to chrysin. The physicochemical properties of the compounds (**4a–4o**) are shown in Table 1.

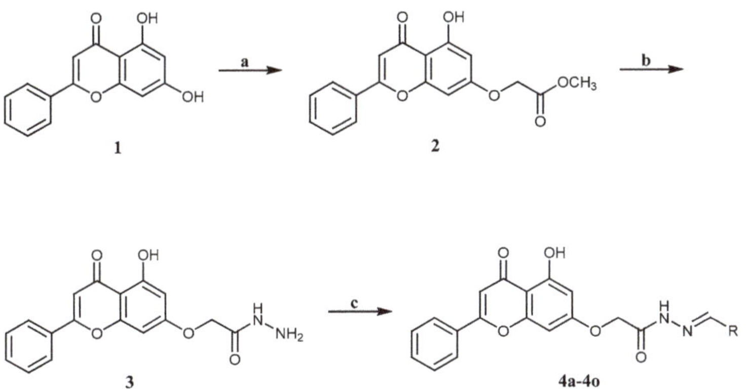

Scheme 1. Reagents and conditions: (**a**) methyl 2-bromoacetate, K_2CO_3, DMF, 0 °C, 3 h; (**b**) hydrazine hydrate 80%, EtOH, 0 °C, HCl (cat.), 1 h; (**c**) different substituted aldehydes, CH_3OH, HCl (cat), rt, 1 h.

Table 1. Physiochemical properties of the compounds **4a–4o** collected from Swiss ADME.

Compound	MW	Solubility	Pharmacokinetics		Drug-Likeness	Medicinal Chemistry		Lipophilicity
		ESOL Class	GI Absorption	BBB Permeant	Lipinski Violations	Lead-likeness Violations	PAINS Alerts	Log P
4a	430.41	Moderately soluble	High	No	0	2	1	3.14
4b	414.41	Moderately soluble	High	No	0	2	0	3.38
4c	444.44	Moderately soluble	High	No	0	3	0	3.62
4d	458.46	Moderately soluble	High	No	0	3	0	3.95
4e	430.41	Moderately soluble	High	No	0	2	1	3.07
4f	444.44	Moderately soluble	High	No	0	3	0	3.62

Table 1. *Cont.*

Compound	MW	Solubility	Pharmacokinetics		Drug-Likeness	Medicinal Chemistry		Lipophilicity
		ESOL Class	GI Absorption	BBB Permeant	Lipinski Violations	Lead-likeness Violations	PAINS Alerts	Log P
4g	446.41	Moderately soluble	Low	No	0	2	2	2.71
4h	474.46	Moderately soluble	High	No	0	3	0	3.65
4i	462.41	Moderately soluble	Low	No	0	2	3	2.38
4j	462.41	Moderately soluble	Low	No	0	2	2	2.43
4k	404.37	Moderately soluble	High	No	0	2	0	2.81
4l	415.4	Moderately soluble	High	No	0	2	0	2.66
4m	415.4	Moderately soluble	High	No	0	2	0	2.72
4n	480.47	Poorly soluble	Low	No	0	2	1	4.04
4o	475.41	Moderately soluble	Low	No	1	3	1	2.52

ESOL Class: Estimated Solubility Class [40]. GI Absorption: Gastrointestinal Absorption. BBB Permeant: Blood Brain Barrier Permeant. Lipinski Violations examines orally active compounds to determine ranges for high probability to be an oral drug. Lead-likeness Violations examines compounds' likeliness to become a lead based on a rule-based method [41]. PAINS Alerts: compounds that give false positives where the compound nonspecifically binds to numerous biological targets, instead of one desired target [42]. Log P: partition coefficient measuring lipophilicity [41].

2.2. *3-(4,5-Dimethylthiazol-2-yl)-2,5-Diphenyltetrazolium Bromide-Based Cytotoxicity Assay*

The synthesized chrysin derivatives were evaluated for cytotoxic efficacy in the human breast cancer cell line, MDA-MB-231, using the 3-(4,5-dimethylthiazol-2yl)-2,5-diphenyltetrazolium bromide (MTT) colorimetric assay and doxorubicin was used as a reference anticancer drug. The IC_{50} values (concentration of compound in μM required to reduce 50% of cell viability) are shown in Table 2.

Table 2. The effects of chrysin derivatives (**4a–4o**) on the survival of the MDA-MB-231 cancer cell line.

Compound	Structure	IC_{50} (μM)
4a	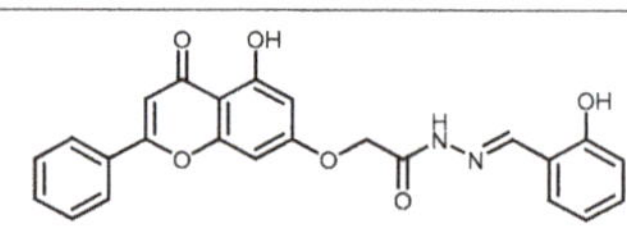	6.8 ± 2.76
4b	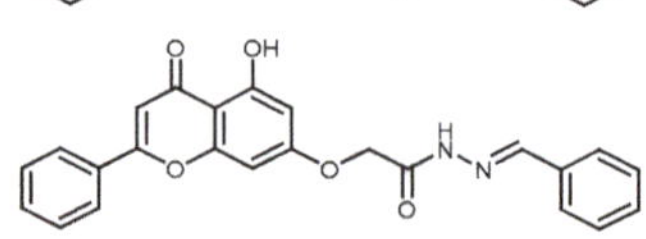	9.4 ± 3.38
4c	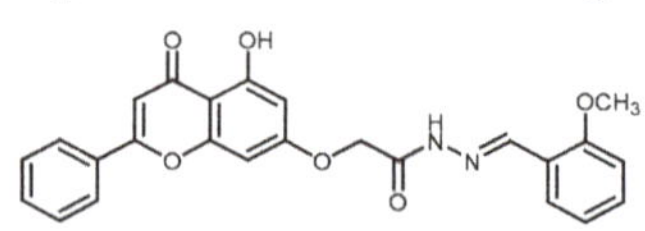	23.3 ± 6.98
4d	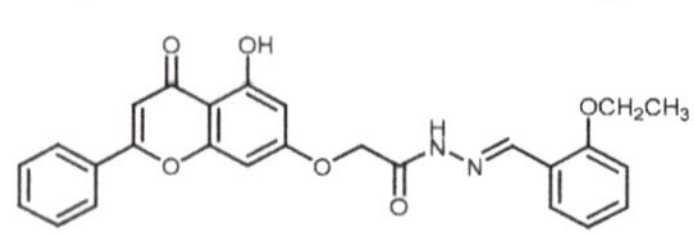	100
4e	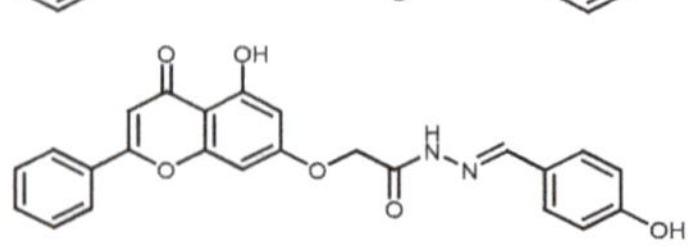	54.8 ± 5.7 [a]

Table 2. *Cont.*

Compound	Structure	IC_{50} (μM)
4f	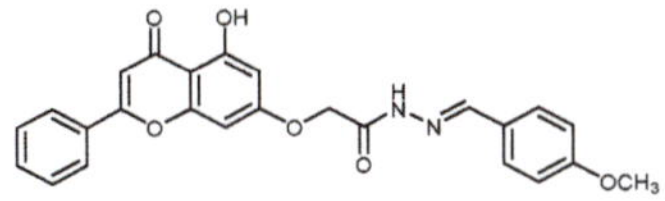	11.9 ± 3.5 [a]
4g	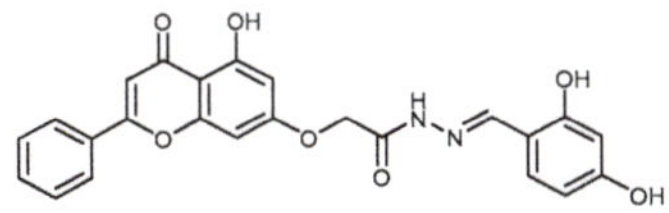	5.98 ± 2.25
4h	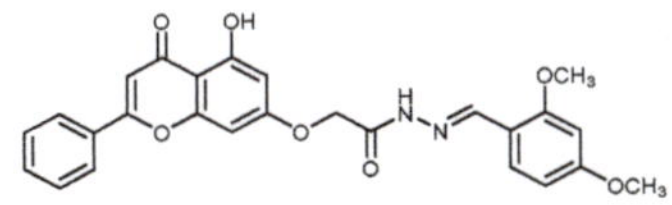	100
4i	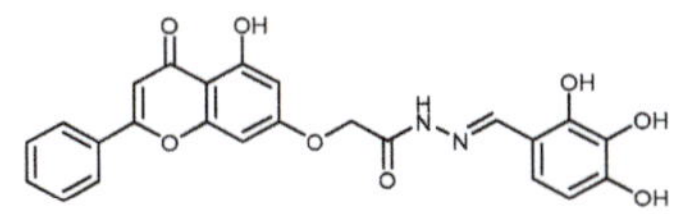	9.40 ± 1.45
4j	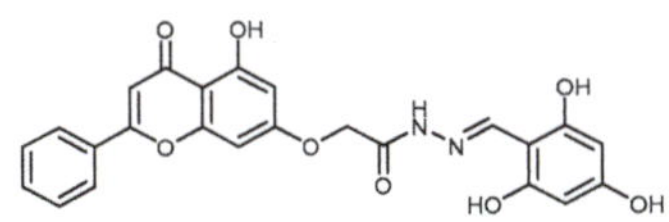	100
4k	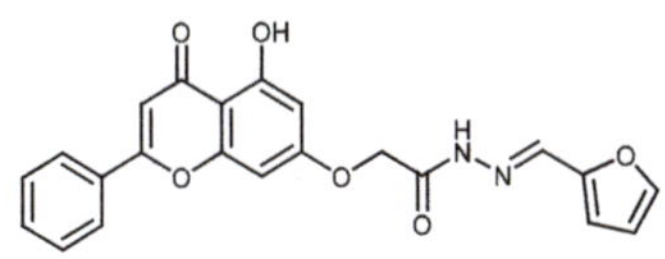	66.65 ± 11.10
4l	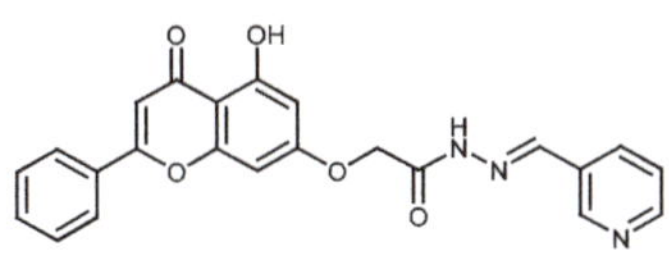	100
4m	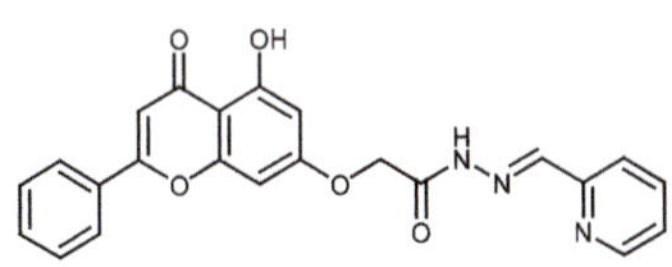	100
4n	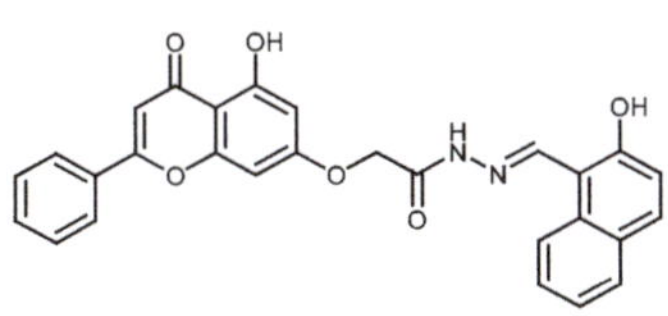	100
4o	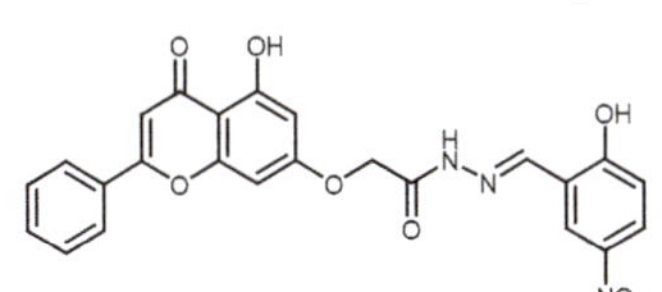	7.90 ± 1.82
Doxorubicin	NA	0.2 ± 0.1

Cell survival was determined by MTT assay as described in materials and methods. The IC_{50} values are represented as mean ± SD of two independent experiments performed in triplicate. [a] The data was taken from [29].

As shown in Table 2, the structure–activity relationship (SAR) results indicated that the cytotoxic efficacy of the synthesized compounds was affected by the modifications on the benzene ring (ring D) of the parent compound **4a**. Compound **4a**, possessing a hydroxyl group at C-2 of ring D, had cytotoxic efficacy, with an IC_{50} value of 6.8 μM. To determine the importance of the hydroxyl group at the C-2 position, compound **4b** was synthesized, and its efficacy was similar to compound **4a**. The methylation of the hydroxyl group in **4a** yielded compound **4c**, which had a lower efficacy than **4a** and **4b**, whereas ethylation of the hydroxyl group, which yielded compound **4d**, produced a significant decrease in cytotoxic efficacy, compared to compound **4a**. Previously, we reported that the shifting of the hydroxyl group from C-2 to C-4 (**4e**) produced a significant reduction in the cytotoxic efficacy (IC_{50} > 50 μM). However, methylation of the hydroxyl group in **4e** yielded compound **4f**, which was ~5 times more efficacious than **4e** [29]. The addition of a second hydroxyl group at the C-4 position in **4a** resulted in compound **4g** (IC_{50} = 5.98 μM), which had cytotoxic efficacy similar to compound **4a**. Interestingly, the methylation of the two hydroxyl groups in **4g**, yielding compound **4h**, significantly decreased the cytotoxic efficacy. The addition of a third hydroxyl group to **4g** at position 3 of ring D, yielding compound **4i**, did not significantly alter the antiproliferative efficacy of the compound, whereas adding a third hydroxyl group at position 6 of ring D yielded a totally inactive compound, **4j**. Next, we determined the effect of ring D on the cytotoxic efficacy of the synthesized compounds. Therefore, compounds **4k–4m** were synthesized, where ring D was replaced with aromatic heterocyclic moieties. Compounds **4k**, **4l**, and **4m**, containing furan, 3-pyridine, and 2-pyridine moieties, respectively, did not have significant cytotoxic efficacy. Furthermore, adding another fused benzene ring to ring D, while keeping the C-2 hydroxyl group (2-hydroxynaphthalene), yielded the inactive compound, **4n**. The addition of a nitro group at the C5-position of ring D in **4a** yielded compound **4o**, which had an efficacy similar to compound **4a** (IC_{50} = 7.9 μM).

Next, the cytotoxicity and selectivity of the most active compounds, **4g** and **4i**, were determined in a panel of cell lines, including the normal cell lines, HMECs, and cancer cell lines, BT-20, U-251, and HCT116, as shown in Figure 2 and Table 3. Compound **4g** had antiproliferative efficacy in the BT-20, U-251, and HCT116, with IC_{50} values of 5.32, 7.64, and 2.68, respectively. In contrast, compound **4i** had IC_{50} values ranging from 10–25 μM. The results indicated that although compound **4g** is more potent than compound **4i** in the three cancer cell lines, compound **4i** is more selective for the cancer cells than the normal cells.

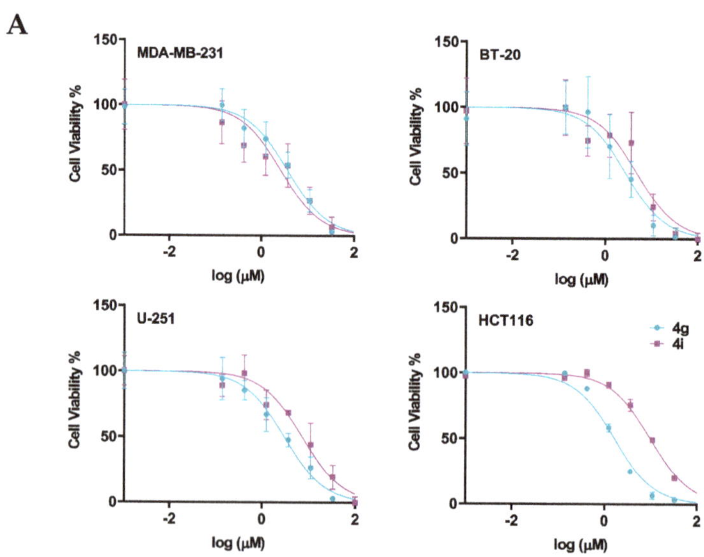

Figure 2. *Cont.*

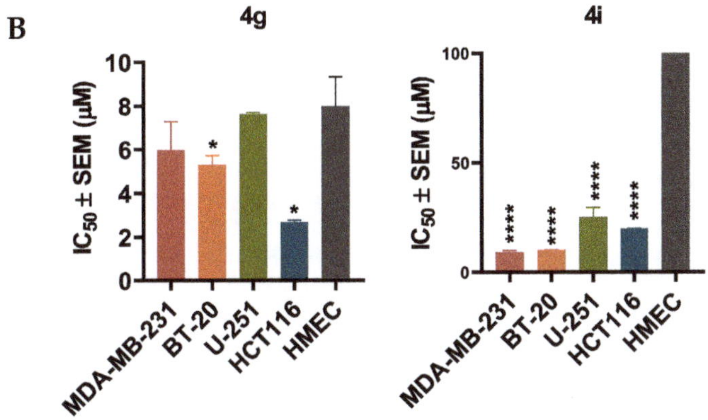

Figure 2. The efficacy and selectivity of **4g** and **4i** in MDA-MB-231, BT-20, U-251, and HCT116, and compared to the normal cell line, HMEC (**A**) the viability curves for cancer cells (MDA-MB-231, BT-20, U-251, HCT116), and the normal cell line, HMEC; (**B**) the IC_{50} values of **4g** and **4i** for these cell lines are also compared to the normal cell line. Cell survival was determined using the 3-(4,5-dimethylthiazol-2yl)-2,5-diphenyltetrazolium bromide (MTT) assay. The IC_{50} values are represented as the means ± SD of three independent experiments performed in triplicate with * $p < 0.05$, **** $p < 0.0001$ vs. control group.

Table 3. The effects of the chrysin-like compounds (**4a–4o**) on the survival of cancer cell lines (breast, glioblastoma, and colon) and a normal non-cancerous cell line (normal human mammary epithelial cells).

Compound	Breast Cancer	Brain Cancer	Colon Cancer	Normal Cells
	BT-20	**U-251**	**HCT116**	**HMEC**
4a	4.41 ± 0.99	8.63 ± 4.86	2.88 ± 0.09	7.12 ± 4.55
4g	5.32 ± 0.72	7.64 ± 0.11	2.68 ± 0.15	8.00 ± 1.33
4i	10.43 ± 0.20	25.36 ± 7.53	20.09 ± 0.13	>100
4o	7.25 ± 1.82	11.27 ± 2.84	3.85 ± 0.34	7.17 ± 4.10

Cell survival was determined by MTT assay as described in the materials and methods. The IC_{50} values (μM) are represented as the mean ± SEM of three independent experiments performed in triplicate. The compounds were screened on breast (MDA-MB-231, BT-20), brain (U-251), and colon (HCT116) cancer cell lines and normal human mammary epithelial cells (HMECs).

2.3. *4g and 4i Induce Apoptosis and G2 Cell Cycle Arrest in a Triple-Negative Breast Cancer Cell Line*

Apoptosis, a type of programmed cell death, is one of the major mechanisms by which chemotherapeutic drugs produce their therapeutic efficacy [43]. Morphologically, apoptosis is characterized by cellular shrinkage, which is accompanied with nuclear chromatin condensation and fragmentation followed by blebbing of the plasma membrane. This leads to the formation of small apoptotic bodies that have an intact cellular membrane and unaltered organelle integrity. These bodies are then released in the extracellular environment and removed by the process of phagocytosis [44,45]. Apoptosis can occur by two pathways: The extrinsic pathway and intrinsic pathway. In either pathway, when the cell is exposed to certain extrinsic or intrinsic stimuli, the integrity of the inner mitochondrial membrane of the cell is compromised, resulting in the loss of the mitochondrial membrane potential, and causing the release of several apoptotic factors, including cytochrome c [46,47]. Numerous studies indicate that during apoptosis, phosphatidylserine (PS), in the cytoplasmic side of the plasma membrane, is translocated to the extracellular cell surface [48]. The flipped anionic PS binds to the Ca^{2+}-dependent phospholipid-binding protein, annexin V [49]. We discovered and reported several potent apoptosis-inducing compounds [50–57]. In this study, the result of our morphological studies in MDA-MB-231 cells after incubation with our lead compounds, **4g** and **4i**, indicated that apoptosis was occurring (Figure 3A). At a concentration of 20 μM, both compounds decreased the number of adherent

MDA-MB-231 cells and induced cellular shrinkage. The cells were rounded and loosely attached, and apoptotic bodies were present. Similarly, the incubation of MDA-MB-231 cells with compounds **4g** or **4i** for 24 h produced a significant loss of the mitochondrial membrane potential. For compound **4g**, the population of cells undergoing apoptosis increased from 14.30% at 0 µM to 26.56% and 58.05% at 5 and 10 µM, respectively (p value < 0.0001; Figure 3B,C). Compound **4i** also produced a significant shift in the apoptotic cell population in quadrant II, from 14.78% at 0 µM to 32.25% and 42.56% at 5 and 10 µM, respectively (p value < 0.0001, Figure 3B,C). Cell cycle analysis indicated that compounds **4g** and **4i** produced a significant disruption in the cell cycle of MDA-MB-231 cells (Figure 3D). Data obtained using flow cytometry indicated that, when incubated with vehicle alone, MDA-MB-231 cells had a normal cell cycle (5.43%, 83.4%, 4.63%, and 4.46% in the subG1, G1, S, and G2 phases, respectively). However, incubation of MDA-MB-231 cells with compound **4g** resulted in a significant shift towards the G2 phase (59.12% and 54.13% for 5 and 10 µM, respectively (p value < 0.0001, Figure 3E).

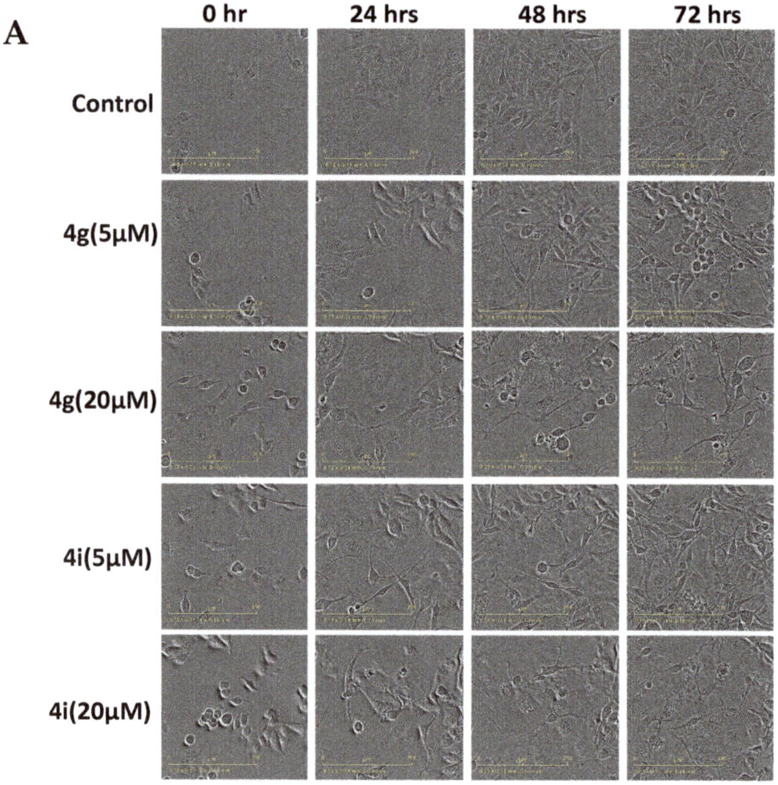

Figure 3. *Cont.*

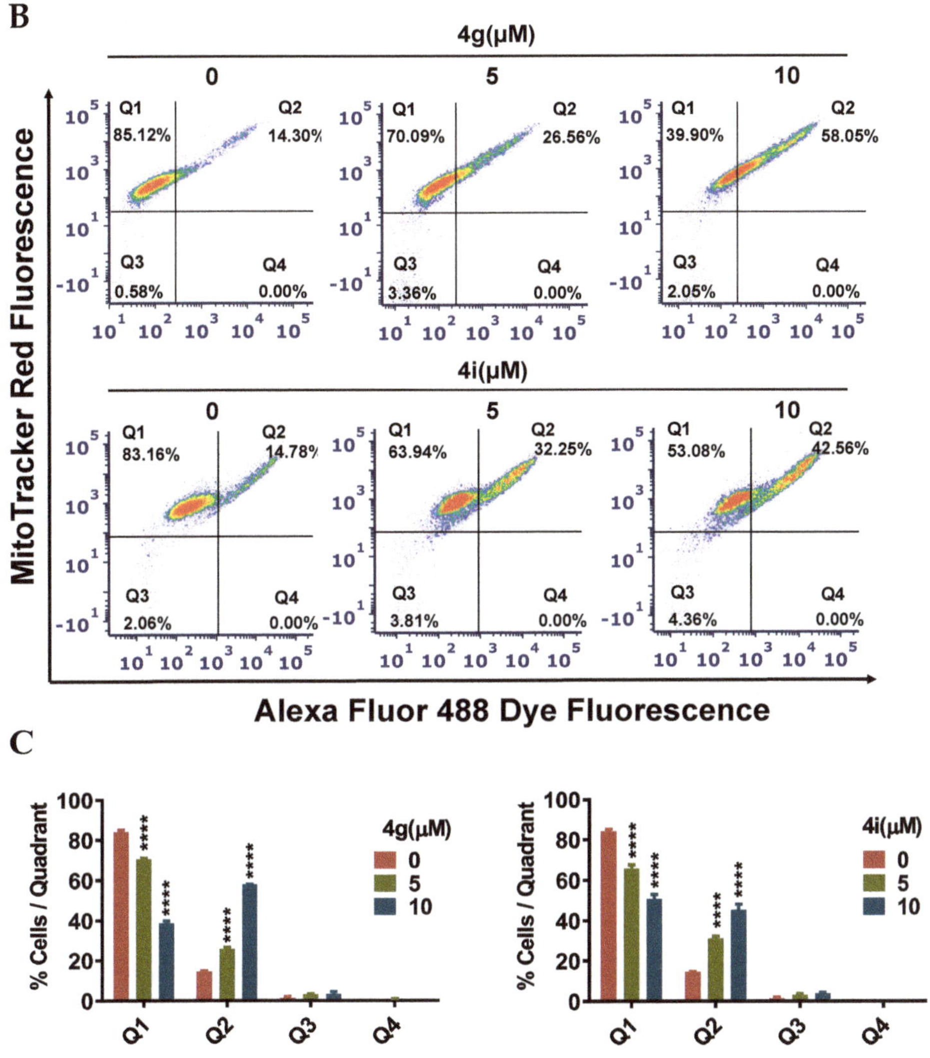

Figure 3. *Cont.*

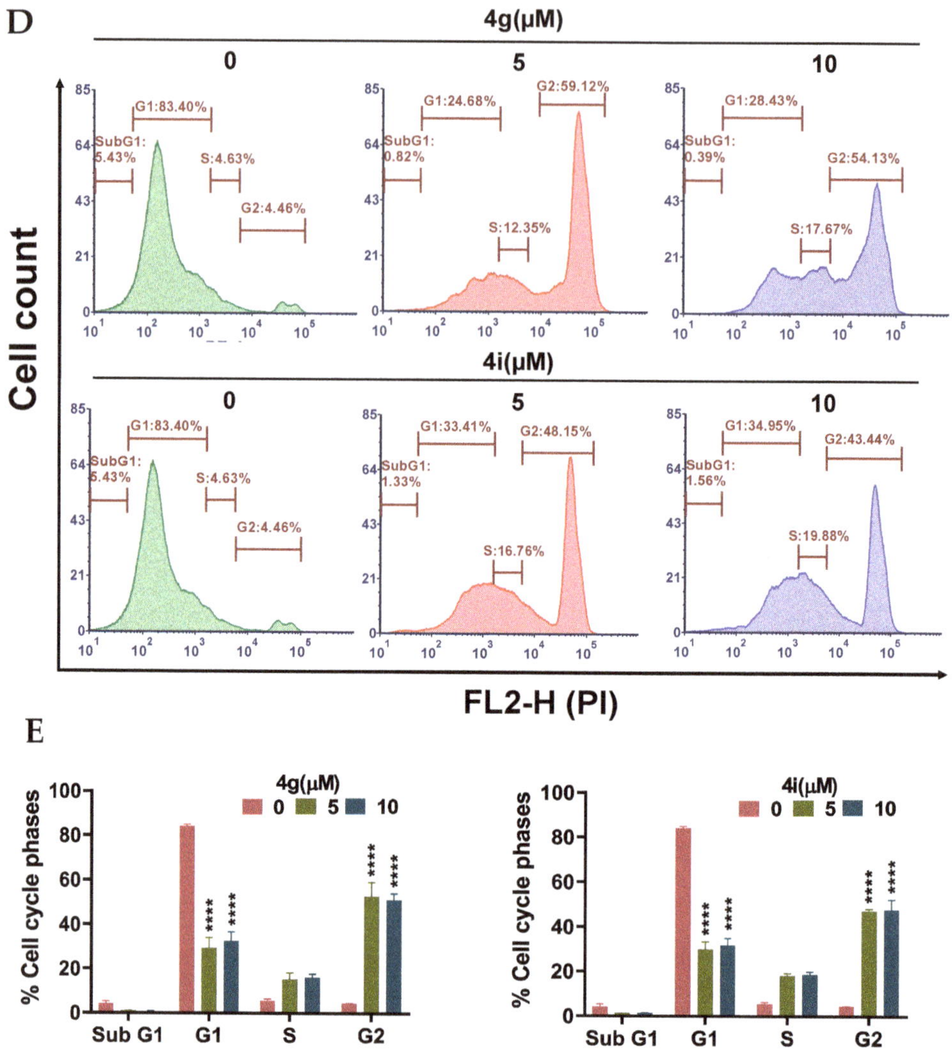

Figure 3. Effects of **4g** and **4i** on cellular morphology, mitochondrial membrane potential, and cell cycle (**A**) Morphological observations of MDA-MB-231 cells incubated with 0, 5, and 20 μM concentrations of **4g** and **4i** at different time intervals of 0, 24, 48, and 72 h, respectively; (**B**) The MDA-MB-231 cells in complete medium were incubated with **4g** and **4i** at 0, 5, or 10 μM for 24 h. Cells were then incubated with the reagents of the MitoTracker Red and Alexa Fluor 488 annexin V kits for flow cytometry. Representative results of MDA-MB-231 cells from two independent experiments, each performed in triplicate, are shown; (**C**) Histograms quantitatively summarize the results following incubation with **4g** and **4i**, respectively; (**D**) The induction of cell cycle arrest in MDA-MB-231 cells by **4g** and **4i** is shown. The MDA-MB-231 cells were incubated with different concentrations (0, 5, and 10 μM) of **4g** and **4i** for 24 h and were subjected to cell cycle analysis by flow cytometry of PI (X axis)/cell counts (Y axis); (**E**) A histogram quantitatively summarizing the change in % of cells in each phase of the cell cycle due to incubation with **4g** and **4i**. The data represents means ± SEM of three independent experiments performed in triplicate with **** $p < 0.0001$ vs. control group.

2.4. *Compounds **4g** and **4i** Activate Apoptosis by Activating the Intrinsic Apoptotic Pathway*

Apoptosis can be induced by the activation of two major pathways: The intrinsic and extrinsic apoptotic pathways [22]. The activation of the intrinsic apoptotic pathway induces the activation of proapoptotic proteins, such as apoptosis regulator Bak (Bcl-2 homologous antagonist/killer) and Bax (Bcl-2-associated X protein) [58]. The activated the Bax and Bak proteins subsequently permeabilize the mitochondrial outer membrane by forming pores on its outer surface [58–60]. Consequently, cytochrome c (Cyt C) is released into the cytosol, where it combines with the adaptor protein (Apaf-1) to form an apoptosome [22]. The initiator caspases (i.e., caspase-2, caspase-8, caspase-9, or caspase-10) are activated and recruited to large protein complexes, resulting in the cleavage of the executioner caspases, caspase-3 or caspase-7 [61].

Since MDA-MB-231 cells incubated with compounds **4g** and **4i** had a decrease in the mitochondrial membrane potential, which is an early event of intrinsic apoptosis, i.e., altered permeability of the inner mitochondrial membrane, we conducted experiments to determine if these compounds altered the expression of key apoptotic proteins, including cytochrome c, in MDA-MB-231 cells using Western blotting analysis. Our results indicated that compounds **4g** at 5 μM, and compound **4i** at 10 μM produced a significant increase in the expression of cytochrome c, compared to cells incubated with vehicle (Figure 4A,B). This may be due to an increase in the expression of Bak following incubation with **4g** and **4i** (Figure 4A,B), compared to cells incubated in the absence of lead compounds. In addition, both compounds (**4g** at 5 μM and **4i** at 10 μM) produced significant cleavage of the initiator caspase, caspase 9, in MDA-MB-231 cells, compared to cells incubated with vehicle (Figure 4A,B). These events activated caspase 7 in breast cancer cells incubated with both concentrations of **4g** and 10 μM of **4i**, compared to cells incubated with vehicle (Figure 4A,B). In contrast, there was no significant change in the mammalian target of rapamycin (mTOR) expression, indicating that cell death induced by **4g** and **4i** in MDA-MB-231 cells is not due to autophagy (Figure 4A,B). Thus, our results suggest that cytochrome c release induces intracellular initiator caspase activation, followed by the activation of executioner caspases, thus activating apoptotic cell death machinery through intrinsic the pathway.

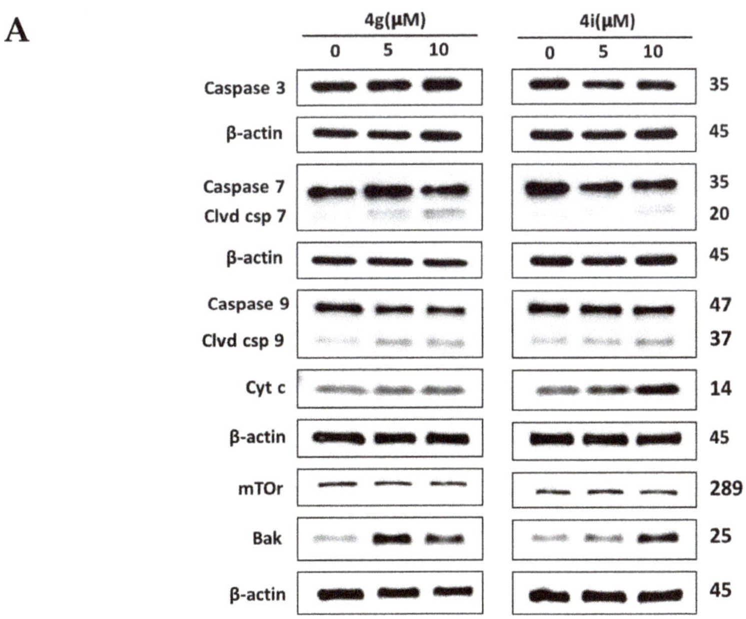

Figure 4. *Cont.*

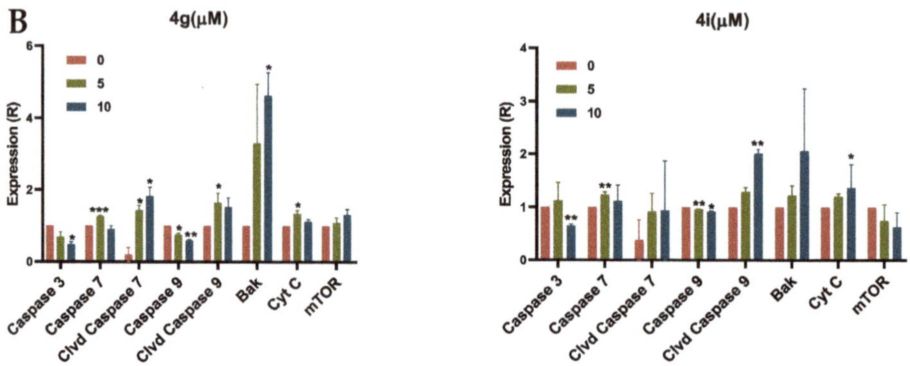

Figure 4. The effect on apoptosis induction at different concentrations of **4g** and **4i** in MDA-MB-231 cells. (**A**) Western blots for the proteins caspase 3, caspase 7, cleaved caspase 7, caspase 9, cleaved caspase 9, Bak, cyt C and mTOR following incubation with **4g** and **4i** at 0, 5, or 10 μM. The values of the proteins were normalized to β-actin levels. (**B**) Histograms summarizing the levels of each protein are also shown. All the data are presented as the means ± SEM of three independent studies with * $p < 0.05$, ** $p < 0.01$, *** $p < 0.001$ vs. control group. Cleaved is abbreviated as Clvd.

3. Materials and Method

3.1. Chemistry

All chemicals and solvents were procured from commercial sources (reagent grade) and were used without further purification. The reaction progress was monitored by thin layer chromatography (TLC) using precoated TLC plates of silica gel 60 F254. ^{1}H-NMR and ^{13}C-NMR spectra were recorded using a 400 MHz Bruker Avance Ultrashield spectrometer. The spectra were obtained in ppm using automatic calibration to the residual proton peak of the solvent, dimethyl-sulphoxide (DMSO-d_6). The ^{1}H NMR data are presented as follows: Chemical shift (δ ppm), multiplicity (s = singlet, d = doublet, t = triplet, q = quartet, m = multiplet), coupling constants (Hz), and integration. The ^{13}C NMR analyses were reported in terms of the chemical shift. The ^{1}H and ^{13}C NMR spectra for all compounds are included in the supporting information (Figure S1). HRMS data were acquired using a Thermo QExactive Plus mass spectrometer equipped with an electrospray ionization source (Thermo Fisher Scientific, Greensboro, NC, USA).

3.1.1. Synthesis of methyl 2-((5-Hydroxy-4-oxo-2-phenyl-4*H*-chromen-7-yl)oxy)acetate (**2**)

The title compound was synthesized as previously described [62].

3.1.2. Synthesis of 2-((5-Hydroxy-4-oxo-2-phenyl-4*H*-chromen-7-yl)oxy)acetohydrazide (**3**)

The title compound was synthesized according to our previously published procedure [29].

3.1.3. General Procedure for the Synthesis of *N*′-arylidene-2-((5-Hydroxy-4-oxo-2-phenyl-4*H*-chromen-7-yl)oxy)acetohydrazide (**4a–4o**)

To a stirred suspension of hydrazide **3** (1.0 g, 3.0 mmol) in anhydrous methanol (60 mL), the appropriate aldehyde (3.0 mmol) was added, along with a few drops of concentrated hydrochloric acid. After one hour, the reaction was completed and the formed precipitate was separated by filtration, washed with methanol, and dried in air to give pure compounds in good yields.

(*E*,*Z*)-2-((5-Hydroxy-4-oxo-2-phenyl-4*H*-chromen-7-yl)oxy)-*N*′-(2-hydroxybenzylidene)acetohydrazide (**4a**)

The product was obtained as a pale-yellow powder. Yield (64%). ^{1}H NMR (DMSO-d_6) (*E*:*Z* = 1:1): δ 12.84–12.81 (m, 2H), 11.84 (s, 1H), 11.62 (s, 1H), 10.99 (s, 1H), 10.05 (s, 1H), 8.57 (s, 1H), 8.33 (s, 1H), 8.12–8.10 (d, *J* = 8 Hz, 4H), 7.77–7.55 (m, 8H), 7.31–7.24 (m, 2H), 7.07–6.85 (m, 8H), 6.51–6.42 (m, 2H), 5.31 (s, 2H), 4.87 (s, 2H). ^{13}C NMR (DMSO-d_6): δ 182.11, 182.06, 167.94, 164.42, 163.65, 163.61, 163.48, 163.37, 161.17, 161.07, 157.36, 157.22, 156.45, 148.27, 141.63, 132.18, 132.12, 131.59, 131.29, 130.57, 130.54, 129.18, 129.15, 129.11, 126.56, 126.47, 120.01, 119.40, 118.65, 116.39, 116.14, 105.44, 105.39, 105.31, 105.09, 98.81, 98.72, 93.62, 93.46, 66.57, 65.36. HRMS (ESI, *m*/*z*): calculated for $C_{24}H_{19}N_2O_6$ $[M + H]^+$ 431.1237; found 431.1238.

(*E*,*Z*)-*N*′-Benzylidene-2-((5-hydroxy-4-oxo-2-phenyl-4H-chromen-7-yl)oxy)acetohydrazide (**4b**)

The synthesis and full characterization of the title compound have been previously reported [29].

(*E*,*Z*)-2-((5-Hydroxy-4-oxo-2-phenyl-4*H*-chromen-7-yl)oxy)-*N*′-(2-methoxybenzylidene)acetohydrazide (**4c**)

The product was obtained as a yellow powder. Yield (55%). ^{1}H NMR (DMSO-d_6) (*E*:*Z* = 1:0.5): δ 12.84–12.80 (m, 1.5H), 11.64 (s, 1.5H), 8.68 (s, 0.5H), 8.37 (s, 1H), 8.11–8.09 (d, *J* = 8 Hz, 3H), 7.91–7.89 (d, *J* = 8 Hz, 1H), 7.82–7.80 (d, *J* = 8 Hz, 0.5H), 7.63–7.55 (m, 4.5H), 7.44–7.4 (m, 1.5H), 7.12–7.0 (m, 4.5H), 6.88–6.84 (m, 1.5H), 6.5–6.42 (m, 1.5H), 5.32 (s, 2H), 4.82 (s, 1H), 3.86 (s, 4.5H). ^{13}C NMR (DMSO-d_6): δ182.09, 182.03, 168.09, 164.43, 163.71, 163.60, 163.48, 163.22, 161.13, 161.05, 157.80, 157.64, 157.21, 143.56, 139.73, 132.15, 132.10, 131.72, 131.48, 130.55, 129.09, 126.45, 125.67, 125.53, 121.94, 120.72, 120.66, 111.84, 111.77, 105.42, 105.31, 105.06, 98.77, 98.70, 93.62, 93.45, 66.65, 65.36, 55.68, 54.87. HRMS (ESI, *m*/*z*): calculated for $C_{25}H_{21}N_2O_6$ $[M + H]^+$ 445.1394; found 445.1392.

(*E*,*Z*)-*N*′-(2-Ethoxybenzylidene)-2-((5-hydroxy-4-oxo-2-phenyl-4*H*-chromen-7-yl)oxy)acetohydrazide (**4d**)

The product was obtained as a light-brown powder. Yield (80%). ^{1}H NMR (DMSO-d_6) (*E*:*Z* = 1:0.5): δ 12.84–12.80 (m, 1.5H), 11.68–11.62 (m, 1.5H), 8.66 (s, 0.5H), 8.40 (s, 1H), 8.11–8.10 (d, *J* = 4 Hz, 3H), 7.90–7.80 (m, 1.5H), 7.60–7.57 (m, 4.5H), 7.41–7.37 (m, 1.5H), 7.10–6.84 (m, 6H), 6.5–6.42 (m, 1.5H), 5.31 (s, 2H), 4.82 (s, 1H), 4.14–4.09 (q, *J* = 8 Hz, 3H), 1.39–1.35 (t, *J* = 8 Hz, 4.5H).^{13}C NMR (DMSO-d_6): δ 182.08, 182.03, 168.03, 164.42, 163.77, 163.57, 163.46, 163.23, 161.14, 161.04, 157.20, 157.13, 156.98, 143.46, 140.01, 132.10, 131.67, 131.42, 130.54, 129.09, 126.45, 125.76, 125.58, 122.14, 122.09, 120.61, 112.75, 105.41, 105.29, 105.05, 98.71, 93.63, 93.45, 66.62, 65.36, 63.80,14.63. HRMS (ESI, *m*/*z*): calculated for $C_{26}H_{23}N_2O_6$ $[M + H]^+$ 459.1550; found 459.1548.

(*E*,*Z*)-2-((5-Hydroxy-4-oxo-2-phenyl-4*H*-chromen-7-yl)oxy)-*N*′-(4-hydroxybenzylidene)acetohydrazide (**3e**)

The synthesis and full characterization of the title compound were previously published [29].

(*E*,*Z*)-2-((5-Hydroxy-4-oxo-2-phenyl-4*H*-chromen-7-yl)oxy)-*N*′-(4-methoxybenzylidene)acetohydrazide (**3f**)

The synthesis and full characterization of the title compound were previously published [29].

(*E*,*Z*)-*N*′-(2,4-Dihydroxybenzylidene)-2-((5-hydroxy-4-oxo-2-phenyl-4*H*-chromen-7-yl)oxy)acetohydrazide (**4g**)

The product was obtained as an off-white powder. Yield (85%). ^{1}H NMR (DMSO-d_6) (*E*:*Z* = 1:0.8): δ 12.84–12.80 (m, 1.8H), 11.67 (s, 1H), 11.43 (s, 0.8H), 11.15 (s, 1H), 9.98 (s, 1.8H), 9.83 (s, 0.8H), 8.42 (s, 1H), 8.20 (s, 0.8H), 8.12–8.10 (d, *J* = 8 Hz, 3.6H), 7.63–7.53 (m, 6.2H), 7.33–7.31 (d, *J* = 8 Hz, 1H), 7.08–7.06 (d, *J* = 8 Hz, 1.8H), 6.89 (d, *J* = 2 Hz, 1H), 6.8 (d, *J* = 2.4 Hz, 0.8H), 6.5 (d, *J* = 2 Hz, 1H), 6.4 (d, *J* = 2 Hz, 0.8H), 6.36–6.30 (m, 3.6H), 5.26 (s, 1.6H), 4.83 (s, 2H). ^{13}C NMR (DMSO-d_6): δ182.10, 182.05, 167.42, 164.44, 163.68, 163.64, 163.50, 162.86, 161.14, 161.04, 160.86, 160.53, 159.35, 158.07, 157.23, 149.28, 142.68, 132.18, 132.12, 131.10, 130.55, 129.15, 129.12, 128.27, 126.47, 111.49, 110.37, 107.84, 107.77, 105.45,

105.37, 105.32, 105.07, 102.60, 102.37, 98.81, 98.72, 93.63, 93.45, 66.59, 65.33. HRMS (ESI, *m/z*): calculated for $C_{24}H_{19}N_2O_7$ [M + H]$^+$ 447.1186; found 447.1187.

(*E,Z*)-*N*′-(2,4-Dimethoxybenzylidene)-2-((5-hydroxy-4-oxo-2-phenyl-4*H*-chromen-7-yl)oxy)acetohydrazide (**4h**)

The product was obtained as a yellow powder. Yield (96%). ^{1}H NMR (DMSO-d_6) (*E:Z* = 1:0.5): δ 12.81 (s, 1.5H), 11.49 (s, 1.5H), 8.58 (s, 0.5H), 8.27 (s, 1H), 8.11–8.10 (m, 3H), 7.84–7.57 (m, 6H), 7.05 (s, 1.5H), 6.88–6.84 (m, 1.5H), 6.63–6.41 (m, 4.5H), 5.29 (s, 2H), 4.79 (s, 1H), 3.86–3.82 (m, 9H). ^{13}C NMR (DMSO-d_6): δ182.04, 167.79, 164.43, 163.69, 163.55, 163.44, 162.91, 162.55, 162.33, 161.09, 161.02, 159.19, 159.02, 157.18, 143.62, 139.82, 132.10, 130.53, 129.09, 126.78, 126.43, 114.76, 106.41, 105.38, 105.28, 105.02, 98.68, 98.24, 98.07, 93.59, 93.42, 66.66, 65.35, 55.74, 55.40.HRMS (ESI, *m/z*): calculated for $C_{26}H_{23}N_2O_7$ [M + H]$^+$ 475.1499; found 475.1499.

(*E,Z*)-2-((5-Hydroxy-4-oxo-2-phenyl-4*H*-chromen-7-yl)oxy)-*N*′-(2,3,4-trihydroxybenzylidene)acetohydrazide (**4i**)

The product was obtained as a yellow powder. Yield (85%). ^{1}H NMR (DMSO-d_6) (*E:Z* = 1:0.5): δ 12.84–12.80 (m, 1.5H), 11.71 (s, 1H), 11.47 (s, 0.5H), 11.18 (s, 1H), 9.57–9.51 (m, 1.5H), 9.37 (s, 0.5H), 8.54–8.50 (m, 1.5H), 8.38 (s, 1H), 8.18–8.10 (m, 3.5H), 7.61–7.59 (m, 4.5H), 7.07–7.0 (m, 2H), 6.90–6.78 (m, 2.5H), 6.51–6.38 (m, 3H), 5.26 (s, 1H), 4.85 (s, 2H). ^{13}C NMR (DMSO-d_6): δ 182.12, 182.07, 167.34, 164.42, 163.68, 163.54, 162.93, 161.16, 161.07, 157.25, 150.45, 148.91, 148.42, 147.47, 146.65, 144.18, 132.76, 132.71, 132.21, 132.16, 130.56, 129.18, 126.49, 121.11, 118.36, 112.11, 110.70, 107.84, 107.73, 105.46, 105.40, 105.34, 105.10, 98.83, 98.75, 93.65, 93.48, 66.59, 65.32. HRMS (ESI, *m/z*): calculated for $C_{24}H_{19}N_2O_8$ [M + H]$^+$ 463.1134; found 463.1133.

(*E,Z*)-2-((5-Hydroxy-4-oxo-2-phenyl-4*H*-chromen-7-yl)oxy)-*N*′-(2,4,6-trihydroxybenzylidene)acetohydrazide (**4j**)

The product was obtained as a brown powder. Yield (76%). ^{1}H NMR (DMSO-d_6) (*E:Z* = 1:0.2): δ 12.83–12.79 (m, 1.2H), 11.65 (s, 1H), 11.48 (s, 0.2H), 10.99 (s, 2H), 10.32 (s, 0.4H), 9.85 (s, 1.2H), 8.72 (s, 1H), 8.41 (s, 0.2H), 8.09–8.08 (m, 2.4H), 7.59–7.58 (m, 3.6H), 7.04 (m, 1.2H), 6.88–6.84 (m, 1.2H), 6.5–6.42 (m, 1.2H), 5.86–5.83 (m, 2.4H), 5.2 (s, 0.4H), 4.82 (s, 2H). ^{13}C NMR (DMSO-d_6): δ 182.08, 166.56, 164.28, 163.61, 163.51, 162.55, 161.74, 161.46, 161.12, 161.04, 159.73, 159.24, 157.20, 147.32, 144.33, 132.15, 130.54, 129.13, 126.45, 105.43, 105.37, 105.11, 98.85, 98.79, 94.37, 93.61, 93.50, 66.58, 65.26. HRMS (ESI, *m/z*): calculated for $C_{24}H_{19}N_2O_8$ [M + H]$^+$ 463.1134; found 463.1134.

(*E,Z*)-*N*′-(Furan-2-ylmethylene)-2-((5-hydroxy-4-oxo-2-phenyl-4*H*-chromen-7-yl)oxy)acetohydrazide(**4k**)

The product was obtained as a yellow powder. Yield (87%). ^{1}H NMR (DMSO-d_6) (*E:Z* = 1:0.5): δ 12.83–12.79 (m, 1.5H), 11.63–11.57 (m, 1.5H), 8.23 (s, 0.5H), 8.11–8.09 (d, *J* = 8 Hz, 3H), 7.92 (s, 1H), 7.85 (s, 1.5H), 7.63–7.55 (m, 4.5H), 7.06–7.05 (m, 1.5H), 6.95–6.83 (m, 3H), 6.64 (m, 1.5H), 6.49–6.39 (m, 1.5H), 5.24 (s, 2H), 4.83 (s, 1H). ^{13}C NMR (DMSO-d_6): δ182.03, 167.97, 164.34, 163.66, 163.59, 163.46, 163.35, 161.13, 161.02, 157.21, 149.12, 148.94, 145.34, 145.10, 137.86, 134.20, 132.11, 130.54, 129.09, 126.45, 113.95, 113.78, 112.16, 105.42, 105.29, 105.08, 98.70, 93.60, 93.38, 66.65, 65.14.HRMS (ESI, *m/z*): calculated for $C_{22}H_{17}N_2O_6$ [M + H]$^+$ 405.1081; found 405.1077.

(*E,Z*)-2-((5-Hydroxy-4-oxo-2-phenyl-4*H*-chromen-7-yl)oxy)-*N*′-(pyridin-3-ylmethylene)acetohydrazide (**4l**)

The product was obtained as a yellow powder. Yield (86%). ^{1}H NMR (DMSO-d_6) (*E:Z* = 1:0.5): δ 12.82(bs, 1.5H), 11.98 (bs, 1.5H), 8.43 (s, 0.5H), 8.30–8.28 (d, *J* = 8 Hz, 3H), 8.13–7.96 (m, 7H), 7.62–7.55 (m, 4.5H), 7.07–7.06 (m, 1.5H), 6.88 (s, 1.5H), 6.5–6.45 (m, 1.5H), 5.39 (s, 2H), 4.9 (s, 1H). ^{13}C NMR (DMSO-d_6): δ 182.12, 168.50, 164.42, 163.67, 163.55, 161.08, 157.27, 150.51, 148.52, 145.40, 141.22, 133.75, 132.20, 130.59, 129.96, 129.16, 126.51, 123.94, 105.36, 105.12, 98.76, 93.55, 66.61, 65.40. HRMS (ESI, *m/z*): calculated for $C_{23}H_{18}N_3O_5$ [M + H]$^+$ 416.1241; found 416.1240.

(*E,Z*)-2-((5-Hydroxy-4-oxo-2-phenyl-4*H*-chromen-7-yl)oxy)-*N*′-(pyridin-2-ylmethylene)acetohydrazide (**4m**)

The product was obtained as a brown powder. Yield (52%). ^{1}H NMR (DMSO-d_6) (*E*:*Z* = 1:0.5): δ 12.84–12.81 (m, 1.5H), 11.89–11.87 (m, 1.5H), 8.61 (m, 1.5H), 8.35 (s, 0.5H), 8.11–8.03 (m, 5H), 7.94–7.87 (m, 2H), 7.62–7.55 (m, 4.5H), 7.44–7.41 (m, 1.5H), 7.07–7.06 (m, 1.5H), 6.88 (m, 1.5H), 6.51–6.45 (m, 1.5H), 5.37 (s, 2H), 4.88 (s, 1H). ^{13}C NMR (DMSO-d_6): δ 182.02, 168.45, 164.34, 163.75, 163.65, 163.59, 163.48, 161.13, 161.05, 157.21, 152.93, 152.78, 149.51, 149.44, 148.26, 144.45, 136.86, 136.75, 132.09, 130.53, 129.07, 126.44, 124.52, 124.34, 119.98, 119.90, 105.42, 105.30, 105.09, 98.70, 93.63, 93.48, 66.61, 65.30. HRMS (ESI, *m*/*z*): calculated for $C_{23}H_{18}N_3O_5$ [M + H]$^+$ 416.1241; found 416.1238.

(*E,Z*)-2-((5-Hydroxy-4-oxo-2-phenyl-4H-chromen-7-yl)oxy)-*N*′-((2-hydroxynaphthalen-1-yl)methylene)acetohydrazide (**4n**)

The product was obtained as a yellow powder. Yield (54%). ^{1}H NMR (DMSO-d_6) (*E*:*Z* = 1:0.5): δ 12.86–12.81 (m, 1.5H), 12.46 (s, 1H), 11.91 (s, 1H), 11.68 (s, 0.5H), 10.77 (s, 0.5H), 9.40 (s, 1H), 8.89 (s, 0.5H), 8.77–8.75 (d, *J* = 8 Hz, 0.5H), 8.30–8.28 (d, *J* = 8 Hz, 1H), 8.12–8.09 (m, 3H), 7.94–7.84 (m, 3H), 7.63–7.58 (m, 6H), 7.42–7.36 (m, 1.5H), 7.24–7.21 (m, 1.5H), 7.08–7.06 (m, 1.5H), 6.94–6.88 (m, 1.5H), 6.55–6.46 (m, 1.5H), 5.38 (s, 1H), 4.94 (s, 2H). ^{13}C NMR (DMSO-d_6): δ182.09, 182.03, 167.52, 164.38, 163.64, 163.54, 163.49, 163.17, 161.17, 161.06, 157.95, 157.23, 156.88, 147.37, 143.29, 132.91, 132.52, 132.16, 132.10, 131.59, 131.25, 130.53, 129.13, 128.89, 128.68, 128.13, 127.80, 127.75, 126.46, 123.54, 123.40, 120.97, 118.75, 118.13, 110.08, 108.45, 105.45, 105.33, 105.10, 98.87, 98.73, 93.68, 93.46, 66.72, 65.59.HRMS (ESI, *m*/*z*): calculated for $C_{28}H_{21}N_2O_6$ [M + H]$^+$ 481.1394; found 481.1394.

(*E,Z*)-2-((5-Hydroxy-4-oxo-2-phenyl-4*H*-chromen-7-yl)oxy)-*N*′-((2-hydroxy-5-nitrobenzylidene)acetohydrazide (**4o**)

The product was obtained as a yellow powder. Yield (91%). ^{1}H NMR (DMSO-d_6) (*E*:*Z* = 1:0.75): δ 12.85–12.80 (m, 1.75H), 11.97 (bs, 2H), 11.78 (s, 1.5H), 8.64–8.54 (m, 2.75H), 8.33 (s, 1H), 8.15–8.10 (m, 5.25H), 7.64–7.55 (m, 5.25H), 7.08–7.04 (m, 3.25H), 6.90–6.86 (m, 1.75H), 6.52–6.44 (m, 1.75H), 5.39 (s, 2H), 4.89 (s, 1.5H). ^{13}C NMR (DMSO-d_6): δ 182.08, 182.03, 168.28, 164.42, 163.71, 163.61, 163.46, 162.04, 161.14, 161.04, 157.20, 144.30, 139.91, 138.65, 132.16, 132.10, 130.55, 129.12, 129.08, 126.73, 126.45, 123.37, 121.68, 120.98, 119.95, 117.10, 116.72, 105.43, 105.37, 105.30, 105.08, 98.78, 98.73, 93.62, 93.46, 66.53, 65.42. HRMS (ESI, *m*/*z*): calculated for $C_{24}H_{18}N_3O_8$ [M + H]$^+$ 476.1088; found 476.1089.

3.2. Biological Studies

3.2.1. Cell Lines and Cell Culture

A panel of cancer cell lines, including breast (MDA-MB-231, BT20), brain (U251), and colon (HCT116), as well as a normal cell line (human mammary epithelial cells: HMECs), were grown as adherent monolayers in flasks with Dulbecco's Modified Eagle Medium (DMEM), supplemented with 10% fetal bovine serum (FBS) and 1% penicillin and streptomycin in a humidified incubator with 5% CO_2 at 37 °C.

3.2.2. MTT Assay

The (3-(4,5-dimethylthiazol-2-yl)-2,5-diphenyltetrazolium bromide) (MTT) assay was used to determine the cytotoxicity of the 15 chrysin derivatives in the above-mentioned cell lines. Briefly, cells were harvested with 0.05% trypsin, 2.21 mM ethylenediaminetetraacetic acid (EDTA), 1× from Corning (Corning, NY, USA), and suspended at a final density of 5 × 10^3 cells/well. Cells were seeded (180 μL/well) into 96-well plates. Initially, four different concentrations of each compound were added to find the compounds with the greatest antiproliferative efficacy in the MDA-MB-231 cell line (0, 1, 10, and 100 μM). Subsequently, eight different concentrations (0.1, 0.3, 1, 3, 10, 30, and 100 μM) of each compound were added to the remaining cell lines mentioned above. After 68 h of incubation,

20 μL of the MTT solution (4 mg/mL) were added to each well, and the plates were incubated for 4 h. This allowed viable cells to biotransform the yellow-colored MTT into dark-blue formazan crystals. Subsequently, the medium was discarded, and 150 μL of DMSO were added to each well to dissolve the formazan crystals. The absorbance was determined at 590 nm using a DTX 880 multimode detector (Beckman Coulter life sciences, IN, USA). The $IC_{50} \pm$ SD concentrations were calculated from three experiments performed in triplicate/duplicate. The IC_{50} values were calculated from the cell survival percentages obtained for each compound tested at different concentrations. Similarly, the cytotoxicity of the test compounds was compared to the normal cell line (HMEC).

3.2.3. Cell Cycle, Apoptosis, and Mitochondrial Membrane Potential Analysis

MDA-MB-231 cells were plated into 6-well plates at 2.5×10^5 cells/well. The cells were incubated with 0, 5, or 10 μM of compounds **4g** or **4i** and incubated for 12 h. Next, the cells were trypsinized with 0.05% trypsin, 2.21 mM EDTA, 1×, washed, counted, and resuspended in 1 mL of ice-cold PBS. The cells then were stained with propidium iodide (PI) dye and incubated for at least 15 min. The distribution of the cells in each cell cycle phase for the different concentrations was measured using a BD Accuri™ C6 flow cytometer from BD Biosciences (Becton-Dickinson, San Jose, CA, USA) and analyzed using FCS Express 5 plus De Novo software (Glendale, CA, USA).

MitoTracker Red and Alexa Fluor 488 annexin V kits for flow cytometry (Molecular Probes Inc., Invitrogen, Eugene, OR) were used to measure the mitochondrial membrane potential and apoptosis in MDA-MB-231 cells. Briefly, cells were seeded into 6-well plates and incubated with 0, 5, or 10 μM of compounds **4g** and **4i** for 12 h. The cells were then lysed using 0.05% trypsin, 2.21 mM EDTA, 1×, counted, and 4 μL of 10 μM of the MitoTracker Red working solution were added to 1 mL of the harvested cells. The cells were incubated at 37 °C with 5% CO_2 for 30 min. The cells were washed once with PBS and resuspended in 100 μL of the annexin binding buffer. The cell suspensions were incubated with 5 μL of Alexa Fluor 488 annexin V for 15 min. This was followed by the addition of 400 μL of the annexin-binding buffer. Finally, flow cytometry was used to detect the fluorescence of stained cells at the following excitation/emission maxima: Alexa Fluor® 488 annexin V: 499/521 nm; MitoTracker® Red: 579/599 nm with the BD Accuri™ C6 flow cytometer from BD Biosciences (Becton-Dickinson, San Jose, CA, USA) and analyzed using FCS express 5 plus De Novo software (Glendale, CA, USA).

3.2.4. Protein Expression Analysis Using Western Blot

To measure the expression of Bak, cytochrome c, caspase-7, caspase-9, and mTOR, Western blotting was performed by lysing MDA-MB-231 cells using a lysis buffer (50 mM Tris–HCl, 150 mM NaCl, 1 mM EDTA, 0.5% NP-40, 1% Triton, 0.1% SDS) containing a protease inhibitor cocktail that consisted of Aprotinin, Bestatin, E-64, Leupeptin, and Pepstatin A (Sigma-Aldrich Life Science, St. Louis, MO, USA). The bicinchoninic acid (BCA) quantification assay was used to determine the protein levels in the cell extracts (G-BIOSCIENCES, St. Louis, MO, USA). The extracted proteins were loaded onto a 10–20% tris-glycine gel. After separation, the proteins were transferred from the gel onto a polyvinylidene difluoride (PVDF) membrane. The membranes were blocked using 5% milk in Tris-buffered saline Tween 20 for 30 min and incubated overnight with primary antibodies against Bak (1:1000), cytochrome C (1:1000), caspase-3 (1:1000), caspase 7 (1:1000), caspase 9 (1:1000), mTOR (1:1000), or B-actin (1:2000) in 5% BSA (bovine serum albumin) at 4 °C. The next day, membranes were washed and incubated with horseradish peroxidase-labelled (HRP) anti-rabbit secondary antibody (1:5000 dilutions). The membrane was incubated with the antibody for an additional 1 h. Subsequently, the membranes were washed and developed by Clarity Western ECL substrate (Bio-Rad; Hercules, CA, USA). Protein was detected using a ChemiDoc Imaging System (Bio-Rad). Densitometry analyses of the blots for the detected protein were quantified using the ImageJ software. Data was calculated as ratios of protein/β-actin.

4. Conclusions

In conclusion, a series of novel chrysin derivatives were designed, synthesized, and characterized. Upon screening these compounds for their antiproliferative efficacy in the TNBC cell line, MDA-MB-231, and normal breast HMEC cells, two compounds, **4g** and **4i**, had the highest efficacy and selectivity towards MDA-MB-231 cells. Upon investigating the mechanism by which these compounds produce cytotoxicity, it was determined that **4g** and **4i** cause the death of MDA-MB-231 cells by inducing apoptosis, producing cell cycle arrest at the G2 phase, and activating the intrinsic apoptotic pathway. Physicochemical characterizations of these compounds suggested that they can be further optimized as potential anticancer compounds for TNBC cells. The compounds were determined to have some solubility issues that need to be overcome in the future design of additional compounds. Overall, our results suggest that **4g** and **4i** could be suitable leads for developing novel compounds to treat TNBC.

Supplementary Materials: The following are available online, Figure S1: Chemical characterization of compounds **4a–4o**.

Author Contributions: Conceptualization, B.A.A.-O., S.A.A. and A.K.T.; methodology, B.A.A.-O., S.A.A., H.R., S.M., N.H. and J.M.L.; software, S.M. and N.H.; validation, S.M. and N.H.; formal analysis, B.A.A.-O.; investigation, H.R., S.M., N.H., J.M.L.; resources, B.A.A.-O. and A.K.T.; data curation, B.A.A.-O., H.R., S.M., N.H. and J.M.L.; writing—original draft preparation, B.A.A. and S.M.; writing—review and editing, B.A.A.-O., S.A.A., S.M., S.K., M.F.B., C.R.A.J. and A.K.T.; visualization, A.K.T.; supervision, A.K.T.; project administration, A.K.T.; funding acquisition, B.A.A.-O., and A.K.T. All authors have read and agreed to the published version of the manuscript.

Funding: This work was funded by the Deanship of Scientific Research at Jordan University of Science and Technology (grant # 20190360 to BAA). This manuscript has been supported, in part, by University of Toledo startup grants (F110760 to AKT) and Susan G. Komen Breast Cancer Foundation (CCR18548498 to AKT).

Acknowledgments: The authors acknowledge the financial support given by the Deanship of Research at the Jordan University of Science and Technology (grant # 20190360 to BAA). The high-resolution mass spectrometry data were acquired from the Triad Mass Spectrometry Laboratory at the University of North Carolina at Greensboro, Greensboro, NC, USA. This manuscript has been supported, in part, by the University of Toledo startup grants (F110760 to AKT) and Susan G. Komen Breast Cancer Foundation (CCR18548498 to AKT).

Conflicts of Interest: The authors declare no conflict of interest.

References

1. Siegel, R.L.; Miller, K.D.; Jemal, A. Cancer statistics, 2019. *CA Cancer J. Clin.* **2019**, *69*, 7–34. [CrossRef]
2. Bianchini, G. Triple-negative breast cancer: Challenges and opportunities of a heterogeneous disease. *Nat. Rev. Clin. Oncol.* **2016**, *13*, 674–690. [CrossRef]
3. Scalbert, A.; Williamson, G. Dietary intake and bioavailability of polyphenols. *J. Nutr.* **2000**, *130*, 2073–2085. [CrossRef] [PubMed]
4. Beecher, G.R. Overview of Dietary Flavonoids: Nomenclature, Occurrence and Intake. *J. Nutr.* **2003**, *133*, 3248–3254. [CrossRef] [PubMed]
5. Hodnick, W.F.; MIlosavljeviĆ, E.B.; Nelson, J.H.; Pardini, R.S. Electrochemistry of flavonoids: Relationships between redox potentials, inhibition of mitochondrial respiration, and production of oxygen radicals by flavonoids. *Biochem. Pharmacol.* **1988**, *37*, 2607–2611. [CrossRef]
6. Namdeo, A.G.; Boddu, S.H.; Amawi, H.; Ashby, C.R., Jr.; Tukaramrao, D.B.; Trivedi, P.; Tiwari, A.K. Flavonoids as Multi-Target Compounds: A Special Emphasis on their Potential as Chemo-adjuvants in Cancer Therapy. *Curr. Pharm. Des.* **2020**, *26*, 1712–1728. [CrossRef] [PubMed]
7. Rapta, P.; Mišík, V.; Staško, A.; Vrábel, I. Redox intermediates of flavonoids and caffeic acid esters from propolis: An EPR spectroscopy and cyclic voltammetry study. *Free Radic. Biol. Med.* **1995**, *18*, 901–908. [CrossRef]
8. Williams, C.A.; Harborne, J.B.; Newman, M.; Greenham, J.; Eagles, J. Chrysin and other leaf exudate flavonoids in the genus Pelargonium. *Phytochemistry* **1997**, *46*, 1349–1353. [CrossRef]
9. Kuang, Y.H.; Patel, J.P.; Sodani, K.; Wu, C.P.; Liao, L.Q.; Patel, A.; Tiwari, A.K.; Dai, C.L.; Chen, X.; Fu, L.W.; et al. OSI-930 analogues as novel reversal agents for ABCG2-mediated multidrug resistance. *Biochem. Pharmacol.* **2012**, *84*, 766–774. [CrossRef]

10. Cherkaoui-Tangi, K.; Lachkar, M.; Wibo, M.; Morel, N.; Gilani, A.; Lyoussi, B. Pharmacological studies on hypotensive, diuretic and vasodilator activities of chrysin glucoside from Calycotome villosa in rats. *Phytother. Res. Int. J. Devoted Pharmacol. Toxicol. Eval. Nat. Prod. Deriv.* **2008**, *22*, 356–361.
11. Wang, J.; Qiu, J.; Dong, J.; Li, H.; Luo, M.; Dai, X.; Zhang, Y.; Leng, B.; Niu, X.; Zhao, S. Chrysin protects mice from Staphylococcus aureus pneumonia. *J. Appl. Microbial.* **2011**, *111*, 1551–1558. [CrossRef]
12. Feng, X.; Qin, H.; Shi, Q.; Zhang, Y.; Zhou, F.; Wu, H.; Ding, S.; Niu, Z.; Lu, Y.; Shen, P. Chrysin attenuates inflammation by regulating M1/M2 status via activating PPARγ. *Biochem. Pharmacol.* **2014**, *89*, 503–514. [CrossRef] [PubMed]
13. Romier, B.; Van De Walle, J.; During, A.; Larondelle, Y.; Schneider, Y.-J. Modulation of signalling nuclear factor-κB activation pathway by polyphenols in human intestinal Caco-2 cells. *Br. J. Nutr.* **2008**, *100*, 542–551. [CrossRef] [PubMed]
14. Wadibhasme, P.G.; Ghaisas, M.M.; Thakurdesai, P.A. Anti-asthmatic potential of chrysin on ovalbumin-induced bronchoalveolar hyperresponsiveness in rats. *Pharm. Biol.* **2011**, *49*, 508–515. [CrossRef]
15. Ahad, A.; Ganai, A.A.; Mujeeb, M.; Siddiqui, W.A. Chrysin, an anti-inflammatory molecule, abrogates renal dysfunction in type 2 diabetic rats. *Toxicol. Appl. Pharmacol.* **2014**, *279*, 1–7. [CrossRef] [PubMed]
16. Zanoli, P.; Avallone, R.; Baraldi, M. Behavioral characterisation of the flavonoids apigenin and chrysin. *Fitoterapia* **2000**, *71*, 117–123. [CrossRef]
17. Cardenas, M.; Marder, M.; Blank, V.C.; Roguin, L.P. Antitumor activity of some natural flavonoids and synthetic derivatives on various human and murine cancer cell lines. *Bioorg. Med. Chem.* **2006**, *14*, 2966–2971. [CrossRef]
18. Amawi, H.; Ashby, C.R.; Samuel, T.; Peraman, R.; Tiwari, A.K. Polyphenolic Nutrients in Cancer Chemoprevention and Metastasis: Role of the Epithelial-to-Mesenchymal (EMT) Pathway. *Nutrients* **2017**, *9*, 911. [CrossRef]
19. Samarghandian, S.; Azimi Nezhad, M.; Mohammadi, G. Role of caspases, Bax and Bcl-2 in chrysin-induced apoptosis in the A549 human lung adenocarcinoma epithelial cells. *Anti-Cancer Agents Med. Chem.* **2014**, *14*, 901–909. [CrossRef]
20. Burke, J.F.; Schlosser, L.; Chen, H.; Kunnimalaiyaan, M. Chrysin induces growth suppression through apoptosis in neuroblastoma cells. *J. Am. Coll. Surg.* **2012**, *215*, S70. [CrossRef]
21. Zhang, T.; Chen, X.; Qu, L.; Wu, J.; Cui, R.; Zhao, Y. Chrysin and its phosphate ester inhibit cell proliferation and induce apoptosis in Hela cells. *Bioorg. Med. Chem.* **2004**, *12*, 6097–6105. [CrossRef] [PubMed]
22. Riedl, S.J.; Shi, Y. Molecular mechanisms of caspase regulation during apoptosis. *Nat. Rev. Mol. Cell Biol.* **2004**, *5*, 897–907. [CrossRef] [PubMed]
23. Shi, Y. Mechanisms of caspase activation and inhibition during apoptosis. *Mol. Cell* **2002**, *9*, 459–470. [CrossRef]
24. Zhu, Z.Y.; Wang, W.X.; Wang, Z.Q.; Chen, L.J.; Zhang, J.Y.; Liu, X.C.; Wu, S.P.; Zhang, Y.M. Synthesis and antitumor activity evaluation of chrysin derivatives. *Eur. J. Med. Chem.* **2014**, *75*, 297–300. [CrossRef]
25. Liu, Y.; Song, X.; He, J.; Zheng, X.; Wu, H. Synthetic derivatives of chrysin and their biological activities. *Med. Chem. Res.* **2014**, *23*, 555–563. [CrossRef]
26. Valdez-Calderón, A.; González-Montiel, S.; Martínez-Otero, D.; Martínez-Torres, A.; Vásquez-Pérez, J.M.; Molina-Vera, C.; Torres-Valencia, J.M.; Alvarado-Rodríguez, J.G.; Cruz-Borbolla, J. Synthesis, structural study and biological activity of new derivatives of chrysin containing a 2-mercaptopyridyl or 5-(trifluoromethyl)-2-mercaptopyridyl fragments. *J. Mol. Struct.* **2016**, *1110*, 196–207. [CrossRef]
27. Patel, R.V.; Mistry, B.; Syed, R.; Rathi, A.K.; Lee, Y.-J.; Sung, J.-S.; Shinf, H.-S.; Keum, Y.-S. Chrysin-piperazine conjugates as antioxidant and anticancer agents. *Eur. J. Pharm. Sci.* **2016**, *88*, 166–177. [CrossRef]
28. Xuan, H.-Z.; Zhang, J.-H.; Wang, Y.-H.; Fu, C.-L.; Zhang, W. Anti-tumor activity evaluation of novel chrysin–organotin compound in MCF-7 cells. *Bioorg. Med. Chem. Lett.* **2016**, *26*, 570–574. [CrossRef]
29. Al-Oudat, B.A.; Alqudah, M.A.; Audat, S.A.; Al-Balas, Q.A.; El-Elimat, T.; Hassan, M.A.; Frhat, I.N.; Azaizeh, M.M. Design, synthesis, and biologic evaluation of novel chrysin derivatives as cytotoxic agents and caspase-3/7 activators. *Drug Des. Deve. Ther.* **2019**, *13*, 423–433. [CrossRef]
30. Srinivasan, R.; Manoharan, S. Chemopreventive Potential of Chrysin in 7, 12-dimethylbenz (A) anthracene induced mammary carcinogenesis in sprague-dawley rats. *J. Cell Tissue Res.* **2011**, *11*, 2909.

31. Lirdprapamongkol, K.; Sakurai, H.; Abdelhamed, S.; Yokoyama, S.; Athikomkulchai, S.; Viriyaroj, A.; Awale, S.; Ruchirawat, S.; Svasti, J.; Saiki, I. Chrysin overcomes TRAIL resistance of cancer cells through Mcl-1 downregulation by inhibiting STAT3 phosphorylation. *Int. J. Oncol.* **2013**, *43*, 329–337. [CrossRef] [PubMed]
32. Yang, B.; Huang, J.; Xiang, T.; Yin, X.; Luo, X.; Huang, J.; Luo, F.; Li, H.; Li, H.; Ren, G. Chrysin inhibits metastatic potential of human triple-negative breast cancer cells by modulating matrix metalloproteinase-10, epithelial to mesenchymal transition, and PI3K/Akt signaling pathway. *J. Appl. Toxicol.* **2014**, *34*, 105–112. [CrossRef] [PubMed]
33. Woo, K.J.; Jeong, Y.-J.; Park, J.-W.; Kwon, T.K. Chrysin-induced apoptosis is mediated through caspase activation and Akt inactivation in U937 leukemia cells. *Biochem. Biophys. Res. Commun.* **2004**, *325*, 1215–1222. [CrossRef] [PubMed]
34. Khoo, B.Y.; Chua, S.L.; Balaram, P. Apoptotic effects of chrysin in human cancer cell lines. *Int. J. Mol. Sci.* **2010**, *11*, 2188–2199. [CrossRef]
35. Putt, K.S.; Chen, G.W.; Pearson, J.M.; Sandhorst, J.S.; Hoagland, M.S.; Kwon, J.-T.; Hwang, S.-K.; Jin, H.; Churchwell, M.I.; Cho, M.-H. Small-molecule activation of procaspase-3 to caspase-3 as a personalized anticancer strategy. *Nat. Chem. Biol.* **2006**, *2*, 543–550. [CrossRef]
36. Peterson, Q.P.; Hsu, D.C.; Goode, D.R.; Novotny, C.J.; Totten, R.K.; Hergenrother, P.J. Procaspase-3 activation as an anti-cancer strategy: Structure– activity relationship of procaspase-activating compound 1 (PAC-1) and Its cellular co-localization with caspase-3. *Eur. J. Med. Chem.* **2009**, *52*, 5721–5731. [CrossRef]
37. Viegas-Junior, C.; Danuello, A.; da Silva Bolzani, V.; Barreiro, E.J.; Fraga, C.A.M. Molecular hybridization: A useful tool in the design of new drug prototypes. *Curr. Med. Chem.* **2007**, *14*, 1829–1852. [CrossRef]
38. Fortin, S.; Bérubé, G. Advances in the development of hybrid anticancer drugs. *Expert Opin. Drug Discov.* **2013**, *8*, 1029–1047. [CrossRef]
39. Zoete, V.; Daina, A.; Bovigny, C.; Michielin, O. *SwissSimilarity: A Web Tool for Low to Ultra High Throughput Ligand-Based Virtual Screening*; ACS Publications: Washington, DC, USA, 2016; pp. 1117–1121.
40. Delaney, J.S. ESOL: Estimating aqueous solubility directly from molecular structure. *J. Chem. Inf. Comput. Sci.* **2004**, *44*, 1000–1005. [CrossRef]
41. Daina, A.; Michielin, O.; Zoete, V. SwissADME: A free web tool to evaluate pharmacokinetics, drug-likeness and medicinal chemistry friendliness of small molecules. *Sci. Rep.* **2017**, *7*, 42717. [CrossRef]
42. Capuzzi, S.J.; Muratov, E.N.; Tropsha, A. Phantom PAINS: Problems with the Utility of Alerts for P an-A ssay IN terference Compound, S.J. *Chem. Inf. Model.* **2017**, *57*, 417–427. [CrossRef] [PubMed]
43. Ricci, M.S.; Zong, W.-X. Chemotherapeutic approaches for targeting cell death pathways. *Oncologist* **2006**, *11*, 342. [CrossRef] [PubMed]
44. Elmore, S. Apoptosis: A review of programmed cell death. *Exp. Toxicol. Pathol.* **2007**, *35*, 495–516. [CrossRef] [PubMed]
45. Levi, C.A.; Ejere, V.C.; Asogwa, C.N.; Iweh, P.; Nwatu, K.U.; Levi, U.E. Apoptosis: Its physiological implication and therapeutic possibilities. *J. Pharm. Biolo Sci.* **2014**, *9*, 38–45. [CrossRef]
46. Yang, J.; Liu, X.; Bhalla, K.; Kim, C.N.; Ibrado, A.M.; Cai, J.; Peng, T.-I.; Jones, D.P.; Wang, X. Prevention of apoptosis by Bcl-2: Release of cytochrome c from mitochondria blocked. *Science* **1997**, *275*, 1129–1132. [CrossRef]
47. Ouyang, L.; Shi, Z.; Zhao, S.; Wang, F.T.; Zhou, T.T.; Liu, B.; Bao, J.K. Programmed cell death pathways in cancer: A review of apoptosis, autophagy and programmed necrosis. *Cell Prolif.* **2012**, *45*, 487–498. [CrossRef]
48. Mariño, G.; Kroemer, G. Mechanisms of apoptotic phosphatidylserine exposure. *Cell Res.* **2013**, *23*, 1247. [CrossRef]
49. Vermes, I.; Haanen, C.; Steffens-Nakken, H.; Reutellingsperger, C. A novel assay for apoptosis flow cytometric detection of phosphatidylserine expression on early apoptotic cells using fluorescein labelled annexin V. *J. Immunol. Methods* **1995**, *184*, 39–51. [CrossRef]
50. Manivannan, E.; Amawi, H.; Hussein, N.; Karthikeyan, C.; Fetcenko, A.; Narayana Moorthy, N.S.H.; Trivedi, P.; Tiwari, A.K. Design and discovery of silybin analogues as antiproliferative compounds using a ring disjunctive—Based, natural product lead optimization approach. *Eur. J. Med. Chem.* **2017**, *133*, 365–378. [CrossRef]

51. Amawi, H.; Hussein, N.; Boddu, S.H.S.; Karthikeyan, C.; Williams, F.E.; Ashby, C.R., Jr.; Raman, D.; Trivedi, P.; Tiwari, A.K. Novel Thienopyrimidine Derivative, RP-010, Induces beta-Catenin Fragmentation and Is Efficacious against Prostate Cancer Cells. *Cancers* **2019**, *11*, 711. [CrossRef]
52. Karthikeyan, C.; Amawi, H.; Viana, A.G.; Sanglard, L.; Hussein, N.; Saddler, M.; Ashby, C.R., Jr.; Moorthy, N.; Trivedi, P.; Tiwari, A.K. lH-Pyrazolo[3,4-b]quinolin-3-amine derivatives inhibit growth of colon cancer cells via apoptosis and sub G1 cell cycle arrest. *Bioorg. Med. Chem. Lett.* **2018**, *28*, 2244–2249. [CrossRef] [PubMed]
53. Amawi, H.; Hussein, N.A.; Karthikeyan, C.; Manivannan, E.; Wisner, A.; Williams, F.E.; Samuel, T.; Trivedi, P.; Ashby, C.R., Jr.; Tiwari, A.K. HM015k, a Novel Silybin Derivative, Multi-Targets Metastatic Ovarian Cancer Cells and Is Safe in Zebrafish Toxicity Studies. *Front. Pharmacol.* **2017**, *8*, 498. [CrossRef]
54. Balaji, N.V.; Ramani, M.V.; Viana, A.G.; Sanglard, L.P.; White, J.; Mulabagal, V.; Lee, C.; Gana, T.J.; Egiebor, N.O.; Subbaraju, G.V.; et al. Design, synthesis and in vitro cell-based evaluation of the anti-cancer activities of hispolon analogs. *Bioorg. Med. Chem.* **2015**, *23*, 2148–2158. [CrossRef] [PubMed]
55. Karthikeyan, C.; Amawi, H.; Ashby, C.R., Jr.; Khare, V.M.; Jones, V.; Hari Narayana Moorthy, N.S.; Trivedi, P.; Tiwari, A.K. Novel 3-((2-chloroquinolin-3-yl)methylene)indolin-2-one derivatives produce anticancer efficacy in ovarian cancer in vitro. *Heliyon* **2019**, *5*, e01603. [CrossRef] [PubMed]
56. Amawi, H.; Karthikeyan, C.; Pathak, R.; Hussein, N.; Christman, R.; Robey, R.; Ashby, C.R., Jr.; Trivedi, P.; Malhotra, A.; Tiwari, A.K. Thienopyrimidine derivatives exert their anticancer efficacy via apoptosis induction, oxidative stress and mitotic catastrophe. *Eur. J. Med. Chem.* **2017**, *138*, 1053–1065. [CrossRef]
57. Amawi, H.; Ashby, C.R., Jr.; Tiwari, A.K. Cancer chemoprevention through dietary flavonoids: What's limiting? *Chin. J. Cancer* **2017**, *36*, 50. [CrossRef]
58. Westphal, D.; Dewson, G.; Czabotar, P.E.; Kluck, R.M. Molecular biology of Bax and Bak activation and action. *BBA-Mol. Cell Res.* **2011**, *1813*, 521–531. [CrossRef]
59. Shamas-Din, A.; Kale, J.; Leber, B.; Andrews, D.W. Mechanisms of action of Bcl-2 family proteins. *CSH Perspect. Biol.* **2013**, *5*, a008714. [CrossRef]
60. Delbridge, A.R.; Grabow, S.; Strasser, A.; Vaux, D.L. Thirty years of BCL-2: Translating cell death discoveries into novel cancer therapies. *Nat. Rev. Cancer* **2016**, *16*, 99. [CrossRef]
61. Lamkanfi, M.; Kanneganti, T.-D. Caspase-7: A protease involved in apoptosis and inflammation. *Intl. J. Biochem. Cell Boil.* **2010**, *42*, 21–24. [CrossRef] [PubMed]
62. Choe, H.; Kim, J.; Hong, S. Structure-based design of flavone-based inhibitors of wild-type and T315I mutant of ABL. *Bioorg. Med. Chem. Lett.* **2013**, *23*, 4324–4327. [CrossRef] [PubMed]

Sample Availability: Samples of the compounds **4a**, **4g**, **4i** and **4o** are available from the authors on request.

molecules

MDPI

Article

Design and Synthesis of Flavonoidal Ethers and Their Anti-Cancer Activity In Vitro

Lu Jin [1,2], Meng-Ling Wang [1], Yao Lv [3], Xue-Yi Zeng [1,2], Chao Chen [1,2], Hai Ren [1,2], Heng Luo [1,2,*] and Wei-Dong Pan [1,2,*]

1 State Key Laboratory of Functions and Applications of Medicinal Plants, Guizhou Medical University, Guiyang 550014, China; m18352807507@163.com (L.J.); WANGMENGLING417@163.com (M.-L.W.); Xueyizeng@126.com (X.-Y.Z.); cc283818640@163.com (C.C.); renh0206@163.com (H.R.)

2 The Key Laboratory of Chemistry for Natural Products of Guizhou Province and Chinese Academy of Sciences, Guiyang 550014, China

3 Bijie Medical College, Bijie 551700, China; Lvyao0918@163.com

* Correspondence: luoheng71050@aliyun.com (H.L.); wdpan@163.com (W.-D.P.)

Academic Editor: Qiao-Hong Chen

Received: 30 March 2019; Accepted: 3 May 2019; Published: 6 May 2019

Abstract: Flavonoids are well-characterized polyphenolic compounds with pharmacological and therapeutic activities. However, most flavonoids have not been developed into clinical drugs, due to poor bioavailability. Herein, we report a strategy to increase the drugability of flavonoids by constructing C(sp^2)-O bonds and stereo- as well as regioselective alkenylation of hydroxyl groups of flavonoids with ethyl-2,3-butadienoate allenes. Twenty-three modified flavonoid derivatives were designed, synthesized, and evaluated for their anti-cancer activities. The results showed that compounds **4b**, **4c**, **4e**, **5e**, and **6b** exhibited better in vitro inhibitory activity against several cancer cell lines than their precursors. Preliminary structure–activity relationship studies indicated that, in most of the cancer cell lines evaluated, the substitution on position 7 was essential for increasing cytotoxicity. The results of this study might facilitate the preparation or late-stage modification of complex flavonoids as anti-cancer drug candidates.

Keywords: flavonoids; allene; E-stereoselective; regioselective; anti-cancer activity

1. Introduction

Consisting of more than 9000 compounds, flavonoids represent the most widely distributed polyphenols in nature [1,2]. In addition, flavonoids are ubiquitous in some medicinal plants and herbal remedies used in traditional medicine around the world, especially in China [2–6]. The characteristic skeleton of flavonoids is a phenylbenzopyrone moiety (C6-C3-C6), which could be further categorized according to the saturation level and the presence or absence of the central pyran ring. Many studies have confirmed that flavonoids are naturally occurring, pharmacologically active molecules. However, most flavonoids have not been developed as clinical drugs because of poor bioavailability (less than 5%), toxicity, and induction or inhibition of some metabolic enzymes [7]. To overcome these problems, structural modifications of the flavonoid skeletons have attracted great interest [8].

Allenes are highly reactive and have been used extensively in organic chemistry [9–15], due to the electronic or steric effects and their 1,2-diene functionality. The transition-metal catalyzed chemistry of allenes has become a recent focus of research [16,17]. We proposed that carbopalladation of allenes would provide a highly convenient method for the formation of a conjugated aryl ether, following β-H elimination by the introduction of a π-allyl palladium species.

In this research, we have developed a friendly and straightforward protocol to access various novel flavonoidal ethers by employing allenes as important multifunctional modules. Notably, both electrophilic groups and aliphatic chains can be embedded in the flavonoid scaffold smoothly with the above mentioned protocol. Therefore, more than 20 flavonoidal ethers were obtained successfully and evaluated for anti-cancer activities.

2. Materials and Methods

2.1. Instruments and Materials

^{1}H- and ^{13}C-NMR spectra were obtained on a 400 MHz (Varian, Inc) or 500 MHz (WIPM, China) spectrometer in $CDCl_3$ or DMSO-d_6 (tetramethylsilane (TMS) as internal standard). Chemical shifts (δ) were expressed in parts per million (ppm), relative to TMS (0 ppm). High resolution mass spectra (HRMS) were recorded on a ThermoFisher QE Focus apparatus. All the solvents were dried using standard methods and distilled before being used. Reagents and solvents were purchased from commercial sources. Solvents were purified according to the guidelines in the Purification of Laboratory Chemicals.

2.2. General Procedure for the Synthesis of Flavonoidal Ether Derivatives

2.2.1. Synthesis of Allenes

Allenes were synthesized according to previously described protocols [16–18].

2.2.2. Optimization of Reaction Conditions

We selected chrysin **2a** and ethyl ester allene **1a** as the model substrates in this study and carried out extensive screening of the reaction conditions. In an initial attempt, a variety of factors including types of Pd catalysts, bases, solvents, and ligands were examined. After extensive optimization, the product (**3a**) was obtained with an isolated yield of 41.7% in the presence of 10 mol% of PPh_3/Pd(dba)$_2$ as a catalyst, K_2CO_3 (2.0 equiv.) as a base, in a solution of MeCN under argon at 80 °C (Table 1, entry 1). Further investigations of the solvent indicated that the yield could be slightly improved to 43.0% by replacing MeCN with DMF (Table 1, entry 6). Furthermore, absence of Pd catalysts and ligands resulted in lower yield (Table 1, entry 14). None of the desired product was obtained when the base was abstracted away (Table 1, entries 15 and 16). Interestingly, only 11.2% yield of the expected product was obtained at lower temperatures (Table 1, entry 17). It was worth noting that **3a** was the only isomer isolated, indicating a highly regio- and stereoselective process, in which the steric effect of the carbonyl or the hydrogen bond effect between the carbonyl and oxygen atom at position 7 may be critical for the highly regio- and stereoselective process.

Table 1. Optimization of reaction conditions.

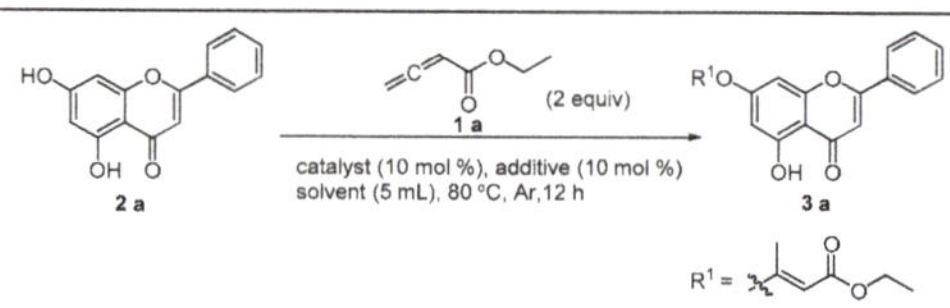

Entry	Catalyst	Base	Ligand	Solvent	Yield (%)	Entry	Catalyst	Base	Ligand	Solvent	Yield (%)
1	Pd(dba)$_2$	K_2CO_3	PPh_3	DMA [a]	<5	10	Pd(dba)$_2$	Cs_2CO_3	PPh_3	DMF	18.4
2	Pd(dba)$_2$	K_2CO_3	PPh_3	EtOH	13.3	11	$PdCl_2$	K_2CO_3	-	DMF	15.8
3	Pd(dba)$_2$	K_2CO_3	PPh_3	MeCN	41.7	12	Pd(OAc)$_2$	K_2CO_3	-	DMF	24.1
4	Pd(dba)$_2$	K_2CO_3	PPh_3	DCM	<5	13	$PdCl_2(PPh_3)_2$	K_2CO_3	-	DMF	13.3
5	Pd(dba)$_2$	K_2CO_3	PPh_3	DMA [b]	32.0	14	-	K_2CO_3	-	DMF	14.9
6	Pd(dba)$_2$	K_2CO_3	PPh_3	DMF	43.0	15	Pd(OAc)$_2$	-	-	DMF	NO.
7	Pd(dba)$_2$	NaH	PPh_3	DMF	14.2	16	Pd(dba)$_2$	-	-	DMF	NO.
8	Pd(dba)$_2$	NH(iPr)$_2$	PPh_3	DMF	<5	17	Pd(dba)$_2$	K_2CO_3	PPh_3	DMF	11.2 [c]
9	Pd(dba)$_2$	Et_3N	PPh_3	DMF	17.2	-	-	-	-	-	-

Conditions: **1a** (0.4 mmol), **2a** (0.2 mmol), isolated yield. [a] *N,N*-Dimethylaniline; [b] *N,N*-Dimethylacetamide; [c] Reaction occurred at rt.

2.2.3. General Procedure for the Synthesis of Target Derivatives **3a–3i**, **4a–4g**, **5a–5e**

Chrysin **2a** (127.12 mg, 0.5 mmol), $Pd(dba)_2$ (5.75 mg, 0.01 mmol), K_2CO_3 (138.21 mg, 1.0 mmol), PPh_3 (13.11 mg, 0.05 mmol), allene (112.13 mg, 1.0 mmol), and anhydrous DMF (5 mL) were added to a 30 mL tube under argon, which was then sealed. The resulting mixture was stirred at 80 °C for 12 h. After completion, the reaction solution was cooled down to room temperature before 80 mL water was added, followed by the addition of 1 N HCl aqueous solution at 0 °C, until the pH value reached 7. Ethyl acetate (100 mL) was added to the reaction solution and the organic layer was washed sequentially with a large amount of water (4 × 200 mL), and then brine, before being dried over anhydrous Na_2SO_4. The solvent was evaporated under reduced pressure. The crude product was purified by silica gel column chromatography (petroleum ether–ethylacetate, 5:1) to give **3a** (78.8 mg, 43% yield). Compounds **3b–3i, 4a–4g,** and **5a–5e** were prepared according to similar procedures in which the double-substitution is a byproduct. The products **4a–4g** were generated in a shorter time compared with the other products (within 10 h).

2.2.4. General Synthetic Procedure for **6a–6b** Target Derivatives

The reaction with 1.0 mmol scale was carried out to assess the scalability of flavonoidal ether formation (Scheme 1, **4a**). Under standard conditions, the yield was lower than that of the small-scale reaction. The reaction solution contained the following components: **4a** (62.8 mg, 0.02 mmol), 1 mL methanol, and 1 N sodium hydroxide solution (2.0 equiv). The solution was then stirred at 60 °C for 5 min and 1 mL water was added before heating at 60 °C for 12 h. After completion, the reaction solution was cooled down to room temperature and 40 mL water as well as 30 mL ethyl acetate was added sequentially. Aqueous HCl (1 N) was added to the water layer at 0 °C until the pH value reached 4. Other post-processing procedures were similar to those performed to synthesize **4a**. The desired product **6a** was finally obtained (41.2 mg, 61% yield). The product **6b** was prepared according to the same general procedure.

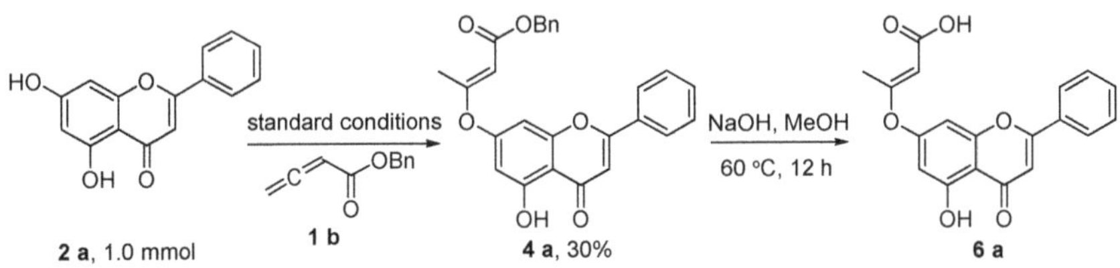

Scheme 1. Synthesis of flavonoidal ether and derivatization.

Ethyl (E)-3-((5-hydroxy-4-oxo-2-phenyl-4H-chromen-7-yl) oxy) but-2-enoate (**3a**); yellow powder; yield 43.0%; HRMS(ESI): calcd. $C_{21}H_{17}O_6$, m/z 365.1031 $[M - H]^-$, found 365.1025; ^{1}H-NMR ($CDCl_3$, 500 MHz) δ(ppm): 7.88 (d, J = 7.0 Hz, 2H), 7.59–7.51 (m, 3H), 6.73 (s, 1H), 6.68 (d, J = 2.0 Hz, 1H), 6.49 (d, J = 2.0 Hz, 1H), 5.16 (s, 1H), 4.12 (q, J = 7.0 Hz, 2H), 2.49 (s, 3H), 1.23 (t, J = 7.0 Hz, 3H); ^{13}C-NMR ($CDCl_3$, 125 MHz) δ(ppm): 182.9, 170.5, 167.1, 164.7, 162.6, 159.4, 157.4, 132.3, 131.0, 129.3, 126.5, 108.6, 106.3, 104.8, 100.0, 99.8, 60.0, 18.2, 14.4.

Ethyl (E)-3-((5,6-dihydroxy-4-oxo-2-phenyl-4H-chromen-7-yl) oxy) but-2-enoate (**3b**); yellow powder; yield 43.9 %; HRMS(ESI): calcd. $C_{21}H_{17}O_7$, m/z 381.0980 $[M - H]^-$, found 381.0970; ^{1}H-NMR (DMSO-d_6, 400 MHz) δ(ppm): 13.02 (s, 1H), 8.04 (d, J = 7.2 Hz, 2H), 7.59–7.52 (m, 3H), 6.97 (s, 1H), 6.69 (s, 1H), 4.80 (s, 1H), 3.97 (q, J = 7.2 Hz, 2H), 2.40 (s, 3H), 1.09 (t, J = 7.2 Hz, 3H); ^{13}C-NMR (DMSO-d_6, 100 MHz) δ(ppm): 182.3, 170.7, 166.6, 163.7, 156.7, 154.2, 152.4, 132.2, 130.7, 129.2, 126.5, 123.8, 105.0, 104.4, 94.8, 93.3, 59.2, 17.6, 14.2.

Diethyl 3,3′-((5-hydroxy-4-oxo-2-phenyl-4H-chromene-6,7-diyl) bis (oxy)) (2E,2′E)-bis (but-2-enoate) (**3c**); yellow powder; yield 29.3%; HRMS(ESI): calcd. $C_{27}H_{27}O_9$, m/z 495.1650 $[M + H]^+$, found 495.1647;

^{1}H-NMR (DMSO-d_6, 500 MHz) δ(ppm): 11.76 (s, 1H), 8.04 (d, *J* = 6.0 Hz, 2H), 7.60–7.57 (m, 3H), 7.16 (s, 1H), 6.78 (s, 1 H), 4.77 (s, 1H), 4.63 (s, 1H), 4.01–3.94 (m, 4H), 2.44 (s, 3H), 2.39 (s, 3H), 1.16–1.03 (m, 6H); ^{13}C-NMR (DMSO-d_6, 125 MHz) δ(ppm): 174.7, 171.6, 170.4, 166.3, 166.2, 161.0, 155.4, 155.3, 143.0, 131.7, 131.3, 130.8, 129.1, 126.3, 109.8, 107.5, 102.7, 94.5, 93.9, 59.3, 59.1, 17.6, 17.3, 14.1.

Ethyl (E)-3-(5-(5,7-dihydroxy-4-oxo-4H-chromen-2-yl)-2-methoxyphenoxy)-2-methylacrylate (**3d**); yellow powder; yield 25.9%; HRMS(ESI): calcd. $C_{22}H_{19}O_8$, *m/z* 411.1085 [M − H]$^-$, found 411.1078; ^{1}H-NMR (DMSO-d_6, 500 MHz) δ(ppm): 12.87 (s, 1H), 10.88 (s, 1H), 8.03 (dd, *J* = 9.0, 2.5 Hz, 1H), 7.87 (d, *J* = 2.5 Hz, 1H), 7.33 (d, *J* = 9 Hz, 1H), 6.95 (s, 1H), 6.52 (d, *J* = 2.0 Hz, 1H), 6.20 (d, *J* = 2.0 Hz, 1H), 4.66 (s, 1H), 3.99 (q, *J* = 7.0 Hz, 2H), 3.88 (s, 3H), 2.43 (s, 3H), 1.10 (t, *J* = 7.0 Hz, 3H); ^{13}C-NMR (DMSO-d_6, 125 MHz) δ(ppm): 181.8, 171.6, 166.3, 164.3, 162.1, 161.4, 157.4, 153.9, 141.1, 126.0, 123.6, 121.1, 113.8, 104.3, 103.8, 99.0, 94.6, 94.2, 59.2, 56.3, 17.7, 14.1.

Ethyl (E)-3-((2-(3-(((E)-4-ethoxy-4-oxobut-2-en-2-yl) oxy)-4-methoxyphenyl)-5-hydroxy-4-oxo-4H-chromen-7-yl) oxy) but-2-enoate (**3e**); yellow powder; yield 21.2%; HRMS(ESI): calcd. $C_{28}H_{29}O_{10}$, *m/z* 525.1755 [M + H]$^+$, found 525.1759; ^{1}H-NMR (DMSO-d_6, 500 MHz) δ(ppm): 12.94 (s, 1H), 8.05 (dd, *J* = 8.5, 2.0 Hz, 1H), 7.86 (d, *J* = 2.0 Hz, 1H), 7.32 (d, *J* = 8.5 Hz, 1H), 7.05 (s, 1H), 6.95 (d, *J* = 2.0 Hz, 1H), 6.51 (d, *J* = 2.0 Hz, 1H), 5.05 (s, 1H), 4.66 (s, 1H), 4.05–3.95 (m, 4H), 3.90 (s, 3H), 2.42 (d, *J* = 3.5 Hz, 6H), 1.21–1.10 (m, 6H). ^{13}C-NMR (DMSO-d_6, 125 MHz) δ(ppm): 181.8, 171.6, 166.3, 164.3, 162.1, 161.4, 157.4, 153.9, 141.1, 126.0, 123.6, 121.1, 113.8, 104.3, 103.8, 99.0, 94.6, 94.2, 59.2, 56.3, 39.7, 39.5, 39.4, 17.7, 14.1.

Ethyl (E)-3-((5-hydroxy-2-(4-hydroxyphenyl)-4-oxo-4H-chromen-7-yl) oxy) but-2-enoate (**3f**); yellow powder; yield 30.3%; HRMS(ESI): calcd. $C_{21}H_{17}O_7$, *m/z* 381.0980 [M − H]$^-$, found 381.0986; ^{1}H-NMR (DMSO-d_6, 400 MHz) δ(ppm): 13.10 (s, 1H), 10.45 (s, 1H), 7.97 (d, *J* = 8.0 Hz, 2H), 6.98–6.91 (m, 4H), 6.56 (s, 1H), 5.05 (s, 1H), 4.03 (q, *J* = 7.2 Hz, 2H), 2.42 (s, 3H), 1.14 (t, *J* = 7.2 Hz, 3H); ^{13}C-NMR (DMSO-d_6, 100 MHz) δ(ppm): 182.3, 170.5, 166.1, 164.7, 161.6, 161.5, 158.4, 156.8, 128.8, 120.8, 116.0, 107.9, 104.0, 103.4, 100.2, 98.7, 59.4, 17.7, 14.1.

Ethyl (E)-3-(4-(5,7-dihydroxy-4-oxo-4H-chromen-2-yl) phenoxy) but-2-enoate (**3g**); yellow powder; yield 28.3%; HRMS(ESI): calcd. $C_{21}H_{17}O_7$, *m/z* 381.0980 [M − H]$^-$, found 381.0976; ^{1}H-NMR (DMSO-d_6, 400 MHz) δ(ppm): 12.82 (s, 1H), 10.96 (s, 1H), 8.17 (d, *J* = 8.8 Hz, 2H), 7.34 (d, *J* = 8.4 Hz, 2H), 6.99 (s, 1H), 6.52 (d, *J* = 2.0 Hz, 1H), 6.22 (d, *J* = 2.0 Hz, 1H), 4.79 (s, 1H), 4.01 (q, *J* = 7.2 Hz, 2H), 2.45 (s, 3H), 1.12 (t, *J* = 7.2 Hz, 3H); ^{13}C-NMR (DMSO-d_6, 100 MHz) δ(ppm): 181.9, 171.7, 166.2, 164.5, 162.4, 161.5, 157.5, 155.6, 128.8, 128.3, 122.2, 105.3, 103.9, 99.1, 96.9, 94.2, 59.3, 17.8, 14.2.

Ethyl 2-(5-(5,7-dihydroxy-4-oxo-4H-chromen-2-yl)-2-methylbenzo [d] [1,3] dioxol-2-yl) acetate (**3h**); yellow powder; yield 30.1%; HRMS(ESI): calcd. $C_{21}H_{17}O_8$, *m/z* 397.0929 [M − H]$^-$, found 397.0923; ^{1}H-NMR ($CDCl_3$, 400 MHz) δ(ppm): 12.62 (s, 1H), 7.43 (dd, *J* = 8.4, 1.6 Hz, 1H), 7.26 (d, *J* = 1.2 Hz, 1H), 6.88 (d, *J* = 8.4 Hz, 1H), 6.52 (s, 1H), 6.49 (d, *J* = 1.2 Hz, 1H), 6.38 (d, *J* = 1.6 Hz, 1H), 4.20 (q, *J* = 7.2 Hz, 2H), 3.06 (s, 2H), δ 1.88 (s, 3H), 1.25 (t, *J* = 7.2 Hz, 3H); ^{13}C-NMR ($CDCl_3$, 100 MHz) δ(ppm): 182.5, 168.3, 164.1, 164.0, 162.1, 157.9, 150.5, 148.1, 124.8, 121.6, 117.6, 108.9, 106.4, 104.9, 104.0, 100.0, 94.6, 61.4, 44.0, 25.0, 14.1.

Ethyl 2-(2-methyl-5-(3,5,7-trihydroxy-4-oxo-4H-chromen-2-yl) benzo [d] [1,3] dioxol-2-yl) acetate (**3i**); yellow powder; yield 30.1%; HRMS(ESI): calcd. $C_{21}H_{19}O_9$, *m/z* 415.1024 [M + H]$^+$, found 415.1018; ^{1}H-NMR (DMSO-d_6, 500 MHz) δ(ppm): 12.40 (s, 1H), 10.83 (s, 1H), 9.57 (s, 1H), 7.74 (dd, *J* = 8.0, 1.5 Hz, 1H), 7.62 (d, *J* = 1.5 Hz, 1H), 7.03 (d, *J* = 8.0 Hz, 1H), 6.47 (d, *J* = 2.0 Hz, 1H), 6.19 (d, *J* = 2.0 Hz, 1H), 4.02 (q, *J* = 7.5 Hz, 2H), 3.13 (s, 2H), 1.78 (s, 3H), 1.10 (t, *J* = 7.5 Hz, 3H); ^{13}C-NMR (DMSO-d_6, 125 MHz) δ(ppm): 176.0, 167.6, 164.1, 160.7, 156.2, 148.2, 147.1, 145.9, 136.3, 124.5, 122.6, 117.3, 108.3, 107.3, 103.1, 98.3, 93.6, 60.3, 43.1, 24.7, 13.9.

Benzyl (E)-3-((5-hydroxy-4-oxo-2-phenyl-4H-chromen-7-yl) oxy) but-2-enoate (**4a**); yellow powder; yield 33.0%; HRMS(ESI): calcd. $C_{26}H_{21}O_6$, *m/z* 429.1333 [M + H]$^+$, found 429.1324; ^{1}H-NMR (DMSO-d_6, 400 MHz) δ(ppm): 12.93 (s, 1 H), 8.12 (d, *J* = 6.8 Hz, 2H), 7.74–7.56 (m, 3H), 7.32 (m, 5H), 7.07 (d,

J = 2.0 Hz, 1H), 6.63 (d, J = 2.0 Hz, 1H), 5.10 (s, 1H), 5.07 (s, 2H), 2.46 (s, 3H); ^{13}C-NMR (DMSO-d_6, 100 MHz) δ(ppm): 182.7, 171.3, 166.1, 164.2, 161.6, 158.7, 157.1, 136.3, 132.5, 130.4, 129.3, 128.5, 128.3, 128.1, 126.8, 108.3, 105.8, 104.4, 100.7, 98.3, 65.3, 17.9.

Dibenzyl 3,3′-((4-oxo-2-phenyl-4H-chromene-5,7-diyl) bis (oxy)) (2E,2′E)-bis (but-2-enoate) (**4b**); white powder; yield 29.8%; HRMS(ESI): calcd. $C_{37}H_{31}O_8$, *m/z* 603.2013 [M + H]$^+$, found 603.2010; ^{1}H-NMR ($CDCl_3$, 400 MHz) δ(ppm): 7.85 (d, J = 6.8 Hz, 2H), 7.52 (d, J = 7.6 Hz, 3H), 7.33 (m, J = 10H), 7.12 (d, J = 2.0 Hz, 1H), 6.71 (d, J = 2.0 Hz, 1H), 6.65 (s, 1H), 5.24 (s, 1H), 5.12 (s, 2H), 5.03 (s, 2H), 4.73 (s, 1H), 2.66 (s, 3H), 2.52 (s, 3H); ^{13}C-NMR ($CDCl_3$, 100 MHz) δ(ppm): 175.6, 174.0, 170.6, 167.0, 166.6, 162.3, 158.9, 157.5, 153.0, 136.3, 136.1 133.1, 131.9, 129.2, 128.7, 128.6, 128.5, 128.4, 128.3, 128.2, 126.3, 114.7, 113.3, 108.9, 108.0, 100.2, 95.2, 66.1, 65.8, 18.6, 18.3.

Dibenzyl 3,3′-((5-hydroxy-4-oxo-2-phenyl-4H-chromene-6,7-diyl) bis (oxy)) (2E,2′E)-bis (but-2-enoate) (**4c**); yellow powder; yield 24.2%; HRMS(ESI): calcd. $C_{37}H_{30}O_9Na$, *m/z* 641.1782 [M + Na]$^+$, found 641.1779; ^{1}H-NMR (DMSO-d_6, 400 MHz) δ(ppm): 13.17 (s, 1H), 8.16-8.11 (m, 2H), 7.76–7.53 (m, 3H), 7.39-7.23 (m, 10H), 7.18 (s, 1H), 5.14 (s, 1H), 5.04 (s, 1H), 5.01 (s, 2H), 4.96 (s, 1H), 2.43 (s, 3H), 2.42 (s, 3H); ^{13}C-NMR (DMSO-d_6, 100 MHz) δ(ppm): 182.9, 170.4, 170.3, 166.1, 165.8, 164.5, 153.7, 152.9, 150.5, 136.1, 130.3, 129.2, 128.4, 128.2, 128.1, 128.0, 126.7, 109.4, 105.4, 101.8, 98.0, 94.3, 65.2, 65.1, 17.5, 17.4.

Benzyl (E)-3-((5,6-dihydroxy-4-oxo-2-phenyl-4H-chromen-7-yl) oxy) but-2-enoate (**4d**); yellow powder; yield 16.0%; HRMS(ESI): calcd. $C_{26}H_{20}O_7Na$, *m/z* 467.1101 [M + Na]$^+$, found 467.1092; ^{1}H-NMR (DMSO-d_6, 500 MHz) δ(ppm): 13.06 (s, 1H), 11.37 (s, 1H), 8.08 (d, J = 6.0 Hz, 2H), 7.62–7.56 (m, 3H), 7.34-7.28 (m, 5H), 7.02 (s, 1H), 6.72 (s, 1H), 5.03 (s, 2H), 4.87 (s, 1H), 2.44 (s, 3H); ^{13}C-NMR (DMSO-d_6, 125 MHz) δ(ppm): 182.3, 171.2, 166.4, 163.7, 156.6, 154.2, 152.4, 136.3, 132.2, 130.7, 129.2, 128.4, 128.3, 128.0, 126.6, 123.7, 105.0, 104.4, 94.8, 92.9, 65.1, 17.7.

Benzyl (E)-3-((5-hydroxy-2-(3-hydroxy-4methoxyphenyl)-4-oxo-4H-chromen-7yl) oxy) but-2-enoate (**4e**); yellow powder; yield 32.5%; HRMS(ESI): calcd. $C_{27}H_{23}O_8$, *m/z* 475.1387 [M + H]$^+$, found 475.1375; ^{1}H-NMR (DMSO-d_6, 400 MHz) δ(ppm): 13.07 (s, 1H), 9.48 (s, 1H), 7.58 (d, J = 8.4 Hz, 1H), 7.46 (d, J = 1.6 Hz, 1H), 7.32 (s, 5H), 7.08 (d, J = 8.4 Hz, 1H), 6.98 (s, 1H), 6.90 (s, 1H), 6.58 (d, J = 1.6 Hz, 1H), 5.10 (s, 1H), 5.06 (s, 2H), 3.87 (s, 3H), 2.45 (s, 3H); ^{13}C-NMR (DMSO-d_6, 100 MHz) δ(ppm): 182.3, 171.3, 166.0, 164.5, 161.6, 158.4, 156.9, 151.5, 146.8, 132.2, 128.4, 128.2, 128.0, 122.6, 119.1, 113.3, 112.1, 108.0, 104.2, 104.1, 100.4, 98.1, 65.2, 55.8, 17.9.

Benzyl (E)-3-(4-(3,5,7-trihydroxy-4-oxo-4H-chromen-2-yl) phenoxy) but-2-enoate (**4f**); yellow powder; yield 23.6%; HRMS(ESI): calcd. $C_{26}H_{20}O_8Na$, *m/z* 483.1050 [M + Na]$^+$, found 483.1047; ^{1}H-NMR (DMSO-d_6, 400 MHz) δ(ppm): 12.24 (s, 1H), 10.96 (s, 1H), 10.40 (s, 1H), 7.78–7.76 (m, 2H), 7.32–7.30 (m, 5H), 6.95–6.93 (m, 2H), 6.48 (d, J = 2.0 Hz, 1H), 6.23 (d, J = 2.0 Hz, 1H), 5.28 (s, 1H), 5.01 (s, 2H), 2.44 (s, 3H); ^{13}C-NMR (DMSO-d_6, 100 MHz) δ(ppm): 175.0, 170.0, 166.3, 164.5, 161.1, 160.8, 156.8, 156.5, 136.2, 131.0, 130.1, 128.4, 128.3, 128.0, 119.5, 115.9, 104.1, 98.9, 94.8, 94.2, 65.1, 17.6.

Benzyl (E)-3-(4-(7-(((E)-3-(benzyloxy)-2-methyl-3-oxoprop-1-en-1-yl) oxy)-5-hydroxy-4-oxo-4H-chromen-2-yl) phenoxy)-2-methylacrylate (**4g**); yellow powder; yield: 64.9%; HRMS(ESI) calcd. $C_{37}H_{31}O_9$, *m/z* 619.1963 [M + H]$^+$, found 619.1954; ^{1}H-NMR ($CDCl_3$, 500 MHz) δ (ppm): 12.75 (s, 1H), 7.91 (d, J = 7.5 Hz, 2H), 7.33 (s, 10H), 7.18 (d, J = 8.0 Hz, 2H), 6.68 (d, J = 14.5 Hz, 2H), 6.50 (s, 1H), 5.20 (s, 1H), 5.11 (d, J = 7.5 Hz, 4H), 5.01 (s, 1H), 2.53 (d, J = 11.5 Hz, 6H); ^{13}C-NMR ($CDCl_3$, 125MHz) δ (ppm):182.7, 172.3, 171.2, 167.0, 166.9, 163.7, 162.6, 159.3, 157.3, 156.5, 136.19, 136.1, 128.6, 128.5, 128.4, 128.3, 122.4, 108.6, 106.2, 105.0, 100.1, 99.1, 97.5, 66.0, 65.9, 18.5, 18.3.

Ethyl (E)-3-((5-hydroxy-4-oxo-2-phenyl-4H-chromen-7-yl) oxy) hex-2-enoate (**5a**); yellow powder; yield 32.0%; HRMS(ESI): calcd. $C_{23}H_{22}O_6Na$, *m/z* 417.1309 [M + Na]$^+$, found 417.1305; ^{1}H-NMR ($CDCl_3$, 400 MHz) δ(ppm): 12.79 (s, 1H), 7.89 (dd, J = 8.0, 2.0 Hz, 2H), 7.57–7.50 (m, 3H), 6.74 (s, 1H), 6.67 (d, J = 2.0 Hz, 1H), 6.49 (d, J = 2.0 Hz, 1H), 5.08 (s, 1H), 4.11 (dd, J = 2H), 2.94–2.90 (m, 2H), 1.74 (m, J = 15.2, 7.6 Hz, 2H), 1.23 (t, J = 7.2 Hz, 3H), 1.05 (t, J = 7.2 Hz, 3H); ^{13}C-NMR ($CDCl_3$, 100 MHz) δ(ppm): 182.9, 174.4, 166.9, 164.7, 162.6, 159.7, 157.5, 132.3, 131.0, 129.3, 126.5, 108.6, 106.3, 105.0, 100.1, 99.2, 60.0, 32.9, 20.9, 14.4, 13.9.

Ethyl (E)-3-((7-hydroxy-4-oxo-2-phenyl-4H-chromen-5-yl) oxy) hex-2-enoate (**5b**); yellow powder; yield 40.0%; HRMS(ESI): calcd. $C_{23}H_{23}O_6$, *m/z* 395.1489 $[M + H]^+$, found 395.1482; ^{1}H-NMR (DMSO-d_6, 400 MHz) δ(ppm): 8.26–8.01 (m, 2H), 7.56 (d, *J* = 7.2 Hz, 3H), 6.98 (d, *J* = 2.2 Hz, 1H), 6.74 (s, 1H), 6.49 (d, *J* = 2.2 Hz, 1H), 4.49 (s, 1H), 3.94 (dd, *J* = 14.4, 7.2 Hz, 2H), 2.94–2.90 (m, 2H), 1.76 (m, *J* = 2H), 1.09–0.99 (m, 6H), 1.00 (t, *J* = 7.2 Hz, 3H); ^{13}C-NMR (DMSO-d_6, 100 MHz) δ(ppm): 176.1, 174.6, 166.2, 162.6, 160.7, 158.8, 151.8, 131.6, 130.9, 129.1, 126.2, 109.5, 108.6, 107.7, 101.5, 93.7, 32.6, 59.1, 19.9, 14.1, 13.8.

Ethyl (E)-3-((7-(((Z)-1-ethoxy-1-oxohex-2-en-3-yl) oxy)-6-hydroxy-4-oxo-2-phenyl-4H-chromen-5-yl) oxy) hex-2-enoate (**5c**); yellow powder; yield 7.0%; HRMS(ESI): calcd. $C_{31}H_{35}O_9$, *m/z* 551.2276 $[M + H]^+$, found 551.2260; ^{1}H-NMR ($CDCl_3$, 400 MHz) δ(ppm): 8.40 (s, 1H), 7.83 (d, *J* = 6.4 Hz, 2H), 7.55–7.48 (m, 3H), 7.11 (s, 1H), 6.60 (s, 1H), 4.90 (s, 1H), 4.70 (s, 1H), 4.10–4.03 (m, 4H), 3.05–3.02 (m, 2H), 2.93–2.90 (m, 2H), 1.87–1.72 (m, 4H), 1.21–1.16 (m, *J* = 6H), 1.07–1.02 (m, 6H); ^{13}C-NMR ($CDCl_3$, 125 MHz) δ(ppm): 176.5, 175.5, 173.6, 167.3, 167.1, 162.5, 156.0, 154.6, 144.1, 132.0, 131.6, 131.0, 129.2, 126.3, 111.4, 107.8, 102.7, 95.6, 94.5, 60.1, 59.9, 33.6, 33.1, 21.2, 20.7, 14.4, 14.2.

Ethyl (E)-3-((5,6-dihydroxy-4-oxo-2-phenyl-4H-chromen-7-yl) oxy) hex-2-enoate (**5d**); yellow powder; yield 11.2%; HRMS(ESI): calcd. $C_{23}H_{21}O_7$, *m/z* 409.1293 $[M - H]^-$, found 409.1289; ^{1}H-NMR (DMSO-d_6, 500 MHz) δ(ppm): 13.03 (s, 1H), 11.36 (s, 1H), 8.07 (d, *J* = 7.5 Hz, 2H), 7.61–7.56 (m, 3H), 7.01 (s, 1H), 6.70 (s, 1H), 4.74 (s, 1H), 3.98 (dd, *J* = 14.5, 6.0 Hz, 2H), 2.86 (t, *J* = 7.0 Hz, 2H), 1.71 (dd, *J* = 15.0, 7.5 Hz, 2H), 1.10 (t, *J* = 7.0 Hz, 3H), 1.00 (t, *J* = 7.5 Hz, 3H); ^{13}C-NMR (DMSO-d_6, 100 MHz) δ(ppm): 182.3, 173.8, 166.3, 163.6, 156.7, 154.1, 152.4, 132.1, 130.7, 129.2, 126.5, 123.7, 104.9, 104.4, 94.7, 92.8, 59.1, 32.3, 20.4, 14.1, 13.5.

Diethyl 3,3′-((5-hydroxy-4-oxo-2-phenyl-4H-chromene-6,7-diyl) bis (oxy)) (2E,2′E)-bis (hex-2-enoate) (**5e**); yellow powder; yield 14.8%; HRMS(ESI): calcd. $C_{31}H_{34}O_9Na$, *m/z* 573.2095 $[M + Na]^+$, found 573.2106; ^{1}H-NMR ($CDCl_3$, 500 MHz) δ(ppm): 12.96 (s, 1H), 7.89 (d, *J* = 7.5 Hz, 2H), 7.60–7.53 (m, 3H), 6.76 (d, *J* = 9.0 Hz, 1H), 5.03 (s, 1H), 4.85 (s, 1H), 4.13–4.06 (m, 4H), 2.93–2.87 (m, 4H), 1.77–1.69 (m, 4H), 1.21 (dd, *J* = 15.2, 7.6 Hz, 6H), 1.06–1.00 (m, 6H); ^{13}C-NMR($CDCl_3$, 125 MHz) δ(ppm): 182.9, 174.0, 173.8, 167.1, 166.7, 165.2, 154.1, 153.8, 151.8, 132.5, 130.9, 129.4, 128.4, 126.6, 109.5, 105.9, 100.7, 98.7, 94.5, 60.0, 59.7, 33.1, 32.8, 21.0, 20.9, 14.4, 14.0, 13.9.

(E)-3-((5-hydroxy-4-oxo-2-phenyl-4H-chromen-7-yl) oxy) but-2-enoic acid (**6a**); yellow powder; yield 69.4%; HRMS(ESI): calcd. $C_{19}H_{13}O_6$, *m/z* 337.0718 $[M + H]^+$, found 337.0711; ^{1}H-NMR (DMSO-d_6, 500 MHz) δ(ppm): 12.93 (s, 1H), 8.14 (d, *J* = 6.4 Hz, 2H), 7.76–7.58 (m, 3H), 7.15 (s, 1H), 7.05 (d, *J* = 2.0 Hz, 1H), 6.61 (d, *J* = 2.0 Hz, 1H), 5.09 (s, 1H), 2.41 (s, 3H); ^{13}C-NMR (DMSO-d_6, 125 MHz) δ(ppm): 182.8, 169.7, 167.6, 164.3, 161.7, 159.3, 157.2, 132.6, 130.6, 129.4, 126.9, 108.1, 105.9, 104.2, 100.7, 100.3, 17.7.

2-(2-methyl-5-(3,5,7-trihydroxy-4-oxo-4H-chromen-2-yl) benzo[d] [1,3] dioxol-2-yl) acetic acid (**6b**); yellow powder; yield 43.7%; HRMS(ESI): calcd. $C_{19}H_{15}O_9$, *m/z* 387.0711 $[M + H]^+$, found 387.0707; ^{1}H-NMR (DMSO-d_6, 500 MHz) δ(ppm): 12.40 (s, 1 H), 7.73 (dd, *J* = 10.5, 1.5 Hz, 1H), 7.61 (d, *J* = 1.5 Hz, 1H), 7.03 (d, *J* = 10.5 Hz, 1H), 6.46 (d, *J* = 2.5 Hz, 1H), 6.19 (d, *J* = 2.5 Hz, 1H), 3.02 (s, 2H), 1.78 (s, 3H); ^{13}C-NMR (DMSO-d_6, 125 MHz) δ(ppm: 217.5, 176.0, 172.1, 169.2, 164.1, 160.7, 156.2, 148.2, 147.1, 146.0, 136.2, 124.8, 122.9, 117.6, 108.4, 107.3, 103.1, 98.3, 93.7, 24.5, 21.1.

2.3. Anti-Cancer Activity Assay

2.3.1. Cell Lines and Cell Culture

The human leukemia cell lines K562 and HEL, the non-small cell lung cancer A549, and the prostate cancer cell line PC3 were obtained from the Key Laboratory of Chemistry for Natural Product of Guizhou Province and Chinese Academy of Science (Guiyang, China). Cells were cultured as a monolayer in DMEM (Hyclone, Germany), supplemented with 10% heat-inactivated research-grade fetal bovine serum (Hyclone, Germany) and penicillin/streptomycin (Sigma, St. Louis, MO, USA) at 37 °C in a humidified atmosphere, containing 5% CO_2.

2.3.2. Cytotoxic Activity Assay

The cytotoxic activity of compounds was measured by MTT assay, using adriamycin as the positive control. Cells were seeded in 96-well microculture plates at a density of 1×10^4 cells/well and left to adhere for 24 h. The cells were then exposed to different concentrations of the compounds for 48 h. MTT was added to each well at a final concentration of 0.5 mg/mL and cells were incubated at 37 °C for an additional 4 h. The medium was then discarded and 200 µL Tris-DMSO solution was added to each well. The dark blue formazan crystals formed were dissolved by slight shaking, and the absorbance was measured at 490 nm, using an ELISA plate reader.

2.3.3. Statistical Analysis

The data were analyzed using SPSS 18.0 and reported as mean ± standard deviation (SD) of the number of experiments indicated. For all the measurements, one-way ANOVA followed by a Student's *t*-test was used to assess the statistical significance of the differences between each group. The statistical significance of the difference between two groups was assessed using the LSD method. $p < 0.05$ was considered to indicate statistical significance. The data are presented as the mean ± standard error of the mean (SEM) of three assays.

3. Results and Discussion

3.1. Synthesis

The optimal reaction conditions were established (Table 1, entry 6). The substrate scope was further extended to other types of allenes (Figure 1). As expected, various substituent groups led to a variety of products. When using either the monoallene (ethyl ester/benzyl ester) or diallene, the Pd catalyst efficiently promoted this C-O functionalization. Intriguingly, the application of triethylamine as a base instead of potassium carbonate was demonstrated to be more efficient for target product purification (**4e**, **4f**). However, completion of the reaction is hard to achieve. Starting flavonoids with OH groups at positions 3′ and 4′ easily generated the 1,3-dioxolane byproducts, instead of the desired ones. The key intermediates **1a**–**1c** were prepared according to reported methods [18–20].

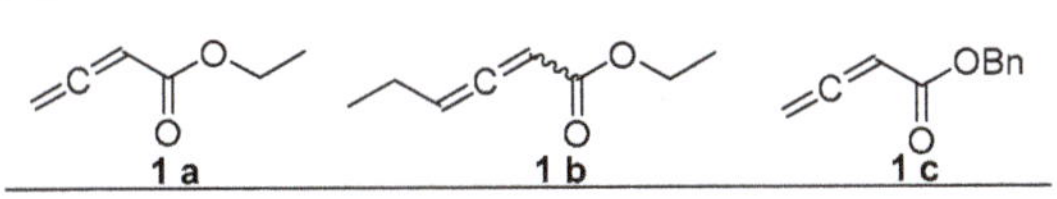

Figure 1. Types of allenes.

Under optimal conditions, as illustrated in Figure 2, a variety of flavonoid substrates was investigated. For instance, flavones and flavonols were well tolerated, providing ample opportunities for further anti-cancer activity evaluation of the derivatives. We found that the property of flavonoid and the substituted phenolic hydroxyl groups had a great impact on the formation of the desired products. Notably, it was more challenging to separate the analog products when more than two hydroxyl groups were presented. Finally, the target products (**3a**–**3i**, **4a**–**4g**, **5a**–**5e**, **6a**, **6b**) were successfully purified by silica gel column chromatography. The configuration of the C=C bond in **3a** and **4a** was determined by the NOE (Nuclear Overhauser Effect) study. The structures of final compounds were characterized by ^{1}H-, ^{13}C-NMR, and MS spectrometry.

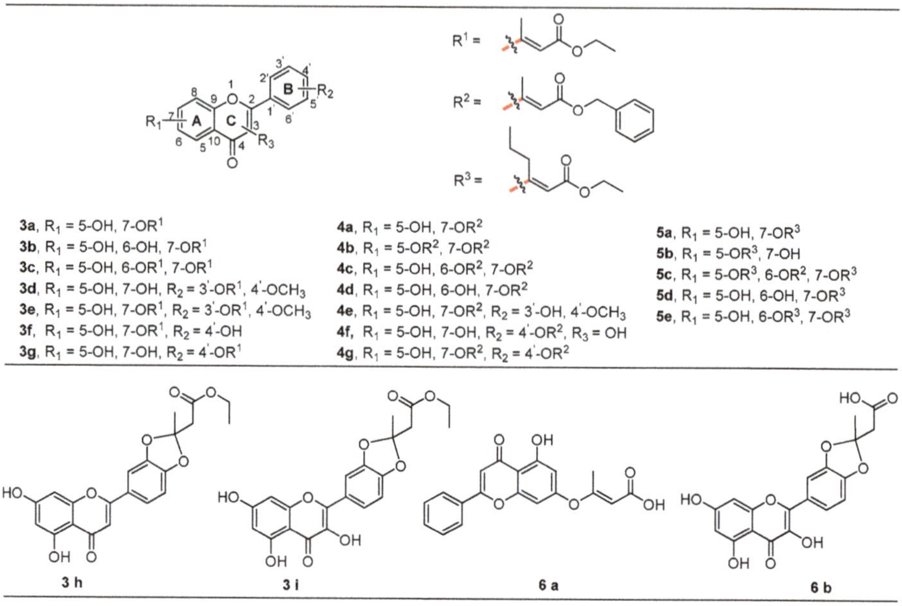

Figure 2. Substrate scope of flavonoids and allenes.

3.2. Anti-Cancer Activity

The anti-tumor activity of all derivatives in vitro was summarized in Table 2. Results showed that the inhibitory effect of compound **4e** on the growth of K562 was six times stronger ($p < 0.01$) than that of the substrate, diosmetin, which indicated that the anti-tumor activity of the diosmetin derivative was associated with the more lipophilic benzyl ester than -OCH_3 moiety at R_6 position of the substrate. Compounds **5e**, **3h**, and **6b** showed better activity ($p < 0.01$) on the proliferation of HEL than that of the substrates, baicalein, kaempferol, and quercetin, respectively. These results suggested that the anti-leukemia activity may be improved by increasing steric hindrance, such as by introducing propyl and 1,3-dioxolane groups onto baicalein. Compound **6b** exhibited an enhanced inhibitory activity on the growth of leukemia cells (K562 and HEL) and non-small cell lung cancer A549 compared with those of **3i**, which can be speculated as the enhanced water solubility associated with the carboxyl group. We then synthesized compounds **3e**, **4b**, and **4c** to improve the anti-cancer activity ($p < 0.01$) on the proliferation of PC3 compared with the substrates, diosmetin, chrysin, and baicalein, respectively. The results suggested that introducing an ethyl and benzyl esters could increase their anti-cancer activity.

Table 2. The anti-cancer activities of the synthetic derivatives.

Compd	Inhibition Rate % (5 μM)			
	K562	A549	HEL	PC3
3a	34.1 ± 4.3	−23.3 ± 2.1	−2.5 ± 3.2	7.1 ± 3.2
3b	28.4 ± 4.9	−14.9 ± 2.8	27.5 ± 4.1	1.5 ± 3.4
3c	23.1 ± 3.2	3.8 ± 1.7	21.2 ± 2.3	16.1 ± 1.2
3d	14.0 ± 1.7	−39.6 ± 2.9	2.7 ± 1.9	36.6 ± 3.6
3e	−45.0 ± 1.9	−20.5 ± 2.5	10.5 ± 2.9	51.7 ± 3.9 **
3f	−13.7 ± 2.2	19.7 ± 2.6	−24.3 ± 2.4	40.4 ± 2.7
3g	26.2 ± 3.1	16.4 ± 2.4	24.9 ± 2.3	38.2 ± 2.5
3h	16.3 ± 3.4	−16.7 ± 2.3	58.6 ± 3.9 **	−15.9 ± 2.6
3i	26.2 ± 3.5	−60.4 ± 2.7	24.9 ± 3.8	42.2 ± 2.1

Table 2. *Cont.*

Compd	Inhibition Rate % (5 μM)			
	K562	A549	HEL	PC3
4a	−33.6 ± 2.3	−36.9±2.0	24.6 ± 2.9	8.9 ± 2.6
4b	−5.0 ± 1.7	−2.7 ± 1.2	−27.1 ± 2.7	56.2 ± 4.0 **
4c	−22.8 ± 2.9	−6.6 ± 1.4	16.2 ± 2.6	51.0 ± 4.7 **
4d	17.3 ± 1.3	−1.9 ± 4.3	18.1 ± 2.5	28.4 ± 2.4
4e	61.9 ± 4.2 **	−3.7 ± 4.3	49.5 ± 2.4	21.9 ± 2.1
4f	−22.6 ± 2.9	−17.5 ± 4.3	10.1 ± 2.1	28.8 ± 2.0
4g	−23.3 ± 2.5	−14.5 ± 1.7	2.7 ± 2.3	36.6 ± 1.9
5a	−8.4 ± 1.2	19.5 ± 1.9	24.6 ± 2.8	21.9± 1.2
5b	18.7 ± 3.5	14.0 ± 2.5	11.4 ± 1.9	32.9± 0.9
5c	19.3 ± 3.1	15.9 ± 2.7	21.3 ± 3.0	31.8 ± 1.2
5d	−10.6 ± 3.0	17.5 ± 2.2	18.7 ± 3.2	30.6± 1.8
5e	−13.4 ± 4.2	21.8 ± 2.1	49.5 ± 2.0 **	39.5 ± 1.7
6a	4.3 ± 1.6	11.7 ± 0.9	28.3 ± 2.2	41.1 ± 1.9
6b	35.7 ± 1.7	38.2 ± 3.5	44.7 ± 1.7 **	35.2 ± 2.6
Chrysin	51.0 ± 4.1	37.5 ± 1.8	21.9 ± 1.3	39.2 ± 2.8
Baicalein	17.7 ± 2.2	29.3 ± 2.1	19.2 ± 3.5	28.3±1.8
Quercetin	−5.0 ± 3.6	8.2 ± 3.0	10.2 ± 3.4	11.3 ± 1.9
Diosmetin	10.9 ± 1.8	7.3 ± 1.2	9.2 ± 3.0	9.5 ± 2.1
Apigenin	−1.5 ± 1.9	5.6 ± 1.1	6.4 ± 2.1	8.3 ± 2.5
Luteolin	19.1 ± 1.7	14.7 ± 1.4	20.4 ± 1.7	16.5 ± 1.7
Kaempferol	−25.3 ± 2.1	8.6 ± 1.3	−24.0 ± 2.4	14.3 ± 2.2

Note: ** represents $p < 0.01$, vs. the inhibition of the substrate to the cancer cell lines. The data represented the average of three independent experiments.

4. Conclusions

Twenty-three flavonoidal ether derivatives were synthesized without the steps of introducing protective groups followed by deprotection. The in vitro tumor growth inhibitory activities of all the derivatives were assayed using four human cancer cell lines, K562, A549, HEL, and PC3. In general, compounds containing 1,3-dioxolane, such as **6b**, possessed broad-spectrum inhibitory activity against the above four cancer cells. Preliminary structure–activity relationship studies indicated that the position-7 substituents were essential for the cytotoxicities of the derivatives. These results provided new insight into developing flavonoid-derived anti-cancer agents.

Author Contributions: Conceptualization, L.J. and M.-L.W.; Methodology, L.J. and X.-Y.Z.; Software, L.J., X.-Y.Z.; Validation, X.-Y.Z. and C.C.; Formal analysis, L.J.; Resources, W.-D.P. and H.L.; Data curation, L.J., Y.L., and M.-L.W.; Writing—original draft preparation, L.J.; Writing—review and editing, L.J., H.R., W.-D.P., and H.L.; Project administration, W.-D.P. and H.L.; Funding acquisition, W.-D.P. and H.L.

Funding: Supported by the National Natural Science Foundation of China (No. 81660580, 81702914) and the Science and Technology Department of Guizhou Province, China (QKHRC[2016]4037, QKHJC[2017]1412).

Acknowledgments: We would like to acknowledge the help of my colleagues Ni Zhang, Xiao-Pan Ma, Chang-Fen Chen, and Sai Jiang.

Conflicts of Interest: The authors declare no conflicts of interest.

References

1. Huang, X.; Liang, J.P.; Hao, B.C. Study on molecular modification and structure-activity relationship of flavonoids. *J. Anhui Arg. Sci.* **2015**, *43*, 57–61.
2. Dhruti, B.; Ronak, S.; Gaurav, K.; Dashora, A. Synthesis and pharmacological activities of flavones: A review. *Indo Am. J. Pharm. Res.* **2016**, *6*, 4345–4363.
3. Craig, W.J. Health-promoting properties of common herbs. *Am. J. Clin. Nutr.* **1999**, *70*, 491S–499S. [CrossRef] [PubMed]

4. Kadarian, C.; Broussalis, A.M.; Mino, J.; Lopez, P.; Gorzalczany, S.; Ferraro, G.; Acevedo, C. Hepatoprotective activity of achyrocline satureioides (Lam) D. C. *Pharmacol. Res.* **2002**, *45*, 57–61. [CrossRef] [PubMed]
5. Pascual, M.E.; Slowing, K.; Carretero, E.; Sánchez Mata, D.; Villar, A. Lippia: Traditional uses, chemistry and pharmacology: A review. *J. Ethnopharmacol.* **2001**, *76*, 201–214. [CrossRef]
6. Samuelsen, A.B. The traditional uses, chemical constituents and biological activities of *Plantago major* L. A review. *J. Ethnopharmacol.* **2000**, *71*, 1–21. [CrossRef]
7. Tang, L.; Feng, Q.; Zhao, J.; Dong, L.; Liu, W.; Yang, C.; Liu, Z. Involvenment of UDP-glucuronosyltranferases and sulfotransferases in the liver and intestinal first- pass metabolism of seven flavones in C57 mice and humans *in vitro*. *Food Chem. Toxicol.* **2012**, *50*, 1460–1467. [CrossRef] [PubMed]
8. Singh, M.; Kaur, M.; Silakari, O. Flavones: An important scaffold for medicinal chemistry. *Eur. J. Med. Chem.* **2014**, *84*, 206–239. [CrossRef] [PubMed]
9. Ma, S.M. Some typical advances in the synthetic applications of allenes. *Chem. Rev.* **2005**, *105*, 2829–2872. [CrossRef] [PubMed]
10. Brasholz, M.; Reissig, H.U.; Zimmer, R. Sugars, alkaloids, and heteroaromatics: Exploring heterocyclic chemistry with alkoxyallenes. *Acc. Chem. Res.* **2009**, *42*, 45–56. [CrossRef] [PubMed]
11. Pfrengle, F.; Reissig, H.U. Amino sugars and their mimetics *Via* 1,2-oxazines. *Chem. Soc. Rev.* **2010**, *39*, 549–557. [CrossRef] [PubMed]
12. Yu, S.C.; Ma, S.M. Allenes in catalytic asymmetric synthesis and natural product syntheses. *Angew. Chem. Int. Ed.* **2012**, *51*, 3074–3112. [CrossRef] [PubMed]
13. Ye, J.T.; Ma, S.M. Palladium-catalyzed cyclization reactions of allenes in the presence of unsaturated carbon-carbon bonds. *Acc. Chem. Res.* **2014**, *47*, 989–1000. [CrossRef] [PubMed]
14. Alcaide, B.; Almendros, P.; Aragoncillo, C. Cyclization reactions of bis(allenes) for the synthesis of polycarbo(hetero)cycles. *Chem. Soc. Rev.* **2014**, *43*, 3106–3135. [CrossRef] [PubMed]
15. Neff, R.K.; Frantz, D.E. Recent applications of chiral allenes in axial-to-central chirality transfer reactions. *Tetrahedron* **2015**, *71*, 7–18. [CrossRef]
16. Jose, L.M.; Lvan, V.; Fernando, L. Allenes and derivatives in gold(I)- and platinum(II)-catalyzed formal cycloadditions. *Acc. Chem. Res.* **2019**, *52*, 465–479.
17. Egle, M.B.; Gianluigi, B.; Michael, S.C.; Giofrè, S. Chapter one—Transition metal- catalyzed intramolecular amination and hydroammination reactions of allenes. *Adv. Organomet. Chem.* **2018**, *69*, 1–71.
18. Campbell, K.A.; House, H.O.; Surber, B.W.; Trahanovsky, W.S. Enones with strained double bonds. 10. use of flash vacuum pyrolysis to obtain bicyclo[3.3.1]non-1-en-3-one. *J. Org. Chem.* **1987**, *52*, 2474–2481. [CrossRef]
19. Rout, L.; Harned, A.M. Allene carboxylates as dipolarophiles in Rh-catalyzed carbonyl ylide cycloadditions. *Chem. Eur. J.* **2009**, *15*, 12926–12928. [CrossRef] [PubMed]
20. Li, R.D.; Leng, P.L.; Liu, B.; Wang, X.; Ge, Z.; Li, R. Efficient and regioselective one-pot synthesis of S-vinyl dithiocarbamates from electron-deficient allenes, amines and CS_2. *Tetrahedron* **2016**, *72*, 5707–5712. [CrossRef]

Sample Availability: Samples of the compounds are available from the authors.

molecules

MDPI

Article

Design, Synthesis, and Mechanism of Dihydroartemisinin–Coumarin Hybrids as Potential Anti-Neuroinflammatory Agents

Haonan Yu [1,†], Zhuang Hou [1,†], Xiaoguang Yang [1], Yanhua Mou [2,*] and Chun Guo [1,*]

1 School of Pharmaceutical Engineering, Shenyang Pharmaceutical University, Shenyang 110016, China; yhna380@hotmail.com (H.Y.); houzhuang8@sina.com (Z.H.); Xiaog_yang@163.com (X.Y.)

2 School of Life Sciences and Biological Pharmacy, Shenyang Pharmaceutical University, Shenyang 110016, China

* Correspondence: mu_hua_jj@sina.com (Y.M.); chunguo@syphu.edu.cn (C.G.); Tel.: +86-24-4352-0226 (C.G.)

† These authors contributed equally to this work.

Received: 6 April 2019; Accepted: 24 April 2019; Published: 28 April 2019

Abstract: Cancer patients frequently suffer from cancer-related fatigue (CRF), which is a complex syndrome associated with weakness and depressed mood. Neuroinflammation is one of the major inducers of CRF. The aim of this study is to find a potential agent not only on the treatment of cancer, but also for reducing CRF level of cancer patients. In this study, total-thirty new Dihydroartemisinin–Coumarin hybrids (DCH) were designed and synthesized. The in vitro cytotoxicity against cancer cell lines (HT-29, MDA-MB-231, HCT-116, and A549) was evaluated. Simultaneously, we also tested the anti-neuroinflammatory activity of DCH. DCH could inhibit the activated microglia N9 release of NO, TNF-α, and IL-6. The docking analysis was shown that MD-2, the coreceptor of TLR4, might be one of the targets of DCH.

Keywords: anticancer; anti-neuroinflammation; coumarin; dihydroartemisinin

1. Introduction

Chemotherapy is an important method in the therapy of cancer, but the adverse side effects of anticancer agents should also be focused on. Gastrointestinal injury induced by chemotherapeutic agents could result in bacterial/endotoxin translocation from the gut to the systemic blood circulation [1,2]. The released endotoxin would cause a systemic inflammatory response including neuroinflammation [3]. Cancer patients frequently suffer from cancer-related fatigue (CRF), which is a complex syndrome associated with weakness and depressed mood. Diana M., Norden et al. demonstrated that the neuroinflammation is one of the major reasons which induce CRF [4]. Currently, there were no effective method to reduce CRF [5]. The aim of this study is to find a potential anti-neuroinflammatory agents which might reduce CRF of cancer patients.

Central nervous system (CNS) consists of two major types of cells, nerve cells and glial cells. Microglia is a major glial cell and plays an important role as the resident macrophage population in the CNS [6,7]. There has been wide recognition that the fully activated microglial cells are neurotoxic. They release reactive oxygen species, nitric oxide (NO), tumor necrosis factor-alpha (TNF-α), and other potentially cytotoxic molecules [8,9]. It means that activation of microglia could induce neuroinflammation.

Lipopolysaccharide (LPS), also known as endotoxin, is a natural Toll-like receptor 4 (TLR4) ligand and it is also a potent microglial activator that can trigger the production of inflammatory mediators. TLR-4, a transmembrane receptor, plays a vital role in the initiation and acceleration of the inflammatory response induced by LPS [10,11]. TLR4 alone does not directly bind LPS and needs the coreceptor MD-2 [12]. MD-2 is linked with the extracellular domain of TLR4 and is indispensable for LPS recognition [13]. MD-2 is a member of the MD-2-related lipid-recognition protein family [14]. MD-2 directly binds to LPS in its hydrophobic cavity with high affinity [15].

Artemisinin and its derivatives have been the first-line antimalarial drug since the late 1990s. Dihydroartemisinin (DHA) is the primary bioactive metabolite of artemisinin and its derivatives, but not artemisinin per se [16]. Additionally, DHA has higher bioavailability and less side effects than artemisinin [17]. Recent research showed that besides antimalarial activity, DHA also exhibits anticancer and anti-inflammatory activity [18–21]. As the anti-inflammatory agent, DHA could decrease LPS-induced protein expression of TLR4 [22].

Coumarins are widely distributed in different parts of plants. There are various pharmacological activities of coumarins, which includes anti-inflammatory [23,24] and anticancer activity [25,26]. As the anticancer agents, coumarins were reported to exhibit negligible or mild side effects [27,28]. Substitution at the C-3 or C-4 position of coumarins exhibit good cytotoxic activity in various cancer cell lines [26,29–31]. Additionally, as anti-inflammatory agents, some kinds of coumarins could also target TLR4/MD-2 complex [32,33].

In our previous study, Dihydroartemisinin–Coumarin hybrids (DCH) were designed and synthesized referring to the principle of hybridization [34,35]. Each of them contains coumarin moiety, DHA moiety and a linker. DCH could inhibit HT-29 cells proliferation and arrest the G_0/G_1 phase of HT-29 cells [35]. They could also suppress cancer cell migration, and induce apoptosis and ferroptosis of HT-29 cancer cells [35]. It also has been confirmed that the DCH having 1,2,3-triazole linker generally exhibit better cytotoxicity exhibition than the others [35].

With this background, total-thirty new DCH were designed and synthesized, and the synthetic approaches were shown in Figure 1. All of them contained 1,2,3-triazole linker. We focused on the modifications of positions 3 and 4 of the coumarin moiety. Due to the new synthesized DCH were for the cancer patients, we evaluated the in vitro cytotoxicity against cancer cell lines (HT-29, MDA-MB-231, HCT-116, and A549). In addition, DCH could inhibit the activated N9 cell release of NO, TNF-α and IL-6. Furthermore, to investigate the mechanism of the anti-neuroinflammatory activity, docking analysis was applied. The results might support that the anti-neuroinflammatory activity was related to inhibiting TLR4/MD-2 complex.

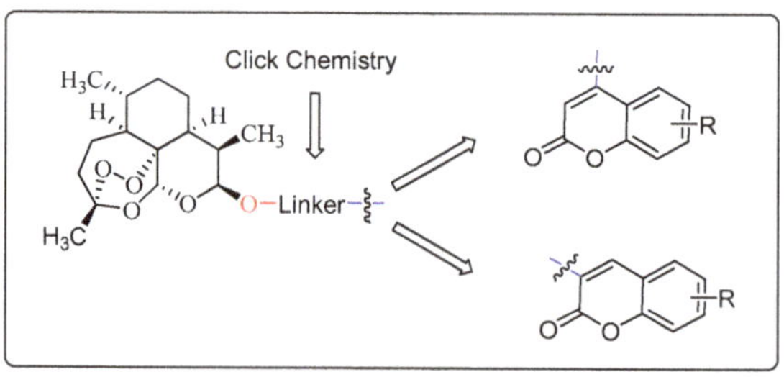

Figure 1. Structures of new designed Dihydroartemisinin–Coumarin hybrids.

2. Results and Discussion

2.1. Chemistry

The synthesis of the intermediates **a–p** and **I–IV** is presented in Scheme 1. The intermediates **I** and **II** were obtained by 2-bromoethanol or 3-bromo-1-propanol, with dihydroartemisinin (DHA), respectively, followed by treating the product with sodium azide. The intermediates **III** and **IV** were synthesized by propargyl alcohol or 3-butyn-1-ol with DHA, respectively. The required 3-methylcoumarin derivatives were obtained by substitution of salicylaldehyde with propionic anhydride in the presence of sodium propionate and triethylamine. The substituted-3-bromomethylcoumarins were prepared by the radical bromination of 3-methylcoumarin derivatives through the reaction with

N-Bromosuccinimide (NBS) in the presence of dibenzoylperoxide [36]. The intermediates **a–e** were synthesized by substituted-3-bromomethylcoumarins via azidation reaction. The required substituted-4-chloromethylcoumarins were prepared by the Pechmann cyclisation [37] of substituted phenols with 4-chloroethylacetoacetate using sulfuric acid as the condensing agent. The intermediates **f–i** were synthesized by substituted-4-chloromethylcoumarin via azidation reaction. To synthesize the intermediates **j–p**, several substituted-4-hydroxycoumarin were prepared by condensing the substituted phenol with malonic acid [38]. Then the products were treated with 3-bromo-1-propyne in the presence of potassium carbonate.

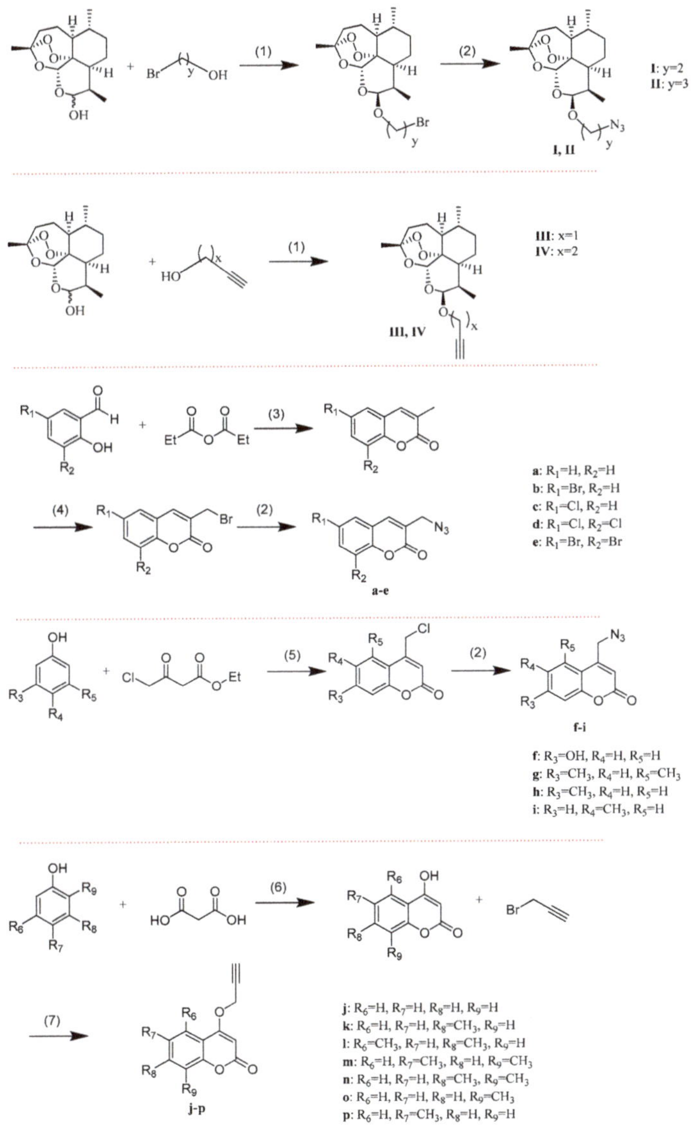

Scheme 1. Synthetic routes of intermediates. Reagents and conditions: (1) $BF_3 \cdot Et_2O$, CH_2Cl_2, 0 °C; (2) NaN_3, DMF, 60 °C; (3) CH_3CH_2COONa, Et_3N, reflux; (4) NBS, BPO, CCl_4, reflux; (5) 70% H_2SO_4, r.t.; (6) $ZnCl_2$, $POCl_3$, 65 °C; and (7) K_2CO_3, DMF, 60 °C.

The synthesis of the desired new compounds was presented in Scheme 2. The target compounds **1a–1e** and **2a–2e** were obtained by the reaction of the intermediates **III** or **IV** with **a–e** via click chemistry, respectively. The target compounds **3f–3i** and **4f–4i** were synthesized by intermediates **III** or **IV** with **f–i** via click chemistry, respectively. The target compounds **5j**, **5l–5o**, and **6j–6p** were prepared by the reaction of the intermediates **I** or **II** with **j–p** via click chemistry, respectively.

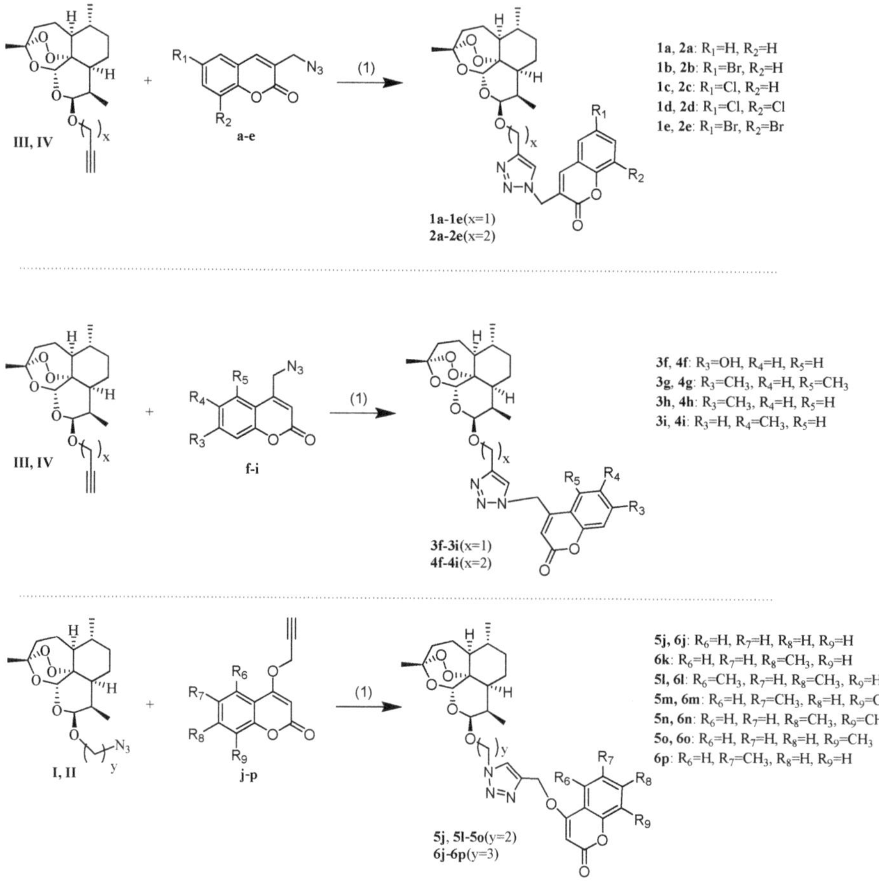

Scheme 2. Synthetic routes of target compounds. Reagents and conditions: (1) CuI, triethylamine, dichloromethane, r.t.

2.2. Biological Assay

2.2.1. In Vitro Cytotoxic Activity of the Compounds

As the anti-neuroinflammatory agents for cancer patients, all newly synthesized compounds were evaluated in vitro for antitumor activity against human breast cancer cell line MDA-MB-231, colorectal cancer cells HT-29 and HCT-116, and lung cancer cell line A549 by using the standard MTT method, respectively. Doxorubicin (DOX) and DHA were used as the reference standard. Additionally, owing to the rapid proliferation, the tumor cells actually was always in hypoxia condition. Therefore, the in vitro cytotoxicity was evaluated in two different conditions (hypoxia and normoxia). All data are summarized in Table 1. Most of the target compounds exhibited moderate activities against the tested cell lines and they showed a general promotion under hypoxia conditions.

The structure–activity relationship was evaluated: (i) the series of compounds **5** and **6** generally exhibited better cytotoxicity activity than that of the series of compounds **3** and **4**, which indicated that the 4-oxygen group in the coumarin moiety as a part of linker could improve the antitumor activity; (ii) although compounds **3** and **4** did not exhibit good activity against three cell lines (MDA-MB-231, HCT-116, and A549), they showed good activity against HT-29 like the other derivatives. Therefore, 4-methyl group in the coumarin moiety could improve the selectivity of DCH against HT-29.

In addition, almost all of the target compounds exhibited good cytotoxicity activity against HT-29. Therefore, HT-29 was selected for the next explorations.

Table 1. IC_{50} (μM) of tested samples in MDA-MB-231, HT-29, HCT-116, and A549 cell lines.

	HT-29		**MDA-MB-231**		**HCT-116**		**A549**	
	Hypoxia	**Normoxia**	**Hypoxia**	**Normoxia**	**Hypoxia**	**Normoxia**	**Hypoxia**	**Normoxia**
DOX	<0.1	0.11	0.69	1.37	>2	1.29	>2	>2
DHA	11.74	51.10	45.93	>100	25.89	10.33	>100	>100
1a	14.29	18.40	30.47	64.97	49.79	48.90	53.87	83.48
1b	13.14	21.35	>100	>100	>100	>100	>100	>100
1c	26.37	35.41	32.26	>100	40.38	60.30	48.70	73.49
1d	13.34	14.94	33.93	68.85	48.61	60.01	45.42	53.34
1e	26.95	15.32	45.46	77.89	>100	54.45	59.75	>100
2a	19.42	>100	>100	>100	>100	>100	>100	>100
2b	12.09	9.75	36.86	37.74	>100	55.99	60.16	>100
2c	19.61	17.46	32.47	43.98	64.37	49.48	66.87	87.15
2d	30.81	19.54	47.92	88.46	46.51	53.19	69.67	96.48
2e	13.92	38.52	44.14	>100	86.49	94.16	79.37	>100
3f	15.46	37.83	63.07	>100	67.74	>100	98.00	>100
3g	15.86	23.89	>100	>100	>100	>100	>100	>100
3h	32.04	>100	>100	>100	>100	>100	>100	>100
3i	8.57	16.36	22.81	>100	>100	64.99	62.27	>100
4f	11.30	32.30	78.79	>100	>100	>100	>100	>100
4g	9.33	13.85	22.71	>100	25.65	34.50	>100	>100
4h	56.35	>100	>100	>100	>100	>100	>100	>100
4i	39.02	>100	>100	>100	>100	>100	>100	>100
5j	12.25	30.03	69.41	100.00	>100	77.20	>100	>100
5l	3.76	2.78	>100	>100	>100	>100	>100	>100
5m	5.89	12.88	13.04	14.17	44.81	62.82	1.282	2.670
5n	8.90	10.19	11.68	11.04	32.92	25.64	2.443	2.107
5o	21.25	16.09	16.54	37.41	38.49	29.69	45.06	50.37
6j	7.42	10.49	33.40	67.42	32.84	25.90	49.03	53.37
6k	5.32	6.85	14.46	38.56	33.70	28.13	9.49	14.92
6l	3.40	8.41	6.85	1.17	27.92	26.90	9.78	6.88
6m	5.90	22.43	18.74	24.64	93.53	42.05	20.14	27.87
6n	4.19	9.16	10.84	13.35	33.74	22.51	0.039	30.40
6o	29.02	81.57	18.57	47.65	42.35	12.09	39.92	78.07
6p	12.48	7.49	10.33	22.08	38.05	35.33	18.82	18.85

2.2.2. Morphological Changes and Effect of Compound 5n on Cell Viability

As shown in A–F of Figure 2, there showed a concentration-dependent cell death after treatment with compound **5n** for 48 h. As the concentration up to 100 μM, the compound **5n** could obviously inhibit the proliferation of HT-29. As shown in the (G) of Figure 2, after HT-29 cells were treated with different concentrations of **5n** for 48 h, the cell viability decreased in a dose-dependent manner.

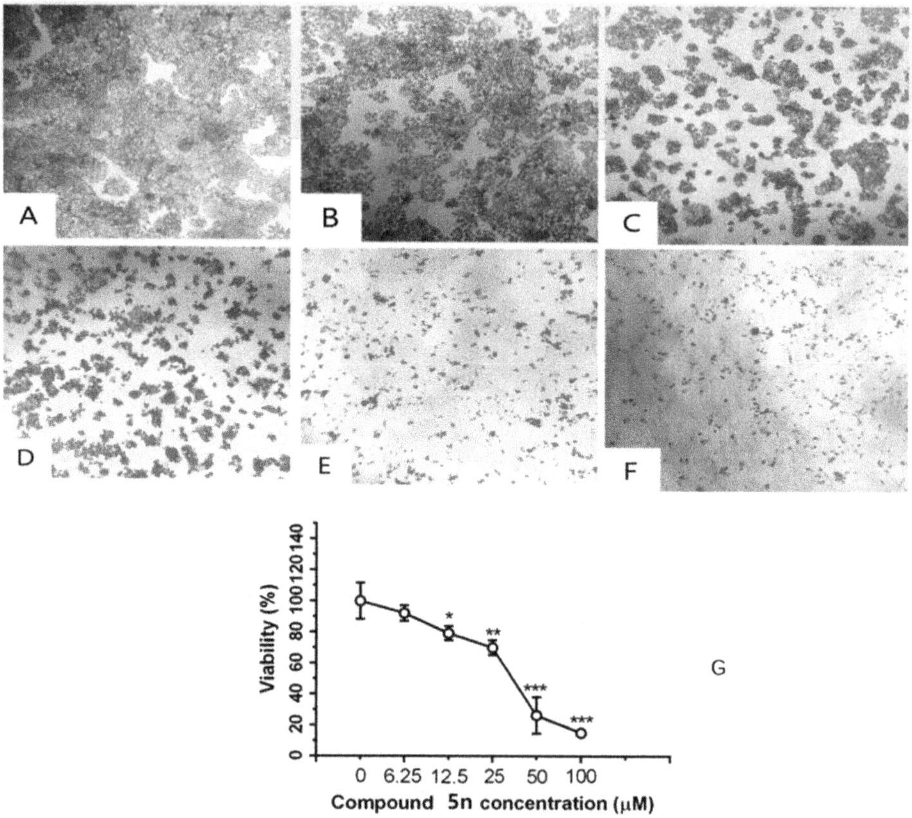

Figure 2. Inhibition of compound **5n** on cell viability in HT-29 cells by MTT staining. Cells were treated with (**A**) 0 μM, (**B**) 6.25 μM, (**C**) 12.5 μM, (**D**) 25.0 μM, (**E**) 50.0 μM, and (**F**) 100.0 μM compound **5n** for 48 h. Representative images were shown; 200×. (**G**) Cells were treated with 6.25, 12.5, 25, 50, and 100 μM compound **5n** for 48 h. Data were shown as mean ± SD. * $p < 0.05$, ** $p < 0.01$ and *** $p < 0.001$ compared with group 0 μM.

2.2.3. Anti-Neuroinflammatory Activity

The anti-neuroinflammatory activity of DCH was evaluated and then the representative compounds were selected for the further study. As shown in Table 2, murine microglial N9 cells were treated with 1μg/mL LPS for 48 h and the NO level in the medium was measured as the preliminary screening. Most of the tested compounds exhibited good anti-inflammatory activity, and especially the IC_{50} of some compounds were even less than 1 μM. Among them, compound **5n** had the best activity and the IC_{50} reached 0.22 μM. In addition, in order to exclude the death influence, MTT-IC20 of all the compounds were measured. The results showed that DCH did not exhibit cytotoxic activity in N9 cells. The exact reason was still unclear, but we supposed that it might be related to the homeostasis of cells. The tumor cells actually were always in hypoxia condition, in which DCH could promote the cytotoxic activity against tumor cells. In brief, DCH could reduce the release of NO caused by LPS-induced microglial cells.

Table 2. IC_{50} of tested samples in LPS-induced N9 cells for the inhibition of NO; IC_{20} of tested samples in N9 cells for cytotoxic activity.

Compound.	NO-IC_{50} (μM)	MTT-IC_{20} (μM)
1a	1.46	>10
1b	>10	>10
1c	5.33	>10
1d	1.60	>10
1e	0.48	>10
2a	0.97	>10
2b	0.64	>10
2c	2.66	>10
2d	1.35	>10
2e	0.94	>10
3f	0.37	>10
3g	>10	>10
3h	>10	>10
3i	0.72	>10
4f	2.03	>10
4g	1.36	>10
4h	5.69	>10
4i	>10	>10
5j	1.59	>10
5l	3.36	7.13
5m	1.08	1.04
5n	0.22	2.44
5o	0.57	>10
6j	0.29	>10
6k	1.91	>10
6l	0.52	>10
6m	5.80	>10
6n	1.13	6.53
6o	1.43	>10
6p	1.42	>10
DHA	1.58	>10
Minocycline	>10	>10

NO Capture Capability

Sodium nitroprusside (SNP) is a NO donor. In this experiment, the reason of the DCH reducing NO level was preliminary explored. As shown in Figure 3, the results showed that the compounds only partially reduced NO levels by direct NO capture. That means the main reason of the NO level reduction is due to species-specific effect.

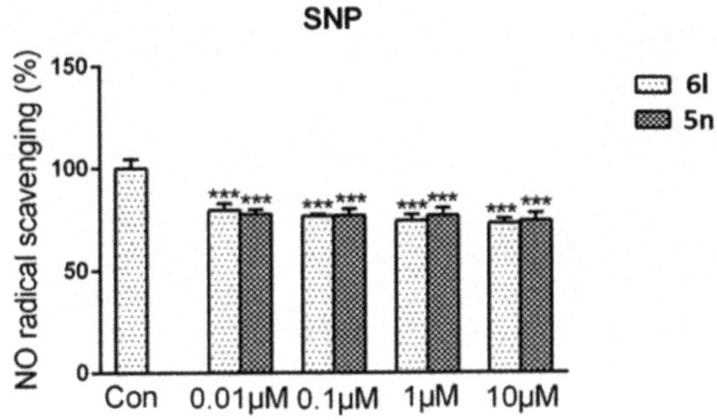

Figure 3. Compound 6l and 5n had NO radical scavenging activity. 6l (0.01 μM, 0.1 μM, 1 μM, and 10 μM) or **5n** (0.01 μM, 0.1 μM, 1 μM, and 10 μM) was added to a concentration of 0.5 mM SNP solution. After reacted for 1 h under normal sun light at room temperature, Griess reagent was added and the optical density was observed at 540 nm. Data were shown as mean ± SD. *** $p < 0.001$ compared with control group.

Effect of Representative Compounds on TNF-α and IL-6 Release

As shown in Table 3, four kinds of DCH were involved to measure the effect on the release of TNF-α and IL-6 from the microglia cells which induced by LPS for 48 h. The results showed that compounds **2b**, **2c**, **5n**, and **6p** could inhibit the release of TNF-α with the inhibition rate of 22% to 32% and the release of IL-6 with the inhibition rate of 26% to 43%. The results indicated that the inhibition effect of DCH on NO release was not only by nonspecific effects, but also by slightly influencing the synthesis and release of upstream inflammatory pathway.

Table 3. The inhibition of compounds (1 μM) on cytokines release (48 h) of the murine microglial cell line N9 induced by lipopolysaccharide (LPS) (1 μg/mL).

Group	TNF-α (pg/mL)	Inhibition (%)	IL-6 (pg/mL)	Inhibition (%)
Con	155.54 ± 79.61	–	0	–
LPS	4455.87 ± 518.24 #	–	1154.44 ± 148.48 #	–
2b	3285.99 ± 1062.40	27.20	797.52 ± 140.74 *	30.92
2c	3077.03 ± 375.48	32.06	850.24 ± 112.47	26.35
5n	3508.08 ± 368.72	22.04	656.75 ± 79.49 **	43.11
6p	3451.29 ± 646.50	23.36	747.80 ± 125.56 *	35.22

# $p < 0.001$ compared with control group, * $p < 0.05$ ** $p < 0.01$ compared with LPS group.

Docking Analysis

Toll-like receptor 4 (TLR4) and its coreceptor—MD-2—are the target of LPS, which could influence innate immune response to release potentially cytotoxic molecules. MD-2 is linked with the extracellular domain of TLR4 and is indispensable for LPS recognition [13]. Therefore, this docking analysis was applied to explore whether or not the target compounds inhibit MD-2 to reduce the release of inflammatory mediators. Umeharu Ohto et al. [39] had revealed the crystal structure of mouse TLR4/MD-2/LPS complex, which was shown in Figure 4. In their study, MD-2 directly bound to LPS in its hydrophobic cavity with high affinity. With this background, compound **5n** was used as the ligand to explore the relationship between DCH and TLR4/MD-2/LPS complex. As shown in Figure 5, compound **5n** could integrate closely with the hydrophobic cavity of MD-2, which is the important TLR4/MD-2/LPS binding position. That means the DCH might disturb the interactions between LPS and TLR4/MD-2 complex. The minimum binding energy of (ΔG) is −10.08 kcal/mol. Given to this result, we supposed TLR4/MD-2 complex is likely to be one of the drug targets of DCH.

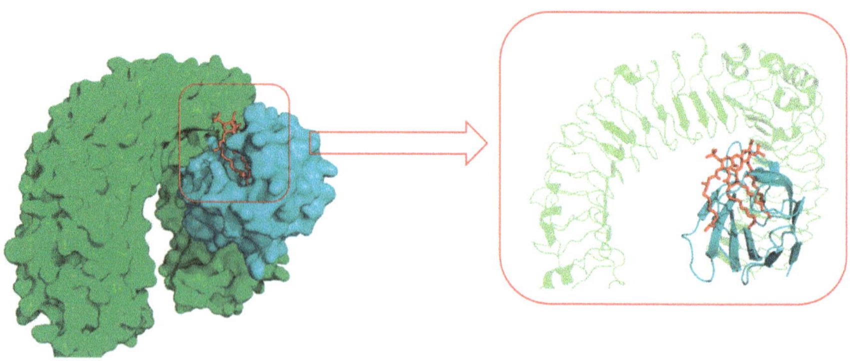

Figure 4. The surface representation of LPS (red) and Toll-like receptor 4 (TLR4) (green)/MD-2 (cyan) binding pocket (PDB: 3VQ2).

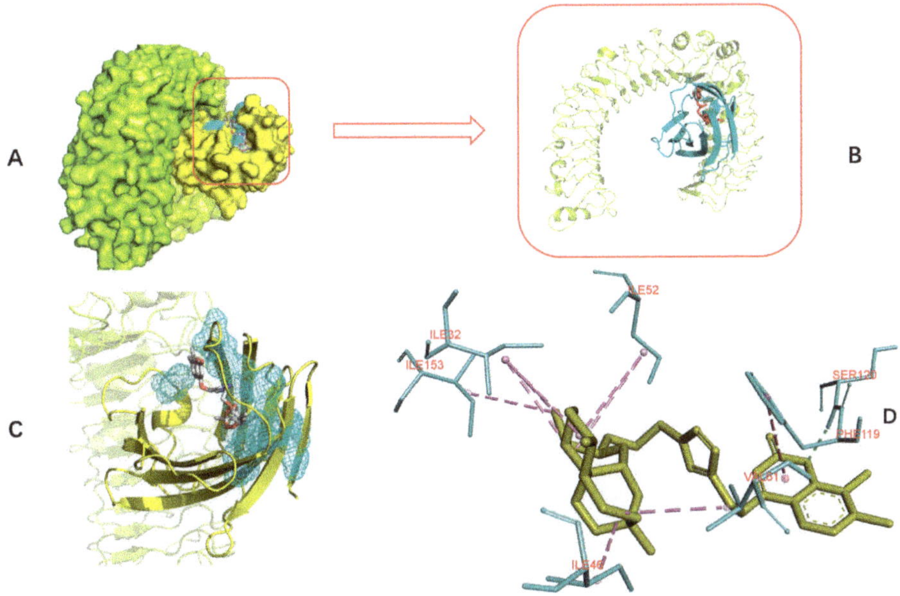

Figure 5. Interaction diagrams of the selected docked conformations of compound 5n to TLR4/MD-2 complex. (**A**) The surface representation of compound **5n** and TLR4 (limon)/MD-2 (yellow) binding pocket. (**B**) The magnified representation of compound **5n** (red) and TLR4 (limon)/MD-2 (cyan) binding pocket. (**C**) The interface of compound **5n** and TLR4/MD-2 complex; (**D**) 3D ligand interactions diagram. Dotted line; pink: alkyl hydrophobic; blue: pi hydrophobic; green: hydrogen bond.

3. Conclusions

Total-thirty new DCH were designed and synthesized. Most of the target compounds exhibited moderate activities against the tested cell lines and they showed a general promotion under hypoxia conditions. Meanwhile, the new potential activity of DCH was found that DCH could exhibit anti-neuroinflammatory activity. DCH could inhibit the release of NO, TNF-α, and IL-6, which were induced by LPS. The docking analysis was shown that MD-2, the coreceptor of TLR4, might be one of the targets of DCH. Additionally, DCH could also reduce NO levels by direct NO capture. In brief, DCH were the potential anti-neuroinflammatory agents which might reduce CRF of cancer patients.

4. Experimental Section

4.1. Chemistry

Unless otherwise specified, all solvents and reagents were commercially available and used without further purification. Analytical TLC was performed using silica gel precoated GF254 plates. The ^{1}H-NMR and ^{13}C-NMR spectra were recorded at 600 MHz and 150 MHZ on a Bruker AV-400 spectrometer (Bruker Bioscience, Billerica, MA, USA), using $CDCl_3$ as solvent with tetramethylsilane as the internal standard. NMR spectra were analyzed using MestReNova. High-resolution mass spectra (HRMS) were measured using an Agilent Accurate-Mass Q-TOF 6530 (Agilent, Santa Clara, CA, USA) instrument in ESI mode. The ^{1}H-NMR and ^{13}C-NMR spectra of synthesized compounds, please see the supplementary materials.

4.1.1. General Procedure for the Synthesis of Compounds **1a–1e** and **2a–2e**

Substituted coumarin (**a–e**) (10 mmol), substituted DHA (**III** or **IV**) (10 mmol), and triethylamine (10 mmol) were dissolved in 20 mL CH_2Cl_2. In addition, CuI (100 mg) was added and the reaction mixture was stirred at room temperature for 8 h under the protection of nitrogen. The mixture was filtered, washed with water, dried over Na_2SO_4 and evaporated to dryness. The crude product was purified through column chromatography.

3-((4-((10S)-dihydroartemisininoxy)methyl-1H-1,2,3-triazol-1-yl)-methyl)-2H-1-chromen-2-one (**1a**) White solid; m.p. 73–75 °C; yield 52%; ^{1}H NMR (600 MHz, $CDCl_3$) δ (ppm): 7.77 (s, 1H), 7.68 (s, 1H), 7.56 (t, *J* = 7.9 Hz, 1H), 7.47 (d, *J* = 7.7 Hz, 1H), 7.34 (d, *J* = 8.4 Hz, 1H), 7.30 (t, *J* = 7.6 Hz, 1H), 5.47 (s, 2H), 5.39 (s, 1H), 4.94 (d, *J* = 12.6 Hz, 1H), 4.92 (d, *J* = 3.5 Hz, 1H), 4.68 (d, *J* = 12.6 Hz, 1H), 2.67–2.60 (m, 1H), 2.38–2.31 (m, 1H), 2.01–1.97 (m, 1H), 1.85–1.81 (m, 1H), 1.77–1.68 (m, 3H), 1.59 (dd, *J* = 13.2, 3.4 Hz, 1H), 1.46–1.43 (m, 1H), 1.41 (s, 3H), 1.31–1.18 (m, 1H), 1.26–1.16 (m, 2H), 0.91 (d, *J* = 6.3 Hz, 3H), 0.88 (d, *J* = 7.3 Hz, 3H); ^{13}C NMR (150 MHz, $CDCl_3$) δ (ppm): 159.64, 152.65, 144.62, 141.31, 131.46, 127.30, 123.92, 122.67, 121.84, 117.53, 115.71, 103.10, 100.77, 86.93, 80.06, 76.22, 76.01, 75.80, 60.70, 51.47, 47.97, 43.33, 36.33, 35.36, 33.52, 29.78, 25.09, 23.59, 23.41, 19.30, 11.99; ESI-HRMS [M + Na]$^+$: (*m/z*) Calcd. for $C_{28}H_{33}N_3O_7Na$: 546.2216. Found: 546.2181.

6-bromo-3-((4-((10S)-dihydroartemisininoxy)methyl-1H-1,2,3-triazol-1-yl)-methyl)-2H-1-chromen-2-one (**1b**) White solid; m.p. 78–80 °C; yield 48%; ^{1}H NMR (600 MHz, $CDCl_3$) δ (ppm): 7.75 (s, 1H), 7.64 (dd, *J* = 8.8, 2.3 Hz, 1H), 7.61 (d, *J* = 2.3 Hz, 1H), 7.55 (s, 1H), 7.24 (d, *J* = 8.8 Hz, 1H), 5.47 (s, 2H), 5.39 (s, 1H), 4.94 (d, *J* = 12.7 Hz, 1H), 4.93 (d, *J* = 3.5 Hz, 1H), 4.69 (d, *J* = 12.8 Hz, 1H), 2.67–2.63 (m, 1H), 2.38–2.33 (m, 1H), 2.03–1.99 (m, 1H), 1.86–1.82 (m, 1H), 1.75–1.70 (m, 2H), 1.62–1.58 (m, 2H), 1.42 (s, 3H), 1.31–1.19 (m, 4H), 0.92 (d, *J* = 6.3 Hz, 3H), 0.89 (d, *J* = 7.4 Hz, 3H); ^{13}C NMR (150 MHz, $CDCl_3$) δ (ppm): 158.90, 151.42, 144.74, 139.67, 134.18, 129.51, 123.17, 122.67, 119.00, 117.43, 116.53, 103.12, 100.87, 86.95, 80.06, 76.20, 75.99, 75.78, 60.76, 51.46, 47.82, 43.32, 36.36, 35.36, 33.52, 29.79, 25.10, 23.62, 23.42, 19.30, 12.00; ESI-HRMS [M + Na]$^+$: (*m/z*) Calcd. for $C_{28}H_{32}BrN_3O_7Na$: 624.1321. Found: 624.1264.

6-chloro-3-((4-((10S)-dihydroartemisininoxy)methyl-1H-1,2,3-triazol-1-yl)-methyl)-2H-1-chromen-2-one (**1c**) White solid; m.p. 93–95 °C; yield 41%; ^{1}H NMR (600 MHz, $CDCl_3$) δ (ppm): 7.75 (s, 1H), 7.56 (s, 1H), 7.51 (dd, *J* = 8.8, 2.5 Hz, 1H), 7.45 (d, *J* = 2.4 Hz, 1H), 7.30 (d, *J* = 8.9 Hz, 1H), 5.47 (s, 2H), 5.39 (s, 1H), 4.95 (d, *J* = 12.7 Hz, 1H), 4.93 (d, *J* = 3.6 Hz, 1H), 4.69 (d, *J* = 12.6 Hz, 1H), 2.68–2.62 (m, 1H), 2.35 (td, *J* = 14.0, 4.0 Hz, 1H), 2.03–1.99 (m, 1H), 1.87–1.82 (m, 1H), 1.75–1.71 (m, 2H), 1.62–1.59 (m, 1H), 1.48–1.43 (m, 2H), 1.42 (s, 3H), 1.31–1.19 (m, 3H), 0.92 (d, *J* = 6.3 Hz, 3H), 0.89 (d, *J* = 7.4 Hz, 3H); ^{13}C NMR (150 MHz, $CDCl_3$) δ (ppm): 158.96, 150.95, 144.73, 139.79, 131.37, 129.27, 126.46, 123.19, 122.67, 118.51, 117.16, 103.12, 100.86, 86.95, 80.06, 76.21, 75.99, 75.78, 60.75, 51.47, 47.84, 43.33, 36.36, 35.36, 33.52, 29.79, 25.10, 23.62, 23.42, 19.30, 12.00; ESI-HRMS [M + Na]$^+$: (*m/z*) Calcd. for $C_{28}H_{32}ClN_3O_7Na$: 580.1826. Found: 580.1788.

6,8-dichloro-3-((4-((10S)-dihydroartemisininoxy)methyl-1H-1,2,3-triazol-1-yl)-methyl)-2H-1-chromen-2-one (**1d**) White solid; m.p. 113–115 °C; yield 60%; ^{1}H NMR (600 MHz, $CDCl_3$) δ (ppm): 7.75 (s, 1H), 7.61 (d, *J* = 2.3 Hz, 1H), 7.55 (s, 1H), 7.37 (d, *J* = 2.4 Hz, 1H), 5.48 (s, 2H), 5.37 (s, 1H), 4.96–4.92 (m, 2H), 4.70 (d, *J* = 12.7 Hz, 1H), 2.69–2.62 (m, 1H), 2.38–2.33 (m, 1H), 2.04–1.99 (m, 1H), 1.87–1.82 (m, 1H), 1.76–1.72 (m, 3H), 1.62–1.59 (m, 1H), 1.42 (s, 3H), 1.32–1.18 (m, 4H), 0.92 (d, *J* = 6.3 Hz, 3H), 0.89 (d, *J* = 7.3 Hz, 3H); ^{13}C NMR (150 MHz, $CDCl_3$) δ (ppm): 157.92, 146.92, 144.86, 139.45, 131.36, 129.12, 125.03, 124.04, 122.68, 121.71, 119.30, 103.13, 100.95, 86.94, 80.04, 76.20, 75.99, 75.78, 60.80, 51.44, 47.63, 43.31, 36.37, 35.35, 33.51, 29.79, 25.09, 23.61, 23.42, 19.28, 12.00; ESI-HRMS [M + Na]$^+$: (*m/z*) Calcd. for $C_{28}H_{31}Cl_2N_3O_7Na$: 614.1437. Found: 614.1428.

6,8-dibromo-3-((4-((10S)-dihydroartemisininoxy)methyl-1H-1,2,3-triazol-1-yl)-methyl)-2H-1-chromen-2-one (**1e**) White solid; m.p. 103–105 °C; yield 61%; ^{1}H NMR (600 MHz, $CDCl_3$) δ (ppm): 7.90 (d, *J* = 2.2 Hz, 1H), 7.75 (s, 1H), 7.56 (d, *J* = 2.2 Hz, 1H), 7.52 (s, 1H), 5.48 (s, 2H), 5.37 (s, 1H), 4.96–4.92 (m, 2H), 4.70 (d, *J* = 12.7 Hz, 1H), 2.67–2.63 (m, 1H), 2.38–2.33 (m, 1H), 2.03–1.99 (m, 1H), 1.87–1.82 (m, 1H),

1.76–1.72 (m, 2H), 1.62–1.58 (m, 4H), 1.42 (s, 3H), 1.25–1.19 (m, 2H), 0.92 (d, *J* = 6.3 Hz, 3H), 0.90 (d, *J* = 7.4 Hz, 3H); ^{13}C NMR (150 MHz, $CDCl_3$) δ (ppm): 158.01, 148.45, 144.87, 139.36, 136.89, 128.75, 123.97, 122.67, 119.74, 116.48, 110.29, 103.13, 100.97, 86.95, 80.04, 76.20, 75.99, 75.78, 60.82, 51.45, 47.56, 43.31, 36.37, 35.35, 33.51, 29.79, 25.09, 23.62, 23.42, 19.30, 12.00; ESI-HRMS [M + Na]$^+$: (*m*/*z*) Calcd. for $C_{28}H_{31}Br_2N_3O_7Na$: 702.0426. Found: 702.0421.

3-((4-(2-((10S)-dihydroartemisininoxy)ethyl)-1H-1,2,3-triazol-1-yl)-methyl)-2H-1-chromen-2-one (**2a**) White solid; m.p. 143–145 °C; yield 66%; ^{1}H NMR (600 MHz, $CDCl_3$) δ (ppm): 7.65 (s, 1H), 7.63 (s, 1H), 7.56 (ddd, *J* = 8.7, 7.3, 1.6 Hz, 1H), 7.47 (dd, *J* = 7.8, 1.6 Hz, 1H), 7.35 (d, *J* = 8.4 Hz, 1H), 7.30 (td, *J* = 7.5, 1.1 Hz, 1H), 5.44 (s, 2H), 5.29 (d, *J* = 9.7 Hz, 1H), 4.78 (d, *J* = 3.6 Hz, 1H), 4.13–4.09 (m, 1H), 3.69–3.65 (m, 1H), 3.07–2.97 (m, 2H), 2.61–2.55 (m, 1H), 2.33 (td, *J* = 14.0, 4.0 Hz, 1H), 2.01–1.97 (m, 1H), 1.85–1.81 (m, 1H), 1.71–1.67 (m, 2H), 1.59–1.56 (m, 1H), 1.41 (s, 3H), 1.40–1.38 (m, 1H), 1.28–1.16 (m, 3H), 0.91 (d, *J* = 6.3 Hz, 3H), 0.89–0.83 (m, 1H), 0.80 (d, *J* = 7.3 Hz, 3H); ^{13}C NMR (150 MHz, $CDCl_3$) δ (ppm): 159.65, 152.64, 144.77, 141.15, 131.43, 127.30, 123.90, 121.98, 121.78, 117.52, 115.70, 103.03, 100.92, 86.84, 80.02, 76.21, 76.00, 75.78, 66.18, 51.47, 47.86, 43.28, 36.34, 35.36, 33.55, 29.79, 25.57, 25.14, 23.62, 23.34, 19.33, 11.93; ESI-HRMS [M + Na]$^+$: (*m*/*z*) Calcd. for $C_{29}H_{35}N_3O_7Na$: 560.2373. Found: 560.2417.

6-bromo-3-((4-(2-((10S)-dihydroartemisininoxy)ethyl)-1H-1,2,3-triazol-1-yl)-methyl)-2H-1-chromen-2-one (**2b**) White solid; m.p. 138–140 °C; yield 52%; ^{1}H NMR (600 MHz, $CDCl_3$) δ (ppm): 7.64 (dd, *J* = 8.8, 2.3 Hz, 1H), 7.61 (d, *J* = 2.3 Hz, 1H), 7.60 (s, 1H), 7.52 (s, 1H), 7.23 (d, *J* = 8.8 Hz, 1H), 5.43 (s, 2H), 5.28 (s, 1H), 4.79 (d, *J* = 3.5 Hz, 1H), 4.13–4.09 (m, 1H), 3.70–3.66 (m, 1H), 3.07–2.98 (m, 2H), 2.62–2.57 (m, 1H), 2.34 (td, *J* = 14.0, 4.0 Hz, 1H), 2.01–1.98 (m, 1H), 1.86–1.81 (m, 1H), 1.71–1.67 (m, 2H), 1.60–1.56 (m, 1H), 1.42 (s, 3H), 1.40–1.37 (m, 1H), 1.27–1.17 (m, 3H), 0.92 (d, *J* = 6.2 Hz, 3H), 0.89–0.85 (m, 1H), 0.82 (d, *J* = 7.3 Hz, 3H); ^{13}C NMR (150 MHz, $CDCl_3$) δ (ppm): 158.90, 151.40, 144.86, 139.50, 134.15, 129.51, 123.31, 121.76, 118.99, 117.41, 116.51, 103.06, 100.92, 86.85, 80.00, 76.20, 75.99, 75.78, 66.18, 51.45, 47.72, 43.26, 36.37, 35.35, 33.55, 29.78, 25.56, 25.14, 23.63, 23.35, 19.32, 11.95; ESI-HRMS [M + Na]$^+$: (*m*/*z*) Calcd. for $C_{29}H_{34}BrN_3O_7Na$: 638.1478. Found: 638.1508.

6-chloro-3-((4-(2-((10S)-dihydroartemisininoxy)ethyl)-1H-1,2,3-triazol-1-yl)-methyl)-2H-1-chromen-2-one (**2c**) White solid; m.p. 138–140 °C; yield 52%; ^{1}H NMR (600 MHz, $CDCl_3$) δ (ppm): 7.60 (s, 1H), 7.53 (s, 1H), 7.50 (dd, *J* = 8.8, 2.5 Hz, 1H), 7.45 (d, *J* = 2.4 Hz, 1H), 7.29 (d, *J* = 8.8 Hz, 1H), 5.43 (d, *J* = 1.1 Hz, 2H), 5.28 (s, 1H), 4.79 (d, *J* = 3.6 Hz, 1H), 4.13–4.09 (m, 1H), 3.70–3.66 (m, 1H), 3.05–2.99 (m, 2H), 2.61–2.58 (m, 1H), 2.37–2.31 (m, 1H), 2.01–1.98 (m, 1H), 1.86–1.81 (m, 1H), 1.70–1.68 (m, 2H), 1.60–1.56 (m, 1H), 1.42 (s, 3H), 1.41–1.36 (m, 1H), 1.26–1.17 (m, 3H), 0.92 (d, *J* = 6.2 Hz, 3H), 0.89–0.85 (m, 1H), 0.82 (d, *J* = 7.3 Hz, 3H); ^{13}C NMR (150 MHz, $CDCl_3$) δ (ppm): 158.97, 150.93, 144.87, 139.62, 131.34, 129.25, 126.47, 123.35, 121.76, 118.51, 117.14, 103.06, 100.93, 86.85, 80.00, 76.20, 75.99, 75.78, 66.19, 51.45, 47.72, 43.27, 36.37, 35.35, 33.56, 29.79, 25.57, 25.14, 23.63, 23.35, 19.32, 11.95; ESI-HRMS [M + Na]$^+$: (*m*/*z*) Calcd. for $C_{29}H_{34}ClN_3O_7Na$: 594.1983. Found: 594.2002.

6,8-dichloro-3-((4-(2-((10S)-dihydroartemisininoxy)ethyl)-1H-1,2,3-triazol-1-yl)-methyl)-2H-1-chromen-2-one (**2d**) White solid; m.p. 101–103 °C; yield 50%; ^{1}H NMR (600 MHz, $CDCl_3$) δ (ppm): 7.60 (d, *J* = 2.2 Hz, 2H), 7.52 (s, 1H), 7.37 (d, *J* = 2.3 Hz, 1H), 5.45 (s, 2H), 5.27 (s, 1H), 4.79 (d, *J* = 3.5 Hz, 1H), 4.13–4.08 (m, 1H), 3.71–3.67 (m, 1H), 3.04–3.01 (m, 2H), 2.61–2.59 (m, 1H), 2.34 (td, *J* = 14.0, 4.0 Hz, 1H), 2.02–1.98 (m, 1H), 1.85–1.82 (m, 1H), 1.71–1.68 (m, 2H), 1.60–1.58 (m, 1H), 1.42 (s, 3H), 1.41–1.36 (m, 1H), 1.26–1.17 (m, 3H), 0.92 (d, *J* = 6.1 Hz, 3H), 0.90–0.85 (m, 1H), 0.82 (d, *J* = 7.3 Hz, 3H); ^{13}C NMR (150 MHz, $CDCl_3$) δ (ppm): 157.93, 146.90, 144.92, 139.29, 131.34, 129.12, 125.04, 124.16, 121.82, 121.70, 119.30, 103.07, 100.94, 86.86, 79.99, 76.20, 75.99, 75.78, 66.17, 51.44, 47.57, 43.26, 36.39, 35.35, 33.55, 29.78, 25.53, 25.13, 23.63, 23.35, 19.32, 11.95; ESI-HRMS [M + Na]$^+$: (*m*/*z*) Calcd. for $C_{29}H_{33}Cl_2N_3O_7Na$: 628.1593. Found: 628.1360.

6,8-dibromo-3-((4-(2-((10S)-dihydroartemisininoxy)ethyl)-1H-1,2,3-triazol-1-yl)-methyl)-2H-1-chromen-2-one (**2e**) White solid; m.p. 93–95 °C; yield 44%; ^{1}H NMR (600 MHz, $CDCl_3$) δ (ppm): 7.83 (d, *J* = 2.1 Hz, 1H), 7.53 (s, 1H), 7.49 (d, *J* = 2.2 Hz, 1H), 7.42 (s, 1H), 5.38 (s, 2H), 5.21 (s, 1H), 4.73 (d, *J* = 3.4 Hz, 1H),

4.06–4.02 (m, 1H), 3.64–3.60 (m, 1H), 2.97–2.94 (m, 2H), 2.56–2.51 (m, 1H), 2.30–2.25 (m, 1H), 1.95–1.91 (m, 1H), 1.79–1.75 (m, 1H), 1.64–1.60 (m, 2H), 1.52 (dd, J = 13.2, 3.3 Hz, 1H), 1.35 (s, 3H), 1.34–1.29 (m, 1H), 1.19–1.11 (m, 3H), 0.85 (d, J = 6.1 Hz, 3H), 0.83–0.78 (m, 1H), 0.75 (d, J = 7.4 Hz, 3H); ^{13}C NMR (150 MHz, $CDCl_3$) δ (ppm): 158.01, 148.41, 144.96, 139.16, 136.85, 128.75, 124.12, 121.77, 119.74, 116.47, 110.26, 103.07, 100.93, 86.86, 80.00, 76.21, 76.00, 75.79, 66.19, 51.44, 47.48, 43.26, 36.39, 35.35, 33.55, 29.78, 25.56, 25.13, 23.63, 23.35, 19.33, 11.96; ESI-HRMS [M + Na]$^+$: (*m*/*z*) Calcd. for $C_{29}H_{33}Br_2N_3O_7Na$: 716.0583. Found: 716.0381.

4.1.2. General Procedure for the Synthesis of Compounds **3f–3i** and **4f–4i**

Substituted coumarin (**f–i**) (10 mmol), substituted DHA (**III** or **IV**) (10 mmol) and triethylamine (10 mmol) were dissolved in 20 mL CH_2Cl_2. In addition, CuI (100 mg) was added and the reaction mixture was stirred at room temperature for 8 h under the protection of nitrogen. The mixture was filtered, washed with water, dried over Na_2SO_4 and evaporated to dryness. The crude product was purified through column chromatography.

7-hydroxy-4-((4-((10S)-dihydroartemisininoxy)methyl-1H-1,2,3-triazol-1-yl)-methyl)-2H-1-chromen-2-one (**3f**) White solid; m.p. 165–167 °C; yield 54%; ^{1}H NMR (600 MHz, $CDCl_3$) δ (ppm): 9.61 (s, 1H), 7.68 (d, J = 8.8 Hz, 1H), 7.67 (s, 1H), 6.99 (dd, J = 8.8, 2.4 Hz, 1H), 6.85 (d, J = 2.4 Hz, 1H), 6.15 (s, 1H), 5.76 (d, J = 15.4 Hz, 1H), 5.57 (d, J = 15.3 Hz, 1H), 5.20 (s, 1H), 4.87 (d, J = 1.9 Hz, 1H), 4.86 (d, J = 7.4 Hz, 1H), 4.68 (d, J = 12.9 Hz, 1H), 2.62–2.60 (m, 1H), 2.34–2.29 (m, 1H), 2.02–1.98 (m, 1H), 1.82–1.78 (m, 1H), 1.66–1.61 (m, 3H), 1.61–1.57 (m, 1H), 1.45–1.42 (m, 1H), 1.40 (s, 3H), 1.20–1.08 (m, 3H), 0.84 (d, J = 7.4 Hz, 3H), 0.82 (d, J = 6.1 Hz, 3H); ^{13}C NMR (150 MHz, $CDCl_3$) δ (ppm): 160.88, 159.75, 154.96, 146.45, 145.19, 124.19, 122.29, 112.78, 111.57, 108.80, 103.21, 103.04, 101.40, 86.91, 79.92, 76.20, 75.99, 75.78, 60.44, 51.32, 50.16, 43.18, 36.28, 35.26, 33.42, 29.74, 25.00, 23.53, 23.32, 19.26, 11.89; ESI-HRMS [M + Na]$^+$: (*m*/*z*) Calcd. for $C_{28}H_{33}N_3O_8Na$: 562.2165. Found: 562.2172.

5,7-dimethyl-4-((4-((10S)-dihydroartemisininoxy)methyl-1H-1,2,3-triazol-1-yl)-methyl)-2H-1-chromen-2-one (**3g**) White solid; m.p. 133~135 °C; yield 57%; ^{1}H NMR (600 MHz, $CDCl_3$) δ (ppm): 7.56 (s, 1H), 7.07 (s, 1H), 6.95 (s, 1H), 5.90 (d, J = 17.0 Hz, 1H), 5.86 (d, J = 17.0 Hz, 1H), 5.51 (s, 1H), 5.41 (s, 1H), 4.98 (d, J = 12.8 Hz, 1H), 4.93 (d, J = 3.5 Hz, 1H), 4.73 (d, J = 12.8 Hz, 1H), 2.68 (s, 3H), 2.40 (s, 3H), 2.35 (dd, J = 14.0, 4.0 Hz, 1H), 2.05–2.01 (m, 1H), 1.88–1.85 (m, 1H), 1.75–1.70 (m, 2H), 1.60 (dd, J = 13.2, 3.4 Hz, 1H), 1.48–1.46 (m, 1H), 1.43 (s, 3H), 1.32–1.20 (m, 5H), 0.93 (d, J = 6.3 Hz, 3H), 0.89 (d, J = 7.4 Hz, 3H); ^{13}C NMR (150 MHz, $CDCl_3$) δ (ppm): 158.67, 154.26, 149.33, 145.35, 142.10, 133.93, 129.26, 122.10, 115.63, 113.36, 112.80, 103.16, 100.93, 86.98, 80.05, 76.21, 76.00, 75.79, 60.80, 52.05, 51.48, 43.31, 36.34, 35.36, 33.50, 29.78, 25.11, 23.61, 23.44, 23.28, 20.24, 19.31, 12.01; ESI-HRMS [M + Na]$^+$: (*m*/*z*) Calcd. for $C_{30}H_{37}N_3O_7Na$: 574.2539. Found: 574.2553.

7-methyl-4-((4-((10S)-dihydroartemisininoxy)methyl-1H-1,2,3-triazol-1-yl)-methyl)-2H-1-chromen-2-one (**3h**) White solid; m.p. 107–109 °C; yield 50%; ^{1}H NMR (600 MHz, $CDCl_3$) δ (ppm): 7.58 (s, 1H), 7.50 (d, J = 8.1 Hz, 1H), 7.19 (s, 1H), 7.11 (d, J = 8.1 Hz, 1H), 6.01 (s, 1H), 5.74 (d, J = 16.3 Hz, 1H), 5.64 (d, J = 16.0 Hz, 1H), 5.30 (s, 1H), 4.92–4.88 (m, 2H), 4.72 (d, J = 12.9 Hz, 1H), 2.65–2.61 (m, 1H), 2.45 (s, 3H), 2.34 (td, J = 14.0, 4.0 Hz, 1H), 2.04–2.00 (m, 1H), 1.86–1.81 (m, 1H), 1.71–1.66 (m, 2H), 1.58–1.55 (m, 1H), 1.42 (s, 3H), 1.26–1.18 (m, 5H), 0.91 (d, J = 5.7 Hz, 3H), 0.86 (d, J = 7.3 Hz, 3H); ^{13}C NMR (150 MHz, $CDCl_3$) δ (ppm): 159.01, 152.86, 146.75, 145.42, 143.16, 125.03, 122.23, 121.95, 116.71, 113.56, 113.41, 103.15, 101.10, 86.93, 80.00, 76.21, 75.99, 75.78, 60.90, 51.41, 49.29, 43.27, 36.34, 35.31, 33.47, 29.77, 25.06, 23.58, 23.38, 20.70, 19.30, 11.96; ESI-HRMS [M + Na]$^+$: (*m*/*z*) Calcd. for $C_{29}H_{35}N_3O_7Na$: 560.2373. Found: 560.2375.

6-methyl-4-((4-((10S)-dihydroartemisininoxy)methyl-1H-1,2,3-triazol-1-yl)-methyl)-2H-1-chromen-2-one (**3i**) White solid; m.p. 88–90°C; yield 60%; ^{1}H NMR (600 MHz, $CDCl_3$) δ (ppm): 7.58 (s, 1H), 7.39 (d, J = 8.8 Hz, 2H), 7.28 (d, J = 8.3 Hz, 1H), 6.01 (s, 1H), 5.75 (d, J = 16.3 Hz, 1H), 5.66 (d, J = 16.3 Hz, 1H), 5.32 (s, 1H), 4.92 (d, J = 12.8 Hz, 1H), 4.90 (d, J = 3.5 Hz, 1H), 4.73 (d, J = 12.8 Hz, 1H), 2.67–2.60 (m,

1H), 2.41 (s, 3H), 2.34 (td, *J* = 14.0, 4.0 Hz, 1H), 2.04–1.99 (m, 1H), 1.86–1.81 (m, 1H), 1.72–1.68 (m, 2H), 1.57 (dd, *J* = 13.2, 3.1 Hz, 1H), 1.42 (s, 3H), 1.26–1.19 (m, 5H), 0.91 (d, *J* = 5.7 Hz, 3H), 0.86 (d, *J* = 7.3 Hz, 3H); ^{13}C NMR (150 MHz, $CDCl_3$) δ (ppm): 158.91, 150.87, 146.72, 145.41, 133.69, 132.71, 122.26, 121.95, 116.32, 115.68, 114.29, 103.15, 101.05, 86.94, 80.00, 76.21, 76.00, 75.78, 60.86, 51.42, 49.17, 43.27, 36.34, 35.31, 33.47, 29.76, 25.07, 23.59, 23.39, 20.01, 19.30, 11.96; ESI-HRMS [M + Na]$^+$: (*m*/*z*) Calcd. for $C_{29}H_{35}N_3O_7Na$: 560.2373. Found: 560.2403.

7-hydroxy-4-((4-(2-((10S)-dihydroartemisininoxy)ethyl)-1H-1,2,3-triazol-1-yl)-methyl)-2H-1-chromen-2-one (**4f**) White solid; m.p. 121–123 °C; yield 54%; ^{1}H NMR (600 MHz, $CDCl_3$) δ (ppm): 9.98 (s, 1H), 7.68 (d, *J* = 8.8 Hz, 1H), 7.49 (s, 1H), 7.01 (dd, *J* = 8.8, 2.4 Hz, 1H), 6.85 (d, *J* = 2.4 Hz, 1H), 6.16 (s, 1H), 5.68–5.59 (m, 2H), 5.20 (s, 1H), 4.71 (d, *J* = 3.5 Hz, 1H), 4.08–4.04 (m, 1H), 3.67–3.63 (m, 1H), 3.03–2.94 (m, 2H), 2.56–2.53 (m, 1H), 2.33 (td, *J* = 14.1, 4.0 Hz, 1H), 2.03–1.99 (m, 1H), 1.86–1.82 (m, 1H), 1.58–1.54 (m, 2H), 1.51–1.48 (m, 1H), 1.40 (s, 3H), 1.40–1.35 (m, 2H), 1.27–1.25 (m, 1H), 1.20–1.16 (m, 2H), 0.88 (d, *J* = 5.6 Hz, 3H), 0.68 (d, *J* = 7.3 Hz, 3H); ^{13}C NMR (150 MHz, $CDCl_3$) δ (ppm): 161.02, 159.72, 155.05, 146.56, 145.44, 124.28, 121.23, 112.79, 111.51, 108.74, 103.16, 103.05, 100.88, 86.87, 79.91, 76.20, 75.99, 75.78, 65.75, 51.37, 50.15, 43.11, 36.37, 35.30, 33.45, 29.66, 25.24, 25.09, 23.62, 23.29, 19.29, 11.73; ESI-HRMS [M + Na]$^+$: (*m*/*z*) Calcd. for $C_{29}H_{35}N_3O_8Na$: 576.2322. Found: 576.2352.

5,7-dimethyl-4-((4-(2-((10S)-dihydroartemisininoxy)ethyl)-1H-1,2,3-triazol-1-yl)-methyl)-2H-1-chromen-2-one (**4g**) White solid; m.p. 135–137 °C; yield 52%; ^{1}H NMR (600 MHz, $CDCl_3$) δ (ppm): 7.41 (s, 1H), 7.06 (s, 1H), 6.94 (s, 1H), 5.84 (s, 2H), 5.54 (s, 1H), 5.28 (s, 1H), 4.80 (d, *J* = 3.4 Hz, 1H), 4.15–4.10 (m, 1H), 3.73–3.69 (m, 1H), 3.11–3.00 (m, 2H), 2.66 (s, 3H), 2.61–2.58 (m, 1H), 2.40 (s, 3H), 2.35 (td, *J* = 14.1, 4.0 Hz, 1H), 2.03–1.99 (m, 1H), 1.89–1.84 (m, 1H), 1.70–1.63 (m, 2H), 1.59–1.55 (m, 1H), 1.49–1.43 (m, 1H), 1.42 (s, 3H), 1.29–1.18 (m, 3H), 0.93 (d, *J* = 6.3 Hz, 3H), 0.87 (dd, *J* = 12.4, 4.6 Hz, 1H), 0.80 (d, *J* = 7.3 Hz, 3H); ^{13}C NMR (150 MHz, $CDCl_3$) δ (ppm): 158.63, 154.30, 149.34, 145.42, 142.09, 133.98, 129.26, 121.15, 115.62, 113.33, 112.98, 103.07, 100.86, 86.87, 80.00, 76.21, 76.00, 75.79, 65.93, 52.03, 51.47, 43.25, 36.36, 35.37, 33.55, 29.76, 25.58, 25.15, 23.66, 23.32, 23.21, 20.24, 19.35, 11.98; ESI-HRMS [M + Na]$^+$: (*m*/*z*) Calcd. for $C_{31}H_{39}N_3O_7Na$: 588.2686. Found: 588.2680.

7-methyl-4-((4-(2-((10S)-dihydroartemisininoxy)ethyl)-1H-1,2,3-triazol-1-yl)-methyl)-2H-1-chromen-2-one (**4h**) White solid; m.p. 100–102 °C; yield 53%; ^{1}H NMR (600 MHz, $CDCl_3$) δ (ppm): 7.48 (d, *J* = 8.1 Hz, 1H), 7.40 (s, 1H), 7.18 (s, 1H), 7.11 (d, *J* = 8.2 Hz, 1H), 6.00 (s, 1H), 5.68–5.62 (m, 2H), 5.29 (d, *J* = 12.6 Hz, 1H), 4.76 (d, *J* = 3.5 Hz, 1H), 4.11–4.08 (m, 1H), 3.69–3.65 (m, 1H), 3.06–2.96 (m, 2H), 2.60–2.54 (m, 1H), 2.45 (s, 3H), 2.34 (td, *J* = 14.0, 4.0 Hz, 1H), 2.05–1.99 (m, 1H), 1.88–1.83 (m, 1H), 1.66–1.63 (m, 2H), 1.60–1.58 (m, 1H), 1.56–1.53 (m, 1H), 1.41 (s, 3H), 1.27–1.17 (m, 3H), 0.93 (d, *J* = 6.1 Hz, 3H), 0.89–0.84 (m, 1H), 0.74 (d, *J* = 7.3 Hz, 3H); ^{13}C NMR (150 MHz, $CDCl_3$) δ (ppm): 158.98, 152.88, 146.91, 145.50, 143.18, 125.06, 122.27, 120.82, 116.69, 113.56, 113.35, 103.08, 100.86, 86.86, 79.97, 76.21, 76.00, 75.78, 65.94, 51.44, 49.21, 43.21, 36.36, 35.35, 33.54, 29.72, 25.55, 25.14, 23.65, 23.31, 20.69, 19.34, 11.86; ESI-HRMS [M + Na]$^+$: (*m*/*z*) Calcd. for $C_{30}H_{37}N_3O_7Na$: 574.2529. Found: 574.2567.

6-methyl-4-((4-(2-((10S)-dihydroartemisininoxy)ethyl)-1H-1,2,3-triazol-1-yl)-methyl)-2H-1-chromen-2-one (**4i**) White solid; m.p. 100–102 °C; yield 43%; ^{1}H NMR (600 MHz, $CDCl_3$) δ (ppm): 7.40 (s, 1H), 7.40 (s, 1H), 7.38 (d, *J* = 1.9 Hz, 1H), 7.28 (d, *J* = 8.3 Hz, 1H), 6.00 (d, *J* = 1.2 Hz, 1H), 5.67 (s, 2H), 5.29 (s, 1H), 4.77 (d, *J* = 3.4 Hz, 1H), 4.13–4.09 (m, 1H), 3.71–3.67 (m, 1H), 3.05–2.99 (m, 2H), 2.61–2.56 (m, 1H), 2.41 (s, 3H), 2.36–2.32 (m, 1H), 2.03–2.00 (m, 1H), 1.88–1.84 (m, 1H), 1.66 (dd, *J* = 13.7, 3.5 Hz, 1H), 1.61 (d, *J* = 4.2 Hz, 1H), 1.58–1.53 (m, 2H), 1.42 (s, 3H), 1.24–1.16 (m, 3H), 0.93 (d, *J* = 6.2 Hz, 3H), 0.88–0.85 (m, 1H), 0.75 (d, *J* = 7.3 Hz, 3H); ^{13}C NMR (150 MHz, $CDCl_3$) δ (ppm): 158.88, 150.89, 146.89, 145.51, 133.70, 132.73, 122.29, 120.86, 116.31, 115.69, 114.22, 103.09, 100.87, 86.86, 79.98, 76.20, 75.99, 75.78, 65.94, 51.45, 49.06, 43.22, 36.37, 35.35, 33.54, 29.73, 25.57, 25.14, 23.65, 23.31, 20.03, 19.34, 11.86; ESI-HRMS [M + Na]$^+$: (*m*/*z*) Calcd. for $C_{30}H_{37}N_3O_7Na$: 574.2529. Found: 574.2558.

4.1.3. General Procedure for the Synthesis of Compounds **5j**,**5l–5o**, and **6j–6p**

Substituted coumarin (**j–p**) (10 mmol), substituted DHA (**I** or **II**) (10 mmol) and triethylamine (10 mmol) were dissolved in 20 mL CH_2Cl_2. In addition, CuI (100 mg) was added and the reaction mixture was stirred at room temperature for 8h under the protection of nitrogen. The mixture was filtered, washed with water, dried over Na_2SO_4 and evaporated to dryness. The crude product was purified through column chromatography.

4-((4-(2-((10S)-dihydroartemisininoxy)ethyl)-1H-1,2,3-triazol-1-yl)-methoxy)-2H-1-chromen-2-one (**5j**) White solid; m.p. 91–93 °C; yield 51%; ^{1}H NMR (600 MHz, $CDCl_3$) δ (ppm): 7.79–7.75 (m, 2H), 7.55 (ddd, *J* = 8.7, 7.3, 1.6 Hz, 1H), 7.33 (d, *J* = 8.3 Hz, 1H), 7.25–7.22 (m, 1H), 5.87 (s, 1H), 5.34 (d, *J* = 2.7 Hz, 2H), 5.16 (s, 1H), 4.77 (d, *J* = 3.6 Hz, 1H), 4.72–4.68 (m, 1H), 4.58–4.54 (m, 1H), 4.32–4.29 (m, 1H), 3.87–3.83 (m, 1H), 2.63–2.60 (m, 1H), 2.33 (td, *J* = 14.0, 4.0 Hz, 1H), 2.01–1.97 (m, 1H), 1.87–1.81 (m, 1H), 1.68–1.64 (m, 1H), 1.58–1.55 (m, 1H), 1.53–1.51 (m, 1H), 1.41 (s, 3H), 1.38 (d, *J* = 11.2 Hz, 1H), 1.26–1.18 (m, 3H), 0.91 (d, *J* = 5.9 Hz, 3H), 0.88–0.83 (m, 1H), 0.78 (d, *J* = 7.4 Hz, 3H); ^{13}C NMR (150 MHz, $CDCl_3$) δ (ppm): 163.90, 161.51, 152.34, 140.45, 131.58, 122.86, 122.85, 122.04, 115.80, 114.40, 103.21, 101.15, 90.15, 86.86, 79.73, 76.20, 75.99, 75.78, 65.36, 61.67, 51.32, 49.57, 42.97, 36.35, 35.25, 33.41, 29.53, 25.06, 23.58, 23.32, 19.29, 11.80; ESI-HRMS $[M + Na]^+$: (*m*/*z*) Calcd. for $C_{29}H_{35}N_3O_8Na$: 576.2322. Found: 576.2336.

5,7-dimethyl-4-((4-(2-((10S)-dihydroartemisininoxy)ethyl)-1H-1,2,3-triazol-1-yl)-methoxy)-2H-1-chromen-2-one (**5l**) White solid; m.p. 111–113 °C; yield 49%; ^{1}H NMR (600 MHz, $CDCl_3$) δ (ppm): 7.74 (s, 1H), 6.98 (s, 1H), 6.83 (s, 1H), 5.75 (s, 1H), 5.28 (s, 2H), 5.14 (s, 1H), 4.76 (d, J = 3.6 Hz, 1H), 4.70–4.66 (m, 1H), 4.58–4.54 (m, 1H), 4.31–4.27 (m, 1H), 3.87–3.84 (m, 1H), 2.84 (s, 1H), 2.61–2.59 (m, 1H), 2.53 (s, 3H), 2.36 (s, 3H), 2.35–2.30 (m, 1H), 2.04–1.97 (m, 2H), 1.87–1.82 (m, 1H), 1.58–1.54 (m, 1H), 1.52–1.50 (m, 1H), 1.41 (s, 3H), 1.25–1.17 (m, 3H), 0.91 (d, *J* = 5.9 Hz, 3H), 0.88–0.85 (m, 1H), 0.76 (d, *J* = 7.4 Hz, 3H); ^{13}C NMR (150 MHz, $CDCl_3$) δ (ppm): 166.97, 161.69, 153.91, 141.76, 140.42, 135.57, 127.92, 122.68, 114.43, 110.62, 103.21, 101.15, 89.15, 86.85, 79.74, 76.21, 76.00, 75.79, 65.38, 61.48, 51.33, 49.59, 42.97, 36.36, 35.25, 33.42, 29.53, 25.05, 23.58, 23.30, 22.49, 20.35, 19.30, 11.80; ESI-HRMS $[M + Na]^+$: (*m*/*z*) Calcd. for $C_{31}H_{39}N_3O_8Na$: 604.2635. Found: 604.2645.

6,8-dimethyl-4-((4-(2-((10S)-dihydroartemisininoxy)ethyl)-1H-1,2,3-triazol-1-yl)-methoxy)-2H-1-chromen-2-one (**5m**) White solid; m.p. 111–113 °C; yield 49%; ^{1}H NMR (600 MHz, $CDCl_3$) δ (ppm): 7.77 (s, 1H), 7.39 (s, 1H), 7.22 (s, 1H), 5.83 (s, 1H), 5.32 (d, *J* = 2.5 Hz, 2H), 5.17 (s, 1H), 4.78 (d, *J* = 3.0 Hz, 1H), 4.72–4.68 (m, 1H), 4.59–4.55 (m, 1H), 4.33–4.29 (m, 1H), 3.87–3.83 (m, 1H), 2.64–2.58 (m, 1H), 2.41 (s, 3H), 2.37–2.33 (m, 1H), 2.33 (s, 3H), 2.02–1.98 (m, 1H), 1.88–1.82 (m, 1H), 1.68–1.63 (m, 1H), 1.58–1.53 (m, 1H), 1.53–1.48 (m, 1H), 1.41 (s, 3H), 1.41–1.38 (m, 1H), 1.28–1.16 (m, 3H), 0.91 (d, *J* = 5.9 Hz, 3H), 0.88–0.84 (m, 1H), 0.78 (d, *J* = 7.4 Hz, 3H); ^{13}C NMR (150 MHz, $CDCl_3$) δ (ppm): 165.31, 162.94, 149.91, 141.55, 134.98, 133.03, 125.90, 123.94, 120.25, 114.82, 104.23, 102.18, 90.77, 87.87, 80.76, 77.24, 77.02, 76.81, 66.39, 62.54, 52.35, 50.58, 44.01, 37.37, 36.28, 34.44, 30.57, 26.07, 24.61, 24.35, 20.82, 20.31, 15.65, 12.84; ESI-HRMS $[M + Na]^+$: (*m*/*z*) Calcd. for $C_{31}H_{39}N_3O_8Na$: 604.2635. Found: 604.2639.

7,8-dimethyl-4-((4-(2-((10S)-dihydroartemisininoxy)ethyl)-1H-1,2,3-triazol-1-yl)-methoxy)-2H-1-chromen-2-one (**5n**) White solid; m.p. 91–93 °C; yield 51%; ^{1}H NMR (600 MHz, $CDCl_3$) δ (ppm): 7.76 (s, 1H), 7.50 (d, *J* = 8.1 Hz, 1H), 7.03 (d, *J* = 8.1 Hz, 1H), 5.79 (s, 1H), 5.32 (d, *J* = 3.0 Hz, 2H), 5.15 (s, 1H), 4.77 (d, *J* = 3.5 Hz, 1H), 4.71–4.67 (m, 1H), 4.58–4.53 (m, 1H), 4.33–4.27 (m, 1H), 3.86–3.82 (m, 1H), 2.63–2.58 (m, 1H), 2.37 (s, 3H), 2.36 (s, 3H), 2.34–2.30 (m, 1H), 2.01–1.97 (m, 1H), 1.86–1.81 (m, 1H), 1.68–1.62 (m, 1H), 1.58–1.53 (m, 1H), 1.51 (dd, *J* = 13.4, 3.5 Hz, 1H), 1.41 (s, 3H), 1.39–1.36 (m, 1H), 1.27–1.15 (m, 3H), 0.91 (d, *J* = 5.8 Hz, 3H), 0.88–0.82 (m, 1H), 0.77 (d, *J* = 7.3 Hz, 3H); ^{13}C NMR (150 MHz, $CDCl_3$) δ (ppm): 165.56, 163.09, 151.58, 142.30, 141.69, 125.34, 124.53, 123.85, 119.71, 113.06, 104.24, 102.18, 89.91, 87.88, 80.78, 77.25, 77.04, 76.82, 66.39, 62.61, 52.37, 50.60, 44.02, 37.37, 36.29, 34.45, 30.58, 26.09, 24.61, 24.35, 20.46, 20.33, 12.85, 11.67; ESI-HRMS $[M + Na]^+$: (*m*/*z*) Calcd. for $C_{31}H_{39}N_3O_8Na$: 604.2635. Found: 604.2646.

8-methyl-4-((4-(2-((10S)-dihydroartemisininoxy)ethyl)-1H-1,2,3-triazol-1-yl)-methoxy)-2H-1-chromen- 2-one (**5o**) White solid; m.p. 84–86 °C; yield 43%; ^{1}H NMR (600 MHz, $CDCl_3$) δ (ppm): 7.77 (s, 1H), 7.61 (d, J = 7.9 Hz, 1H), 7.39 (d, J = 7.4 Hz, 1H), 7.13 (t, J = 7.7 Hz, 1H), 5.85 (s, 1H), 5.33 (d, J = 2.8 Hz, 2H), 5.15 (s, 1H), 4.77 (d, J = 3.5 Hz, 1H), 4.71–4.67 (m, 1H), 4.58–4.54 (m, 1H), 4.33–4.27 (m, 1H), 3.86–3.82 (m, 1H), 2.62–2.59 (m, 1H), 2.45 (s, 3H), 2.33 (td, J = 14.1, 4.0 Hz, 1H), 2.01–1.97 (m, 1H), 1.86–1.81 (m, 1H), 1.65 (dd, J = 14.0, 3.6 Hz, 1H), 1.58–1.54 (m, 1H), 1.51 (dd, J = 13.4, 3.5 Hz, 1H), 1.41 (s, 3H), 1.40–1.35 (m, 1H), 1.27–1.17 (m, 3H), 0.90 (d, J = 5.8 Hz, 3H), 0.88–0.84 (m, 1H), 0.77 (d, J = 7.3 Hz, 3H); ^{13}C NMR (150 MHz, $CDCl_3$) δ (ppm): 165.30, 162.70, 151.74, 141.60, 133.84, 126.28, 123.84, 123.42, 120.66, 115.15, 104.24, 102.18, 90.88, 87.89, 80.77, 77.25, 77.03, 76.82, 66.39, 62.71, 52.36, 50.60, 44.01, 37.38, 36.28, 34.45, 30.57, 26.09, 24.61, 24.35, 20.33, 15.76, 12.84; ESI-HRMS [M + Na]$^+$: (m/z) Calcd. for $C_{30}H_{37}N_3O_8Na$: 590.2478. Found: 590.2477.

4-((4-(3-((10S)-dihydroartemisininoxy)propyl)-1H-1,2,3-triazol-1-yl)-methoxy)-2H-1-chromen-2-one (**6j**) White solid; m.p. 74–76 °C; yield 47%; ^{1}H NMR (600 MHz, $CDCl_3$) δ (ppm): 7.79 (dd, J = 8.0, 1.6 Hz, 1H), 7.72 (s, 1H), 7.55 (ddd, J = 8.7, 7.4, 1.6 Hz, 1H), 7.32 (dd, J = 8.4, 1.1 Hz, 1H), 7.26–7.23 (m, 1H), 5.86 (s, 1H), 5.41 (s, 1H), 5.34 (s, 2H), 4.79 (d, J = 3.6 Hz, 1H), 4.56–4.46 (m, 2H), 3.93–3.89 (m, 1H), 3.44–3.41 (m, 1H), 2.69–2.63 (m, 1H), 2.39–2.34 (m, 1H), 2.27–2.20 (m, 2H), 2.05–2.01 (m, 1H), 1.91–1.86 (m, 1H), 1.79–1.75 (m, 1H), 1.67–1.64 (m, 1H), 1.51–1.46 (m, 2H), 1.42 (s, 3H), 1.39–1.33 (m, 1H), 1.28–1.22 (m, 2H), 0.96 (d, J = 6.4 Hz, 3H), 0.94 (d, J = 7.4 Hz, 3H); ^{13}C NMR (150 MHz, $CDCl_3$) δ (ppm): 163.96, 161.59, 152.33, 140.41, 131.55, 122.89, 122.40, 122.13, 115.78, 114.42, 103.18, 101.19, 90.16, 86.93, 79.93, 76.21, 76.00, 75.79, 63.62, 61.66, 51.47, 46.73, 43.23, 36.45, 35.33, 33.53, 29.78, 29.43, 25.12, 23.64, 23.54, 19.33, 12.07; ESI-HRMS [M + Na]$^+$: (m/z) Calcd. for $C_{30}H_{37}N_3O_8Na$: 590.2478. Found: 590.2463.

7-methyl-4-((4-(3-((10S)-dihydroartemisininoxy)propyl)-1H-1,2,3-triazol-1-yl)-methoxy)-2H-1-chromen-2-one (**6k**) White solid; m.p. 80–82 °C; yield 51%; ^{1}H NMR (600 MHz, $CDCl_3$) δ (ppm): 7.71 (s, 1H), 7.65 (d, J = 8.1 Hz, 1H), 7.12 (s, 1H), 7.05 (d, J = 8.1 Hz, 1H), 5.80 (s, 1H), 5.41 (s, 1H), 5.32 (s, 2H), 4.79 (d, J = 3.6 Hz, 1H), 4.53–4.46 (m, 2H), 3.93–3.89 (m, 1H), 3.44–3.40 (m, 1H), 2.69–2.64 (m, 1H), 2.44 (s, 3H), 2.37 (td, J = 14.0, 4.0 Hz, 1H), 2.27–2.21 (m, 2H), 2.05–2.01 (m, 1H), 1.91–1.86 (m, 1H), 1.80–1.75 (m, 2H), 1.68–1.64 (m, 1H), 1.51–1.46 (m, 2H), 1.42 (s, 3H), 1.28–1.24 (m, 3H), 0.96 (d, J = 6.4 Hz, 3H), 0.94 (d, J = 7.3 Hz, 3H); ^{13}C NMR (150 MHz, $CDCl_3$) δ (ppm): δ 164.21, 161.95, 152.44, 142.81, 140.51, 124.11, 122.39, 121.82, 115.88, 111.91, 103.19, 101.18, 89.25, 86.93, 79.94, 76.20, 75.99, 75.78, 63.62, 61.55, 51.47, 46.73, 43.24, 36.44, 35.33, 33.53, 29.78, 29.42, 25.12, 23.63, 23.53, 20.72, 19.33, 12.07; ESI-HRMS [M + Na]$^+$: (m/z) Calcd. for $C_{31}H_{39}N_3O_8Na$: 604.2635. Found: 604.2617.

5,7-dimethyl-4-((4-(3-((10S)-dihydroartemisininoxy)propyl)-1H-1,2,3-triazol-1-yl)-methoxy)-2H-1-chromen-2-one (**6l**) White solid; m.p. 86–88 °C; yield 42%; ^{1}H NMR (600 MHz, $CDCl_3$) δ (ppm): 7.68 (s, 1H), 6.98 (s, 1H), 6.83 (s, 1H), 5.74 (s, 1H), 5.40 (s, 1H), 5.28 (s, 2H), 4.78 (d, J = 3.7 Hz, 1H), 4.53–4.48 (m, 2H), 3.91–3.87 (m, 1H), 3.42–3.38 (m, 1H), 2.69–2.64 (m, 1H), 2.53 (s, 3H), 2.40–2.33 (m, 4H), 2.25–2.19 (m, 2H), 2.05–2.01 (m, 1H), 1.91–1.86 (m, 1H), 1.80–1.77 (m, 1H), 1.76–1.73 (m, 1H), 1.67–1.64 (m, 1H), 1.51–1.47 (m, 2H), 1.42 (s, 3H), 1.30–1.21 (m, 3H), 0.96 (d, J = 6.4 Hz, 3H), 0.94 (d, J = 7.4 Hz, 3H); ^{13}C NMR (150 MHz, $CDCl_3$) δ (ppm): 166.99, 161.73, 153.90, 141.72, 140.46, 135.57, 127.92, 122.26, 114.43, 110.63, 103.18, 101.15, 89.14, 86.91, 79.93, 76.21, 76.00, 75.78, 63.49, 61.58, 51.46, 46.66, 43.23, 36.46, 35.33, 33.53, 29.78, 29.42, 25.11, 23.64, 23.54, 22.46, 20.35, 19.33, 12.08; ESI-HRMS [M + Na]$^+$: (m/z) Calcd. for $C_{32}H_{41}N_3O_8Na$: 618.2791. Found: 618.2827.

6,8-dimethyl-4-((4-(3-((10S)-dihydroartemisininoxy)propyl)-1H-1,2,3-triazol-1-yl)-methoxy)-2H-1-chromen-2-one (**6m**) White solid; m.p. 90–92 °C; yield 55%; ^{1}H NMR (600 MHz, $CDCl_3$) δ (ppm): 7.71 (s, 1H), 7.40 (s, 1H), 7.21 (s, 1H), 5.82 (s, 1H), 5.41 (s, 1H), 5.32 (s, 2H), 4.79 (d, J = 3.6 Hz, 1H), 4.55–4.46 (m, 2H), 3.94–3.90 (m, 1H), 3.44–3.40 (m, 1H), 2.69–2.63 (m, 1H), 2.40 (s, 3H), 2.39–2.34 (m, 1H), 2.33 (s, 3H), 2.27–2.21 (m, 2H), 2.06–2.01 (m, 1H), 1.91–1.86 (m, 1H), 1.79–1.77 (m, 1H), 1.76–1.73 (m, 1H), 1.67–1.63 (m, 1H), 1.51–1.45 (m, 2H), 1.42 (s, 3H), 1.37–1.35 (m, 1H), 1.28–1.22 (m, 2H), 0.95 (d, J = 6.4 Hz, 3H), 0.94 (d, J = 7.4 Hz, 3H); ^{13}C NMR (150 MHz, $CDCl_3$) δ (ppm): 165.37, 163.02, 149.90, 141.55,

134.97, 133.07, 125.88, 123.45, 120.35, 114.83, 104.21, 102.21, 90.79, 87.96, 80.97, 77.25, 77.04, 76.83, 64.68, 62.56, 52.51, 47.77, 44.27, 37.47, 36.37, 34.56, 30.82, 30.47, 26.15, 24.67, 24.57, 20.83, 20.36, 15.66, 13.11; ESI-HRMS [M + Na]$^+$: (*m*/*z*) Calcd. for $C_{32}H_{41}N_3O_8Na$: 618.2791. Found: 618.2808.

7,8-dimethyl-4-((4-(3-((10S)-dihydroartemisininoxy)propyl)-1H-1,2,3-triazol-1-yl)-methoxy)-2H-1-chromen-2-one (**6n**) White solid; m.p. 115–117 °C; yield 44%; ^{1}H NMR (600 MHz, $CDCl_3$) δ (ppm): 7.71 (s, 1H), 7.52 (d, *J* = 8.1 Hz, 1H), 7.04 (d, *J* = 8.1 Hz, 1H), 5.80 (s, 1H), 5.40 (s, 1H), 5.32 (s, 2H), 4.79 (d, *J* = 3.5 Hz, 1H), 4.56–4.45 (m, 2H), 3.93–3.89 (m, 1H), 3.44–3.40 (m, 1H), 2.69–2.64 (m, 1H), 2.39–2.34 (m, 7H), 2.27–2.19 (m, 2H), 2.06–2.01 (m, 1H), 1.92–1.86 (m, 1H), 1.81–1.77 (m, 1H), 1.74 (dd, *J* = 13.4, 3.5 Hz, 1H), 1.67–1.63 (m, 1H), 1.52–1.45 (m, 2H), 1.42 (s, 3H), 1.39–1.34 (m, 1H), 1.27–1.24 (m, 2H), 0.96 (d, *J* = 6.4 Hz, 3H), 0.94 (d, *J* = 7.4 Hz, 3H); ^{13}C NMR (150 MHz, $CDCl_3$) δ (ppm): 165.61, 163.15, 151.58, 142.28, 141.66, 125.37, 124.51, 123.38, 119.78, 113.07, 104.21, 102.21, 89.92, 87.96, 80.97, 77.25, 77.04, 76.82, 64.66, 62.60, 52.51, 47.76, 44.27, 37.47, 36.37, 34.56, 30.82, 30.46, 26.15, 24.67, 24.57, 20.46, 20.37, 13.11, 11.67; ESI-HRMS [M + Na]$^+$: (*m*/*z*) Calcd. for $C_{32}H_{41}N_3O_8Na$: 618.2791. Found: 618.2793.

8-methyl-4-((4-(3-((10S)-dihydroartemisininoxy)propyl)-1H-1,2,3-triazol-1-yl)-methoxy)-2H-1-chromen-2-one (**6o**) White solid; m.p. 143–145°C; yield 38%; ^{1}H NMR (600 MHz, $CDCl_3$) δ (ppm): 7.71 (s, 1H), 7.63 (d, *J* = 8.0 Hz, 1H), 7.39 (d, *J* = 7.3 Hz, 1H), 7.14 (t, *J* = 7.7 Hz, 1H), 5.85 (s, 1H), 5.40 (s, 1H), 5.33 (s, 2H), 4.79 (d, *J* = 3.7 Hz, 1H), 4.55–4.46 (m, 2H), 3.93–3.89 (m, 1H), 3.44–3.40 (m, 1H), 2.70–2.63 (m, 1H), 2.45 (s, 3H), 2.37 (td, *J* = 14.0, 3.9 Hz, 1H), 2.28–2.19 (m, 2H), 2.05–2.01 (m, 1H), 1.92–1.86 (m, 1H), 1.81–1.72 (m, 2H), 1.67–1.64 (m, 1H), 1.53–1.46 (m, 2H), 1.42 (s, 3H), 1.39–1.33 (m, 1H), 1.30–1.22 (m, 2H), 0.96 (d, *J* = 6.4 Hz, 3H), 0.94 (d, *J* = 7.4 Hz, 3H); ^{13}C NMR (150 MHz, $CDCl_3$) δ (ppm): 165.35, 162.77, 151.73, 141.56, 133.82, 126.25, 123.45, 123.40, 120.73, 115.17, 104.22, 102.21, 90.89, 87.96, 80.97, 77.24, 77.03, 76.82, 64.65, 62.69, 52.51, 47.76, 44.27, 37.48, 36.37, 34.56, 30.82, 30.46, 26.15, 24.67, 24.57, 20.37, 15.76, 13.11; ESI-HRMS [M + Na]$^+$: (*m*/*z*) Calcd. for $C_{31}H_{39}N_3O_8Na$: 604.2635. Found: 604.2646.

6-methyl-4-((4-(3-((10S)-dihydroartemisininoxy)propyl)-1H-1,2,3-triazol-1-yl)-methoxy)-2H-1-chromen-2-one (**6p**) White solid; m.p. 80–82 °C; yield 45%; ^{1}H NMR (600 MHz, $CDCl_3$) δ (ppm): 7.72 (s, 1H), 7.56 (s, 1H), 7.35 (dd, *J* = 8.5, 2.0 Hz, 1H), 7.21 (d, *J* = 8.4 Hz, 1H), 5.84 (s, 1H), 5.41 (s, 1H), 5.33 (s, 2H), 4.80 (d, *J* = 3.6 Hz, 1H), 4.55–4.47 (m, 2H), 3.94–3.90 (m, 1H), 3.45–3.41 (m, 1H), 2.70–2.64 (m, 1H), 2.40–2.33 (m, 4H), 2.27–2.21 (m, 2H), 2.06–2.01 (m, 1H), 1.91–1.87 (m, 1H), 1.80–1.73 (m, 2H), 1.65 (dd, *J* = 13.3, 3.4 Hz, 1H), 1.53–1.46 (m, 2H), 1.42 (s, 3H), 1.38–1.34 (m, 1H), 1.28–1.22 (m, 2H), 0.96 (d, *J* = 6.4 Hz, 3H), 0.94 (d, *J* = 7.3 Hz, 3H); ^{13}C NMR (150 MHz, $CDCl_3$) δ (ppm): 165.02, 162.88, 151.52, 141.46, 133.69, 133.59, 123.52, 122.80, 116.56, 115.08, 104.22, 102.22, 91.11, 87.97, 80.97, 77.24, 77.03, 76.82, 64.68, 62.60, 52.51, 47.80, 44.27, 37.48, 36.37, 34.57, 30.82, 30.48, 26.15, 24.67, 24.58, 20.90, 20.37, 13.12; ESI-HRMS [M + Na]$^+$: (*m*/*z*) Calcd. for $C_{31}H_{39}N_3O_8Na$: 604.2635. Found: 604.2621.

4.2. Biology

4.2.1. Storage and Preparation of Samples

All the target compounds were dissolved in dimethylsulfoxide and storage under −20 °C. They get to be diluted to different concentration when they will be used.

4.2.2. Cell Culture

After recovery, the cells were cultured in 96-well plates for 24 h at 37 °C in a humidified atmosphere with 95% air and 5% CO_2. After treated with different tested compounds, the hypoxia groups were placed in a sealed hypoxia incubator chamber (Stemcell Technologies, Inc., Vancouver, BC, Canada) filled with 5% CO_2 and 95% N_2 for 24 h, and then transferred to the incubator chamber filled with air for 72 h. On the contrary, the normoxia groups were cultured under air condition for 96h.

Cancer cells HT-29 (Human Colorectal Adenocarcinoma cell line), MDA-MB-231 (Human Breast Cancer cell line), HCT-116 (Human Colorectal Carcinoma cell line), and A549 (Human Lung Adenocarcinomic cell line) were from ATCC.

4.2.3. MTT Assay

When the adherent cells reached 80% confluence, the culture medium was discarded. The cells were digested by trypsin and collected after centrifugation. The fresh culture medium was gently blown into it to form single-cell suspension. Cell suspension will be diluted to 1.5–3 × 10^4 cells/mL. Each hole of 96-well plates was added 100 μL cell suspension and incubated for 24 h (5% CO_2; 37 °C). Then the holes were added different concentrations of tested compounds. The early screening concentration is set to 100 μM, 50 μM, 25 μM, 12.5 μM, and 6.25 μM. Three replicates were made for each concentration of the tested compounds. After the cells were grown for 96h, 20 μL MTT (5 mg/mL) was added to each well and incubated for 4 h. The medium was discarded and each well was added 100 μL DMSO to dissolve the formazan blue. Absorbance was measured at 570 nm with a microplate reader (Synergy-HT, BioTek Instruments, Winooski, VT, USA).

Hypoxia condition: The cells were treated with different concentration of tested compounds, placed in hypoxia chamber (Catalog Number 27310, Stemcell Technologies, Inc., Vancouver, BC, Canada), and incubated for 24 h (5% air; 95% N_2; 37 °C). Then the cells were placed in normoxia condition (5% CO_2; 37 °C) and incubated for 72 h.

4.2.4. Preparation of N9 Cells

The murine microglial cell line N9 was a kind gift from Dr. P. Ricciardi-Castagnoli (Universita Degli Studi di Milano-Bicocca, Milan, Italy).

N9 cells, which were in the logarithmic phase, were incubated for 24 h by adherent culture. Subsequently, the medium was changed to new one without serum. The cells were treated with different concentration of tested compounds. After specific time in the LPS condition, the supernatants were collected and analyzed.

4.2.5. Nitrite Measurement

The nitrite levels in medium were determined by Griess reaction. The absorbance was measured at 540 nm using a microplate reader.

4.2.6. NO Capture Analysis

SNP was dissolved in PBS to prepare the 100 mM stock solution. In this experiment, SNP solution of 25 μL was added to 975 μL PBS solution which included different concentration of tested compounds. After 60 min under r.t. condition, the concentration of NO_2^- was tested using Griess assay.

4.2.7. Evaluation of Inflammatory Mediator

The secreted level of TNF-α and IL-6 was measured using mouse Th1/Th2/Th17 Cytokine Kit, purchased from BD Pharningen. The data was analyzed by FCAP Array v3.0. IL-2, IL-4, IL-10, IL-17A, and IFN-γ were not detected in the experiment.

4.2.8. Molecular Docking Simulations

The crystallographic structure of TLR4/MD-2 complex was retrieved from the Protein DataBank (PDB ID: 3VQ2), which was optimized by removing water molecules, cofactors and heteroatoms. Receptor grid was generally around the MD-2 active site. Docking calculations were accomplished using AutoDock4. The docking results were further analyzed and visually optimized by Discovery Studio 4.0 and PyMOL.

Supplementary Materials: The H and 13 C NMR spectra of synthesized compounds are available online.

Author Contributions: H.Y. performed experiments, analyzed data, and drafted the manuscript. Z.H. performed experiments, analyzed data, and revised the manuscript. X.Y. performed experiments. Y.M. and C.G. conceived the work, gave critical comments, and revised the manuscript.

Funding: We greatly appreciate the funding support for this research provided by the National Natural Science Foundation of China (Grant No. 81573292).

Conflicts of Interest: The authors declare no conflict of interest.

Abbreviations

DHA	Dihydroartemisinin
DCH	Dihydroartemisinin–Coumarin hydrids
CRF	Cancer-related fatigue
DOX	Doxorubicin
CNS	Central nervous system
SNP	Sodium nitroprusside
LPS	Lipopolysaccharide
TLR4	Toll-like receptor 4

References

1. Tsuji, E.; Hiki, N.; Nomura, S.; Fukushima, R.; Kojima, J.; Ogawa, T.; Mafune, K.; Mimura, Y.; Kaminishi, M. Simultaneous onset of acute inflammatory response, sepsis-like symptoms and intestinal mucosal injury after cancer chemotherapy. *Int. J. Cancer* **2003**, *107*, 303–308. [CrossRef] [PubMed]
2. Cerci, C.; Ergin, C.; Eroglu, E.; Agalar, C.; Agalar, F.; Cerci, S.; Bulbul, M. Effects of granulocyte-colony stimulating factor on peritoneal defense mechanisms and bacterial translocation after administration of systemic chemotherapy in rats. *World J. Gastroenterol.* **2007**, *13*, 2596–2599. [CrossRef] [PubMed]
3. Rivest, S. Molecular insights on the cerebral innate immune system. *Brain Behav. Immun.* **2003**, *17*, 13–19. [CrossRef]
4. Norden, D.M.; Bicer, S.; Clark, Y.; Jing, R.; Henry, C.J.; Wold, L.E.; Reiser, P.J.; Godbout, J.P.; McCarthy, D.O. Tumor growth increases neuroinflammation, fatigue and depressive-like behavior prior to alterations in muscle function. *Brain Behav. Immun.* **2015**, *43*, 76–85. [CrossRef] [PubMed]
5. Bower, J.E.; Lamkin, D.M. Inflammation and cancer-related fatigue: Mechanisms, contributing factors, and treatment implications. *Brain Behav. Immun.* **2013**, *30*, S48–S57. [CrossRef]
6. Perry, V.H.; Gordon, S. Macrophages and microglia in the nervous system. *Trends Neurosci.* **1988**, *11*, 273–277. [CrossRef]
7. Kreutzberg, G.W. Microglia: A sensor for pathological events in the CNS. *Trends Neurosci.* **1996**, *19*, 312–318. [CrossRef]
8. Colton, C.A.; Gilbert, D.L. Production of superoxide anions by a CNS macrophage, the microglia. *FEBS Lett.* **1987**, *223*, 284–288. [CrossRef]
9. Banati, R.B.; Gehrmann, J.; Schubert, P.; Kreutzberg, G.W. Cytotoxicity of microglia. *Glia* **1993**, *7*, 111–118. [CrossRef]
10. Lissauer, M.E.; Johnson, S.B.; Bochicchio, G.V.; Feild, C.J.; Cross, A.S.; Hasday, J.D.; Whiteford, C.C.; Nussbaumer, W.A.; Towns, M.; Scalea, T.M. Differential expression of toll-like receptor genes: Sepsis compared with sterile inflammation 1 day before sepsis diagnosis. *Shock* **2009**, *31*, 238–244. [CrossRef]
11. Steiner, A.A.; Chakravarty, S.; Rudaya, A.Y.; Herkenham, M.; Romanovsky, A.A. Bacterial lipopolysaccharide fever is initiated via Toll-like receptor 4 on hematopoietic cells. *Blood* **2006**, *107*, 4000–4002. [CrossRef]
12. Shimazu, R.; Akashi, S.; Ogata, H.; Nagai, Y.; Fukudome, K.; Miyake, K.; Kimoto, M. MD-2, a Molecule that Confers Lipopolysaccharide Responsiveness on Toll-like Receptor 4. *J. Exp. Med.* **1999**, *189*, 1777–1782. [CrossRef] [PubMed]
13. Nagai, Y.; Akashi, S.; Nagafuku, M.; Ogata, M.; Iwakura, Y.; Akira, S.; Kitamura, T.; Kosugi, A.; Kimoto, M.; Miyake, K. Essential role of MD-2 in LPS responsiveness and TLR4 distribution. *Nat. Immunol.* **2002**, *3*, 667–672. [CrossRef] [PubMed]
14. Inohara, N.; Nuñez, G. ML—A conserved domain involved in innate immunity and lipid metabolism. *Trends Biochem. Sci.* **2002**, *27*, 219–221. [CrossRef]
15. Viriyakosol, S.; Tobias, P.S.; Kitchens, R.L.; Kirkland, T.N. MD-2 binds to bacterial lipopolysaccharide. *J. Biol. Chem.* **2001**, *276*, 38044–38051. [PubMed]

16. Navaratnam, V.; Mansor, S.M.; Sit, N.W.; Grace, J.; Li, Q.; Olliaro, P. Pharmacokinetics of artemisinin-type compounds. *Clin. Pharmacokinet.* **2000**, *39*, 255–270. [CrossRef] [PubMed]
17. Balint, G.A. Artemisinin and its derivatives: An important new class of antimalarial agents. *Pharmacol. Ther.* **2001**, *90*, 261–265. [CrossRef]
18. Chen, H.; Gu, S.; Dai, H.; Li, X.; Zhang, Z. Dihydroartemisinin Sensitizes Human Lung Adenocarcinoma A549 Cells to Arsenic Trioxide via Apoptosis. *Biol. Trace Elem. Res.* **2017**, *179*, 203–212. [CrossRef]
19. Cao, L.; Duanmu, W.; Yin, Y.; Zhou, Z.; Ge, H.; Chen, T.; Tan, L.; Yu, A.; Hu, R.; Fei, L.; et al. Dihydroartemisinin exhibits anti-glioma stem cell activity through inhibiting p-AKT and activating caspase-3. *Die Pharm.* **2014**, *69*, 752–758.
20. Zhang, Z.; Guo, M.; Zhao, S.; Shao, J.; Zheng, S. ROS-JNK1/2-dependent activation of autophagy is required for the induction of anti-inflammatory effect of dihydroartemisinin in liver fibrosis. *Free Radic. Biol. Med.* **2016**, *101*, 272–283. [CrossRef]
21. Jiang, L.B.; Meng, D.H.; Lee, S.M.; Liu, S.H.; Xu, Q.T.; Wang, Y.; Zhang, J. Dihydroartemisinin inhibits catabolism in rat chondrocytes by activating autophagy via inhibition of the NF-kappaB pathway. *Sci. Rep.* **2016**, *6*, 38979. [CrossRef]
22. Huang, X.; Xie, Z.; Liu, F.; Han, C.; Zhang, D.; Wang, D.; Bao, X.; Sun, J.; Wen, C.; Fan, Y. Dihydroartemisinin inhibits activation of the Toll-like receptor 4 signaling pathway and production of type I interferon in spleen cells from lupus-prone MRL/lpr mice. *Int. Immunopharmacol.* **2014**, *22*, 266–272. [CrossRef]
23. Witaicenis, A.; de Oliveira, E.C.S.; Tanimoto, A.; Zorzella-Pezavento, S.F.G.; de Oliveira, S.L.; Sartori, A.; Di Stasi, L.C. 4-methylesculetin, a coumarin derivative, ameliorates dextran sulfate sodium-induced intestinal inflammation. *Chem. Biol. Interact.* **2018**, *280*, 59–63. [CrossRef] [PubMed]
24. Chougala, B.M.; Samundeeswari, S.; Holiyachi, M.; Naik, N.S.; Shastri, L.A.; Dodamani, S.; Jalalpure, S.; Dixit, S.R.; Joshi, S.D.; Sunagar, V.A. Green, unexpected synthesis of bis-coumarin derivatives as potent anti-bacterial and anti-inflammatory agents. *Eur. J. Med. Chem.* **2018**, *143*, 1744–1756. [CrossRef] [PubMed]
25. Emami, S.; Dadashpour, S. Current developments of coumarin-based anti-cancer agents in medicinal chemistry. *Eur. J. Med. Chem.* **2015**, *102*, 611–630. [CrossRef] [PubMed]
26. Basanagouda, M.; Jambagi, V.B.; Barigidad, N.N.; Laxmeshwar, S.S.; Devaru, V.; Narayanachar. Synthesis, structure-activity relationship of iodinated-4-aryloxymethyl-coumarins as potential anti-cancer and anti-mycobacterial agents. *Eur. J. Med. Chem.* **2014**, *74*, 225–233. [CrossRef]
27. Devji, T.; Reddy, C.; Woo, C.; Awale, S.; Kadota, S.; Carrico-Moniz, D. Pancreatic anticancer activity of a novel geranylgeranylated coumarin derivative. *Bioorg. Med. Chem. Lett.* **2011**, *21*, 5770–5773. [CrossRef] [PubMed]
28. Bronikowska, J.; Szliszka, E.; Jaworska, D.; Czuba, Z.P.; Krol, W. The coumarin psoralidin enhances anticancer effect of tumor necrosis factor-related apoptosis-inducing ligand (TRAIL). *Molecules* **2012**, *17*, 6449–6464. [CrossRef] [PubMed]
29. Reddy, N.S.; Gumireddy, K.; Mallireddigari, M.R.; Cosenza, S.C.; Venkatapuram, P.; Bell, S.C.; Reddy, E.P.; Reddy, M.V. Novel coumarin-3-(N-aryl)carboxamides arrest breast cancer cell growth by inhibiting ErbB-2 and ERK1. *Bioorg. Med. Chem.* **2005**, *13*, 3141–3147. [CrossRef]
30. Harada, K.; Kubo, H.; Tomigahara, Y.; Nishioka, K.; Takahashi, J.; Momose, M.; Inoue, S.; Kojima, A. Coumarins as novel 17beta-hydroxysteroid dehydrogenase type 3 inhibitors for potential treatment of prostate cancer. *Bioorg. Med. Chem. Lett.* **2010**, *20*, 272–275. [CrossRef]
31. Vijay Avin, B.R.; Thirusangu, P.; Lakshmi Ranganatha, V.; Firdouse, A.; Prabhakar, B.T.; Khanum, S.A. Synthesis and tumor inhibitory activity of novel coumarin analogs targeting angiogenesis and apoptosis. *Eur. J. Med. Chem.* **2014**, *75*, 211–221. [CrossRef]
32. Jin, J.; Yu, X.; Hu, Z.; Tang, S.; Zhong, X.; Xu, J.; Shang, P.; Huang, Y.; Liu, H. Isofraxidin targets the TLR4/MD-2 axis to prevent osteoarthritis development. *Food Funct.* **2018**, *9*, 5641–5652. [CrossRef]
33. Liu, J.; Chen, Q.; Jian, Z.; Xiong, X.; Shao, L.; Jin, T.; Zhu, X.; Wang, L. Daphnetin Protects against Cerebral Ischemia/Reperfusion Injury in Mice via Inhibition of TLR4/NF-kappaB Signaling Pathway. *Biomed. Res. Int.* **2016**, *2016*, 2816056. [CrossRef]
34. Tian, Y.; Liang, Z.; Xu, H.; Mou, Y.; Guo, C. Design, Synthesis and Cytotoxicity of Novel Dihydroartemisinin-Coumarin Hybrids via Click Chemistry. *Molecules* **2016**, *21*, 758. [CrossRef]
35. Yu, H.; Hou, Z.; Tian, Y.; Mou, Y.; Guo, C. Design, synthesis, cytotoxicity and mechanism of novel dihydroartemisinin-coumarin hybrids as potential anti-cancer agents. *Eur. J. Med. Chem.* **2018**, *151*, 434–449. [CrossRef]

36. Tan, Y.; Yang, X.-D.; Liu, W.-J.; Sun, X.-W. Novel one-pot asymmetric cascade approach toward densely substituted enantioenriched α-methylene-γ-lactams. *Tetrahedron Lett.* **2014**, *55*, 6105–6108. [CrossRef]
37. Pechmann, H.V. Berichte der deutschen chemischen. *Gesellschaft* **1884**, *17*, 929.
38. Ji, Q.; Ge, Z.; Ge, Z.; Chen, K.; Wu, H.; Liu, X.; Huang, Y.; Yuan, L.; Yang, X.; Liao, F. Synthesis and biological evaluation of novel phosphoramidate derivatives of coumarin as chitin synthase inhibitors and antifungal agents. *Eur. J. Med. Chem.* **2016**, *108*, 166–176. [CrossRef]
39. Ohto, U.; Fukase, K.; Miyake, K.; Shimizu, T. Structural basis of species-specific endotoxin sensing by innate immune receptor TLR4/MD-2. *Proc. Natl. Acad. Sci. USA* **2012**, *109*, 7421–7426. [CrossRef]

Sample Availability: Not available.

molecules

MDPI

Article

A Comparative Study of the Anticancer Activity and PARP-1 Inhibiting Effect of Benzofuran–Pyrazole Scaffold and Its Nano-Sized Particles in Human Breast Cancer Cells

Manal M. Anwar [1], Somaia S. Abd El-Karim [1], Ahlam H. Mahmoud [1], Abd El-Galil E. Amr [2,3,*] and Mohamed A. Al-Omar [2]

1. Department of Therapeutic Chemistry, National Research Centre, Dokki, Cairo 12622, Egypt
2. Pharmaceutical Chemistry Department, Drug Exploration & Development Chair (DEDC), College of Pharmacy, King Saud University, Riyadh 11451, Saudi Arabia
3. Applied Organic Chemistry Department, National Research Center, Cairo, Dokki 12622, Egypt

* Correspondence: aamr@ksu.edu.sa; Tel.: +966-565-148-750

Academic Editor: Qiao-Hong Chen
Received: 26 May 2019; Accepted: 26 June 2019; Published: 29 June 2019

Abstract: Breast cancer is considered the most common and deadly cancer among women worldwide. Nanomedicine has become extremely attractive in the field of cancer treatment. Due to the high surface to volume ratio and other unique properties, nanomaterials can be specifically targeted to certain cells and tissues to interact with the living systems. The strategic planning of this study is based on using the nanoprecipitation method to prepare nanoparticles **BZP-NPs** (3.8–5.7 nm) of the previously prepared benzofuran–pyrazole compound (**IV**) **BZP** which showed promising cytotoxic activity. The capacity of **BZP** and **BZP-NPs** to suppress the growth of human breast tumor MCF-7 and MDA-MB-231 cells was evaluated using MTT assay. The IC_{50} doses of **BZP** and **BZP-NPs** targeting normal breast cells MCF-12A exceeded those targeting the cancer cells by >1000-fold, demonstrating their reasonable safety profiles in normal cells. Furthermore, cell cycle analysis, apoptosis induction detection, assessment of p53, Bcl-2, caspase-3, and PARP-1 levels of **BZP** and its nano-sized-**BZP-NPs** particles were also evaluated. Although the obtained results were in the favor of compound **IV** in its normal-sized particles, **BZP-NPs** appeared as a hit compound which showed improved cytotoxicity against the tested human breast cancer cells associated with the induction of pre-G1 apoptosis as well as cell cycle arrest at G2/M phase. The increase in caspase-3 level, upregulation of p53, and downregulation of Bcl-2 protein expression levels confirmed apoptosis. Furthermore, ELISA results exhibited that **BZP-NPs** produced a more favorable impact as a PARP-1 enzyme inhibitor than the parent **BZP**.

Keywords: breast cancer; benzofuran–pyrazole; nanoparticles; cytotoxic activity; apoptosis; PARP-1 inhibition

1. Introduction

Breast cancer is the most common malignancy in women, accounting for about 18% of female cancers and over half a million new cases are diagnosed worldwide each year. Its incidence increases with age and is currently rising. Although earlier diagnosis has improved the survival rates, saving lives and elevating treatment rates, metastatic breast cancer is still considered as the major factor of breast cancer-related mortality [1–4]. Despite the continuous development in the treatment of cancer disease, the strategy for cancer management has remained essentially unchanged: surgical resection of the malignant tumor followed by either chemotherapeutic administration, radiotherapy, or a combination of the two. In fact, both of these therapies cause unselective and undesirable damage to the healthy tissues. In addition, a number of factors can lead to treatment failure, such as the remaining of some residual cells after the surgery, resistance to chemotherapies, physiological obstacles against the treatments, such as the blood–brain barrier and cellular barriers which hamper the access to drug targets, debilitating systemic toxicities, and poor pharmacokinetics of the chemotherapeutic [5–7].

Nanomedicine is defined as the use of nanotechnology for different medical purposes. Nanotechnology deals with research of materials of dimensions ranges between 1 to 100 nm (National Nanotechnology Initiative). This active protocol is applied in various science applications including cancer chemotherapeutics [8]. Deep studies have shed light on the combination of nanotechnology with cancer biology advances to gain novel techniques for cancer care. The concept that the strategy of nanomedicines is based on improving the therapeutic index of anticancer drugs by optimizing their pharmacokinetics and tissue distribution to facilitate and fasten delivery to the site of action is well known and has been investigated clinically [9–11]. Smaller (sub-100 nm) nanomedicine systems and lower molecular weight macromolecules have been shown to extravasate to a greater extent and/or penetrate farther from the vasculature than larger systems. This size effect has also been associated with improved efficacy [11,12]. Because of their sizes, the chemical properties and biodistribution of the nanomaterials are different from bulky materials. Thus, in recent years, nanomedicine has been considered as one of the most promising and important tools to defeat the problems obtained due to the administration of the traditional antitumor drugs. In addition, nanoparticle formulations can reduce or prevent systemic toxicities by specific delivery of the drugs to the cancer cells via size-mediated passive targeting and physiologically mediated active targeting. They can overcome drug resistance by the delivery of complimentary treatments and they can improve early detection of the disease using targeted delivery of molecular imaging agents to tumors in order to improve the diagnostic imaging of the tumor tissues, thus beginning the treatment before the onset of metastasis [13,14].

Inspired by the literature studies mentioned above and in continuation with our previous efforts in developing new effective agents of significant anticancer activity [15–17], this study deals with generating the previously prepared 1-(5-(3-(benzofuran-2-yl)-1-phenyl-1*H*-pyrazol-4-yl)-4,5-dihydro-3-(1*H*-pyrrol-2-yl)pyrazol-1-yl)ethanone **(IV) BZP** in nanoparticles **BZP-NPs** of sizes 3.8–5.7 nm (Figure 1).

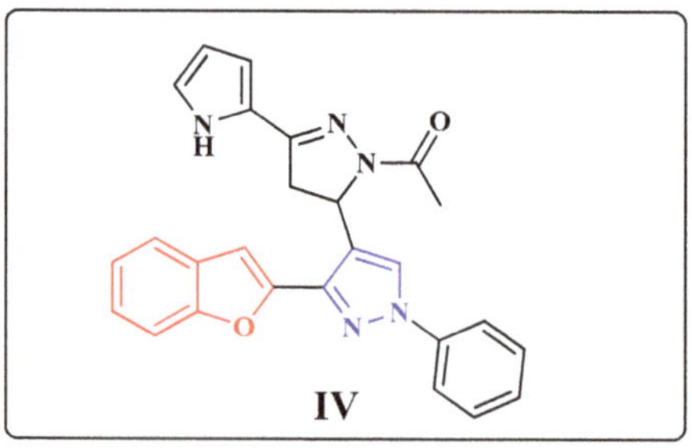

Figure 1. The chemical structure of the benzofuran-pyrazole compound **IV** (**BZP**).

In our previous research, compound **IV** (**BZP**) was subjected, among other eight different benzofuran-pyrazole derivatives, to NCI for *in vitro* anticancer evaluation targeting full 60 human cancer cell lines using a single high dose concentration (10^{-5} M) under the drug discovery program of the NCI [15]. The derivatives were chosen depending upon the degree of structural variations and computer modeling techniques in NCI. Fortunately, compound **IV** (**BZP**) exhibited promising cytotoxic potency against various cancer cell lines, so it was further evaluated by NCI team at five different minimal concentrations (0.01, 0.1, 1, 10, and 100 µM). It displayed cell growth inhibition of different breast cancer lines in the range of 45.95–55.44%. These data motivated the authors to convert compound **IV** (**BZP**) to nano-sized **BZP-NPs** to study the influence of the nanorange and whether nano-sized particles enhance the cytotoxic potency of the benzofuran compound.

The anticancer activity of **BZP** compound **IV** was assessed in comparison with its nano-sized **BZP-NPs** against MCF-7 and MDA-MB-231cancer cell lines. Various cellular mechanisms of action were also studied, such as apoptosis, cell cycle analysis, detection of caspase-3, p53, and Bcl-2 intensities, in addition to the efficiency of PARP-1 enzyme inhibition in the two types of the tested breast cancer cell lines

2. Results and Discussion

2.1. Chemistry

The preparation approach of the benzofuran–pyrazole derivative **IV** was outlined in Scheme 1 according to the reported method [15]. Using the Vilsmeier–Haach reaction, the key starting 1-(benzofuran-2-yl)ethanone (**I**) was converted to the intermediate pyrazole-4-carbaldehyde (**II**). The chalcone analogue **III** was obtained in a good yield by Claisen–Schmidt condensation of **II** with 2-acetylpyrrole in ethanolic sodium hydroxide solution. Cyclocondensation of **III** with hydrazine hydrate in acetic acid yielded the target compound **IV** in 85% yield (Scheme 1).

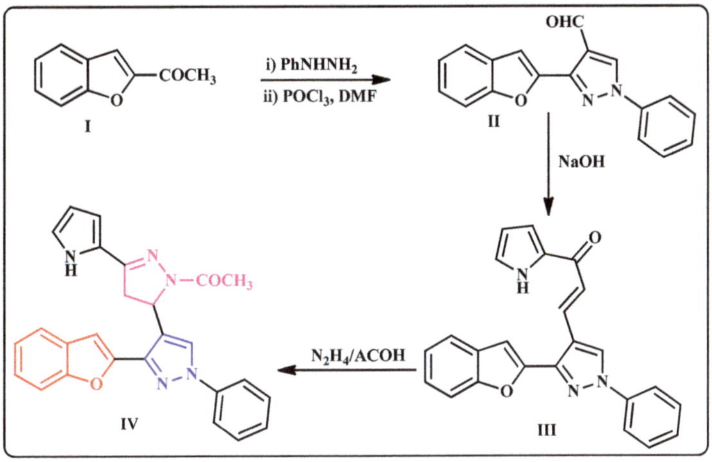

Scheme 1. Synthetic route of the benzofuran–pyrazole derivative (**IV**).

The nano-sized benzofuran–pyrazole **BZP-NPs** of different sizes (3.8–5.7 nm) were synthesized using the nanoprecipitation method [18]. The sizes and morphology of the nanobenzofuran–pyrazole hybrid **BZP-NPs** were examined by dynamic light scattering (DLS) and transmission electron microscopy (TEM). The results showed that nanoparticles were spherical in shape and their average size was 3.8–5.7 nm (Figure 2). The stability of the **BZP-NPs** was further investigated by X-ray diffraction (XRD) using a Pananalylical Empyrean X-ray Diffractometer and thermal analysis using a SDT Q600 V20.9 Build 20 thermal gravimetric instrument (Figures S1 and S2, Supplementary material).

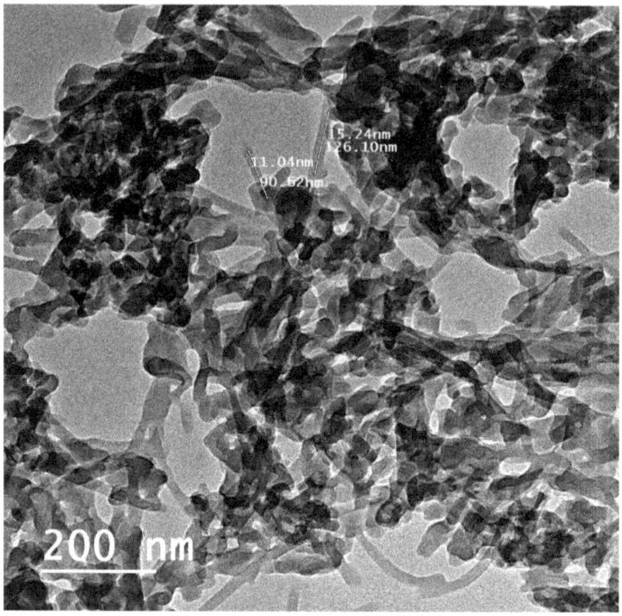

Benzofuran–pyrazole **IV** (**BZP**)

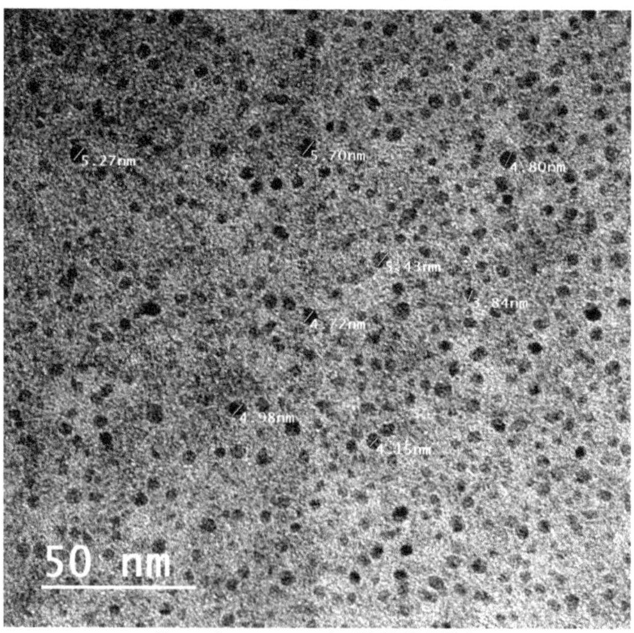

Benzofuran–pyrazole **IV** (**BZP-NPs**)

Figure 2. Electron micrograph of the **BZP** and **BZP-NPs**. The bar marker represents 50 nm.

Surface charge and stability of the nanoparticles were analyzed using the Malvern Zetasizer nano Zs instrument (MAL1074157) and the zeta potential was −27.3 mV with a polydispersity index (PDI) of 0.77 (Figure 3).

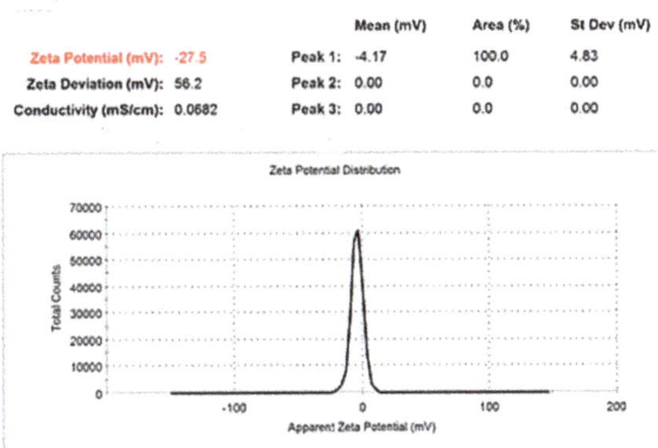

Figure 3. Zeta potential distribution of **BZP-NPs**.

2.2. Biological Analysis

2.2.1. In Vitro Anticancer Activity

The sensitivity of two human breast cancer cell lines, MCF-7 and MDA-MB-231, was evaluated against the benzofuran–pyrazole compound **BZP** and the target nano-sized benzofuran–pyrazole nanoparticles **BZP-NPs** using MTT assay. Doxorubicin served as a standard drug [17]. The resultant data were expressed as IC_{50} (nM) values which are the average of at least three independent experiments and are tabulated in Table 1. The obtained results showed that compound **IV** (**BZP**) produced significant cytotoxic activity against both breast cancer cell lines, with about 85- and 62-fold, respectively, greater potency than that of doxorubicin. Dramatic increase in the activity was observed by about 620 and 1000-fold for targeting both types of cancer cells by **BZP-NPs** compared to the reference drug doxorubicin. It could be detected that MDA-MB-231 cancer cells represented significant sensitivity against the nano-sized particles **BZP-NPs** more than their sensitivity against **BZP**.

Table 1. In vitro cytotoxic activity of compound **IV** (**BZP**) and **BZP-NPs**.

Compound Name	IC_{50} (nM)		
	MCF-7	MDA-MB-231	MCF-12A
Compound IV (**BZP**)	7 ± 1	10 ± 1	87600 ± 335
Compound IV (**BZP-NPs**)	1 ± 0.4	0.6 ± 0.1	21540 ± 66
Doxorubicin	620 ± 31	620 ± 31	

Despite the obvious benefits of chemotherapeutic drugs, there are several treatment-related damages to the normal cells that should be considered before finalizing the cancer treatment strategy. This study investigated the impact of compound **IV** (**BZP**) and **BZP-NPs** on normal breast cells (MRC-12A) using MTT assay [16]. Interestingly, a significant increase in the IC_{50} doses of **IV BZP** and **BZP-NPs** against the normal breast cells was detected when compared to their IC_{50} doses against both cancer cell lines (>1000-fold) (Table 1). This result confirmed the significant safety profile of the benzofuran-pyrazole compound **IV** either in the normal size particles or in its nano-sized particles **BZP-NPs**.

2.2.2. Cell Cycle Analysis

Due to the antiproliferative efficacy of compound **IV** (**BZP**) and **BZP-NPs**, it was of interest to study its modes of action in both tested types of cancer cells, including cell cycle progression and apoptosis induction. Cell death occurs via different pathways, including apoptosis or type I cell-death, and autophagy or type II cell-death, which are both forms of programmed cell death, whereas necrosis is a nonphysiological process resulting from an infection or injury [19,20]. Apoptosis rate in MCF-7 and MDA-MB-231 cells was detected by flow cytometry, using propidium iodide (PI) and an annexin-V–FITC double staining assay [21]. After incubation of both types of the tested cancer cells for 24 h with BZP and BZP-NPs at their IC_{50} concentrations of 7 nM and 1 nM for MCF-7 cells and at 10 nM and 0.6 nM for MDA-MB-231 cells, they were labeled with the two dyes. The corresponding red (PI) and green (FITC) fluorescence was detected using flow cytometry and the results were compared to DMSO-treated cells which served as a negative control. Marked alterations in cell cycle phases have occurred. There was a great enhancement in the percentage of apoptotic cells at the pre-G phase. The tested particles (**BZP**) and (**BZP-NPs**) induced total apoptotic cells (annexin V^+/PI^- and annexin V^+/PI^+) of percentages 9.18%, 21.54%, respectively, in MCF-7 cells vs. 2.64% in the control MCF-7 cells. They also induced total apoptotic percentages of 11.09% and 23.17%, respectively, in MDA-MB-231 cells vs. 2.82% in the control MDA-MB-231cells. It is observable that the **BZP-NPs** produced a more favorable impact about two-fold more potent than **BZP** particles against both types of the tested cancer cells, especially MDA-MB-231 cells, which was consistent with the cytotoxicity assay results (Figures 4 and 5). Also, exposure of MCF-7 and MDA-MB-231 cells to **BZP** and **BZP-NPs** led to an interference with the cell cycle distribution, inducing a pronounced elevation in the percentage of cells at the G2/M phase, reaching 11.26% and 17.52%, respectively, in MCF-7 vs. 6.28% in the control cells and to 12.11% and 19.24% in MDA-MB-231 cells, respectively, vs. 4.92% in the negative control (Table 2). Accordingly, it can be concluded that the compound **IV** (**BZP**) inhibits the cancer cells' proliferation with a synchronous significant arrest at the G2/M phase. The inhibition potency was signified by the **BZP-NPs** (Figures 6 and 7). Accumulation of cells at G2/M phase is a remarkable hallmark of the apoptotic role of **BZP** and **BZP-NPs** in both tested cancer cell lines.

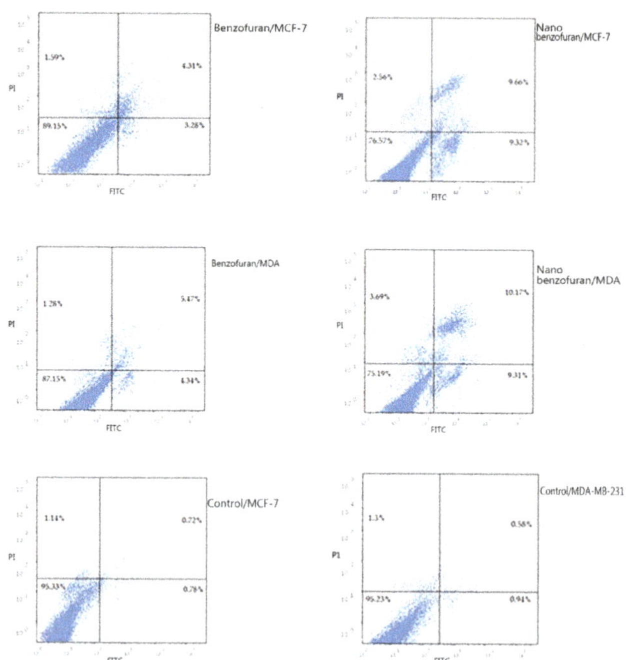

Figure 4. Representative dot plots of MCF-7 and MDA-MB-231 cells treated with compound **IV** (**BZP**) and **BZP-NPs** at their IC_{50} (μM) for 24 h, analyzed by flow cytometry after double staining of the cells with annexin-V FITC and PI.

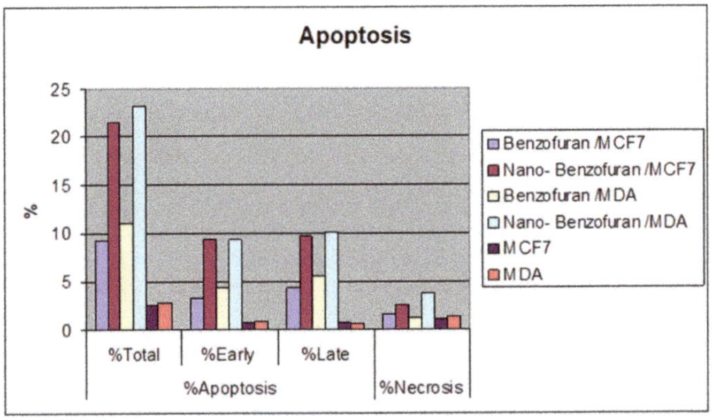

Figure 5. Percentage of compound **IV** (**BZP**) and **BZP-NPs** in MCF-7 and MDA-MB-231 cancer cells.

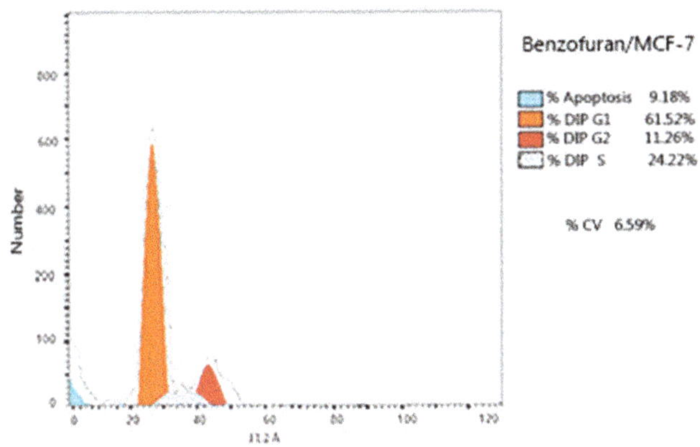

(**A**): The effect of compound **IV** (**BZP**) on MCF-7 cancer cells

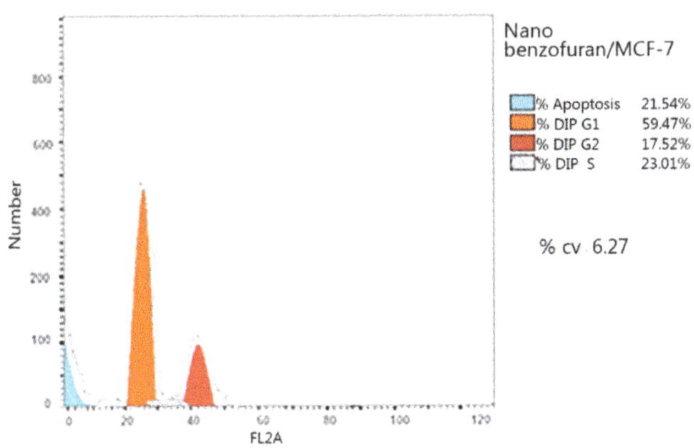

(**B**): The effect of compound **IV** (**BZP-NPs**) on MCF-7 cancer cells

Figure 6. *Cont.*

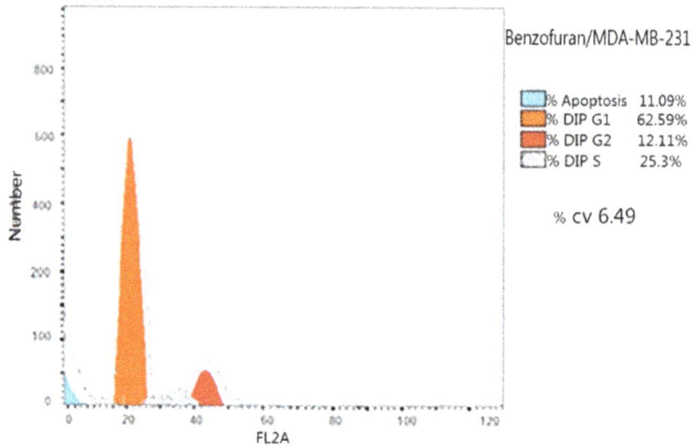

(**C**): The effect of compound **IV** (**BZP**) on MDA-MB-231cancer cells

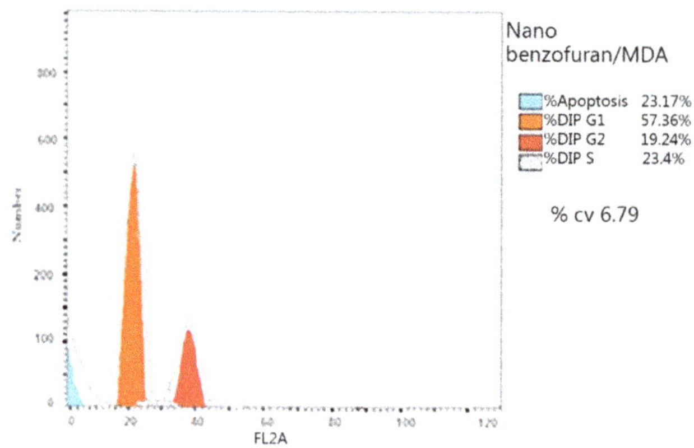

(**D**): The effect of compound **IV** (**BZP-NPs**) on MDA-MB-231cancer cells

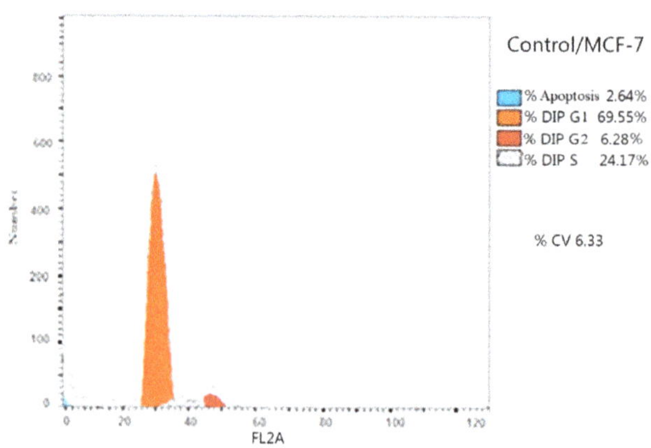

(**E**): The negative control of MCF-7 cancer cells

Figure 6. *Cont.*

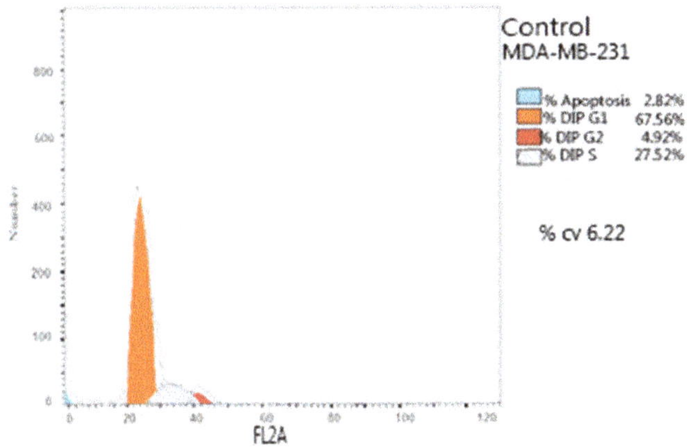

(**F**): The negative control of MDA-MB-231 cancer cells

Figure 6. Flow cytometric analysis of compound **IV** (**BZP**) and **BZP-NPs** on MCF-7 and MDA-MB-231 cells. The orange color represents G1 phase percentage and red color represents G2/M phase percentage.

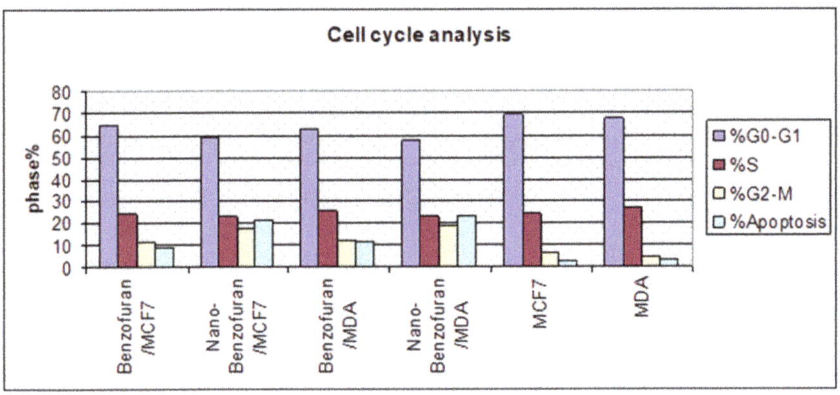

Figure 7. Cycle analysis of compound **IV** (**BZP**) and **BZP-NPs** in MCF-7 and MDA-MB-231 cancer cells.

Table 2. Determination of cell cycle inhibition of MCF-7 and MDA-MB-231 cancer cells by **BZP** and **BZP-NPs**.

Compound Name	Conc. (nM)	%G0-G1	%S	%G2-M	%Pre-G1	Comment
BZP/MCF-7	7	64.52	24.22	11.26	9.18	PreG1apoptosis&Cell growth arrest@ G2/M
BZP-NPs/MCF-7	1	59.47	23.01	17.52	21.54	PreG1apoptosis&Cell growth arrest@ G2/M
BZP/MDA-MB-231	10	62.59	25.3	12.11	11.09	PreG1apoptosis&Cell growth arrest@ G2/M
BZP-NPs/MDA-MB-231	0.6	57.36	23.4	19.24	23.17	PreG1apoptosis&Cell growth arrest@ G2/M
MCF-7		69.55	24.17	6.28	2.64	
MDA-MB-231		67.56	27.52	4.92	2.82	

2.2.3. Effect Compound **IV** (**BZP**) and **BZP-NPs** on the Levels of Caspase-3/p53/Bax/Bcl-2

Caspases are cysteine protease enzymes in humans. Their presence is critical in starting the phase of programmed cell death (apoptosis). Some caspases initiate the intracellular cascade, whereas others (effector caspases) produce their activities downstream by controlling the cellular break via splitting of the structural proteins [19–21]. Caspase-3 displays an important role in the apoptotic process which includes cell shrinkage, chromatin condensation, and DNA fragmentation [22,23]. Enzyme Linked Immuno-Sorbent Assay (ELISA) was used to analyze the apoptotic events of both types of the tested breast cancer cells [16]. Table 3 shows that 24 h treatment of MCF-7 with compound **IV** (**BZP**) and **BZP-NPs** at concentrations of 7 nM and 1 nM and MDA-MB-231 cells at concentrations of 10 nM and 0.6 nM led to significant overexpression of caspase-3 compared to the doxorubicin-treated cells. **BZP** elevated the level of caspase-3 by six and five-fold compared to the untreated cells. A detectable enhancement in the level of caspase-3 occurred upon treatment of the tested cells with **BZP-NPs** by 14 and 17-fold compared to the untreated MCF-7 and MDA-MB-231 cells (Table 3).

Table 3. Determination of caspase-3, p53, Bax, and Bcl-2 levels in the tested cancer cells.

	Results (Fold Change)			
Compound Name	**Caspase-3**	**p53**	**Bax**	**Bcl.2**
BZP/MCF-7	6.383836	7.453852	5.745321	0.272695
BZP-NPs/MCF-7	14.56524	12.51432	9.149760	0.131011
BZP/MDA-MB-231	5.399087	7.792609	7.553853	0.181989
BZP-NPs/MDA-MB-231	17.915	14.60536	13.19230	0.134738
MCF-7	1	1	1	1
MDA-MB-231	1	1	1	1

The tumor suppressor protein p53 serves as a transcription factor. It induces the expression of several downstream targets which are very important in regulation of the cell cycle, apoptosis, and DNA repair, among other mechanisms [24,25]. Cellular stress leads to the activation of the p53 pathway, compromising tumor development and preventing the proliferation of the damaged cells of oncogenic potential. p53 is considered as one of the most relevant tumor suppressor genes [26]. In addition, the B-cell lymphoma protein 2 (Bcl-2) plays a key role in tumor progression via inhibition of the intrinsic apoptotic pathway triggered by mitochondrial dysfunction. Cancer cells can resist apoptosis by modulating the expression of Bcl-2 family proteins which in turn regulate the mitochondrial apoptotic pathway via production Bcl-2 or downregulating pro-apoptotic proteins, such as Bax [26]. Accordingly, in this study, the impact **of IV** (**BZP**) and **BZP-NPs** was assessed on the intrinsic apoptotic pathway via measuring the levels of p53, Bax, and Bcl-2 after treatment of MCF-7 and MDA-MB-231 cells with **BZP** and **BZP-NPs** at their IC_{50} concentrations for 24 h. In comparison to the untreated control, p53 level increased seven-fold in both types of the tested cancer cells upon **BZP** treatment, while the level was doubled to 14-fold by the **BZP-NPs**. On the other hand, **BZP** and **BZP-NPs** elevated the level of the proapoptotic protein Bax by 5.7–13.1-fold with concurrent reduction in the expression levels of the antiapoptotic protein Bcl-2 by four to seven-fold in both tested cancer cell lines in comparison with the untreated control (Table 3).

2.2.4. PARP-1 Cleavage Assay

Breast cancer is among the targets of a new class of drugs known as Poly (ADP-ribose) polymerase-1 (PARP-1) inhibitors. PARP-1 is a nuclear enzyme plays a role in the repair of single-stranded DNA (ss DNA) breaks [26]. The rationale for the therapeutic benefit for the pharmacological inhibition of PARP-1 in breast cancer comes from the following points: (a) sensitization of tumor cells to anticancer therapies such as radiation and cytotoxic agents [27]; (b) certain polymorphisms in PARP-1 can lead to breast cancer and negatively affect the efficacy of the hormone therapies; and (c) breast tumors with deficiencies in DNA-repair genes such as BRCA-1 or BRCA-2 represent acute sensitivity in response to the inhibition of PARP-1. Interestingly, clinical evidence investigates that the usage of PARP-1-inhibiting candidates are not limited to BRCA-1 or BRCA-2 mutated cancers, but they also target non-BRCA mutated breast and ovarian cancers and produce a valuable impact in combination therapy [28,29]. Thus, it was of interest to study the inhibitory effects of **BZP** and **BZP-NPs** against PARP-1 enzyme in MCF-7 and MDA-MB-231 cancer cells using staurosporine as a standard drug. The resulting data were expressed as IC_{50} (nM) values and are summarized in (Table 4). It should be noted that **BZP** produced a slightly weaker inhibitory effect against PARP-than the reference drug, with an IC_{50} of 40 nM vs. 10 nM for staurosporine in MCF-7 cells. A dramatic decrease, about 13-fold, in the sensitivity was noticed in the case of MDA-MB-231 cancer cells against **BZP** which produced an IC_{50} of 60 nM vs. 8 nM for staurosporine. On the other hand, an interesting increase in the inhibitory potency was observed for the **BZP-NPs**, exhibiting an IC_{50} value of 10 nM, which is equal to that obtained by the standard drug in MCF-7 cells. The suppression activity was intensified against PARP-1 in MDA-MB-231 cells, producing an IC_{50} of 6 nM vs. 8 nM for staurosporine.

Table 4. In vitro PARP-1 inhibitory assay of compound **IV (BZP)** and **BZP-NPs**.

Compound Name	IC_{50} (nM)	
	MCF-7	MDA-MB-231
BZP	40 ± 1	60 ±1
BZP-NPs	10 ± 4	6 ± 3
Staurosporine	10 ± 1	8 ± 1

3. Experimental

3.1. *Synthesis of 1-(5-(3-(Benzofuran-2-yl)-1-phenyl-1H-pyrazol-4-yl)-4,5-dihydro-3-(1H-pyrrol-2-yl) pyrazol-1-yl)ethanone* (IV).

Compound **IV** was synthesized according to the previously reported procedure [15].

3.2. *Preparation of Nanobenzofuran–Pyrazole* BZP-NPs

The nanoparticles were prepared by the nanoprecipitation method [18]. The sizes and morphology of the nanoparticles **BZP-NPs** were examined by transmission electron microscopy (TEM) (H-7600; Hitachi Ltd., Tokyo, Japan). The results exhibited that the nanoparticles were spherical in shape and their average size was 3.8–5.7 nm (Figure 2).

3.3. *Physicochemical Characterization of the Nanobenzofuran–Pyrazole Compound* BZP-NPs

3.3.1. Particle Size and Zeta Potential Using Photon Correlation Spectroscopy

Particle size was measured by dynamic light scattering (DLS) using a Zetasizer NANO-ZS (Ver. 7.04, Serial Number: MAL 1074157, Malvern Instruments Ltd., London, United Kingdom) at a wavelength of 633 nm with a 4.0 mW light source for collecting data at a fixed scattering angle of 173°. The electrophoretic mobility (zeta potential) measurements were made using a Zetasizer NANO-ZS (Ver. 7.04, Serial Number: MAL 1074157, Malvern Instruments Ltd., United Kingdom) at 25 °C. **BZP-NPs** morphology was determined using JEOL Transmission Electron Microscope (JEM-1230, Tokyo, Japan) with 500,000 × magnification power, 100 kV acceleration voltage, and 0.5 nm resolving power.

3.3.2. In Vitro Anticancer Activity

In vitro evaluation of the anticancer activity of the **BZP** compound and **BZP-NPs** targeting MCF-7 and MDA-MB-231 cells was performed using MTT assay according to a previously reported method [19]. Each experiment was performed at least three times.

3.4. Cell Cycle Analysis and Apoptosis Detection

Cell cycle analysis and apoptosis detection was carried out by flow cytometry (Beckman Coulter, Brea, CA, USA) [19–21]. Apoptosis detection was performed using a FITC Annexin-V/PI commercial kit (Becton Dickenson, Franklin Lakes, NJ, USA) following the manufacturer's protocol.

3.5. Caspases-3 Assays

Caspase-3 activity was measured using a Caspase-3 (Active) (human) ELISA kit, Catalog # KHO1091 (96 tests) (Invitrogen Corporation, Carlsbad, CA, USA) according to the manufacturer's instructions [16].

3.6. In Vitro Determination of p53, Bax, and Bcl-2 Levels

The levels of p53, Bax, and Bcl-2 markers were assessed using a BIORAD iScript TM One-Step RT-PCR kit with SYBR® Green according to the manufacturer's instructions [26,30].

3.7. In Vitro PARP-1 Assay

The procedure was done according to the supplied protocol of ab119690 Cleaved PARP Human ELISA (Enzyme-Linked Immunosorbent Assay) kit for the quantitative measurement of the 89 kDa fragment of Human PARP-1 in cell and tissue lysates [31].

4. Conclusions

This study demonstrates that the conversion of the benzofuran-pyrazole compound **IV** (**BZP**) to nanoparticles **BZP-NPs** greatly intensified its cytotoxic activity against two breast cancer cell lines, MCF-7 and MDA-MB-231, with respective IC_{50} values of 7 nM, 10 nM vs. nanoparticle IC_{50} values of 1 nM, 0.6 nM. The IC_{50} value of DOX was 620 nM. Furthermore, the IC_{50} doses of BZP and BZP-NPs against normal breast cells were >1000-fold greater than those against cancer cells, suggesting acceptable safety profiles in normal cells. The resultant data of cell cycle and apoptosis determination revealed that the tested derivative in both forms induced G2/M phase arrest, accompanied by an increase in apoptosis in the tested cancer cells. Further modes of action of the target compound were also predicted in both types of breast cancer cells. The biological results revealed that **BZP** significantly increased p53, caspase-3, and Bax levels and decreased Bcl-2 levels, and their levels were intensified upon treating the tested cancer cells with (**BZP-NPs**). The PARP1 enzyme assay showed that the efficiency of PARP-1 inhibition by (**BZP**) was slightly less than that of staurosporine, while **BZP-NPs** inhibited the enzyme efficiently as staurosporine in MCF-7 or to a greater extent in case of MDA-MB-231 cancer cells. It has been detected that the nanoparticles were more effective as an anticancer agent against MDA-MB-231 cells than against MCF-7 cancer cells.

Supplementary Materials: The following are available online, Figure S1: Diffraction (XRD) of BZP-NPs, Figure S2: Analysis of **BZP-NPs**.

Author Contributions: S.S.A.E.-K., M.M.A. performed most of the experiments; A.E.-G.E.A., M.A.A.-O., analyzed the data; A.H.M. the contributed to the anticancer activity assays; All authors read and approved the final manuscript.

Funding: This work was supported financially by National Research Centre, Dokki, Cairo, Egypt, under the project No. 11010317, entitled "Development of Novel Poly (ADP-ribose) Polymerase-1 Inhibitors as Anticancer and Chemo-sensitizers Targeting Breast Cancer Disease". Also, the authors extend their appreciation and thanking to Essam Rashwan, the head of confirmatory diagnostic unit, Vacsera-Egypt, for helping in performing the pharmacological screening.

Acknowledgments: The authors are grateful to the Deanship of Scientific Research, king Saud University for funding through Vice Deanship of Scientific Research Chairs.

Conflicts of Interest: The authors declare no conflict of interest.

References

1. Giordano, M.C.; Rovitoa, D.; Baroneb, I.; Mancusoc, R.; Bonofigliob, D.; Giordanob, F.; Catalanob, S.; Gabrielec, B.; Andòa, S. Benzofuran-2-acetic ester derivatives induce apoptosis in breastcancer cells by upregulating p21Cip/WAF1gene expression inp53-independent manner. *DNA Repair.* **2017**, *51*, 20–30. [CrossRef] [PubMed]
2. Ferlay, J.; Soerjomataram, I.; Dikshit, R.; Eser, S.; Mathers, C.; Rebelo, M.; Parkin, D.M.; Forman, D.; Bray, F. Cancer incidence and mortality worldwide: sources, methods and majorpatterns in GLOBOCAN. *Int. J. Cancer* **2015**, *136*, 359–386. [CrossRef] [PubMed]
3. Kassab, A.E.; Gedawy, E.M.; El-Nassan, H.B. Synthesis of 4-heteroaryl-quinazoline derivatives as potential anti-breast cancer agents. *J. Heterocycl. Chem.* **2017**, *54*, 624–633. [CrossRef]
4. Amin, K.M.; Syam, Y.M.; Anwar, M.M.; Ali, H.I.; Abdel-Ghani, T.M.; Serry, A.M. Synthesis and molecular docking study of new benzofuran and furo[3,2-*g*]chromone-based cytotoxic agents against breast cancer and p38$^{\alpha}$ MAP kinase inhibitors. *Bioorg. Chem.* **2018**, *76*, 487–500. [CrossRef] [PubMed]
5. Hull, L.C.; Farrell, D.; Grodzinski, P. Highlights of recent developments and trends in cancer nanotechnology research-View from NCI Alliance for Nanotechnology in Cancer. *Biotechnol. Adv.* **2014**, *32*, 666–678. [CrossRef] [PubMed]
6. Zamboni, W.C.; Torchilin, V.; Patri, A.K.; Hrkach, J.; Stern, S.; Lee, R.; Nel, A.; Panaro, N.J.; Grodzinski, P. Best practices in cancer nanotechnology: Perspective from NCI nanotechnology alliance. *Clin. Cancer. Res.* **2012**, *18*, 3229–3241. [CrossRef] [PubMed]
7. Hare, J.I.; Lammers, T.; Ashford, M.B.; Puri, S.; Storm, G.; Barry, S.T. Challenges and strategies in anti-cancer nanomedicine development: An industry perspective. *Adv. Drug Deliv. Rev.* **2017**, *108*, 25–38. [CrossRef] [PubMed]
8. Salata, O.V. Applications of nanoparticles in biology and medicine. *J. Nano Biotechnol.* **2004**, *2*, 1–6.
9. Dyawanapelly, S.; Mehrotra, P.; Ghosh, G.; Jagtap, D.D.; Dandekar, P.; Jain, R. How the surface functionalized nanoparticles affect conformation and activity of proteins: Exploring through protein-nanoparticle interactions. *Bioorg. Chem.* **2019**, *82*, 17–25. [CrossRef]
10. Saraiva, C.; Praça, C.; Ferreira, R.; Santos, T.; Ferreira, L.; Bernardino, L. Nanoparticle-mediated brain drug delivery: Overcoming blood–brain barrier to treat neurodegenerative diseases. *J. Control Release* **2016**, *235*, 34–47. [CrossRef]
11. Popovic, Z.; Liu, W.; Chauhan, V.P.; Lee, J.; Wong, C.; Greytak, A.B.; Insin, N.; Nocera, D.G.; Fukumura, D.; Jain, R.K.; et al. A nanoparticle size series for in vivo fluorescence imaging. *Angew. Chem. Int. Ed. Eng.* **2010**, *49*, 8649–8652. [CrossRef] [PubMed]
12. Cabral, H.; Matsumoto, Y.; Mizuno, K.; Chen, Q.; Murakami, M.; Kimura, M.; Terada, Y.; Kano, M.R.; Miyazono, K.; Uesaka, M.; et al. Accumulation of sub-100 nm polymeric micelles in poorly permeable tumors depends on size. *Nat. Nanotechnol.* **2011**, *6*, 815–823. [CrossRef] [PubMed]
13. Wang, J.; Mao, W.; Lock, L.L.; Tang, J.; Sui, M.; Sun, W.; Cui, H.; Xu, D.; Shen, Y. The role of micelle size in tumor accumulation, penetration, and treatment. *ACS Nano.* **2015**, *9*, 7195–7206. [CrossRef] [PubMed]
14. Thakur, S.; Pramod, K.S.; Malviya, R. Utilization of Polymeric Nanoparticle in Cancer Treatment: A Review. *J. Pharma. Care Health Sys.* **2017**, *4*, 2.
15. Abd El-Karim, S.S.; Anwar, M.M.; Mohamed, N.A.; Nasr, T.; Elseginy, S.A. Design, synthesis, biological evaluation and molecular docking studies of novel benzofuran-pyrazole derivatives as anticancer agents. *Bioorg. Chem.* **2015**, *63*, 1–12. [CrossRef] [PubMed]
16. Amin, K.M.; Syam, Y.M.; Anwar, M.M.; Ali, H.I.; Abdel-Ghani, T.M.; Serry, A.M. Synthesis and molecular docking studies of new furochromone derivatives as p38α MAPK inhibitors targeting human breast cancer MCF-7 cells. *Bioorg. Med. Chem.* **2017**, *25*, 2423–2436. [CrossRef] [PubMed]
17. Abd El-Karim, S.S.; Anwar, M.M.; Zaki, E.R.; Elseginy, S.A.; Nofal, Z.M. Synthesis and molecular modeling of new benzimidazoles as glutathione S-transferase inhibitors and anticancer agents. *Future Med. Chem.* **2018**, *10*, 157–181. [CrossRef]
18. Cherian, A.M.; Snima, K.S.; Kamath, C.R.; Nair, S.V.; Lakshmanan, V.K. Effect of Baliospermummontanumnanomedicine apoptosis induction and anti-migration of prostate cancer cells. *Biomed. Pharm.* **2015**, *71*, 201–209. [CrossRef]

19. Coskun, D.; Erkisa, M.; Ulukaya, E.; Coskun, M.F.; Ari, F. Novel 1-(7-ethoxy-1-benzofuran-2-yl) substituted chalcone derivatives: synthesis, characterization and anticancer activity. *Eur. J. Med. Chem.* **2017**, *136*, 212–222. [CrossRef]
20. Zhang, L.; Ren, W.; Wang, X.; Zhang, J.; Liu, J.; Zhao, L.; Zhang, X. Discovery of novel polycyclic spiro-fused carbocyclicoxindole-based anticancer agents. *Eur. J. Med. Chem.* **2017**, *126*, 1071–1082. [CrossRef]
21. Labib, M.B.; Philoppes, J.N.; Lamie, P.F.; Ahmed, E.R. Azole-hydrazone derivatives: Design, synthesis, in vitro biological evaluation, dual EGFR/HER2 inhibitory activity, cell cycle analysis and molecular docking study as anticancer agents. *Bioorg. Chem.* **2018**, *76*, 67–80. [CrossRef] [PubMed]
22. Van Raam, B.J.; Salvesen, G.S. Handbook of Proteolytic Enzymes, 3rd ed.Elsevier Ltd.: Amsterdam, The Netherlands, 2013; pp. 2252–2255.
23. Ghorab, M.M.; Alsaid, M.S.; Samir, N.; Abdel-Latif, G.A.; Soliman, A.M.; Ragab, F.A.; Abou El Ella, D.A. Aromatase inhibitors and apoptotic inducers: Design, synthesis, anticancer activity and molecular modeling studies of novel phenothiazine derivatives carrying sulfonamide moiety as hybrid molecules. *Eur. J. Med. Chem.* **2017**, *134*, 304–315. [CrossRef] [PubMed]
24. Taguchi, T.; Kato, Y.; Baba, Y.; Nishimura, G.; Tanigaki, Y.; Horiuchi, C.; Mochimatsu, I.; Tsukuda, M. Protein levels of p21, p27, cyclin E and Bax predict sensitivity to cisplatin and paclitaxel in head and neck squamous cell carcinomas. *Oncol. Rep.* **2004**, *11*, 421–426. [CrossRef] [PubMed]
25. Fridman, J.S.; Lowe, S.W. Control of apoptosis by p53. *Oncogene* **2003**, *22*, 9030–9040. [CrossRef] [PubMed]
26. Brandao, P.; Loureiro, J.B.; Carvalho, S.; Hamadou, M.H.; Cravo, S.; Moreira, J.; Pereira, D.; Palmeira, A.; Pinto, M.; Saraiva, L.; et al. Targeting the MDM2-p53 protein-protein interaction with prenylchalcones: Synthesis of a small library and evaluation of potential antitumor activity. *Eur. J. Med. Chem.* **2018**, *156*, 711–721. [CrossRef] [PubMed]
27. Griguolo, G.; Vittoria Dieci, M.; Guarneri, V.; Conte, P.F. Olaparib for the treatment of breast cancer. *Expert Rev. Anticancer Ther.* **2018**, *18*, 519–530. [CrossRef] [PubMed]
28. Amin, K.M.; Anwar, M.M.; Syam, Y.M.; Khedr, M.; Kamel, M.M.; Kassem, E.M.M. A novel class of substituted spiro[quinazoline-2,1′-cyclohexane] derivatives as effective PARP-1 inhibitors: Molecular modeling, synthesis, cytotoxic and enzyme assay evaluation. *Acta Poloni. Pharm. Drug Res.* **2013**, *70*, 687–708.
29. Livraghi, L.J.; Garber, E. PARP inhibitors in the management of breast cancer: Current data and future prospects. *BMC Med.* **2015**, *13*, 188–203. [CrossRef]
30. Abdelhaleem, E.F.; Abdelhameid, M.K.; Kassab, A.E.; Kandeel, M.M. Design and synthesis of thienopyrimidine urea derivatives with potential cytotoxic and proapoptotic activity against breast cancer cell line MCF-7. *Eur. J. Med. Chem.* **2018**, *143*, 1807–1825. [CrossRef]
31. Jagtap, P.G.; Southan, G.J.; Baloglu, E.; Ram, S.; Mabley, J.G.; Marton, A.; Salzman, A.; Szabó, C. The Discovery and Synthesis of Novel Adenosine Substituted 2,3-Dihydro-1H-isoindol-1-ones: Potent Inhibitors of Poly(ADP-ribose) Polymerase-1 (PARP-1). *Bioorg. Med. Chem. Lett.* **2004**, *14*, 81–85. [CrossRef]

Sample Availability: Samples of the compounds are available from the authors.

molecules

MDPI

Article

Synthesis of New Derivatives of Benzofuran as Potential Anticancer Agents

Mariola Napiórkowska [1,*], Marcin Cieślak [2,*], Julia Kaźmierczak-Barańska [2], Karolina Królewska-Golińska [2] and Barbara Nawrot [2]

1 Chair and Department of Biochemistry, Medical University of Warsaw, 1 Banacha Str., 02-097 Warsaw, Poland
2 Centre of Molecular and Macromolecular Studies, Polish Academy of Sciences, 112 Sienkiewicza Str., 90-363 Łódź, Poland; julia@cbmm.lodz.pl (J.K.-B.); kkrolews@cbmm.lodz.pl (K.K.-G.); bnawrot@cbmm.lodz.pl (B.N.)
* Correspondence: mariola.napiorkowska@wum.edu.pl (M.N.); marcin@cbmm.lodz.pl (M.C.); Tel.: +48-22-572-06-93 or +48-22-572-06-39 (M.N.); +48-22-681-89-52 (M.C.); Fax: +48-22-572-06-79 (M.N.); +48-22-648-71-26 (M.C.)

Academic Editor: Qiao-Hong Chen
Received: 28 March 2019; Accepted: 16 April 2019; Published: 18 April 2019

Abstract: The results of our previous research indicated that some derivatives of benzofurans, particularly halogeno-derivatives, are selectively toxic towards human leukemia cells. Continuing our work with this group of compounds we here report new data on the synthesis as well as regarding the physico-chemical and biological characterization of fourteen new derivatives of benzofurans, including six brominated compounds. The structures of all new compounds were established by spectroscopic methods (^{1}H- and, ^{13}C-NMR, ESI MS), and elemental analyses. Their cytotoxicity was evaluated against K562 (leukemia), MOLT-4 (leukemia), HeLa (cervix carcinoma), and normal cells (HUVEC). Five compounds (**1c**, **1e**, **2d**, **3a**, **3d**) showed significant cytotoxic activity against all tested cell lines and selectivity for cancer cell lines. The SAR analysis (structure-activity relationship analysis) indicated that the presence of bromine introduced to a methyl or acetyl group that was attached to the benzofuran system increased their cytotoxicity both in normal and cancer cells.

Keywords: benzofurans; chemical synthesis; cytotoxic properties; HeLa; MOLT-4; K562

1. Introduction

Benzofuran skeleton holds an important position in organic chemistry and it is considered to be one of the most important heterocyclic systems because of its diverse profile of biological activity. This structural unit is a central part of a variety of biologically active compounds. Natural and synthetic benzofuran derivatives have been reported to possess wide therapeutic properties, including antiviral, immunosuppressive, antioxidant, antifungal, anti-inflammatory, antimicrobial, analgesic, antihyperglycemic, and antitumor activities [1–6]. *Cicerfuran*, *Conocarpan*, and *Ailanthoidol* are the best known biologically active natural benzofurans (Figure 1). Specifically, the *Cicerfuran* shows antifungal activity, *Conocarpan* has been reported as an antifungal and antitrypanosomal agent, and *Ailanthoidol* exhibits anticancer, antiviral, immunosuppressive, antioxidant, and antifungal activity [1,2,7]. The synthetic benzofuran derivatives are represented by *Amiodarone* (Figure 1), being used in the treatment of ventricular and supraventricular arrhythmias, and by *Bufuralol*, which is a non-specific β-adrenergic blocker with an affinity for β1 and β2-adrenergic receptors [3,4,7].

Nowadays, when cancer, after cardiovascular diseases, is the second most common cause of death and still constitutes an unresolved problem of clinical medicine and pharmacology, extensive research regarding new anticancer compounds is especially important. These new drugs should possess improved pharmacokinetics and specifically destroy cancer cells, without causing negative side effects. Research in the group of benzofuran derivatives is justified, especially by the fact that one can find many examples of data in the literature on benzofurans with anticancer activity. In many cases, the benzofuran skeleton is fused with other heterocyclic or aromatic moieties (Figure 2).

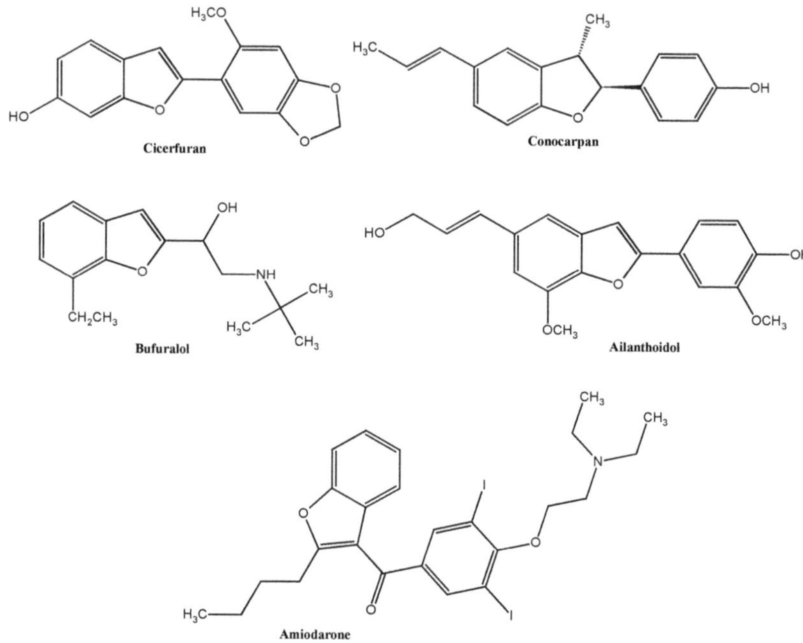

Figure 1. Structures of natural and synthetic benzofuran derivatives with biological activity.

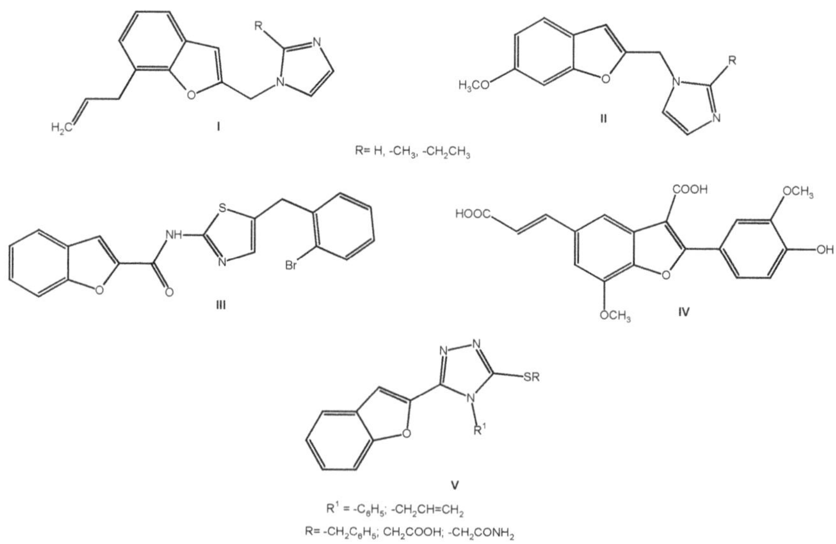

Figure 2. Structures of synthetic benofuran derivatives **I–V** with anticancer activity [7].

There are several benzofuranyl imidazole derivatives among them (**I** and **II**), which were found to be cytotoxic towards an ovarian carcinoma cell line (Skov-3). The study of *N*-(5-(2-bromobenzyl) thiazole-2-yl) benzofuran-2-carboxamide (**III**) showed that this compound inhibited the growth of HCC (human hepatocellular carcinoma) cells and induced their apoptosis. The synthetic derivative **IV** was found to have antitumor activity and it was an effective chemopreventive and chemotherapeutic agent against malignant T cells. Moreover, a series of triazole derivatives **V** showed moderate antitumor activity. Recent data reported this type of benzofuran derivatives as potential therapeutic agents for breast cancer [7].

These are only a few examples from a large group of benzofurans with anticancer activity. Moreover, examples of compounds with cytotoxic activity were found among the simple derivatives of benzofuran like 2- and 3-benzofuranocarboxylic acid derivatives **VI–VII** (Figure 3). The above-mentioned compounds exhibit significant cytotoxic activity against human cancer cell lines [8].

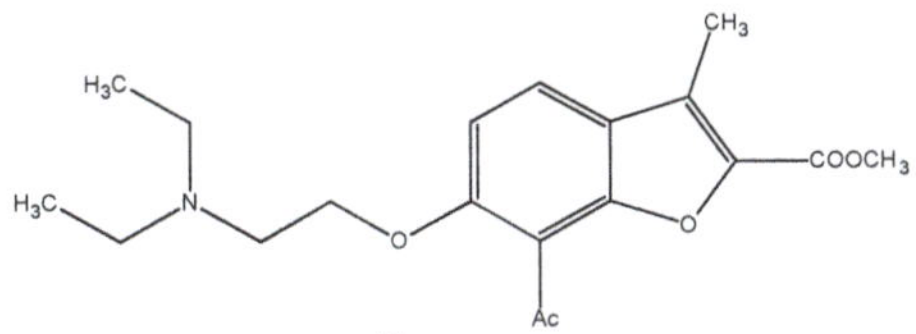

VI

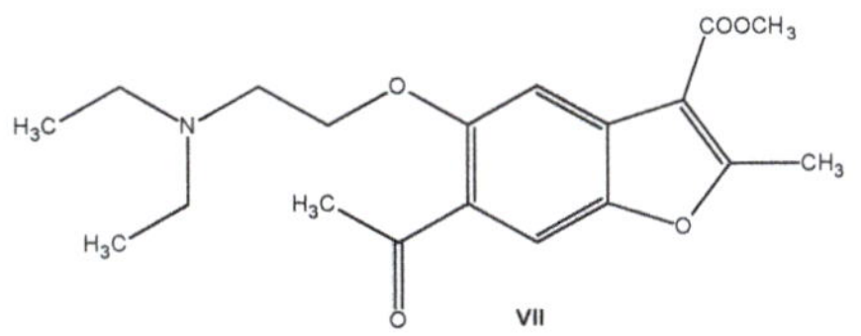

VII

Figure 3. Structures of 2- and 3-benzofurancarboxylic acid derivatives **VI–VII** with cytotoxic activity.

The literature survey shows that benzofurans containing halogens in their structure constitute an important group of compounds, with antitumor, cytotoxic, spasmolytic, antiarrhythmic, and antifungal activity [9–20]. Thus, this group of compounds is interesting for researchers, especially because the presence of halogen can increase the activity and selectivity of derivatives. This is probably related to the ability of halogens to create a "halogen bond", which results from the formation of the σ-hole. Although the halogen bonds are weaker than hydrogen bonds, they have specific effects and can lead to significant gains in binding affinity. These interactions can be found in protein-receptor complexes as well as in small molecules [21–24].

Furthermore, we have identified three bromo derivatives **VIII–X** (Figure 4) that showed selective toxicity towards human leukemia cells in our previous studies [25,26]. Compound **VIII** is especially cytotoxic towards K562 and HL-60 leukemic cell lines (IC_{50} 5.0 and 0.1 μM, respectively), however it is not toxic towards HeLa cancer cells and healthy endothelial cells (HUVEC) (IC_{50} > 1 mM). Moreover, the observed remarkable cytotoxicity of **VIII** towards K562 cells resulted from cells apoptosis. Compounds **IX** and **X** proved to be highly toxic towards cancer cells (IC_{50} in a few μM range) and non-toxic towards endothelial cells (HUVEC) [25–27]. Unfortunately, these compounds are poorly soluble in water, which limits their use in the cell culture or animal studies.

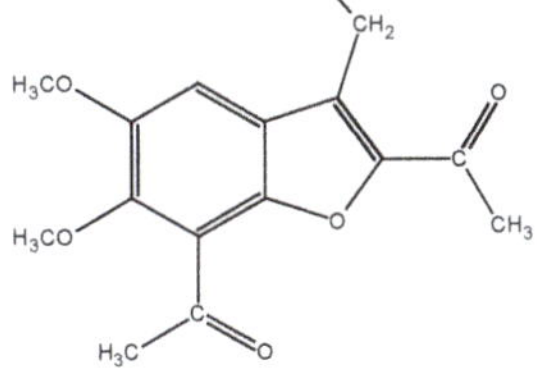

VIII

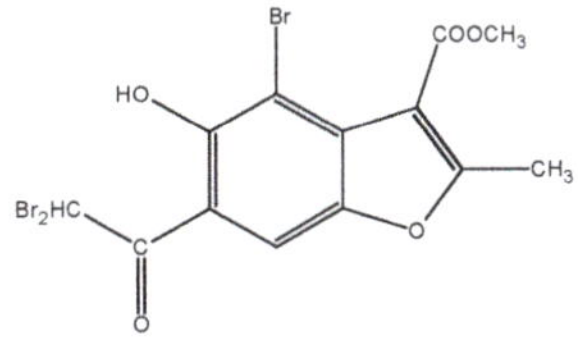

IX

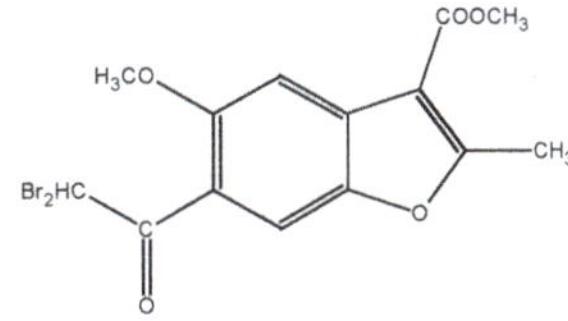

X

Figure 4. Structures of the benzofuran derivatives **VIII–X**, lead compounds used in the present studies.

Using **VIII–X** as the lead compounds, we designed and synthesized fourteen new derivatives with hopes for their better solubility in aqueous solutions (of lower lipophilicity when compared to **VIII–X**). The biological activity (i.e., cytotoxicity, activation of apoptosis, interaction with DNA) of these new derivatives was also evaluated.

2. Results

2.1. *Synthesis*

Our goal was to obtain a small library of new, less lipophilic derivatives/analogs of lead compounds **VIII–X**. We designed the synthesis of a set of compounds containing a carboxyl (**1**), formamide (**1a**), and methoxycarbonyl groups (**1b**), instead of an acetyl group in the position 2 of the parent benzofuran ring to obtain new benzofuran **VIII** analogs.

Thus, the starting acid **1**, which was obtained by the multistep synthesis according to the previously reported procedures [28] was submitted either to oxalyl chloride and ammonium solution treatment or methylated with dimethyl sulphate, delivering the amide derivative **1a** and methyl ester **1b**, respectively (Scheme 1). In the next step, compounds **1** and **1b** were submitted to bromination. For this purpose, ester **1b** was reacted with molecular bromine in chloroform. Under these conditions, hydrogen in the methyl group at position 3 was substituted by a bromine atom to give compound **1c**, which only differed by the substituent in position 2 (methoxycarbonyl versus acetyl). During bromination of the acid **1** using bromine in chloroform or NBS in CCl_4, a mixture of products was obtained, which was difficult to separate. Thus, the reaction conditions were changed and ethanol, instead of CCl_4, was used as a solvent in bromination reaction that was carried out in the presence of the NBS, while acetic acid was used as a solvent in the respective reaction that was carried out in the presence of bromine. Under these conditions, we managed to isolate the bromo-derivative **1d**, with satisfactory yield. Moreover, bromo-derivative **1e** was also obtained, but only in the reaction that was facilitated by NBS. The analyses of nuclear magnetic resonance spectra (^{1}H- and ^{13}C-NMR), mass spectra, and elemental analysis showed that the structures of the received compounds were different from the assumed ones (bromination of the methyl group at position 3). Instead, the derivatives in which the carboxyl group was replaced by the bromine atom at the position 2 were isolated. Moreover, we confirmed the formation of **1e**, in which one bromine atom substituted the hydrogen atom in the acetyl group of the benzene moiety of benzofuran ring. The use of polar protic solvents (acetic acid, ethanol) could explain this substitution.

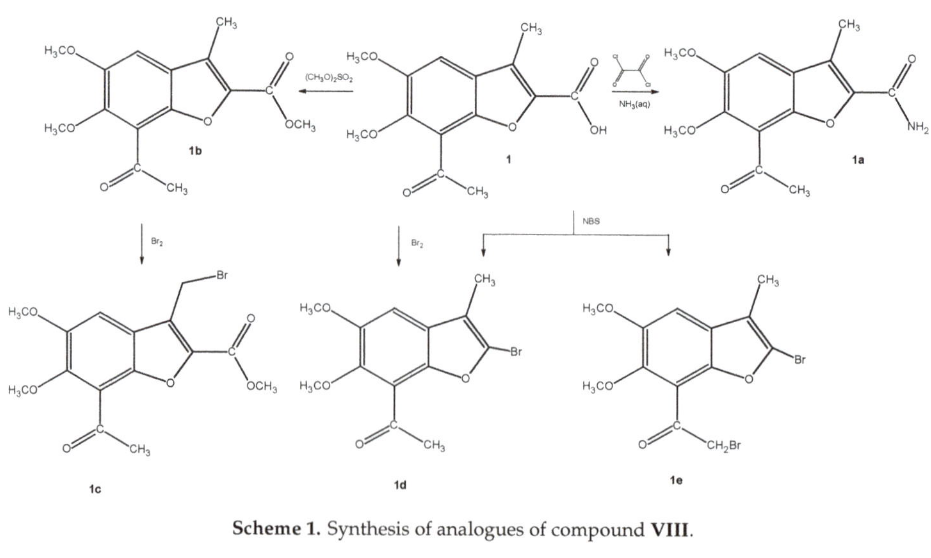

Scheme 1. Synthesis of analogues of compound **VIII**.

Analysis of the calculated log*P* values (Table 1) has shown that carboxyl and formamide analogs of lead compound **VIII** (**1** and **1a**, respectively) are much less lipophilic, while methoxycarbonyl analogs **1b** and **1c** exhibit similar properties as **VIII**. In contrast, an introduction of the bromine atom at position 2 of the furane ring resulted in significant increase of the benzofuran system hydrophobicity.

Table 1. Theoretical log*P* values (clog*P*) for obtained compounds calculated by the OSIRIS Property Explorer program.

Compound	clog*P*
VIII	2.4327
1	1.7254
1a	1.3276
1b	2.1533
1c	2.4745
1d	3.0089
1e	3.3301
IX	3.5663
2a	1.1219
2b	1.8471
2d	2.2688
2e	2.2449
X	3.1168
3a	2.9350
3b	1.7954
3c	1.3972
3d	2.5445

Schemes 2 and 3 show the syntheses of analogs of compounds **IX** and **X**, respectively. The starting material in both cases was 6-acetyl-5-hydroxy-2-methylbenzofuran-3-carboxylic acid (**2**), which was subjected to multidirectional transformations (Scheme 2). In the first approach, the amide-derivative **2a** was obtained in the reaction of the acid **2** with oxalyl chloride and ammonium hydroxide. Next, the bromo-derivative **2b** was obtained by the bromination of **2a** with bromine in acetic acid as a solvent. The nuclear magnetic resonance (^{1}H- and ^{13}C-NMR), mass spectrometry and elemental analyses confirmed the substitution of hydrogen by bromine in aromatic ring in the position 4. We assume that the presence of the OH group in position 5 of the benzene ring assisted in the electrophilic substitution of bromide cation in its ortho position. In the second path, the acid **2** was brominated in the same conditions and the bromo-derivative **2e**, also with a bromine substitution to the benzene ring, was obtained. In the third approach, an ester-derivative **2c**, which was obtained in the reaction of the acid **2** with dimethyl sulphate, was brominated by using NBS in CCl_4 to give the derivative **2d**, with a bromomethyl group in the position 2. Interestingly, all of the obtained derivatives **2** (**2a**–**2e**) exhibited lower clog*P* values, confirming the better water solubility of derivatives compared to lead compound **IX**, and the most pronounced occurred primary carboxamides **2a** and **2b**.

To obtain analogs of compound **X**, the starting acid **2** was reacted with an excess of dimethyl sulphate and the obtained derivative **3** was subjected to a multidirectional synthesis (Scheme 3). In the first case, bromine was introduced into the methyl group to give a compound **3d**, by reaction with NBS in CCl_4. In the reaction of the compound **3** with a bromine in acetic acid, the lead compound **X** was obtained and then finally reduced to provide a hydroxyl-derivative **3a**. In the third path, ester **3** was hydrolyzed in alkaline conditions to acid **3b**, and finally this derivative was converted to an amide **3c** by reaction with oxalyl chloride and ammonium hydroxide. Importantly, all of the new benzofuran derivatives related to **X** are characterized by lower clog*P* values when compared to the lead compound, indicating their improved solubility in aqueous media (Table 1).

The introduced substituents significantly affected the lipophilicity of the obtained benzofurans. In most cases, the new derivatives had a lower clog*P* value in comparison with the lead compounds. The exception are three derivatives **1c**, **1d**, **1e**, where the substitution of bromine in the furan ring (compounds **1d** and **1e**) or in the methyl group caused the clog*P* to increase (Table 2).

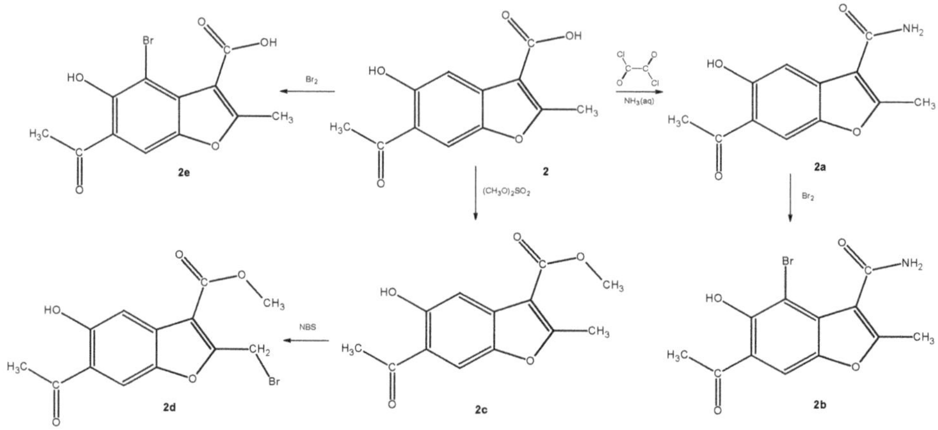

Scheme 2. Synthesis of analogues of compound **IX**.

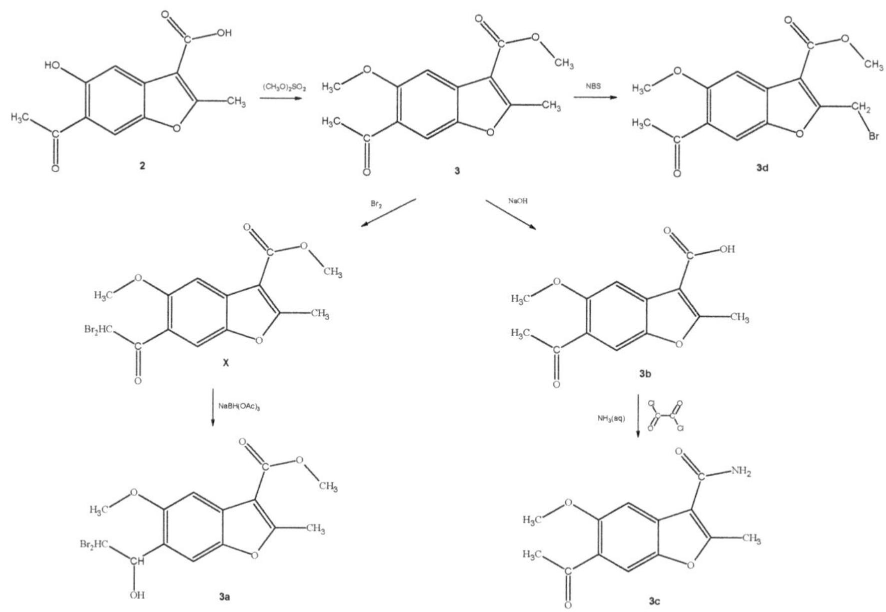

Scheme 3. Synthesis of analogues of compound **X**.

2.2. MTT Cytotoxicity Studies

Fourteen new benzofuran derivatives were tested for their cytotoxic properties in K562, MOLT-4 (leukemia, suspension cells), HeLa (cervix carcinoma, adherent cells), and normal endothelial cells (HUVEC). First, we measured the viability of cells after 48 h incubation with the given compound at the concentration of 100 μM. Next, for compounds that reduced cancer cells survival for more than 50%, we determined IC_{50} values. Cells that were exposed to 1% DMSO (a vehicle) served as the control with 100% survival. Cells treated with 1 μM staurosporine served as the internal control of the cytotoxicity experiments.

We have identified five compounds **1c**, **1e**, **2d**, **3a**, and **3d** in the initial screening, which, at the concentration of 100 μM, reduced the viability of all tested cancer cells K562, HeLa and MOLT-4 for more than 50% (data not shown). These compounds were also cytotoxic against human normal endothelial cells, so these compounds did not show any selectivity between the cancer and normal cells.

Next, for compounds **1c**, **1e**, **2d**, **3a**, and **3d**, the IC_{50} values were calculated (data given in Table 2). The test compounds were similarly toxic toward both cancer and normal cells, with IC_{50} values in the range of 20–85 μM. The exceptions were compounds **1c** and **3d**, which show IC_{50} out of this range (180 μM for MOLT-4 and 6 μM for HUVEC cells, respectively). We did not observe any significant differences in susceptibility between adherent and suspension cell lines.

Table 2. The IC_{50} values [μM] after 48 h incubation with cells.

Compound	HeLa	K562	MOLT-4	HUVEC
1c	50	25	180	30
1e	28	41	70	30
2d	35	20	35	30
3a	80	85	85	67
3d	35	28	55	6

For compounds **1c**, **1e**, **2d**, and **3d**, that exhibited the highest toxicity for K562 leukemia cells (IC_{50} below 50 μM), we investigated whether they induce apoptosis in these cells. We have measured the activity of caspases 3 and 7 (caspase 3/7), which are markers of programmed cell death. The K562 cells were treated with 1% DMSO (negative control), 1 μM staurosporine (positive control), or a test compound at the concentration of 5 × IC_{50} for 18 h. The activity of caspase 3/7 was measured using pro-fluorescent peptide substrate.

As shown in Figure 5, staurosporine, which is a strong inducer of apoptosis significantly increased the activity of caspase 3/7 in K562 cells. On the other hand, 1% DMSO had no effect on the activation of caspases. Interestingly, the incubation of cells with compound **1e** resulted in nearly five-fold increase in the activity of caspase 3/7, while compounds **1c** and **2d** activated caspase 3/7 to a lesser extent (about two-fold increase). In the presence of compound **3d**, the activation of caspases was minimal, if any. Altogether, this result suggests that the cytotoxic activity of test benzofurans **1c**, **1e**, and **2d** in K562 cells may be due to the induction of death by apoptosis.

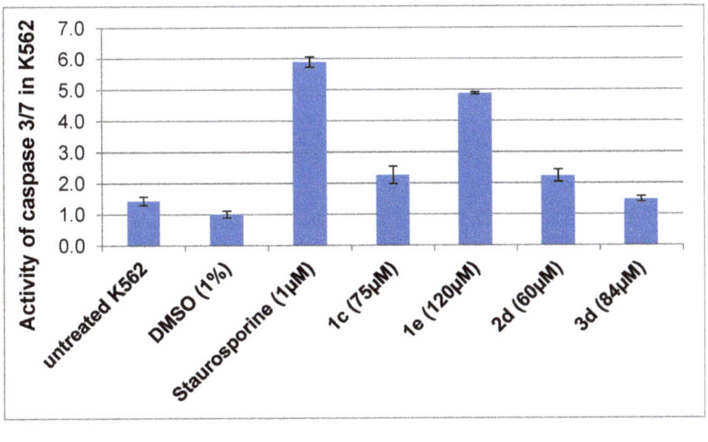

Figure 5. Activity of caspase 3 and 7 in K562 cells treated with the test benzofurans **1c**, **1e**, **2d**, **3d**, or staurosporine for 18 h. Apoptosis was determined by Apo-ONE® Homogeneous Caspase-3/7 Assay (Promega, Madison, WI, USA). Abbreviations: DMSO—K562 cells treated with 1% DMSO. The caspase activation level in cells exposed to 1% DMSO was normalized to 1.0. Mean values +/− SD are shown.

2.3. Interaction with DNA

The results of MTT cytotoxicity experiments indicated that compounds **1c**, **1e**, **2d**, and **3d** were highly toxic towards the used cell lines. We hypothesized that a possible explanation of observed cytotoxicity might be due to an interaction of test benzofurans with genomic DNA (e.g., by intercalation). To verify this hypothesis, we investigated whether the test benzofurans have any effect on digestion of a plasmid DNA (pcDNA3.1 HisC) with endonuclease *BamH1*. pcDNA3.1 HisC contains a unique *BamH1* restriction site which allows for plasmid linearization. Plasmid DNA exists in linear, superhelical, and circular forms that differ in electrophoretic mobility (Figure 6 lane 1). Plasmid DNA was converted to a linear form upon digestion with *BamH1* (lane 2). Daunorubicin, which is a strong intercalator to double-stranded DNA, was used as a control in this experiment and it completely inhibited the digestion of plasmid DNA with *BamH1* (lane 3). In the presence of test compounds, pcDNA3.1 HisC was partially digested with *Bam H1* restriction enzyme (Figure 6 lanes 4–7). Most of the plasmid DNA was converted to a linear form, however there is a circular form still present. These results suggest that test benzofurans, to some extent, interact with DNA (especially compounds **1c**, **1e**, **2d**), and this interaction inhibits the digestion of double stranded DNA chain with restriction endonuclease.

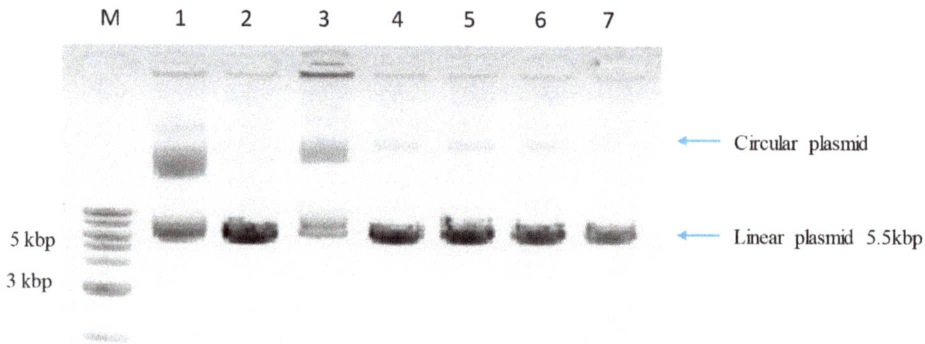

Figure 6. Digestion of pcDNA3.1HisC (total length 5.5kbp) with *BamH1* endonuclease. M—marker DNA; 1—not digested plasmid DNA; 2—plasmid DNA digested with *BamH1* (DNA present in linear form); 3—plasmid DNA + daunorubicin + *BamH1*; 4—plasmid DNA + **1c** + *BamH1*; 5—plasmid DNA + **2d** + *BamH1*; 6—plasmid DNA + **1e** + *BamH1*; and, 7—plasmid DNA + **3d** + *BamH1*.

3. Discussion

We have previously identified benzofurans **VIII**, **IX**, and **X** (lead benzofurans), which efficiently killed cancer cells and were not toxic toward normal endothelial cells [25–27]. Moreover, lead compound **VIII** demonstrated selective toxicity toward leukemia cell lines. However, these compounds were poorly soluble in aqueous solutions. Based on their structure, we have synthesized 14 new derivatives with decreased lipophilicity. The polarity of new compounds was predicted based on the calculated log*P* values. We tested their cytotoxic properties in human cells of cancer and normal origin. Five compounds, **1c**, **1e**, **2d**, **3a**, and **3d**, displayed the highest cytotoxicity toward cancer cell lines. However, these compounds were less toxic than lead compounds **VIII**, **IX**, **X**, and did not demonstrate any selectivity toward leukemia cells (Table 2). Moreover, new derivatives exhibited significant toxicity in normal endothelial cells. Cells death is usually carried out in one of the two major mechanisms: apoptosis or necrosis. Apoptosis is a highly regulated and controlled process that does not elicit an inflammation response at the site of cell death. Necrosis leads to sudden and uncontrolled cell disintegration that is associated with release of the cellular content and massive inflammation [29]. Therefore, in the next experiments, we investigated whether the cellular toxicity of new benzofurans is the result of apoptosis or necrosis. Our data demonstrate that the activity of caspase 3/7 (an apoptosis marker) is significantly increased (1.5- to 5-fold) in the presence of benzofurans (Figure 5). It suggests that these derivatives induce apoptosis in cancer cells. In the search of cellular targets for testing benzofurans, we examined whether DNA may be such a target. Using biochemical assay, we found out that the incubation of test compounds with plasmid DNA inhibited its cleavage with selected endonuclease (*BamH1*). A similar result was obtained with daunorubicin, which is a strong DNA intercalating agent. The presence of undigested plasmid DNA suggests that benzofurans intercalate to DNA (or bind DNA in other way). However, a comparison of DNA digestion products clearly indicates that the binding of benzofurans to DNA is much weaker than daunorubicin (Figure 6).

The presence of a bromine substituent in the alkyl chain attached to the furan ring is most likely to be responsible for cytotoxic activity of compounds **1c**, **2d**, and **3d**. The activity of compound **1e** is probably related to the presence of a bromoacetyl substituent in a benzene ring. Whilst the presence of a halogen (bromine) directly substituted to the benzene ring or the furan skeleton does not seem to increase the cytotoxic activity of the tested compounds, for example, **2e**, **2b**, and **1d**. The amide derivatives of benzofurans (compounds **2a**, **3c**, **1a**) that lack halogen-containing alkyl substituents (a bromine atom) did not show the cytotoxic properties toward cancer cell lines. A similar effect is observed for derivatives with a free acidic group (compounds **1**, **3b**) and ester derivatives (**1b**).

We can observe a marked decrease in the activity and selectivity of these derivatives when comparing the activity of bromo-derivatives **1c** and **1e** with the activity of the lead compound **VIII**. This effect is probably due to the absence of the acetyl group at the 2-position of the furan ring. The derivative **1c** has an ester group and the compound **1e** a bromine atom in this position. Thus, it can be concluded that the arrangement of substituents: the acetyl group at the 2-position and the bromomethyl at the three-position determines the activity and selectivity of the lead compound.

Analysis of the results for the active **2d** derivative in comparison to its lead compound **IX** also indicates that the structural modifications of **2d** resulted in a loss of selectivity and decreased activity. In this case, the derivatives differ in the location of the halogen atom. The **2d** derivative contains the bromomethyl substituent in the two-position and the acetyl group in the six-position of the benzofuran system, while the **IX** contains the methyl group in the two-position and the bromoacetyl substituent in the six-position of the benzofuran system. It can again be assumed that the presence of a halogen atom substituted to an alkyl/acetyl moiety determines the activity of the derivatives, but the appropriate positioning of substituents is important in their selectivity. Finally, by comparing the active derivatives **3a** and **3d** with their lead compound **X**, we also observe a decrease in activity and selectivity. The **3a** compound differs from the leading compound by the presence of a hydroxyl group. It can be hypothesized that the reduction of the keto group and the possibility of creating additional hydrogen bonds, as well as an increase in the hydrophilicity could affect the activity of this derivative.

Compound **3d** contains a bromomethyl substituent at the two-position and an acetyl group at the six-position, while **X** contains a bromoacetyl group at the six-position and a methyl at the two-position. Both of the compounds exhibit cytotoxicity, but the absence of the bromoacetyl substituent in compound **3d** eliminated its selectivity and decreased cytotoxicity to the cancer cells.

4. Materials and Methods

4.1. Chemistry

All of the solvents, reagents, and chemicals used in these studies were purchased from Aldrich Chemical (Saint Louis, MO, USA) and Merck AG (Saint Louis, MO, USA). The melting points were determined with Electrothermal 9100 capillary apparatus and they are uncorrected. The nuclear magnetic resonance spectra (University of Warsaw, Warsaw, Poland) were recorded in DMSO-d_6 or $CDCl_3$ on VMNRS300 operating at 300 MHz (^{1}H-NMR) and 75 MHz (^{13}C-NMR). Chemical shifts (δ) are expressed in parts per million relative to tetramethylsilane used as the internal reference. The coupling constants (J) values are given in hertz (Hz) and spin multiples are given as s (singlet), d (dublet), t (triplet), and m (multiplet). Mass spectral ESI (Electrospray Ionization) measurements were carried out on a MicrOTOF II, Bruker instrument with a TOF detector (Jagiellonian Univeristy in Krakov, Poland). The spectra were obtained in the positive ion mode. Elemental analyses were recorded with CHNS micro analyzer elementary model Vario Micro Cube with electronic microbalance (Jagiellonian Univeristy in Krakow, Poland). Flash chromatography was performed on Merck Kieselgel 0.05–0.2 mm reinst (70–325 mesh ASTM, Saint Louis, MO, USA) silica gel using chloroform as eluent. TLC monitored progress of the reactions described in the experimental section on silica gel (plates with fluorescent indicator 254 nm, layer thickness 0.2 mm, Kieselgel G. Merck, Saint Louis, MO, USA), using chloroform-methanol as an eluent system at the *v*/*v* ratio of 9.8:0.2 or 9.5:0.5.

4.2. General Synthetic Procedures

Procedure 1. Procedure for Synthesis of Amides.

An appropriate carboxylic acid (0.004 mol) was suspended in anhydrous dichlorometane (DCM) (10 mL). Next, oxalyl chloride (0.43 mL, 0.005 mol) and the one drop of dimethylformamide (DMF) were added to the solution. The reaction mixture was stirred at room temperature for 24 h. Then, ammonium solution (aq. 30%, 5 mL) was added drop by drop and the mixture was stirred at room temperature for additional 12 h. When the reaction was complete (TLC control) the resulting mixture was diluted with water (50 mL) and extracted with DCM (3 × 50 mL). The organic extracts were dried with magnesium sulfate and concentrated under reduced pressure. The resulting solid was purified by a silica gel column chromatography (eluent: chloroform or chloroform:methanol; 50:0.2, *v*/*v*).

Procedure 2. Procedure for the Preparation of Methyl ester.

Procedure according to the method described earlier [11]. Thus, a mixture of appropriate carboxylic acid (0.02 mol), K_2CO_3 (0.1 mol) and $(CH_3O)_2SO_2$ (0.02 mol) in acetone was refluxed for 48 h. When the reaction was complete, the mixture was filtered and the solvent was removed on rotary evaporator [11]. The residue was purified by a silica gel column chromatography (eluent: chloroform or chloroform:methanol; 50:0.2 *v*/*v*).

Procedure 3. Procedure for Bromination by Using N-Bromosuccinimide (NBS).

In this method, the procedure was used, as described earlier [11]. Briefly, *N*-bromosuccinimide (NBS) (0.02 mol) and the catalytic amount of benzoyl peroxide were added to a solution of the appropriate ester or acid (0.02 mol) in dry carbon tetrachloride or alternatively in ethanol (50 mL). The reaction mixture was refluxed for 24 h. When the reaction was complete (TLC monitoring), the mixture was filtered and the solvent was removed under reduced pressure. Silica gel column chromatography purified the residue (eluent: chloroform or chloroform:methanol; 50:0.2 *v*/*v*).

Procedure 4. Procedure for Bromination by Using Br_2.

Method a. Procedure according to the method that was described earlier [11]. Thus, an appropriate ester, amide, or acid (0.02 mol) was dissolved in $CHCl_3$ (20 mL), and then a solution of bromine in $CHCl_3$ (0.02 mol in 10 mL) was added dropwise with stirring for 1 h. The obtained mixture was stirred at room temperature for 24 h. When the reaction was finished, the solvent was removed under reduced pressure. The residue was purified by a silica gel column chromatography (eluent: chloroform or chloroform:methanol; 50:0.2 *v*/*v*).

Method b. Procedure according to the method described earlier [11]. Thus, an appropriate ester, amide, or acid (0.02 mol) was dissolved in CH_3COOH (80%, 20 mL), and then a solution of bromine in CH_3COOH (0.02 mol in 10 mL) was added dropwise with stirring for 1 h. The obtained mixture was stirred at room temperature for 24 h. When the reaction was complete, the resulting mixture was diluted by $Na_2S_2O_3$ solution (10 mL) and extracted with DCM (3 × 50 mL). The obtained organic extracts were dried with calcium chloride, filtered, and concentrated under reduced pressure. Silica gel column chromatography purified the residue (eluent: chloroform or chloroform:methanol; 50:0.2 *v*/*v*).

Procedure 5. Procedure for Reduction.

A starting ketone (0.0024 mol) was dissolved in the peroxides-free dioxane (20 mL), and then $NABH(OAc)_3$ (0.0048 mol) was added. The mixture was stirred at room temperature for 24–48 h. When the reaction was complete, the solvent was removed under reduced pressure. The solid residue was dissolved in $CHCl_3$ (50 mL) and then washed with water (3 × 20 mL). The organic solution was dried with magnesium sulfate, filtered, and concentrated under reduced pressure. Finally, silica gel column chromatography purified the residue (eluent: chloroform or chloroform:methanol; 50:0.2 *v*/*v*).

4.2.1. Synthesis of Analogues of Compound **VIII**

Synthesis of 7-Acetyl-5,6-Dimethoxy-3-Methylbenzofuran-2-Carboxylic Acid (**1**)

7-Acetyl-5,6-dimethoxy-3-methylbenzofuran-2-carboxylic acid was obtained in the multistep reaction according to the method described earlier [28].

M.W. = 278.2573; $C_{14}H_{14}O_6$; Yield: 30%; white powder, m.p. 212–214 °C; ^{1}H-NMR (300 MHz, DMSO, δ/ppm): 2.50 (3H, s, -CH_3), 2.62 (3H, s, -$COCH_3$), 3.84 (3H, s, -OCH_3), 3.92 (3H, s, -OCH_3), 7.47 (1H, s, Ar-H), 13.41 (1H, br.s, -COOH); ^{13}C-NMR: δ 9.15, 32.13, 56.43, 61.755, 105.50, 119.64, 124.39, 124.68, 142.19, 144.27, 147.40, 150.07, 160.76, 197.33;.HRMS (*m/z*): calculated value for [M + Na] 100% = 301.0683; found 100% = 301.0681$^+$; Anal. Calc. for $C_{14}H_{14}O_6$: 60.43% C; 5.07% H, found 59.25% C; 4.92% H.

Synthesis of 7-Acetyl-5,6-Dimethoxy-3-Methylbenzofuran-2-Carboxamide (**1a**)

7-Acetyl-5,6-dimethoxy-3-methylbenzofuran-2-carboxamide was obtained according to Procedure 1.

M.W. = 277.2726; $C_{14}H_{15}NO_5$, Yield: 37%; white powder, m.p. 203–205 °C; ^{1}H-NMR (300 MHz, $CDCl_3$, δ/ppm): 2.50 (3H, s, -CH_3), 2.68 (3H, s, -$COCH_3$), 3.80 (3H, s, -OCH_3), 3.90 (3H, s, -OCH_3), 7.41 (1H, s, Ar-H), 7.70 (2H, br.m, -NH_2); ^{13}C-NMR: δ 8.73, 32.47, 56.04, 61.85, 104.99, 120.02, 121.07, 125.07, 143.14, 144.08, 146.34, 150.07, 160.93, 197.55; HRMS (*m/z*): calculated value for [M + Na] 100% = 300.0842, found 100% = 300.0842$^+$. Anal. Calc. for $C_{14}H_{15}NO_5$: 60.64% C; 5.45% H, 5.05% N, found 60.04% C; 4.537% H, 4.81% N.

Synthesis of Methyl 7-Acetyl-5,6-Dimethoxy-3-Methylbenzofuran-2-Carboxylate (**1b**)

Methyl 7-acetyl-5,6-dimethoxy-3-methyl-1-benzofuran-2-carboxylate was obtained according to Procedure 2. M.W. = 292.2839; $C_{15}H_{16}O_6$; Yield: 60%; white powder, m.p. 98–100 °C; ^{1}H-NMR (300 MHz, $CDCl_3$, δ/ppm): 2.55 (3H, s, -CH_3), 2.73 (3H, s, -$COCH_3$), 3.94 (3H, s, -OCH_3), 3.95 (3H, s, -OCH_3), 3.95 (3H, s, -$COOCH_3$), 7.10 (1H, s, Ar-H); ^{13}C-NMR: δ 9.22, 32.34, 51.84, 56.38, 62.40, 104.42, 120.28, 124.84, 125.43, 141.68, 145.57, 148.67, 150.58, 160.41, 197.50; HRMS (*m/z*): calculated value for [M + Na] 100% = 315.0839, found 100% = 315.0839. Anal. Calc. for $C_{15}H_{16}O_6$: 61.64% C; 5.52% H, found 61.35% C; 5.516% H.

Synthesis of Methyl 7-Acetyl-3-(Bromomethyl)-5,6-Dimethoxybenzofuran-2-Carboxylate (**1c**)

Methyl 7-acetyl-3-(bromomethyl)-5,6-dimethoxybenzofuran-2-carboxylate was obtained according to Procedure 4 (method a). M.W. = 371.1800; $C_{15}H_{15}BrO_6$; Yield: 20%; white powder, m.p. 124–125 °C; ^{1}H-NMR (300 MHz, $CDCl_3$, δ/ppm): 2.72 (3H, s, -$COCH_3$), 3.97 (9H, m, -OCH_3, -OCH_3, -$COOCH_3$), 4.90 (2H, -CH_2Br), 7.33 (1H, s, Ar-H); ^{13}C-NMR: δ 20.46, 32.30, 52.35, 56.43, 62.41, 104.32, 120.53, 122.56, 124.99, 141.66, 145.71, 149.11, 151.01, 159.61, 197.15; HRMS (*m/z*): calculated value for [M + Na] 100% = 392.9944, 99% = 394.9927, found 100% = 392.9945, 99% = 394.9926. Anal. Calc. for $C_{15}H_{14}$ BrO_6: 48.54% C; 4.07% H, found 48.82% C; 4.15% H.

Synthesis of 1-(2-Bromo-5,6-Dimethoxy-3-Methylbenzofuran-7-yl)ethanone (**1d**)

1-(2-Bromo-5,6-dimethoxy-3-methylbenzofuran-7-yl)ethanone was obtained according to Procedure 3 (in ethanol) as well as Procedure 4 (method b). Yield: M.W. = 313.1439; $C_{13}H_{13}BrO_4$; Yield: 27%; white powder, m.p. 94–95 °C; ^{1}H-NMR (300 MHz, $CDCl_3$, δ/ppm): 2.16 (3H, s, -CH_3), 2.69 (3H, s, -$COCH_3$), 3.90 (3H, s, -OCH_3), 3.93 (3H, s, -OCH_3), 6.98 (1H, s, Ar-H); ^{13}C-NMR: δ 8.69, 32.26, 56.47, 62.38, 103.39, 114.99, 119.83, 125.37, 126.39, 145.20, 1454.74, 150.22, 197.82; HRMS (*m/z*): calculated value for [M + Na] 100% = 334.9889, 99% = 336.9870, found 100% = 334.9897, 99% = 336.9869. Anal. Calc. for $C_{13}H_{13}BrO_4$: 49.86% C; 4.18% H, found 49.76% C; 4.159% H.

Synthesis of 2-Bromo-1-(2-Bromo-5,6-Dimethoxy-3-Methylbenzofuran-7-yl]ethanone (**1e**)

2-Bromo-1-(2-bromo-5,6-dimethoxy-3-methylbenzofuran-7-yl)ethanone was obtained according to Procedure 3 (in ethanol). M.W. = 392.0399; $C_{13}H_{12}Br_2O_4$; Yield: 27%; white powder, m.p. 128–129 °C; ^{1}H-NMR (300 MHz, $CDCl_3$, δ/ppm): 2.17 (3H, s, -CH_3), 3.94 (6H, s, -OCH_3, -OCH_3), 4.58 (2H, s, -$COCH_2Br$), 7.03 (1H, s, Ar-H); ^{13}C-NMR: δ 8.69, 36.49, 56.53, 62.49, 104.60, 115.16, 116.09, 125.46, 126.66, 145.84, 145.95, 150.10, 190.29; HRMS (*m/z*): calculated value for [M + Na] 50% = 412.8995, 100% = 414.8975, 49% = 416.8956, found 50% = 412.8991, 100% = 414.8973, 49% = 416.8944. Anal. Calc. for $C_{13}H_{12}Br_2O_4$: 39.83% C; 3.09% H, found 40.21% C; 3.066% H.

4.2.2. Synthesis of Analogues of Compound **IX**

Synthesis of 6-Acetyl-5-Hydroxy-2-Methylbenzofuran-3-Carboxamide (**2a**)

6-Acetyl-5-hydroxy-2-methylbenzofuran-3-carboxamide was obtained according to Procedure 1. M.W. = 233.2200; $C_{12}H_{11}NO_4$; Yield: 50%; white powder, m.p. 268–267 °C; ^{1}H-NMR (300 MHz, DMSO, δ/ppm): 2.65 (3H, s, -$COCH_3$), 2.68 (3H, s, -CH_3), 7.22 (1H, s, Ar-H), 7.48 (2H, br.s, -NH_2), 8.11 (1H, s, Ar-H), 11.97 (1H, s, -OH); ^{13}C-NMR: δ 14.20, 27.52, 107.03, 112.69, 112.74, 116.38, 133.39, 146.00, 157.39, 163.86, 164.22, 204.26; HRMS (*m/z*): calculated value for [M + Na] 100% = 256.0580, found 100% = 256.0582. Anal. Calc. for $C_{12}H_{11}NO_4$: 61.80% C; 4.75% H, 6.01% N, found 60.85% C; 4.766% H, 5.83% N.

Synthesis of 6-Acetyl-4-Bromo-5-Hydroxy-2-Methylbenzofuran-3-Carboxamide (**2b**)

6-Acetyl-4-bromo-5-hydroxy-2-methylbenzofuran-3-carboxamide was obtained according to Procedure 4 (method b). M.W. = 312.1161; $C_{12}H_{10}BrNO_4$; Yield: 40%; white powder, m.p. 249–248 °C; ^{1}H-NMR (300 MHz, DMSO, δ/ppm): 2.50 (3H, s, -$COCH_3$), 2.68 (3H, s, -CH_3), 7.69 (1H, br.s, -NH_2), 7.94 (1H, br.s, -NH_2), 8.23 (1H, s, Ar-H), 12.88 (1H, s, -OH); ^{13}C-NMR: δ 13.20, 27.05, 99.21, 112.59, 115.82, 115.86, 133.19, 145.62, 154.37, 160.33, 163.79, 204.99; HRMS (*m/z*): calculated value for [M + Na] 100% = 333.9685, 98% = 335.9666, found 100% = 333.9685, 98% = 335.9669. Anal. Calc. for $C_{12}H_{10}BrNO_4$: 46.18% C; 3.23% H, 4.49% N, found 46.33% C; 3.265% H, 4.35% N.

Synthesis of Methyl 6-Acetyl-5-Hydroxy-2-Methylbenzofuran-3-Carboxylate (**2c**)

Methyl 6-acetyl-5-hydroxy-2-methylbenzofuran-3-carboxylate (**2c**) was obtained according to the method described previously [11].

Synthesis of Methyl 6-Acetyl-2-(Bromomethyl)-5-Hydroxybenzofuran-3-Carboxylate (**2d**)

Methyl 6-acetyl-2-(bromomethyl)-5-hydroxybenzofuran-3-carboxylate was obtained according to Procedure 3 (in CCl_4). M.W. = 327.1274; $C_{13}H_{11}BrO_5$; Yield: 30%; white powder, m.p. 94–95 °C (chyba 138–140); ^{1}H-NMR (300 MHz, $CDCl_3$, δ/ppm): 2.70 (3H, s, -$COCH_3$), 3.99 (3H, s, -$COOCH_3$), 4.94 (2H, s, -CH_2Br), 7.53 (1H, s, Ar-H), 7.88 (1H, s, Ar-H), 12.11 (1H, s, -OH); ^{13}C-NMR: δ 14.19, 26.80, 52.08, 110.51, 112.63, 117.59, 132.64, 146.73, 155.99, 161.21, 162.63, 164.00, 203.35; HRMS (*m/z*): calculated value for [M + Na] 100% = 348.9682, 99% = 350.9663, found 100% = 348.9683, 99% = 350.9663. Anal. Calc. for $C_{13}H_{11}BrO_5$: 47.73% C; 3.39% H, found 47.33% C; 3.265% H.

Synthesis of 6-Acetyl-4-Bromo-5-Hydroxy-2-Methylbenzofuran-3-Carboxylic Acid (**2e**)

6-Acetyl-4-bromo-5-hydroxy-2-methylbenzofuran-3-carboxylic acid was obtained according Procedure 4 (method b). M.W. = 313.1008; $C_{12}H_9BrO_5$; Yield: 30%; white powder, m.p. 196–197 °C; ^{1}H-NMR (300 MHz, $CDCl_3$, δ/ppm): 2.48 (3H, s, -$COCH_3$), 2.69 (3H, s, -CH_3), 7.72 (1H, s, Ar-H), 12.89 (1H, s, -OH); ^{13}C-NMR: δ 13.20, 26.70, 94.45, 100.68, 111.33, 116.11, 132.08, 145.99, 155.30, 159.72, 203.35;

HRMS (*m/z*): calculated value for [M + Na] 100% = 334.9526, 99% = 336.9506, found 100%= 334.9525, 99% = 336.9505. Anal. Calc. for $C_{12}H_9BrO_5$: 46.03% C; 2.90% H, found 46.33% C; 2.265% H.

4.2.3. Synthesis of Analogues of Compound **X**

Synthesis of Methyl 6-Acetyl-5-Methoxy-2-Methylbenzofuran-3-Carboxylate (**3**) and Methyl 6-(Dibromoacetyl)-5-Methoxy-2-Methyl-1-Benzofuran-3-Carboxylate (**X**)

Methyl 6-acetyl-5-methoxy-2-methylbenzofuran-3-carboxylate (**3**) and methyl 6-(dibromoacetyl)-5-methoxy-2-methylbenzofuran-3-carboxylate (**X**) were obtained according to the method described previously [11].

Synthesis of Methyl 6-(2,2-Dibromo-1-Hydroxyethyl)-5-Methoxy-2-Methylbenzofuran-3-Carboxylate (**3a**)

Methyl 6-(2,2-dibromo-1-hydroxyethyl)-5-methoxy-2-methylbenzofuran-3-carboxylate (**3a**) was obtained according to Procedure 5. M.W. = 422.0659; $C_{14}H_{14}Br_2O_5$; Yield: 70%; white powder, m.p. 170–172 °C; ^{1}H-NMR (300 MHz, DMSO, δ/ppm): 2.74 (3H, s, -COOCH$_3$), 3.18 (1H, br.s, -CH-), 3.93 (3H, s, -OCH$_3$), 3.94 (3H, s, -CH$_3$), 5.34 (1H, br.s, –OH), 6.14 (1H, d, -CH-, *J* = 3 Hz), 7.41 (1H, s, Ar-H), 7.59 (1H, s, Ar-H); ^{13}C-NMR: δ 14.73, 51.46, 51.77, 55.93, 75.00, 102.26, 108.96, 110.78, 123.97, 126.92, 148.14, 153.17, 164.71, 164.75; HRMS (*m/z*): calculated value for [M + Na] 50% = 442.9100, 100% = 444.9081, 50% = 446.9063, found 50% = 442.9094, 100% = 444.9079, 50% = 446.9065. Anal. Calc. for $C_{14}H_{14}Br_2O_6$: 39.84% C; 3.34% H, found 40.20% C; 3.37% H.

Synthesis of 6-Acetyl-5-Methoxy-2-Methylbenzofuran-3-Carboxylic Acid (**3b**)

A mixture of methyl 6-acetyl-5-methoxy-2-methylbenzofuran-3-carboxylate (0.0008 mol) and 2 M NaOH (0.6 mL, 0.0012 mol) in ethanol (1.2 mL) was heated for 1 h. The bulk of the solvent was evaporated and the residue was acidified with 2 M HCl (1.2 mL) to give a fine precipitate. Next, the mixture was cooled to room temperature and then filtered to give the product. M.W. = 248.2313; $C_{13}H_{12}O_5$; Yield: 30%; white powder, m.p. 249–250 °C; ^{1}H-NMR (300 MHz, DMSO, δ/ppm): 2.55 (3H, s, -COCH$_3$), 2.71 (3H, s, -CH$_3$), 3.90 (3H, s, -OCH$_3$), 7.45 (1H, s, Ar-H), 7.69 (1H, s, Ar-H); ^{13}C-NMR: δ 14.41, 31.61, 56.03, 103.27, 109.23, 111.32, 124.90, 130.79, 147.06, 155.84, 164.66, 166.58, 197.99; HRMS (*m/z*): calculated value for [M + Na] 100% = 271.0577, found 100% = 270.0737. Anal. Calc. for $C_{13}H_{12}O_5 * \frac{1}{2} H_2O$: 60.50% C; 5.07% H, found 60.05% C; 4.715% H.

Synthesis of 6-Acetyl-5-Methoxy-2-Methylbenzofuran-3-Carboxamide (**3c**)

6-Acetyl-5-methoxy-2-methylbenzofuran-3-carboxamide was obtained according to Procedure 1.

M.W. = 247.2466; $C_{13}H_{13}NO_4$; Yield: 30%; white powder, m.p. 223–224 °C; ^{1}H-NMR (300 MHz, DMSO, δ/ppm): 2.55 (3H, s, -COCH$_3$), 2.68 (3H, s, -CH$_3$), 3.98 (3H, s, -OCH$_3$), 7.22 (1H, s, Ar-H), 7.53 (2H, br.s, -NH$_2$), 7.70 (1H, s, Ar-H); ^{13}C-NMR: δ 14.11, 31.61, 56.17, 103.10, 111.14, 112.81, 124.65, 130.56, 146.94, 155.49, 162.02, 164.42, 198.08; HRMS (*m/z*): calculated value for [M + Na] 100% = 270.0737, found 100% = 270.0737. Anal. Calc. for $C_{13}H_{13}NO_4$: 63.15% C; 5.30% H, 5.67% N, found 62.90% C; 5.245% H, 5.63% N.

Synthesis of Methyl 6-Acetyl-2-(Bromomethyl)-5-Methoxybenzofuran-3-Carboxylate (**3d**)

Methyl 6-acetyl-2-(bromomethyl)-5-methoxybenzofuran-3-carboxylate was obtained according to Procedure 3 (in CCl_4). M.W. = 341.1540; $C_{14}H_{13}BrO_5$; Yield: 30%; white powder, m.p. 148–150 °C; ^{1}H-NMR (300 MHz, CDCl$_3$, δ/ppm): 2.65 (3H, s, -COCH$_3$), 3.98 (3H, s, -OCH$_3$), 4.01 (3H, s, -COOCH3), 4.91 (2H, s, -CH2Br), 7.50 (1H, s, Ar-H), 7.86 7.70 (1H, s, Ar-H); ^{13}C-NMR: δ 20.94, 31.08, 52.07, 56.03, 103.76, 110.48, 112.98, 127.44, 129.80, 148.49, 156.56, 161.91, 163.30, 199.04; HRMS (*m/z*): calculated value for [M + Na] 100% = 362.9839, 99% = 364.9820, found 100% = 362.9839, 99% = 364.9820. Anal. Calc. for $C_{14}H_{13}BrO_5$: 49.29% C; 3.84% H, found 48.87% C; 3.755% H.

4.3. Anticancer Activity

4.3.1. Cells and Cytotoxicity Assay

Human umbilical vein endothelial cells (Life Technologies, Waltham, MA, USA) were cultured (according to the manufacturer instructions) in Medium 200 supplemented with Low Serum Growth Supplement. 1×10^4 HUVEC cells were seeded on each well on a 96-well plate (Nunc). The HeLa (human cervix carcinoma) K562 and MOLT-4 (leukemia) cells were cultured in RPMI 1640 medium supplemented with antibiotics and 10% fetal calf serum (HeLa, K562) in a 5% CO_2-95% air atmosphere. 7×10^3 HeLa, K562, or MOLT-4 cells were seeded on each well on 96-well plate (Nunc). 24 h later cells were treated with the test compounds and then incubated for an additional 48 hours. Stock solutions of test compounds were freshly prepared in DMSO (dimethylsulfoxide). The final concentrations of compounds that were tested in the cell cultures were: 2×10^{-1}, 1×10^{-1}, 5×10^{-2}, 1×10^{-2}, 1×10^{-3} and 1×10^{-4} mM. The concentration of DMSO in the cell culture medium was 1%.

The values of IC_{50} (the concentration of test compound that is required to reduce the cell survival fraction to 50% of the control) were calculated from dose-response curves and used as a measure of cellular sensitivity to a given treatment.

The MTT [3-(4,5-dimethylthiazol-2-yl)-2,5-diphenyltetrazolium bromide; Sigma, St. Louis, MO, USA] assay determined the cytotoxicity of all the compounds, as described previously [30]. Briefly, after 24 h or 48 h of incubation with the drug, the cells were treated with the MTT reagent, and incubation was continued for 2 h. MTT-formazan crystals were dissolved in 20% SDS and 50% DMF at pH 4.7 and absorbance was read at 570 and 650 nm on an ELISA-PLATE READER (FLUOstar Omega, BMG LABTECH GmbH, Ortenberg, Germany). As a control (100% viability), cells that were grown in the presence of medium vehicle only with 1% DMSO were used.

4.3.2. Induction of Cell Apoptosis Analyzed by Caspase-3/7 Assay

20×10^3 K562 cells were seeded on each well of 96-well plate in RPMI 1640 medium supplemented with 10% fetal calf serum and antibiotics. Cells were grown for 24 h at 37 °C and 5% CO_2. The test compounds were dissolved in DMSO and added to the cell culture. The concentration of tested benzo[b]furans in cell culture was $5 \times IC_{50}$.

Cells treated with 1% DMSO served as a negative control, while cells incubated with staurosporine (a strong inducer of apoptosis) were used as a positive control. Cells were exposed to test compounds for 18 h at 37 °C and 5% CO_2. Subsequently, Apo-ONE® Homogeneous Caspase-3/7 Assay (Promega, Madison, WI, USA) measured the activity of caspase 3 and 7, according to the manufacturer's instructions. Briefly, the cells were lysed and incubated for 1.5 h with profluorescent substrate for caspase 3 and 7. Next, fluorescence was read at an excitation wavelength of 485 nm and emission of 520 nm with FLUOStar Omega plate reader (BMG-Labtech, Ortenberg, Germany).

4.3.3. Digestion of Plasmid DNA with BamHI Restriction Nuclease

0.5 μg of plasmid DNA (pcDNAHisC, total length 5.5 kbp) containing a unique *BamHI* restriction site was dissolved in a 1× *BamHI* reaction buffer and then incubated overnight at 37 °C with the test compounds or daunorubicin, a strong intercalating agent, which was used as a positive control. The concentration of the test compounds and daunorubicin samples was 100 μM. In the next step, the reaction mixtures were digested with *BamHI* restriction endonuclease (2 U/μL) for 3 h at 37 °C. The total reaction volume was 10 μL. Products of the reaction were subjected to the 1% agarose gel electrophoresis in TBE buffer. The gel was stained with ethidium bromide and DNA fragments were visualized under a UV lamp (GBox, Syngene, Cambridge, UK).

5. Conclusions

We synthesized and tested a group of new benzofuran derivatives. The presence of bromine in the alkyl group in the furan ring is most likely responsible for the cytotoxic properties of the tested derivatives (compounds **1c**, **2d**, **3d**). Compound **1e** shows the cytotoxic property, and contains an acetyl halide substituent (bromine) in the benzene ring and a bromine atom that is directly attached to the furan ring. The most active compounds **2d** and **3d**, showed increased polarity when compared to the lead compounds **VIII-X**, but their cytotoxicity against human cancer cells decreased by 5–10 folds and the toxicity against normal cells increased. The formation of amide derivatives of benzofurans (compounds **1a**, **2a**, **2b**, **3c**) and the lack of a halogen-containing alkyl substituent in their structure resulted in better water solubility but loss of cytotoxic properties towards the cancer cells studied. A reduction of the bromoacetyl group in compound **X** increased its polarity but also eliminated the selectivity of the compound and diminished its toxicity towards tumor cells.

Author Contributions: Conceptualization, M.N.; Methodology, M.N. and M.C.; Performed the experiments M.N., M.C., J.K.-B., K.K.-G. Writing—Original Draft Preparation, M.N.; Writing—Review & Editing, M.N., M.C. and B.N.; Visualization, M.N. and M.C.; Supervision, B.N.; Project Administration, M.N. and M.C.; Funding Acquisition, M.N. and B.N.

Funding: This work was supported by the Polish Ministry of Science, project NCN OPUS UMO-2014/15/B/NZ7/00966.

Acknowledgments: The cytotoxicity, activation of caspases and DNA interaction studies were performed in the Screening Laboratory at the Division of Bioorganic Chemistry, Centre of Molecular and Macromolecular Studies of the Polish Academy of Sciences.

Conflicts of Interest: The authors declare no conflict of interest.

References

1. Habtemarian, S. Antiinflammatory activity of the antirheumatic herbal drug, gravel root (Eupatorium purpureum): Further biological activities and constituents. *Phytoter. Res.* **2001**, *15*, 687–690. [CrossRef] [PubMed]
2. Pauletti, M.P.; Araujo, A.R.; Young, M.C.; Giesbrecht, A.M.; Bolzani, V.D. nor-Lignans from the leaves of Styrax ferrugineus (Styracaceae) with antibacterial and antifungal activity. *Phytochemistry* **2000**, *55*, 597–601. [CrossRef]
3. Masubuchi, M.; Kawasaki, K.; Ebiike, H.; Ikeda, Y.; Tsujii, S.; Sogabe, S.; Fujii, T.; Sakata, K.; Shiratori, Y.; Aoki, Y.; et al. Design and synthesis of novel benzofurans as new class of antifungal agents targeting fungal N-myristoyltransferase. Part 1. *Bioorg. Med. Chem. Lett.* **2001**, *11*, 1833–1837. [CrossRef]
4. Wróbel, J.E.; Dietrich, A.J.; Antane, M.M. Benzotiophenes, Benzofurans, and Indoles useful in the treatment of insulin resistance and hyperglycemia. U.S. Patent 6,251,936, 26 June 2001.
5. Kayser, O.; Chen, M.; Kharazmi, A.; Kiderlen, A.F. Aurones Interfere with *Leismania major* mitochondrial fumarate reductase. *Z. Naturforsch. C* **2002**, *57*, 717–720. [CrossRef]
6. Hayakawa, I.; Shioya, R.; Agatsuma, T.; Furukawa, H.; Naruto, S.; Sugano, Y. 4-Hydroxy-3-methyl-6-phenylbenzofuran-2-carboxylic acid ethyl ester derivatives as potent anti-tumor agents. *Bioorg. Med. Chem. Lett.* **2004**, *14*, 455–458. [CrossRef] [PubMed]
7. Dawood, K.M. Benzofuran derivatives: A patent review. *Expert Opin. Ther. Pat.* **2013**, *23*, 1133–1156. [CrossRef] [PubMed]
8. Kossakowski, J.; Ostrowska, K.; Hejchman, E.; Wolska, I. Synthesis and structural characterization of derivatives of 2- and 3-benzo[b]furan carboxylic acids with potential cytotoxic activity. *Il Farmaco* **2005**, *60*, 519–527. [CrossRef] [PubMed]
9. Graves, A.P.; Brenk, R.; Shoichet, B.K. Decoys for Docking. *J. Med. Chem.* **2005**, *48*, 3714–3728. [CrossRef]
10. Repolles, M.J.; Pubill, C.F.; Cabeza, L.L.; Carbo, B.M.; Cerda, R.J.A.; Negrie, R.C. Benzofuran, dihydrobenzofuran, dihydrobenzopyran and benzopyran derivatives as antidepressant agents. Spanish Patent ES2131020 A1, 1 July 1999.
11. Kossakowski, J.; Krawiecka, M.; Kuran, B.; Stefańska, J.; Wolska, I. Synthesis and preliminary evaluation of the antimicrobial activity of selected 3-benzofurancarboxylic acid derivatives. *Molecules* **2010**, *15*, 4737–4749. [CrossRef]
12. Kossakowski, J.; Ostrowska, K. Synthesis of new derivatives of 2,3-dihydro-7-benzo[b]furanol with potential pharmacological activity. *Acta Pol. Pharm.* **2006**, *63*, 271–275.

13. Kossakowski, J.; Ostrowska, K.; Struga, M.; Stefańska, J. Synthesis of new derivatives of 2,2-dimethyl-2,3-dihydro-7-benzo[b]furanol with potential antimicrobial activity. *Med. Chem. Res.* **2009**, *18*, 555–565. [CrossRef]
14. Kodama, I.; Kamiya, K.; Toyama, J. Amiodarone: Ionic and cellular mechanisms of action of the most promising class III agent. *Am. J. Cardiol.* **1999**, *84*, 20R–28R. [CrossRef]
15. Courchesne, W.E. Characterization of novel, broad-based fungicidal activity for anti-arrhythmic drug amiodarone. *J. Pharmacol. Exp. Ther.* **2002**, *300*, 195–199. [CrossRef]
16. Courchesne, W.E.; Ozturk, S. Amiodarone induces a caffeine-inhibited, MID1-dependent rise in free cytoplasic calcium in *Saccharomyces cerevisiae*. *Mol. Microbiol.* **2003**, *47*, 223–234. [CrossRef]
17. Gill, J.; Heel, R.C.; Fitton, A. Amiodarone. An overview of its pharmacological properties, and review of its therapeutic use in cardiac arrhythmias. *Drugs* **1992**, *43*, 69–110. [CrossRef]
18. Pizzichini, M.; Aleo, M.F.; Marcolongo, R.; Marinello, E. The mechanism of benziodarone activity. *Quad. Sclavo. Diagn.* **1982**, *18*, 203–208.
19. Heel, R.C.; Brogden, R.N.; Speight, T.M.; Avery, G.S. Benzbromarone: A review of its pharmacological properties and therapeutic use in gout and hyperuricaemia. *Drugs* **1977**, *14*, 349–366. [CrossRef]
20. Masbernard, A.; Giudicelli, C.P. Ten years' experience with benzbromarone in the management of gout and hyperuricaemia. *S. Afr. Med. J.* **1981**, *59*, 701–706.
21. Lu, Y.; Shi, T.; Wang, Y.; Yang, H.; Yan, X.; Luo, X.; Jiang, H.; Zhu, W. Halogen Bonding-A Novel Interaction for Rational Drug Design? *J. Med. Chem.* **2009**, *52*, 2584–2862. [CrossRef]
22. Bissantz, C.; Kuhn, B.; Stahl, M. A Medicinal Chemist's Guide to Molecular Interaction. *J. Med. Chem.* **2010**, *53*, 5061–5084. [CrossRef]
23. Wilcken, R.; Zimmermann, M.O.; Lange, A.; Joerger, A.C.; Boeckler, F.M. Principles and Applications of Halogen Bonding in Medicinal Chemistry and Chemical Biology. *J. Med. Chem.* **2013**, *56*, 1363–1388. [CrossRef]
24. Ford, C.M.; Shing, H.P. Computational Tools To model Halogen Bonds in Medicinal Chemistry. *J. Med. Chem.* **2016**, *59*, 1655–1670. [CrossRef] [PubMed]
25. Krawiecka, M.; Kuran, B.; Kossakowski, J.; Cieślak, M.; Kazmierczak-Barańska, J.; Królewska, K.; Nawrot, B. Synthesis and cytotoxic properties of halogen and aryl-/heteroarylpiperazinyl derivatives of benzofurans. *Anti Cancer Agents Med. Chem.* **2015**, *15*, 115–121. [CrossRef]
26. Kossakowski, J.; Kuran, B.; Kazmierczak-Baranska, J.; Królewska, K.; Nawrot, B.; Krawiecka, M.; Cieslak, M. Halogen derivatives of benzo[b]furans useful as anti-neoplastic or anti-proliferative drugs. Spanish Patent EP 2631232 A1, 9 January 2013.
27. Królewska-Golińska, K.; Cieślak, M.J.; Sobczak, M.; Dolot, R.; Radzikowska-Cieciura, E.; Napiórkowska, M.; Wybrańska, I.; Nawrot, B. Novel benzo[b]furans with anti-microtubule activity upregulate expression of apoptotic genes and arrest leukemia cells in G2/M phase. *Anticancer Agents Med. Chem.* **2018**. [CrossRef] [PubMed]
28. Zawadowski, T.; Suski, S.; Rump, S.; Borkowska, G. Synthesis of new aminoalkanoles derivatives of benzofurans with an expected β-adrenolityc activity. *Acta Polon. Pharm.* **1989**, *XLVI*, 201–208.
29. Fink, S.L.; Cookson, B.T. Apoptosis, Pyroptosis, and Necrosis: Mechanistic Description of Dead and Dying Eukaryotic Cells. *Infect. Immun.* **2005**, *73*, 1907–1916. [CrossRef]
30. Maszewska, M.; Leclaire, J.; Cieslak, M.; Nawrot, B.; Okruszek, A.; Caminade, A.M.; Majoral, J.P. Water-soluble polycationic dendrimers with a phosphoramidothioate backbone: Preliminary studies of cytotoxicity and oligonucleotide/plasmid delivery in human cell culture. *Oligonucleotides* **2003**, *13*, 193–205. [CrossRef]

Sample Availability: Not available.

molecules

MDPI

Article

In Vitro and In Vivo Anti-Breast Cancer Activities of Some Newly Synthesized 5-(thiophen-2-yl)thieno-[2,3-d]pyrimidin-4-one Candidates

Abd El-Galil E. Amr [1,2,*], Alhussein A. Ibrahimd [2], Mohamed F. El-Shehry [3,4], Hanaa M. Hosni [3], Ahmed A. Fayed [2,5] and Elsayed A. Elsayed [6,7]

1 Pharmaceutical Chemistry Department, Drug Exploration & Development Chair (DEDC), College of Pharmacy, King Saud University, Riyadh 11451, Saudi Arabia

2 Applied Organic Chemistry Department, National Research Center, Cairo, Dokki 12622, Egypt; alhusseina62@yahoo.com (A.A.I.); dr_ahmedfayed14@yahoo.com (A.A.F.)

3 Pesticide Chemistry Department, National Research Center, Dokki 12622, Cairo, Egypt; hanaanrc@yahoo.com (M.F.E.-S.); hanaahosni434@yahoo.com (H.M.H.)

4 Chemistry Department, Al-Zahrawy University College, Karbala 56001, Iraq

5 Respiratory Therapy Department, College of Medical Rehabilitation Sciences, Taibah University, Madinah Munawara, 22624, Saudi Arabia

6 Zoology Department, Bioproducts Research Chair, Faculty of Science, King Saud University, Riyadh 11451, Saudi Arabia; eaelsayed@ksu.edu.sa

7 Chemistry of Natural and Microbial Products Department, National Research Centre, Dokki 12622, Cairo, Egypt

* Correspondence: aamr@ksu.edu.sa; Tel.: +966-543074312

Academic Editor: Qiao-Hong Chen
Received: 29 May 2019; Accepted: 14 June 2019; Published: 17 June 2019

Abstract: In this study, some of new thiophenyl thienopyrimidinone derivatives **2–15** were prepared and tested as anti-cancer agents by using thiophenyl thieno[2,3-d]pyrimidinone derivative **2** as a starting material, which was prepared from cyclization of ethyl ester derivative **1** with formamide. Treatment of **2** with ethyl- chloroacetate gave thienopyrimidinone *N*-ethylacetate **3**, which was reacted with hydrazine hydrate or anthranilic acid to afford acetohydrazide **4** and benzo[d][1,3]oxazin-4-one **5**, respectively. Condensation of **4** with aromatic aldehydes or phenylisothiocyanate yielded Schiff base derivatives **6,7**, and thiosemicarbazise **10**, which were treated with 2-mercaptoacetic acid or chloroacetic acid to give the corresponding thiazolidinones **8**, **9**, and phenylimino-thiazolidinone **11**, respectively. Treatment of **4** with ethylacetoacetate or acetic acid/acetic anhydride gave pyrazole **12** and acetyl acetohydrazide **13** derivatives, respectively. The latter compound **13** was reacted with ethyl cycno-acetate or malononitrile to give **14** and **15**, respectively. In this work, we have studied the anti-cancer activity of the synthesized thienopyrimidinone derivatives against MCF-7 and MCF-10A cancer cells. Furthermore, in vivo experiments showed that the synthesized compounds significantly reduced tumor growth up to the 8th day of treatment in comparison to control animal models. Additionally, the synthesized derivatives showed potential inhibitory effects against pim-1 kinase activities.

Keywords: thiopene; thienopyrimidinone; thiazolidinone; anticancer activity

1. Introduction

Cancer is a major health problem acting as a global killer, so synthesizing new compounds, which may act as potent antitumor agents, is a great target for chemists working in this field. In this study, we are interested in synthesizing and studying biological activities of thieno[2,3-d]pyrimidinone derivatives [1–11]. Thienopyrimidinones are very important moieties that act as keys for pharmacological and pharmaceutical properties. They are reported to cause antiviral [12], antimicrobial [13], antihypertensive [14], analgesic, and anti-inflammatory activities [15]. They also inhibit various protein kinase enzymes, such as CK2 involved in particular anticancer activity [16]. Additionally, the nitrogenous ring system was associated with some types of biological activities such as: anti-inflammatory [17], insecticidal [18], antimicrobial and antituberculosis [19,20] activities. On the other hand, thienopyrimidinones contain a thiophene ring fused with a pyrimidinone nucleus. In general, this system was thought to be interesting in development of pharmaceutical compounds [21,22], and was not only evaluated as cGMP phosphodiesterase inhibitors [23], anti-viral [24], anti-inflammatory [25], anti-microbial agents [26], but also as kinase inhibitors and potential anti-cancer agents [27,28]. In continuation to our previous work, and to extend our research [1–11], from the above points, we have studied the anticancer activity of the newly synthesized substituted thienopyrimidinone derivatives against MCF-7 and MCF-10A cancer cells. Furthermore, the work was extended to evaluate the effects of synthesized derivatives on the inhibition of tumor growth in an in vivo animal model. Finally, we evaluated the inhibitory effects of our synthesized compounds against pim-1 kinase activity as a possible mechanism of their action.

2. Results and Discussion

2.1. Chemistry

A series of thiophenyl thienopyrimidinone derivatives **2–15** were prepared and tested as anti-cancer agents. Cyclization of ethyl 5′-amino-[2,3′-bithiophene]-4′-carboxylate (**1**) with formamide gave the corresponding thiophenylthieno[2,3-d]pyrimidinone derivative (**2**), which was treated with ethylchloroacetate to give thienopyrimidinone N-ethylacetate **3**. Reaction of **3** with hydrazine hydrate or anthranilic acid afforded the corresponding hydrazide **4** and benzooxazinone **5** derivatives, respectively (Scheme 1).

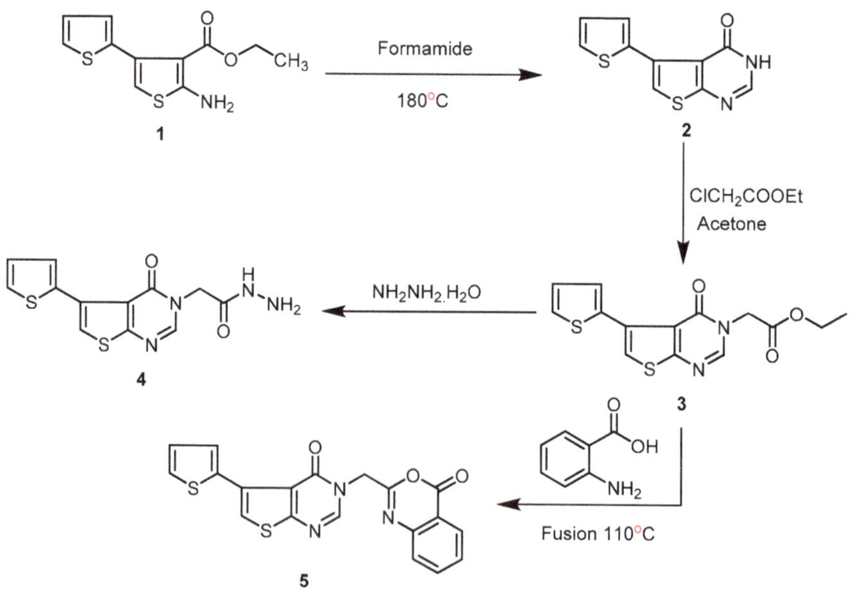

Scheme 1. Synthetic route for compounds **2–5**.

Condensation of **4** with aromatic aldehydes, namely, 2,3-dimethoxybenzaldehyde or 4-chlorobenzaldehyde gave the corresponding Schiff base derivatives **6** and **7**, which were cyclized via reaction with 2-mercaptoacetic acid in dry benzene to give the corresponding thiazolidinone derivatives **8** and **9**, respectively. Treatment of **4** with phenylisothiocyanate gave thiosemicarbazide **10**, which was condensed with chloroacetic acid to afford phenyliminothiazolidinone derivative **11** (Scheme 2).

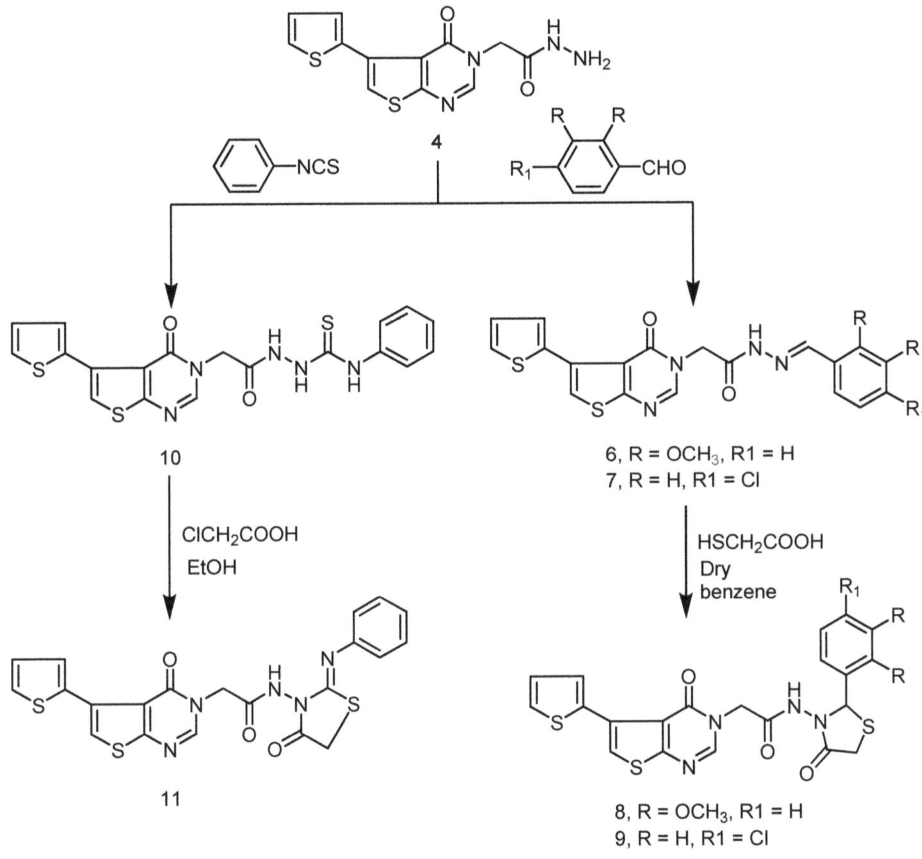

Scheme 2. Synthetic route for compounds **6–11**.

Finally, treatment of **4** with ethylacetoacetate or acetic acid/acetic anhydride gave the corresponding pyrazolyl derivative **12** and N-acetyl hydrazide **13**, respectively. The latter compound **13** was reacted with ethylcycnoacetate or malononitrile to give pyridine derivatives **14** and **15**, respectively (Scheme 3).

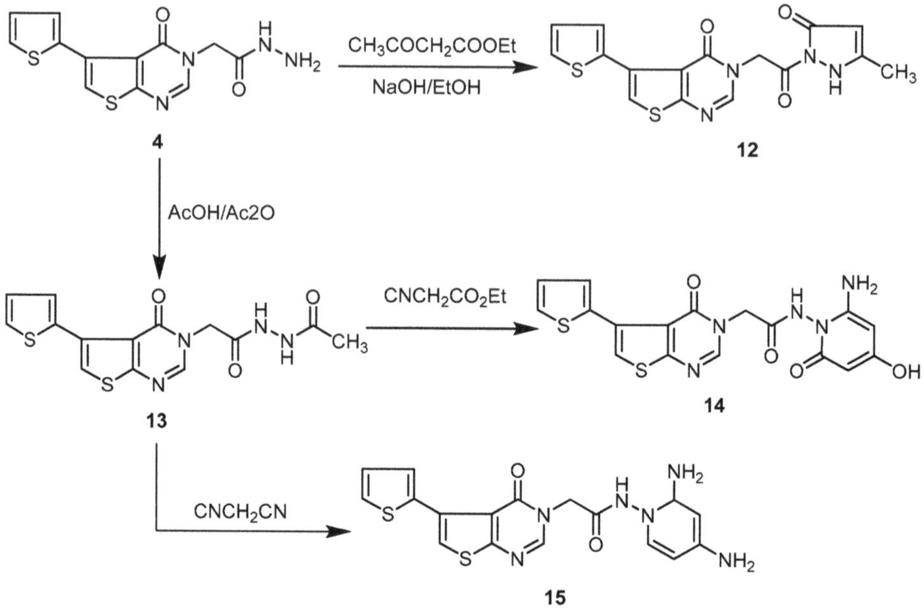

Scheme 3. Synthetic route for compounds **12–15**.

2.2. Biological Evaluation

MCF-7 cells were used to investigate the potential in vitro anti-proliferative potential of the synthesized compounds. With the exception of Cpd. **2** (data not shown), we found that all compounds have promising activities when used in µM concentration. On the other hand, Cisplatin and Milaplatin showed higher IC_{50} values (13.34 ± 0.11 and 18.43 ± 0.13 µM, respectively). DMSO at concentrations of 0.1% and 0.5%, had little or no toxicity, whereas higher concentrations inhibited the growth of MCF-7cells. Therefore, it seems DMSO could be solvents of choice acceptable to be used at concentrations < 0.5% (*v*/*v*) towards the examined cells and possibly for other cell lines. Also, the effect on cell viability was proportional to the concentration applied. From Figure 1, we can see that Cpd. **15, 14** and **8** (IC_{50}, 1.18 ± 0.032, 1.19 ± 0.042, 1.26 ± 0.052 µM, respectively) followed by **9** and **11** (IC_{50}, 2.37 ± 0.053 and 2.48 ± 0.054 µM respectively) produced the highest effect on cell viability. Secondly, compounds **12, 10** and **13**, showed moderate activities (IC_{50}, 3.36 ± 0.063, 3.55 ± 0.065 and 3.64 ± 0.074 µM, respectively). Compounds **7, 6, 5, 4** and **3** were the least active ones (IC_{50}, 4.33 ± 0.076, 4.52 ± 0.085, 4.76 ± 0.087, 4.87 ± 0.098 and 5.98 ± 0.099 µM, respectively). The order of activities can be arranged as **15** > **14** > **8** > **9 > 11** > **12** > **10** > **13** > **7** > **6** > **5** > **4** > **3**.

Results revealed that the substitution with pyridine moiety at the terminal NH improved the cytotoxic effect than the pyrimidone derivatives. In contrast, substitution with 5-membered di-heterocyclic ring system with aryl moiety decreased the obtained activities (methoxy phenyl > chlorophenyl). Attaching five membered pyrazolinone ring system bearing no aryl moiety at terminal NH (compound **12** decreased the activities than those containing aryl substitutions (compounds **9** and **11**). Compounds **10, 7** and **6** that contain aromatic *N*-substitution still have more potent activity. The increased effect of the aromatic ring may be attributed to ring aromaticity and electron resonance. On the other hand, aliphatic side chains (compounds **4** and **3**) or methylene bridges (Compound **5**) have less potent activities.

Additionally, results against non-tumorigenic MCF-10A proved that our derivatives have higher degrees of safety towards normal cells.

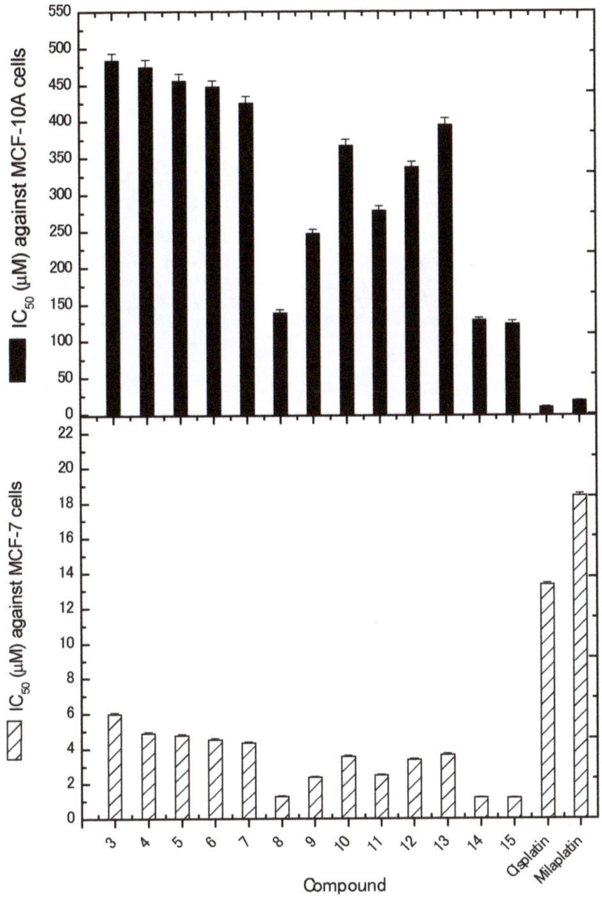

Figure 1. Obtained IC_{50} values for MCF-7 and MCF-10A cells.

In Vivo Xenograft Model

The in vivo anti-breast cancer activities of different synthesized derivatives were evaluated using a breast cancer mouse xenograft model. Figure 2 shows the increase in percentage of inhibition in tumor growth with treatment time when animals were exposed to different compounds. This was also compared with tumor development in control animals. It can be seen, that our derivatives reduced tumor growth starting day 2. The maximal effect was obtained after 8 days. Furthermore, the in vivo effect showed also the same inhibitory pattern obtained in the in vitro experiments. The average weight of each group of mice treated with drug and the control group summarized in Table 1.

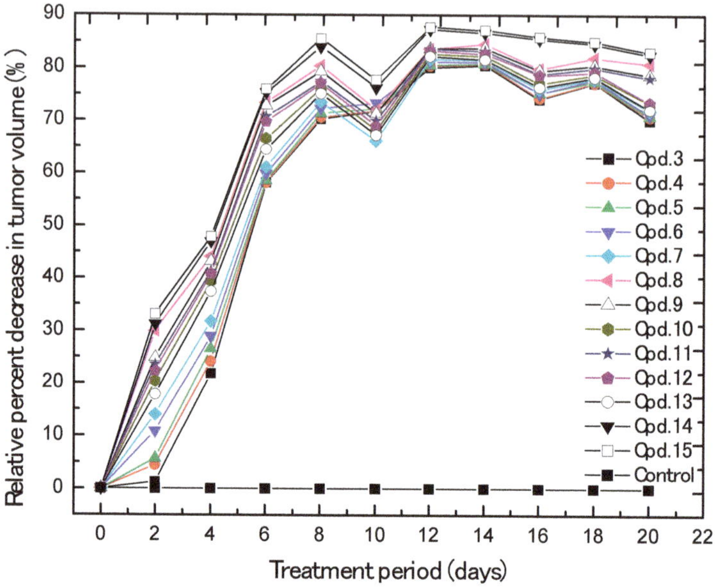

Figure 2. Relative percentage of decrease in tumor volume in response to prepared compounds.

Table 1. The average weight of each group of mice treated with drug and the control group.

Drugs	Average Weight of Animals in Grams after Days											
	0	2	4	6	8	10	12	14	16	18	20	22
Control	28	28	28	28	28.2	28.	28.3	28.4	28.4	28.4	28.4	28.4
3	28	28	28	28	28.2	27.9	27.8	27.7	27.7	27.6	27.7	27.7
4	24.2	24.2	24.1	24.0	23.9	23.9	23.7	23.7	23.6	23.6	23.6	236.
5	22.9	22.9	22.9	22.8	22.8	22.7	22.8	22.7	22.9	22.6	22.6	22.5
6	23.7	23.7	23.6	23.6	23.5	23.5	23.5	23.4	23.4	23.5	23.5	23.5
7	27.3	27.3	27.2	27.2	27.2	27.1	27.1	27.1	27.0	27.0	27.0	27.0
8	25.3	25.3	25.2	25.2	25.2	25.1	25.1	24.8	24.7	24.6	24.5	24.2
9	24.1	24.1	24.0	24.0	24.0	24.0	23.7	23.7	23.6	23.6	23.6	23.6
10	24.9	24.9	24.9	24.9	24.8	24.8	24.8	24.4	24.4	24.4	24.4	24.4
11	26.6	26.6	26.6	26.5	26.6	26.6	26.4	26.3	26.3	26.3	26.3	263.
12	27.4	27.4	27.4	27.3	27.3	27.3	27.2	27.2	27.2	27.1	27.1	27.1
13	25.4	25.4	25.4	25.4	25.4	25.3	25.3	25.3	25.3	25.3	25.3	25.3
14	26.5	26.4	26.3	26.2	26.1	25.9	25.9	25.9	25.8	25.8	25.7	25.7
15	26.1	26.1	26.1	25.8	25.8	25.7	25.7	25.6	25.6	25.5	25.5	25.2

The Provirus Integration in Maloney (Pim) kinases represents a family of constitutively active serine/threonine kinases and includes three subtypes (pim-1, pim-2 and pim-3). Pim kinases regulate many biological processes such as cell cycle, cell proliferation, apoptosis and drug resistance [29–32]. Being expressed in many types of solid and hematological cancers and almost absent in benign lesions, pim kinases proved to be a successful anti-cancer drug target of low toxicity [33–40]. Results obtained in Figure 3 showed that all synthesized compounds were showed potent inhibitory effects against pim-1 kinase.

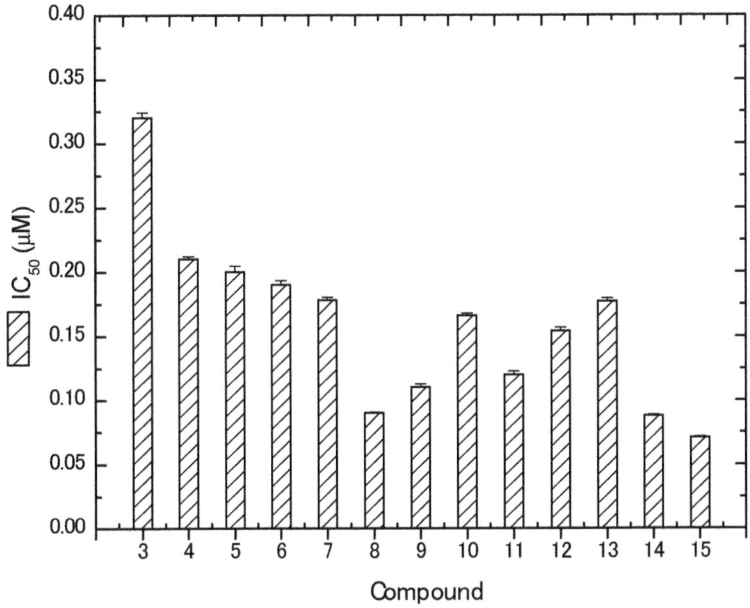

Figure 3. IC_{50} of the tested compounds against pim-1 Kinase.

3. Materials and Methods

3.1. Chemistry

"Melting points were determined in open glass capillary tubes with an Electro Thermal Digital melting point apparatus (model: IA9100) and are uncorrected. Elemental microanalyses were carried out in the microanalysis unit of NRC and were found within the acceptable limits of the calculated values. Infrared spectra (KBr) were recorded on a Nexus 670 FTIR Nicolet, Fourier Transform infrared spectrometer. ^{1}H- and ^{13}C NMR spectra were run in (DMSO-d_6) on Jeol 500 MHz instruments. Mass spectra were run on a MAT Finnigan SSQ 7000 spectrometer, using the electron impact technique (EI)."

Synthesis of 5-(thiophen-2-yl)thieno[2,3-d]pyrimidin-4(3H)-one **(2).** A mixture of compound **1** (1 mmol, 253 mg) and formamide (20 mL) was heated at 180 °C in oil bath for 2 h. The formed solid was collected by filtration, washed with cold methanol, dried and crystallized from EtOH to give compound **2**. Yield 80%, M.p 192–194 °C; IR (KBr, cm^{-1}): ῡ 3323 (NH), 1659 (C=O). ^{1}H NMR (DMSO-d_6) δ_H: 7.11–7.72 (m, 4H, thiophene-H), 8.50 (s, 1H, CH-pyrimidine), 13.30 (s, 1H, NH, disappeared with D_2O). ^{13}C NMR: 119.98, 122.01, 122.17, 126.84, 127.75, 128.74, 131.26, 136.42, (8C, thiophene-C), 157.05 (1C, pyrimidine-C), 165.56 (C=O). Mass spectrum, *m/z* (EI, %): 234 (M^+, 100), 235 (M^+ + 1, 11), 236 (M^+ + 2, 9). Analysis for $C_{10}H_6N_2OS_2$ (234.29): Calculated: C, 51.27; H, 2.58; N, 11.96; S, 27.37. Found: C, 51.20; H, 2.50; N, 11.90; S, 27.30.

Synthesis of ethyl 2-(4-oxo-5-(thiophen-2-yl)thieno[2,3-d]pyrimidin-3(4H)-yl)acetate **(3).** A mixture of **2** (1 mmol, 234 mg), ethylchloroacetate (1 mmol, 122 mg) and anhydrous potassium carbonate (8 mmol) in dry acetone (30 mL) was heated under reflux for 4h. The obtained solid was removed by filtration, the filtrate was concentrated, the precipitate solid was filtered off, dried, and crystallized from EtOH to give the ester derivative **3**. Yield 70%, m.p 135–137 °C. IR (KBr, cm^{-1}): ν 1753 (C=O, ester), 1655 (CO); ^{1}H NMR (DMSO-d_6), δ: 1.24 (t, 3H, CH_3), 4.20 (s, 2H, CH_2), 4.85 (q, 2H, CH_2-ethyl), 7.10–7.72 (m, 4H, thiophene-H), 8.50 (s, 1H, pyrimidine-H). ^{13}C-NMR (DMSO)-d_6) δc: 14.5 (CH_3), 40.2 (CH_2), 47.8 (CH_2), 119.9, 122.2, 126.9, 127.8, 128.7, 128.9, 131.3, 136.4 (8C, thiophene-C), 157.0 (1C, pyrimidine-C), 165.6,

168.3 (2C, 2CO). Mass spectrum, *m/z* (EI, %): 320 (M^+, 100), 321 (M^+ + 1, 18). Analysis for $C_{14}H_{12}N_2O_3S_2$ (320.38): Calculated: C, 52.49; H, 3.78; N, 8.74; S, 20.01. Found: C, 52.40; H, 3.70; N, 8.68; S, 19.86.

Synthesis of 2-(4-oxo-5-(thiophen-2-yl)thieno[2,3-d]pyrimidin-3(4H)-yl)acetohydrazide **(4).** To a solution of **3** (1 mmol, 320 mg) in ethanol (50 mL), hydrazine hydrate (4 mmol, 85%) was added and refluxed for 8 h. The precipitated solid was collected by filteration, dried and crystallized from EtOH to give compound **4**. Yield 75%, m.p. 205–207 °C, IR (KBr, cm^{-1}): ν 3322 (NH), 3246 (NH_2), 1659 (C=O). ^{1}H-NMR (DMSO-d_6) δ: 3.39 (s, 2H, CH_2), 4.65 (s, 2H, NH_2, disappeared with D_2O), 7.10–7.65 (m, 4H, thiophene-H), 8.17 (s, 1H, pyrimidine-H), 12.58 (s, 1H, NH, disappeared with D_2O). ^{13}C-NMR (DMSOd$_6$) δc: 40.1 (CH_2), 120.5, 120.8, 126.6, 127.8, 128.7, 131.4, 133.5, 136.8 (8C, thiophene-C), 157.9 (1C, pyrimidine-C), 166.3, 169.4 (2C, 2CO). Mass spectrum, m/z (EI, %): 306 (M^+, 100), 307 (M^+ + 1, 14). Analysis for $C_{12}H_{10}N_4O_2S_2$ (306.36): Calculated: C, 47.05; H, 3.29; N, 18.29; S, 20.93. Found: C, 46.85; H, 3.20; N, 18.20; S, 20.85.

Synthesis of 2-((4-oxo-5-(thiophen-2-yl)thieno[2,3-d]pyrimidin-3(4H)-yl)methyl)-4H-benzo[d]-[1,3] *oxazin-4-one* **(5).** A mixture of **3** (1 mmol, 320 mg) and anthranilic acid (1 mmol, 137 mg) was fused together at 110 °C in an oil bath for 3hr. The residue was boiled with ethanol, the formed solid was removed by filtration, the solid formed was filtered off, and crystallized from EtOH to give **5**. Yield 60%, m.p. 225–227 °C. IR (KBr, Cm^{-1}): ν 1750 (C=O), 1684 (C=O). ^{1}H-NMR (DMSO d_6) $δ_H$: 4.58 (s, 2H, CH_2), 7.10–7.54 (m, 4H, thiophene-H), 7.68-8.16 (m, 4H, Ph-H), 8.64 (s, 1H, pyrimidine-H). ^{13}C-MNR (DMSO-d_6) $δ_c$: 43.0 (CH_2), 120.0, 120.1, 121.3, 121.7, 126.7, 126.8, 127.7, 128.7, 131.3, 136.5, 136.6, 149.5, 149.7, 158.2 (14C, thiophene + Ph-C), 157.2 (1C, pyrimidine-C), 160.1, 165.6, 166.5 (3C, 3C=O). Mass spectrum, *m/z* (EI, %): 393 (M^+, 100). Analysis for $C_{19}H_{11}N_3O_3S_2$ (393.44): Calculated: C, 58.00; H, 2.82; N, 10.68; S, 16.30. Found: C, 57.90; H, 2.78; N, 10.60; S, 16.25.

Synthesis of hydrazone derivatives **6** *and* **7**. To a mixture of **4** (1 mmol, 306 mg) and aromatic aldehydes, namely 3,4-dimethoxybenazaldehyed or 4-chlorobenzaldehyde (1 mmol) in ethanol (50 mL), few drops of piperidine were added and refluxed for 5 h, with stirring. After cooling, the formed solid was filtered off and recrystallized from dioxan to give the corresponding derivatives **6** and **7** respectively.

N′-(2,3-Dimethoxybenzylidene)-2-(4-oxo-5-(thiophen-2-yl)thieno[2,3-d]pyrimidin-3(4H)-yl)-acetohydrazide **(6).** Yield 68%, m.p. 248–250 °C. IR (KBr, cm^{-1}): ν 3388 (NH), 1660 (C=O). ^{1}H-NMR (DMSO-d_6) $δ_H$: 3.72, 3.86 (2s, 6H, 2OCH_3), 4.11 (s, 2H, CH_2), 6.98-7.61 (m, 7H, thiophene + Ph-H), 8.60 (s, 1H, CH=N), 9.05 (s, 1H, pyrimidine-H), 10.51 (s, 1H, NH, disappeared with D_2O). ^{13}C-NMR (MDSO-d_6) δc: 44.1 (1C, CH_2), 56.1, 60.1 (2C, OCH_3), 114.3, 116.1, 119.5, 121.8, 124.0, 126.7, 127.7, 128.7, 129.3, 130.6, 131.3, 136.47, 149.07, 149.77 (14C, thiophene-C + Ph-C), 148.56 (1C, CH=N), 157.19 (1C, pyrimidine-C), 163.66, 169.74 (2C, 2C=O). Mass spectrum, *m/z* (EI, %): 454 (M^+, 100). Analysis for $C_{21}H_{18}N_4O_4S_2$ (454.52): Calculated: C, 55.49; H, 3.99; N, 12.33; S, 14.11. Found: C, 55.40; H, 3.90; N, 12.25; S, 13.96.

N′-(4-Chlorobenzylidene)-2-(4-oxo-5-(thiophen-2-yl)thieno[2,3-d]pyrimidin-3(4H)-yl)acetohydrazide **(7).** Yield 65%, m.p. 250–252 °C. IR (KBr, Cm^{-1}): ν 3408 (NH), 1670 (CO), 1659 (CO). ^{1}H-NMR (DMSO-d_6) δH: 4.10 (s, 2H, CH_2), 7.10–7.80 (m, 9H, Ar-H + CH=N), 9.05 (s, 1H, pyrimidine-H), 10.56 (s, 1H, NH, disappeared with D_2O). ^{13}C-NMR (MDSO-d_6) δc: 44.1 (1C, CH_2), 145.2 (1C, CH=N), 119.5, 121.9, 124.0, 126.8, 127.8, 128.1, 129.3, 130.6, 131.3, 136.5, 149.1, 149.8 (14C, thiophene-C + Ph-C), 157.5 (1C, pyrimidine-C), 162.7, 169.9 (2C, 2C=O). Mass spectrum, *m/z* (EI, %): 428 (M^+, 100), 430 (M^+ + 2, 40). Analysis for $C_{19}H_{13}ClN_4O_2S_2$ (428.91): Calculated: C, 53.21; H, 3.06; N, 13.06; S, 14.95. Found: C, 53.12; H, 3.00; N, 13.00; S, 14.88.

Synthesis of thiazolidinone derivatives **8** *and* **9**. To a stirred solution of **6** or **7** (1 mmol) in dry benzene (40 mL), thioglycollic acid (1 mmol, 92 mg) in dry benzene (10 mL) was added and refluxed for 12 h. The solvent was evaporated to dryness. The formed product was collected, and crystallized with dioxan to obtain the corresponding products **8** and **9**, respectively.

N-(2-(2,3-Dimethoxyphenyl)-4-oxothiazolidin-3-yl)-2-(4-oxo-5-(thiophen-2-yl)thieno[2,3-d]pyrimidin-3(4H)-yl)acetamide **(8).** Yield 60%, m.p. 280–282 °C. IR (KBr, cm^{-1}): ν 3417 (NH), 1670, 1680, 1630 (3 C=O). ^{1}H-NMR (DMSO-d_6) δ_H: 3.65, 3.90 (2s, 6H, $2OCH_3$), 4.66 (s, 2H, CH_2), 4.77 (s, 2H, CH_2), 5.86 (s, 1H, CH), 6.95-7.65 (m, 7H, thiophene + Ph-H), 8.49 (s, 1H, pyrimidine-H), 10.84 (s, 1H, NH, disappeared with D_2O). ^{13}C-NMR (DMSO-d_6) δ_c: 35.9, 47.4 (2C, $2CH_2$), 56.5, 58.42 (2C, $2OCH_3$), 59.2 (1C, CH), 113.4, 117.9, 118.9, 120.7, 121.8, 126.8, 127.5, 128.7, 130.7, 131.0, 136.5, 145.3, 149.5, 149.9 (14C, thiophene-C + Ph-C), 156.9 (1C, pyrimidine-C), 162.5, 165.4, 169.2 (3C, 3C=O). Mass spectrum, *m*/*z* (EI, %): 528 (M^+, 100), 529 (M^+ + 1, 30). Analysis for $C_{23}H_{20}N_4O_5S_3$ (528): Calculated: C, 52.26; H, 3.81; N, 10.60; S, 18.19. Found: C, 52.18; H, 3.75; N, 10.52; S, 18.10.

N-(2-(4-Chlorophenyl)-4-oxothiazolidin-3-yl)-2-(4-oxo-5-(thiophen-2-yl)thieno[2,3-d]-pyrimidin-3(4H)-yl)-acetamide **(9).** Yield 75%, m.p. 175-177 °C. IR (KBr, cm^{-1}): ν 3417 (NH), 1720, 1630, 1660 (3C=O). ^{1}H-NMR (DMSO-d_6) δ_H: 3.81, 5.16 (2s, 4H, $2CH_2$), 5.90 (s, 1H, CH), 7.08–7.72 (m, 8H, thiophene-H + Ph-H), 8.50 (s, 1H, pyrimidine-H), 10.92 (s, 1H, NH, disappeared with D_2O). ^{13}CNMR (DMSO-d_6) δc: 40.1, 48.2 (2C, $2CH_2$), 65.2 (1C, CH), 120.0, 121.8, 127.7, 128.7, 129.3, 129.4, 131.3, 133.3, 135.0, 136.5, 143.5, 149.7 (14C, thiophene-C + Ph-C), 157.2 (1C, pyrimidine-C), 163.8, 165.6, 169.9 (3C, 3C=O). Mass spectrum, *m*/*z* (EI, %): 503 (M^+, 100), 505 (M^+ + 2, 34). Analysis for $C_{21}H_{15}ClN_4O_3S_3$ (503.01): Calculated: C, 50.14; H, 3.01; N, 11.14; S, 19.12. Found: C, 50.02; H, 3.00; N, 11.04; S, 19.06.

Synthesis of 2-(2-(4-oxo-5-(thiophen-2-yl)thieno[2,3-d]pyrimidin-3(4H)-yl)acetyl)-N-phenylhydrazine-1-carbothioamide **(10).** A mixture of **4** (1mmol, 306 mg) and phenylisothiocynate (1 mmol, 135 mg) in dry dioxan (50 mL) was refluxed for 6 h. The obtained solid was filtered off, washed with ether, dried and recrystallized from ethanol to give thiosemicarbazide **10**. Yield 60%, m.p. 240–242 °C. IR (KBr, cm^{-1}): ν 3414-3323 (NH), 1680, 1660 (2CO). ^{1}H-NMR (DMSO-d_6) δ_H: 4.66 (s, 2H, CH_2), 6.95-7.58 (m, 9H, thiophene + Ph-H), 8.49 (s, 1H, pyrimidine-H), 8.70, 10.71, 12.78 (3s, 3H, 3NH, disappeared with D_2O). ^{13}CNMR (DMSO-d_6) δc: 40.16 (CH_2), 119.9, 121.8, 126.8, 127.9, 128.8, 129.1, 130.2, 131.3, 134.1, 136.5, 137.9, 149.9 (14C, thiophene + Ph-C), 156.5 (1C, pyrimimidine-C), 166.5, 169.1 (2C, 2C=O), 171.0 (1C, C=S). Mass spectrum, *m*/*z* (EI, %): 441 (M^+, 100), 442 (M^+ + 1, 26). Analysis for $C_{19}H_{15}N_5O_2S_3$ (441.54): Calculated: C, 51.68; H, 3.42; N, 15.86; S, 21.78. Found: C, 51.60; H, 3.40; N, 15.80; S, 21.70.

Synthesis of N-(4-oxo-2-(phenylimino)thiazolidin-3-yl)-2-(4-oxo-5-(thiophen-2-yl)thieno[2,3-d]-pyrimidin-3(4H)-yl)acetamide **(11).** A mixture of 10 (1 mmol, 441 mg) and chloroacetic acid (1 mmol, 94 mg) in absolute ethanol (30 mL) was heated under reflux for 8 h. The solid formed was filtered off and crystallized with dioxane to give thiazole derivative 11. Yield 60%, m.p. 255–257 °C. IR (KBr, cm^{-1}): ν 3420 (NH), 1720, 1630 (2C=O). ^{1}H-NMR (DMSO-d_6) δ_H: 3.76 (s, 2H, CH_2), 4.85 (s, 2H, CH_2), 6.95-7.65 (m, 9H, thiophene-H + Ph-H), 8.50 (s, 1H, pyrimidine-H), 11.10 (s, 1H, NH, disappeared with D_2O). ^{13}CNMR (DMSO-d_6) δc: 40.2 (CH_2), 56.8 (CH_2), 120.0, 122.0, 126.7, 128.7, 130.7, 131.3, 132.5, 136.4, (8C, thiophene-C), 145.2, 149.3, 150.8, 151.9 (6C, Ph-C), 156.6 (1C, pyrimidine-C), 158.1 (1C, C=N), 163.4, 165.7, 169.6 (3C, 3C=O). Mass spectrum, *m*/*z* (EI, %): 481 (M^+. 100), 482 (M^+ + 1, 24). Analysis for $C_{21}H_{15}N_5O_3S_3$ (481.56): Calculated: C, 52.38; H, 3.14; N, 14.54; S, 19.97. Found: C, 52.30; H, 3.10; N, 14.50; S, 19.90.

Synthesis of 3-(2-(3-methyl-5-oxo-2,5-dihydro-1H-pyrazol-1-yl)-2-oxoethyl)-5-(thiophen-2-yl)thieno-[2,3-d]pyrimidin-4(3H)-one **(12).** A mixture of compound 4 (1 mmol, 306 mg) and ethylacetoacetate (1 mmol, 130 mg) in ethanolic sodium hydroxide (0.5 mmol/50 mL) was refluxed with stirring for 6 h. The precipitate was collected by filtration and crystallized from dioxane to give pyrazole derivative 12. Yield 80%, m.p. 225–227 °C. IR (KBr, cm^{-1}): ν 3417 (NH), 1650, 1630 (2C=O). ^{1}H-NMR (DMSOd$_6$) δ_H: 1.70 (s, 3H, CH_3), 4.35 (s, 2H, CH_2), 5.65 (s, 1H, pyrazole-CH), 7.51–7.69 (m, 4H, thiophene-H), 8.46 (s, 1H, pyrimidine-H), 12.93 (s, 1H, NH, disappeared with D_2O). ^{13}C-NMR (DMSO-d_6) δc: 34.4 (CH_3), 47.0 (CH_2), 120.0, 123.8, 127.7, 128.7, 129.4, 130.9, 132.6, 136.5 (8C, thiophene), 98.3, 151.9 (2C, Pyrazole-C), 156.6 (1C, pyrimidine-C), 163.4, 166.5, 169.7 (3C, 3C=O). Mass spectrum, *m*/*z* (EI, %): 372

(M^+, 100), 373 (M^+ + 1, 18). Analysis for $C_{16}H_{12}N_4O_3S_2$ (372.42): Calculated: C, 51.60; H, 3.25; N, 15.04; S, 17.22. Found: C, 51.50; H, 3.20; N, 15.00; S, 17.16.

Synthesis of N′-acetyl-2-(4-oxo-5-(thiophen-2-yl)thieno[2,3-d]pyrimidin-3(4H)-yl)aceto-hydrazide **(13).** A solution of **4** (1 mmol, 306 mg) in a mixture of AcOH acid and Ac_2O (50 m, 1:1 *v*/*v*) was refluxed with stirring for 8 h. The reaction mixture was dropped onto iced-water. The obtained precipitate was filtered off, washed with water, and recrystallized from ethanol to give N-acetyl derivative **13**. Yield 70%, m.p. 235–237 °C. IR (KBr, cm^{-1}): ν 3369-3232 (NH, NH), 1732 (C=O). ^{1}H-NMR (DMSOd$_6$) δ_H: 1.86 (s, 3H, CH_3), 4.68 (s, 2H, CH_2), 7.10–7.70 (m, 4H, thiophene-H), 8.44 (s, 1H, pyrimidine-H), 10.70, 10.82 (2s, 2NH, disappeared with D_2O). ^{13}C-NMR (DMSO-d$_6$) δc: 20.1 (CH_3), 50.1 (CH_2), 119.9, 122.0, 122.2, 126.8, 127.8, 128.7, 131.3, 136.4 (8C, thiophene-C), 157.0 (1C, pyrimidine-C), 162.8, 165.6, 169.1 (3C, 3C=O). Mass spectrum, *m*/*z* (EI, %): 348 (M^+, 100), 349 (M^+ + 1, 16). Analysis for $C_{14}H_{12}N_4O_3S_2$ (348.40): Calculated: C, 48.27; H, 3.47; N, 16.08; S, 18.40. Found: C, 48.20; H, 3.40; N, 16.00; S, 18.32.

Synthesis of compounds **14** *and* **15.** To a mixture of **13** (1 mmol, 348 mg) and ethylcyanoacetate or malononitrile (1 mmol) in EtOH (40 mL), a few drops of triethylamine were refluxed for 8 h, poured into iced-water. The precipitate was filtered off, and crystallized from EtOH to obtain compounds 14 and **15**, respectively.

N-(6-Amino-4-hydroxy-2-oxopyridin-1(2H)-yl)-2-(4-oxo-5-(thiophen-2-yl)thieno[2,3-d]-pyrimidin-3(4H)-yl)acetamide **(14).** Yield 75%, m.p. 280–282 °C. IR (KBr, cm^{-1}): ν 3492-3196 (OH, NH_2, NH), 1420, 1680, 1653 (3 C=O). ^{1}H-NMR (DMSO-d$_6$) δ_H: 4.15 (s, 2H, CH_2), 4.95, 5.70 (2s, 2H, 2CH), 6.50 (s, 2H, NH_2, disappeared with D_2O), 7.15–7.74 (m, 4H, thiophene-H), 8.50 (s, 1H, pyrimidine-H), 10.25 (s, 1H, OH, disappeared with D_2O), 10.65 (s, 1H, NH, disappeared with D_2O). ^{13}C-NMR (DMSO-d$_6$) δc: 49.00 (CH_2), 116.1, 120.2, 121.8, 126.7, 127.9, 128.9, 131.3, 136.5 (8C, thiophene-C), 86.5, 100.2, 145.5, 158.7 (4C, pyridine-C), 156.2 (1C, pyrimidine-C), 164.1, 165.5, 169.5 (3C, 3CO). Mass spectrum, *m*/*z* (EI, %): 415 (M^+, 75). Analysis for $C_{17}H_{13}N_5O_4S_2$ (415.44): Calculated: C, 49.15; H, 3.15; N, 16.86; S, 15.43. Found: C, 49.05; H, 3.10; N, 16.80; S, 15.35.

N-(2,4-Diaminopyridin-1(2H)-yl)-2-(4-oxo-5-(thiophen-2-yl)thieno[2,3-d]-pyrimidin-3(4H)-yl)acetamide **(15).** Yield 75%, m.p. 290–292 °C, IR (KBr, cm^{-1}). ν 3460-3345 (NH, NH2), 1680, 1653 (2C=O). ^{1}H-NMR (DMSO-d$_6$) δ_H: 4.13 (s, 2H, CH_2), 4.60 (s, 2H, NH_2, exchangeable with D_2O), 5.60–6.10 (m, 4H, 4CH), 7.10–8.72 (m, 4H, thiophene-H), 8.47 (s, 1H, pyrimidine-H), 9.12 (s, 2H, NH_2, disappeared with D_2O), 10.32 (s, 1H, NH, disappeared with D_2O). ^{13}C-NMR (DMSO-d$_6$) δc: 48.00 (CH_2), 115.1, 120.0, 121.8, 126.8, 127.7, 128.7, 131.3, 136.5 (8C, thiophene-C), 78.5, 105.1, 118.5, 139.7, 150.0 (5C, pyridine-C), 157.0 (1C, pyrimidine-C), 165.6, 169.3 (2C, 2CO). Mass spectrum, *m*/*z* (EI, %): 400 (M^+, 50). Analysis for $C_{17}H_{16}N_6O_2S_2$ (400.48): Calculated: C, 50.99; H, 4.03; N, 20.99; S, 16.01. Found: C, 50.90; H, 4.00; N, 20.90; S, 15.95.

3.2. Biological Evaluation

3.2.1. Cytotoxic Assay

"Human breast cancer cells (MCF-7) and normal non-tumorigenic MCF-10A cells were used throughout the work. Cells were obtained from ATCC, Gaithersburg, MD, USA. Standard MTT assay was used to explore the possible cytotoxic effects of the synthesized compounds [41,42]. Medium composition, cultivation conditions and assay performance were exactly the same as our previous work [43,44]. Cells were treated with varying concentrations (0–1 μM) of the compounds prepared in DMSO. After MTT addition, the absorbance of the dissolved formazan crystals was read at 570 nm [45]. The IC_{50} values were obtained with linear regression equations using Origin® 6.1 software (Origin Lab Corporation, Northampton, MA, USA)".

3.2.2. Human Breast Cancer Xenograft Animal Model

"In this work, MCF-7 mouse xenograft model was used. The animal protocol was approved by the Institutional Animal Use Ethics and Care Committee of the University of Alabama at Birmingham (50-01-05-08B). Female athymic pathogen-free nude mice (nu/nu, 4–6 weeks) were purchased from Frederick Cancer Research and Development Center (Frederick, MD, USA). To establish MCF-7 human breast cancer xenografts, each of the female nude mice was first implanted with a 60-day (subcutaneously, s.c.) slow release estrogen pellet (SE-121, 1.7 mg 17α-estradiol/pellet; Innovative Research of America, Sarasota, FL, USA). After 24 h, grown cells were harvested, washed twice with serum-free medium, resuspended, and injected subcutaneously (5 million cells/0.2 mL) into the left inguinal area of the mice. During the experiment, animals were checked periodically and the percentages of tumor growth, as well as animal weights, were recorded. Every 48 h, the size of the tumor was recorded by measuring two perpendicular diameters of the tumor and tumor volume was calculated according to Wang et al. [46]".

"Treated animals and control groups (7–10 mice/group) received different compounds and vehicles, respectively. The tested compounds were dissolved in PEG400:ethanol:saline (57.1:14.3:28.6, *v*/*v*/*v*), and injected intraperitoneal (i.p.) at doses of 5 and 10 µM/kg/d, 3 d/wk for 3 weeks. The higher dose (10 µM/kg/d, 3 d/wk) inhibited MCF-7 xenograft tumor growth".

3.2.3. Pim-1 Kinase Inhibitory Activity

Materials and Methods

"The kinase inhibitory activity of the synthesized compounds was determined using the Kinexus compound profiling service, Canada. Compounds were tested at 50 nM concentration. The kinase used was cloned, expressed and purified using proprietary methods. Quality control testing is routinely performed to ensure compliance to acceptable standards. ^{33}P-ATP was purchased from PerkinElmer. All other materials were of standard laboratory grade".

Pim-1 Kinase Protein Assay

"The protein kinase target profiling was executed via employing a radioisotope assay format. All the assays were performed in a prepared radioactive working area. The protein kinase profiling assays were performed at room temperature for 20–30 min in a final volume of 25 µL according to the reported method [47]".

4. Conclusions

During the current work, different new **14** thiophenyl thienopyrimidinone derivatives were synthesized using variable cyclization and condensation routes. The synthesized derivatives showed promising potential biological potentials for their use in the pharmaceutical industry. They revealed higher in vitro cytotoxic activities against breast cancer cell line MCF-7 in comparison to known drugs, e.g., Cisplatin and Milaplatin. Furthermore, the prepared derivatives proved to be less toxic against the non-tumorigenic MCF-10A cell line. In vivo studies also showed potential reduction in tumor growth in animal models for all synthesized derivatives compared to control animals. Finally, mechanism of action studies showed that the newly synthesized derivatives exert their anticancer effects through the inhibition of pim-1 kinase enzymes.

Author Contributions: M.F.E.-S., A.A.I., A.A.F. and H.M.H. performed most of the experiments; A.E.-G.E.A. and M.A.A. analyzed the data; E.A.E. contributed to the anticancer activity assays; All authors read and approved the final manuscript.

Funding: The authors are grateful to the Deanship of Scientific Research, King Saud University for funding through Vice Deanship of Scientific Research Chairs.

Acknowledgments: The authors are grateful to the Deanship of Scientific Research, King Saud University for funding through Vice Deanship of Scientific Research Chairs.

Conflicts of Interest: The authors declare no conflict of interest.

References

1. Amr, A.E.; Mohamed, A.M.; Mohamed, S.F.; Abdel-Hafez, N.A.; Hammam, A.G. Anticancer activities of some newly synthesized pyridine, pyrane and pyrimidine derivatives. *Bioorg. Med. Chem.* **2006**, *14*, 5481–5488. [CrossRef] [PubMed]
2. Amr, A.E.; Abdalla, M.M. Anticancer activities of some synthesized 2,4,6-trisubstituted pyridine candidates. *Biomed. Res.* **2016**, *27*, 731–736.
3. Mohamed, S.F.; Flefel, E.M.; Amr, A.E.; Abd El-Shafy, D.N. Anti-HSV-1 activity and mechanism of action of some new synthesized substituted pyrimidine, thiopyrimidine and thiazolopyrimidine derivatives. *Eur. J. Med. Chem.* **2010**, *45*, 1494–1501. [CrossRef] [PubMed]
4. Ouf, N.H.; Amr, A.E. Synthesis and anti-inflammatory activity of some pyrimidines and thienopyrimidines using 1-(2-benzo[d][1,3]dioxol-5-yl)vinyl)-4-mercapto-6-methyl- pyrimidine-5-yl)- ethan-2-one as a starting material. *Mon. Chem.* **2008**, *139*, 579–585. [CrossRef]
5. Abdel-Hafez, N.A.; Mohamed, A.M.; Amr, A.E.; Abdalla, M.M. Antiarrhythmic activities of some new synthesized tricyclic and tetracyclic thienopyridine derivatives. *Sci. Pharm.* **2009**, *77*, 539–553. [CrossRef]
6. Abdulla, M.M.; Amr, A.E.; Al-Omar, M.A.; Hussain, A.A.; Shalaby, A.F.A. Anti- inflammatory activity and acute toxicity (LD_{50}) of some new synthesized pyridine-2-yl- phenyl)-2-methoxybenzamide and thieno[2,3-b]pyridine derivatives. *Life Sci. J.* **2013**, *10*, 286–297.
7. Fayed, A.A.; Amr, A.E.; Al-Omar, M.A.; Mostafa, E.E. Synthesis and antimicrobial activity of some new substituted pyrido[3′,2′:4,5]thieno[3,2-d]pyrimidinone derivatives. *Russ. J. Bioorg. Chem.* **2014**, *40*, 308–313. [CrossRef]
8. Ouf, N.H.; Sakran, M.I.; Amr, A.E. Anti-inflammatory activities of some newly synthesized substituted thienochromene and Schiff base derivatives. *Res. Chem. Intermed.* **2015**, *41*, 2521–2536. [CrossRef]
9. Said, S.A.; El-Sayed, H.A.; Amr, A.E.; Abdalla, M.M. Selective and orally bioavailable CHK1 inhibitors of some synthesized substituted thieno[2,3-b]pyridine candidates. *Int. J. Pharm.* **2015**, *11*, 659–671.
10. Amr, A.E.; Al-Omar, M.A.; Abdalla, M.M. Biological evaluations of some synthesized pyrimidothieno[2,3-b]pyrimidine candidates as antiulcer agents. *Int. J. Pharm.* **2015**, *11*, 840–845. [CrossRef]
11. Amr, A.E.; Abdalla, M.M.; Ouf, N.H. Anti-angiogenic effects of some (5-hydroxy-4-methyl-2-((1-methyl-1H-indol-3-yl)methyl)thieno[2,3-d]pyrimidine derivatives. *J. Comput. Nanosci.* **2017**, *14*, 448–453. [CrossRef]
12. Nasr, M.N.; Gineinah, M.M. Pyrido[2,3-d]pyrimidines and pyrimido[5,4-5,6]pyrido[2,3-d] pyrimidines as new antiviral agents, synthesis and biologicalactivity. *Arch. Pharm. Pharm. Med. Chem.* **2002**, *335*, 289–295. [CrossRef]
13. Chambhare, R.V.; Khadse, B.G.; Bobde, A.S.; Bahekar, R.H. Synthesis and preliminary evaluation of some N-[5-(2-furanyl)-2-methyl-4-oxo-4H-thieno[2,3-d]pyrimidine-3-yl]- carboxamide and 3-substituted-5-(2-furanyl)-2-methyl-3H-thieno[2,3-d]pyrimidine-4-ones as antimicrobial agents. *Eur. J. Med. Chem.* **2003**, *38*, 89–100. [CrossRef]
14. Russell, R.K.; Press, J.B.; Rampulla, R.A.; McNally, J.J.; Falotico, R.; Keiser, J.A.; Bright, D.A.; Tobia, A. Thiophene systems. 9. Thienopyrimidinedione derivatives as potential antihypertensive agents. *J. Med. Chem.* **1988**, *31*, 1786–1793. [CrossRef]
15. Alagarsamy, V.; Meena, S.; Ramseshu, K.V.; Solomon, V.R.; Thirumurugan, K.; Dhanabal, K.; Murugan, M. Synthesis, analgesic, anti-inflammatory, ulcerogenic index and antibacterial activities of novel 2-methylthio-3-substituted-5,6,7,8-tetrahydrobenzo thieno [2,3-d]pyrimidin- 4(3h)-ones. *Eur. J. Med. Chem.* **2006**, *41*, 1293–1300. [CrossRef] [PubMed]
16. Petrie, C.R.; Cottam, H.B.; Mckernan, P.A.; Robins, R.K.; Revankar, G.R. Synthesis and biological activity of 6-azacadeguomycin and certain 3,4,6-trisubstituted pyrazolo-[3,4-d]pyrimidine ribonuleosi. *J. Med. Chem.* **1985**, *28*, 1010–1016. [CrossRef]
17. Mullican, M.D.; Wilson, M.W.; Connor, D.T.; Kostlan, C.R.; Schrier, D.J.; Dyer, R.D. Design of 5-(3,5-di-tert-butyl-4-hydroxyphenyl)-1,3,4-thiadiazoles-1,3,4-oxadiazoles, and 1,2,4-triazoles as orally-active, nonulcerogenic antiinflammatory agents. *J. Med. Chem.* **1993**, *36*, 1090–1099. [CrossRef] [PubMed]

18. Shi, W.; Qian, X.; Zhang, R.; Song, G. Synthesis and quantitative structure-activity relationships of new 2,5-disubstituted-1,3,4-oxadiazoles. *J. Agric. Food Chem.* **2001**, *49*, 124–130. [CrossRef] [PubMed]
19. Gaonkar, S.L.; Rai, K.M.L.; Prabhuswamy, B. Synthesis and antimicrobial studies of a new series of 2-{4-[2-(5-ethylpyridin-2-yl)ethoxy]phenyl}-5-substituted-1,3,4-oxadiazoles. *Eur. J. Med. Chem.* **2006**, *41*, 841–846. [CrossRef] [PubMed]
20. Patel, R.V.; Pate, P.K.; Kumari, P.; Rajani, D.P.; Chikhalia, K.H. Synthesis of benzimida zolyl-1,3,4-oxadiazol-2ylthio-n-phenyl (benzothiazolyl) acetamides as antibacterial, antifungal and antituberculosis agents. *Eur. J. Med. Chem.* **2012**, *53*, 41–51. [CrossRef] [PubMed]
21. Varvounis, G.; Giannopoulos, T. Synthesis, Chemistry, and Biological Properties of Thienopyrimidines. In *Advances in Heterocyclic Chemistry*; Alan, R.K., Ed.; Academic Press: Cambridge, MA, USA, 1996; pp. 193–283.
22. Litvinov, V.P. The Chemistry of Thienopyrimidines. In *Advances in Heterocyclic Chemistry*; Alan, R.K., Ed.; Academic Press: Cambridge, MA, USA, 2006; pp. 83–143.
23. Dumaître, B.; Dodic, N. Synthesis and cyclic GMP phosphodiesterase inhibitory activity of a series of 6-phenylpyrazolo[3,4-d]pyrimidines. *J. Med. Chem.* **1996**, *39*, 1635–1644. [CrossRef] [PubMed]
24. El-Sherbeny, M.A.; El-Ashmawy, M.B.; El-Subbagh, H.I.; El-Emam, A.A.; Badria, F.A. Synthesis, antimicrobial and antiviral evaluation of certain thienopyrimidine derivatives. *Eur. J. Med. Chem.* **1995**, *30*, 445–449. [CrossRef]
25. Rizk, O.H.; Shaaban, O.G.; El-Ashmawy, I.M. Design, synthesis and biological evaluation of some novel thienopyrimidines and fused thienopyrimidines as anti-inflammatory agents. *Eur. J. Med. Chem.* **2012**, *55*, 85–93. [CrossRef] [PubMed]
26. Aly, H.M.; Saleh, N.M.; Elhady, H.A. Design and synthesis of some new thiophene, thienopyrimidine and thienothiadiazine derivatives of antipyrine as potential antimicrobial agents. *Eur. J. Med. Chem.* **2011**, *46*, 4566–4572. [CrossRef] [PubMed]
27. Elrazaz, E.Z.; Serya, R.A.T.; Ismail, N.S.M.; Abou El Ella, D.A.; Abouzid, K.A.M. Thieno[2,3-d]pyrimidine based derivatives as kinase inhibitors and anticancer agents. *Future Journal of Pharmaceutical Sciences* **2015**, *1*, 33–41. [CrossRef]
28. Munchhof, M.J.; Beebe, J.S.; Casavant, J.M.; Cooper, B.A.; Doty, J.L.; Higdon, R.C.; Hillerman, S.M.; Soderstrom, C.I.; Knauth, E.A.; Marx, M.A.; et al. Design and SAR of thienopyrimidine and thienopyridine inhibitors of VEGFR-2 kinase activity. *Bioorg. Med. Chem. Lett.* **2004**, *14*, 21–24. [CrossRef] [PubMed]
29. Le, B.T.; Kumarasiri, M.; Adams, J.R.; Yu, M.; Milne, R.; Sykes, M.J.; Wang, S. Targeting Pim kinases for cancer treatment: Opportunities and challenges. *Future Med. Chem.* **2015**, *7*, 35–53. [CrossRef]
30. Narlik-Grassow, M.; Blanco-Aparicio, C.; Carnero, A. The PIM family of serine/threonine kinases in cancer. *Med. Res. Rev.* **2014**, *34*, 136–159. [CrossRef]
31. Nawijn, M.C.; Alendar, A.; Berns, A. For better or for worse: The role of PIM oncogenes in tumorigenesis. *Nat. Rev. Cancer* **2011**, *11*, 23–34. [CrossRef]
32. Cuypers, H.T.; Selten, G.; Quint, W.; Zijlstra, M.; Maandag, E.R.; Boelens, W.; van Wezenbeek, P.; Melief, C.; Berns, A. Murine leukemia virus induced T-cell lymphomagenesis: Integration of proviruses in a distinct chromosomal region. *Cell* **1984**, *37*, 141–150. [CrossRef]
33. Tursynbay, Y.; Zhang, J.; Li, Z.; Tokay, T.; Zhumadilov, Z.; Wu, D.; Xie, Y. PIM-1 kinase as cancer drug target: An update (Review). *Biomed. Rep.* **2016**, *4*, 140–146. [CrossRef] [PubMed]
34. Keane, N.A.; Reidy, M.; Natoni, A.; Raab, M.S.; O'Dwyer, M. Targeting the PIM kinases in multiple myeloma. *Blood Cancer J.* **2015**, *5*, e325. [CrossRef] [PubMed]
35. Foulks, J.M.; Carpenter, K.J.; Luo, B.; Xu, Y.; Senina, A.; Nix, R.; Chan, A.; Clifford, A.; Wilkes, M.; Vollmer, D.; et al. A small-molecule inhibitor of pim kinases as a potential treatment for urothelial carcinomas. *Neoplasia* **2014**, *16*, 403–412. [CrossRef] [PubMed]
36. Decker, S.; Finter, J.; Forde, A.J.; Kissel, S.; Schwaller, J.; Mack, T.S.; Kuhn, A.; Gray, N.; Follo, M.; Jumaa, H.; et al. PIM kinases are essential for chronic lymphocytic leukemia cell survival (PIM2/3) and CXCR4-mediated microenvironmental interactions (PIM1). *Mol. Cancer* **2014**, *13*, 1231–1245. [CrossRef] [PubMed]
37. Lu, J.; Zavorotinskaya, T.; Dai, Y.; Niu, X.H.; Castillo, J.; Sim, J.; Yu, J.; Wang, Y.; Langowski, J.L.; Holash, J.; et al. PIM2 is required for maintaining multiple myeloma cell growth through modulating TSC2 phosphorylation. *Blood* **2013**, *122*, 1610–1620. [CrossRef] [PubMed]

38. Drygin, D.; Haddach, M.; Pierre, F.; Ryckman, D.M. Potential use of selective and nonselective pim kinase inhibitors for cancer therapy. *J. Med. Chem.* **2012**, *55*, 8199–8208. [CrossRef] [PubMed]
39. Guo, S.; Mao, X.; Chen, J.; Huang, B.; Jin, C.; Xu, Z.; Qiu, S. Overexpression of Pim-1 in bladder cancer. *J. Exp. Clin. Cancer Res.* **2010**, *29*, 161–167. [CrossRef] [PubMed]
40. Brault, L.; Gasser, C.; Bracher, F.; Huber, K.; Knapp, S.; Schwaller, J. PIM serine/threonine kinases in the pathogenesis and therapy of hematologic malignancies and solid cancers. *Haematologica* **2010**, *95*, 1004–1015. [CrossRef] [PubMed]
41. Elsayed, E.A.; Sharaf-Eldin, M.A.; Wadaan, M. In vitro evaluation of cytotoxic activities of essential oil from Moringa oleifera seeds on HeLa, HepG2, MCF-7, CACO-2 and L929 cell lines. *Asian Pac. J. Cancer Prev.* **2015**, *16*, 4671–4675. [CrossRef]
42. Elsayed, E.A.; Farooq, M.; Dailin, D.; El-Enshasy, H.A.; Othman, N.Z.; Malek, R.; Danial, E.; Wadaan, M. In vitro and in vivo biological screening of kefiran polysaccharide produced by lactobacillus kefiranofaciens. *Biomed. Res.* **2017**, *28*, 594–600.
43. Amr, A.E.; Elsayed, E.A.; Al-Omar, M.A.; Badr Eldin, H.O.; Nossier, E.S.; Abdallah, M.M. Design, synthesis, anticancer evaluation and molecular modeling of novel estrogen derivatives. *Molecules* **2019**, *24*, 416. [CrossRef]
44. Amr, A.E.; El-Naggar, M.; Al-Omar, M.A.; Elsayed, E.A.; Abdalla, M.M. In vitro and in vivo anti-breast cancer activities of some synthesized pyrazolinyl-estran-17-one candidates. *Molecules* **2018**, *23*, 1572. [CrossRef]
45. McCauley, J.; Zivanovic, A.; Skropeta, D. Bioassays for anticancer activities. *Methods Mol. Biol.* **2013**, *1055*, 191–205.
46. Wang, H.; Yu, D.; Agrawal, S.; Zhang, R. Experimental therapy of human prostate cancer by inhibiting MDM2 expression with novel mixed-backbone antisense oligonucleotides: In vitro and in vivo activities and mechanisms. *Prostate* **2003**, *54*, 194–205. [CrossRef]
47. Naguib, B.H.; El-Nassan, H.B.; Abdelghany, T.M. Synthesis of new pyridothieno- pyrimidinone derivatives as Pim-1 inhibitors. *J. Enzyme Inhibit. Med. Chem.* **2017**, *32*, 457–467. [CrossRef]

Sample Availability: Samples of the all compounds are available from the authors.

molecules

MDPI

Article

Cytotoxic Effects of Newly Synthesized Heterocyclic Candidates Containing Nicotinonitrile and Pyrazole Moieties on Hepatocellular and Cervical Carcinomas

Amira A. El-Sayed [1,*], Abd El-Galil E. Amr [2,3,*], Ahmed K. EL-Ziaty [1] and Elsayed A. Elsayed [4,5]

1 Laboratory of Synthetic Organic Chemistry, Chemistry Department, Faculty of Science, Ain Shams University, Abbassia, Cairo 11566, Egypt; ahm512@gmail.com
2 Pharmaceutical Chemistry Department, Drug Exploration & Development Chair (DEDC), College of Pharmacy, King Saud University, Riyadh 11451, Saudi Arabi
3 Applied Organic Chemistry Department, National Research Center, Cairo, Dokki 12622, Egypt
4 Zoology Department, Bioproducts Research Chair, Faculty of Science, King Saud University, Riyadh 11451, Saudi Arabiap; eaelsayed@ksu.edu.sa
5 Chemistry of Natural and Microbial Products Department, National Research Centre, Dokki 12622, Cairo, Egypt
* Correspondence: aamr@ksu.edu.sa (A.E.-G.E.A.); amira_aa47@hotmail.com (A.A.E.-S.); Tel.: +966-543074312 (A.E.-G.E.A.); +201-006532767 (A.A.E.-S.)

Academic Editor: Qiao-Hong Chen
Received: 28 April 2019; Accepted: 16 May 2019; Published: 22 May 2019

Abstract: In this study, a series of newly synthesized substituted pyridine **9, 11–18**, naphthpyridine derivative **10** and substituted pyrazolopyridines **19–23** by using cycnopyridone **8** as a starting material. Some of the synthesized candidates are evaluated as anticancer agents against different cancer cell lines. In vitro cytotoxic activities against hepatocellular and cervical carcinoma cell lines were evaluated using standard MTT assay. Different synthesized compounds exhibited potential in vitro cytotoxic activities against both HepG2 and HeLa cell lines. Furthermore, compared to standard positive control drugs, compounds **13** and **19** showed the most potent cytotoxic effect with IC_{50} values of 8.78 ± 0.7, 5.16 ± 0.4 μg/mL, and 15.32 ± 1.2 and 4.26 ± 0.3 μg/mL for HepG2 and HeLa cells, respectively.

Keywords: cyanopyridone; substituted pyridine; pyridotriazine; pyrazolopyridine; thioxotriazopyridine; anticancer activity; HepG2; HeLa

1. Introduction

Multicomponent reactions (MCR) "in which three or more starting materials react to form a product" play a significant role in the synthesis of heterocyclic compounds with pharmaceutical and chemical importance [1]. Several nicotinonitriles have been constructed via (MCR) and showed antitumor [2], antimicrobial [3], and antioxidant [4] activities. Also nicotinonitriles have been utilized as a scaffold for the synthesis of heterocyclic compounds containing a pyridine moiety with antimicrobial and antiviral activities [5]. A series of nicotinonitriles **1–3** (Figure 1) and have been synthesized and anti-proliferative [6], anti-Alzheimer's [7], and anti-inflammatory [8] activities.

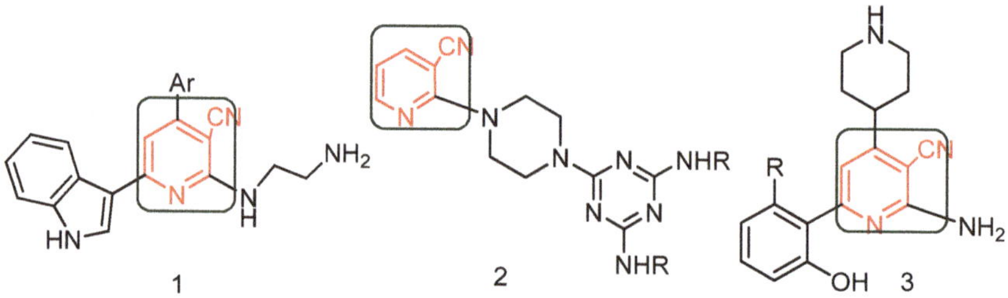

Figure 1. Nicotinonitriles with anti-proliferative, anti-Alzheimer's anti-inflammatory activities.

The pyrazole moiety is both pharmacologically and medicinally significant [9]. A series of pyrazoles **4–7** (Figure 2) has been reported as anti-inflammatory activity by Bekhit et al. [10], they observed that the synthesized pyrazoles showed more anti-inflammatory activity than the standard indomethacin [11]. Trisubstituted pyrazoles have been constructed by Christodoulou et al. (2010) [11] and evaluated as anti-angiogenic agents; these derivatives showed a potent anti-angiogenic efficacy and moreover inhibited the growth of Mammary gland breast cancer (MCF-7) and cervical carcinoma (Hela) [12]. Recently novel derivatives of pyrazoles **5,6** have been prepared as antimicrobial [13] and anticonvulsant [14] agents. The pyrazole **7** has been prepared by Bonesi et al. (2010) [15] and showed effective Angiotensin -1-Converting Enzyme (ACE) inhibitor activity [15].

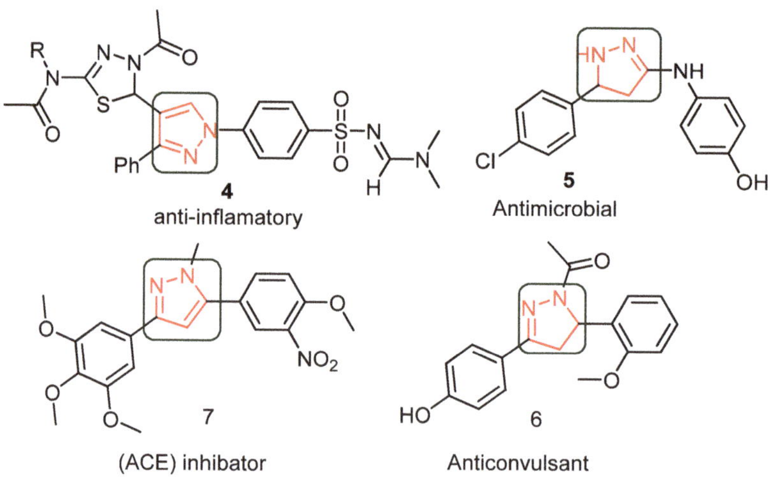

Figure 2. Pyrazoles as anti-inflammatory antimicrobial and anticonvulsant activities.

Based on the previous facts about the importance of pyrazoles and nicotinonitriles in medicinal chemistry, we have herein synthesized of some novel heterocyclic candidates containing nicotinonitrile and pyrazole moieties and tested their anticancer activity.

2. Results

2.1. Chemistry

The nicotinonitriles were obtained by two different ways, from the reaction of chalcone with ethylcyanoacetate, ammonium acetate and drops of piperidine as a base and from one pot four components reaction of methylketone, aldehyde, ethylcyanoacetate, ammonium acetate and drops of piperidine as a base [15]. In prolongation of our work in the synthesis of heterocyclic compounds and evaluation of their medicinal importance [16–27] and based on the literature survey about the pharmacological and medicinal importance of pyrazoles and nicotinonitriles, we have devoted our efforts to design and synthesize novel heterocyclic compounds containing pyrazol and nicotine-nitrile moieties, 4-(3-(4-fluorophenyl)-1-phenyl-1*H*-pyrazol-4-yl)-2-hydroxy-6-(naphthalen-1-yl)-nicotinenitrile **8** has been obtained by reacting of 1-acetylnaphthalene (**A**), 3-(4-fluorophenyl)-1-phenyl-1*H*-pyrazole-4-carbaldehyde (**B**), ethyl 2-cyanoacetate, ammonium acetate and piperidine (Scheme 1).

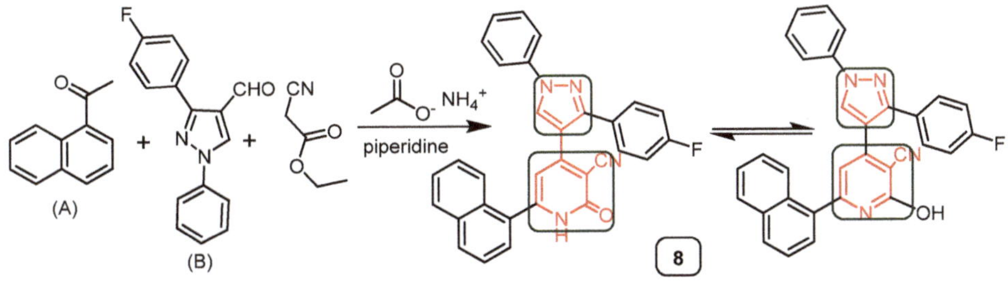

Scheme 1. Synthesis of compound **8** as starting material.

The structure of the nicotinonitrile **8** has been confirmed from its spectral data. IR spectrum showing absorption frequencies at ν 3159 cm^{-1}, 2220 cm^{-1} and ν 1647 cm^{-1} for OH, C≡N and C=N groups, respectively. Also, ^{1}H-NMR spectrum of the assigned compound displayed signals at δ 12.89 ppm (disappeared with D_2O) corresponding to acidic OH. A compelling evidence for the structure of **8** was provided by ^{13}C-NMR spectrum that showed a singlet signal at δ 149.8, 139.3 and 139.3 ppm for C-OH, C=N and C≡N groups respectively. Mass spectra of **8** showed [M^+] at *m*/*z* (%) 482 (22). Treatment of **8** with ethylchloroacetate afforded compound **9**, which was hydrazinolysis with NH_2NH_2 to give the corresponding cyclized product **10**.

Remediation of the nicotinonitrile derivative **8** with malononitrile in the presence of few drops of piperidine afforded 1,8-naphthyridine-3-carbonitrile derivative **11**. Chlorination of **8** by a mixture of ($POCl_3$/PCl_5) afforded 2-chloronicotinonitrile derivative **12**, which was reacted with malono nitrile as a carbon nucleophile gave the nicotinonitrile derivative **13**. Reaction of **12** with primary and secondary amines, namely, *o*-aminothiophenol, morpholine, 1-methylpiperazine and hydrazine hydrate gave novel nicotinonitriles **14**, **15a**, **b** and **16** (Scheme 2). The mechanism formation route of compound **11** has been shown in Figure 3.

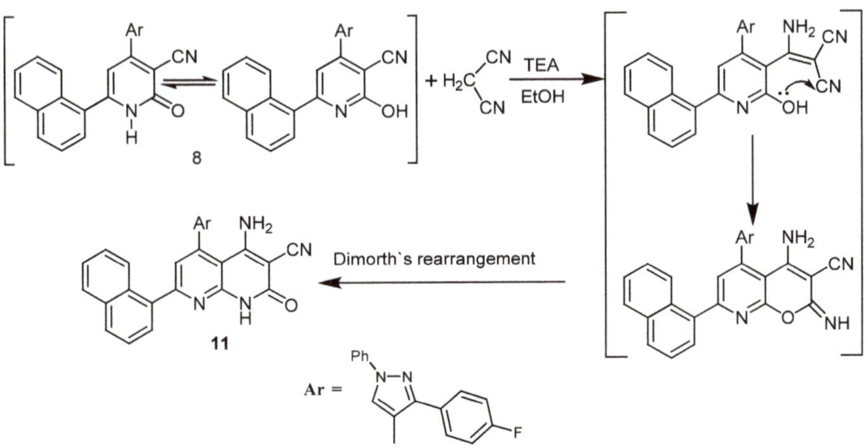

Figure 3. The mechanism formation route of compound **11**.

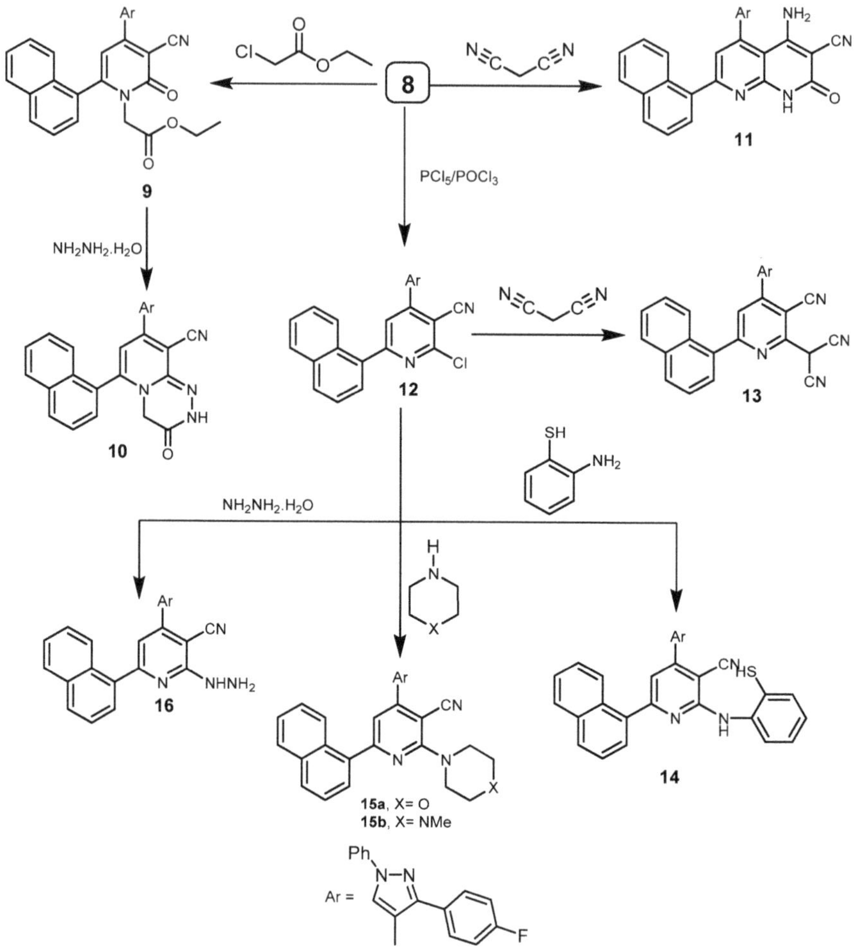

Scheme 2. Synthetic route for compounds **9–16**.

Compound **16** was utilized as a building block for novel nicotinonitriles containing two pyrazole moieties. 2-Pyrazolyl nicotinonitrile derivatives **17** and **18** were prepared by treatment of **16** with acetyl acetone and 4,4,4,-trifluoro-1-(thiophen-2-yl)butane-1,3-dione, respectively. Treatment of **16** with acetic anhydride and acetic acid afforded pyrazolopyridine derivative **19**. The derivative **16** was treated with acetic anhydride to afford the *N*-acetyl pyrazolopyridine as a sole product **20**. The structure of compound **20** was confirmed chemically by acetylation of the amino pyrazopyridine **19** (Scheme 3).

Treatment of **16** with 4-chlorobenzaldehyde and/or tetrachlorophthalic anhydride in the presence of acetic acid afforded the cyclized **19** followed by condensation to give the Schiff's base **21** and tetra chloroisoindoline **22**, respectively. The structures of **21** and **22** were confirmed chemically by condensation of compound **19** with 4-chlorobenzaldehyde and/or tetrachlorophthalic anhydride to provide compounds **21** and **22**, respectively. Treatment of hydrazinyl derivative **16** with CS_2 in the presence of alcoholic KOH provided thioxotriazolo pyridine derivative **23** (Scheme 3).

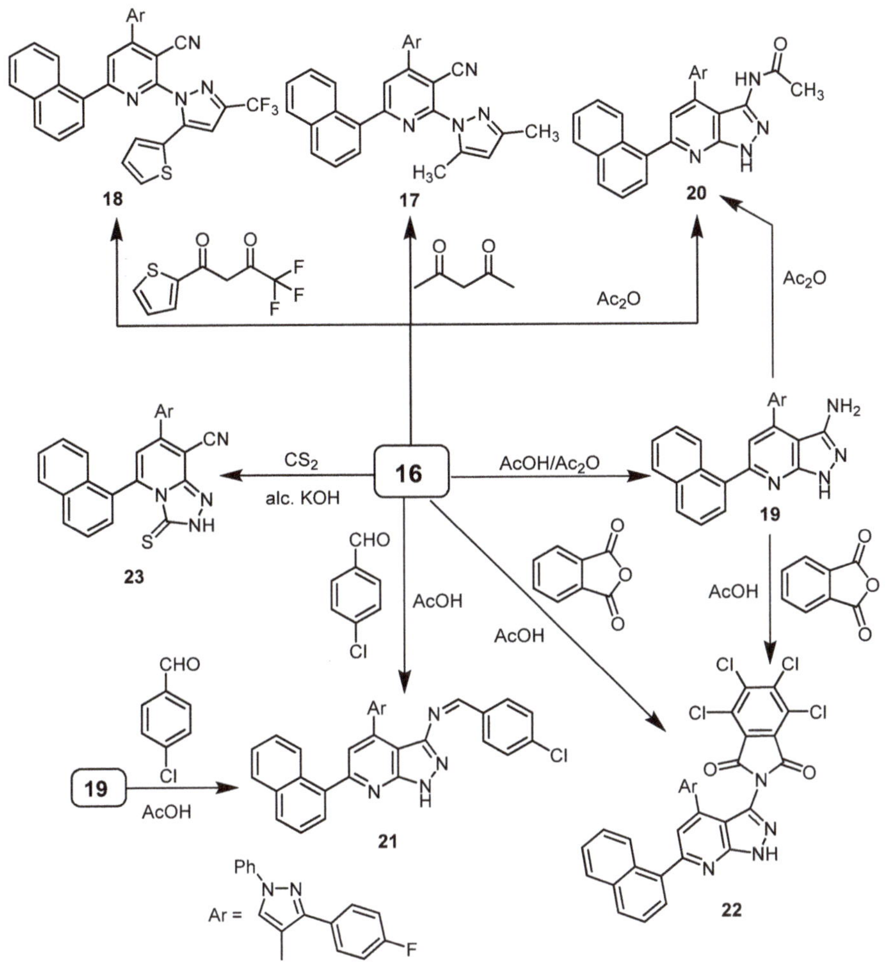

Scheme 3. Synthetic route for compounds **17–23**.

2.2. *Cytotoxic Activity*

The newly synthesized compounds were screened for their anticancer potentials against hepatocellular carcinoma HepG2 and cervical carcinoma HeLa. The cytotoxicity of the compounds was determined using MTT assay and DOX as a positive control [28–31].

The cytotoxic activities of the novel synthesized compounds **8–23** were estimated and the obtained results are presented in Figure 4. In general, it can be seen that all synthesized compounds exhibited cytotoxic activities against both tested cancer cell lines. Moreover, it can be seen that both cells reacted in a dose-dependent manner toward the applied concentrations. Additionally, both tested cell lines varied in their response toward different synthesized compounds. Furthermore, based on the IC_{50} values (Table 1) obtained for the tested compounds, it can be seen that cytotoxic activities ranged from very strong to non-cytotoxic. Compounds **13** and **19** exhibited the most potent cytotoxic effect (very strong activity) with IC_{50} 8.78 ± 0.7, 5.16 ± 0.4 µg/mL, and 15.32 ± 1.2 and 4.26 ± 0.3 µg/mL for HepG2 and HeLa cells, respectively. Furthermore, it can be noticed that **Cpd. 19** exhibited more or less stronger activity similar to DOX towards HepG2 cells, (IC_{50} 5.16 ± 0.4 and 4.50 ± 0.2 µg/mL, respectively). On the other hand, it was stronger by about 23.5% than DOX against HeLa cells (4.50 ±

0.2 and 5.57 ± 0.4 µg/mL, respectively). Additionally, **Cpd. 18** showed very strong activity towards HeLa cells with IC_{50}value of 7.67 ± 0.6 µg/mL, while it exhibited strong activity towards HepG2 cells (IC_{50} 16.70 ± 1.3 µg/mL). Moreover, **Cpd. 14** showed strong cytotoxic activities towards both tested cell lines (IC_{50}values 12.20 ± 1.0 and 19.44 ± 1.4 µg/mL for HepG2 and HeLa cells, respectively). Meanwhile, **Cpds. 16** and **22** showed moderate and strong activities towards both cell lines. **Cpd. 16** showed IC_{50}value of 33.45 ± 2.3 and 10.37 ± 0.9 µg/mL against HepG2 and HeLa cells, respectively. Also, **Cpd. 22** showed IC_{50} of 26.64 ± 1.9 and 9.33 ± 0.8 µg/mL for HepG2 and HeLa cells, respectively. On the other hand, **Cpd. 17** showed strong activity towards HepG2 cells (IC_{50} 20.00 ± 1.7 µg/mL) and moderate activity towards HeLa cells (IC_{50} 35.58 ± 2.6 µg/mL). Finally, **Cpds. 9, 10, 11, 12, 15a, b, 17, 20, 21** and **23** showed activities ranging from moderate to non-cytotoxic, with IC_{50} values ranging from 24.83 ± 1.8 to >100 µg/mL.

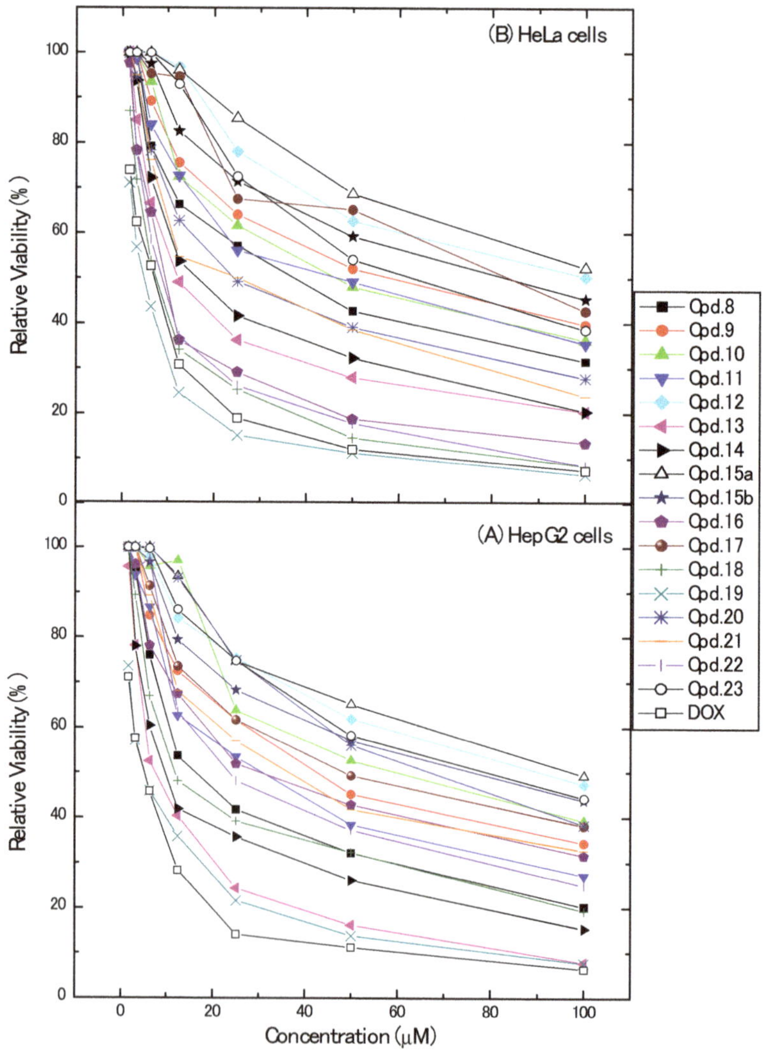

Figure 4. Relative viabilities of HepG2 and HeLa cells as affected by different synthesized compounds.

Table 1. IC_{50} values obtained for the tested compounds against both HepG2 and HeLa cell lines.

Compound	IC_{50} (μM) *	
	HepG2	HeLa
8	20.00 ± 1.7	35.58 ± 2.6
9	42.95 ± 3.2	55.00 ± 3.7
10	56.57 ± 3.4	47.02 ± 3.4
11	30.22 ± 2.1	43.64 ± 3.3
12	83.82 ± 4.5	89.72 ± 4.7
13	8.87 ± 0.70	15.32 ± 1.2
14	12.20 ± 1.0	19.44 ± 1.4
15a	90.05 ± 5.1	>100
15b	68.19 ± 3.7	75.05 ± 4.5
16	33.45 ± 2.3	10.37 ± 0.9
17	49.66 ± 3.2	65.91 ± 4.1
18	16.70 ± 1.3	7.67 ± 0.60
19	5.16 ± 0.40	4.26 ± 0.30
20	64.39 ± 3.6	28.15 ± 2.2
21	37.42 ± 2.5	24.83 ± 1.8
22	26.64 ± 1.9	9.33 ± 0.80
23	73.48 ± 4.0	62.07 ± 3.9
Doxorubicin	4.50 ± 0.20	5.57 ± 0.40

* IC_{50}: 1–10 is (very strong), 11–20 is (strong), 21–50 is (moderate), 51–100 is (weak) and above is 100 (non-cytotoxic).

3. Discussion

During current work, multi-component reaction strategy was used to synthesize of compound **8**, which was used as a building block for preparing **16** new derivatives. The cytotoxic potential of the new prepared compounds has been evaluated against HepG2 and HeLa cells. Results obtained showed potential cytotoxic activities against both cell lines. Compounds **13** and **19** showed the most cytotoxic effects (IC_{50} 8.78 ± 0.7 and 5.16 ± 0.4 μg/mL, for HepG2 cells, and 15.32 ± 1.2 and 4.26 ± 0.3 μg/mL for HeLa cells, respectively). Also, results showed that both tested cell lines varied in their response toward different synthesized compounds. This can be attributed to the inherent differences in both cell lines in terms of membrane structure and organization, hence different cell lines react differently towards different compounds [32–35].

Different activities of the prepared compounds may be attributed to the structure–activity relationship of these compounds. It can be seen that conversion of **Cpd. 12** to **13**, **14** and **16**, **18**, **19** and **22** altered the cytotoxicity from weak to moderate and strong activity towards two cell lines. This explained due to the introduction of two more nitrile groups, which significantly increased the activity. Compound **14** exhibited very strong activity due to the entity of the SH and NH groups, which may be added to any unsaturated group in DNA (thia or aza Michael addition) or the formation of hydrogen bonds with either one of the nucleo-bases of the DNA, thus causing DNA damage. Furthermore, the cytotoxicity of **Cpd. 16** may be due to the intermolecular hydrogen bonding of NH and NH_2 groups with DNA moieties. Additionally, conversion of **Cpd. 16** to **18**, **19** and **22** increased their cytotoxic activities against both cell lines. Introducing thiophene ring increases the cytotoxic effect of **Cpd. 18** beside the effect of the pyrazole ring and the trifluoromethyl group. Additionally, introducing pyrazole ring bearing NH_2 group to **Cpd. 16** increases the cytotoxic effect of **Cpd. 19** to very strong effect against both cell lines. The introduction of chloroiso- indoline-1,3-dione increases the cytotoxic effects of **Cpd. 22**. The chloro- group, with more electron withdrawing properties, may be the crucial for tumor cell inhibition beside the effect of the isoindoline-1,3-dioneas moderate cytokine inhibitor in cancer cells.

4. Materials and Methods

4.1. Chemistry

"Melting points reported are inaccurate. IR spectra were registered on Shimadzu FT-IR 8300 E (Shimadzu Corporation, Kyoto, Japan) spectrophotometer using the (KBr) disk technique. ^{1}H-NMR spectra were determined on a Varian Spectrophotometer at 400 MHz using (TMS) as an internal reference and DMSO-d_6 as solvent using (TMS) as internal standard. All chemical shifts (δ) are uttered in ppm. The mass spectra were determined using (MP) model MS-5988 and Shimadzu single focusing mass spectrophotometer (70 eV). Elemental analysis was investigated by Elemental analyzer Vario EL III".

4.1.1. Synthesis of 4-(3-(4-fluorophenyl)-1-phenyl-1*H*-pyrazol-4-yl)-2-hydroxy-6-(naphthalen-1-yl)-nicotinenitrile (**8**)

A mixture of 1-acetyl naphthalene (**A**) (1.7 g, 0.01 mol), ethyl cyanoacetate (1.3 g, 0.01 mol), aldehyde (**B**) (3.6 g, 0.01 mol), ammonium acetate (5.40 g, 0.07 mol) and three drops of piperidine in ethanol (20 mL) was heated under reflux for 3 h. The obtained precipitate was filtered off, washed with cold water, dried and crystallized from ethanol/dioxane to give compound **8**. Yield 75%, yellow powder, m.p. > 300 °C; IR (KBr): ν (cm^{-1}) 3159 (OH), 2220 (C≡N), 1647 (C=N); ^{1}H-NMR (DMSO-d_6): δ (ppm) 12.89 (s, 1H, OH, disappeared by D_2O), 9.80 (s, 1H, pyrazole-H), 8.39–7.78 (m, 7H, Ar-H for naphthalene), 7.75–7.37 (m, 10H, Ar-H). ^{13}C NMR (DMSO-d_6): δ (ppm) 149.8 (C-OH), 139.3 (C=N), 119.3 (C≡N), 139.4, 134.3, 133.8, 133.5, 131.6, 131.2, 131.0, 130.9, 130.4, 130.3, 130.2, 129.9, 129.4, 129.3, 129.2, 129.1, 128.9, 128.2, 127.8, 127.6, 127.0, 125.6, 125.1, 117.4, 114.8 (Ar-CH), 40.6, 39.9 (aliph-C); MS *m/z* (ESI): 482 [M$^+$] (22), 465 (21), 440 (12), 237 (100), 204; Anal. Calcd. for $C_{31}H_{19}FN_4O$ (482.50): C, 77.17; H, 3.97; N, 11.61. Found C, 76.98; H, 3.78; N, 11.52%.

4.1.2. Synthesis of ethyl 2-(3-cyano-4-(3-(4-fluorophenyl)-1-phenyl-1*H*-pyrazol-4-yl)-6-(naphthalene-1-yl)-2-oxopyridin-1(2*H*)-yl)acetate (**9**)

A mixture of **8** (4.84 g, 0.01 mol), ethylchloroacetate (1.22 g, 0.01 mol) and K_2CO_3 (2.2 g, 0.015 mol) in $(CH_3)_2O$ (40 mL) was heated under reflux for 24 h, concentrated and poured on water; the obtained precipitate was collected by filteration off, dried and crystallized from EtOH/dioxane to give **9**. Yield 74%, m.p. 158–160 °C; IR (KBr): ν (cm^{-1}) 2204 (C≡N), 1751 (C=O ester), 1651 (C=O pyridine); ^{1}H-NMR (DMSO-d_6): δ (ppm) 9.15 (s, 1H, pyrazole-5H), 8.10–7.49 (m, 7H, Ar-H for naphthalene), 7.48–7.33 (m, 10H, Ar-H), 4.16 (q, 2H, -CH_2 ester), 3.40 (s, 2H, -CH_2), 1.20 (t, 3H, -CH_3, ester); MS *m/z* (ESI): 568 [M$^+$] (2.5), 495 (65), 237 (80), 127 (100); Anal. Calcd. for $C_{35}H_{25}FN_4O_3$ (568.60): C, 73.93; H, 4.43, N, 9.85. Found C, 73.80; H, 4.21; N, 9.64%.

4.1.3. Synthesis of 8-(3-(4-fluorophenyl)-1-phenyl-1*H*-pyrazol-4-yl)-6-(naphthalen-1-yl)-3-oxo-3,4-dihydro-2*H*-pyrido[2,1-c][1,2,4]triazine-9-carbonitrile (**10**)

A mixture of **9** (5.7 g, 0.01 mol), $NH_2NH_2\eta H_2O$ (2 mL, 0.04 mol) and EtOH (20 mL) was heated under reflux for 3 h. The outward appearance solid was filtered off, dried and crystallized from EtOH/dioxane to give **10**. Yield 71%, yellow powder, m.p. > 300 °C; IR (KBr): ν (cm^{-1}) 3209 (NH), 2218 (C≡N), 1647 (C=O); ^{1}H-NMR (DMSO-d_6): δ (ppm) 12.38 (s, 1H, NH, disappeared in D_2O), 9.13 (s, 1H, pyrazole-5H), 8.87–7.65 (m, 7H, Ar-H for naphthalene), 7.63–6.85 (m, 10H, Ar-H), 6.10 (s, 2H, CH_2). ^{13}C-NMR (DMSO-d_6): δ (ppm) 165.8 (C=O), 139.7 (C=N), 136.1 (C=N), 133.8, 133.4, 131.7, 130.9, 130.8, 130.7, 130.6, 130.3, 130.2, 130.1, 129.9, 129.7, 129.2, 129.1, 128.8, 128.5, 128.1, 127.3, 126.8, 125.8, 125.6, 119.2, 119.1, 118.9, 118.5, 117.6 (Ar-CH), 119.3 (C≡N), 40.5, 39.9 (2CH), 17.6 (CH_2); MS *m/z* (ESI): 519 [M$^+$ − OH] (82), 393 (64), 284 (100), 237 (68), 127 (56); Anal. Calcd. for $C_{33}H_{21}FN_6O$ (536.50): C, 73.87; H, 3.94; N, 15.66. Found C, 73.68; H, 3.24; N, 15.06%.

4.1.4. Synthesis of 5-(3-(4-fluorophenyl)-1-phenyl-1*H*-pyrazol-4-yl)-7-(naphthalen-1-yl)-2-oxo-1,2-dihydro-1,8-naphthyridine-3-carbonitrile (**11**)

Refluxing of compound **8** (4.84 g, 0.01 mol) with malononitrile (0.015 mol) in ethanol (20 mL) in the presence of drops of TEA for 5 h, then cooled, poured on ice/water, neutralized with drops of conc. HCl. The obtained solid was collected by filtration, crystallized from EtOH/dioxane to afford **11**. Yield 71%, pale brown powder, m.p. > 300 °C; IR (KBr): ν (cm^{-1}) 3386, 3273 (NH_2), 3158 (NH), 2218 (C≡N), 1646 (C=O), ^{1}H-NMR (DMSO-d_6): δ (ppm) 12.89 (s, 1H, NH, disappeared by D_2O), 9.08 (s, 1H, pyrazole-5H), 8.07–7.61 (m, 7H, Ar-H for naphthalene), 7.60–7.37 (m, 10H, Ar-H), 6.22 (s, 2H, NH_2, disappeared in D_2O). ^{13}C-NMR (DMSO-d_6): δ (ppm) 149.9 (C=O), 139.3 (C=N), 133.8, 133.5, 131.2, 131.1, 131.00 (2), 130.9, 130.4, 130.3 (2), 130.2, 129.9 (2), 129.4, 129.1, 128.9 (2), 128.2, 127.8(2), 127.6, 127.1 (2), 125.6, 125.2 (2), 117.4, 116.8, 110.0 (Ar-CH), 119.3 (C≡N), 40.6, 39.9 (2CH); MS *m/z* (ESI): 532 [M^+ – NH_3] (82), 516 (76), 440 (28), 310 (20), 237 (100); Anal. Calcd. for $C_{34}H_{21}FN_6O$ (548.50): C, 74.44; H, 3.89; N, 15.32. Found C, 74.24; H, 3.25; N, 14.98%.

4.1.5. Synthesis of 2-chloro-4-(3-(4-fluorophenyl)-1-phenyl-1*H*-pyrazol-4-yl)-6-(naphthalen-1-yl)-nicotinenitrile (**12**)

A mixture of **8** (4.82 g, 0.01 mol), PCl_5 (3 g, 0.03 mol) and $POCl_3$ (5 mL, 0.03 mol) was heated under reflux for 8 h, then it was poured on crushed ice. The formed solid was filtered off, dried and crystallized from EtOH/dioxane to give **12**. Yield 61%, yellow powder, m.p. 164–166 °C; IR (KBr): ν (cm^{-1}) 2227 (C≡N), 1628 (C=N); ^{1}H-NMR (DMSO-d_6): δ (ppm) 9.16 (s, 1H, pyrazole-5H), 8.35–7.63 (m, 7H, Ar-H for naphthalene), 7.61–7.39 (m, 10H, Ar-H). ^{13}C-NMR (DMSO-d_6): δ (ppm) 152.7, 150.0, 148.4, 139.2 (C=N), 135.3(C=N), 133.8, 131.5, 131.0, 130.4, 130.3, 130.2, 129.8, 129.5, 129.2 (2), 129.1, 127.9, 127.6, 126.9, 125.8 (2), 125.4, 125.1, 119.3 (C≡N), 116.6, 115.5, 107.8 (Ar-CH), 40.6, 39.9 (2CH); MS *m/z* (ESI): 503 [M^+ + 2] (6), 501 [M^+] (50), 465 (100), 237 (82); Anal. Calcd. for $C_{31}H_{18}ClFN_4$ (500.90): C, 74.32; H, 3.62; N, 11.84. Found C, 74.12; H, 3.26; N, 11.42%.

4.1.6. Synthesis of 2-[4-(3-(4-fluorophenyl)-1-phenyl-1*H*-pyrazol-4-yl)-6-(naphthalen-1-yl)-3-cyano-pyridinyl]malononitrile (**13**)

To a solution of **12** (5.0 g, 0.01 mol) in EtOH (20 mL), malononitrile (0.01 mol) and TEA (1 mL) were added. The reaction mixture was heated under for 3 h. After cooling, it was poured on water and neutralized with diluted HCl. The obtained solid was separated by filtration, washed with water, dried and crystallized from EtOH/dioxane to yield **13**. Yield 76%, pale brown powder, m.p. 194–196 °C; IR (KBr): ν (cm^{-1}) 2203 (C≡N), ^{1}H-NMR (DMSO-d_6): δ (ppm) 9.15 (s, 1H, pyrazole-5H), 8.11–7.66 (m, 7H, Ar-H for naphthalene), 7.65–7.36 (m, 10H, Ar-H), 7.07 (s, 1H, CH of $CH(CN)_2$), MS *m/z* (ESI): 530 [M^+] (12), 440 (100), 237 (76), 204 (31); Anal. Calcd. for $C_{34}H_{19}FN_6$ (530.50): C, 76.97; H, 3.61; N, 15.84. Found C, 76.78; H, 3.42; N, 15.24%.

4.1.7. Synthesis of **14** and **15a,b**

A mixture of 2-chloronicotinonitrile **12** (5.0 g, 0.01 mol) and the appropriate amine, namely, o-aminothiophenol, morpholine or 2-methylpiperidine (0.01 mol) in EtOH (20 mL) was heated under reflux for 3 h, then it was poured on cold water, filtered off and crystallized from EtOH/dioxane to afford **14** and **15a,b**, respectively.

4-(3-(4-Fluorophenyl)-1-phenyl-1*H*-pyrazol-4-yl)-2-(2-mercaptophenylamino)-6-(naphthalen-1-yl) nicotinonitrile (**14**). Yield 74%, brown powder, m.p. 108–110 °C; IR (KBr): ν (cm^{-1}) 3330 (NH), 2208 (C≡N), ^{1}H-NMR (DMSO-d_6): δ (ppm) 9.29 (s, 1H, pyrazole-5H), 9.06–8.54 (m, 4H, Ar-H, thionyl-H), 8.26–7.66 (m, 7H, Ar-H for naphthalene), 7.60–6.66 (m, 10H, Ar-H), 3.34 (s, 1H, NH, disappeared in D2O), 1.20 (s, 1H, SH, disappeared in D_2O). MS *m/z* (ESI): 589 [M^+] (32), 465 (82), 441 (62), 237 (100), 127(12), 124 (20); Anal. Calcd. for $C_{37}H_{24}FN_5O$ (589.60): C, 75.36, H, 4.10; N, 11.88. Found C, 75.18; H, 4.05; N, 11.73%.

4-(3-(4-Fluorophenyl)-1-phenyl-1*H*-pyrazol-4-yl)-2-morpholino-6-(naphthalen-1-yl)nicotinonitrile (**15a**). Yield 65%, pale brown powder, m.p. 130–133 °C; IR (KBr): ν (cm^{-1}) 2226 (C≡N), ^{1}H-NMR (DMSO-d_6): δ (ppm) 9.16 (s, 1H, pyrazole-5H), 8.71–7.56 (m, 7H, Ar-H for naphthalene), 7.55–7.15 (m, 10H, Ar-H), 3.76 (t, 4H, *J* = 8.8 Hz), 3.05 (t, 4H, *J* = 8.8 Hz), MS *m/z* (ESI): 552 [M^+] (52), 465 (28), 237 (100), 230 (7), 127 (12), 87 (22); Anal. Calcd. for $C_{35}H_{26}FN_5O$ (551.60): C, 76.21; H, 4.75; N, 12.70. Found C, 75.98; H, 4.26; N, 12.31%.

4-(3-(4-Fluorophenyl)-1-phenyl-1*H*-pyrazol-4-yl)-2-(4-methylpiperazin-1-yl)-6-(naphthalen-1-yl) nicotinonitrile (**15b**). Yield 61%, brown powder, m.p. 156–158 °C; IR (KBr): ν (cm^{-1}) 2918 (aliph-H), 2227 (C≡N), ^{1}H-NMR (DMSO-d_6): δ (ppm) 9.18 (s, 1H, pyrazole-5H), 8.71–7.65 (m, 7H, Ar-H for naphthalene), 7.64–7.12 (m, 10H, Ar-H), 3.30–3.25 (m, 4H, $2CH_2$), 2.43–2.23 (m, 4H, $2CH_2$), 2.24 (s, 3H, CH_3), MS *m/z* (ESI): 564 [M^+] (27), 538 (25), 439 (12), 237 (100), 100 (23); Anal. Calcd. for $C_{35}H_{29}FN_6$ (564.60): C, 76.58, H, 5.18; N, 14.88. Found C, 75.98; H, 4.92; N, 14.72%.

4.1.8. Synthesis of 4-(3-(4-Fluorophenyl)-1-phenyl-1*H*-pyrazol-4-yl)-2-hydrazinyl-6-(naphthalen-1-yl) nicotinonitrile (**16**)

A mixture of the 2-chloronicotinonitrile **12** (5.0 g, 0.01 mol) and $NH_2NH_2{\cdot}H_2O$ (0.04 mol) in EtOH (20 mL) was heated under reflux for 4h. The obtained solid was collected by filtration, dried and crystallized from EtOH/dioxane to yield **16**. Yield 86%, yellow powder, m.p. 164–168 °C; IR (KBr): ν (cm^{-1}) 3417, 3310 (NH_2), 3199 (NH), 2206 (C≡N), ^{1}H-NMR (DMSO-d_6): δ (ppm) 9.16 (s, 1H, pyrazole-5H), 8.35–7.97 (m, 7H, Ar-H for naphthalene), 7.96–6.88 (m, 10H, Ar-H), 4.82 (s, 1H, NH, disappeared in D_2O), 3.43 (s, 2H, NH_2, disappeared in D_2O). ^{13}C-NMR (DMSO-d_6): δ (ppm) 149.3 (C-$NHNH_2$), 148.3, 139.7 (C≡N), 139.2, 138.5, 136.1 (C=N), 135.3, 134.0, 133.8, 131.7, 131.5, 131.0, 130.9, 130.4, 130.2, 130.1, 129.5, 129.1, 128.1, 127.9, 127.6, 127.3, 126.9, 126.7, 126.4, 125.8, 125.4, 119.3 (C≡N), 118.2 (Ar-CH), 40.6, 40.0 (2CH); MS *m/z* (ESI): 496 [M^+] (12), 465 (81), 440 (100), 237 (20), 204 (76); Anal. Calcd. for $C_{31}H_{21}FN_6$ (496.55): C, 74.99; H, 4.26; N, 16.93. Found C, 74.86; H, 4.12; N, 16.78%.

4.1.9. Synthesis of **17** and **18**

A mixture of **16** (4.9 g, 0.01 mol), acetylacetone or 4,4,4-trifluoro-1-(thiophen-2-yl)butane-1,3-dione (0.01 mol) in EtOH (10 mL) and AcOH (4 mL) was heated reflux for 3 h. After cooling, the solid obtained was filtered off, dried and crystallized from EtOH/dioxane to afford **17** and **18**, respectively.

2-(3,5-Dimethyl-1*H*-pyrazol-1-yl)-4-(3-(4-fluorophenyl)-1-phenyl-1*H*-pyrazol-4-yl)-6-(naphthalen-1-yl)nicotinonitrile (**17**). Yield 85%, pale orange powder, m.p. 270–272 °C; IR (KBr): ν (cm^{-1}) 2209 (C≡N), 1620 (C=N), ^{1}H-NMR (DMSO-d_6): δ (ppm) 9.24 (s, 1H, pyrazole-5H), 8.17–7.96 (m, 7H, Ar-H for naphthalene), 7.66–7.35 (m, 10H, Ar-H), 7.25 (s, 1H, pyrazole-4H), 2.48 (s, 6H, 2 CH_3); MS *m/z* (ESI): 560 [M^+] (13), 533 (26), 438 (62), 237 (15), 95 (100); Anal. Calcd. for $C_{36}H_{25}FN_6$ (560.60): C, 77.13; H, 4.49; N, 14.99. Found C, 76.92; H, 4.32; N, 14.81%.

4-(3-(4-Fluorophenyl)-1-phenyl-1*H*-pyrazol-4-yl)-6-(naphthalen-1-yl)-2-(5-(thiophen-2-yl)-3-(trifluoromethyl)-1*H*-pyrazol-1-yl)nicotinonitrile (**18**). Yield 82%, dark yellow powder, m.p. 117–119 °C; IR (KBr): ν (cm^{-1}) 2209 (C≡N), ^{1}H-NMR (DMSO-d_6): δ (ppm) 8.92 (s, 1H, pyrazole-5H), 8.03–7.89 (m, 7H, Ar-H for naphthalene), 7.59–7.54 (m, 3H, thionyl-H), 7.53–7.33 (m, 10H, Ar-H), 6.88 (s, 1H, pyrazole-4H); MS *m/z* (ESI): 583 [M^+] (10), 465 (72), 237 (100), 299 (8), 217 (5); Anal. Calcd. for $C_{39}H_{22}F_4N_6S$ (682.60): C, 68.61; H, 3.25; N, 12.31. Found C, 68.02; H, 3.12; N, 12.03%.

4.1.10. Synthesis of **19** and **20**

A solution of **16** (4.9 g, 0.01 mol) in a mixture of AcOH/Ac_2O (10 mL) or in glacial AcOH (10 mL) was refluxed for 2 h, poured on ice/water, filtered off and crystallized from EtOH/dioxane to give **19** and **20**, respectively. Also, refluxing of **19** (0.5 g, 0.01 mol) in acetic anhydride (7 mL) afforded compound **20**.

4-(3-(4-Flurophenyl)-1-phenyl-1*H*-pyrazol-4-yl)-6-(naphthalen-1-yl)-1*H*-pyrazolo[3,4-b]pyridin-3-amine (**19**). Yield 84%, pale yellow powder, m.p. 140–143 °C; IR (KBr): ν (cm^{-1}) 3425–3354 (NH_2),

3198 (NH), ^{1}H-NMR (DMSO-d_6): δ (ppm) 8.92 (s, 1H, pyrazole-5H), 8.22–7.90 (m, 7H, Ar-H for naphthalene), 7.66–7.34 (m, 10H, Ar–H), 5.02 (s, 2H, NH2, disappeared in D_2O), 4.63 (s, 1H, NH, disappeared in D_2O); MS *m/z* (ESI): 496 [M^+] (28), 479 (76), 244 (50), 237 (100); Anal. Calcd. for $C_{31}H_{21}FN_6$ (496.52): C, 74.99; H, 4.26; N, 16.93. Found C, 74.76; H, 4.15; N, 16.82%.

N-(4-(3-(4-Flurophenyl)-1-phenyl-1*H*-pyrazol-4-yl)-6-(naphthalen-1-yl)-1*H*-pyrazolo-[3,4-b] pyridin-3-yl)acetamide (**20**). Yield 78%, yellow powder, m.p. 138–140 °C; IR (KBr): ν (cm^{-1}) 3196 (NH), 1690 (C=O), ^{1}H-NMR (DMSO-d_6): δ (ppm) 12.37 & 10.31 (s, NH, OH), 8.88 (s, 1H, pyrazole- 5H), 7.98–7.59 (m, 7H, Ar-H for naphthalene), 7.57–6.88 (m, 10H, Ar-H), 4.82 (s, 1H, NH, disappeared in D_2O), 2.73 (s, 3H, acetyl); MS *m/z* (ESI): 538 [M^+] (20), 479 (36), 244 (20), 237 (100); Anal. Calcd. for $C_{33}H_{23}FN_6O$ (538.59): C, 73.59; H, 4.30; N, 15.60. Found C, 73.28; H, 4.19; N, 15.32%.

4.1.11. Synthesis of *N*-(4-chlorobenzylidene)-4-(3-(4-fluorophenyl)-1-phenyl-1*H*-pyrazol-4-yl)-6-(naphthalen-1-yl)-1*H*-pyrazolo[3,4-b]pyridine-3-amine (**21**)

A solution of **16** or **19** (0.01 mol) in AcOH (10 mL) in the presence of 4-chlorobenzaldehyde (0.01 mol) was heated under reflux for 2 h, left to precipitate, filtered and crystallized from EtOH/ dioxane to afford **21**. Yield 58%, yellow powder, m.p. 158–160 °C; IR (KBr): ν (cm^{-1}) 3192 (NH), ^{1}H-NMR (DMSO-d_6): δ (ppm) 9.89 (s, 1H, pyrazole-5H), 9.06 (s, 1H, N=C-H), 8.87–7.56 (m, 7H, Ar-H for naphthalene), 7.52–6.88 (m, 14H, Ar-H), 4.82 (s, 1H, NH, disappeared in D_2O); MS *m/z* (ESI): 621 [M^+] (15), 619 (48), 479 (20), 237 (80), 139 (35), 137 (100); Anal. Calcd. for $C_{38}H_{24}ClFN_6$ (619.10): C, 73.72; H, 3.91; N, 13.57. Found C, 73.25; H, 3.82; N, 13.27%.

4.1.12. Synthesis of 2-(4-(3-(4-fluorophenyl)-1-phenyl-1*H*-pyrazol-4-yl)-6-(naphthalen-1-yl)-1*H*-pyrazolo[3,4-b]-pyridin-3-yl)isoindoline-1,3-dione (**22**)

A mixture of **16** or **19** (0.01 mol) and tetrachlorophthalic anhydride (0.01 mol) in glacial acetic acid (10 mL) was refluxed for 1 h, poured on ice water, filtered off and crystallized from EtOH/dioxane to yield **22**. Yield 94%, yellow powder, m.p. 115–117 °C; IR (KBr): ν (cm^{-1}) 3196 (NH), 1785, 1731 (C=O); ^{1}H-NMR (DMSO-d_6): δ (ppm) 8.87 (s, 1H, pyrazole-5H), 8.04–7.56 (m, 7H, Ar-H for naphthalene), 7.55–7.33 (m, 10H, Ar-H), 4.28 (s, 1H, NH, disappeared in D_2O); Anal. Calcd. for $C_{39}H_{19}Cl_4FN_6O_2$ (764.42): C, 61.28; H, 2.51; N, 10.99. Found C, 61.00; H, 2.42; N, 10.89%.

4.1.13. Synthesis of 7-(3-(4-fluorophenyl)-1-phenyl-1*H*-pyrazol-4-yl)-5-(naphthalen-1-yl)-3-thioxo-2,3-dihydro[1,2,4]triazolo[4,3-a]pyridine-8-carbonitrile (**23**)

Solution of hydrazinyl derivative **16** (4.9 g, 0.01 mol) in alcoholic KOH (10%, 20 mL) and CS_2 (0.01 mol) was refluxed for 2 h, lift overnight, then poured on ice water, filtered off the solid obtained and crystallized from EtOH/dioxane to afford **23**. Yield 47% yellow powder, m.p. 288–290 °C; IR (KBr): ν (cm^{-1}) 3192 (NH), 2218 (C≡N), 1240 (C=S); ^{1}H-NMR (DMSO-d_6): δ (ppm) 8.73 (s, 1H, pyrazole-5H), 7.97–7.63 (m, 7H, Ar-H for naphthalene), 7.53–6.77 (m, 10H, Ar-H), 3.76 (s, 1H, NH, disappeared in D_2O). ^{13}C-NMR (DMSO-d_6): δ (ppm) 148.1 (C=S), 142.3, 138.7 (C=N), 133.8 (2), 133.4 (C=N), 131.7 (2), 131.2, 130.6 (2), 130.1, 129.9 (2), 129.4, 129.2 (2), 128.9, 128.4 (2), 126.9, 126.4 (2), 126.3 (2), 125.9 (2), 119.1 (C≡N), 110.0 (Ar-CH), 40.5, 39.9 (2CH); MS *m/z* (ESI): 538 [M^+] (45), 494 (18), 479 (10), 453 (50), 237 (100); Anal. Calcd. for $C_{32}H_{19}FN_6S$ (538.60): C, 71.36; H, 3.56; N, 15.60. Found C, 71.31; H, 3.52; N, 15.58%.

4.2. *Cytotoxicity Assay*

4.2.1. Materials and Cell Lines

Hepatocellular carcinoma (HepG2) and cervical Carcinoma (HeLa) cell lines, ATCC, VA, USA, were used throughout the work. All used chemicals and reagents were of high purity-cell culture grade.

4.2.2. MTT Assay

Cytotoxic assay depends on the formation of purple formazan crystals by the action of dehydrogenase in living cells. Cells were cultured in RPMI-1640 medium supplemented with 10% fetal bovine serum, antibiotic solution (100 units/mL penicillin, 100 μg/mL streptomycin) at 37 °C in a 5% CO2 incubator. Cells were seeded in a 96-well plate (10^4 cells/well), and the plates were incubated for 48 h. Afterwards, cells were exposed to variable concentrations of prepared derivatives and incubation proceeded for further 24 h. After treatment, 20 μL of MTT solution (5 mg/mL) was added and incubated for 4 h. DMSO (100 μL/well) is added and the developed color density was measured at 570 nm using a plate reader (ELx 800, BioTek, Winuski, VT, USA). Relative cell viability was calculated as (Atreated/Auntreated) ×100 [36,37]. Results were compared with doxorubicin as a positive control.

5. Conclusions

During the current investigation, we synthesized a new building block; namely 4-(3-(4-fluorophenyl)-1-phenyl-1*H*-pyrazol-4-yl)-2-hydroxy-6-(naphthalen-1-yl)nicotinonitril, with the help of multicomponent reaction systems. From that compound, a series of **16** different nicotinonitril derivatives were synthesized, and their structural and spectral data were elucidated. Furthermore, in vitro cytotoxic activities against hepatocellular and cervical carcinoma cell lines were investigated. Obtained results revealed that different synthesized compounds showed promising in vitro cytotoxic activities against both HepG2 and HeLa cell lines. Compounds **13** and **19** showed the most potent cytotoxic effect (IC_{50}: 8.78 ± 0.7, 5.16 ± 0.4 μg/mL, and 15.32 ± 1.2 and 4.26 ± 0.3 μg/mL for HepG2 and HeLa cells, respectively.

Author Contributions: The listed authors contributed to this work as described in the following: A.A.E.-S. and A.K.E.-Z. synthesis, and interpreted the spectroscopic identification of the synthesized compounds, A.E.-G.E.A. and E.A.E. are interpreted the results, the experimental part and E.A.E. performed the revision before submission. All authors read and approved the final manuscript.

Funding: The authors are grateful to the Deanship of Scientific Research, king Saud University for funding through Vice Deanship of Scientific Research Chairs.

Acknowledgments: The authors are appreciative to Faculty of Science, Ain Shams University where the experimental part carried out in its laboratories and Faculty of Pharmaceutical, El-Masoura University to carry the anticancer activity in it.

Conflicts of Interest: The authors declare no conflict of interest.

References

1. Rajeswari, M.; Saluja, P.; Khurana, J.M. A facile and green approach for the synthesis of spiro[naphthalene-2,50-pyrimidine]-4-carbonitrile via a one-pot three-component condensation reaction using DBU as a catalyst. *Rsc. Adv.* **2016**, *6*, 1307–1312. [CrossRef]
2. El-Sayed, H.A.; Moustafa, A.H.; Haikal, A.Z.; Abu-El-Halawa, R.; El Ashry, E.H. Synthesis, antitumor and antimicrobial activities of 4-(4-chlorophenyl)-3-cyano-2-(b-o-glycosyloxy)-6-(thien-2-yl)nicotine- nitrile. *Eur. J. Med. Chem.* **2011**, *46*, 2948–2954. [CrossRef]
3. Kotb, E.R.; El-Hashash, M.A.; Salama, M.A.; Kalf, H.S.; Abdel Wahed, N.A.M. Synthesis and reactions of some novel nicotinonitrile derivatives for anticancer and antimicrobial evaluation. *Acta Chim. Slov.* **2009**, *56*, 908–919.
4. Hamdy, N.A.; Anwar, M.M.; Abu-Zied, K.M.; Awad, H.M. Synthesis, tumor inhibitory and antioxidant activity of new polyfunctionally 2-substituted 5,6,7,8-tetrahydronaphthalene derivatives containing pyridine, thioxopyridine and pyrazolopyridine moieties. *Acta Polo. Pharm. Drug Res.* **2013**, *70*, 987–1001.
5. Salem, M.S.; Sakr, S.I.; El-Senousy, W.M.; Madkour, H.M.F.; El-Senousy, W.M. Synthesis, Antibacterial, and Antiviral Evaluation of New Heterocycles Containing the Pyridine Moiety. *Arch. der Pharm.* **2013**, *346*, 766–773. [CrossRef]

6. El-Sayed, N.S.; Shirazi, A.N.; El-Meligy, M.G.; El-Ziaty, A.K.; Rowley, D.; Sun, J.; Nagib, Z.A.; Parang, K. Synthesis of 4-aryl-6-indolylpyridine-3-carbonitriles and evaluation of their anti-proliferative activity. *Tetra. Lett.* **2014**, *55*, 1154–1158. [CrossRef]
7. Ruiz, J.F.M.; Kedziora, K.; Keogh, B.; Maguire, J.; Reilly, M.; Windle, H.; Kelleher, D.P.; Gilmer, J.F. A double prodrug system for colon targeting of benzenesulfonamide COX-2 inhibitors. *Bioorganic Med. Chem. Lett.* **2011**, *21*, 6636–6640. [CrossRef]
8. Balsamo, A.; Coletta, I.; Guglielmotti, A.; Landolfi, C.; Mancini, F.; Martinelli, A.; Milanese, C.; Minutolo, F.; Nencetti, S.; Orlandini, E.; et al. Synthesis of heteroaromatic analogues of (2-aryl-1-cyclopentenyl-1-alkylidene)-(arylmethyloxy)amine COX-2 inhibitors: effects on the inhibitory activity of the replacement of the cyclopentene central core with pyrazole, thiophene or isoxazole ring. *Eur. J. Med. Chem.* **2003**, *38*, 157–168. [CrossRef]
9. Karrouchi, K.; Radi, S.; Ramli, Y.; Taoufik, J.; Mabkhot, Y.N.; Al-Aizari, F.A.; Al-Aizari, F.; Ansar, M.; A Al-Aizari, F.; Ansar, M. Synthesis and Pharmacological Activities of Pyrazole Derivatives: A Review. *Molecules* **2018**, *23*, 134. [CrossRef]
10. Bekhit, A.A.; Ashour, H.M.; Ghany, Y.S.A.; Bekhit, A.E.-D.A.; Baraka, A. Synthesis and biological evaluation of some thiazolyl and thiadiazolyl derivatives of 1H-pyrazole as anti-inflammatory antimicrobial agents. *Eur. J. Med. Chem.* **2008**, *43*, 456–463. [CrossRef]
11. Christodoulou, M.S.; Liekens, S.; Kasiotis, K.M.; Haroutounian, S.A. Novel pyrazole derivatives: Synthesis and evaluation of anti-angiogenic activity. *Bioorganic Med. Chem.* **2010**, *18*, 4338–4350. [CrossRef]
12. Bondock, S.; Fadaly, W.; Metwally, M.A. Synthesis and antimicrobial activity of some new thiazole, thiophene and pyrazole derivatives containing benzothiazole moiety. *Eur. J. Med. Chem.* **2010**, *45*, 3692–3701. [CrossRef] [PubMed]
13. Chimenti, F.; Bolasco, A.; Manna, F.; Secci, D.; Chimenti, P.; Befani, O.; Turini, P.; Giovannini, V.; Mondovi, B.; Cirilli, R.; et al. Synthesis and Selective Inhibitory Activity of 1-Acetyl-3,5-diphenyl-4,5-dihydro-(1H)-pyrazole Derivatives against Monoamine Oxidase. *J. Med. Chem.* **2004**, *47*, 2071–2074. [CrossRef]
14. Rashad, A.E.; Hegab, M.I.; Abdel-Megeid, R.E.; Micky, J.A.; Abdel-Megeid, F.M. Synthesis and antiviral evaluation of some new pyrazole and fused pyrazolopyrimidine derivatives. *Bioorganic Med. Chem.* **2008**, *16*, 7102–7106. [CrossRef]
15. Bonesi, M.; Loizzo, M.R.; Statti, G.A.; Michel, S.; Tillequin, F.; Menichini, F. The synthesis and Angiotensin Converting Enzyme (ACE) inhibitory activity of chalcones and their pyrazole derivatives. *Bioorganic Med. Chem. Lett.* **2010**, *20*, 1990–1993. [CrossRef]
16. Mahmoud, M.R.; El-Ziaty, A.K.; Abu El-Azm, F.S.M.; Ismail, M.F.; Shiba, S.A. Utility of Cyano-N-(2-oxo-1,2-dihydroindol-3-ylidene)acetohydrazide in the Synthesis of Novel Heterocycles. *J. Chem.* **2013**, *37*, 80–85. [CrossRef]
17. El-Sayed, N.S.; Shirazi, A.N.; El-Meligy, M.G.; El-Ziaty, A.K.; Nagieb, Z.A.; Parang, K.; Tiwari, R.K. Design, synthesis, and evaluation of chitosan conjugated GGRGDSK peptides as a cancer cell-targeting molecular transporter. *Int. J. Boil. Macromol.* **2016**, *87*, 611–622. [CrossRef]
18. El-Ziaty, A.K.; Shiba, S.A. Antibacterial activities of new (E) 2-cyano-3-(3,4-dimethoxyphenyl) -2-propenoylamide derivatives. *Synth. Commun.* **2007**, *37*, 4043–4057. [CrossRef]
19. Mahmoud, M.R.; Shiba, S.A.; El-Ziaty, A.K.; Abu El-Azm, F.S.M.; Ismail, M.F. Synthesis and reactions of novel 2,5-disubistituted 1,3,4-thiadiazoles. *Synth. Commun.* **2014**, *44*, 1094–1102. [CrossRef]
20. El-Shahawi, M.M.; El-Ziaty, A.K. Enaminonitrile as Building Block in Heterocyclic Synthesis: Synthesis of Novel 4H -Furo[2,3-d][1,3]oxazin-4-one and Furo[2,3- d]pyrimidin-4 (3H) -one Derivatives. *J. Chem.* **2017**, *2017*, 1–6. [CrossRef]
21. Mahmoud, M.R.; El-Ziaty, A.K.; Hussein, A.M. Synthesis and Spectral Characterization of Novel Thiazolopyridine and Pyrimidine Derivatives. *Synth. Commun.* **2013**, *43*, 961–978. [CrossRef]
22. Ismail, M.F.; El-Sayed, A.A. Synthesis and in-vitro antioxidant and antitumor evaluation of novel pyrazole-based heterocycles. *Iran. Chem. Soc.* **2019**, *16*, 921–937. [CrossRef]
23. Fahmy, A.F.M.; Rizk, S.A.; Hemdan, M.M.; El-Sayed, A.A.; Hassaballah, A.I. Efficient Green Synthesis and Computational Chemical Study of Some Interesting Heterocyclic Derivatives as Insecticidal Agents. *J. Chem.* **2018**, *55*, 2545–2555. [CrossRef]
24. Rizk, S.A.; El-Sayed, A.A.; Mounier, M.M.; El-Sayed, A.A. Synthesis of Novel Pyrazole Derivatives as Antineoplastic Agent. *J. Chem.* **2017**, *54*, 3358–3371. [CrossRef]

25. Fahmy, A.F.M.; El-Sayed, A.A.; Hemdan, M.M. Multicomponent synthesis of 4-arylidene-2-phenyl-5(4H)-oxazolones (azlactones) using a mechanochemical approach. *Chem. Central J.* **2016**, *10*, 59. [CrossRef]
26. Hemdan, M.M.; El-Sayed, A.A. Use of phthalimidoacetylisothiocyanate as a scaffold in synthesis of target heterocyclic systems with their antimicrobial assessment. *Chem. Pharm. Bull.* **2016**, *64*, 483–489. [CrossRef]
27. Hemdan, M.M.; El-Sayed, A.A. Synthesis of some new heterocycles derived from novel 2-(1,3-dioxisoindolin-2-yl)benzoyl isothiocyanate. *J. Heterocycl. Chem.* **2016**, *53*, 487–492. [CrossRef]
28. Metwally, M.; Gouda, M.; Harmal, A.N.; Khalil, A. Synthesis, antitumor, cytotoxic and antioxidant evaluation of some new pyrazolotriazines attached to antipyrine moiety. *Eur. J. Med. Chem.* **2012**, *56*, 254–262. [CrossRef] [PubMed]
29. Hossan, A.; Abu-Melha, H. Synthesis, mass spectroscopic studies, cytotoxicity evaluation and quantitative structure activity relationship of novel isoindolin-1,3-dione derivatives. *Chem. Process Eng. Res.* **2014**, *21*, 60–71.
30. Eissa, I.H.; El-Naggar, A.M.; El-Hashash, M.A. Design, synthesis, molecular modeling and biological evaluation of novel 1H-pyrazolo[3,4-b]pyridine derivatives as potential anticancer agents. *Bioorganic Chem.* **2016**, *67*, 43–56. [CrossRef]
31. Shaaban, S.; Negm, A.; Sobh, M.A.; Wessjohann, L.A. Organoselenocyanates and symmetrical diselenides redox modulators: Design, synthesis and biological evaluation. *Eur. J. Med. Chem.* **2015**, *97*, 190–201. [CrossRef]
32. Elsayed, E.A.; Farooq, M.; Dailin, D.; El-Enshasy, H.A.; Othman, N.Z.; Malek, R.; Danial, E.; Wadaan, M. In vitro and in vivo biological screening of kefiran polysaccharide produced by Lactobacillus kefiranofaciens. *Biomed. Res.* **2017**, *28*, 594–600.
33. Amr, A.E.-G.E.; El-Naggar, M.; Al-Omar, M.A.; Elsayed, E.A.; Abdalla, M.M. In Vitro and In Vivo Anti-Breast Cancer Activities of Some Synthesized Pyrazolinyl-estran-17-one Candidates. *Molecules* **2018**, *23*, 1572. [CrossRef]
34. Amr, A.E.-G.E.; Abo-Ghalia, M.H.; Moustafa, G.O.; Al-Omar, M.A.; Nossier, E.S.; Elsayed, E.A. Design, Synthesis and Docking Studies of Novel Macrocyclic Pentapeptides as Anticancer Multi-Targeted Kinase Inhibitors. *Molecules* **2018**, *23*, 2416. [CrossRef]
35. Dailin, D.J.; Elsayed, E.A.; Othman, N.Z.; Malek, R.; Phin, H.S.; Aziz, R.; Wadaan, M.; El Enshasy, H.A. Bioprocess development for kefiran production by *Lactobacillus kefiranofaciens* in semi industrial scale bioreactor. *Saudi J. Biol. Sci.* **2016**, *23*, 495–502. [CrossRef]
36. Mosmann, T. Rapid colorimetric assay for cellular growth and survival: Application to proliferation and cytotoxicity assays. *J. Immunol. Methods* **1983**, *65*, 55–63. [CrossRef]
37. Denizot, F.; Lang, R. Rapid colorimetric assay for cell growth and survival. Modifications to the tetrazolium dye procedure giving improved sensitivity and reliability. *J. Immunol. Methods* **1986**, *89*, 271–277. [CrossRef]

Sample Availability: Samples of the compounds are available from the authors.

molecules

MDPI

Article

Design, Synthesis and Biological Evaluation of a New Series of 1-Aryl-3-{4-[(pyridin-2-ylmethyl)thio]phenyl}urea Derivatives as Antiproliferative Agents

Chuanming Zhang [1], Xiaoyu Tan [1], Jian Feng [1], Ning Ding [1], Yongpeng Li [1], Zhe Jin [1], Qingguo Meng [2], Xiaoping Liu [1,*] and Chun Hu [1,*]

[1] Key Laboratory of Structure-Based Drug Design & Discovery, Ministry of Education, Shenyang Pharmaceutical University, Shenyang 110016, China; chuanming_zhang@yeah.net (C.Z.); tanxiaoyuaikaoyan@163.com (X.T.); mr.fengjian@foxmail.com (J.F.); dingning2216@163.com (N.D.); yongpengli1993@163.com (Y.L.); jinzheln@163.com (Z.J.)

[2] Department of Pharmacy, Yantai University, Yantai 264005, China; qinggmeng@163.com

[*] Correspondence: lxp19730107@163.com (X.L.); chunhu@syphu.edu.cn (C.H.); Tel.: +86-24-43520246 (X.L. & C.H.)

Academic Editor: Qiao-Hong Chen
Received: 30 April 2019; Accepted: 30 May 2019; Published: 4 June 2019

Abstract: To discover new antiproliferative agents with high efficacy and selectivity, a new series of 1-aryl-3-{4-[(pyridin-2-ylmethyl)thio]phenyl}urea derivatives (**7a–7t**) were designed, synthesized and evaluated for their antiproliferative activity against A549, HCT-116 and PC-3 cancer cell lines in vitro. Most of the target compounds demonstrated significant antiproliferative effects on all the selective cancer cell lines. Among them, the target compound, 1-[4-chloro-3-(trifluoromethyl)phenyl]-3-{4-{{[3-methyl-4-(2,2,2-trifluoroethoxy)pyridin-2-yl]methyl}thio}phenyl}urea (**7i**) was identified to be the most active one against three cell lines, which was more potent than the positive control with an IC_{50} value of 1.53 ± 0.46, 1.11 ± 0.34 and 1.98 ± 1.27 μM, respectively. Further cellular mechanism studies confirmed that compound **7i** could induce the apoptosis of A549 cells in a concentration-dependent manner and elucidated compound **7i** arrests cell cycle at G1 phase by flow cytometry analysis. Herein, the studies suggested that the 1-aryl-3-{4-[(pyridin-2-ylmethyl)thio]phenyl}urea skeleton might be regarded as new chemotypes for designing effective antiproliferative agents.

Keywords: antiproliferative agent; urea; synthesis; antiproliferative activity; apoptosis

1. Introduction

Cancer is a major public health problem in developed countries and will become the most serious life-threatening disease worldwide in the near future [1]. Some advances in cancer treatment by molecule-targeted drugs, such as imatinib, gefitinib, and trastuzumab, were expected to improve cancer cure rates and also to reduce severe adverse reactions because of the high specificity of the targeted molecules, which are expressed and have critical roles in cancer cells, but not in normal cells. However, the clinical effect was found to be limited and did not last for a long time period because of the acquired resistance of the tumor cells. Furthermore, these molecules often cause on-target and/or off-target severe toxicity [2]. Therefore, the development of more target-specific therapy, with minimum toxicity, is warranted to extend disease-free survival and improve the quality of life of cancer patients.

In recent years, proton pump inhibitors (PPIs) as potential anticancer agents were intensively studied in cancer treatment. Lugini et al. compared the anti-tumor efficacy of different PPIs, including omeprazole, esomeprazole, lansoprazole, rabeprazole and pantoprazole in vitro and in vivo. The result indicated that all the PPIs have shown different degrees of antitumor efficacy and lansoprazole showed a higher anti-tumor effect when compared to the other PPIs. [3]. Recently, the research by Zeng and Zheng et al. indicated that T-cell originated protein kinase (TOPK) activities were inhibited by pantoprazole and ilaprazole with high affinity and selectivity [4,5]. TOPK (also known as PBK or PDZ-binding kinase) was first reported by Abe et al. in 2000 [6], and it is a Ser/Thr protein kinase overexpressed in hematologic tumors, breast cancer, melanoma, colorectal cancer, prostate cancer, cervical cancer, bladder cancer and lung cancer [7–14]. The results of their studies demonstrated that pantoprazole can suppress the growth of colorectal cancer cells as a TOPK inhibitor both in vitro and in vivo, and also showed that the TOPK activities were inhibited by ilaprazole in HCT-116, ES-2, A549, SW1990 cancer cells in vitro [4,5]. As shown in Figure 1, all of the PPIs molecules contain thiomethylpyridine fragments. It can be predicted that these fragments should play an important role in the antiproliferative activity of proton pump inhibitors.

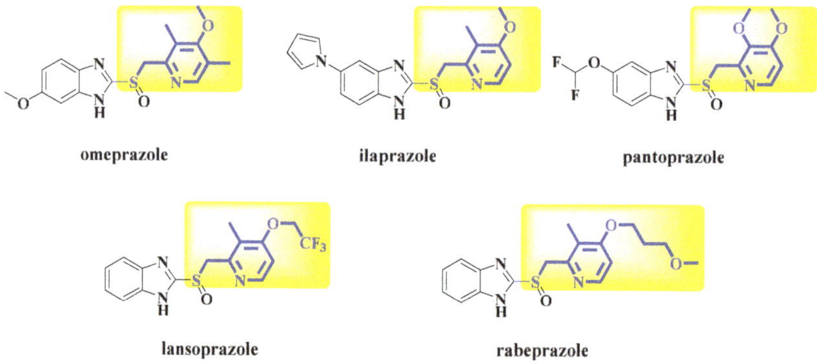

Figure 1. Chemical structures of proton pump inhibitors (PPIs).

As known, the diaryl urea is a fragment of great importance in medicinal chemistry and can be used for the synthesis of numerous heterocyclic compounds with diversified biological activities, including antithrombotic [15], antimalarial [16], antibacterial [17,18] and anti-inflammatory [19] properties, and it is characterized by its ability to form hydrogen bond interactions with drug targets [20–22]. The carbonyl oxygen atom acts as a proton acceptor while the two amide nitrogen atoms are proton donors (Figure 2). This unique type of structure endows urea derivatives with the ability to bind a variety of enzymes and receptors in the biological systems. Remarkably, the diaryl urea moiety is widely used in the design of anticancer drugs, such as sorafenib, regorafenib, linifanib and tivozanib (Figure 3).

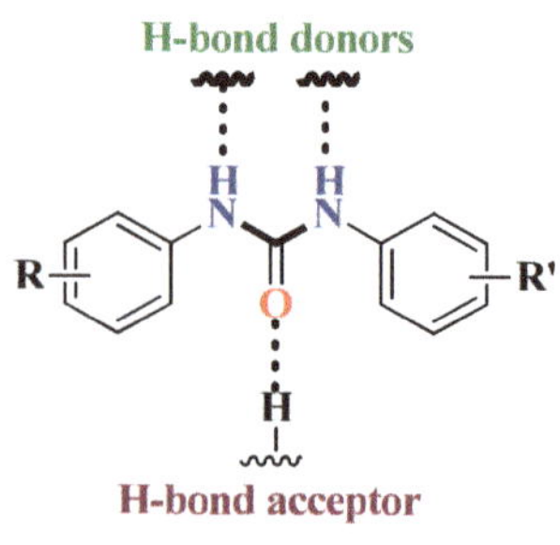

Figure 2. H-bond acceptor and donors within the diaryl urea scaffold.

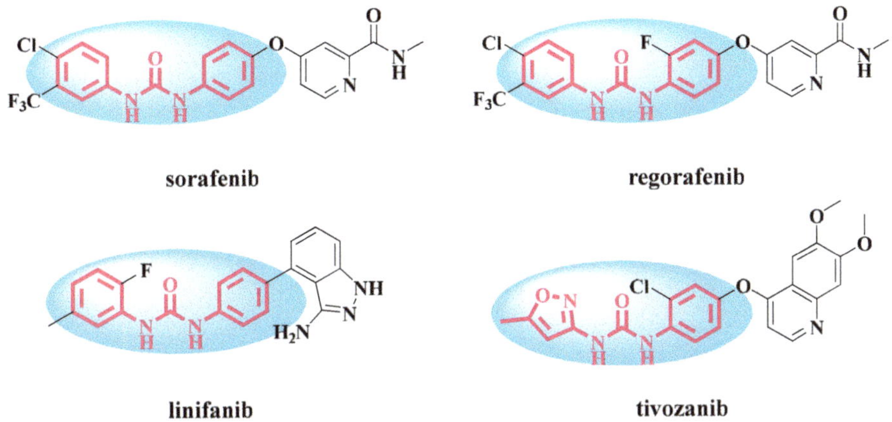

Figure 3. Some anticancer drugs of the diaryl urea moiety.

Molecular hybridization strategy is a useful concept in drug design and development based on the combination of pharmacophoric moieties of different bioactive substances to produce a new structure, the affinity and efficacy would be improved, when compared to the parent drugs [23]. These above interesting findings and our continuous quest to identify more potent antiproliferative agents led to the molecular hybridization of diaryl urea and thiomethylpyridine to integrate them in one molecular platform to generate a new hybrid, as shown in Figure 4, and expected that taking this way could get the antiproliferative agents with highly inhibitory activity.

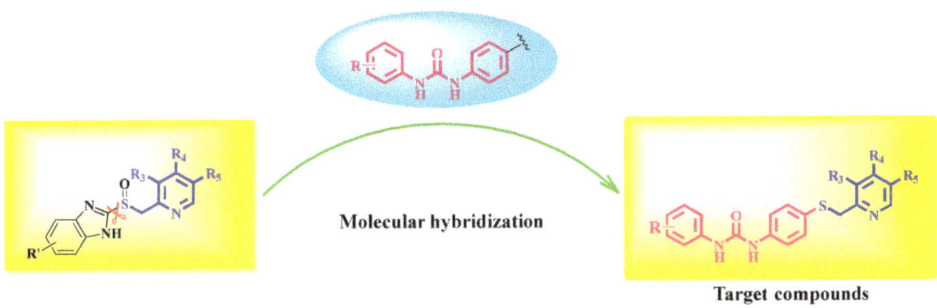

Figure 4. Rational design of the target compounds based on molecular hybridization strategy.

2. Results and Discussion

2.1. Chemistry

The general synthetic route is illustrated in Scheme 1. The reaction of the commercially available 4-nitrobenzenethiol (**1**) with 2-(chloromethyl)pyridine derivatives (**2**) in ethanol at r.t. (room temperature) obtained compounds **3a–3d** [24], which converted to key intermediates **4a–4d** via Pd-C catalytic hydrogenation reduction [25]. The aryl isocyanates **6a–6e** were prepared by reaction between aromatic amines and bis(trichloromethyl)carbonate (BTC) [26]. Finally, treatment of **4a–4d** with aryl isocyanates **6a–6e** in methylene dichloride yielded 1-aryl-3-{4-[(pyridin-2-ylmethyl)thio]phenyl}urea derivatives (**7a–7t**) as the target compounds [26]. The structures of the target compounds were characterized by infraredspectra (IR), proton nuclear magnetic resonance spectra (^{1}H-NMR), carbon nuclear magnetic resonance spectra (^{13}C-NMR), electrospray ionization mass spectra (ESI-MS) and high-resolution mass spectra (HRMS).

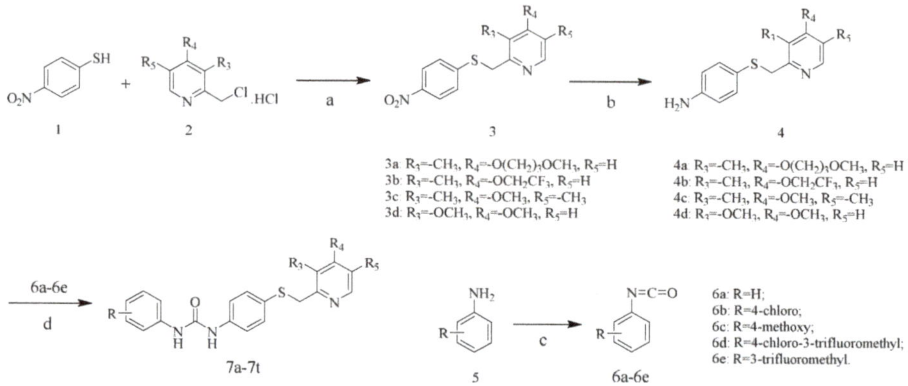

Scheme 1. Synthetic route of the target compounds **7a–7t.** Reagents and conditions: (a) NaOH (aq. 2M), EtOH, r.t.; (b) H_2, 1 atm, 10% Pd-C, MeOH, r.t.; (c) BTC, Et_3N, CH_2Cl_2, r.t.; (d) intermediate **4**, aryl isocyanates **6a–6e**, CH_2Cl_2, r.t.

2.2. *Biological Evaluation*

2.2.1. Antiproliferative Activity

Using sorafenib as a positive control, all of the target compounds were evaluated for the antiproliferative activity in vitro against cancer cell lines, including A549 (lung cancer), HCT-116 (colorectal cancer), and PC-3 (prostate cancer) cell lines by MTT assay. The antiproliferative assay results evaluated as IC_{50} value (Table 1) and demonstrated that several target compounds have shown moderate to excellent potency against A549, HCT-116, and PC-3 cancer cell lines. Among the target compounds**7i** showed the more potent inhibitory effect against three cancer cell lines than positive control with IC_{50} values of 1.53 ± 0.46, 1.11 ± 0.34 and 1.98 ± 1.27 μM, respectively.

All the target compounds could be divided into four classes according to different substituents on the pyridine ring (Figure 5). The analyses of the structure-activity relationships (SARs) were summarized as follows: (1) The results of cytostatic activity assay showed that the substitutions of the 4 (R_4) and 5 (R_5) positions of the C ring had a weak effect on the inhibitory activity. However, if the 3-position (R_3) hydrogen atom of the C ring was substituted by a methoxy group, the inhibitory activity was significantly decreased. At the same time, it could be seen that the inhibitory activity was better than other classes when the 4-position (R_4) of the C ring was occupied by the trifluoroethoxy group. (2) The substituents on the A ring had a significant effect on the inhibitory activity of each class. When the substituents on C ring were the same, if there was no substituent on A ring, the inhibitory activity was worst in each class, such as compound **7a**, **7f**, **7k** and **7p**. Moreover, when the substituents in A ring were electron-withdrawing groups, such as 4-Cl or 3-CF_3, the inhibitory activity was better than that substitution of the electron-donating groups, such as 4-OCH_3 in each class. Furthermore, when the two electron-withdrawing groups coexist on the A ring, the target compounds displayed the strongest inhibitory activity, such as compound **7d**, **7i**, **7n** and **7s**.

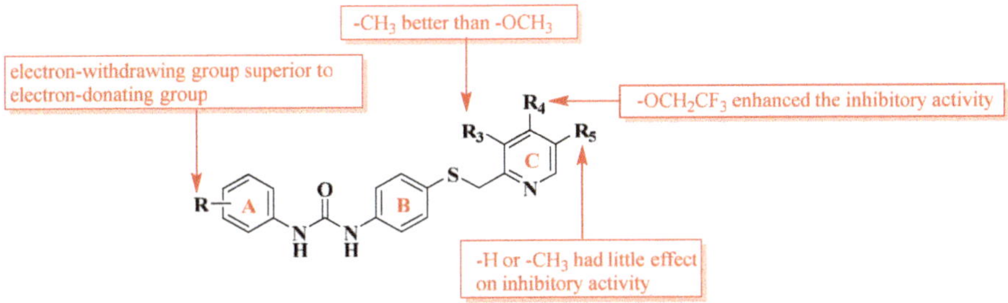

Figure 5. SARs summary for the target compounds.

Table 1. The chemical structures and inhibitory activities of the target compounds.

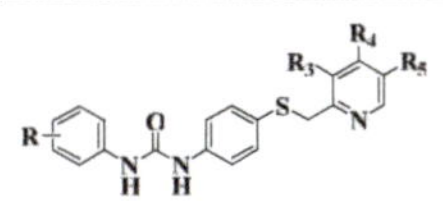

7a–7t

Compound	R	R_3	R_4	R_5	IC_{50} (μM) [a]		
					A549	HCT-116	PC-3
7a	H	$-CH_3$	$-O(CH_2)_3OCH_3$	H	12.31 ± 1.90	29.26 ± 4.53	27.22 ± 3.36
7b	4-chloro	$-CH_3$	$-O(CH_2)_3OCH_3$	H	3.03 ± 2.79	4.80 ± 1.57	6.00 ± 0.22
7c	4-methoxy	$-CH_3$	$-O(CH_2)_3OCH_3$	H	6.35 ± 0.51	5.29 ± 0.22	6.95 ± 1.24
7d	4-chloro-3-trifluoromethyl	$-CH_3$	$-O(CH_2)_3OCH_3$	H	2.02 ± 2.20	1.94 ± 3.45	3.97 ± 1.02
7e	3-trifluoromethyl	$-CH_3$	$-O(CH_2)_3OCH_3$	H	2.90 ± 0.36	3.78 ± 1.41	11.48 ± 0.98
7f	H	$-CH_3$	$-OCH_2CF_3$	H	14.29 ± 1.77	19.31 ± 3.64	20.40 ± 2.89
7g	4-chloro	$-CH_3$	$-OCH_2CF_3$	H	2.23 ± 1.27	3.04 ± 0.37	6.78 ± 0.23
7h	4-methoxy	$-CH_3$	$-OCH_2CF_3$	H	4.71 ± 0.11	12.09 ± 1.46	15.65 ± 0.69
7i	4-chloro-3-trifluoromethyl	$-CH_3$	$-OCH_2CF_3$	H	1.53 ± 0.46	1.11 ± 0.34	1.98 ± 1.27
7j	3-trifluoromethyl	$-CH_3$	$-OCH_2CF_3$	H	4.22 ± 0.99	10.69 ± 0.87	14.33 ± 3.24
7k	H	$-CH_3$	$-OCH_3$	$-CH_3$	13.37 ± 0.81	>100	>100
7l	4-chloro	$-CH_3$	$-OCH_3$	$-CH_3$	2.23 ± 1.38	3.20 ± 2.75	5.97 ± 0.55
7m	4-methoxy	$-CH_3$	$-OCH_3$	$-CH_3$	5.27 ± 1.01	3.49 ± 0.78	6.95 ± 0.35
7n	4-chloro-3-trifluoromethyl	$-CH_3$	$-OCH_3$	$-CH_3$	2.63 ± 1.25	2.51 ± 0.15	6.32 ± 1.68
7o	3-trifluoromethyl	$-CH_3$	$-OCH_3$	$-CH_3$	4.88 ± 1.02	3.50 ± 0.13	7.18 ± 1.58
7p	H	$-OCH_3$	$-OCH_3$	H	26.98 ± 4.12	45.93 ± 6.65	30.95 ± 5.41
7q	4-chloro	$-OCH_3$	$-OCH_3$	H	14.52 ± 2.67	5.15 ± 1.01	18.57 ± 2.34
7r	4-methoxy	$-OCH_3$	$-OCH_3$	H	16.47 ± 4.51	33.10 ± 2.90	22.51 ± 3.07
7s	4-chloro-3-trifluoromethyl	$-OCH_3$	$-OCH_3$	H	6.23 ± 0.60	5.61 ± 0.66	10.05 ± 2.23
7t	3-trifluoromethyl	$-OCH_3$	$-OCH_3$	H	14.13 ± 1.82	17.37 ± 1.69	19.77 ± 0.74
sorafenib					2.12 ± 0.18	2.25 ± 0.71	3.60 ± 1.08

[a] Inhibitory activity was assayed by exposure for 72 h to substance and expressed as the concentration required to inhibit tumor cell proliferation by 50% (IC_{50}). Data are presented as the means ± SEMs of three independent experiments.

2.2.2. Cell Apoptosis Assay

The acceptable antiproliferative activity of compound **7i** promoted us to investigate its effect on cell apoptosis. To explore the effect of compound **7i** on cell apoptosis, the apoptotic analysis was performed with Annexin V-FITC/PI double staining and analyzed with flow-cytometry calculation. Treatment of A549 cells with compound **7i** resulted in a concentration-dependent apoptosis increase, as shown in Figure 6. Specifically, the percentage of early/primary apoptotic cells was about 4.33% for the low concentration (1 μM) of compound **7i**. When treated with high concentration (10 μM) of compound **7i**, around 29.47% of early/primary apoptosis rate was observed. While the late apoptosis rate of A549 cells was not changed significantly with increasing concentrations.

2.2.3. Cell Cycle Analysis

The effect of compound **7i** on the cell cycle was also evaluated. After treatment of A549 cells with compound **7i** for 24 h at indicated concentrations (1, 5, 10 μM), the percentage of cells in G1 phase were 60.77%, 78.05% and 90.65%, respectively (Figure 7), suggesting that compound **7i** caused an obvious

G1 arrest in a concentration-dependent manner with a concomitant decrease in terms of the number of cells in other phases of the cell cycle.

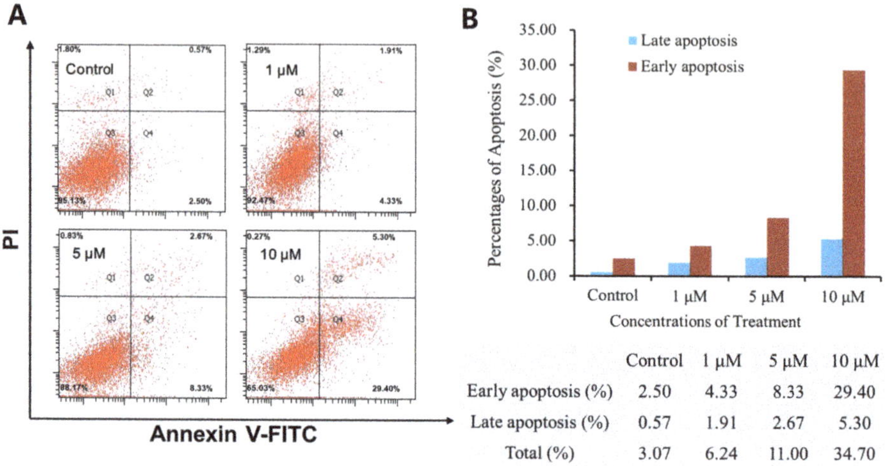

	Control	1 μM	5 μM	10 μM
Early apoptosis (%)	2.50	4.33	8.33	29.40
Late apoptosis (%)	0.57	1.91	2.67	5.30
Total (%)	3.07	6.24	11.00	34.70

Figure 6. Compound **7i** induced apoptosis of A549 cells. (**A**) Apoptosis effect on A549 cell line induced by compound **7i** for 24 h using Annexin V-FITC/PI double staining and flow-cytometry calculation. The lower left quadrant represents live cells, the lower right is for early/primary apoptotic cells, upper right is for late/secondary apoptotic cells, and the upper left represents cells damaged during the procedure; (**B**) Quantitative analysis of apoptotic cells. The experiments were performed three times, and a representative experiment is shown.

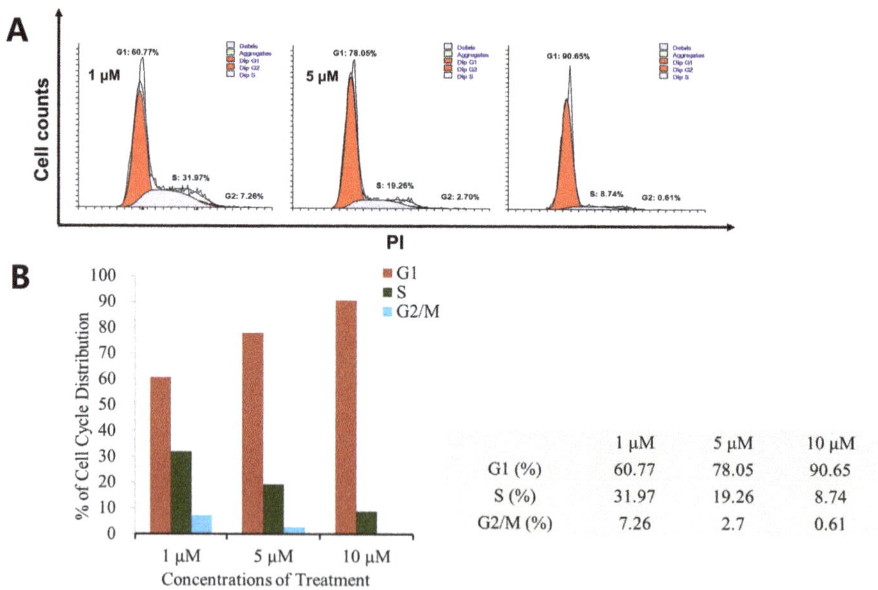

	1 μM	5 μM	10 μM
G1 (%)	60.77	78.05	90.65
S (%)	31.97	19.26	8.74
G2/M (%)	7.26	2.7	0.61

Figure 7. Effects of compound **7i** on A549 cell cycle progress for 24 h. (**A**) Treatment of A549 cells with compound **7i** at different concentrations (1 μM, 5 μM, 10 μM) for 24 h. (**B**) Quantitative analysis of cell cycle. The experiments were performed three times, and a representative experiment is shown.

3. Materials and Methods

3.1. Synthesis

All reagents were obtained from commercial suppliers and used without further purification. Reaction progress was monitored by thin layer chromatography (TLC) on silica gel plates. The spots were visualized by ultraviolet (UV) light (254 nm). The column chromatography was performed using 200–300 mesh silica gel (Qingdao PUKE, Qingdao, China). Melting points were obtained by X-5 micro-melting point apparatus (Beijing Zhongyi Boteng Technology Co., Ltd., Beijing, China) and were uncorrected. ^{1}H-NMR and ^{13}C-NMR spectra were recorded on Bruker NMR spectrophotometers (Karlsruhe, Germany) using DMSO-d_6 as the solvent and TMS as the internal standard. Mass spectra were measured with an electrospray (ESI-MS) on a Waters spectrometer (Waters Corporation, Milford, MA, USA). High resolution mass spectrometry (HRMS) analyses were performed on an Agilent Technologies 6530 Accurate-Mass Q-TOF Mass Spectrometer (Santa Clara, CA, USA). The purities were determined by high-performance liquid chromatography (HPLC) using an Agilent 1100 series HPLC (Santa Clara, CA, USA).

The original figures of ^{1}H-NMR, ^{13}C-NMR, MS and HRMS of all the target compounds as the Supplementary Materials are available online.

3.1.1. General Procedure for the Preparation of 2-{[(4-nitrophenyl)thio]methyl}pyridine Derivatives (**3a–3d**)

4-Nitrobenzenethiol **1** (1.55 g, 0.01 mol), and 2-(chloromethyl)pyridine hydrochloride derivatives **2** (0.01 mol) were dissolved in EtOH (100 mL), then aqueous NaOH (2M) was added dropwise. After the addition completed, the solution was stirred for 8 h at room temperature. Upon completion, the excess ethanol was evaporated to give the residue. A large number of white solids have been precipitated when 200 mL of water was added. The Precipitate was filtered off and washed with water to obtain the intermediates (**3a–3d**), which was used for next step without further purification.

4-(3-Methoxypropoxy)-3-methyl-2-{[(4-nitrophenyl)thio]methyl}pyridine (**3a**) by using compound **1** (1.55 g, 0.01 mol) and 2-(chloromethyl)-4-(3-methoxypropoxy)-3-methylpyridine hydrochloride (2.66 g, 0.01 mol), obtained a yellow solid (3.12 g) in 89.7% yield. ESI-MS (*m/z*): 349.3 ([M + H]$^+$).

3-Methyl-2-{[(4-nitrophenyl)thio]methyl}-4-(2,2,2-trifluoroethoxy)pyridine (**3b**) by using compound **1** (1.55 g, 0.01 mol) and 2-(chloromethyl)-3-methyl-4-(2,2,2-trifluoroethoxy)pyridine hydrochloride (2.76 g, 0.01 mol), obtained a yellow solid (3.26 g) in 91.2% yield. ESI-MS (*m/z*): 359.1 ([M + H]$^+$).

4-Methoxy-3,5-dimethyl-2-{[(4-nitrophenyl)thio]methyl}pyridine (**3c**) by using compound **1** (1.55 g, 0.01 mol) and 2-(chloromethyl)-4-methoxy-3,5-dimethylpyridine hydrochloride (2.22 g, 0.01 mol), obtained a yellow solid (2.69 g) in 88.5% yield. ESI-MS (*m/z*): 305.0 ([M + H]$^+$).

3,4-Dimethoxy-2-{[(4-nitrophenyl)thio]methyl}pyridine (**3d**) by using compound **1** (1.55 g, 0.01 mol) and 2-(chloromethyl)-3,4-dimethoxypyridine hydrochloride (2.24 g, 0.01 mol), obtained a yellow solid (2.86 g) in 93.5% yield. ESI-MS (*m/z*): 307.4 ([M + H]$^+$).

3.1.2. General Procedure for the Preparation of 4-{[(pyridin-2-yl)methyl]thio}aniline Derivatives (**4a–4d**)

A mixture of **3a–3d** (5 mmol) and 0.1 g of preequilibrated 10% palladium/carbon in MeOH (50 mL) was hydrogenated at room temperature and atmospheric pressure. The reaction was completely monitored by TLC. When the reaction has completed, the mixture was filtered, and the filtrate was evaporated to yield intermediate (**4a–4d**) as yellowish oil, which was used for the next step without further purification.

4-{{[4-(3-Methoxypropoxy)-3-methylpyridin-2-yl]methyl}thio}aniline (**4a**) by using compound **3a** (1.74 g, 5 mmol), H_2 and 10% Pd-C, obtained a yellowish oil (1.52 g) in 95.4% yield. ESI-MS (*m/z*): 319.3 ([M + H]$^+$).

4-{{[3-Methyl-4-(2,2,2-trifluoroethoxy)pyridin-2-yl]methyl}thio}aniline (**4b**) by using compound **3b** (1.79 g, 5 mmol), H_2 and 10% Pd-C, obtained a yellowish oil (1.58 g) in 96.1% yield. ESI-MS (*m/z*): 329.6 ([M + H]$^+$).

4-{[(4-Methoxy-3,5-dimethylpyridin-2-yl)methyl]thio}aniline (**4c**) by using compound **3c** (1.52 g, 5 mmol), H_2 and 10% Pd-C, obtained a yellowish oil (1.30 g) in 94.8% yield. ESI-MS (*m/z*): 275.2 ([M + H]$^+$).

4-{[(3,4-Dimethoxypyridin-2-yl)methyl]thio}aniline (**4d**) by using compound **3d** (1.53 g, 5 mmol), H_2 and 10% Pd-C, obtained a yellowish oil (1.30 g) in 94.2% yield. ESI-MS (*m/z*): 276.1 ([M + H]$^+$).

3.1.3. General Procedure for the Preparation of the Target Compounds (**7a–7t**)

To a solution of BTC (1 mmol) in CH_2Cl_2 (20 mL) was added dropwise to primary aromatic amine **5** (1 mmol) in CH_2Cl_2 (20 mL) followed by the dropwise addition of triethylamine (1 mL) in CH_2Cl_2 (10 mL). The solvent was evaporated. The resulting residue was dissolved in CH_2Cl_2 (20 mL), and intermediates (**4a–4d**) (1 mmol) in CH_2Cl_2 (10 mL) was added dropwise. The mixture was stirred for about 3 h, monitored by TLC. After the reaction completed, the solvent was washed with water and brine, then dried over anhydrous magnesium sulfate. The mixture was filtered, the filtrate was evaporated and purified by silica gel chromatography (CH_2Cl_2/MeOH = 60/1, *v/v*) to obtain target compounds.

1-{4-{{[4-(3-Methoxypropoxy)-3-methylpyridin-2-yl]methyl}thio}phenyl}-3-phenylurea (**7a**)

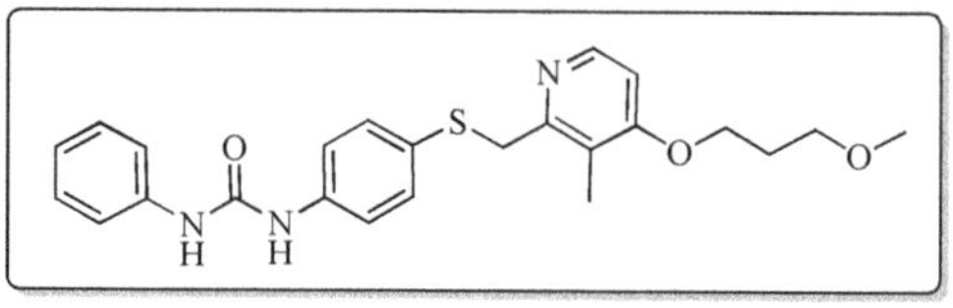

Compound **7a** was prepared according to the general procedure by using compound **4a** (0.32 g, 1 mmol) and aniline (0.10 g, 1 mmol), obtained a white solid (0.20 g) in 45.1% yield. m.p. 105.2–106.8 °C. IR (KBr, cm^{-1}): υ 3421.1, 2922.7, 2852.4, 1596.1, 1545.1, 1492.4, 1460.8, 1440.3, 1398.2, 1385.2, 1309.3, 1231.3, 1174.2, 1092.1, 1006.7, 894.6, 832.0, 799.2, 751.9, 693.4, 617.3, 507.5. ^{1}H-NMR (400 MHz, DMSO-d_6) δ 8.74 (s, 1H), 8.69 (s, 1H), 8.17 (d, *J* = 5.6 Hz, 1H), 7.46 (s, 1H), 7.44 (s, 1H), 7.41 (s, 1H), 7.39 (s, 1H), 7.32 (s, 1H), 7.31-7.29 (m, 1H), 7.28 (s, 1H), 7.26 (s, 1H), 6.97 (t, *J* = 7.3 Hz, 1H), 6.90 (d, *J* = 5.7 Hz, 1H), 4.22 (s, 2H), 4.09 (t, *J* = 6.2 Hz, 2H), 3.48 (t, *J* = 6.2 Hz, 2H), 3.25 (s, 3H), 2.12 (s, 3H), 2.02–1.94 (m, 2H). ^{13}C-NMR (101 MHz, DMSO-d_6) δ 163.17, 156.31, 152.87, 147.91, 140.07, 131.77, 129.23, 128.07, 122.34, 120.30, 119.09, 118.69, 106.49, 68.79, 65.48, 58.44, 31.14, 29.16, 10.88. ESI-MS (*m/z*): 438.4 ([M + H]$^+$), 460.2 ([M + Na]$^+$). HRMS (ESI) (*m/z*): Calcd. for $C_{24}H_{27}N_3O_3S$, 438.1846 ([M + H]$^+$), found: 438.1856 ([M + H]$^+$). Purity (HPLC): 99.27%.

1-(4-Chlorophenyl)-3-{4-{{[4-(3-methoxypropoxy)-3-methylpyridin-2-yl]methyl}thio}phenyl}urea (**7b**)

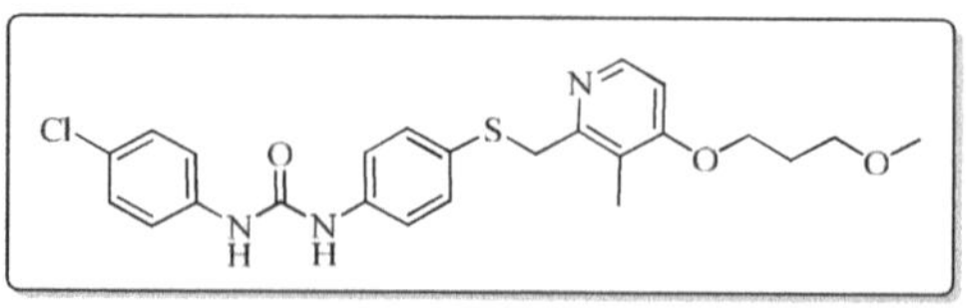

Compound **7b** was prepared according to the general procedure by using compound **4a** (0.32 g, 1 mmol) and 4-chloroaniline (0.13 g, 1 mmol), obtained a white solid (0.36 g) in 75.3% yield. m.p. 191.7–192.5 °C.

IR (KBr, cm^{-1}): υ 3428.1, 2923.1, 2852.9, 1631.8, 1490.8, 1398.9, 1384.8, 1298.9, 1273.5, 1237.0, 1174.2, 1121.4, 1086.2, 1008.0, 881.2, 832.1, 702.8, 619.7, 506.0. ^{1}H-NMR (400 MHz, DMSO-d_6) δ 8.83 (s, 1H), 8.77 (s, 1H), 8.17 (d, *J* = 5.6 Hz, 1H), 7.49 (d, *J* = 2.2 Hz, 1H), 7.47 (d, *J* = 2.1 Hz, 1H), 7.40 (d, *J* = 2.0 Hz, 1H), 7.39 (d, *J* = 2.1 Hz, 1H), 7.34 (s, 1H), 7.33 (s, 1H), 7.32 (d, *J* = 2.1 Hz, 1H), 7.31 (s, 1H), 6.90 (d, *J* = 5.7 Hz, 1H), 4.22 (s, 2H), 4.08 (t, *J* = 6.2 Hz, 2H), 3.48 (t, *J* = 6.2 Hz, 2H), 3.25 (s, 3H), 2.12 (s, 3H), 2.00–1.94 (m, 2H). ^{13}C-NMR (101 MHz, DMSO-d_6) δ 163.09, 156.35, 152.77, 147.99, 139.09, 138.88, 131.62, 129.07, 128.41, 125.86, 120.22, 119.24, 106.47, 68.80, 65.45, 58.43, 31.14, 29.16, 10.89. ESI-MS (*m/z*): 473.3 ([M + H]$^+$), 495.2 ([M + Na]$^+$). HRMS (ESI) (*m/z*): Calcd. for $C_{24}H_{26}ClN_3O_3S$, 472.1456 ([M + H]$^+$), found: 472.1467 ([M + H]$^+$). Purity (HPLC): 98.66%.

1-(4-Methoxyphenyl)-3-{4-{{[4-(3-methoxypropoxy)-3-methylpyridin-2-yl]methyl}thio}phenyl}urea (**7c**)

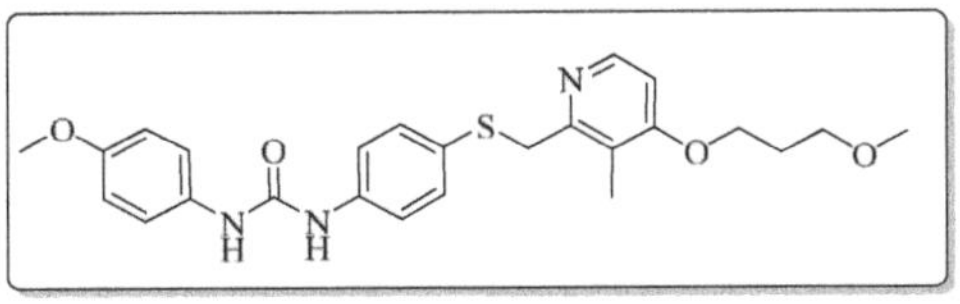

Compound **7c** was prepared according to the general procedure by using compound **4a** (0.32 g, 1 mmol) and 4-methoxyaniline (0.12 g, 1 mmol), obtained a white solid (0.22 g) in 46.3% yield. m.p. 144.8–146.6 °C. IR (KBr, cm^{-1}): υ 3428.6, 2984.7, 2923.0, 2852.7, 1635.5, 1599.5, 1562.6, 1510.7, 1492.7, 1461.8, 1441.3, 1398.1, 1289.8, 1245.2, 1173.5, 1120.3, 1093.5, 1035.2, 1005.6, 800.0, 617.1, 548.4, 522.7. ^{1}H-NMR (400 MHz, DMSO-d_6) δ 8.64 (s, 1H), 8.47 (s, 1H), 8.16 (d, *J* = 5.7 Hz, 1H), 7.39 (d, *J* = 1.9 Hz, 1H), 7.37 (d, *J* = 2.2 Hz, 1H), 7.35 (d, *J* = 2.2 Hz, 1H), 7.33 (d, *J* = 2.3 Hz, 1H), 7.30 (d, *J* = 2.1 Hz, 1H), 7.29 (d, *J* = 2.0 Hz, 1H), 6.89 (d, *J* = 5.6 Hz, 1H), 6.87 (d, *J* = 2.2 Hz, 1H), 6.86 (d, *J* = 2.2 Hz, 1H), 4.21 (s, 2H), 4.08 (t, *J* = 6.2 Hz, 2H), 3.71 (s, 3H), 3.48 (t, *J* = 6.2 Hz, 2H), 3.25 (s, 3H), 2.12 (s, 3H), 2.00–1.94 (m, 2H). ^{13}C-NMR (101 MHz, DMSO-d_6) δ 163.06, 156.41, 154.97, 153.07, 148.01, 139.37, 133.09, 131.78, 127.82, 120.52, 120.22, 118.98, 114.44, 106.44, 68.79, 65.42, 58.43, 55.63, 31.14, 29.16, 10.88. ESI-MS (*m/z*): 468.4 ([M + H]$^+$), 490.2 ([M + Na]$^+$). HRMS (ESI) (*m/z*): Calcd. for $C_{25}H_{29}N_3O_4S$, 468.1952 ([M + H]$^+$), found: 468.1959 ([M + H]$^+$). Purity (HPLC): 98.91%.

1-[4-Chloro-3-(trifluoromethyl)phenyl]-3-{4-{{[4-(3-methoxypropoxy)-3-methylpyridin-2-yl]methyl}thio}phenyl}urea (**7d**)

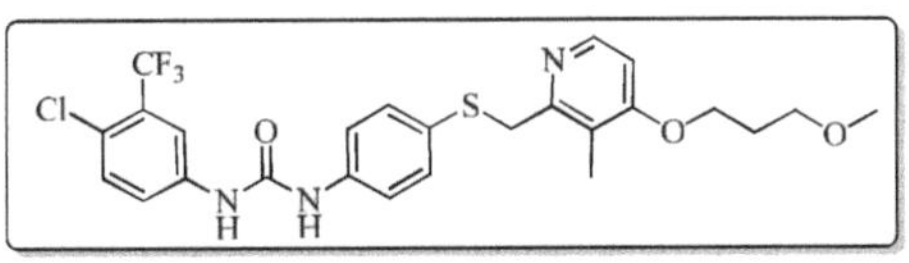

Compound **7d** was prepared according to the general procedure by using compound **4a** (0.32 g, 1 mmol) and 3-chloro-4-(trifluoromethyl)aniline (0.20 g, 1 mmol), obtained a white solid (0.24 g) in 43.8% yield. m.p. 136.0–137.2 °C. IR (KBr, cm^{-1}): υ 3425.2, 2922.0, 2852.7, 1590.1, 1546.1, 1482.2, 1463.1, 1384.5, 1306.6, 1175.4, 1117.7, 1034.4, 820.6. ^{1}H-NMR (400 MHz, DMSO-d_6) δ 9.16 (s, 1H), 8.89 (s, 1H), 8.16 (d, *J* = 5.6 Hz, 1H), 8.10 (d, *J* = 2.2 Hz, 1H), 7.63 (d, *J* = 2.2 Hz, 1H), 7.62 (s, 1H), 7.42 (d, *J* = 2.0 Hz, 1H), 7.40 (d, *J* = 2.2 Hz, 1H), 7.33 (d, *J* = 2.1 Hz, 1H), 7.32 (d, *J* = 2.0 Hz, 1H), 6.89 (d, *J* = 5.7 Hz, 1H), 4.23 (s, 2H), 4.09 (t, *J* = 6.2 Hz, 2H), 3.48 (t, *J* = 6.2 Hz, 2H), 3.25 (s, 3H), 2.13 (s, 3H), 2.00–1.94 (m, 2H). ^{13}C-NMR (101 MHz, DMSO-d_6) δ 163.08, 156.34, 152.76, 148.01, 139.76, 138.48, 132.45, 131.46, 128.91, 123.55, 122.80, 120.24, 119.57, 117.23, 106.48, 68.80, 65.44, 58.43, 31.14, 29.16, 10.89. ESI-MS (*m/z*): 540.2 ([M + H]$^+$), 562.0 ([M + Na]$^+$). HRMS (ESI) (*m/z*): Calcd. for $C_{25}H_{25}ClF_3N_3O_3S$, 540.1330 ([M + H]$^+$), found: 540.1320 ([M + H]$^+$). Purity (HPLC): 97.33%.

1-{4-{{[4-(3-Methoxypropoxy)-3-methylpyridin-2-yl]methyl}thio}phenyl}-3-[3-(trifluoromethyl)phenyl]urea (**7e**)

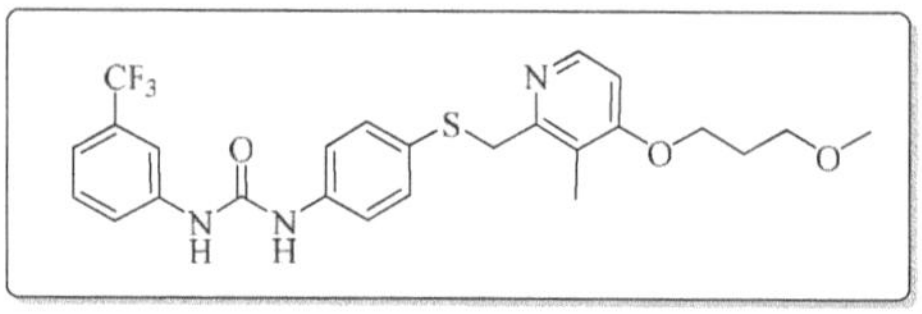

Compound **7e** was prepared according to the general procedure by using compound **4a** (0.32 g, 1 mmol) and 3-(trifluoromethyl)aniline (0.16 g, 1 mmol), obtained a white solid (0.27 g) in 53.1% yield. m.p. 136.1–137.9 °C. IR (KBr, cm^{-1}): υ 3327.8, 2958.7, 2927.8, 2859.0, 2377.4, 2350.2, 2311.0, 1724.0, 1648.5, 1585.5, 1552.2, 1492.5, 1465.2, 1397.5, 1338.6, 1295.8, 1230.8, 1166.2, 1116.1, 1092.4, 1068.9, 1005.4, 890.0, 804.1, 732.9, 699.2, 602.3, 505.8. ^{1}H-NMR (400 MHz, DMSO-d_6) δ 9.05 (s, 1H), 8.84 (s, 1H), 8.17 (d, *J* = 5.6 Hz, 1H), 8.09 (s, 0H), 8.00 (d, *J* = 2.3 Hz, 1H), 7.57 (d, *J* = 8.4 Hz, 1H), 7.51 (t, *J* = 7.9 Hz, 1H), 7.42 (d, *J* = 2.0 Hz, 1H), 7.40 (s, 1H), 7.33 (d, *J* = 2.1 Hz, 1H), 7.32 (d, *J* = 2.1 Hz, 1H), 7.30 (s, 1H), 6.90 (d, *J* = 5.7 Hz, 1H), 4.23 (s, 2H), 4.09 (t, *J* = 6.2 Hz, 2H), 3.48 (t, *J* = 6.2 Hz, 2H), 3.25 (s, 3H), 2.13 (s, 3H), 2.01–1.94 (m, 3H). ^{13}C-NMR (101 MHz, DMSO-d_6) δ 163.11, 156.32, 152.85, 147.97, 140.98, 138.68, 131.55, 130.34, 129.10, 128.64, 122.30, 120.25, 119.40, 118.53, 106.46, 68.79, 65.44, 58.42, 31.13, 29.16, 10.88. ESI-MS (*m*/*z*): 506.3 ([M + H]$^+$). HRMS (ESI) (*m*/*z*): Calcd. for $C_{25}H_{26}F_3N_3O_3S$, 506.1720 ([M + H]$^+$), found: 506.1728 ([M + H]$^+$). Purity (HPLC): 97.09%.

1-{4-{{[3-Methyl-4-(2,2,2-trifluoroethoxy)pyridin-2-yl]methyl}thio}phenyl}-3-phenylurea (**7f**)

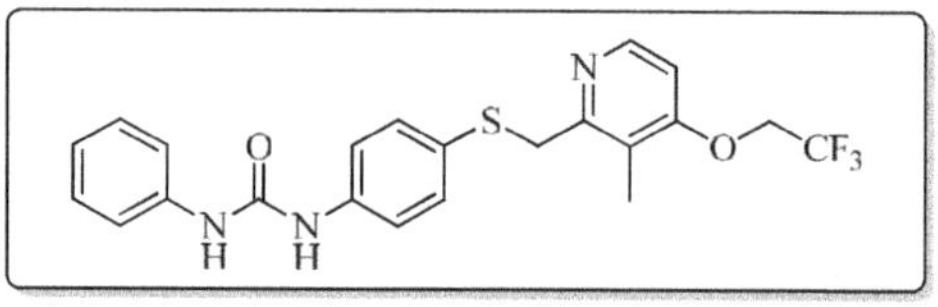

Compound **7f** was prepared according to the general procedure by using compound **4b** (0.33 g, 1 mmol) and aniline (0.10 g, 1 mmol), obtained a white solid (0.18 g) in 39.9% yield. m.p. 143.3–145.1 °C. IR (KBr, cm^{-1}): υ 3424.1, 2923.9, 2852.6, 1687.8, 1639.9, 1600.0, 1548.5, 1495.9, 1441.2, 1399.4, 1384.7, 1307.8, 1284.4, 1266.4, 1232.1, 1176.6, 1112.2, 970.6, 915.9, 854.7, 836.1, 801.5, 783.1, 751.0, 696.2, 657.1, 618.8, 574.4. ^{1}H-NMR (400 MHz, DMSO-d_6) δ 8.73 (s, 1H), 8.67 (s, 1H), 8.24 (d, *J* = 5.7 Hz, 1H), 7.46 (s, 1H), 7.44 (s, 1H), 7.41 (s, 1H), 7.39 (s, 1H), 7.32 (s, 1H), 7.30 (s, 1H), 7.28 (s, 1H), 7.26 (s, 1H), 7.03 (d, *J* = 5.7 Hz, 1H), 6.97 (t, *J* = 7.3 Hz, 1H), 4.89 (q, *J* = 8.7 Hz, 2H), 4.25 (s, 2H), 2.16 (s, 3H). ^{13}C-NMR (101 MHz, DMSO-d_6) δ 161.62, 157.24, 152.87, 148.00, 140.05, 139.22, 131.90, 129.23, 127.85, 125.66, 122.90, 122.35, 120.44, 119.10, 118.71, 107.07, 64.92, 31.13, 10.74. ESI-MS (*m*/*z*): 448.4 ([M + H]$^+$), 470.2 ([M + Na]$^+$). HRMS (ESI) (*m*/*z*): Calcd. for $C_{22}H_{20}F_3N_3O_2S$, 448.1301 ([M + H]$^+$), found: 448.1295 ([M + H]$^+$). Purity (HPLC): 97.04%.

1-(4-Chlorophenyl)-3-{4-{{[3-methyl-4-(2,2,2-trifluoroethoxy)pyridin-2-yl]methyl}thio}phenyl}urea (**7g**)

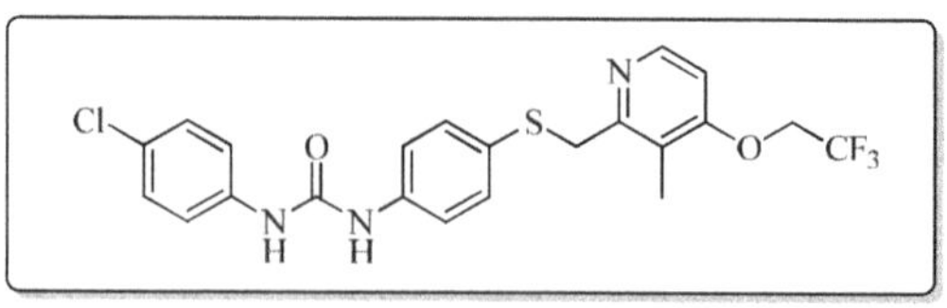

Compound **7g** was prepared according to the general procedure by using compound **4b** (0.33 g, 1 mmol) and 4-chloroaniline (0.13 g, 1 mmol), obtained a white solid (0.29 g) in 61.0% yield. m.p. 203.6–205.2 °C. IR (KBr, cm^{-1}): υ 3424.1, 2984.9, 2923.1, 2851.9, 2350.0, 2311.0, 1611.4, 1548.6, 1491.9, 1440.3, 1399.6, 1384.9, 1370.1, 1311.1, 1268.3, 1172.6, 1111.7, 1051.4, 1004.4, 897.2, 798.3, 668.5, 615.4.

^{1}H-NMR (400 MHz, DMSO-d_6) δ 8.81 (s, 1H), 8.75 (s, 1H), 8.23 (d, J = 5.7 Hz, 1H), 7.48 (d, J = 2.1 Hz, 1H), 7.47 (d, J = 2.2 Hz, 1H), 7.40 (d, J = 2.0 Hz, 1H), 7.38 (s, 1H), 7.33 (d, J = 2.1 Hz, 1H), 7.32 (d, J = 2.2 Hz, 1H), 7.31 (s, 1H), 7.30 (d, J = 1.9 Hz, 1H), 7.03 (d, J = 5.7 Hz, 1H), 4.88 (q, J = 8.7 Hz, 2H), 4.25 (s, 2H), 2.16 (s, 3H). ^{13}C-NMR (101 MHz, DMSO-d_6) δ 161.62, 157.22, 152.77, 148.00, 139.08, 138.98, 131.80, 129.07, 128.11, 125.87, 122.90, 120.43, 120.23, 119.23, 107.08, 65.09, 31.14, 10.74. ESI-MS (*m/z*): 482.6 ([M + H]$^+$), 504.3 ([M + Na]$^+$). HRMS (ESI) (*m/z*): Calcd. for $C_{22}H_{19}ClF_3N_3O_2S$, 482.0911 ([M + H]$^+$), found: 482.0916 ([M + H]$^+$). Purity (HPLC): 99.19%.

1-(4-Methoxyphenyl)-3-{4-{{[3-methyl-4-(2,2,2-trifluoroethoxy)pyridin-2-yl]methyl}thio}phenyl}urea (**7h**)

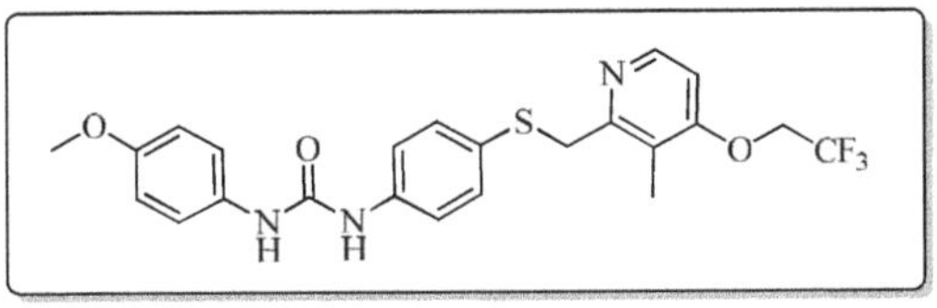

Compound **7h** was prepared according to the general procedure by using compound **4b** (0.33 g, 1 mmol) and 4-methoxyaniline (0.12 g, 1 mmol), obtained a white solid (0.22 g) in 45.9% yield. m.p. 171.3–172.1 °C. IR (KBr, cm^{-1}): υ 3383.8, 2922.1, 2851.4, 2377.6, 2349.6, 1703.0, 1656.7, 1619.2, 1591.3, 1546.4, 1511.1, 1492.7, 1465.5, 1399.3, 1312.1, 1264.5, 1231.2, 1175.1, 1112.8, 1040.3, 1006.7, 970.2, 918.1, 897.2, 831.5, 799.7, 658.3. ^{1}H-NMR (400 MHz,) δ 8.64 (s, 1H), 8.47 (s, 1H), 8.16 (d, J = 5.7 Hz, 1H), 7.39 (d, J = 1.9 Hz, 1H), 7.37 (d, J = 2.2 Hz, 1H), 7.35 (d, J = 2.2 Hz, 1H), 7.33 (d, J = 2.3 Hz, 1H), 7.30 (d, J = 2.1 Hz, 1H), 7.29 (d, J = 2.0 Hz, 1H), 6.89 (d, J = 5.6 Hz, 1H), 6.87 (d, J = 2.2 Hz, 1H), 6.86 (d, J = 2.2 Hz, 1H), 4.91-4.85 (m, 2H), 4.21 (s, 2H), 3.71 (s, 3H), 2.12 (s, 3H). ^{13}C-NMR (101 MHz, DMSO-d_6) δ 161.84, 156.03, 154.81, 153.88, 153.39, 148.09, 133.72, 133.38, 125.65, 121.84, 120.37, 120.33, 115.40, 114.43, 108.04, 65.10, 55.63, 31.13, 10.44. ESI-MS (*m/z*): 478.3 ([M + H]$^+$). HRMS (ESI) (m/z): Calcd. for $C_{23}H_{22}F_3N_3O_3S$, 478.1407 ([M + H]$^+$), found: 478.1408 ([M + H]$^+$). Purity (HPLC): 99.66%.

1-[4-Chloro-3-(trifluoromethyl)phenyl]-3-{4-{{[3-methyl-4-(2,2,2-trifluoroethoxy)pyridin-2-yl]methyl}thio}phenyl}urea (**7i**)

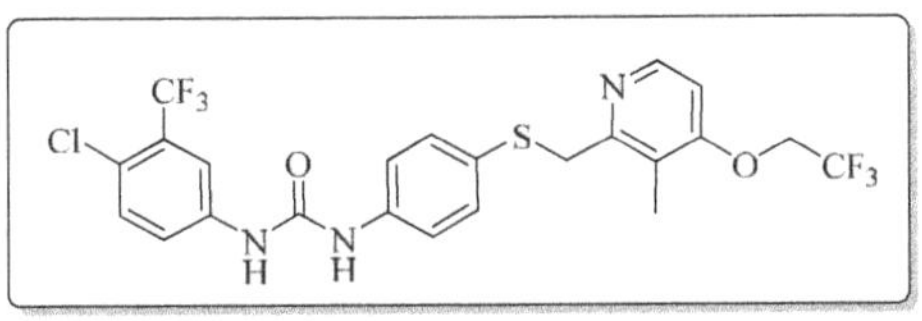

Compound **7i** was prepared according to the general procedure by using compound **4b** (0.33 g, 1 mmol) and 3-chloro-4-(trifluoromethyl)aniline (0.20 g, 1 mmol), obtained a white solid (0.27 g) in 49.5% yield. m.p. 142.0–143.0 °C. IR (KBr, cm^{-1}): υ 3422.3, 2922.1, 2852.6, 1587.4, 1547.6, 1480.8, 1419.0, 1309.8, 1263.9, 1177.2, 1111.0, 1035.5, 974.7, 819.3, 618.3. ^{1}H-NMR (400 MHz, DMSO-d_6) δ 9.17 (s, 1H), 8.90 (s, 1H), 8.24 (d, J = 5.7 Hz, 1H), 8.10 (d, J = 2.2 Hz, 1H), 7.64 (dd, J = 8.9, 2.2 Hz, 1H), 7.61 (d, J = 8.7 Hz, 1H), 7.42 (d, J = 2.0 Hz, 1H), 7.40 (d, J = 2.2 Hz, 1H), 7.33 (d, J = 2.2 Hz, 1H), 7.32 (d, J = 2.1 Hz, 1H), 7.04 (d, J = 5.7 Hz, 1H), 4.89 (q, J = 8.7 Hz, 2H), 2.16 (s, 3H). ^{13}C-NMR (101 MHz, DMSO-d_6) δ 161.61, 157.18, 152.75, 148.00, 139.74, 138.60, 132.42, 131.64, 128.58, 127.33, 127.02, 125.65, 123.53, 122.80, 120.44, 119.55, 117.28, 117.22, 107.07, 64.79, 39.69, 10.72. ESI-MS (*m/z*): 550.1, 552.1, 553.1 ([M + H]$^+$). HRMS (ESI) (*m/z*): Calcd. for $C_{23}H_{18}ClF_6N_3O_2S$, 550.0785 ([M + H]$^+$), found: 550.0769 ([M + H]$^+$). Purity (HPLC): 99.97%.

1-{4-{{[3-Methyl-4-(2,2,2-trifluoroethoxy)pyridin-2-yl]methyl}thio}phenyl}-3-[3-(trifluoromethyl)phenyl] urea (**7j**)

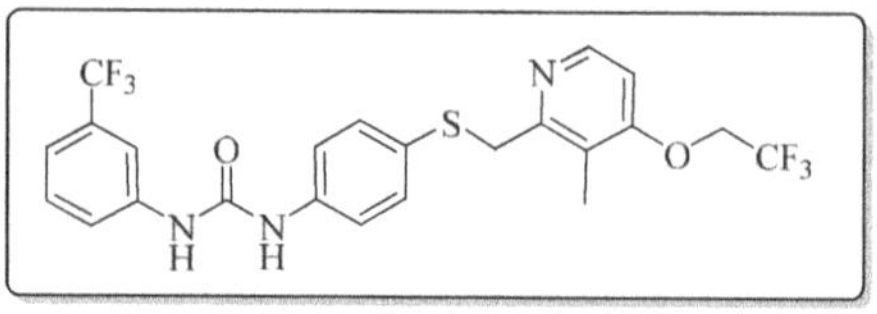

Compound **7j** was prepared according to the general procedure C by using compound **4b** (0.33 g, 1 mmol) and 3-(trifluoromethyl)aniline (0.16 g, 1 mmol), obtained a white solid (0.34 g) in 66.1% yield. m.p. 174.7–176.4 °C. IR (KBr, cm^{-1}): υ 3421.4, 2985.6, 2924.1, 2852.9, 2349.2, 2311.0, 1614.9, 1491.8, 1445.1, 1399.1, 1339.8, 1313.1, 1288.0, 1264.6, 1231.2, 1173.2, 1114.6, 1071.2, 1006.3, 976.0, 832.4, 798.2, 700.6, 616.4. ^{1}H-NMR (400 MHz, DMSO-d_6) δ 9.07 (s, 1H), 8.87 (s, 1H), 8.24 (d, J = 5.7 Hz, 1H), 8.01 (d, J = 2.0 Hz, 1H), 7.60–7.54 (m, 1H), 7.51 (t, J = 7.9 Hz, 1H), 7.43 (d, J = 2.0 Hz, 1H), 7.41 (d, J = 2.1 Hz, 1H), 7.33 (d, J = 2.1 Hz, 1H), 7.33–7.31 (m, 1H), 7.30 (d, J = 1.7 Hz, 1H), 7.04 (d, J = 5.7 Hz, 1H), 4.89 (q, J = 8.7 Hz, 2H), 4.26 (s, 2H), 2.16 (s, 3H). ^{13}C-NMR (101 MHz, DMSO-d_6) δ 161.66, 157.16, 152.86, 147.96, 140.97, 138.80, 131.76, 130.35, 130.15, 129.84, 128.31, 122.30, 120.47, 119.40, 118.54, 114.59, 107.09, 65.09, 49.05, 31.13, 10.73. ESI-MS (m/z): 516.2 ([M + H]$^+$). HRMS (ESI) (m/z): Calcd. for $C_{23}H_{19}F_6N_3O_2S$, 516.1175 ([M + H]$^+$), found: 516.1174 ([M + H]$^+$). Purity (HPLC): 97.29%.

1-{4-{[(4-Methoxy-3,5-dimethylpyridin-2-yl)methyl]thio}phenyl}-3-phenylurea (**7k**)

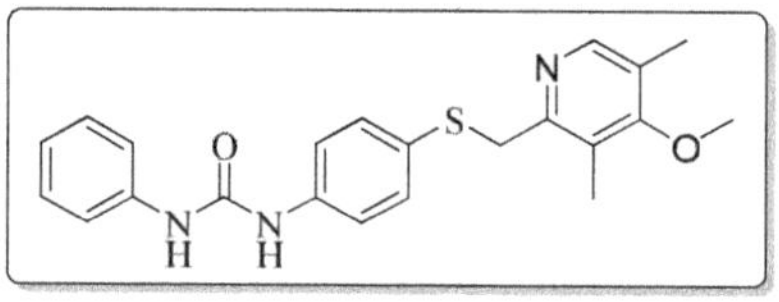

Compound **7k** was prepared according to the general procedure by using compound **4c** (0.27 g, 1 mmol) and aniline (0.10 g, 1 mmol), obtained a white solid (0.23 g) in 57.3% yield. m.p. 188.1–188.9 °C. IR (KBr, cm^{-1}): υ 3422.4, 2923.8, 2852.4, 2351.0, 2321.9, 1644.0, 1597.4, 1553.7, 1494.2, 1441.5, 1398.0, 1312.9, 1270.7, 1237.5, 1173.3, 1127.7, 1073.5, 1002.5, 798.1, 755.7, 738.0, 694.0, 616.4. ^{1}H-NMR (400 MHz, DMSO-d_6) δ 8.72 (s, 1H), 8.67 (s, 1H), 8.12 (s, 1H), 7.45 (d, J = 1.3 Hz, 1H), 7.44-7.42 (m, 1H), 7.40 (d, J = 2.1 Hz, 1H), 7.39 (d, J = 2.1 Hz, 1H), 7.31 (d, J = 2.2 Hz, 1H), 7.29 (d, J = 2.1 Hz, 1H), 7.28 (s, 1H), 7.26 (d, J = 1.6 Hz, 1H), 6.97 (t, J = 7.4 Hz, 1H), 4.21 (s, 2H), 3.70 (s, 3H), 2.18 (s, 6H). ^{13}C-NMR (101 MHz, DMSO-d_6) δ 163.86, 155.80, 152.86, 148.97, 140.05, 139.16, 131.86, 129.24, 127.98, 125.19, 125.03, 122.35, 119.11, 118.70, 60.17, 31.15, 13.38, 11.34. ESI-MS (m/z): 394.6 ([M + H]$^+$), 416.3 ([M + Na]$^+$). HRMS (ESI) (m/z): Calcd. for $C_{22}H_{23}N_3O_2S$, 394.1584 ([M + H]$^+$), found: 394.1586 ([M + H]$^+$). Purity (HPLC): 99.89%.

1-(4-Chlorophenyl)-3-{4-{[(4-methoxy-3,5-dimethylpyridin-2-yl)methyl]thio}phenyl}urea (**7l**)

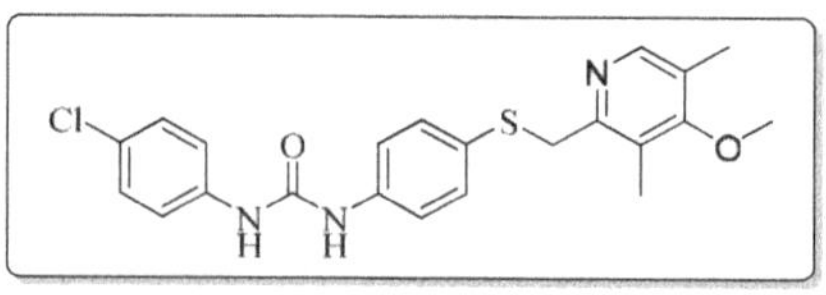

Compound **7l** was prepared according to the general procedure by using compound **4c** (0.27 g, 1 mmol) and 4-chloroaniline (0.13 g, 1 mmol), obtained a white solid (0.28 g) in 66.2% yield. m.p. 206.8–208.2 °C. IR (KBr, cm^{-1}): υ 3422.5, 2923.0, 2852.0, 2377.1, 2349.6, 2310.8, 1630.4, 1547.7, 1491.7, 1439.7, 1399.2, 1385.1, 1309.9, 1270.9, 1235.5, 1173.0, 1124.1, 1051.3, 1004.6, 832.1, 798.2, 702.1, 668.3, 617.0. ^{1}H-NMR (400 MHz, DMSO-d_6) δ 8.81 (s, 1H), 8.75 (s, 1H), 8.11 (s, 1H), 7.48 (d, J = 2.1 Hz, 1H), 7.46 (d, J = 2.2 Hz, 1H), 7.40 (d, J = 2.0 Hz, 1H), 7.38 (d, J = 2.2 Hz, 1H), 7.33 (d, J = 2.1 Hz, 1H), 7.32 (s, 1H), 7.31 (s,

1H), 7.30 (d, J = 2.1 Hz, 1H), 4.21 (s, 2H), 3.70 (s, 3H), 2.18 (s, 3H), 2.18 (s, 3H). ^{13}C-NMR (101 MHz, DMSO-d_6) δ 163.86, 155.79, 152.77, 148.97, 139.08, 138.94, 131.76, 129.07, 127.98, 128.25, 125.87, 125.19, 125.03, 120.23, 119.25, 60.17, 31.14, 13.37, 11.33. ESI-MS (m/z): 428.7 ([M + H]$^+$). HRMS (ESI) (m/z): Calcd. for $C_{22}H_{22}ClN_3O_2S$, 428.1194 ([M + H]$^+$), found: 428.1199 ([M + H]$^+$). Purity (HPLC): 99.53%.

1-{4-{[(4-Methoxy-3,5-dimethylpyridin-2-yl)methyl)]thio}phenyl}-3-(4-methoxyphenyl)urea (**7m**)

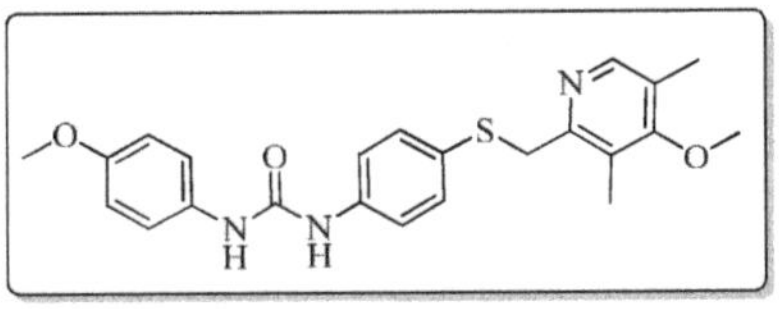

Compound **7m** was prepared according to the general procedure by using compound **4c** (0.27 g, 1 mmol) and 4-methoxyaniline (0.12 g, 1 mmol), obtained a white solid (0.21 g) in 49.2% yield. m.p. 171.4–172.6 °C. IR (KBr, cm^{-1}): υ 3422.5, 2921.1, 2850.5, 1642.5, 1593.2, 1547.5, 1493.7, 1468.2, 1439.0, 1397.7, 1311.5, 1292.4, 1270.1, 1240.4, 1173.4, 1073.2, 1053.2, 1031.3, 1003.9, 828.2, 797.9, 616.3. ^{1}H-NMR (400 MHz, DMSO-d_6) δ 8.68 (s, 1H), 8.50 (s, 1H), 8.15 (s, 1H), 7.39 (d, J = 1.9 Hz, 1H), 7.37 (d, J = 2.1 Hz, 1H), 7.35 (d, J = 2.0 Hz, 1H), 7.33 (d, J = 2.2 Hz, 1H), 7.29 (d, J = 2.1 Hz, 1H), 7.27 (d, J = 1.9 Hz, 1H), 6.87 (d, J = 2.3 Hz, 1H), 6.86 (d, J = 2.2 Hz, 1H), 4.21 (s, 2H), 3.73 (s, 3H), 3.71 (s, 3H), 2.20 (s, 3H), 2.17 (s, 3H). ^{13}C-NMR (101 MHz, DMSO-d_6) δ 164.47, 155.40, 154.98, 153.08, 148.27, 139.64, 133.09, 132.28, 127.19, 125.70, 125.46, 125.41, 120.49, 118.95, 118.40, 114.46, 60.30, 55.65, 31.14, 13.45, 11.35. ESI-MS (m/z): 424.3 ([M + H]$^+$). HRMS (ESI) (m/z): Calcd. for $C_{23}H_{25}N_3O_3S$, 424.1689 ([M + H]$^+$), found: 424.1698 ([M + H]$^+$). Purity (HPLC): 96.88%.

1-[4-Chloro-3-(trifluoromethyl)phenyl]-3-{4-{[(4-methoxy-3,5-dimethylpyridin-2-yl)methyl]thio}phenyl}urea (**7n**)

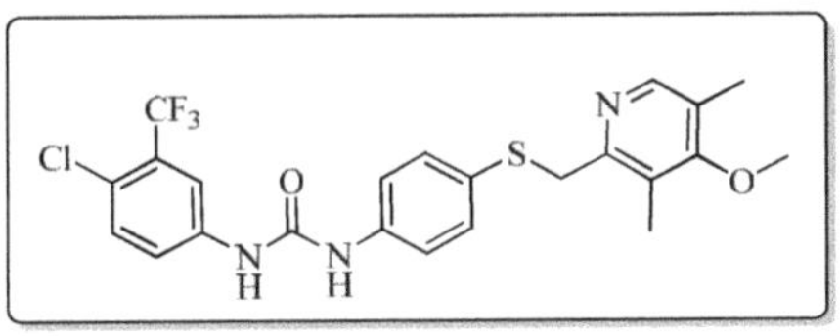

Compound **7n** was prepared according to the general procedure by using compound **4c** (0.27 g, 1 mmol) and 3-chloro-4-(trifluoromethyl)aniline (0.20 g, 1 mmol), obtained a white solid (0.35 g) in 70.1% yield. m.p. 152.3–153.1 °C. IR (KBr, cm^{-1}): υ 3422.2, 2921.6, 2852.2, 1719.2, 1593.8, 1546.4, 1480.4, 1419.8, 1384.6, 1311.1, 1265.2, 1229.0, 1174.6, 1130.8, 1073.5, 1031.7, 823.3, 619.9. ^{1}H-NMR (400 MHz, DMSO-d_6) δ 9.18 (s, 1H), 8.91 (s, 1H), 8.12 (s, 1H), 8.10 (d, J = 2.0 Hz, 1H), 7.64 (d, J = 8.9 Hz, 1H), 7.62 (s, 1H), 7.42 (d, J = 2.1 Hz, 1H), 7.40 (d, J = 2.1 Hz, 1H), 7.33 (s, 1H), 7.31 (d, J = 1.9 Hz, 1H), 4.22 (s, 2H), 3.70 (s, 3H), 2.19 (s, 3H), 2.18 (s, 3H). ^{13}C-NMR (101 MHz, DMSO-d_6) δ 164.07, 154.69, 154.49, 153.03, 149.00, 140.01, 132.84, 132.38, 126.45, 126.36, 124.20, 123.34, 122.49, 121.03, 115.40, 60.18, 31.13, 13.43, 11.00. ESI-MS (m/z): 496.1; 497.1; 498.1; 499.1 ([M + H]$^+$). HRMS (ESI) (m/z): Calcd. for $C_{23}H_{21}ClF_3N_3O_2S$, 496.1068 ([M + H]$^+$), found: 496.1066 ([M + H]$^+$). Purity (HPLC): 98.56%.

1-{4-{[(4-Methoxy-3,5-dimethylpyridin-2-yl)methyl]thio}phenyl}-3-[3-(trifluoromethyl)pHenyl]urea (**7o**)

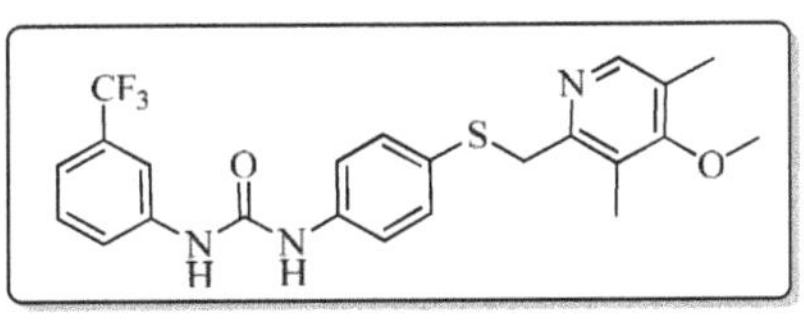

Compound **7o** was prepared according to the general procedure by using compound **4c** (0.27 g, 1 mmol) and 3-(trifluoromethyl)aniline (0.16 g, 1 mmol), obtained a white solid (0.30 g) in 64.7% yield. m.p. 156.9–158.1 °C. IR (KBr, cm^{-1}): υ 3420.6, 2984.8, 2922.8, 2851.8, 2350.3, 2321.1, 1609.8, 1491.8, 1443.2, 1398.4, 1369.9, 1338.2, 1311.7, 1271.2, 1229.2, 1172.1, 1124.2, 1072.1, 1002.9, 797.9, 698.2, 616.0. ^{1}H-NMR (400 MHz, DMSO-d_6) δ 9.04 (s, 1H), 8.84 (s, 1H), 8.12 (s, 1H), 8.00 (d, *J* = 2.0 Hz, 1H), 7.57 (d, *J* = 8.8 Hz, 1H), 7.51 (t, *J* = 7.8 Hz, 1H), 7.42 (d, *J* = 1.9 Hz, 1H), 7.40 (d, *J* = 2.2 Hz, 1H), 7.33 (s, 1H), 7.32 (s, 1H), 7.30 (d, *J* = 2.6 Hz, 1H), 4.22 (s, 2H), 3.70 (s, 3H), 2.19 (s, 3H), 2.18 (s, 3H). ^{13}C-NMR (101 MHz, DMSO-d_6) δ 163.88, 155.76, 152.85, 148.95, 140.97, 138.73, 131.69, 130.35, 128.51, 125.21, 125.05, 123.31, 122.32, 119.43, 118.58, 114.64, 60.16, 31.13, 13.36, 11.33. ESI-MS (*m/z*): 462.3 ([M + H]$^+$). HRMS (ESI) (*m/z*): Calcd. for $C_{23}H_{22}F_3N_3O_2S$, 462.1458 ([M + H]$^+$), found: 462.1469 ([M + H]$^+$). Purity (HPLC): 99.79%.

1-{4-{[(3,4-Dimethoxypyridin-2-yl)methyl]thio}phenyl}-3-phenylurea (**7p**)

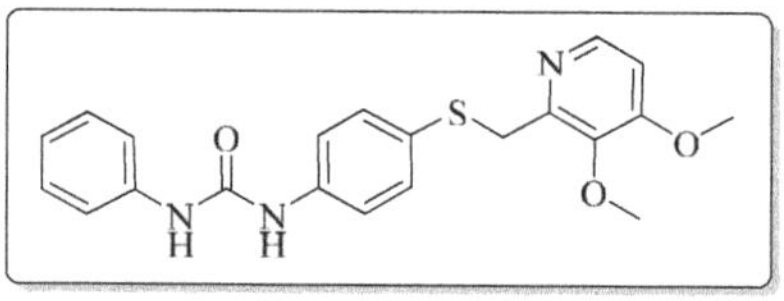

Compound **7p** was prepared according to the general procedure by using compound **4d** (0.28 g, 1 mmol) and aniline (0.10 g, 1 mmol), obtained a white solid (0.18 g) in 45.8% yield. m.p. 127.7–128.5 °C. IR (KBr, cm^{-1}): υ 3287.2, 2937.3, 1654.0, 1593.7, 1548.0, 1487.0, 1442.7, 1421.2, 1379.4, 1297.9, 1270.4, 1231.6, 1175.0, 1071.7, 997.3, 932.8, 829.0, 782.9, 742.9, 692.4, 618.5, 516.5. ^{1}H-NMR (400 MHz, DMSO-d_6) δ 8.72 (s, 1H), 8.67 (s, 1H), 8.12 (d, *J* = 5.5 Hz, 1H), 7.49–7.45 (m, 1H), 7.44 (s, 1H), 7.41 (d, *J* = 2.0 Hz, 1H), 7.40 (d, *J* = 2.2 Hz, 1H), 7.33 (d, *J* = 2.0 Hz, 1H), 7.31 (d, *J* = 1.9 Hz, 1H), 7.29 (d, *J* = 7.7 Hz, 1H), 7.28–7.25 (m, 1H), 7.03 (d, *J* = 5.5 Hz, 1H), 6.97 (t, *J* = 7.3 Hz, 1H), 4.17 (s, 2H), 3.87 (s, 3H), 3.74 (s, 3H). ^{13}C-NMR (101 MHz, DMSO-d_6) δ 158.52, 152.88, 151.53, 145.72, 143.40, 138.98, 131.39, 129.24, 128.54, 122.33, 119.17, 118.69, 108.29, 60.99, 56.34, 36.37, 31.14. ESI-MS (*m/z*): 396.3 ([M + H]$^+$), 418.2 ([M + Na]$^+$). HRMS (ESI) (*m/z*): Calcd. for $C_{21}H_{21}N_3O_3S$, 396.1376 ([M + H]$^+$), found: 396.1380 ([M + H]$^+$). Purity (HPLC): 99.90%.

1-(4-Chlorophenyl)-3-{4-{[(3,4-dimethoxypyridin-2-yl)methyl]thio}phenyl}urea (**7q**)

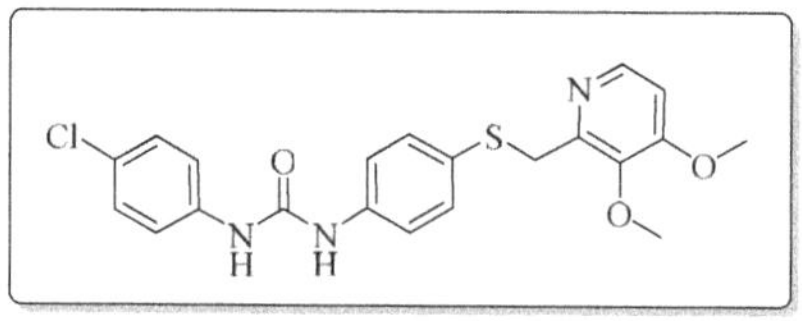

Compound **7q** was prepared according to the general procedure by using compound **4d** (0.28 g, 1 mmol) and 4-chloroaniline (0.13 g, 1 mmol), obtained a white solid (0.21 g) in 49.1% yield. m.p. 141.7–142.9 °C. IR (KBr, cm^{-1}): υ 3345.3, 3096.8, 2924.2, 2852.2, 1711.6, 1631.2, 1590.8, 1535.1, 1490.0, 1449.2, 1427.9, 1399.4, 1300.6, 1284.5, 1237.1, 1195.2, 1174.0, 1087.1, 1067.2, 996.9, 828.3, 703.0, 509.1. ^{1}H-NMR (400 MHz, DMSO-d_6) δ 8.83 (s, 1H), 8.76 (s, 1H), 8.11 (d, *J* = 5.5 Hz, 1H), 7.49 (s, 1H), 7.47 (s, 1H), 7.41 (s, 1H), 7.39 (s, 1H), 7.34-7.31 (m, 2H), 7.03 (d, *J* = 5.5 Hz, 1H), 4.17 (s, 2H), 3.87 (s, 3H), 3.74 (s, 3H). ^{13}C-NMR (101 MHz, DMSO-d_6) δ 158.52, 152.78, 151.50, 145.71, 143.40, 139.10, 138.75, 131.29, 129.07, 128.79, 125.85, 120.21, 119.30, 108.30, 60.99, 56.34, 36.29, 31.14. ESI-MS (*m/z*): 430.6 ([M + H]$^+$), 452.1 ([M + Na]$^+$). HRMS (ESI) (*m/z*): Calcd. for $C_{21}H_{20}ClN_3O_3S$, 430.0987 ([M + H]$^+$), found: 430.0993 ([M + H]$^+$). Purity (HPLC): 99.33%.

1-{4-{[(3,4-Dimethoxypyridin-2-yl)methyl]thio}phenyl}-3-(4-methoxyphenyl)urea (**7r**)

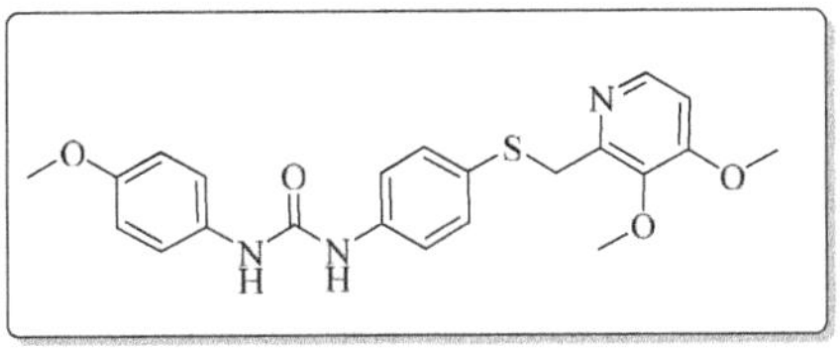

Compound **7r** was prepared according to the general procedure by using compound **4d** (0.28 g, 1 mmol) and 4-methoxyaniline (0.12 g, 1 mmol), obtained a white solid (0.20 g) in 47.9% yield. m.p. 179.0–180.6 °C. IR (KBr, cm^{-1}): υ 3428.5, 2985.2, 2923.2, 2851.3, 1630.7, 1587.2, 1557.0, 1510.3, 1490.9, 1442.6, 1398.6, 1299.7, 1270.7, 1232.4, 1173.6, 1072.2, 1033.0, 1000.9, 934.0, 829.1, 799.5, 617.4, 549.0, 523.3. ^{1}H-NMR (400 MHz, DMSO-d_6) δ 8.62 (s, 1H), 8.46 (s, 1H), 8.11 (d, *J* = 5.5 Hz, 1H), 7.39 (d, *J* = 2.0 Hz, 1H), 7.38 (d, *J* = 2.2 Hz, 1H), 7.35 (d, *J* = 2.2 Hz, 1H), 7.33 (d, *J* = 2.2 Hz, 1H), 7.31 (d, *J* = 2.2 Hz, 1H), 7.30 (d, *J* = 2.0 Hz, 1H), 7.03 (d, *J* = 5.5 Hz, 1H), 6.87 (d, *J* = 2.2 Hz, 1H), 6.85 (d, *J* = 2.2 Hz, 1H), 4.15 (s, 2H), 3.87 (s, 3H), 3.74 (s, 3H), 3.71 (s, 3H). ^{13}C-NMR (101 MHz, DMSO-d_6) δ 158.51, 154.98, 153.07, 151.55, 145.73, 143.40, 139.22, 133.08, 131.45, 128.24, 120.54, 119.06, 114.46, 108.30, 60.99, 56.35, 55.65, 36.43, 31.15. ESI-MS (*m/z*): 426.3 ([M + H]$^+$). HRMS (ESI) (*m/z*): Calcd. for $C_{22}H_{23}N_3O_4S$, 426.1482 ([M + H]$^+$), found: 426.1489 ([M + H]$^+$). Purity (HPLC): 98.84%.

1-[4-Chloro-3-(trifluoromethyl)phenyl]-3-{4-{[(3,4-dimethoxypyridin-2-yl)methyl]thio}pHenyl}urea (**7s**)

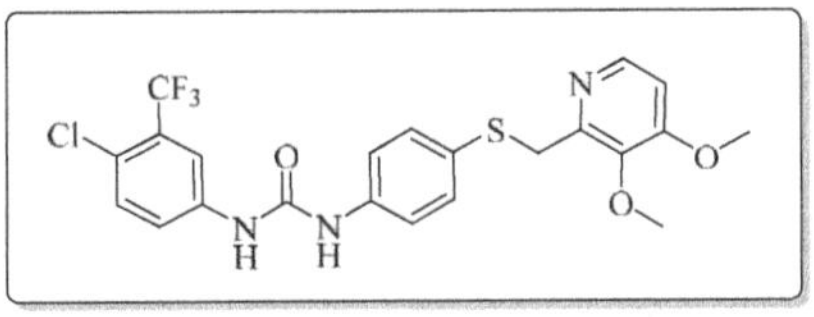

Compound **7s** was prepared according to the general procedure by using compound **4d** (0.28 g, 1 mmol) and 3-chloro-4-(trifluoromethyl)aniline (0.20 g, 1 mmol), obtained a white solid (0.32 g) in 64.5% yield. m.p. 188.1–189.2 °C. IR (KBr, cm^{-1}): υ 3425.5, 2921.9, 2852.4, 1589.9, 1545.2, 1485.2, 1419.2, 1384.4, 1306.1, 1229.2, 1175.6, 1132.0, 1068.8, 1033.0, 824.9. ^{1}H-NMR (400 MHz, DMSO-d_6) δ 9.15 (s, 1H), 8.88 (s, 1H), 8.11 (d, *J* = 5.5 Hz, 1H), 8.10 (d, *J* = 2.2 Hz, 1H), 7.64 (d, *J* = 8.8 Hz, 1H), 7.62–7.58 (m, 1H), 7.42 (d, *J* = 2.0 Hz, 1H), 7.41 (d, *J* = 2.2 Hz, 1H), 7.34 (d, *J* = 2.2 Hz, 1H), 7.33 (d, *J* = 2.0 Hz, 1H), 7.03 (d, *J* = 5.5 Hz, 1H), 4.17 (s, 2H), 3.88 (s, 3H), 3.74 (s, 3H). ^{13}C-NMR (101 MHz, DMSO-d_6) δ 158.52, 152.76, 151.47, 145.73, 143.40, 139.76, 138.36, 132.44, 131.12, 129.28, 123.53, 122.78, 119.62, 117.24, 108.32, 61.00, 56.35, 36.17, 31.14. ESI-MS (*m/z*): 498.2 ([M + H]$^+$). HRMS (ESI) (*m/z*): Calcd. for $C_{22}H_{19}ClF_3N_3O_3S$, 498.0861 ([M + H]$^+$), found: 498.0844 ([M + H]$^+$). Purity (HPLC): 98.10%.

1-{4-{[(3,4-Dimethoxypyridin-2-yl)methyl]thio}phenyl}-3-[3-(trifluoromethyl)phenyl]urea (**7t**)

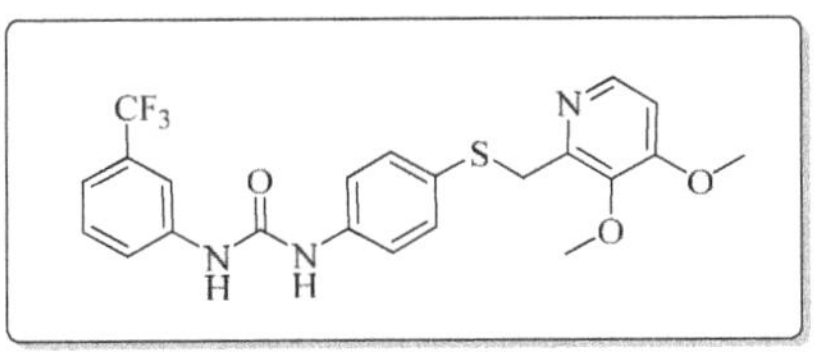

Compound **7t** was prepared according to the general procedure by using compound **4d** (0.28 g, 1 mmol) and 3-(trifluoromethyl)aniline (0.16 g, 1 mmol), obtained a white solid (0.21 g) in 44.3% yield. m.p. 198.4–199.8 °C. IR (KBr, cm^{-1}): υ 3422.2, 2985.4, 2377.5, 2349.8, 2320.7, 2024.8, 1712.9, 1594.1, 1564.4, 1537.2, 1491.3, 1445.8, 1399.4, 1370.2, 1316.3, 1273.6, 1230.1, 1173.8, 1124.9, 1068.3, 1002.1, 932.4, 892.8, 828.2, 798.3, 743.3, 697.8, 615.6. ^{1}H-NMR (400 MHz, DMSO-d_6) δ 9.04 (s, 1H), 8.83 (s, 1H), 8.11 (d,

J = 5.5 Hz, 1H), 8.01 (d, J = 2.0 Hz, 1H), 7.60–7.54 (m, 1H), 7.51 (t, J = 7.9 Hz, 1H), 7.43 (d, J = 2.0 Hz, 1H), 7.41 (d, J = 2.2 Hz, 1H), 7.34 (d, J = 2.2 Hz, 1H), 7.32 (d, J = 2.5 Hz, 1H), 7.30 (s, 1H), 7.03 (d, J = 5.6 Hz, 1H), 4.17 (s, 2H), 3.88 (s, 3H), 3.75 (s, 3H). ^{13}C-NMR (101 MHz, DMSO-d_6) δ 158.52, 152.87, 151.50, 145.72, 143.41, 140.98, 138.55, 131.22, 130.34, 129.08, 122.31, 119.49, 118.56, 114.65, 108.31, 60.99, 56.34, 36.24, 31.12. ESI-MS (*m/z*): 464.2 ([M + H]$^+$). Purity (HPLC): 98.85%.

3.2. Biological Evaluation

3.2.1. Antiproliferative Activity Assays

The antiproliferative activities of target compounds were determined using a standard MTT assay [27–30]. Exponentially growing cells A549 (3 × 10^3 cells/well), HCT-116 (1 × 10^4 cells/well) and PC-3 (8 × 10^3 cells/well) were seeded into 96-well plates and incubated for 24 h to allow the cells to attach. After 24 h of incubation, the culture medium was removed and fresh medium containing various concentrations of the candidate compounds was added to each well. The cells were then incubated for 72 h, thereafter MTT assays were performed and cell viability was assessed at 570 nm by a microplate reader (ThermoFisher Scientific (Shanghai) Instrument Co., Ltd., Shanghai, China).

3.2.2. Cell Apoptosis Assay

A549 cells were seeded into a 6-well plate (2 × 10^5/well) and incubated for 24 h. Then the cells were treated with different concentrations of the tested compound **7i** for 24 h. Thereafter, the cells were collected and the Annexin-V-FITC/PI apoptosis kit (Biovision, Milpitas, CA, USA) was used according to the manufacturer's protocol. The cells were analyzed by Accuri C6 flow cytometric (Becton Dickinson, Franklin Lakes, NJ, USA) [31].

3.2.3. Cell Cycle Analysis

For flow cytometric analysis of DNA content, 5 × 10^5 A549 cells in exponential growth were treated with different concentrations of the compound **7i** for 24 or 48 h. After an incubation period, the cells were collected, centrifuged and fixed with ice cold ethanol (70%). The cells were then treated with buffer containing RNAse A and 0.1% Triton X-100 and then stained with the propidium iodide (PI). The samples were analyzed on Accuri C6 flow cytometer (Becton Dickinson). [32].

4. Conclusions

In summary, a new series of 1-aryl-3-{4-[(pyridin-2-ylmethyl)thio]phenyl}urea derivatives were designed and synthesized based on molecular hybridization strategy. Majority of target compounds showed moderate to good growth inhibition against the tested cancer cells. Particularly, compound **7i** exhibited more potent antiproliferative activity than well-known anticancer drug sorafenib against all three cancer cell lines (A549, HCT-116 and PC-3). The preliminary mechanism investigation showed that compound **7i** could induce A549 cells to apoptosis, and halted cell cycle progression at the G1 phase. The SARs illustrated that these target compounds in this work might serve as bioactive fragments, and compound **7i** could be used as a lead compound for the development of potent cancer chemotherapeutic agents in the drug discovery process.

Supplementary Materials: The following are available online. ^{1}H-NMR, ^{13}C-NMR, ESI-MS and HRMS of the target compounds, respectively.

Author Contributions: C.Z., X.T., J.F., Y.L., N.D. and Z.J. contributed to the synthetic work and the characterization of all target compounds. C.Z. and Z.J. the preparation of the manuscript. C.Z., X.T. and Q.M. performed the biological assays. X.L. and C.H. proposed the studies and contributed to their design, as well as to the writing of the manuscript. All authors have read and approved the final manuscript.

Funding: This work was supported by the National Science Foundation of China (Grant No. 21342006), the Program for Innovative Research Team of the Ministry of Education of China (Grant No. IRT_14R36), the Natural

Science Foundation of Liaoning Province, China (Grant No. 201602695), and the Scientific Research Foundation of Department of Education of Liaoning Province, China (Grant No. L2015517).

Conflicts of Interest: The authors confirm that this article content has no conflict of interest.

References

1. Siegel, R.; Naishadham, D.; Jemal, A. Cancer statistics, 2013. *CA Cancer J. Clin.* **2013**, *63*, 11–30. [CrossRef] [PubMed]
2. Keefe, D.M.; Bateman, E.H. Tumor control versus adverse events with targeted anticancer therapies. *Nat. Rev. Clin. Oncol.* **2011**, *9*, 98–109. [CrossRef] [PubMed]
3. Matsuo, Y.; Park, J.H.; Miyamoto, T.; Yamamoto, S.; Hisada, S.; Alachkar, H.; Nakamura, Y. TOPK inhibitor induces complete tumor regression in xenograft models of human cancer through inhibition of cytokinesis. *Sci. Transl. Med.* **2014**, *6*, 259. [CrossRef] [PubMed]
4. Zeng, X.Y.; Lin, L.; Zheng, M.Z.; Sun, H.M.; Xiao, J.J.; Lu, T.; Huang, G.Q.; Chen, P.P.; Zhang, J.M.; Zhu, F.; et al. Pantoprazole, an FDA-approved proton-pump inhibitor, suppresses colorectal cancer growth by targeting T-cell-originated protein kinase. *Oncotarget* **2016**, *7*, 22460–22473. [CrossRef] [PubMed]
5. Zheng, M.Z.; Luan, S.S.; Gao, S.Y.; Cheng, L.; Hao, B.; Li, J.C.; Chen, Y.; Hou, X.M.; Chen, L.X.; Li, H. Proton pump inhibitor ilaprazole suppresses cancer growth by targeting T-cell-originated protein kinase. *Oncotarget* **2017**, *8*, 39143–39153. [CrossRef] [PubMed]
6. Abe, Y.; Matsumoto, S.; Kito, K.; Ueda, N. Cloning and Expression of a Novel MAPKK-like Protein Kinase, Lymphokine-activated Killer T-cell-originated Protein Kinase, Specifically Expressed in the Testis and Activated Lymphoid Cells. *J. Biol. Chem.* **2000**, *275*, 21525–21531. [CrossRef] [PubMed]
7. Park, J.H.; Lin, M.L.; Nishidate, T.; Nakamura, Y.; Katagiri, T. PDZ-binding kinase/T-LAK cell-originated protein kinase, a putative cancer/testis antigen with anoncogenic activity in breast cancer. *Cancer Res.* **2006**, *66*, 9186–9195. [CrossRef]
8. Simons-Evelyn, M.; Bailey-Dell, K.; Toretsky, J.A.; Ross, D.D.; Fenton, R.; Kalvakolanu, D.; Rapoport, A.P. PBK/TOPK is a novel mitotic kinase which is upregulated in Burkitt's lymphoma and other highly proliferative malignant cells. *Blood Cells, Mol., Dis.* **2001**, *27*, 825–829. [CrossRef]
9. Nandi, A.; Tidwell, M.; Karp, J.; Rapoport, A.P. Protein expression of PDZ-binding kinase is up-regulated in hematologic malignancies and strongly downregulated during terminal differentiation of HL-60 leukemic cells. *Blood Cells Mol. Dis.* **2004**, *32*, 240–245. [CrossRef]
10. Zykova, T.A.; Zhu, F.; Lu, C.; Higgins, L.; Tatsumi, Y.; Abe, Y.; Bode, A.M.; Dong, Z. Lymphokine-activated killer T-cell-originated protein kinase phosphorylation of histone H2AX prevents arsenite-induced apoptosis in RPMI7951 melanoma cells. *Clin. Cancer Res.* **2006**, *12*, 6884–6893. [CrossRef]
11. Wei, D.C.; Yeh, Y.C.; Hung, J.J.; Chou, T.Y.; Wu, Y.C.; Lu, P.J.; Cheng, H.C.; Hsu, Y.L.; Kuo, Y.L.; Chen, K.Y.; et al. Overexpression of T-LAK cell-originated protein kinase predicts poor prognosis in patients with stage I lung adenocarcinoma. *Cancer Sci.* **2012**, *103*, 731–738. [CrossRef] [PubMed]
12. Shih, M.C.; Chen, J.Y.; Wu, Y.C.; Jan, Y.H.; Yang, B.M.; Lu, P.J.; Cheng, H.C.; Huang, M.S.; Yang, C.J.; Hsiao, M.; et al. TOPK/PBK promotes cell migration via modulation of the PI3K/PTEN/AKT pathway and is associated with poor prognosis in lung cancer. *Oncogene* **2012**, *31*, 2389–2400. [CrossRef] [PubMed]
13. Luo, Q.; Lei, B.; Liu, S.; Chen, Y.; Sheng, W.; Lin, P.; Li, W.; Zhu, H.; Shen, H. Expression of PBK/TOPK in cervical cancer and cervical intraepithelial neoplasia. *Int. J. Clin. Exp. Pathol.* **2014**, *7*, 8059–8064. [PubMed]
14. Dou, X.; Wei, J.; Sun, A.; Shao, G.; Childress, C.; Yang, W.; Lin, Q. PBK/TOPK mediates geranylgeranylation signaling for breast cancer cell proliferation. *Cancer Cell Int.* **2015**, *15*, 27. [CrossRef] [PubMed]
15. Qiao, J.X.; Wang, T.C.; Ruel, R.; Thibeault, C.; L'Heureux, A.; Schumacher, W.A.; Spronk, S.A.; Hiebert, S.; Bouthillier, G.; Lloyd, J.; et al. Conformationally constrained *ortho*anilino diaryl ureas, discovery of 1-(2-(1′-neopentylspiro[indoline-3,4′-piperidine]-1-yl)phenyl)-3-(4-(trifluoro-methoxy) phenyl)urea, a potent, selective, and bioavailable P2Y1 antagonist. *J. Med. Chem.* **2013**, *56*, 9275–9295. [CrossRef] [PubMed]
16. Anderson, J.W.; Sarantakis, D.; Terpinski, J.; Kumar, T.R.; Tsai, H.C.; Kuo, M.; Ager, A.L.; Jacobs, W.R., Jr.; Schiehser, G.A.; Ekins, S.; et al. Novel diaryl ureas with efficacy in a mouse model of malaria. *Bioorg. Med. Chem. Lett.* **2013**, *23*, 1022–1025. [CrossRef] [PubMed]

17. Keche, A.P.; Hatnapure, G.D.; Tale, R.H.; Rodge, A.H.; Kamble, V.M. Synthesis, anti-inflammatory and antimicrobial evaluation of novel 1-acetyl-3,5-diaryl-4,5-dihydro (1H) pyrazole derivatives bearing urea, thiourea and sulfonamide moieties. *Bioorg. Med. Chem. Lett.* **2012**, *22*, 6611–6615. [CrossRef] [PubMed]
18. Keche, A.P.; Hatnapure, G.D.; Tale, R.H.; Rodge, A.H.; Birajdar, S.S.; Kamble, V.M. A novel pyrimidine derivatives with aryl urea, thiourea and sulfonamide moieties, synthesis, anti-inflammatory and antimicrobial evaluation. *Bioorg. Med. Chem. Lett.* **2012**, *22*, 3445–3448. [CrossRef] [PubMed]
19. Kulkarni, R.G.; Laufer, S.; Mangannavar, C.; Garlapati, A. Design, synthesis and characterization of N′, N″-diaryl ureas as p38 kinase inhibitors. *Med. Chem.* **2013**, *9*, 213–221. [CrossRef]
20. Xuan, W.; Ding, W.; Hui, H.X. Synthesis and cytotoxic activity of diaryl urea derivatives with a 4-methylpiperazinylcarbonyl moiety. *Med. Chem. Res.* **2013**, *22*, 3857–3862. [CrossRef]
21. Lu, C.; Tang, K.; Li, Y.; Li, P.; Lin, Z.; Yin, D.; Chen, X.; Huang, H. Design, synthesis and evaluation of novel diaryl urea derivative as potent antitumor agents. *Eur. J. Med. Chem.* **2014**, *77*, 351–360. [CrossRef] [PubMed]
22. Kim, H.J.; Cho, H.J.; Kim, H.; El-Gamal, M.I.; Oh, C.H.; Lee, S.H.; Sim, T.; Hah, J.M.; Yoo, K.H. New diarylureas and diarylamides possessing acet(benz)amidophenyl scaffold, design, synthesis, and antiproliferative activity against melanoma cell line. *Bioorg. Med. Chem. Lett.* **2012**, *22*, 3269–3273. [CrossRef] [PubMed]
23. Claudio, V.J.; Amanda, D.; Vanderlan da Silva, B.; Eliezer, J.B.; Carlos alberto manssour, F. Molecular hybridization: a useful tool in the design of new drug prototypes. *Curr. Med. Chem.* **2007**, *14*, 1829–1852. [CrossRef]
24. Seto, M.; Miyamoto, N.; Aikawa, K.; Aramaki, Y.; Kanzaki, N.; Iizawa, Y.; Babab, M.; Shiraishia, M. Orally active CCR5 antagonists as anti-HIV-1 agents. Part 3: Synthesis and biological activities of 1-benzazepine derivatives containing a sulfoxide moiety. *Bioorg. Med. Chem.* **2005**, *13*, 363–386. [CrossRef] [PubMed]
25. Nguyen, T.; Yang, T.M.; Go, M.L. Functionalized acridin-9-yl phenylamines protected neuronal HT22 cells from glutamate-induced cell death by reducing intracellular levels of free radical species. *Bioorg. Med. Chem. Lett.* **2014**, *24*, 1830–1838. [CrossRef] [PubMed]
26. Liu, D.Z.; Tian, Z.; Yan, Z.H.; Wu, L.X.; Ma, Y.; Wang, Q.; Liu, W.; Zhou, H.G.; Yang, C. Design, synthesis and evaluation of 1,2-benzisothiazol-3-one derivatives as potent caspase-3 inhibitors. *Bioorg. Med. Chem.* **2013**, *21*, 2960–2967. [CrossRef] [PubMed]
27. Mosmann, T. Rapid colorimetric assay for cellular growth and survival: Application to proliferation and cytotoxicity assays. *J. Immun. Methods* **1983**, *65*, 55–63. [CrossRef]
28. Liu, C.M.; Zhang, M.; Zhang, Z.H.; Zhang, S.B.; Yang, S.M.; Zhang, A.; Yin, L.J.; Swarts, S.; Vidyasagar, S.; Zhang, L.R.; et al. Synthesis and anticancer potential of novel xanthone derivatives with 3,6-substituted chains. *Bioorg. Med. Chem.* **2016**, *24*, 4263–4271. [CrossRef] [PubMed]
29. Zhang, L.; Deng, X.S.; Zhang, C.; Meng, G.P.; Wu, J.F.; Li, X.S.; Zhao, Q.C.; Hu, C. Design, synthesis and cytotoxic evaluation of a novel series of benzo[*d*]thiazole-2-carboxamide derivatives as potential EGFR inhibitors. *Med. Chem. Res.* **2017**, *26*, 2180–2189. [CrossRef]
30. Ke, J.; Lu, Q.; Wang, X.; Sun, R.; Jin, Z.; Zhan, X.; Hu, J.; Wan, D.C.; Hu, C. Discovery of 4,5-Dihydro-1*H*-thieno[2′,3′:2,3]thiepino [4,5-c]pyrazole-3-carboxamide Derivatives as the Potential Epidermal Growth Factor Receptors for Tyrosine Kinase Inhibitors. *Molecules* **2018**, *23*, 1980. [CrossRef]
31. Yan, Q.; Li, R.X.; Xin, A.Y.; Han, Y.; Zhang, Y.X.; Liu, J.X.; Li, W.G.; Di, D.L. Design, synthesis, and anticancer properties of isocorydine derivatives. *Bioorg. Med. Chem.* **2017**, *25*, 6542–6553. [CrossRef] [PubMed]
32. Xu, Y.M.; Jing, D.W.; Chen, R.; Rashid, U.H.; Jiang, J.; Liu, X.; Wang, L.S.; Xie, P. Design, synthesis and evaluation of novel sophoridinic imine derivatives containing conjugated planar structure as potent anticancer agents. *Bioorg. Med. Chem.* **2018**, *26*, 4136–4144. [CrossRef] [PubMed]

Sample Availability: Samples of all the target compounds are available from the authors.

molecules

MDPI

Article

Potent Cytotoxicity of Novel L-Shaped Ortho-Quinone Analogs through Inducing Apoptosis

Sheng-You Li [1,2], Ze-Kun Sun [2,3], Xue-Yi Zeng [2,4], Yue Zhang [2,5], Meng-Ling Wang [2,4], Sheng-Cao Hu [4], Jun-Rong Song [2,4], Jun Luo [4], Chao Chen [2,4,*], Heng Luo [2,4,*] and Wei-Dong Pan [1,2,4,*]

1 College of Pharmacy, Guizhou University, Huaxi Avenue South, Guiyang 550025, China; 13118517665@163.com
2 State Key Laboratory of Functions and Applications of Medicinal Plants, Guizhou Medical University, 3491 Baijin Road, Guiyang 550014, China; xueyizeng@126.com (X.-Y.Z.); menglingwang@yahoo.com (M.-L.W.); 18275365116@163.com (J.-R.S.); 18798628024@163.com (J.L.)
3 School of Medicine, Guizhou University, Huaxi Avenue South, Guiyang 550025, China; zekunsun@163.com
4 The Key Laboratory of Chemistry for Natural Products of Guizhou Province and Chinese Academy of Sciences, 3491 Baijin Road, Guiyang 550014, China; hushengcao0221@163.com
5 College of Agriculture, Guizhou University, Huaxi Avenue South, Guiyang 550025, China; zhangyueinsect@163.com
* Correspondence: cc283818640@163.com (C.C.); luoheng@gzcnp.cn (H.L.); wdpan@163.com (W.D.P.); Tel.: +86-15597724842 (C.C.); +86-0851-83876210 (H.L.); +86-18985130307 (W.D.P.)

Academic Editor: Qiao-Hong Chen
Received: 10 October 2019; Accepted: 11 November 2019; Published: 15 November 2019

Abstract: Twenty-seven L-shaped ortho-quinone analogs were designed and synthesized using a one pot double-radical synthetic strategy followed by removing methyl at C-3 of the furan ring and introducing a diverse side chain at C-2 of the furan ring. The synthetic derivatives were investigated for their cytotoxicity activities against human leukemia cells K562, prostate cancer cells PC3, and melanoma cells WM9. Compounds **TB1, TB3, TB4, TB6, TC1, TC3, TC5, TC9, TC11, TC12, TC14, TC15, TC16,** and **TC17** exhibited a better broad-spectrum cytotoxicity on three cancer cells. **TB7** and **TC7** selectively displayed potent inhibitory activities on leukemia cells K562 and prostate cancer cells PC3, respectively. Further studies indicated that **TB3, TC1, TC3, TC7,** and **TC17** could significantly induce the apoptosis of PC3 cells. **TC1** and **TC17** significantly induced apoptosis of K562 cells. **TC1, TC11,** and **TC14** induced significant apoptosis of WM9 cells. The structure-activity relationships evaluation showed that removing methyl at C-3 of the furan ring and introducing diverse side chains at C-2 of the furan ring is an effective strategy for improving the anticancer activity of L-shaped ortho-quinone analogs.

Keywords: ortho-quinones; antitumor activity; beta-lapachone; tanshione IIA

1. Introduction

Over several decades, cancer continues to be the most awful disease due to its uncontrolled cell growth and the fact that it is a dominate killer of human beings worldwide [1]. Especially in China, millions of deaths have been caused by tumor. The common cancer types in Chinese male, in 2018, were lung, stomach, colorectum, liver, and esophageal cancer. Additionally, breast, lung, colorectum, thyroid, and stomach cancer were the common types in Chinese female [2]. The incidence of colorectal cancer in males and females has increased, however, the incidence of esophageal, stomach, and liver cancer has decreased between 2000 and 2011 [3]. Meanwhile, the incidence and mortality of prostate cancer and bladder cancer in males, together with obesity and hormonal exposure-related cancers, namely thyroid, breast, and ovarian cancer in females have shown a rising trend [3]. However, the standardized treatments of cancer, including surgery, chemotherapy, and radiation therapy, show many limitations, such as severe adverse effects, recurrence, and increasing drug resistance [4].

Currently, phytochemicals have become a valuable source of anticancer drugs. Actually, over 75% of nonbiological anticancer drugs approved are either plant-derived natural products or developed based on these products [5]. Therefore, natural products have continued to be a hot research topic for the development of new antitumor drugs [6–9].

Tanshinone IIA is a natural ortho-quinone isolated from the rhizome of *Salvia miltiorrhiza Bunge* with antineoplastic activity, such as gastric cancer, breast cancer, osteosarcoma, etc. [10–13]. These various properties demonstrate that tanshinone IIA is a potential antitumor drug candidate. Furthermore, beta-lapachone is another natural ortho-quinone which has been reported to selectively kill many human cancer cells [14], however, the pyran ring of beta-lapachone has been found to be unstable during metabolism in the human body, and may led to side effects on normal tissues [15,16]. Recently, studies have revealed that some tanshinone analogs show similar or stronger antitumor activity when the ring-A is removed but the furan ring is retained [17,18]. You et al. [19,20] discovered that the binding site for quinone oxidoreductase-1 (NQO1) substrates was an L-shaped pocket (Figure 1B) which binds well with tanshinone analogs, and showed higher antitumor activities than the planar compound **1** and beta-lapachone. Therefore, we surmise that removing methyl at C-3 of the furan ring is more suitable for the binding site, and we anticipate that a novel L-shaped molecule without methyl at C-3 of the furan ring could provide better antitumor activities. Considering that some nitrogen, oxygen-substituted, and amino acid substrates can improve aqueous solubility and antitumor activities [21–25], we have attempted to introduce a great diversity of oxygen-substituted, nitrogen-containing groups and amino acids. Thus, in this work, we developed quinone-directed agents by removing methyl at C-3 of the furan ring and introducing a diverse side chain at C-2 of the furan ring, culminating in the discovery of a promising scaffold. The inhibitory activity was assessed in vitro using three cell lines including K562, PC3, and WM9.

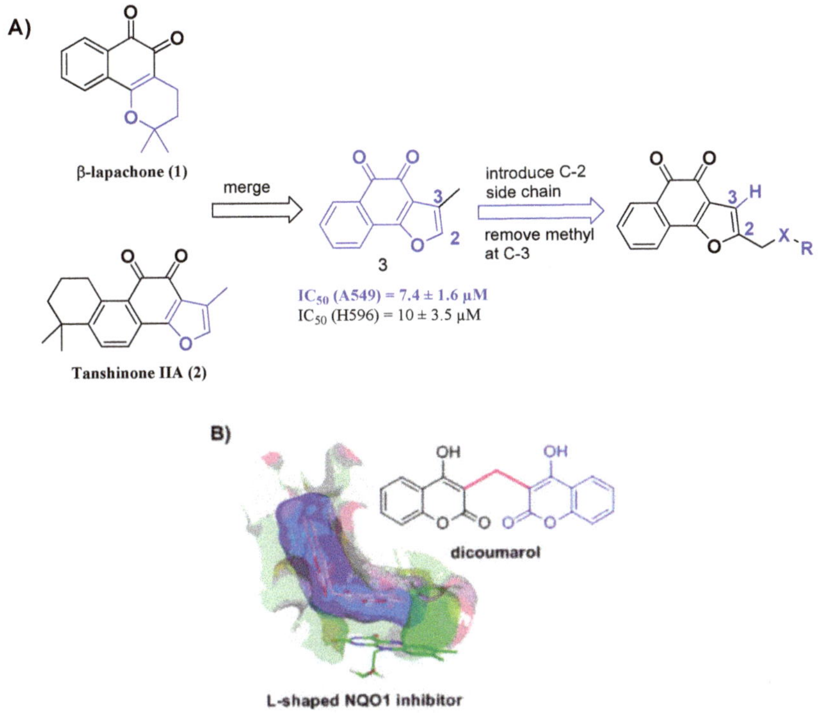

Figure 1. (**A**) Structural design strategy and (**B**) L-shaped pocket. The figure is available in reference [19].

2. Discussion and Results

2.1. Chemistry

The synthesis of two substituted naphtho[1,2-b]furan-4,5-diones is outlined in Scheme 1. Briefly, treatment of lawsone **6** with allyl bromide followed by subsequent Claisen rearrangement afforded **7**, which was then cyclized to get the ortho-quinone **8** by using Lewis acid $NbCl_5$ at room temperature [26].

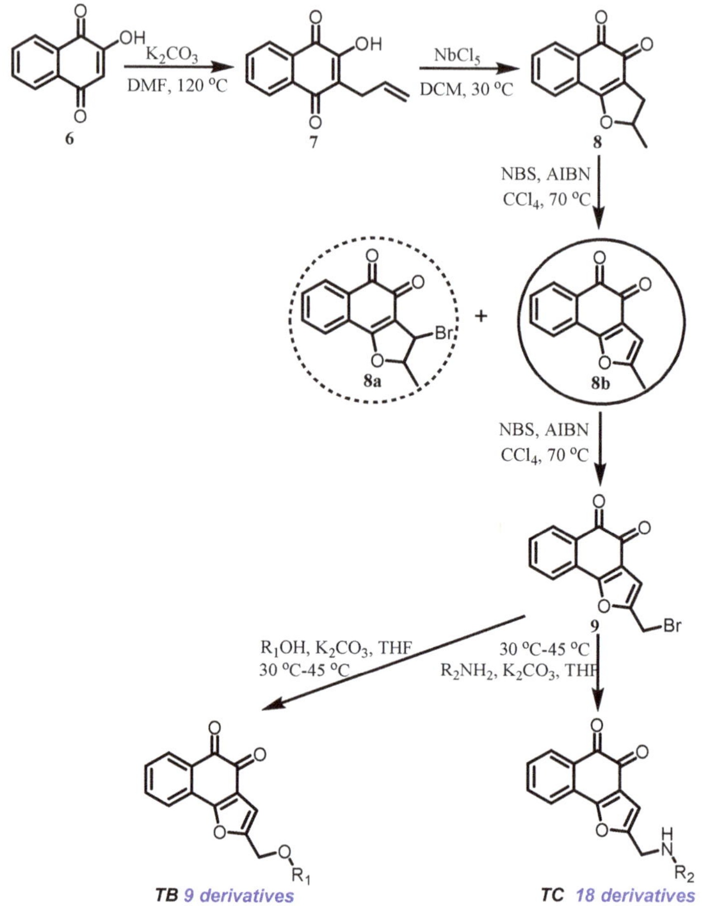

Scheme 1. Synthesis of L-shaped ortho-quinone analogs.

Initially, dealing **8** with *N*-bromosuccinimide (NBS) and 2,2′-azobis(2-methylpropionitrile) (AIBN) afforded only trace amounts of **8a**. Another intermediate, **8b**, was obtained by Nelson's method [27] as shown in Scheme 1. Then, compound **9** was obtained from **8b** through a second radical reaction. Considering the same reaction condition, we successfully got **9** from **8** through a bis-radical reaction. The brominated intermediate **9** was reacted with substituted phenol or amine to provide ortho-quinone derivatives **TB1–TB9** and **TC1–TC18**, respectively. All the structures of ortho-quinone derivatives were identified through ^{1}H, ^{13}C, and HRMS.

In summary, we successfully established an effective synthetic strategy, which removed the methyl at C-3 of the furan ring and introduced diverse side chains at C-2 of the furan ring. In addition, we replaced the bromide of **9** with a variety of oxygen-substituted, nitrogen-containing group, and amino acid by a nucleophilic substitution.

2.2. *In Vitro Cytotoxicity Assay*

The cytotoxic activities of 5 μmol/L of the synthesized L-shaped ortho-quinone analogs were determined by using three cancer cell lines (Table 1). The results revealed that compounds **TB1, TB3, TB4, TB6, TC1, TC3, TC5, TC9, TC11, TC12, TC15, TC16,** and **TC17** showed a broad-spectrum potent inhibitory activity on the proliferation of the cancer cell lines, with a more than 70% inhibition rate, and **TB7** showed better inhibitory activity on K562 cells as compared with other cells. Moreover, we observed that **TC7** inhibited the growth of PC3 cells more efficiently than other cells.

Table 1. The structures and inhibitory rates after treating cancer cell lines with 5 μmol/L of target compounds, respectively. Data was presented as the mean ± SD of three independent experiments.

Compounds	R	Inhibition (%)		
		PC3	K562	WM9
TB1	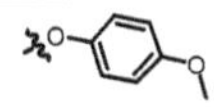	92.078 ± 1.885	88.641 ± 3.055	80.287 ± 6.354
TB2	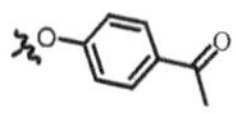	58.700 ± 29.309	20.642 ± 16.695	9.216 ± 2.449
TB3	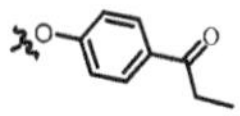	91.861 ± 2.125	83.613 ± 10.448	54.153 ± 3.948
TB4	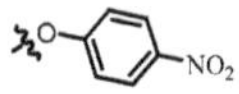	92.224 ± 1.811	91.192 ± 1.479	87.963 ± 2.430
TB5	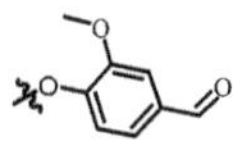	30.673 ± 54.356	49.127 ± 33.985	64.870 ± 2.894
TB6	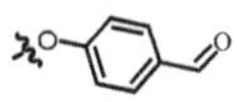	87.165 ± 1.953	82.901 ± 1.484	89.843 ± 2.010
TB7	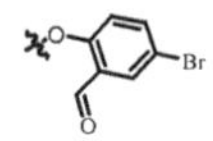	−7.664 ± 10.055	81.835 ± 1.553	31.754 ± 6.422
TB8		9.692 ± 11.981	7.191 ± 4.705	49.307 ± 3.791
TB9	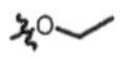	−17.125 ± 11.619	15.334 ± 9.484	−0.591 ± 1.055
TC1	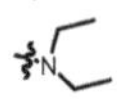	91.027 ± 0.553	83.717 ± 3.469	84.117 ± 2.686
TC2	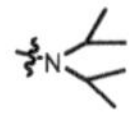	−0.437 ± 1.129	25.032±2.579	16.431±1.583
TC3	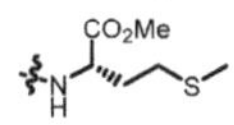	78.849 ± 13.221	83.518 ± 12.045	81.670 ± 0.994
TC4	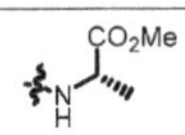	24.242 ± 18.544	0.082 ± 15.067	15.453 ± 1.508
TC5	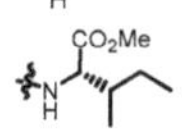	89.676 ± 0.331	81.950 ± 12.469	72.452 ± 8.039
TC6	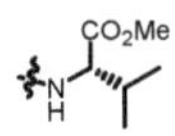	43.133 ± 11.878	31.137 ± 16.045	63.384 ± 8.949
TC7	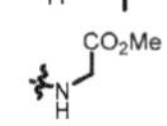	82.402 ± 4.585	30.087 ± 20.307	16.191 ± 2.699
TC8	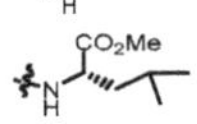	44.842 ± 25.172	28.448 ± 30.220	0.468 ± 5.166

Table 1. *Cont.*

Compounds	R	Inhibition (%) PC3	K562	WM9
TC9	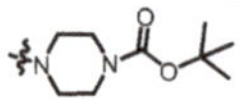	89.869 ± 1.839	81.545 ± 6.968	83.003 ± 2.806
TC10	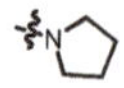	−6.375 ± 8.094	−9.749 ± 17.889	1.005 ± 2.601
TC11	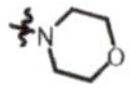	90.214 ± 0.520	85.766 ± 1.737	85.807 ± 3.752
TC12	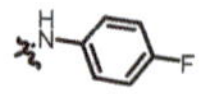	82.522 ± 9.039	83.688 ± 8.252	61.839 ± 3.448
TC13	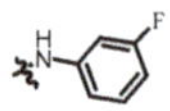	74.681 ± 2.470	84.251 ± 1.430	39.955 ± 6.425
TC14	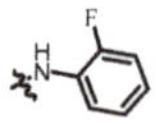	4.453 ± 5.002	84.497 ± 0.876	90.717 ± 1.184
TC15	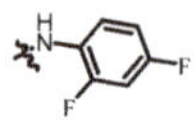	84.916 ± 1.761	84.185 ± 0.419	90.135 ± 1.602
TC16	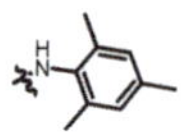	78.720 ± 7.560	84.323 ± 1.273	90.520 ± 2.108
TC17	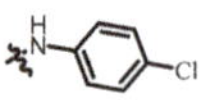	86.637 ± 2.482	83.999 ± 0.943	72.021 ± 6.850
TC18	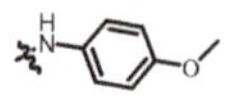	−5.220 ± 13.979	8.854 ± 12.236	1.410 ± 5.093
tanshinone IIA		89.458 ± 1.987	82.215 ± 4.069	85.236 ± 3.654
Paclitaxel		81.589 ± 1.763	91.315 ± 2.467	78.369 ± 6.380

The concentration inhibition curves (Figure 2) were analyzed to calculate the IC_{50} values of the selected active compounds. The results indicated there was a dose-dependent trend of the inhibitory response of all active compounds on three cancer cells for treating 48 h. The IC_{50} values were summarized in Table 2 and show that the cytotoxicity of compounds **TB3, TC1, TC3, TC7, TC9,** and **TC17** on PC3 were better ($P < 0.05$) than that of the positive control (tanshinone IIA and paclitaxel), and another active compound exhibited similar activity to that of the positive control. The inhibition activity of **TC1** against the growth of K562 was better than that of the positive control, paclitaxel, and tanshinone IIA. Compounds **TB6, TC1, TC11, TC14,** and **TC15** inhibited the growth of WM9 better ($P < 0.05$) than that of tanshinone IIA and paclitaxel. In summary, most of novel L-shaped ortho-quinone analogs exhibited relatively better cytotoxicity activity as compared with the two positive controls, which indicated that the analogs containing L-shaped ortho-quinone as the core structure, possessed stronger anticancer activity. This result provided a preliminary biological activity basis for the investigation of anticancer candidate agents.

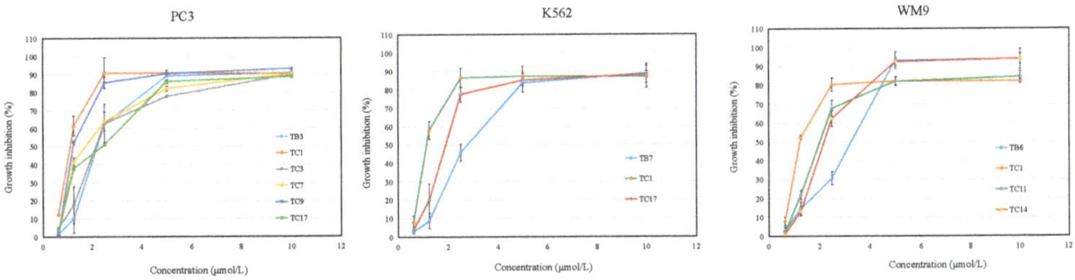

Figure 2. Growth inhibition induced by the active L-shaped ortho-quinone analogs on PC3, K562, and WM9 cells by MTT assay. The IC_{50} values (μM) of the compounds were determined according to these curves at different incubation times. The 100 μL tested compounds were added to 96-well microculture plates and 100 μL cells (a final concentration of 5×10^4/well) were incubated for 48 h at 37 °C. Cell survival was evaluated by MTT assay. The inhibition ratio (%) was calculated as described in the Methods section. Data was presented as mean ± SD of three independent experiments.

Table 2. IC_{50} values of selected compounds in vitro.

Compounds	IC_{50}/μM		
	PC3	K562	WM9
TB1	2.809 ± 0.413	3.157 ± 0.947 **	4.841 ± 0.301
TB3	1.121 ± 0.731 **	2.580 ± 0.285 **	NA [a]
TB4	3.348 ± 0.347	3.103 ± 0.702 **	3.358 ± 0.297
TB6	3.249 ± 0.464	2.964 ± 0.168 *	2.774 ± 0.299 **
TB7	NA	2.981 ± 0.368 **	NA
TC1	0.347 ± 0.290 **	0.379 ± 0.138	0.406 ± 0.117 **
TC3	1.778 ± 0.835 **	4.647 ± 0.647 **	4.990 ± 0.360
TC5	3.018 ± 0.452	3.448 ± 0.224 **	NA
TC7	1.507 ± 0.369 **	NA	NA
TC9	0.469 ± 0.281 **	4.194 ± 0.139 **	4.027 ± 0.341
TC11	2.578 ± 0.957	3.565 ± 0.344 **	2.127 ± 0.582 **
TC12	2.963 ± 0.261	4.157 ± 0.677 **	NA
TC13	3.433 ± 0.444	4.719 ± 0.984	NA
TC14	NA	3.100 ± 0.320 **	2.261 ± 0.111 **
TC15	3.696 ± 0.492	3.644 ± 0.524 **	3.050 ± 0.230 *
TC16	3.874 ± 0.557	2.640 ± 0.642 **	4.324 ± 0.292
TC17	1.914 ± 0.224 **	1.927 ± 0.414	NA
tanshinone IIA	3.162 ± 3.160	4.638 + 1.270	4.261 ± 0.182
Paclitaxel	4.323 ± 0.929	2.149 ± 0.406	4.835 ± 0.359

Note: * represents $p < 0.05$ and ** represents $p < 0.01$, vs. the inhibition of the positive control to the cancer cell lines. The data represented the average of three independent experiments.

2.3. Structure-Activity Relationships Study

To obtain two series of analogs, we successfully built an effective synthetic strategy by removing the methyl at C-3 of the furan ring and introducing diverse side chains at C-2 of the furan ring. On the basis of the cytotoxicity results (Tables 1 and 2), a preliminary structure-activity relationships could be established. The TB series molecules bearing electron-withdrawing groups or multi-substituted groups such as compounds **TB3**, **TB4**, and **TB6** showed a better inhibitory effect on PC3 cell lines, K562 cell lines, and WM9 cell lines, whereas the TB series molecules bearing alkane groups at the 2-position showed decreased cytotoxicity in PC3 cell lines, K562 cell lines, and WM9 cell lines, such as compounds **TB9**. The TC series molecules with electron-withdrawing groups, saturate six-membered rings, or multi-substituted groups emerged greater inhibitory effects on three cancer cell lines, such as **TC11**, **TC12**, **TC15**, and **TC16**, whereas the TC series molecules bearing donating groups or alkane groups at the 2-position showed reduced cytotoxicity in three cancer cell lines. The structure-activity relationships evaluation also showed that removing methyl at C-3 of the furan ring and introducing diverse side chains at C-2 of the furan ring were good strategies for improving the anticancer activity of L-shaped ortho-quinone analogs.

2.4. *Effects of Active Compounds on Cell Apoptosis*

According to the above IC_{50} values of all active compounds, we selected six active compounds (**TB3**, **TC1**, **TC3**, **TC7**, **TC9**, and **TC17**) for PC3, three active compounds (**TB6**, **TC1**, and **TC17**) for K562, and four active compounds (**TB6**, **TC1**, **TC11**, and **TC14**) for WM9, based on their higher activities than that of the positive control and better selectivity and, then, studied their effects on cell apoptosis by microscope observation (Figure 3) and flow cytometry (Figure 4). The microscopic observations (Figure 3A) showed that the number of PC3 cells was significantly reduced by treatments with 2.5 μmol/L of **TB3**, **TC1**, **TC3**, and **TC7**; the apoptotic bodies and cell fragments were significantly observed as compared with the control group. The PC3 cells treated with **TC9** showed that the number of cells were significantly reduced, while fewer cells died and there were no significant apoptotic bodies. The PC3 cells treated with **TC7** showed a significant decrease in the number of cells, meanwhile, some cells died, apoptotic bodies appeared obviously, and the morphology of some cells became an irregular shape of spindle length. Above all, the inhibitory activity of **TB3**, **TC1**, **TC3**, and **TC7** may be through inducing apoptosis, another two compounds may be through different types.

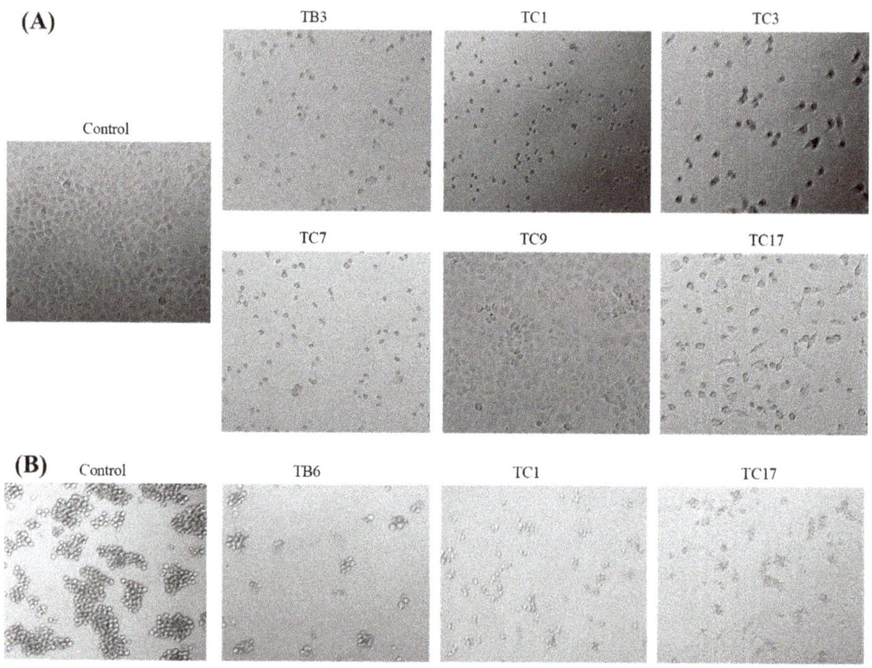

Figure 3. *Cont.*

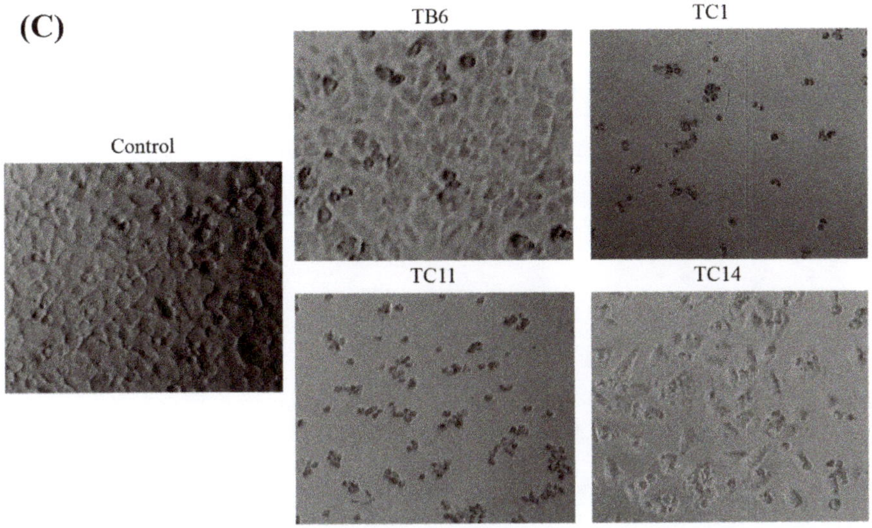

Figure 3. Effects of the active compounds on PC3 (**A**), K562 (**B**), and WM9 (**C**) cell growth and apoptosis. Cell number and morphological appearance of the two types of cell lines treated with 2.5 μmol/L of active compounds, then, it was observed by a fluorescent inverted microscope after 24 h. Scale bar = 100 μM in all images. All experiments were performed in triplicate.

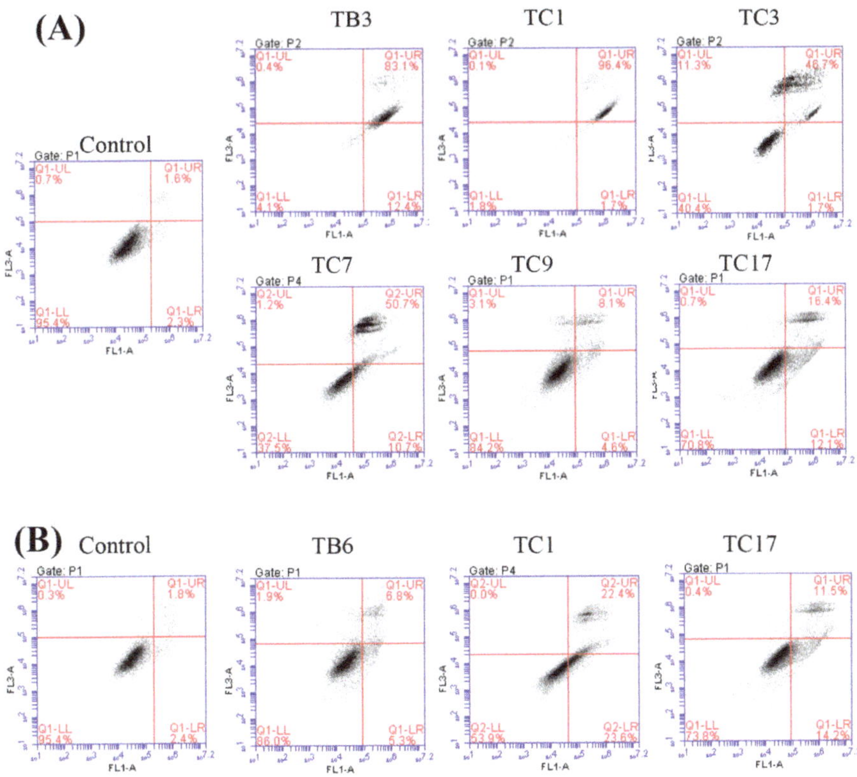

Figure 4. *Cont.*

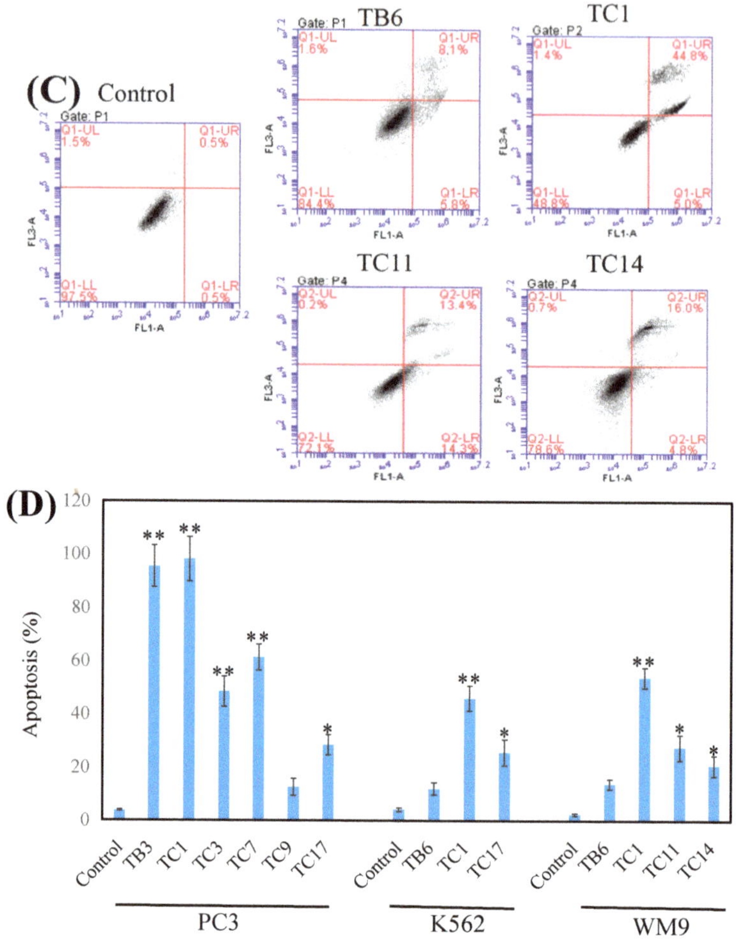

Figure 4. Effects of the active compounds on PC3 (**A**), K562 (**B**), and WM9 (**C**) cell growth and apoptosis. Cell apoptosis induced by the compounds and tested by flow cytometry and the date was analyzed with Origin Pro 9.0 (**D**) and presented as means ± SEM from at least three independent experiments. * $p < 0.05$, ** $p < 0.01$ ($n = 3$) as compared with the control.

The K562 cells treated with **TC1** were obviously dead and dispersed, with the appearance of apoptotic bodies as comparing with the control group (Figure 3B). The cells treated with **TB6** had a significantly reduced number of cells and most cells clumped growth similar to the control cells. For the cells treated with **TC17** we observed both dead cells and fewer clumps of cells. Furthermore, for the WM9 cell lines treated with **TB6**, **TC1**, **TC11**, and **TC14** (Figure 3C), we observed that the cells treated with **TC1** and **TC11** were obviously dead with a large number of apoptotic bodies and dispersed cells; the cells treated with **TB6** showed a significant decrease in the number of cells and fewer dead cells. Observation of the cells treated with **TC14** showed that the number of cells was significantly reduced, while some cells were obviously dead with apoptotic bodies appearing, and the morphology of some cells also became an irregular shape of spindle length. The above results indicated that **TC1** can induce apoptosis for K562 and WM9 cells to inhibit the growth; **TB6**, **TC11**, **TC14**, and **TC17** can jointly inhibit the proliferation of cell through a variety of mechanisms.

Flow cytometry analyzed results (Figure 4) confirmed that **TB3** ($p < 0.01$), **TC1** ($p < 0.01$), **TC3** ($p < 0.01$), **TC7** ($p < 0.01$), and **TC17** ($p < 0.05$) could significantly induce the apoptosis of PC3 cells (Figure 4A), while **TC9** did not. **TC1** ($p < 0.01$) and **TC17** ($p < 0.05$) significantly induced apoptosis of K562 cells (Figure 4B), while **TB6** had no significant effect on apoptosis of K562 and WM9 cells. **TC1** ($p < 0.01$), **TC11** ($p < 0.05$), and **TC14** ($p < 0.01$) could potently induce apoptosis for WM9 cells (Figure 4C).

3. Materials and Methods

3.1. Instruments and Materials

High-resolution mass spectra (HRMS) were obtained on an electrospray ionization (ESI) mode on a Bruker ESI-QTOF mass spectrometry. Nuclear magnetic resonance (NMR) spectra were recorded on a Bruker Avance NEO (^{1}H NMR, 600 MHz; ^{13}C NMR, 150 MHz, Bruker, Switzerland) with TMS as an internal standard. The IR spectra were recorded by using a FTIR Spectrometer (IR 200 Fourier Energy Spectrum Technology Co., Ltd., TianJin, China) and the KBr disk method was adopted. The melting points (mp) were determined on an WRX-4 microscope melting point apparatus. The column chromatography was performed on silica gel (Qingdao, 200–300 mesh) and the thin-layer (0.25 mm) chromatography (TLC) analysis was carried out on silica gel plates (Qingdao, China). Other reagents were analytical grade or guaranteed reagent commercial product and used without further purification, unless otherwise noted.

3.2. Methods of Synthesis

3.2.1. Synthesis of 2-Allyl-3-hydroxy-1,4-naphthoquinone (7)

A mixture of lawsone **6** (10.0 g, 57.42 mmol) and anhydrous K_2CO_3 (7.94 g, 57.42 mmol) in anhydrous DMF (100 mL) were stirred for 15 min at room temperature. Allyl bromide (17.37 g, 143.55 mmol) in DMF (5 mL) was added dropwise and stirred for 15 min at 0 °C. The mixture was refluxed at 120 °C for 3 h and then cooled to room temperature before it was poured into water and extracted with EA. The organic phase was washed with brine, dried over Na_2SO_4, filtered, and concentrated in vacuo. The crude product was purified by column chromatography on silica gel (eluent: petroleum ether/EtOAc 15:1) to afford **7** (7.8 g, 63% yield) as a light yellow solid. Other data was found in reference [26].

3.2.2. Synthesis of 2-Methyl-2,3-dihydrolnaphthol[1,2-*b*]furan-4,5-dione (8)

$NbCl_5$ (18.92 g, 70.02 mmol) was added into **7** (3.0 g, 14.00 mmol) in anhydrous DCM (50 mL) at 0 °C. After stirring for 45 min at 30 °C, the mixture was poured into ice water and extracted with DCM. The organic phase was washed with brine, dried over Na_2SO_4, filtered, and concentrated in vacuo. The crude product was purified by column chromatography on silica gel (eluent: petroleum ether/EtOAc 4:1) to afford **8** (2.16 g, 72% yield) as red solid. Other data was found in reference [26].

3.2.3. Synthesis of 2-Bromomethyl-naphtho[1-*b*]furan-4,5-dione (9)

A mixture of **8** (1.5 g, 7.00 mmol), anhydrous *N*-bromosuccinimide (2.49 g, 1.40mmol), and 2,2′-azobis(2-methylpropionitrile) (114.98 mg, 1.40 mmol) in anhydrous CCl_4 (50 mL) was stirred under argon at 70 °C, until **8** were disappeared. Then, the mixture was cooled to room temperature, and anhydrous N-bromosuccinimide (2.49 g, 1.40 mmol) and 2,2′-azobis(2-methylpropionitrile) (114.98 mg, 1.40 mmol) were added and stirred at 70 °C for 2 h. The mixture was cooled to room temperature, and poured into water, extracted with EA, washed with brine, dried over Na_2SO_4, filtered, and concentrated in vacuo. The crude product was purified by column chromatography on silica gel (eluent: petroleum ether/EtOAc 12:1) to afford **9** (1.0 g, 67% yield) as red solid. Mp: 169–170 °C. ^{1}H NMR (600 MHz, $CDCl_3$) δ 8.09 (d, J = 7.8 Hz, 1H), 7.77 (d, J = 7.6 Hz, 1H), 7.69 (t, J = 7.6 Hz, 1H), 7.51 (t, J = 7.6 Hz, 1H), and 6.83 (s, 1H), 4.55 (s, 2H). ^{13}C NMR (150 MHz, $CDCl_3$) δ 180.06, 174.13, 160.94, 153.46, 135.56, 130.74, 130.69, 129.03, 127.98, 122.69, 122.34, 108.04, and 21.87. IR (ν, cm^{-1}): 3118.33, 2920.28, 2339.32, 1670.84, 1551.16, and 691.42. HRMS (ESI) calcd. for [M + Na]$^+$ $C_{13}H_7O_3BrNa^+$: 312.9471, found 312.9460.

3.2.4. Synthesis of **TB1–9** and **TC1–18**

A mixture of the corresponding amines or alcohols (0.52 mmol), K_2CO_3 (142 mg, 1.03 mmol), and **9** (100 mg, 0.34 mmol) in THF (5 mL) was stirred at 30 °C to 50 °C for 4 h. After cooling, the mixture was poured into water and extracted with EA. The combined organic layer was washed with brine and dried over anhydrous Na_2SO_4, filtered, and concentrated to afford a crude product which was purified through column chromatography on silica gel.

TB1: *2-(((4-methoxyphenyl)oxy)methyl)naphtho[1-b]furan-4,5-dione.* Red solid, yield: 34%. Mp: 112–113 °C. ^{1}H NMR (600 MHz, $CDCl_3$) δ 8.09 (d, J = 7.6 Hz, 1H), 7.75 (d, J = 7.6 Hz, 1H), 7.66 (t, J = 7.5 Hz, 1H), 7.48 (t, J = 7.6 Hz, 1H), 6.94–6.92 (m, 2H), 6.87–6.85 (m, 2H), 6.83 (s, 1H), 5.04 (s, 2H), and 3.78 (s, 3H). ^{13}C NMR (150 MHz, $CDCl_3$) δ 180.34, 174.38, 160.88, 154.72, 153.82, 151.95, 135.47, 130.66, 130.50, 128.98, 128.28, 122.59, 122.12, 116.34, 114.81, 108.37, 63.03, and 55.73. IR (ν, cm^{-1}): 3445.32, 2358.40, 2339.32, 1671.47, 1598.48, 1253.20, 1219.81, 1161.58, and 1057.34. HRMS (ESI) calcd. for [M + Na]$^+$ $C_{20}H_{14}O_5Na^+$: 357.0733, found 357.0723.

TB2: *2-(((4-acetylphenyl)oxy)methyl)naphtho[1,2-b]furan-4,5-dione.* Light orange solid, yield: 40%. Mp: 190–191 °C. ^{1}H NMR (600 MHz, $CDCl_3$) δ 8.13 (d, J = 6.4 Hz, 1H), 8.00 (d, J = 8.9 Hz, 2H), 7.78 (d, J = 9.1 Hz, 1H), 7.69 (t, J = 7.6 Hz, 1H), 7.53 (t, J = 7.6 Hz, 1H), 7.06 (d, J = 8.9 Hz, 2H), 6.94 (s, 1H), 5.19 (s, 2H), and 2.60 (s, 3H). ^{13}C NMR (150 MHz, $CDCl_3$) δ 196.71, 180.20, 174.31, 161.58, 161.10, 152.60, 135.53, 131.28, 130.74, 130.70, 129.02, 128.11, 122.64, 122.08, 114.48, 108.98, 61.92, and 26.43. IR (ν, cm^{-1}): 3445.93, 2358.51, 2341.16, 1671.86, 1599.84, 1249.41, 1217.01, 1178.57, and 1008.47. HRMS (ESI) calcd. for [M + Na]$^+$ $C_{21}H_{14}O_5Na^+$: 369.0733, found 369.0721.

TB3: *2-(((4-propiophenyl)oxy)methyl)naphtho[1,2-b]furan-4,5-dione.* Orange solid, yield: 37%. Mp: 179–180 °C. ^{1}H NMR (600 MHz, $CDCl_3$) δ 8.11 (d, J = 7.6 Hz, 1H), 8.00 (d, J = 8.9 Hz, 2H), 7.77 (d, J = 6.4 Hz, 1H), 7.71–7.68 (m, 1H), 7.53–7.50 (m, 1H), 7.06 (d, J = 8.9 Hz, 2H), 6.93 (s, 1H), 5.18 (s, 2H), 2.99 (q, J = 7.2 Hz, 2H), and 1.24 (t, J = 7.3 Hz, 3H). ^{13}C NMR (150 MHz, $CDCl_3$) δ 199.42, 180.20, 174.30, 161.40, 161.06, 152.68, 135.53, 130.98, 130.72, 130.68, 130.36, 129.01, 128.11, 122.63, 122.08, 114.47, 108.92, 61.90, 31.53, and 8.38. IR (ν, cm^{-1}): 3447.03, 2358.62, 2341.16, 1669.65, 1601.07, 1222.31, 1180.35, and 1002.86. HRMS (ESI) calcd. for [M + Na]$^+$ $C_{22}H_{16}O_5Na^+$: 383.0890, found 383.0876.

TB4: *2-(((4-nitrophenyl)oxy)methyl)naphtho[1,2-b]furan-4,5-dione.* Red solid, yield: 48%. Mp: 205–206 °C. ^{1}H NMR (600 MHz, DMSO-d_6) δ 8.25 (d, J = 9.3 Hz, 2H), 7.96 (d, J = 7.6 Hz, 1H), 7.77–7.74 (m, 2H), 7.59–7.55 (m, 1H), 7.34 (d, J = 9.3 Hz, 2H), 7.18 (s, 1H), and 5.42 (s, 2H). ^{13}C NMR (150 MHz, DMSO-d_6) δ 179.58, 174.56, 163.29, 160.07, 152.42, 141.83, 135.43, 130.84, 130.17, 129.83, 127.89, 126.41, 122.50, 122.36, 115.94, 110.32, and 62.45. IR (ν, cm^{-1}): 3445.75, 2358.70, 2341.16, 1681.37,1592.17, 1507.95, 1384.15, 1340.19, 1277.67, and 1110.13. HRMS (ESI) calcd. for [M + Na]$^+$ $C_{19}H_{11}O_6NNa^+$: 372.0479, found 372.0465.

TB5: *2-(((2-methoxyl-4-formyl)phenyl)oxy)methyl)naphtho[1,2-b]furan-4,5-dione.* Red solid, yield: 34%. Mp: 203–204 °C. ^{1}H NMR (600 MHz, $CDCl_3$) δ 9.91 (s, 1H), 8.13 (d, J = 6.4 Hz, 1H), 7.77 (d, J = 7.6 Hz, 1H), 7.72–7.68 (m, 1H), 7.54–7.48 (m, 3H), 7.15 (d, J = 8.0 Hz, 1H), 6.96 (s, 1H), 5.28 (s, 2H), and 3.97 (s, 3H). ^{13}C NMR (150 MHz, $CDCl_3$) δ 190.88, 180.19, 174.31, 161.15, 152.50, 152.42, 150.30, 135.52, 131.28, 130.75, 129.67, 129.03, 128.10, 122.68, 122.09, 115.30, 112.93, 109.87, 109.40, 62.85, and 56.09. IR (ν, cm^{-1}): 3446.32, 2358.18, 2341.16, 1702.84, 1676.79, 1586.53, 1508.23, 1267.05, 1236.25, 1137.10, and 999.76. HRMS (ESI) calcd. for [M + Na]$^+$ $C_{21}H_{14}O_6Na^+$: 385.0683, found 385.0668.

TB6: *2-(((4-formylphenyl)oxy)methyl)naphtho[1,2-b]furan-4,5-dione.* Orange solid, yield: 30%. Mp: 212–213 °C. ^{1}H NMR (600 MHz, $CDCl_3$) δ 9.95 (s, 1H), 8.13 (d, J = 7.8 Hz, 1H), 7.92 (d, J = 8.9 Hz, 2H), 7.78 (d, J = 7.8 Hz, 1H), 7.73–7.69 (m, 1H), 7.56–7.51 (m, 1H), 7.14 (d, J = 8.7 Hz, 2H), 6.96 (s, 1H), and 5.21 (s, 2H). ^{13}C NMR (150 MHz, $CDCl_3$) δ 190.71, 180.17, 174.30, 162.67, 161.14, 152.36, 135.53, 132.10, 130.82, 130.77, 130.74, 129.05, 128.09, 122.64, 122.08, 115.06, 109.11, and 61.99. IR (ν, cm^{-1}): 3446.21,

2358.24, 2337.30, 1687.41, 1671.45, 1598.48, 1253.19, 1219.95, 1161.49, and 1057.40. HRMS (ESI) calcd. for [M + Na]$^+$ $C_{20}H_{12}O_5Na^+$: 355.0577, found 355.0565.

TB7: *2-(((4-bromo-2-formyl)phenyl)oxy)methyl)naphtho[1,2-b]furan-4,5-dione.* Light orange solid, yield: 33%. Mp: 201–202 °C. ^{1}H NMR (600 MHz, $CDCl_3$) δ 10.43 (s, 1H), 8.14 (d, *J* = 7.6 Hz, 1H), 7.99 (d, *J* = 2.7 Hz, 1H), 7.76 (d, *J* = 7.6 Hz, 1H), 7.73–7.69 (m, 2H), 7.57–7.51 (m, 1H), 7.06 (d, *J* = 8.7 Hz, 1H), 6.96 (s, 1H), and 5.24 (s, 2H). ^{13}C NMR (150 MHz, $CDCl_3$) δ 187.86, 180.06, 174.25, 161.30, 158.94, 151.80, 138.27, 135.59, 131.52, 130.87, 130.82, 129.07, 127.95, 126.84, 122.64, 121.99, 115.01, 114.95, 109.43, and 62.80. IR (ν, cm^{-1}): 3445.63, 2358.34, 2337.30, 1671.90, 1599.56, 1556.29, 1249.42, 1217.50, 1178.60, and 1008.51. HRMS (ESI) calcd. for [M + Na]$^+$ $C_{20}H_{11}O_5BrNa^+$: 432.9682, found 432.9673.

TB8: *2-(methoxymethyl)naphtho[1,2-b]furan-4,5-dione.* Red solid, yield: 12%. Mp: 53–54 °C. ^{1}H NMR (600 MHz, $CDCl_3$) δ 8.11 (dd, *J* = 7.8, 1.5 Hz, 1H), 7.78 (dd, *J* = 7.7, 1.4 Hz, 1H), 7.70–7.66 (m, 1H), 7.52–7.48 (m, 1H), 6.80 (s, 1H), 4.51 (s, 2H), and 3.46 (s, 3H). ^{13}C NMR (150 MHz, $CDCl_3$) δ 180.43, 174.46, 160.91, 154.77, 135.45, 130.64, 130.44, 128.96, 128.34, 122.59, 122.05, 107.97, 66.02, and 58.32. IR (ν, cm^{-1}): 3446.10, 2358.55, 2337.96, 1677.60, 1276.65, 1216.21, 1153.22, and 1082.89. HRMS (ESI) calcd. for [M + Na]$^+$ $C_{14}H_{10}O_4Na^+$: 265.0471, found 265.0463.

TB9: *2-(ethoxymethyl)naphtho[1,2-b]furan-4,5-dione.* Red solid, yield: 11%. Mp: 60–61 °C. ^{1}H NMR (600 MHz, $CDCl_3$) δ 8.10 (dd, *J* = 8.2, 1.3 Hz, 1H), 7.77 (dd, *J* = 7.6, 1.2 Hz, 1H), 7.71–7.65 (m, 1H), 7.52–7.46 (m, 1H), 6.78 (s, 1H), 4.55 (s, 2H), 3.63 (q, *J* = 7.0 Hz, 2H), and 1.29 (t, *J* = 7.0 Hz, 3H). ^{13}C NMR (150 MHz, $CDCl_3$) δ 180.47, 174.45, 160.81, 155.23, 135.45, 130.61, 130.37, 128.90, 128.39, 122.59, 122.08, 107.66, 66.26, 64.25, and 15.10. IR (ν, cm^{-1}): 3446.08, 2358.74, 2342.78, 1681.54, 1275.43, 1215.49, 1159.01, and 1083.47. HRMS (ESI) calcd. for [M + Na]$^+$ $C_{15}H_{12}O_4Na^+$: 279.0628, found 279.0621.

TC1: *2-(diethylaminomethyl)naphtho[1,2-b]furan-4,5-dione.* Red solid, yield: 51%. Mp: 78–79 °C. ^{1}H NMR (600 MHz, $CDCl_3$) δ 8.07 (d, *J* = 7.6 Hz, 1H), 7.72 (d, *J* = 7.6 Hz, 1H), 7.65 (t, *J* = 7.0 Hz, 1H), 7.46 (t, *J* = 7.6 Hz, 1H), 6.66 (s, 1H), 3.77 (s, 2H), 2.62 (q, *J* = 7.2 Hz, 4H), and 1.14 (t, *J* = 7.2 Hz, 6H). ^{13}C NMR (150 MHz, $CDCl_3$) δ 180.65, 174.55, 160.34, 156.44, 135.41, 130.55, 130.12, 128.74, 128.58, 122.45, 122.21, 107.11, 48.69, 47.10, and 12.01. IR (ν, cm^{-1}): 3445.24, 2953.88, 2358.48, 2339.23, 1700.91, 1676.52, 1216.10, and 1111.39. HRMS (ESI) calcd. for [M + Na]$^+$ $C_{17}H_{18}O_3Na^+$: 284.1281, found 284.1271.

TC2: *2-(diisopropylaminomethyl)naphtho[1,2-b]furan-4,5-dione.* Red solid, yield: 18%. Mp: 69–70 °C. ^{1}H NMR (600 MHz, $CDCl_3$) δ 8.06 (d, *J* = 7.8 Hz, 1H), 7.68 (d, *J* = 6.2 Hz, 1H), 7.64 (t, *J* = 7.5 Hz, 1H), 7.44 (t, *J* = 6.7 Hz, 1H), 6.66 (s, 1H), 3.72 (s, 2H), 3.13 (p, *J* = 6.5 Hz, 2H), and 1.08 (d, *J* = 6.7 Hz, 12H). ^{13}C NMR (150 MHz, $CDCl_3$) δ 180.88, 174.66, 161.17, 159.76, 135.37, 130.50, 129.81, 128.91, 128.65, 122.50, 122.09, 105.12, 49.12, 42.36, and 20.81. IR (ν, cm^{-1}): 3445.80, 2966.49, 2358.61, 2337.30, 1676.07, 1558.32, 1215.85, and 1149.51. HRMS (ESI) calcd. for [M + Na]$^+$ $C_{19}H_{22}O_3Na^+$: 312.1594, found 312.1583.

TC3: *2-((L-methionine methyl ester-1-yl)methyl)naphtho[1,2-b]furan-4,5-dione.* Red solid, yield: 12%. Mp: 52–53 °C. ^{1}H NMR (600 MHz, $CDCl_3$) δ 8.08 (d, *J* = 7.8 Hz, 1H), 7.72 (d, *J* = 7.6 Hz, 1H), 7.66 (t, *J* = 7.6 Hz, 1H), 7.47 (t, *J* = 7.6 Hz, 1H), 6.66 (s, 1H), 3.95 (d, *J* = 15.1 Hz, 1H), 3.79 (d, *J* = 15.1 Hz, 1H), 3.74 (s, 3H), 3.52 (dd, *J* = 8.4, 5.0 Hz, 1H), 2.64 (t, *J* = 7.2 Hz, 2H), 2.10 (s, 3H), 2.02–1.97 (m, 1H) and 1.89–1.82 (m, 1H). ^{13}C NMR (150 MHz, $CDCl_3$) δ 180.55, 175.18, 174.44, 160.36, 157.00, 135.44, 130.58, 130.19, 128.80, 128.47, 122.35, 122.17, 106.00, 59.14, 52.14, 44.65, 32.68, 30.48, and 15.38. IR (ν, cm^{-1}): 3446.14, 2923.56, 2358.62, 2335.37, 1698.61, 1670.40, 1215.45, and 1147.65. HRMS (ESI) calcd. for [M + Na]$^+$ $C_{19}H_{19}O_5NSNa^+$: 396.0876, found 396.0865.

TC4: *2-((L-alanine methyl ester-1-yl)methyl)naphtho[1,2-b]furan-4,5-dione.* Red solid, yield: 27%. Mp: 83–84 °C. ^{1}H NMR (600 MHz, $CDCl_3$) δ 8.07 (d, *J* = 6.9 Hz, 1H), 7.73 (d, *J* = 4.9 Hz, 1H), 7.65 (d, *J* = 8.6 Hz, 1H), 7.46 (t, *J* = 6.6 Hz, 1H), 6.66 (s, 1H), 3.94 (d, *J* = 14.1 Hz, 1H), 3.81 (d, *J* = 14.9 Hz, 1H), 3.74 (s, 3H), 3.46 (q, *J* = 6.9 Hz, 1H), and 1.37 (d, *J* = 6.6 Hz, 3H). ^{13}C NMR (150 MHz, $CDCl_3$) δ 180.52, 175.63, 174.42, 160.36, 156.93, 135.40, 130.56, 130.18, 128.80, 128.46, 122.39, 122.18, 105.99, 55.69, 52.05, 44.26, and 19.13. IR (ν, cm^{-1}): 3328.35, 2958.60, 2358.44, 2337.30, 1735.12, 1676.39, 1216.30, and 1139.72. HRMS (ESI) calcd. for [M + Na]$^+$ $C_{17}H_{15}O_5NNa^+$: 336.0842, found 336.0831.

TC5: *2-((L-isoleucinate methyl ester-1-yl)methyl)naphtho[1,2-b]furan-4,5-dione.* Red solid, yield: 39%. Mp: 112–113 °C. ^{1}H NMR (600 MHz, $CDCl_3$) δ 8.07 (d, *J* = 7.7 Hz, 1H), 7.71 (d, *J* = 7.7 Hz, 1H), 7.67–7.62

(m, 1H), 7.48–7.43 (m, 1H), 6.65 (s, 1H), 3.92 (d, *J* = 15.1 Hz, 1H), 3.72 (d, *J* = 16.4 Hz, 4H), 3.17 (d, *J* = 5.8 Hz, 1H), 1.57–1.50 (m, 1H), 1.26–1.16 (m, 2H), and 0.93–0.88 (m, 6H). ^{13}C NMR (150 MHz, $CDCl_3$) δ 180.60, 175.16, 174.46, 160.27, 157.37, 135.45, 130.55, 130.15, 128.78, 128.52, 122.32, 122.19, 105.82, 65.31, 51.64, 45.08, 38.47, 25.39, 15.66, and 11.49. IR (ν, cm^{-1}): 3445.72, 2924.70, 2358.43, 2341.16,1732.42, 1682.86, 1209.15, and 1150.10. HRMS (ESI) calcd. for $[M + Na]^+$ $C_{20}H_{21}O_5NNa^+$: 378.1312, found 378.1299.

TC6: *2-((L-valine methyl ester-1-yl)methyl)naphtho[1,2-b]furan-4,5-dione*. Red solid, yield: 41%. Mp: 54–55 °C. ^{1}H NMR (600 MHz, $CDCl_3$) δ 8.09 (d, *J* = 6.2 Hz, 1H), 7.73 (d, *J* = 7.6 Hz, 1H), 7.70–7.64 (m, 1H), 7.50–7.45 (m, 1H), 6.67 (s, 1H), 3.95 (d, *J* = 15.3 Hz, 1H), 3.77–3.72 (m, 4H), 3.11 (d, *J* = 5.8 Hz, 1H), 2.02–1.95 (m, 1H), and 0.98 (t, *J* = 6.3 Hz, 7H). ^{13}C NMR (150 MHz, $CDCl_3$) δ 180.62, 175.22, 174.49, 160.28, 157.39, 135.43, 130.59, 130.14, 128.82, 128.56, 122.32, 122.22, 105.83, 66.36, 51.70, 45.16, 31.75, 19.28, and 18.35. IR (ν, cm^{-1}): 3425.42, 2923,62, 2358.56, 2337.30, 1698.57, 1670.37, 1187.10, and 1118.00. HRMS (ESI) calcd. for $[M + Na]^+$ $C_{19}H_{19}O_5NNa^+$: 364.1155, found 364.1141.

TC7: *2-((L-glycine methyl ester-1-yl)methyl)naphtho[1,2-b]furan-4,5-dione*. Red solid, yield: 17%. Mp: 55–56 °C. ^{1}H NMR (600 MHz, $CDCl_3$) δ 8.06 (d, *J* = 7.6 Hz, 1H), 7.71 (d, *J* = 6.4 Hz, 1H), 7.68–7.62 (m, 1H), 7.49–7.43 (m, 1H), 6.67 (s, 1H), 3.93 (s, 2H), 3.75 (s, 3H), and 3.50 (s, 2H). ^{13}C NMR (150 MHz, $CDCl_3$) δ 180.49, 174.42, 172.45, 160.49, 156.62, 135.44, 130.57, 130.25, 128.79, 128.39, 122.41, 122.14, 106.25, 52.03, 49.50, and 45.38. IR (ν, cm^{-1}): 3328.36, 2958.26, 2358.57, 2337.30, 1735.10, 1676.24, 1216.29, and 1180.25. HRMS (ESI) calcd. for $[M + Na]^+$ $C_{16}H_{13}O_5NNa^+$: 322.0686, found 322.0680.

TC8: *2-((L-leucinate methyl ester-1-yl)methyl)naphtho[1,2-b]furan-4,5-dione*. Red solid, yield: 19%. Mp: 54–55 °C. ^{1}H NMR (600 MHz, $CDCl_3$) δ 8.09 (d, *J* = 7.6 Hz, 1H), 7.73 (d, *J* = 7.6 Hz, 1H), 7.67 (t, *J* = 7.6 Hz, 1H), 7.47 (t, *J* = 7.6 Hz, 1H), 6.66 (s, 1H), 3.94 (d, *J* = 15.1 Hz, 1H), 3.77 (d, *J* = 15.1 Hz, 1H), 3.73 (s, 3H), 3.38 (t, *J* = 7.2 Hz, 1H), 1.82–1.77 (m, 1H), 1.52 (t, *J* = 7.4 Hz, 2H), 0.95 (d, *J* = 6.7 Hz, 3H), and 0.90 (d, *J* = 6.7 Hz, 3H). ^{13}C NMR (150 MHz, $CDCl_3$) δ 180.59, 176.01, 174.47, 160.32, 157.18, 135.42, 130.59, 130.17, 128.84, 128.51, 122.32, 122.20, 105.94, 59.08, 51.88, 44.63, 42.75, 24.89, 22.78, and 22.09. IR (ν, cm^{-1}): 3434.68, 2958.49, 2358.68, 2339.23, 1670.06, 1518.72, 1211.01, and 1107.62. HRMS (ESI) calcd. for $[M + Na]^+$ $C_{20}H_{21}O_5NNa^+$: 378.1312, found 378.1302.

TC9: *2-((4-boc-piperazin-1-yl)methyl)naphtho[1,2-b]furan-4,5-dione*. Red solid, yield: 26%. Mp: 56–57 °C. ^{1}H NMR (600 MHz, $CDCl_3$) δ 8.10 (d, *J* = 7.4 Hz, 1H), 7.76 (d, *J* = 7.6 Hz, 1H), 7.67 (t, *J* = 7.6 Hz, 1H), 7.48 (t, *J* = 7.6 Hz, 1H), 6.70 (s, 1H), 3.68 (s, 2H), 3.49 (s, 4H), 2.52 (s, 4H), and 1.47 (s, 9H). ^{13}C NMR (150 MHz, $CDCl_3$) δ 180.53, 174.48, 160.57, 155.01, 154.68, 135.44, 130.64, 130.29, 128.81, 128.46, 122.53, 122.17, 107.66, 79.88, 54.60, 52.60, and 28.42. IR (ν, cm^{-1}): 3434.73, 2358.58, 2339.23, 1669.96, 1518.77, 1211.18, and 1107.93. HRMS (ESI) calcd. for $[M + H]^+$ $C_{22}H_{25}O_5N_2^+$: 397.1758, found 397.1751.

TC10: *2-((pyrrolidin-1-yl)methyl)naphtho[1,2-b]furan-4,5-dione*. Red solid, yield: 24%. Mp: 62–63 °C. ^{1}H NMR (600 MHz, $CDCl_3$) δ 8.08 (d, *J* = 7.8 Hz, 1H), 7.76 (d, *J* = 7.6 Hz, 1H), 7.65 (t, *J* = 7.6 Hz, 1H), 7.46 (t, *J* = 7.6 Hz, 1H), 6.68 (s, 1H), 3.76 (s, 2H), 2.69–2.63 (m, 4H), and 1.89–1.83 (m, 4H). ^{13}C NMR (150 MHz, $CDCl_3$) δ 180.64, 174.54, 160.39, 156.44, 135.40, 130.56, 130.14, 128.80, 128.56, 122.55, 122.24, 106.71, 54.01, 51.84, and 23.53. IR (ν, cm^{-1}): 3388.30, 3110.62, 2358.68, 2337.30, 1660.65, 1510.49, 1222.52, and 1091.51. HRMS (ESI) calcd. for $[M + H]^+$ $C_{17}H_{16}O_3N^+$: 282.1125, found 282.1115.

TC11: *2-(morpholinomethyl)naphtho[1,2-b]furan-4,5-dione*. Red solid, yield: 38%. Mp: 98–99 °C. ^{1}H NMR (600 MHz, $CDCl_3$) δ 8.09 (d, *J* = 7.6 Hz, 1H), 7.76 (d, *J* = 7.6 Hz, 1H), 7.69–7.64 (m, 1H), 7.51–7.45 (m, 1H), 6.70 (s, 1H), 3.78–3.74 (m, 4H), 3.66 (s, 2H), and 2.61–2.55 (m, 4H). ^{13}C NMR (150 MHz, $CDCl_3$) δ 180.50, 174.46, 160.50, 155.01, 135.36, 130.59, 130.23, 128.86, 128.47, 122.46, 122.21, 107.64, 66.79, 54.93, and 53.28. IR (ν, cm^{-1}): 3438.84, 2807.27, 2358.54, 2342.76, 1676.47, 1557.77, 1215.99, 1111.32, and 1006.63. HRMS (ESI) calcd. for $[M + Na]^+$ $C_{17}H_{15}O_4NNa^+$: 320.0893, found 320.0886.

TC12: *2-(((4-fluorophenyl)amino)methyl)naphtho[1,2-b]furan-4,5-dione*. Dark red solid, yield: 51%. Mp: 174–175 °C. ^{1}H NMR (600 MHz, DMSO-d_6) δ 7.92 (d, *J* = 7.3 Hz, 1H), 7.73 (t, *J* = 7.5 Hz, 1H), 7.65 (d, *J* = 7.6 Hz, 1H), 7.52 (t, *J* = 7.5 Hz, 1H), 6.94 (t, *J* = 8.9 Hz, 2H), 6.74 (s, 1H), 6.73–6.68 (m, 2H), 6.20 (t, *J* = 6.4 Hz, 1H), and 4.37 (d, *J* = 6.0 Hz, 2H). ^{13}C NMR (150 MHz, DMSO-d_6) δ 179.86, 174.62, 159.03, 157.32, 155.16 (d, *J* = 231.0 Hz), 145.06, 135.47, 130.37, 129.85, 129.69, 128.27, 122.42, 122.06, 115.77 (d,

J = 21.0 Hz), 113.88 (d, J = 6.0 Hz), and 105.93. IR (ν, cm^{-1}): 3378.05, 2923.56, 2358.52, 2335.37, 1662.70, 1514.18, 1215.45, and 1161.45. HRMS (ESI) calcd. for [M + Na]$^+$ $C_{19}H_{12}O_3NFNa^+$: 344.0693, found 344.0681.

TC13: *2-(((3-fluorophenyl)amino)methyl)naphtho[1,2-b]furan-4,5-dione*. Dark red solid, yield: 45%. Mp: 169–170 °C. ^{1}H NMR (600 MHz, DMSO-d_6) δ 7.92 (d, J = 7.6 Hz, 1H), 7.74 (t, J = 7.5 Hz, 1H), 7.65 (d, J = 7.6 Hz, 1H), 7.53 (t, J = 7.6 Hz, 1H), 7.10 (q, J = 8.0 Hz, 1H), 6.78 (s, 1H), 6.61 (t, J = 6.3 Hz, 1H), 6.54 (d, J = 8.2 Hz, 1H), 6.50 (d, J = 12.2 Hz, 1H), 6.35 (t, J = 8.4 Hz, 1H), and 4.41 (d, J = 6.2 Hz, 2H). ^{13}C NMR (150 MHz, DMSO-d_6) δ 179.83, 174.63, 163.90 (d, J = 238.5 Hz), 159.09, 156.86, 150.51 (d, J = 10.5 Hz), 135.46, 130.79 (d, J = 9.0 Hz), 130.40, 129.85, 129.73, 128.25, 122.42, 122.04, 109.34, 106.10, 102.99 (d, J = 21.0 Hz), and 99.24 (d, J = 27.0 Hz). IR (ν, cm^{-1}): 3390.68, 3105.83, 2360.44, 2337.30, 1665.28, 1618.38, 1220.09, and 1152.73. HRMS (ESI) calcd. for [M + Na]$^+$ $C_{19}H_{12}O_3NFNa^+$: 344.0693, found 344.0688.

TC14: *2-(((2-fluorophenyl)amino)methyl)naphtho[1,2-b]furan-4,5-dione*. Dark red solid, yield: 46%. Mp: 170–171 °C. ^{1}H NMR (600 MHz, $CDCl_3$) δ 8.08 (d, J = 7.8 Hz, 1H), 7.69 (d, J = 7.4 Hz, 1H), 7.66 (t, J = 7.4 Hz, 1H), 7.47 (t, J = 7.5 Hz, 1H), 7.05–7.00 (m, 2H), 6.79 (t, J = 8.5 Hz, 1H), 6.75–6.72 (m, 1H), 6.71 (s, 1H), and 4.51 (d, J = 6.4 Hz, 2H). ^{13}C NMR (150 MHz, $CDCl_3$) δ 180.39, 174.38, 160.36, 155.98, 151.74 (d, J = 237.0 Hz), 135.45, 135.22 (d, J = 12.0 Hz), 130.63, 130.29, 128.79, 128.36, 124.67 (d, J = 4.5 Hz), 122.26 (d, J = 15.0 Hz), 118.16 (d, J = 6.0 Hz), 114 (d, J = 19.5 Hz), 112.52, 112.50, 106.03, and 40.74. IR (ν, cm^{-1}): 3425.04, 2923.94, 2358.97, 2854,13, 1670.34, 1513.50, 1186.96, and 1117.57. HRMS (ESI) calcd. for [M + Na]$^+$ $C_{19}H_{12}O_3NFNa^+$: 344.0693, found 344.0684.

TC15: *2-(((2,4-difluorophenyl)amino)methyl)naphtho[1,2-b]furan-4,5-dione*. Red solid, yield: 33%. Mp: 154–155 °C. ^{1}H NMR (600 MHz, $CDCl_3$) δ 8.10 (d, J = 7.6 Hz, 1H), 7.71 (d, J = 7.6 Hz, 1H), 7.67 (t, J = 7.4 Hz, 1H), 7.49 (t, J = 7.4 Hz, 1H), 7.14 (t, J = 8.1 Hz, 1H), 6.77 (d, J = 8.0 Hz, 1H), 6.71 (s, 2H), 6.59 (d, J = 8.2 Hz, 1H), and 4.46 (d, J = 6.4 Hz, 2H). ^{13}C NMR (150 MHz, $CDCl_3$) δ 180.36, 174.38, 160.42, 155.83 (d, J = 9.0 Hz), 154.24 (d, J = 10.5 Hz), 151.95 (d, J = 12.0 Hz), 150.34 (d, J = 12.0 Hz), 135.49, 131.73 (d, J = 12.0 Hz), 130.52 (d, J = 46.5 Hz), 129.67, 128.55 (d, J = 73.5 Hz), 122.24 (d, J = 24 Hz), 115.33, 112.73 (dd, J = 12.0 Hz), 110.86 (dd, J = 25.5 Hz), 106.09, 103.90 (dd, J = 49.5 Hz), and 41.22. IR (ν, cm^{-1}): 3434.72, 2358.46, 2337.30, 1689.86, 1518.53, 1210.93, 1107.68, and 957.02. HRMS (ESI) calcd. for [M + Na]$^+$ $C_{19}H_{11}O_3NF_2Na^+$: 362.0599, found 362.0589.

TC16: *2-(((2,4,6-trimethylphenyl)amino)methyl)naphtho[1,2-b]furan-4,5-dione*. Red solid, yield: 33%. Mp: 173–174 °C. ^{1}H NMR (600 MHz, $CDCl_3$) δ 8.10 (d, J = 7.6 Hz, 1H), 7.67 (d, J = 3.8 Hz, 2H), 7.50–7.46 (m, 1H), 6.85 (s, 2H), 6.60 (s, 1H), 4.21 (s, 2H), 2.29 (s, 6H), and 2.25 (s, 3H). ^{13}C NMR (150 MHz, $CDCl_3$) δ 180.53, 174.47, 160.18, 157.50, 141.61, 135.47, 132.42, 130.65, 130.23, 130.13, 129.64, 128.84, 128.47, 122.23, 122.18, 105.72, 44.94, 20.62, and 18.23. IR (ν, cm^{-1}): 3445.76, 2357.38, 2327.66, 1670.28, 1557.44, 1215.32, 1147.47, and 1025.94. HRMS (ESI) calcd. for [M + Na]$^+$ $C_{22}H_{19}O_3NNa^+$: 368.1257, found 368.1250.

TC17: *2-(((4-chlorophenyl)amino)methyl)naphtho[1,2-b]furan-4,5-dione*. Dark red solid, yield: 28%. Mp: 205–206 °C. ^{1}H NMR (600 MHz, DMSO-d_6) δ 7.92 (d, J = 6.8 Hz, 1H), 7.74 (t, J = 7.5 Hz, 1H), 7.65 (d, J = 7.6 Hz, 1H), 7.52 (t, J = 7.1 Hz, 1H), 7.12 (d, J = 8.9 Hz, 2H), 6.75 (s, 1H), 6.72 (d, J = 8.9 Hz, 2H), 6.49 (t, J = 6.3 Hz, 1H), and 4.40 (d, J = 6.2 Hz, 2H). ^{13}C NMR (150 MHz, DMSO-d_6) δ: 179.82, 174.61, 159.06, 156.95, 147.33, 135.46, 130.39, 129.84, 129.72, 129.09, 128.24, 122.41, 122.05, 120.26, 114.42, and 106.08. IR (ν, cm^{-1}): 3388.22, 3110.62, 2358.84, 2342.68, 1660.69, 1510.19, 1222.68 and 1118.65. HRMS (ESI) calcd. for [M + Na]$^+$ $C_{19}H_{12}O_3NClNa^+$, 360.0398, found 360.0384.

TC18: *2-(((4-methoxyphenyl)amino)methyl)naphtho[1,2-b]furan-4,5-dione*. Dark solid, yield: 64%. Mp: 112–113 °C. ^{1}H NMR (600 MHz, $CDCl_3$) δ 8.08 (d, J = 6.4 Hz, 1H), 7.70 (d, J = 7.6 Hz, 1H), 7.69–7.63 (m, 1H), 7.50–7.44 (m, 1H), 6.82 (d, J = 8.9 Hz, 2H), 6.70–6.67 (m, 3H), 4.42 (s, 2H), and 3.77 (s, 3H). ^{13}C NMR (150 MHz, $CDCl_3$) δ 180.49, 174.43, 160.22, 156.83, 152.98, 140.82, 135.43, 130.62, 130.21, 128.77, 128.46, 122.27, 115.00, 114.74, 105.84, 55.77, and 42.13. IR (ν, cm^{-1}): 3370.45, 3105.23, 2358.89, 2337.30, 1660.16, 1514.41, 1234.80, and 1040.25. HRMS (ESI) calcd. for [M + Na]$^+$ $C_{20}H_{15}O_4NNa^+$: 356.0893, found 356.0883.

3.3. *In Vitro Cytotoxicity Assay*

The *human cancer cell lines*, including prostate cancer cells PC3, leukemia cells K562, and melanoma cells WM9, were stored in the biology laboratory of the Key Laboratory of Chemistry for Natural Products of Guizhou Province and Chinese Academy of Sciences (Guiyang, China). All cells were cultured in DMEM supplemented with 10% fetal bovine serum (FBS) and 1% penicillin and streptomycin (Sijiqing, Hangzhou, China) and incubated at 37 °C under 5% CO_2, 95% air, and 95% humidity. Cytotoxicity was evaluated by performing the MTT assay [24]. Briefly, the cells were seeded in 96-well microculture plates at a density from 4×10^3 to 8×10^3 cells/well. Cells were then exposed to different concentrations of the assayed compounds for 48 h. Then, 20 μL of MTT solution (5 mg/mL) was added to each well and incubated at 37 °C for an additional 4 h. The medium was then removed and 200 μL Tris-DMSO solution was added. Plates were lightly shaking up to dissolve the dark blue formazan crystals and the absorbance was measured in an ELISA plate reader at 570 nm.

3.4. *Flow Cytometry Assay*

Cell apoptosis was determined by an inverted fluorescence microscope observation and flow cytometry as describe in our previous study [28]. Briefly, the cancer cells treated with compounds were harvested for centrifugation at 1000 rpm for 5 min at room temperature, washed twice with PBS and resuspended with binding buffer, and then PI (Sigma, St. Louis, MO, USA) was added to a final concentration of 20 mg/mL. The cell lines were analyzed by flow cytometry (Becton Dickinson, Franklin Lakes, NJ, USA).

3.5. *Statistical Analysis*

The IC_{50} values were calculated from the semilogarithmic dose-response curves. The data were analyzed using SPSS 18.0 and reported as mean ± SD of the number of experiments indicated. For all measurements, one-way ANOVA followed by Student's t-test was used to assess the statistical significance of the difference between each group. The LSD method was used to assess the statistical significance of the difference between the two groups. A statistically significant difference was considered at the level of $P < 0.05$. The data are presented as the mean ± SEM of three assays.

4. Conclusions

In this study, 27 novel L-shaped ortho-quinone analogs were synthesized and evaluated for their anti-cancer activities. Compounds **TB1, TB3, TB4, TB6, TC1, TC3, TC5, TC9, TC11, TC12, TC14, TC15, TC16**, and **TC17** possessed broad-spectrum potent cytotoxicity against PC3, K562, and WM9 cells. With more than a 70% inhibitory rate, **TB7** showed better inhibitory activity of K562 cells as compared with other cells. Moreover, we observed that **TC7** inhibited the growth of PC3 cells more efficiently than other cells. Some of the active compounds such as **TB3, TC1, TC3,** and **TC7** inhibited cell proliferation mainly through inducing apoptosis. The structure-activity relationships evaluation showed that removing methyl at C-3 of the furan ring and introducing diverse side chains at C-2 of the furan ring is an effective strategy for improving the anticancer activity of L-shaped ortho-quinone analogs.

Author Contributions: W.-D.P. and H.L. conceived and designed the experiments; S.-Y.L. and X.-Y.Z. performed part of chemical experiment; Z.-K.S., Y.Z., M.-L.W. performed the biology experiment; S.-C.H., J.L., J.-R.S. and C.C. contributed reagents and materials and revised the paper; S.-Y.L. and H.L. wrote the paper.

Funding: This work was supported by the Science and Technology Department of Guizhou Province (no. QKHJC (2017)1412, QKHRC (2016)4037, QKHZC (2019)2757, QKHJC (2016)1099, and QKHPTRC (2017) 5737), the National Science Foundation of China (NSFC no. 81660580 and 81702914), and Financial support from Guizhou Provincial Engineering Research Center for Natural Drugs.

Conflicts of Interest: The authors declare no conflict of interest.

References

1. Ferlay, J.; Colombet, M.; Soerjomataram, I.; Mathers, C.; Parkin, D.M.; Piñeros, M.; Znaor, A.; Bray, F. Estimating the global cancer incidence and mortality in 2018: GLOBOCAN sources and methods. *Int. J. Cancer* **2019**, *144*, 1941–1953. [CrossRef] [PubMed]
2. Feng, R.M.; Zong, Y.N.; Cao, S.M.; Xu, R.H. Current cancer situation in China: Good or bad news from the 2018 Global Cancer Statistics? *Cancer Commun.* **2019**, *39*, 22. [CrossRef] [PubMed]
3. Chen, W.; Zheng, R.; Baade, P.D.; Zhang, S.; Zeng, H.; Bray, F.; Jemal, A.; Yu, X.Q.; He, J. Cancer statistics in China, 2015. *CA Cancer J. Clin.* **2016**, *66*, 115–132. [CrossRef] [PubMed]
4. Weerink, L.B.; Gant, C.M.; Leeuwen, B.L.V.; De Bock, G.H.; Kouwenhoven, E.A.; Faneyte, I.F. Long-term survival in octogenarians after surgical treatment for colorectal cancer: Prevention of postoperative complications is key. *Ann. Surg. Oncol.* **2018**, *25*, 3874–3882. [CrossRef]
5. Newman, D.J.; Cragg, G.M. Natural products as sources of new drugs over the Last 25 years. *J. Nat. Prod.* **2007**, *70*, 461–477. [CrossRef]
6. Tan, Y.H.; Xiao, X.; Yao, J.N.; Han, F.; Lou, H.Y.; Luo, H.; Liang, G.Y.; Ben-David, Y.; Pan, W.D. Syntheses and Anti-cancer Activities of Glycosylated Derivatives of Diosgenin. *Chem. Res. Chin. Univ.* **2017**, *33*, 80–86. [CrossRef]
7. Lan, J.J.; Huang, L.; Lou, H.Y.; Chen, C.; Liu, T.J.J.; Hu, S.C.; Yao, Y.; Song, J.R.; Luo, J.; Liu, Y.Z.; et al. Design and synthesis of novel C-14-urea-tetrandrine derivatives with potent anti-cancer activity. *Eur. J. Med. Chem.* **2018**, *143*, 1968–1980. [CrossRef]
8. Lan, J.J.; Wang, N.; Huang, L.; Liu, Y.Z.; Ma, X.P.; Lou, H.Y.; Chen, C.; Feng, Y.P.; Pan, W.D. Design and synthesis of novel tetrandrine derivatives as potential anti-tumor agents against human hepatocellular carcinoma. *Eur. J. Med. Chem.* **2019**, *127*, 554–566. [CrossRef]
9. Song, J.R.; Lan, J.J.; Chen, C.; Hu, S.C.; Song, J.L.; Liu, W.L.; Zeng, X.Y.; Lou, H.Y.; Ben-David, Y.; Pan, W.D. Design, synthesis and bioactivity investigation of tetrandrine derivatives as potential anti-cancer agents. *MedChemComm* **2018**, *9*, 1131–1141. [CrossRef]
10. Liu, F.; Yu, G.; Wang, G.; Liu, H.; Wu, X.; Wang, Q.; Liu, M.; Liao, K.; Wu, M.; Cheng, X.; et al. An NQO1-initiated and p53-independent apoptotic pathway determines the anti-tumor effect of tanshinone IIA against non-small cell lung cancer. *PLoS ONE* **2012**, *7*, e42138. [CrossRef]
11. Xu, Z.Y.; Chen, L.; Xiao, Z.G.; Zhu, Y.H.; Jiang, H.; Jin, Y.; Gu, C.; Wu, Y.L.; Wang, L.; Zhang, W.; et al. Potentiation of the anticancer effect of doxorubicinin drug-resistant gastric cancer cells by tanshinone IIA. *Phytomedicine* **2018**, *51*, 58–67. [CrossRef] [PubMed]
12. Lin, C.Y.; Wang, L.; Wang, H.; Yang, L.Q.; Guo, H.J.; Wang, X.J. Tanshinone IIA inhibits breast cancer stem cells growth in vitro and in vivo through attenuation of IL-6/STAT3/NF-kB signaling pathways. *J. Cell Biochem.* **2013**, *114*, 2061–2070. [CrossRef] [PubMed]
13. Huang, S.T.; Huang, C.C.; Huang, W.L.; Lin, T.K.; Liao, P.L.; Wang, P.W.; Liou, C.W.; Chuang, J.H. Tanshinone IIA induces intrinsic apoptosis in osteosarcoma cells both in vivo and in vitro associated with mitochondrial dysfunction. *Sci. Rep.* **2017**, *7*, 40382. [CrossRef] [PubMed]
14. Bentle, M.S.; Reinicke, K.E.; Bey, E.A.; Spitz, D.R.; Boothman, D.A. Calcium-dependent modulation of poly (ADP-ribose) polymerase-1 alters cellular metabolism and DNA repair. *J. Biol. Chem.* **2006**, *281*, 33684–33696. [CrossRef]
15. Bey, E.A.; Bentle, M.S.; Reinicke, K.E.; Dong, Y.; Yang, C.R.; Girard, L.; Minna, J.D.; Bornmann, W.G.; Gao, J.M.; Boothman, D.A. An NQO1- and PARP-1-mediated cell death pathway induced in non-small-cell lung cancer cells by β-lapachone. *Proc. Natl. Acad. Sci. USA* **2007**, *104*, 11832–11837. [CrossRef]
16. Cheng, X.F.; Liu, F.; Yan, T.T.; Zhou, X.Y.; Wu, L.; Liao, K.; Wang, G.J.; Hao, H.P. , Metabolic profile, enzyme kinetics, and reaction phenotyping of β-lapachone metabolism in human liver and intestine in vitro. *Mol. Pharm.* **2012**, *9*, 3476–3485. [CrossRef]
17. Huang, W.G.; Li, J.Y.; Zhang, W.; Zhou, Y.Y.; Xie, C.M.; Luo, Y.; Li, Y.F.; Wang, J.L.; Li, J.; Lu, W. Synthesis of miltirone analogues as inhibitors of Cdc25 phosphatases. *Bioorg. Med. Chem. Lett.* **2006**, *16*, 1905–1908. [CrossRef]
18. Huang, W.G.; Jiang, Y.Y.; Li, Q.; Li, J.; Li, J.Y.; Lu, W.; Cai, J.C. Synthesis and biological evaluation of (±)-cryptotanshinone and its simplified analogues as potent CDC25 inhibitors. *Tetrahedron* **2005**, *61*, 1863–1870. [CrossRef]

19. Bian, J.L.; Deng, B.; Xu, L.L.; Xu, X.L.; Wang, N.; Hu, T.H.; Yao, Z.Y.; Du, J.Y.; Yang, L.; Lei, Y.H.; et al. 2-Substituted 3-methylnaphtho[1,2-*b*]furan-4,5-diones as novel L-shaped ortho-quinone substrates for NAD(P)H: Quinone oxidoreductase (NQO1). *Eur. J. Med. Chem.* **2014**, *82*, 56–67. [CrossRef]
20. Bian, J.L.; Li, X.; Wang, N.; Wu, X.S.; You, Q.D.; Zhang, X.J. Discovery of quinone-directed antitumor agents selectively bioactivated by NQO1 over CPR with improved safety profile. *Eur. J. Med. Chem.* **2017**, *129*, 27–40. [CrossRef]
21. Deniz, N.G.; Ozyurek, M.; Tufan, A.N.; Apak, R. One-pot synthesis, characterization, and antioxidant capacity of sulfur-and oxygen-substituted 1,4-naphthoquinones and a structural study. *Monatshefte für Chemie-Chemical Monthly* **2015**, *146*, 2117–2126. [CrossRef]
22. Arenas, P.; Peña, A.; Rios, D.; Benites, J.; Muccioli, G.G.; Calderon, P.B.; Valderrama, J.A. Eco-friendly synthesis and antiproliferative evaluation of some oxygen substituted diaryl ketones. *Molecules* **2013**, *18*, 9818–9832. [CrossRef]
23. Li, X.; Bian, J.L.; Wang, N.; Qian, X.; Gu, J.; Mu, T.; Fan, J.; Yang, X.W.; Li, S.Z.; Yang, T.T.; et al. Novel naphtho[2,1-*d*]oxazole-4,5-diones as NQO1 substrates with improved aqueous solubility: Design, synthesis, and in vivo antitumor evaluation. *Bioorg. Med. Chem.* **2016**, *24*, 1006–1013. [CrossRef] [PubMed]
24. Jain, M.; Nilsson, R.; Sharma, S.; Madhusudhan, N.; Kitami, T.; Souza, A.L.; Kafri, R.; Kirschner, M.W.; Clish, C.B.; Mootha, V.K. Metabolite profiling identifies a key role for glycine in rapid cancer cell proliferation. *Science* **2012**, *336*, 1040–1044. [CrossRef]
25. Hu, K.Z.; Wang, H.; Huang, T.; Tang, G.; Liang, X.; He, S.; Tang, X. Synthesis and biological evaluation of *N*-(2-[(18)F]Fluoropropionyl)-L-methionine for tumor imaging. *Nucl. Med. Biol.* **2013**, *40*, 926–932. [CrossRef]
26. Kongkathip, N.; Kongkathip, B.; Siripong, P.; Sangma, C.; Luangkamin, S.; Niyomdecha, M.; Pattanapa, S.; Piyaviriyagul, S.; Kongsaeree, P. Potent antitumor activity of synthetic 1,2-Naphthoquinones and 1,4-Naphthoquinones. *Bioorg. Med. Chem.* **2003**, *11*, 3179–3191. [CrossRef]
27. Weerawarna, S.A.; Guha-Biswas, M.; Nelson, W.L. Improved Syntheses of Bufuralol, 7-Ethyl-2-(2-tertbutylamino-1-hydroxyethyl)benzofuran, and 1 Oxobufuralol, 7-Acetyl-2-(2-tert-butylamino-1-hydroxyethyl)benzofuran. *Heterocycl* **1991**, *28*, 1395–1403. [CrossRef]
28. Wen, Z.H.; Zhang, Y.Q.; Wang, X.H.; Zeng, X.P.; Hu, Z.X.; Liu, Y.; Xie, Y.X.; Liang, G.Y.; Zhu, J.G.; Luo, H.; et al. Novel 3′,5′-diprenylated chalcones inhibited the proliferation of cancer cells in vitro by inducing cell apoptosis and arresting cell cycle phase. *Eur. J. Med. Chem.* **2017**, *133*, 227–239. [CrossRef]

Sample Availability: Samples of the compounds are available from the authors.

molecules

MDPI

Article

Synthesis, Antiproliferative, and Antioxidant Evaluation of 2-Pentylquinazolin-4(3*H*)-one(thione) Derivatives with DFT Study

Amira A. El-Sayed [1], Mahmoud F. Ismail [1], Abd El-Galil E. Amr [2,3,*] and Ahmed M. Naglah [2,4]

1 Department of Chemistry, Faculty of Science, Ain Shams University, 11566 Abbassia, Cairo 11566, Egypt; amira_aa47@hotmail.com (A.A.E.-S.); fawzy2010@sci.asu.edu.eg (M.F.I.)
2 Pharmaceutical Chemistry Department, Drug Exploration & Development Chair (DEDC), College of Pharmacy, King Saud University, Riyadh 11451, Saudi Arabia; amnaglah@gmail.com
3 Applied Organic Chemistry Department, National Research Center, Cairo, Dokki 12622, Egypt
4 Peptide Chemistry Department, Chemical Industries Research Division, National Research Centre, Dokki, Cairo 12622, Egypt
* Correspondence: aamr@ksu.edu.sa; Tel.: +966-543074312

Academic Editor: Qiao-Hong Chen
Received: 5 October 2019; Accepted: 20 October 2019; Published: 21 October 2019

Abstract: The current study was chiefly designed to examine the antiproliferative and antioxidant activities of some novel quinazolinone(thione) derivatives **6–14**. The present work focused on two main points; firstly, comparing between quinazolinone and quinazolinthione derivatives. Whereas, antiproliferative (against two cell lines namely, HepG2 and MCF-7) and antioxidant (by two methods; ABTS and DPPH) activities of the investigated compounds, the best quinazolinthione derivatives were **6** and **14,** which exhibited excellent potencies comparable to quinazolinone derivatives **5** and **9**, respectively. Secondly, we compared the activity of four series of Schiff bases which included the quinazolinone moiety (**11a–d**). In addition, the antiproliferative and antioxidant activities of the compounds with various aryl aldehyde hydrazone derivatives (**11a–d**) analogs were studied. The compounds exhibited potency that increased with increasing electron donating group in *p*-position (OH > OMe > Cl) due to extended conjugated systems. Noteworthy, most of antiproliferative and antioxidant activities results for the tested compounds are consistent with the DFT calculations.

Keywords: quinazolin-4(3*H*)-one; quinazolin-4(3*H*)-thione; Schiff base; antiproliferative activity; antioxidant activity; DFT study

1. Introduction

Cancer is the second leading cause of death globally, and the contribution of cancer disease to the overall mortality rate is increasing. Economically, the total annual cost of cancer in 2010 was estimated at approximately US$ 1.16 trillion [1]. So that, more rational design, synthesis, and evaluation of new compounds as anticancer, with higher efficiency is considered as urgent mission in the medicinal chemistry field.

Quinazoline and quinazolinone derivatives are considered as tremendous targets for the medicinal chemists, due to the fact that they are the scaffold of different potent anticancer drugs, such as Gefitinib (trade name Iressa®), Erlotinib (trade name Tarceva®) [2–4], Methaqualone [5], Afloqualone (as anticonvulsant activity) [6,7], Chloroqualone (as antitussive), and Diproqualone (as sedative-hypnotic agents) [8] (Figure 1).

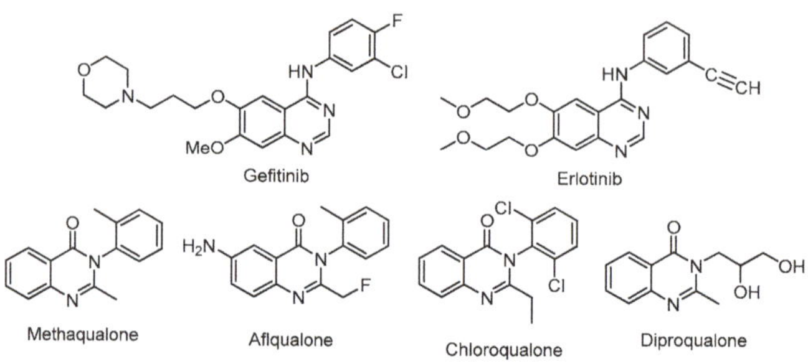

Figure 1. Some structures of synthetic drugs scaffold quinazoline and quinazolinone derivatives.

In the last decades and until now, various compounds including quinazolinone moiety conspicuously exhibited broad spectrum in numerous pharmacological activities such as anticancer [9–14], anticonvulsants [15], antiproliferative [16], anti-inflammatory [17], antihypertensive [18], antifungal [19], antibacterial, antioxidant [20], antimicrobial [21], anti-allergic [22], antimalarial [23], antileishmanial [24], and treatment of Alzheimer's disease (AD) [25].

Generally, the natural products are considered as one of the most interesting sources of biologically active compounds. Among them, naturally occurring quinazolin-4(3*H*)-one derivatives, which can be isolated from various plants and microorganisms such as Luotonin A (sources; *Peganum nigellastrum*) [26], 2-(heptan-3-yl)quinazolinone (sources; *Bacillus cereus*) [27], Dictyoquinazol A (sources; *Dictyophora indusiata*) [28], and Echinozolinone (sources; *Echinops echinatus*) [29] (Figure 2).

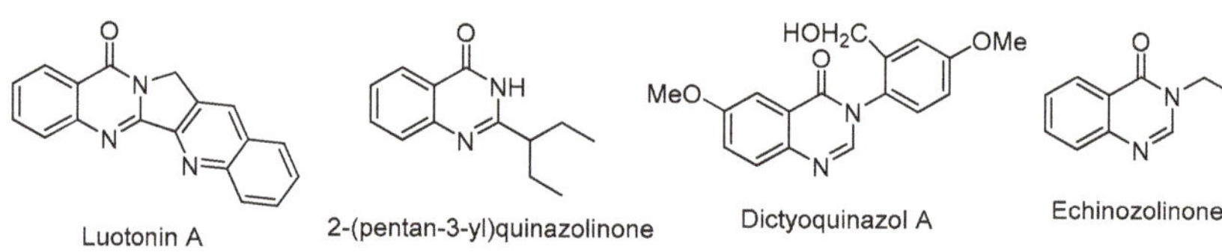

Figure 2. Some structures of naturally occurring quinazolin-4(3*H*)-one derivatives.

Quinazolinones have been synthesized by different methodologies [28,30–37], in the present study, the conventional methodology to construct novel qunizolinone compounds has been adopted, followed by the study of the antiproliferative activity, antioxidant activity, and DFT calculations for the synthesized compounds.

2. Results and Discussion

2.1. Chemistry

In this interesting work, curing of anthranilic acid **1** with hexanoyl chloride **2** in dry pyridine afforded the corresponding *N*-hexanoyl derivative **3** [38], which was cyclized by heating in distilled acetic anhydride to give 2-pentyl-4*H*-benzo[*d*][1,3]oxazin-4-one **4** [39,40] (Scheme 1).

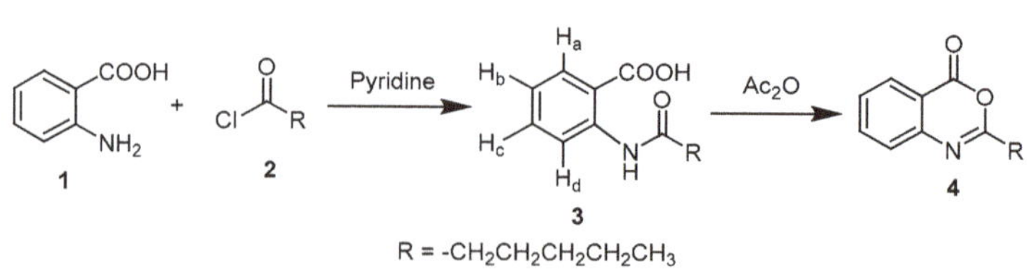

Scheme 1. The strategy for synthesis of compound **4**.

Benzoxazinone derivative **4** was utilized in situ as a precursor to construct new quinazolinone derivatives. For instance, reaction of benzoxazinone derivative **4** with formamide afforded 2-pentylquinazolin-4(3*H*)-one **5** [41] (Scheme 2). The ^{1}H NMR spectrum of **5** exhibited a singlet peak at 12.13 ppm exchangeable with D_2O corresponding to NH proton, two doublet and two triplet peaks in the aromatic region at 8.05–7.42 ppm corresponding to four aromatic protons, and four characteristic peaks upfield at 2.56–0.84 ppm for *n*-pentyl protons.

Afterwards, sulfuration of 2-pentylquinazolin-4(3*H*)-one **5** by utilizing of phosphorus pentasulfide in dry toluene afforded 2-pentylquinazoline-4(3*H*)-thione **6** (Scheme 2). The formation of compound **6** was unambiguously elaborated by the presence of intense band at 1236 cm^{-1} corresponding to $\upsilon_{C=S}$ and the absence of the stretching band of $\upsilon_{C=O}$ in the IR spectrum. On the other hand, the incorporation of β-D-glucose pentaacetate with quinazolinone derivative **5** at the nitrogen atom of the later awarded *N*-(β-D-glucopyranosyl-2,3,4,6-tetraacetate)-2-pentyl quinazolin-4(3*H*)-one **7** (Scheme 2), via attacking of the lone pair of nitrogen atom of quinazolinone derivative **5** at the anomeric carbon (C_1) of β-D-glucose pentaacetate, followed by ring opening and then ring closure with expulsion of acetate as a leaving group.

The chemical structure of compound **7** was explained by the IR spectrum, whereas it showed a band at 1746 cm^{-1} compatible with $\upsilon_{C=O}$ of the acetate groups and lacked the absorption band for the NH group. Moreover, this structure was also interpreted by the ^{1}H-NMR spectrum which revealed seven signals at 5.92–3.51 ppm and four singlet signals at 1.97–1.91 ppm all of them corresponding to the protons of β-D-glucopyranosyl-2,3,4,6-tetraacetate moiety.

Curing of the benzoxazinone derivative **4** with ethanolamine under reflux for 3 h afforded 3-(2-hydroxyethyl)-2-pentylquinazolin-4(3*H*)-one **8** as the sole product. The IR spectrum of compound **8** showed a broad band at 3395 cm^{-1} corresponding to OH functionality. Furthermore, the ^{1}H-NMR spectrum appreciably emerged a triplet peak at 4.95 ppm exchangeable with D_2O corresponding to OH proton, triplet, and quartet peaks at 4.11 and 3.65 ppm, respectively, compatible with ethyl protons of 2-hydroxyethyl moiety. As well, the ^{13}C-NMR spectrum exhibited two peaks at 58.8 and 46.1 ppm corresponding to the two carbons of 2-hydroxyethyl moiety.

3-Amino-2-pentylquinazolin-4(3*H*)-one **9** was commenced by refluxing of compound **4** with hydrazine monohydrate in absolute ethanol for 4 h (Scheme 2). The formation of compound **9** was confirmed by spectroscopic and elemental data. In particular, the ^{1}H-NMR spectrum of compound **9** manifested a singlet signal commutable in D_2O at 5.70 ppm corresponding to NH_2 protons.

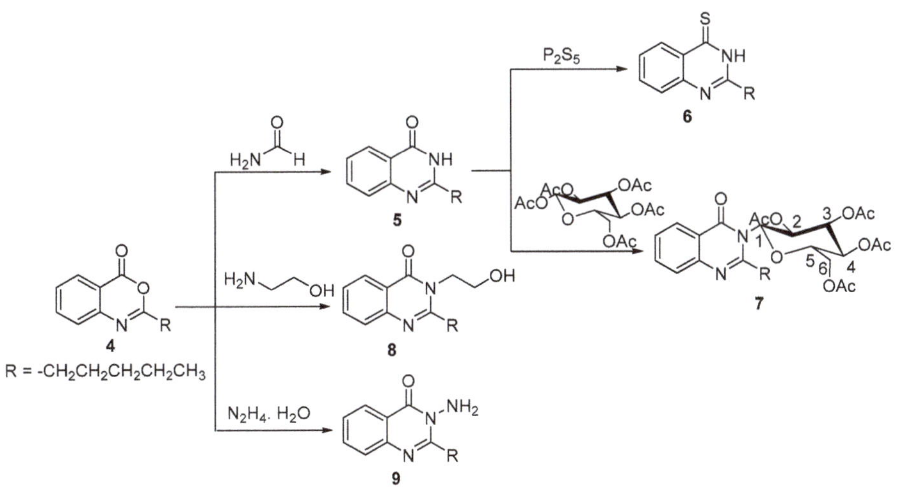

Scheme 2. Synthetic route to compounds **5–9**.

Reaction of 3-amino-2-pentylquinazolin-4(3*H*)-one **9** with various aldehydes **10a–d** gave Schiff bases **11a–d** as the sole product in each case (Scheme 3). The ^{1}H-NMR spectra of compounds **11a–d** exhibited the appearance of a singlet signal in the region between 8.81–8.69 ppm compatible with methine proton of N=CH group.

The thiazolidin-4-one moiety **12** was constructed by the reaction of Schiff base **11a** with methyl thioglycolate in absolute ethanol including a small amount of piperidine as a catalyst for 3 h (Scheme 3). The prospective structure **12** is in keeping with its spectral and elemental analyses.

Additionally, the nucleophilicity of the amino group of compound **9** was also estimated by fusion of it with 4,5,6,7-tetrachloroisobenzofuran-1,3-dione in oil bath for an hour and that afforded phthalimido derivative **13** in an excellent yield (Scheme 3). The foreseeable structure of compound **13** was elucidated by their spectral data and elemental analysis. Obviously, its IR spectrum showed stretching absorption bands at 1788, and 1746 cm^{-1} corresponding to the carbonyl groups of phthalimido moiety and at 1707 cm^{-1} corresponding to carbonyl group of the quinazolinone moiety. The ^{1}H-NMR spectrum exhibited four peaks for four aromatic protons and another four peaks for n-pentyl protons. Furthermore, its ^{13}C-NMR spectrum emerged variant peaks, all of them fit with the proposed structure.

Eventually, the thione derivative **14** was obtained via sulfuration of compound **9** by utilizing phosphorus pentasulfide as the above pervious method (Scheme 3). The structure of **14** was unequivocally explained via the existence of a peak in the ^{13}C NMR spectrum at 182.1 ppm compatible with the carbon of the thione functional group.

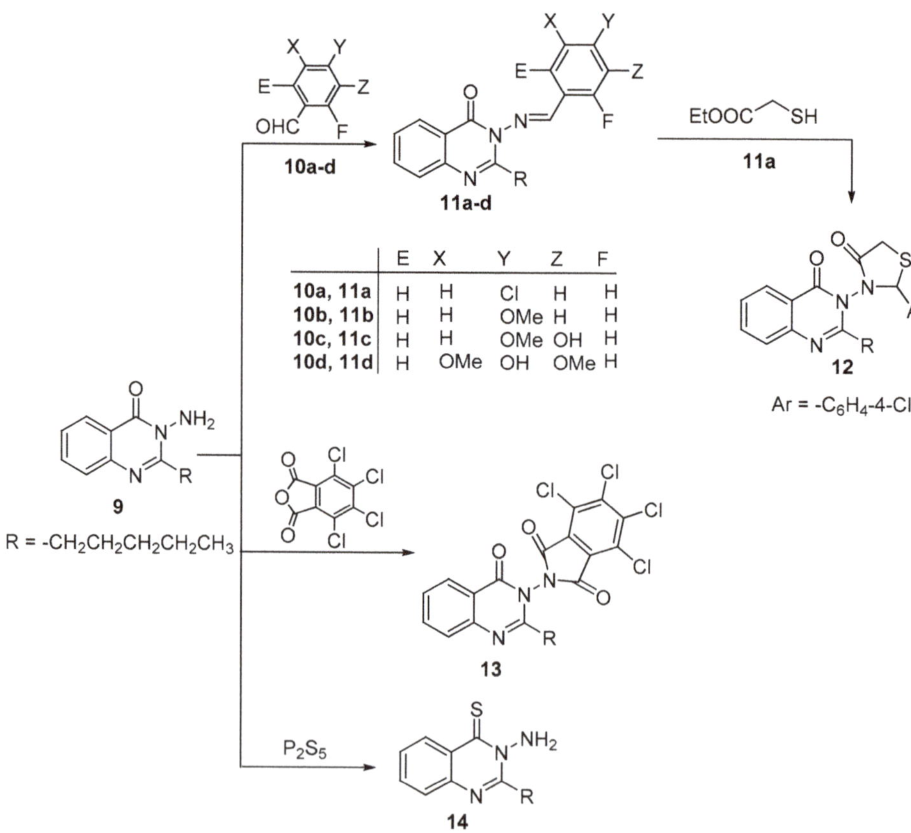

Scheme 3. Synthetic route to compounds **11–14**.

2.2. Biological Evaluation

2.2.1. Antiproliferative Screening

Twelve compounds possessing quinazolinone(thione) moieties **5–14** along with compound **3** were screened against two cell lines, namely hepatocellular carcinoma (HepG2) and mammary gland (MCF-7) in vitro by utilizing MTT assay [42,43]. The latter assay is a colorimetric test based on the change of the yellow MTT (3-(4,5-dimethylthiazolyl-2)-2,5-diphenyltetrazolium bromide) to a purple formazan derivative by mitochondrial succinate dehydrogenase in viable cells and the Doxorubicin (DOX) was used as a standard reference.

The results listed in Table 1 and illustrated in Figure 3, demonstrate that compounds **6** and **11d** have a very strong efficacy against HePG2 cell line with IC_{50} values at 5.20 ± 0.5 and 7.63 ± 0.6 μM, respectively. Meanwhile, compounds **6, 11d,** and **14** have a very strong efficacy against the MCF-7 cell line with IC_{50} values at 6.88 ± 0.4, 8.60 ± 0.7, and 10.78 ± 0.9 μM, respectively. Compounds **11b, 11c** have a strong efficacy against both cell lines with IC_{50} values in the range (12.54 ± 1.1–19.68 ± 1.6 μM). For the HePG2 cell line, compounds **5, 9, 11a,** and **14** have a moderate efficacy with IC_{50} values in the range (23.75 ± 1.9–41.92 ± 2.8 μM). Where, for the MCF-7 cell line, compounds **3, 5, 9,** and **11a** have a moderate efficacy with IC_{50} in the range (21.98 ± 1.8–47.53 ± 2.9 μM). Ultimately, the remaining compounds in both cases have weak efficacies with IC_{50} values > 50 μM.

Table 1. Cytotoxic efficacy of thirteen compounds against hepatocellular carcinoma (HePG2) and mammary gland (MCF-7) cell lines.

Compounds	In Vitro Cytotoxicity IC_{50} (μM)	
	HePG2	MCF-7
DOX	4.50 ± 0.3	4.17 ± 0.2
3	52.01 ± 3.3	47.53 ± 2.9
5	23.75 ± 1.9	21.98 ± 1.8
6	5.20 ± 0.5	6.88 ± 0.4
7	66.84 ± 4.0	54.23 ± 3.2
8	85.55 ± 4.5	70.86 ± 4.1
9	33.27 ± 2.5	28.69 ± 2.2
11a	41.92 ± 2.8	33.39 ± 2.5
11b	17.27 ± 1.4	19.68 ± 1.6
11c	12.54 ± 1.1	14.10 ± 1.3
11d	7.63 ± 0.6	8.60 ± 0.7
12	76.14 ± 4.3	59.15 ± 3.8
13	60.34 ± 3.8	56.28 ± 3.5
14	27.39 ± 2.3	10.78 ± 0.9

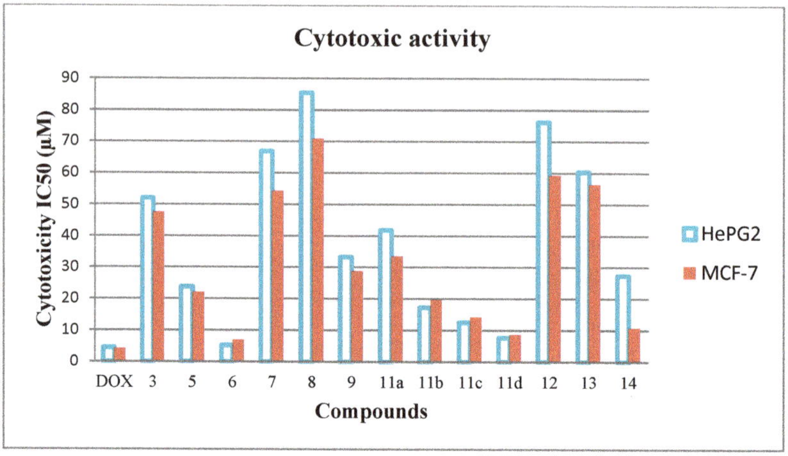

Figure 3. Cytotoxic efficacy of thirteen compounds against HePG2 and MCF-7 cell lines.

Through our screening of the antiproliferative efficacy of the synthesized compounds, it was determined that the average of relative viability of cells (%) with different concentrations such as 100, 50, 25, 12.5, 6.25, 3.125, and 1.56 µM against two cell lines (HePG2 and MCF-7) as shown in Figures 4 and 5.

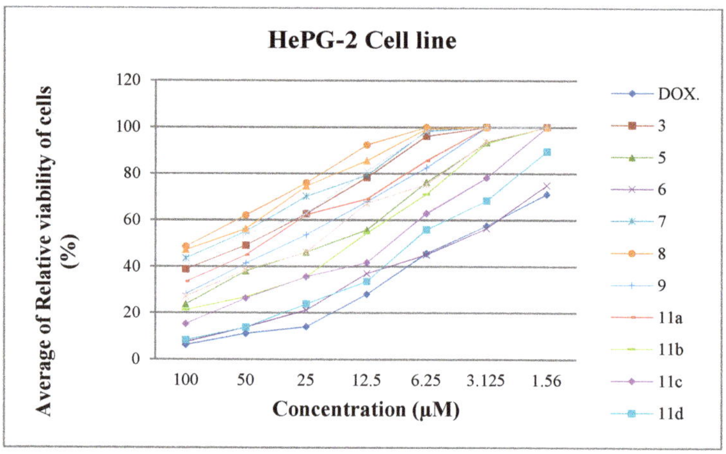

Figure 4. Average of relative viability of HePG-2 cell line (%) with different concentrations.

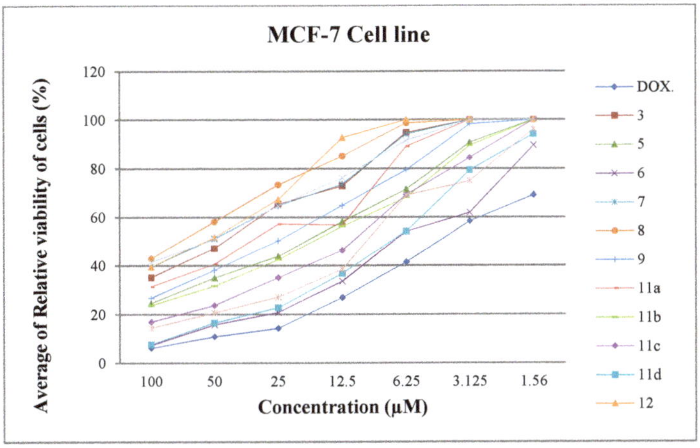

Figure 5. Average of relative viability of MCF-7 cell line (%) with different concentrations.

Structure Activity Relationship (SAR)

By comparing the antiproliferative efficacy of the thirteen synthesized compounds in this study to their chemical structures, it was concluded that the following structure activity relationship's (SAR's) is hypothesized:

1. Conversion of quinazolin-4(3*H*)-one derivative **5** to quinazolin-4(3*H*)-thione derivative **6** enhanced the antiproliferative activity against both cell lines from moderate activity to very strong activity.

2. Similarly, conversion of 3-amino-2-pentylquinazolin-4(3*H*)-one **9** to 3-amino-2-pentylquinazoline-4(3*H*)-thione **14** enhanced the antiproliferative activity against both cell lines.

3. Reaction of **9** with various aryl aldehydes afforded hydrazone derivatives **(11a–d)** analoges with variable potencies according to the following sequence: 3,5-$(OMe)_2$-4-OH-C_6H_2 **11d** > 3-OH-4-(OMe)-C_6H_3 **11c** > 4-(OMe)-C_6H_4 **11b** > 4-Cl-C_6H_4 **11a**, whereas, the OH group in *p*-position is more electron donating group than the OMe group and Cl atom (i.e., the delocalization of n-π electrons decreased in the above sequence).

4. Construction of the thiazolidinone ring in compound **12** decreased the antiproliferative activity comparable with the hydrazone derivative **11a**, due to decreasing of the delocalization of n-π electrons after replacement of the C=N group (electron attracting group) by the thiazolidinone ring.

2.2.2. Antioxidant Activity Screening

One of the aims of this work is the screening of all synthesized compounds for antioxidant activity using two different methods, namely ABTS [2,2′-azino-bis(3-ethyl benzothiazoline-6-sulfonic acid)] and DPPH assays. DPPH (2,2-diphenyl-1-picryl-hydrazyl-hydrate) free radical assay based on electron-transfer that produces a violet solution in ethanol. This free radical is stable at ambient temperature and reduced in the presence of an antioxidant molecule, leading to colorless ethanol solution. After investigation of these results as listed in Table 2 and Figure 6, it was realized that, compounds **6** and **11d** have promising activity through using ABTS assay. Meanwhile, in the case of using DPPH assay, compounds **6**, **11d** and **14** have also very high activity. Ascorbic acid was used as a reference through the antioxidant activity screening.

The results depicted in Table 2 and Figure 6 demonstrated that, DPPH assay findings are very approximately related to those of ABTS assay with only one exception, compound **14** has an excellent antioxidant activity against DPPH (IC_{50} = 26.87 ± 0.23 μM) than that of the ABTS method (IC_{50} = 71.42 ± 0.52 μM). Noteworthy, all the screened compounds in the case of the DPPH method exhibited IC_{50}

smaller than the corresponding ones of the same compounds in the case of the ABTS method, and it proposed that these compounds are more promising scavengers of the DPPH radical than those of the ABTS radical.

By comparing the antioxidant efficacy of the thirteen synthesized compounds in this study to their chemical structures, it was concluded that the following structure antioxidant activity relationship's (SAR's) is hypothesized:

1. The presence of C=S enhanced antioxidant activity than the presence of C=O, as shown in compounds **6** and **14** comparable with compounds **5** and **9**, respectively.

2. The hydrazone derivatives **(11a–d)** analogs have variable potencies according to the following sequence: 3,5-$(OMe)_2$-4-OH-C_6H_2 **11d** > 3-OH-4-(OMe)-C_6H_3 **11c** > 4-(OMe)-C_6H_4 **11b** > 4-Cl-C_6H_4 **11a**, whereas, OH group in *p*-position is a more electron donating group (has more conjugated system) than OMe group and Cl atom.

3. In compound **12**, replacement of C=N group by the thiazolidinone ring decreased the antioxidant activity comparable with **11a**, because of the lack of the conjugated system.

Table 2. Antioxidant activities of all synthesized compounds by using 2,2′-azino-bis(3-ethyl benzothiazoline-6-sulfonic acid (ABTS) and 2,2-diphenyl-1-picryl-hydrazyl-hydrate (DPPH) methods.

Compounds	ABTS IC_{50} (μM)	DPPH IC_{50} (μM)
Ascorbic acid	31.26 ± 0.20	16.83 ± 0.15
3	93.24 ± 0.70	52.14 ± 0.65
5	65.13 ± 0.46	41.16 ± 0.42
6	35.48 ± 0.23	19.25 ± 0.18
7	114.63 ± 0.73	59.43 ± 0.68
8	160.92 ± 0.94	92.36 ± 0.76
9	77.38 ± 0.56	46.23 ± 0.48
11a	89.10 ± 0.64	50.12 ± 0.54
11b	58.03 ± 0.41	38.47 ± 0.37
11c	52.87 ± 0.36	32.69 ± 0.29
11d	46.25 ± 0.28	22.91 ± 0.21
12	154.51 ± 0.85	73.03 ± 0.72
13	131.95 ± 0.77	65.58 ± 0.66
14	71.42 ± 0.52	26.87 ± 0.23

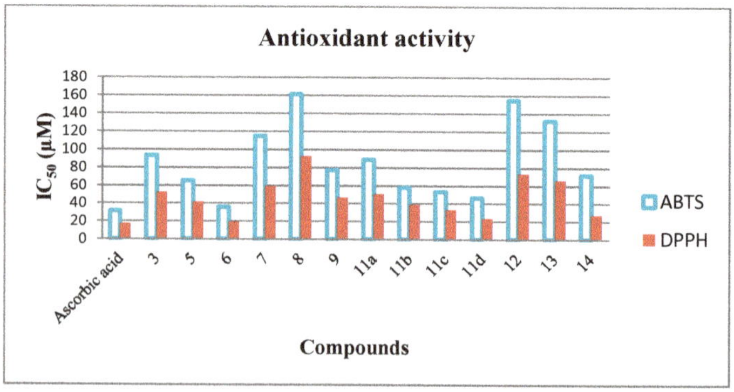

Figure 6. Antioxidant activities of all synthesized compounds by using ABTS and DPPH methods.

Previous reports of structurally similar compounds (in quinazoline ring) but with different substituents have demonstrated different results in antiproliferative and antioxidant activities from our results [9,33,44].

2.3. Density Functional Theory

According to the frontier molecular orbital (FMO) theory, the highest occupied molecular orbital (HOMO) acts as an electron-donor and the lowest unoccupied molecular orbital (LUMO) acts as an electron-acceptor [45]. Meanwhile, both play remarkable roles in the electronic studies by using quantum chemical calculations and they are also of significant importance in modern biochemistry and molecular biology [46]. A molecule is considered as a softer and has an excellent chemical reactivity when it has a smaller energy gap. Meanwhile, a molecule is considered to have a higher chemical hardness and assumed to have good stability when it has a larger energy gap [47–51].

The quantum chemical calculations were implemented by the density functional theory (DFT) method by using the Gaussian(R) 09 program at the B3LYP level in conjunction with 6-31G(d,p) basis set and computed parameters are summarized in Table 3.

By computing and using the energy gap ($\Delta E = E_{LUMO} - E_{HOMO}$) and dipole moment values beside another quantum chemical parameters such as ionization energy ($I = -E_{HOMO}$), electron affinity ($A = -E_{LUMO}$) [52], chemical hardness ($\eta = (I - A)/2$), chemical softness ($S = 1/\eta$) [53], and binding energy, we can rationally explicate the relation between the chemical structure and the antiproliferative activity (SAR's). Whereas, the energy gap of compound **6** (ΔE = 3.98 eV) is smaller than that corresponding of compound **5** (ΔE = 4.85 eV) and also compound **6** has a higher chemical softness value (S = 0.50 eV^{-1}) than that corresponding of compound **5** (S = 0.41 eV^{-1}). These results are matching with the results of the antiproliferative screening whereas, compound **6** has a higher potency comparable with compound **5** for both cell lines (HepG2 and MCF-7) as shown in Table 1 and Figure 3. Similarly, compound **14** has a smaller energy gap and a higher chemical softness than that corresponding to compound **9** as listed in Table 2. In addition, in vitro compound **14** showed a remarkable higher efficacy comparable with compound **9** as shown in Table 1 and Figure 3. Notably, the dipole moment values of compounds **6** (μ = 3.4641 D) and **14** (μ = 1.852 D) are higher than that of compounds **5** (μ = 3.2867 D) and **9** (μ = 1.764 D), respectively.

On the other hand, compounds **11a–d** possess antiproliferative activity in the following order **11d** > **11c** > **11b** > **11a**, meanwhile, the energy gaps of these compounds increase in the following order **11a** (ΔE = 2.99 eV) < **11d** (ΔE = 3.05 eV) < **11c** (ΔE = 3.10 eV) < **11b** (ΔE = 3.13 eV). The lower of the antiproliferative activity of compound **11a** may be explained by values of the dipole moment whereas; the dipole moment of compound **11a** is smaller than that of compounds **11b–d** as shown in Table 3.

Table 3. Quantum chemical parameters of the selected compounds with Density Functional Theory (DFT) at B3LYP/6-31G (d,p) basis set.

Comp. No.	5	6	9	14	11a	11b	11c	11d
E HOMO (eV)	−5.9432	−5.6352	−5.9405	−4.7724	−5.7277	−5.6363	−5.6717	−5.6602
E LUMO (eV)	−1.0917	−1.6515	−1.1298	−1.6836	−2.7301	−2.4983	−2.5709	−2.6009
(ΔE) Energy gap (eV)	4.8515	3.9837	4.8107	3.0888	2.9976	3.1380	3.1008	3.0593
(I) Ionization energy (eV)	5.9432	5.6352	5.9405	4.7724	5.7277	5.6363	5.6717	5.6602
(A) Electron affinity (eV)	1.0917	1.6515	1.1298	1.6836	2.7301	2.4983	2.5709	2.6009
(η) Chemical hardness (eV)	2.4258	1.9919	2.4054	1.5444	1.49881	1.56901	1.5504	1.52969
(S) Chemical softness (eV^{-1})	0.4122	0.5020	0.4157	0.6475	0.6672	0.6374	0.6450	0.6537
(E_T) Binding energy (a.u)	−689.79	−1012.73	−745.11	−1068.05	−1473.81	−1128.73	−1203.94	−1318.44
(μ) Dipole moment (D)	3.2867	3.4641	1.764	1.852	3.2722	4.4472	4.1944	6.232

The distributions of the HOMO and LUMO orbitals of the selected compounds are computed at the same level of the DFT theory and are provided in Figures 7 and 8. The results manifested that possible reactive sites exist as shown below:

1. The HOMO of compounds **5** and **9** are nearly similar and the distribution of orbitals are mainly situated on the quinazolinone moiety, also, the LUMO of these compounds are situated on the same moiety.
2. The HOMO of compounds **6** and **14** are nearly similar and the distribution of orbitals are mainly situated on C=S, while, the LUMO of these compounds are mainly situated on the quinazolinthione moiety.
3. The HOMO of compounds **11a–d** are nearly similar and the distribution of orbitals are mainly situated on the quniazolinone moiety, meanwhile, the LUMO of these compounds are mainly situated on the aryl aldehyde hydrazone system.

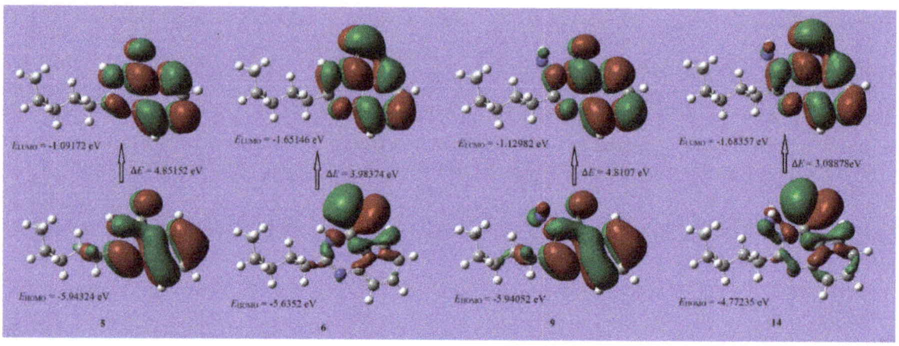

Figure 7. Schematic representation of HOMO and LUMO coefficient distribution of compounds **5**, **6**, **9**, and **14**.

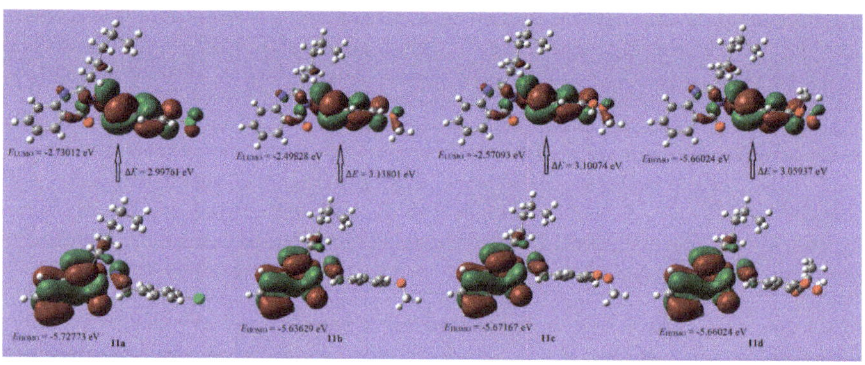

Figure 8. Schematic representation of highest occupied molecular orbital (HOMO) and loest unoccupied molecular orbital (LUMO) coefficient distribution of compounds **11a–d**.

3. Materials and Methods

3.1. Chemistry

The melting point is uncorrected and was measured on a Stuart SMP 30 advanced digital electric melting point apparatus (Cole-Parmer, Staffordshire, UK). All reactions were monitored by TLC (Kieselgel 60 F_{254}, Merck, Munchen, Germany) and spots were visualized using UV (254 nm), In the region (400–4000 cm^{-1}), the IR spectrum was measured in the KBr phase by using the Nicolet iS10 FT-IR spectrometer (Shimadzu Corporation, Kyoto, Japan). The ^{1}H-NMR (at 400 MHz) and ^{13}C-NMR (at 100 MHz) spectra were performed at chemical warfare labs, Egypt, with a Varian Gemini spectrometer (Metrohim, California, United States) in DMSO-d_6 as a solvent by using tetramethylsilane (TMS) as a reference. Perkin-Elmer 2400 CHN elemental analyzer (Waltham, MA, USA) was used to record CHN elemental analysis at the Faculty of Science, Cairo University, Egypt. The mass spectrum was measured on Shimadzu GC-MS QP1000EX apparatus (Shimadzu Corporation, Kyoto, Japan) at the central analytical lab, Ain Shams University, Cairo, Egypt.

3.1.1. 2-Hexanamidobenzoic Acid **3**

Hexanoyl chloride **2** (1.39 mL, 0.01 mol) was added dropwise to anthranilic acid **1** (1.37 g, 0.01 mol) dissolved in dry pyridine (20 mL) at ambient temperature with stirring. The stirring was continued for an hour, and then the resulting emulsion was acidified with cold 10% HCl solution. The white solid which separated was collected by filtration and then recrystallized from benzene to give **3** [38] as white crystals; m.p.: 92–95 °C (Lit. m.p.: 93–95 °C) [38], yield: 92%. IR (KBr, cm^{-1}): 3426–2463 (br) (OH), 3206 (NH), 2959, 2934, 2861 ($CH_{aliph.}$), 1691, 1637 (C=O). ^{1}H-NMR (400 MHz, DMSO-d_6) δ (ppm): 13.51 (br.s, 1H, OH, exchangeable with D_2O), 11.09 (s, 1H, NH, exchangeable with D_2O), 8.48 (d, 1H, Ar-H, H_a, J = 8.8 Hz), 7.95 (d, 1H, Ar-H, H_d, J = 8.0 Hz), 7.55 (t, 1H, Ar-H, H_c, J = 7.8 Hz, J = 8.0 Hz), 7.11 (t, 1H, Ar-H, H_b, J = 7.4 Hz, J = 7.8 Hz), 2.35 (t, 2H, $COCH_2$, J = 7.2 Hz, J = 7.6 Hz), 1.60 (quintet, 2H, $COCH_2\underline{CH_2}$, J = 7.2 Hz, J = 7.6 Hz), 1.31–1.26 (m, 4H, $CH_3\underline{CH_2CH_2}$), 0.85 (t, 3H, CH_3, J = 6.8 Hz, J = 7.2 Hz), MS m/z (%): 235 ($M^{\cdot+}$; 29.4). Anal. Calcd. for $C_{13}H_{17}NO_3$ (235.28): C, 66.36; H, 7.28; N, 5.95. Found: C, 66.36; H, 7.28; N, 5.95.

3.1.2. 2-Pentyl-4*H*-benzo[*d*][1,3]oxazin-4-one **4**

A suspension of 2-hexanamidobenzoic acid **3** (2.35 g, 0.01 mol) in freshly distilled acetic anhydride (10 mL) was heated in water bath for an hour followed by a concentration of the mixture in vacuo and used in situ [39,40].

3.1.3. 2-Pentylquinazolin-4(3*H*)-one **5**

A solution of benzoxazinone **4** (2.17 g, 0.01 mol) in formamide (15 mL) was refluxed for 7 h. After cooling, the reaction mixture was poured onto ice cold water, the obtained solid was filtered off, dried, and recrystallized from petroleum ether 60–80 °C to give **5** [41] as white crystals; m.p.: 142–144 °C (Lit. m.p.: 153–154 °C) [41], yield: 92%. IR (KBr, cm^{-1}): 3171 (NH), 2958, 2928, 2860 ($CH_{aliph.}$), 1680 (C=O), 1614 (C=N or C=C). ^{1}H-NMR (400 MHz, DMSO-d_6) δ (ppm): 12.13 (s, 1H, NH, exchangeable with D_2O), 8.05 (d, 1H, Ar-H, H_a, J = 8.0 Hz), 7.74 (t, 1H, Ar-H, H_c, J = 7.6 Hz, J = 7.8 Hz), 7.56 (d, 1H, Ar-H, H_d, J = 8 Hz), 7.42 (t, 1H, Ar-H, H_b, J = 7.6 Hz), 2.56 (t, 2H, N=CCH_2, J = 7.6 Hz, J = 8.0 Hz), 1.70 (quintet, 2H, N=$CCH_2\underline{CH_2}$, J = 7.6 Hz, J = 7.2 Hz), 1.30–1.26 (m, 4H, $CH_3\underline{CH_2CH_2}$), 0.84 (t, 3H, CH_3, J = 6.8 Hz, J = 7.2 Hz). ^{13}C-NMR (100 MHz, DMSO-d_6) δ (ppm): 162.2, 157.9, 149.4, 134.7, 127.2, 126.3, 126.1, 121.2, 34.9, 31.1, 26.9, 22.2, 14.2. MS m/z (%): 216 ($M^{\cdot+}$; 26.3). Anal. Calcd. for $C_{13}H_{16}N_2O$ (216.28): C, 72.19; H, 7.46; N, 12.95. Found: C, 72.26; H, 7.49; N, 12.86.

3.1.4. 2-Pentylquinazoline-4(3*H*)-thione **6**

To a solution of quinazolinone **5** (2.16 g, 0.01 mol) in dry toluene (30 mL), P_2S_5 (2.22 g, 0.01 mol) was added. The reaction mixture was refluxed for 1 h, and then filtered off. The obtained filtrate was evaporated under reduced pressure, the formed solid was collected by filtration, dried, and recrystallized from ethanol to give **6** as light brown crystals; m.p.: 101–103 °C, yield: 76%. IR (KBr, cm^{-1}): 3184, 3141 (NH), 2967, 2935, 2852 ($CH_{aliph.}$), 1618 (C=N), 1604 (C=C), 1236 (C=S). ^{1}H-NMR (400 MHz, DMSO-d_6) δ (ppm): 13.69 (s, 1H, NH, exchangeable with D_2O), 8.52 (d, 1H, Ar-H, H_d, J = 8.4 Hz), 7.83 (t, 1H, Ar-H, H_c, J = 7.6 Hz), 7.63 (d, 1H, Ar-H, H_a, J = 8.4 Hz), 7.52 (t, 1H, Ar-H, H_b, J = 7.4 Hz, J = 7.8 Hz), 2.70 (t, 2H, N=CCH_2, J = 7.6 Hz, J = 8.0 Hz), 1.72 (quintet, 2H, N=$CCH_2\underline{CH_2}$, J = 7.6 Hz, J = 7.2 Hz), 1.31–1.26 (m, 4H, $CH_3\underline{CH_2CH_2}$), 0.85 (t, 3H, CH_3, J = 6.8 Hz). MS m/z (%): 232 ($M^{\cdot+}$; 16.7). Anal. Calcd. for $C_{13}H_{16}N_2S$ (232.35): C, 67.20; H, 6.94; N, 12.06; S, 13.80. Found: C, 67.31; H, 7.03; N, 12.01; S, 13.85.

3.1.5. N-(β-D-Glucopyranosyl-2,3,4,6-tetraacetate)-2-pentylquinazolin-4(3H)-one **7**

Quinazolinone **5** (2.16 g, 0.01 mol) was refluxed with β-D-glucose pentaacetate (3.90 g, 0.01 mol) in absolute ethanol (50 mL) for 3 h. the solid obtained after slow evaporation of the resulting solution was collected and recrystallized from ethanol to give **7** as white crystals; m.p.: 135–137 °C, yield: 62%. IR (KBr, cm^{-1}): 2955, 2924, 2854 ($CH_{aliph.}$), 1746 ($C{=}O_{ester}$), 1678 ($C{=}O_{quinazolinone}$), 1613 (C=N). ^{1}H-NMR (400 MHz, DMSO-d_6) δ (ppm): 8.05 (d, 1H, Ar-H, H_a, J = 8.0 Hz), 7.74 (t, 1H, Ar-H, H_c, J = 8.4 Hz, J = 6.8 Hz), 7.56 (d, 1H, Ar-H, H_d, J = 8.4 Hz), 7.43 (t, 1H, Ar-H, H_b, J = 8.0 Hz, J = 7.2 Hz), 5.92 (d, 1H, C_1-H, J = 8.4 Hz), 5.39 (t, 1H, C_2-H, J = 9.6 Hz), 4.93 (t, 1H, C_3-H, J = 9.6 Hz), 4.90 (t, 1H, C_4-H, J = 8.4 Hz, J = 10.0 Hz), 4.14, 412 (d,d, 1H, C_6-H, J = 10.4 Hz, J = 5.6 Hz), 3.97 (d, 1H, C_6-H, J = 10.4 Hz), 3.51 (m, 1H, C_5-H), 2.56 (t, 2H, N=CCH_2, J = 8.0 Hz, J = 7.6 Hz), 1.978 (s, 3H, CH_3), 1.973 (s, 3H, CH_3), 1.961 (s, 3H, CH_3), 1.917 (s, 3H, CH_3), 1.69 (quintet, 2H, N=$CCH_2\underline{CH_2}$, J = 7.6 Hz, J = 6.8 Hz), 1.31–1.26 (m, 4H, $CH_3\underline{CH_2CH_2}$), 0.84 (t, 3H, CH_3, J = 6.8 Hz, J = 7.2 Hz). MS m/z (%): 546 (M^+; 32.4). Anal. Calcd. for $C_{27}H_{34}N_2O_{10}$ (546.57): C, 59.33; H, 6.27; N, 5.13. Found: C, 59.18; H, 6.21; N, 5.08.

3.1.6. 3-(2-Hydroxyethyl)-2-pentylquinazolin-4(3H)-one **8**

A solution of benzoxazinone **4** (2.17 g, 0.01 mol) in ethanolamine (15 mL) was heated under reflux for 3 h. The reaction mixture was poured onto ice cold water, the obtained solid was filtered off, dried, and then recrystallized from ethanol to give **8** as white crystals; m.p.: 84–85 °C, yield: 47%. IR (KBr, cm^{-1}): 3395 (OH), 2953, 2931, 2872 ($CH_{aliph.}$), 1648 (C=O), 1611 (C=N). ^{1}H-NMR (400 MHz, DMSO-d_6) δ (ppm): 8.07 (d, 1H, Ar-H, H_a, J = 8.0 Hz), 7.75 (t, 1H, Ar-H, H_c, J = 7.8 Hz, J = 7.6 Hz), 7.57 (d, 1H, Ar-H, H_d, J = 8.0 Hz), 7.44 (t, 1H, Ar-H, H_b, J = 7.6 Hz, J = 7.2 Hz), 4.95 (t, 1H, OH, exchangeable with D_2O, J = 5.6 Hz), 4.11 (t, 2H, $\underline{CH_2}CH_2OH$, J = 5.6 Hz, J = 6.0 Hz), 3.65 (q, 2H, $\underline{CH_2}OH$, J = 6.0 Hz, J = 5.6 Hz), 2.93 (t, 2H, N=$C\underline{CH_2}$, J = 7.6 Hz, J = 8.0 Hz), 1.75 (quintet, 2H, N=$CCH_2\underline{CH_2}$, J = 7.6 Hz, J = 7.6 Hz), 1.40–1.32 (m, 4H, $CH_3\underline{CH_2CH_2}$), 0.88 (t, 3H, CH_3, J = 7.2 Hz). ^{13}C-NMR (100 MHz, DMSO-d_6) δ (ppm): 161.7, 158.4, 147.4, 134.6, 127.1, 126.5, 126.4, 120.4, 58.8, 46.1, 34.6, 31.3, 26.3, 22.4, 14.3. MS m/z (%): 260 (M^+; 41.2). Anal. Calcd. for $C_{15}H_{20}N_2O_2$ (260.34): C, 69.20; H, 7.74; N, 10.76. Found: C, 69.17; H, 7.68; N, 10.81.

3.1.7. 3-Amino-2-pentylquinazolin-4(3H)-one **9**

A mixture of benzoxazinone **4** (2.17 g, 0.01 mol) and hydrazine hydrate (1.5 mL) in absolute ethanol (20 mL) was refluxed for 3 h. The mixture was poured onto ice cold water, the formed solid was filtered off, and recrystallized from ethanol to give **9** as buff crystals; m.p.: 58–60 °C, yield: 43%. IR (KBr, cm^{-1}): 3306, 3263 (NH_2), 2954, 2931, 2910, 2856 ($CH_{aliph.}$), 1673 (C=O), 1630 (C=N). ^{1}H NMR (400 MHz, DMSO-d_6) δ (ppm): 8.08 (d, 1H, Ar-H, H_a, J = 7.8 Hz), 7.75 (t, 1H, Ar-H, H_c, J = 7.4 Hz, J = 7.8 Hz), 7.59 (d, 1H, Ar-H, H_d, J = 7.6 Hz), 7.45 (t, 1H, Ar-H, H_b, J = 7.2 Hz, J = 7.6 Hz), 5.70 (s, 2H, NH_2, exchangeable with D_2O), 2.90 (t, 2H, N=CCH_2, J = 7.2 Hz, J = 8.0 Hz), 1.74 (quintet, 2H, N=$CCH_2\underline{CH_2}$, J = 7.6 Hz, J = 7.2 Hz), 1.37–1.30 (m, 4H, $CH_3\underline{CH_2CH_2}$), 0.87 (t, 3H, CH_3, J = 6.4 Hz, J =7.2 Hz). ^{13}C-NMR (400 MHz, DMSO-d_6) δ (ppm): 160.9, 158.8, 147.0, 134.3, 127.2, 126.39, 126.31, 120.2, 34.0, 31.4, 26.0, 22.3, 14.3. MS m/z (%): 231 (M^+; 41.1). Anal. Calcd. for $C_{13}H_{17}N_3O$ (231.30): C, 67.51; H, 7.41; N, 18.17. Found: C, 67.39; H, 7.34; N, 18.24.

3.1.8. General Procedure for Synthesis of **11a–d**

A mixture of compound **9** (2.31 g, 0.01 mol) and the appropriate aldehydes **10a–d** (0.01 mol) in absolute ethanol (30 mL) was refluxed for 4–6 h. The reaction mixture was evaporated under reduced pressure; the obtained residue was collected and recrystallized from the proper solvent to give the corresponding benzylidene derivatives **11a–d**, respectively.

3-((4-Chlorobenzylidene)amino)-2-pentylquinazolin-4(3*H*)-one **11a**

Yellow crystals; m.p.: 176–178 °C (ethanol), yield: 72%. IR (KBr, cm^{-1}): 2943, 2866 ($CH_{aliph.}$), 1667 (C=O), 1624 (C=N). ^{1}H-NMR (400 MHz, DMSO-d_6) δ (ppm): 8.69 (s, 1H, N=CH), 7.95 (d, 1H, Ar-H, H_a, J = 7.8 Hz), 7.88 (d, 2H, Ar-H, $H_E + H_F$, J = 8.8 Hz), 7.66 (t, 1H, Ar-H, H_c, J = 8.4 Hz), 7.57 (d, 3H, Ar-H, $H_d + H_X + H_Z$), 7.46 (t, 1H, Ar-H, H_b, J = 8.4 Hz), 2.34 (t, 2H, N=CCH_2, J = 7.6 Hz), 1.60 (quintet, 2H, N=$CCH_2\underline{CH_2}$, J = 7.2 Hz), 1.31−1.26 (m, 4H, $CH_3\underline{CH_2CH_2}$), 0.85 (t, 3H, CH_3, J = 6.8 Hz). MS *m/z* (%): 353 (M^+; 4.0). Anal. Calcd. for $C_{20}H_{20}ClN_3O$ (353.85): C, 67.89; H, 5.70; Cl, 10.02; N, 11.88. Found: C, 67.78; H, 5.62; Cl, 9.89; N, 11.79.

3-((4-Methoxybenzylidene)amino)-2-pentylquinazolin-4(3*H*)-one **11b**

White crystals; m.p.: 83–84 °C (petroleum ether 60–80 °C), yield: 64%. IR (KBr, cm^{-1}): 2946, 2912, 2882, 2843 ($CH_{aliph.}$), 1669 (C=O), 1606 (C=N or C=C). ^{1}H-NMR (400 MHz, DMSO-d_6) δ (ppm): 8.81 (s, 1H, N=CH), 8.12 (d, 1H, Ar-H, H_a, J = 7.8 Hz), 7.89 (d, 2H, Ar-H, $H_E + H_F$, J = 8.8 Hz), 7.80 (t, 1H, Ar-H, H_c, J = 8.2, Hz, J = 7.4 Hz), 7.65 (d, 1H, Ar-H, H_d, J = 8.0 Hz), 7.50 (t, 1H, Ar-H, H_b, J = 7.6, Hz, J = 7.4 Hz), 7.12 (d, 2H, Ar-H, $H_X + H_Z$, J = 8.8 Hz), 3.85 (s, 3H, OCH_3), 2.80 (t, 2H, N=CCH_2, J = 7.6 Hz, J = 8.0 Hz), 1.71 (quintet, 2H, N=$CCH_2\underline{CH_2}$, J = 7.6 Hz, J = 7.2 Hz), 1.33−1.26 (m, 4H, $CH_3\underline{CH_2CH_2}$), 0.81 (t, 3H, CH_3, J = 7.2 Hz). MS *m/z* 7(%): 349 (M^+; 11.). Anal. Calcd. for $C_{21}H_{23}N_3O_2$ (349.43): C, 72.18; H, 6.63; N, 12.03. Found: C, 72.29; H, 6.69; N, 11.88.

3-((3-Hydroxy-4-methoxybenzylidene)amino)-2-pentylquinazolin-4(3*H*)-one **11c**

White crystals; m.p.: 150–152 °C (ethanol), yield: 57%. IR (KBr, cm^{-1}): 3277 (OH), 2956, 2927, 2892, 2863, 2845 ($CH_{aliph.}$), 1678 (C=O), 1603 (C=N or C=C). ^{1}H-NMR (400 MHz, DMSO-d_6) δ (ppm): 9.49 (s, 1H, OH, exchangeable with D_2O), 8.70 (s, 1H, N=CH), 8.12 (d, 1H, Ar-H, H_a, J = 8.0 Hz), 7.79 (t, 1H, Ar-H, H_c, J = 8.0 Hz, J =8.4 Hz), 7.65 (d, 1H, Ar-H, H_d, J = 7.6 Hz), 7.49 (t, 1H, Ar-H, H_b, J = 8.0 Hz, J = 7.2 Hz), 7.42 (d, 1H, H_F, J_m = 2 Hz), 7.30, 7.28 (d,d, 1H, Ar-H, H_E, J_o = 8.4 Hz, J_m = 2 Hz), 7.07 (d, 1H, Ar-H, H_X, J = 8.4 Hz), 3.85 (s, 3H, OCH_3), 2.78 (t, 2H, N=CCH_2, J = 7.6 Hz), 1.71 (quintet, 2H, N=$CCH_2\underline{CH_2}$, J = 7.6 Hz, J = 7.2 Hz), 1.31−1.28 (m, 4H, $CH_3\underline{CH_2CH_2}$), 0.81 (t, 3H, CH_3, J = 6.8 Hz, J = 7.2 Hz). MS *m/z* (%): 365 (M^+; 23.4). Anal. Calcd. for $C_{21}H_{23}N_3O_3$ (365.43): C, 69.02; H, 6.34; N, 11.50. Found: C, 68.88; H, 6.28; N, 11.62.

3-((4-Hydroxy-3,5-dimethoxybenzylidene)amino)-2-pentylquinazolin-4(3*H*)-one **11d**

White crystals; m.p.: 148–150 °C (benzene), yield: 61%. IR (KBr, cm^{-1}): 3408 (OH), 2952, 2911, 2844 ($CH_{aliph.}$), 1668 (C=O), 1591 (C=N or C=C). ^{1}H-NMR (400 MHz, DMSO-d_6) δ (ppm): 9.36 (br.s, 1H, OH, exchangeable with D_2O), 8.72 (s, 1H, N=CH), 8.12 (d, 1H, Ar-H, H_a, J = 8.2 Hz), 7.79 (t, 1H, Ar-H, H_c, J = 8.0 Hz, J = 7.4 Hz), 7.65 (d, 1H, Ar-H, H_d, J = 7.6 Hz), 7.50 (t, 1H, Ar-H, H_b, J = 8.0 Hz, J = 7.2 Hz), 7.23 (s, 2H, $H_E + H_F$), 3.82 (s, 6H, $2OCH_3$), 2.81 (t, 2H, N=CCH_2, J = 7.6 Hz, J = 8.0 Hz), 1.72 (quintet, 2H, N=$CCH_2\underline{CH_2}$, J = 7.6 Hz, J = 7.2 Hz), 1.36−1.26 (m, 4H, $CH_3\underline{CH_2CH_2}$), 0.81 (t, 3H, CH_3, J = 6.8 Hz, J =7.2 Hz). ^{13}C-NMR (100 MHz, DMSO-d_6) δ (ppm): 169.8, 158.0, 156.5, 148.6 (2), 146.7, 140.8, 134.6, 127.4, 127.0, 126.7, 122.8, 121.3, 106.8 (2), 56.5 (2), 34.5, 31.3, 26.0, 22.2, 14.2. MS *m/z* (%): 395 (M^+; 62.1), Anal. Calcd. for $C_{22}H_{25}N_3O_4$ (395.46): C, 66.82; H, 6.37; N, 10.63. Found: C, 66.95; H, 6.41; N, 10.58.

3.1.9. 2-(4-Chlorophenyl)-3-(4-oxo-2-pentylquinazolin-3(4*H*)-yl)thiazolidin-4-one **12**

A mixture of compound **11a** (3.53 g, 0.01 mol) and methyl thioglycolate (0.89 mL, 0.01 mol) in absolute ethanol (30 mL) containing piperidine (0.5 mL) was refluxed for 3 h. The obtained solid after evaporation of the solvent was collected and recrystallized from petroleum ether 60–80 °C to give **12** as pale yellow crystals; m.p.: 78–80 °C, yield: 47%. IR (KBr, cm^{-1}): 2951, 2925, 2868 ($CH_{aliph.}$), 1736 ($C{=}O_{thiazolidinone}$), 1671 ($C{=}O_{quinazolinone}$), 1608 (C=N or C=C). ^{1}H-NMR (100 MHz, DMSO-d_6) δ (ppm): 8.13 (d, 1H, Ar-H, H_a, J = 8.2 Hz), 7.96 (d, 2H, Ar-H, $H_E + H_F$, J = 8.0 Hz), 7.80 (t, 1H, Ar-H,

H_c, J = 7.6 Hz), 7.65 (d, 1H, Ar-H, H_d, J = 8.0 Hz), 7.64 (d, 2H, Ar-H, $H_X + H_Z$, J = 8.4 Hz), 7.51 (t, 1H, Ar-H, H_b, J = 7.6 Hz, J = 7.8 Hz), 5.70 (s, 1H, SCH), 3.75, 3.67 (d,d, 2H, $CH_{2(thiazolidinone)}$, J = 23.6 Hz, J = 23.2 Hz), 2.81 (t, 2H, N=CCH_2, J = 8.0 Hz, J = 7.6 Hz), 1.71 (quintet, 2H, N=$CCH_2\underline{CH_2}$, J = 7.6 Hz, J = 8.0 Hz), 1.35–1.17 (m, 4H, $CH_3\underline{CH_2CH_2}$), 0.80 (t, 3H, CH_3, J = 7.2 Hz). MS *m/z* (%): 427 (M^+; 11.8). Anal. Calcd. for $C_{22}H_{22}ClN_3O_2S$ (427.95): C, 61.75; H, 5.18; Cl, 8.28; N, 9.82; S, 7.49. Found: C, 61.66; H, 5.12; Cl, 8.31; N, 9.75; S, 7.55.

3.1.10. 4,5,6,7-Tetrachloro-2-(4-oxo-2-pentylquinazolin-3(4*H*)-yl)isoindoline-1,3-dione **13**

Compound **9** (2.31 g, 0.01 mol) was fused with 4,5,6,7-tetrachloroisobenzofuran-1,3-dione (2.85 g, 0.01 mol) in oil bath for an hour. The resulting solid was recrystallized from ethanol to give **13** as orange crystals; m.p.: 178–180 °C, yield: 86%. IR (KBr, cm^{-1}): 2943, 2856 ($CH_{aliph.}$), 1788, 1746 ($C{=}O_{imide}$), 1705 ($C{=}O_{quinazolinone}$), 1606 (C=N or C=C). ^{1}H-NMR (400 MHz, DMSO-d_6) δ (ppm): 8.08 (d, 1H, Ar-H, H_a, J = 8 Hz), 7.94 (t, 1H, Ar-H, H_c, J = 8.0 Hz, J = 7.2 Hz), 7.76 (d, 1H, Ar-H, H_d, J = 8.0 Hz), 7.60 (t, 1H, Ar-H, H_b, J = 7.6 Hz), 2.73 (t, 2H, N=CCH_2, J = 6.8 Hz, J = 8.0 Hz), 1.70–1.60 (m, 2H, N=$CCH_2\underline{CH_2}$), 1.29–1.27 (m, 4H, $CH_3\underline{CH_2CH_2}$), 0.81 (t, 3H, CH_3, J = 6.8 Hz, J =7.2 Hz). ^{13}C-NMR (100 MHz, DMSO-d_6) δ (ppm): 161.5, 161.3, 157.9, 157.7, 147.4, 146.7, 140.0, 138.8, 136.6 (2), 128.2 (2), 128.0, 127.1, 126.8, 119.8, 32.6, 30.9, 26.0, 22.2, 14.2. MS *m/z* (%): 231 (M^+; 41.1). Anal. Calcd. for $C_{21}H_{15}C_{14}N_3O_3$ (499.17): C, 50.53; H, 3.03; Cl, 28.41; N, 8.42. Found: C, 50.61; H, 3.09; Cl, 28.37; N, 8.53.

3.1.11. 3-Amino-2-pentylquinazoline-4(3*H*)-thione **14**

A mixture of compound **9** (2.31 g, 0.01 mol) and P_2S_5 (2.22 g, 0.01 mol) in dry toluene (15 mL) was heated under reflux for 4 h. The mixture was filtered off, the filtrate was evaporated under reduced pressure, the obtained solid was collected, dried, and recrystallized from ethanol to give **14** as yellow crystals; m.p.: 57–59 °C, yield: 53%. IR (KBr, cm^{-1}): 3240, 3200 (NH_2), 2925, 2855 ($CH_{aliph.}$), 1591 (C=N or C=C), 1238 (C=S). ^{1}H-NMR (400 MHz, DMSO-d_6) δ (ppm): 8.51 (d, 1H, Ar-H, H_a, J = 8.2 Hz), 7.82 (t, 1H, Ar-H, H_c, J = 7.6 Hz, J = 7.8 Hz), 7.69 (d, 1H, Ar-H, H_d, J = 7.6 Hz), 7.57 (t, 1H, Ar-H, H_b, J = 7.6 Hz), 7.04 (s, 2H, NH_2, exchangeable with D_2O), 3.06 (t, 2H, N=CCH_2, J = 7.2 Hz, J = 8.0 Hz), 1.81 (quintet, 2H, N=$CCH_2\underline{CH_2}$, J = 7.6 Hz, J = 7.2 Hz), 1.42–1.32 (m, 4H, $CH_3\underline{CH_2CH_2}$), 0.88 (t, 3H, CH_3, J = 6.8 Hz, J =7.2 Hz). ^{13}C NMR (100 MHz, DMSO-d_6) δ (ppm): 182.1, 155.5, 142.0, 134.5, 130.6, 128.1 (2), 127.4, 34.4, 31.3, 25.5, 22.4, 14.3. MS *m/z* (%): 247 (M^+; 74.3). Anal. Calcd. for $C_{13}H_{17}N_3S$ (247.36): C, 63.12; H, 6.93; N, 16.99; S, 12.96. Found: C, 63.19; H, 6.96; N, 17.11; S, 12.82.

3.2. *Cytotoxicity and Antiproliferative Evaluation*

MTT Assay

The implement of MTT methodology for the antiproliferative screening of quinazolinone derivatives **5–14** along with compound **3** against two cell lines, namely, hepatocellular carcinoma (HepG2) and mammary gland (MCF-7) were obtained from ATCC through the Holding company for biological products and vaccines (VACSERA), Cairo, Egypt. The reference anticancer drug used was Doxorubicin. The MTT assay was carried out at the pharmacology department, Faculty of pharmacy, Mansoura University, Egypt according to the reported literatures [42,43,54]. The cells were cultured in a RPMI-1640 medium with 10% fetal bovine serum, followed by the addition of antibiotics (100 units/mL penicillin and 100 μg/mL streptomycin) at 37 °C in a 5% CO_2 incubator. The cells were seeded in a 96-well plate at a density of (1.0×10^4 cells/well) at 37 °C for 48 h under 5% CO_2. Treatment of cells with different concentrations of compounds such as 100, 50, 25, 12.5, 6.25, 3.125, and 1.56 μM was carried out and placed in the incubator for 24 h. Then, 20 μL of MTT solution at 5 mg/mL was added and incubated for 4 h. DMSO (100 μL) was added into each well to dissolve the purple formazan formed. At 570 nm absorbance the colorimetric assay was measured and recorded by using a plate reader (BioTek EL ×800 Microplate Reader, BioTek Instruments, Inc, Winooski, VT, USA).

Calculation of the relative cell viability (%) = (A of treated samples /A of untreated sample) × 100.

3.3. *Antioxidant Assay*

3.3.1. Antioxidant Activity Screening Assay

ABTS Method

By the bleaching of ABTS derived radical cations, the detections of antioxidant activities were estimated. The radical cation was prepared by the reaction of ABTS [2,2′-azino-bis(3-ethyl benzothiazoline-6-sulfonic acid)] (60 µL) with MnO_2 (3 mL, 25 mg/mL) in a phosphate buffer solution (10 µM, pH 7, 5 mL). The solution was shaken for 3 min, centrifuged, filtered, and recorded at λ_{max} 734 nm the absorbance $A_{(control)}$ of the resulting ABTS radical solution (green-blue). Upon the addition of the tested sample solution (20 µl) with different concentrations of compounds such as 200, 100, 50, 25, and 12.5 µM in spectroscopic grade MeOH/buffer (1:1 *v*/*v*) to the ABTS solution, the absorbance $A_{(test)}$ was measured. The decreasing in the absorbance is expressed as % inhibition which was calculated according to the following equation [55]:

$$\% \text{ Inhibition} = [A_{(control)} - A_{(test)}/A_{(control)}] \times 100 \quad (1)$$

where; the reference and standard antioxidant compound in this test is the ascorbic acid solution (20 µL, 2 mM) and the blank sample was performed by the solvent without ABTS.

DPPH Method

According to the methodology described by Brand-Williams et al. [56], the measurement of the DPPH radical scavenging activity was implemented. The samples with different concentrations of compounds such as 200, 100, 50, 25, and 12.5 µM were allowed to react with the stable DPPH radical in ethanol solution. Whereas, the reaction mixture consisted of sample (0.5 mL), absolute ethanol (3 mL), and DPPH radical solution (0.3 mL) 0.5 mM in ethanol. DPPH is reduced when it reacts with an antioxidant compound, which can donate hydrogen. The changes in color (from deep violet to light yellow) were recorded [absorbance (*Abs*)] at λ_{max} 517 nm after 100 min of reaction using a UV-Vis spectrophotometer (Schimadzu Co., Tokyo, Japan). The blank solution was prepared by mixing ethanol (3.3 mL) and the sample (0.5 mL). Meanwhile, the mixture of ethanol (3.5 mL) and DPPH radical solution (0.3 mL) serve as a positive control.

The scavenging activity percentage (*AA* %) was determined according to Mensor et al. [57]:

$$AA\ \% = 100 - [(Abs_{(sample)} - Abs_{(blankl)}/Abs_{(control)}) \times 100] \quad (2)$$

3.4. *Computational Procedures*

All theoretical calculations and results of the studied compounds were implemented by utilizing Gaussian(R) 09 D.01 [58] (Semichem Inc., Shawnee Mission, KS, USA) by applying the DFT operation with the hybrid functional B3LYP level [59,60] in conjunction with the 6–31G(d,p) basis set. The visualization of these results was achieved using GaussView 6.0.16 software (Semichem Inc., Shawnee Mission, KS, USA).

4. Conclusions

In conclusion, this work focused on the study of the antiproliferative and antioxidant activities in vitro in addition to the theoretical calculation of the DFT theory of some novel quinazolinone(thione) derivatives **6**–**14**. Two main points were the principal targets; firstly, by comparing the activities of quinazolinone and quinazolinthione derivatives. Secondly, comparing the activities of four series of Schiff bases, that have quinazolinone moiety. The results of this study imply that the quinazolinthione derivatives **6** and **14** have promising potent antiproliferative activity comparable with quinazolinone derivatives **5** and **9**, respectively. According to the DFT study, compounds **6** and **14** have a smaller energy gap and a higher chemical softness than that of compounds **5** and **9**, respectively. Additionally, screening of various aryl aldehyde hydrazone derivatives **(11a–d)** analogs exhibited that the potency increased with increasing the electron donating group in *p*-position due to increasing of the conjugated system, and that was supported by the DFT study.

On the other hand, compounds **6** and **11d** showed promising antioxidant activity using ABTS assay. While in the DPPH assay, compounds **6, 11d,** and **14** have showed potent activities comparable to the ascorbic acid which was used as a reference drug. Noteworthy, the results of both antiproliferative and antioxidant activities for each compound individually are nearly the same.

Author Contributions: The listed authors contributed to this work as described in the following: A.A.E.-S., M.F.I., and A.E.-G.E.A. designed the research idea, implemented the synthesis and characterization of novel compounds, and contributed to the data interpretation. A.E.-G.E.A. and A.M.N. contributed to discuss the results, writing the original draft manuscript, and revisions. All authors read and approved the final manuscript.

Funding: The authors are grateful to the Deanship of Scientific Research, King Saud University for funding this work through research group project "RGP-172".

Conflicts of Interest: The authors declare no conflict of interest.

References

1. Stewart, B.W.; Wild, C.P. (Eds.) *World Cancer Report*; International Agency for Research on Cancer: Lyon, France, 2014.
2. Spanò, V.; Montalbano, A.; Carbone, A.; Parrino, B.; Diana, P.; Cirrincione, G.; Castagliuolo, I.; Brun, P.; Issinger, O.G.; Tisi, S.; et al. Synthesis of a new class of pyrrolo[3,4-h]quinazolines with antimitotic activity. *Eur. J. Med. Chem.* **2014**, *74*, 340–357. [CrossRef] [PubMed]
3. Sordella, R.; Bell, D.W.; Haber, D.A.; Settleman, J. Gefitinib-sensitizing EGFR mutations in lung cancer activate anti-apoptotic pathways. *Science* **2004**, *305*, 1163–1167. [CrossRef] [PubMed]
4. Raymond, E.; Faivre, S.; Armand, J.P. Epidermal growth factor receptor tyrosine kinase as a target for anticancer therapy. *Drugs* **2000**, *60*, 15–23. [CrossRef] [PubMed]
5. Ko, H.C.; Wang, Y.H.; Liou, K.T.; Chen, C.M.; Chen, C.H.; Wang, W.Y.; Chang, S.; Hou, Y.C.; Chen, K.T.; Chen, C.F.; et al. Antiinflammatory effects and mechanisms of the ethanol extract of Evodia rutaecarpa and its bioactive components on neutrophils and microglial cells. *Eur. J. Pharmacol.* **2007**, *555*, 211–217. [CrossRef] [PubMed]
6. Keller, T.L.; Zocco, D.; Sundrud, M.S.; Hendrick, M.; Edenius, M.; Yum, J.; Kim, Y.J.; Lee, H.K.; Cortese, J.F.; Wirth, D.F.; et al. Halofuginone and other febrifugine derivatives inhibit prolyl-tRNA synthetase. *Nat. Chem. Biol.* **2012**, *8*, 311–317. [CrossRef]
7. El-Azab, A.S.; Eltahir, K.E. Synthesis and anticonvulsant evaluation of some new 2,3,8-trisubstituted-4(3*H*)-quinazoline derivatives. *Bioorg. Med. Chem. Lett.* **2012**, *22*, 327–333. [CrossRef]
8. Shcherbakova, I.; Balandrin, M.F.; Fox, J.; Ghatak, A.; Heaton, W.L.; Conklin, R.L. 3*H*-Quinazolin-4-ones as a new calcilytic template for the potential treatment of osteoporosis. *Bioorg. Med. Chem. Lett.* **2005**, *15*, 1557–1560. [CrossRef]
9. Reddy, A.G.; Babu, V.H.; Rao, Y.J.P. A review on quinazolines as anticancer agents. *J. Chem. Pharm.Sci.* **2017**, *10*, 1492–1504.
10. Mohamed, M.A.; Ayyad, R.R.; Shawer, T.Z.; Abdel-Aziz, A.A.-M.; El-Azab, A.S. Synthesis and antitumor evaluation of trimethoxyanilides based on 4(3*H*)-quinazolinone scaffolds. *Eur. J. Med. Chem.* **2016**, *112*, 106–113. [CrossRef]
11. Chinigo, G.M.; Paige, M.; Grindrod, S.; Hamel, E.; Dakshanamurthy, S.; Chruszcz, M.; Minor, W.; Brown, M.L. Asymmetric synthesis of 2,3-dihydro-2-arylquinazolin-4-ones: methodology and application to a potent fluorescent tubulin inhibitor with anticancer activity. *J. Med. Chem.* **2008**, *51*, 4620–4631. [CrossRef]
12. Kubo, K.; Shimizu, T.; Ohyama, S.; Murooka, H.; Iwai, A.; Nakamura, K.; Hasegawa, K.; Kobayashi, Y.; Takahashi, N.; Takahashi, K.; et al. Novel potent orally active selective VEGFR-2 tyrosine kinase inhibitors: synthesis, structure-activity relationships, and antitumor activities of *N*-phenyl-*N*′-{4-(4-quinolyloxy)phenyl}ureas. *J. Med. Chem.* **2005**, *48*, 1359–1366. [CrossRef] [PubMed]

13. Hour, M.-J.; Huang, L.-J.; Kuo, S.-C.; Xia, Y.; Bastow, K.; Nakanishi, Y.; Hamel, E.; Lee, K.-H. 6-Alkylamino- and 2,3-Dihydro-3′-methoxy-2-phenyl-4-quinazolinones and related compounds: Their synthesis, cytotoxicity, and inhibition of tubulin polymerization. *J. Med. Chem.* **2000**, *43*, 4479–4487. [CrossRef] [PubMed]
14. Takase, Y.; Saeki, T.; Watanabe, N.; Adachi, H.; Souda, S.; Saito, I. Cyclic GMP Phosphodiesterase inhibitors. 2. requirement of 6-substitution of quinazoline derivatives for potent and selective inhibitory activity. *J. Med. Chem.* **1994**, *37*, 2106–2111. [CrossRef] [PubMed]
15. Khodarahmi, G.; Jafari, E.; Hakimelahi, G.; Abedi, D.; Rahmani, K.M.; Hassanzadeh, F. Synthesis of some new quinazolinone derivatives and evaluation of their antimicrobial activities. *Iran, J. Pharm. Res.* **2012**, *11*, 789–797.
16. Venkatesh, R.; Kasaboina, S.; Jain, N.; Janardhan, S.; Holagunda, U.D.; Nagarapu, L. Design and synthesis of novel sulphamide tethered quinazolinone hybrids as potential antitumor agents. *J. Mol. Struct.* **2019**, *1181*, 403–411. [CrossRef]
17. Patel, M.B.; Kumar, S.P.; Valand, N.N.; Jasrai, Y.T.; Menon, S.K. Synthesis and biological evaluation of cationic fullerene quinazolinone conjugates and their binding mode with modeled Mycobacterium tuberculosis hypoxanthine-guanine phosphoribosyltransferase enzyme. *J. Mol. Model.* **2013**, *19*, 3201–3217. [CrossRef]
18. Mhaske, S.B.; Argade, N.P. the chemistry of recently isolated naturally occurring quinazolinone alkaloids. *Tetrahedron* **2006**, *62*, 9787–9826. [CrossRef]
19. Song, F.; Ren, B.; Yu, K.; Chen, C.; Guo, H.; Yang, N.; Gao, H.; Liu, X.; Liu, M.; Tong, Y.; et al. Quinazolin-4-one coupled with pyrrolidin-2-iminium alkaloids from marine-derived fungus Penicillium aurantiogriseum. *Mar Drugs.* **2012**, *10*, 1297–1306. [CrossRef]
20. Obafemi, C.A.; Fadare, O.A.; Jasinski, J.P.; Millikan, S.P.; Obuotor, E.M.; Iwalewa, E.O.; Famuyiwa, S.O.; Sanusi, K.; Yilmaz, Y.; Ceylan, Ü. Microwave-assisted synthesis, structural characterization, DFT studies, antibacterial and antioxidant activity of 2-methyl-4-oxo-1,2,3,4- tetrahydroquinazoline-2-carboxylic acid. *J. Mol. Struct.* **2018**, *1155*, 610–622. [CrossRef]
21. Patel, N.B.; Patel, V.N. New 2,3-disubstituted quinazolin-4 (3*H*)-ones as antimicrobial agents. *Ind. J. Heterocycl. Chem.* **2007**, *16*, 247–250.
22. Peet, N.P.; Baugh, L.E.; Sunder, S.; Lewis, J.E.; Matthews, E.H.; Olberding, E.L.; Shah, D.N. 3-(1*H*-Tetrazol-5-yl)-4(3*H*)-quinazolinone sodium salt (MDL 427): A new antiallergic agent. *J. Med. Chem.* **1986**, *29*, 2403–2409. [CrossRef] [PubMed]
23. Patil, A.; Barge, M.; Rashinkar, G.; Salunkhe, R. Aqueous hydrotrope: An efficient and reusable medium for a green one-pot, diversity-oriented synthesis of quinazolinone derivatives. *Mol. Divers.* **2015**, *19*, 435–445. [CrossRef] [PubMed]
24. Khattab, S.N.; Haiba, N.S.; Asal, A.M.; Bekhit, A.A.; Guemei, A.A.; Amer, A.; El-Faham, A. Study of antileishmanial activity of 2-aminobenzoyl amino acid hydrazides and their quinazoline derivatives. *Bioorg. Med. Chem. Lett.* **2017**, *27*, 918–921. [CrossRef] [PubMed]
25. Haghighijoo, Z.; Firuzi, O.; Hemmateenejad, B.; Emami, S.; Edraki, N.; Miri, R. Synthesis and biological evaluation of quinazolinone-based hydrazones with potential use in Alzheimer's disease. *Bioorg. Chem.* **2017**, *74*, 126–133. [CrossRef] [PubMed]
26. Mhaske, S.B.; Argade, N.P. Regioselective quinazolinone-directed ortho lithiation of quinazolinoylquinoline: practical synthesis of naturally occurring human DNA topoisomerase I poison luotonin a and luotonins B and E. *J. Organomet. Chem.* **2004**, *69*, 4563–4566. [CrossRef]
27. Houck, D.R.; Ondeyka, J.; Zink, D.L.; Inamine, E.; Goetz, M.A.; Hensens, O.D. On the biosynthesis of asperlicin and the directed biosynthesis of analogs in Aspergillus alliaceus. *J. Antibiot. (Tokyo)* **1988**, *41*, 882–891. [CrossRef]
28. He, L.; Li, H.; Chen, J.; Wu, X. Recent advances in 4(3*H*)-quinazolinone syntheses. *RSC Adv.* **2014**, *4*, 12065–12077. [CrossRef]
29. Chaudhuri, P.K. Echinozolinone, an alkaloid from Echinops echinatus. *Phytochemistry* **1987**, *26*, 587–589. [CrossRef]
30. Ramanathan, M.; Hsu, M.T.; Liu, S.T. Preparation of 4(3*H*)-quinazolinones from aryldiazonium salt, nitriles and 2-aminobenzoate via a cascade annulation. *Tetrahedron* **2019**, *75*, 791–796. [CrossRef]
31. Sales, Z.S.; Mani, N.S.; Allison, B.D. The synthesis of 2-amino-4(3*H*)-quinazolinones and related heterocycles via a mild electrocyclization of aryl guanidines. *Tetrahedron Lett.* **2018**, *59*, 1623–1626. [CrossRef]

32. Ismail, M.F.; El-sayed, G.A. Dodecanoyl isothiocyanate and *N'*-(2-cyanoacetyl)dodecane- hydrazide as precursors for the synthesis of different heterocyclic compounds with interesting antioxidant and antitumor activity. *Synth. Commun.* **2018**, *48*, 892–905. [CrossRef]
33. Ajani, O.O.; Audu, O.Y.; Aderohunmu, D.V.; Owolabi, F.E.; Olomieja, A.O. Review Article Undeniable Pharmacological Potentials of Quinazoline Motifs in Therapeutic Medicine. *Am. J. Drug Discov. Dev.* **2017**, *7*, 1–24. [CrossRef]
34. Abbas, S.Y.; El-Bayouki, K.A.M.; Basyouni, W.M. Utilization of isatoic anhydride in the syntheses of various types of quinazoline and quinazolinone derivatives. *Synth. Commun.* **2016**, *46*, 993–1035. [CrossRef]
35. Maiden, T.M.M.; Harrity, J.P.A. Recent developments in transition metal catalysis for quinazolinone synthesis. *Org. Biomol. Chem.* **2016**, *14*, 8014–8025. [CrossRef]
36. Rohokale, R.S.; Kshirsagar, U.A. Advanced Synthetic Strategies for Constructing Quinazolinone Scaffolds. *Synthesis* **2016**, *48*, 1253–1268. [CrossRef]
37. Youssef, Y.M.; El-Sayed, A.A.; Azab, M.E. Utility of Benzoxazin-4-one and 3-amino- quinazolin-4-one Derivatives as Precursors for Construction of Potent Insecticidal Heterocycles. *J. Heterocyclic Chem.* **2019**. [CrossRef]
38. Park, W.J.; Ma, E. Inhibition of PCAF histone acetyltransferase and cytotoxic effect of *N*-acylanthranilic acids. *Pharmacal. Res.* **2012**, *35*, 1379–1386. [CrossRef]
39. Li, W.; Wu, X.-F. Palladium-catalyzed carbonylative synthesis of benzoxazinones from *N*-(*o*-Bromoaryl)amides using paraformaldehyde as the carbonyl source. *J. Org. Chem.* **2014**, *79*, 10410–10416. [CrossRef]
40. Mahindroo, N.; Ahmed, Z.; Bhagat, A.; Bedi, K.L.; Khajuria, R.K.; Kapoor, V.K.; Dhar, K.L. Synthesis and structure-activity relationships of vasicine analogues as bronchodilatory agents. *Med. Chem. Res.* **2006**, *14*, 347–368. [CrossRef]
41. Zhang, W.; Meng, C.; Liu, Y.; Tang, Y.; Li, F. Auto-tandem catalysis with ruthenium: From o-aminobenzamides and allylic alcohols to quinazolinones via redox isomerization/acceptorless dehydrogenation. *Adv. Synth. Catal.* **2018**, *360*, 3751–3759. [CrossRef]
42. Mosmann, T. Rapid colorimetric assay for cellular growth and survival: application to proliferation and cytotoxicity assays. *J. Immunol. Methods* **1983**, *65*, 55–63. [CrossRef]
43. Denizot, F.; Lang, R. Rapid colorimetric assay for cell growth and survival. Modifications to the tetrazolium dye procedure giving improved sensitivity and reliability. *J. Immunol. Methods* **1986**, *89*, 271–277. [CrossRef]
44. He, D.; Wang, M.; Zhao, S.; Shu, Y.; Zeng, H.; Xiao, C.; Lu, C.; Liu, Y. Pharmaceutical prospects of naturally occurring quinazolinone and its derivatives. *Fitoterapia* **2017**, *119*, 136–149. [CrossRef] [PubMed]
45. Karunakaran, V.; Balachandran, V. FT-IR, FT-Raman spectra, NBO, HOMO-LUMO and thermodynamic functions of 4-chloro-3-nitrobenzaldehyde based on ab initio HF and DFT calculations. *Spectrochim. Acta A* **2012**, *98*, 229–239. [CrossRef] [PubMed]
46. Ayyamperumal, N.; Balachandran, V.; Thangavel, K. Molecular structure, vibrational spectra, first hyperpolarizability and HOMO-LUMO analysis of p-acetylbenzonitrile using quantum chemical calculation. *J. Mol. Struct.* **2013**, *1038*, 134–144. [CrossRef]
47. Prashanth, J.; Ramesh, G.; Naik, J.L.; Ojha, J.K.; Reddy, B.V. Molecular geometry, NBO analysis, Hyperpolarizability and HOMO-LUMO energies of 2-azido-1-phenylethanone using Quantum chemical calculations. *Mater. Today Proc.* **2016**, *3*, 3761–3769. [CrossRef]
48. Al-Omary, F.A.M.; Mary, Y.S.; Panicker, C.Y.; El-Emam, A.A.; Al-Swaidan, I.A.; Al-Saadi, A.A.; Alsenoy, C.V. Spectroscopic investigations, NBO, HOMO-LUMO, NLO analysis molecular docking of 5-(adamantan-1-yl)-3anilinomethyl-2,3-dihydro-1,3,4-oxadiazole-2-thione, a potential bioactive agent. *J. Mol. Struct.* **2015**, *1096*, 1–14. [CrossRef]
49. Koparir, M.; Orek, C.; Koparir, P.; Sarac, K. Synthesis, experimental, theoretical characterization and biological activities of4-ethyl-5-(2-hydroxyphenyl)-2*H*-1,2,4-triazole- 3(4*H*)-thione. *Spectrochim. Acta, Part A* **2013**, *105*, 522–531. [CrossRef]
50. Fleming, I. *Frontier Orbitals and Organic Chemical Reactions*; John Wiley & Sons: New York, NY, USA, 1976.
51. Şahin, Z.S.; Kantar, G.K.; Şaşmaz, S.; Büyükgüngör, O. Synthesis, molecular structure, spectroscopic analysis, thermodynamic parameters and molecular modeling studies of (2-methoxyphenyl)oxalate. *J. Mol. Struct.* **2015**, *1087*, 104–112. [CrossRef]
52. Koopmans, T. Über die Zuordnung von Wellenfunktionen und Eigenwerten zu den Einzelnen Elektronen Eines Atoms. *Physica* **1934**, *1*, 104–113. [CrossRef]

53. Pearson, R.G. Absolute electronegativity and hardness correlated with molecular orbital theory. *Proc. Natl. Acad. Sci. USA.* **1986**, *83*, 8440–8441. [CrossRef] [PubMed]
54. Ismail, M.F.; El-sayed, A.A. Synthesis and in-vitro antioxidant and antitumor evaluation of novel pyrazole-based heterocycles. *J. Iran. Chem. Soc.* **2019**, *16*, 921–937. [CrossRef]
55. Lissi, E.A.; Modak, B.; Torres, R.; Escobar, J.; Urzua, A. Total antioxidant potential of resinous exudates from Heliotropium species, and a comparison of the ABTS and DPPH methods. *Free Radic. Res.* **1999**, *30*, 471. [CrossRef] [PubMed]
56. Brand-Williams, W.; Cuvelier, M.E.; Berset, C. use of a free radical method to evaluate antioxidant activity. *Lebensm. Wiss. Technol.* **1995**, *28*, 25–30. [CrossRef]
57. Mensor, L.L.; Menezes, F.S.; Leitao, G.G.; Reis, A.S.; dos Santos, T.C.; Coube, C.S.; Leitão, S.G. Screening of Brazilian plant extracts for antioxidant activity by the use of DPPH free radical method. *Phytother. Res.* **2001**, *15*, 127–130. [CrossRef]
58. Frisch, M.J.; Trucks, G.W.; Schlegel, H.B.; Scuseria, G.E.; Robb, M.A.; Cheeseman, J.R.; Scalmani, G.; Barone, V.; Mennucci, B.; Petersson, G.A.; et al. *Gaussian 09, Revision D.01*; Gaussian Inc.: Wallingford, CT, USA, 2009.
59. Becke, A.D. Density-functional exchange-energy approximation with correct asymptotic behavior. *Phys. Rev. A* **1988**, *38*, 3098–3100. [CrossRef]
60. Lee, C.; Yang, W.; Parr, R.G. Development of the Colle-Salvetti correlation-energy formula into a functional of the electron density. *Phys. Rev. B* **1988**, *37*, 785–789. [CrossRef]

Sample Availability: Samples of the compounds are available from the authors.

MDPI
St. Alban-Anlage 66
4052 Basel
Switzerland
Tel. +41 61 683 77 34
Fax +41 61 302 89 18
www.mdpi.com

Molecules Editorial Office
E-mail: molecules@mdpi.com
www.mdpi.com/journal/molecules

www.ingramcontent.com/pod-product-compliance
Lightning Source LLC
Chambersburg PA
CBHW061452220926
51850CB00004B/72
9783036501406